Canine Medicine and Therapeutics

Fourth Edition

Edited by

Neil T. Gorman

BVSc, PhD, FRCVS, DipACVIM (Oncology)

for the British Small Animal Veterinary Association

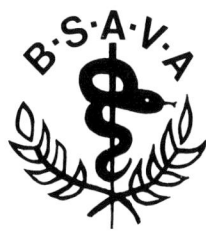

Blackwell Science

© 1979, 1984, 1991, 1998 by
Blackwell Science Ltd
Editorial Offices:
Osney Mead, Oxford OX2 0EL
25 John Street, London WC1N 2BL
23 Ainslie Place, Edinburgh EH3 6AJ
350 Main Street, Malden
    MA 02148 5018, USA
54 University Street, Carlton
    Victoria 3053, Australia
10, rue Casimir Delavigne
    75006 Paris, France

Other Editorial Offices:

Blackwell Wissenschafts-Verlag GmbH
Kurfürstendamm 57
10707 Berlin, Germany

Blackwell Science KK
MG Kodenmacho Building
7-10 Kodenmacho Nihombashi
Chuo-ku, Tokyo 104, Japan

First published 1979
Second edition 1984
Reprinted 1986, 1987, 1989
Spanish edition 1984
Japanese edition 1984
Italian edition 1985
Portuguese edition 1986
Third edition 1991
Reissued in paperback 1994
Reprinted in 1995
Fourth edition 1998

Set in 9 on 10.5 point Ehrhardt
by Best-set Typesetter Ltd, Hong Kong
Printed and bound in Spain
by T.G. Hostench, S.A.

DISTRIBUTORS

Marston Book Services Ltd
PO Box 269
Abingdon
Oxon OX14 4YN
(*Orders*: Tel: 01235 465500
        Fax: 01235 465555)

USA
Blackwell Science, Inc.
Commerce Place
350 Main Street
Malden, MA 02148 5018
(*Orders*: Tel: 800 759 6102
             781 388 8250
        Fax: 781 388 8255)

Canada
Login Brothers Book Company
324 Saulteaux Crescent
Winnipeg, Manitoba R3J 3T2
(*Orders*: Tel: 204 224-4068)

Australia
Blackwell Science Pty Ltd
54 University Street
Carlton, Victoria 3053
(*Orders*: Tel: 03 9347 0300
        Fax: 03 9347 5001)

A catalogue record for this title
is available from the British Library

ISBN 0-632-04045-9

Library of Congress
Cataloging-in-Publication Data
Canine medicine and therapeutics. – 4th ed. / edited by Neil T.
    Gorman for the British Small Animal Veterinary Association.
        p.   cm.
    Includes bibliographical references and index.
    ISBN 0-632-04045-9 (HB)
    1. Dogs – Diseases.   I. Gorman, Neil T.   II. British Small
Animal Veterinary Association.
    [DNLM: 1. Dog Diseases.   SF 991 C2232 1998]
SF991.C24   1998
636.7′0896 – dc21
DNLM/DLC
for Library of Congress   97-27105
                                                                CIP

To the memory of my father, who always had faith in me

Contents

Section Editors

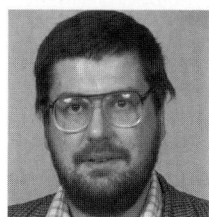

Malcolm Bennett
BVSc, PhD, MRCVS
Senior Lecturer, Department of
    Veterinary Pathology and
    Centre for Comparative
    Infectious Diseases, The
    University of Liverpool,
    Leahurst, Chester High Road,
    Neston, South Wirral L64 7TE

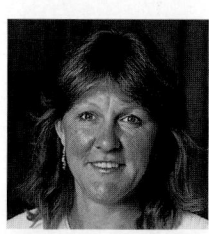

Jane M. Dobson
MA, DVetMed, MRCVS
Lecturer, Department of Clinical
    Veterinary Medicine,
    University of Cambridge,
    Madingley Road, Cambridge
    CB3 0ES

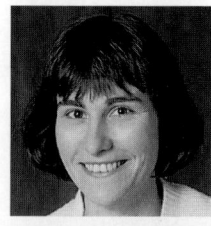

Katie Dunn
MAVetMB, CertSAM, MRCVS
Resident, Department of Clinical
    Veterinary Medicine,
    University of Cambridge,
    Madingley Road, Cambridge
    CB3 0ES

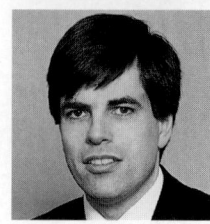

Jonathan Elliott
MAVetMB, PhD, CertSAC,
    MRCVS
Lecturer, Department of
    Veterinary Basic Sciences,
    Royal Veterinary College,
    University of London, Royal
    College Street, London NW1
    0UT

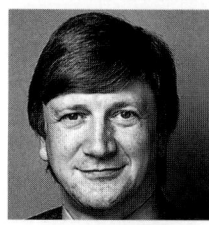

Neil T. Gorman (Editor)
BVSc, PhD, FRCVS, DipACVIM
    (Oncology)
Vice President R&D, Mars
    Petcare Europe, Mill Street,
    Melton Mowbray LE13 1BB

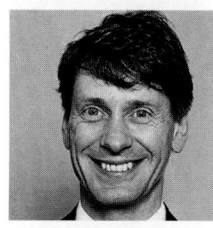

Richard Harvey
BVetMed, CIBiol, MIBiol, DVD,
    DipECVD, MRCVS
The Veterinary Centre, 207
    Daventry Road, Coventry CV3
    5HH

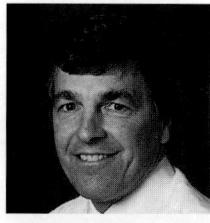

Michael E. Herrtage
MA, BVSc, DVR, DVD, DSAM,
    MRCVS, DipECVDI,
    DipECVIM
Lecturer, Department of Clinical
    Veterinary Medicine,
    University of Cambridge,
    Madingley Road, Cambridge
    CB3 0ES

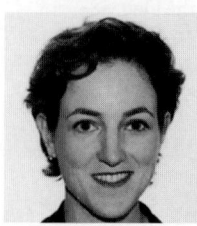

Virginia Luis Fuentes
MAVetMB, PhD, DVC, MRCVS
Assistant Professor, College of
    Veterinary Medicine,
    Veterinary Medical Teaching
    Hospital, Clydesdale Hall,
    University of Missouri-
    Columbia, Columbia, MO
    65211, USA

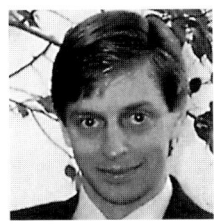
Christopher May
MAVetMB, CertSAO, PhD,
    MRCVS
Grove Veterinary Hospital,
    Hibbert Street, New Mills,
    Stockport, Cheshire SK12 3JJ

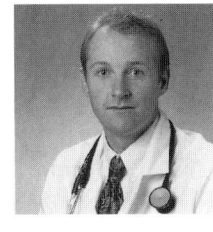
Kenneth W. Simpson
BVM&S, PhD, DipACVIM,
    MRCVS
Assistant Professor, Department
    of Clinical Sciences, College of
    Veterinary Medicine, Cornell
    University, Ithaca, NY 14853-
    6401, USA

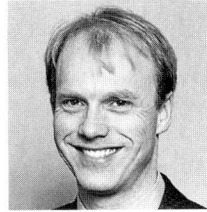
Simon Petersen-Jones
DVetMed, PhD, DVO, MRCVS
Department of Small Animal
    Clinical Sciences, College of
    Veterinary Medicine, Michigan
    State University, East Lansing,
    MI 48824-1314, USA

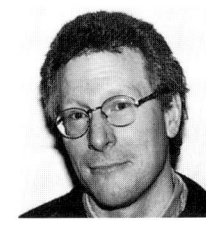
Richard A. Squires
BVSc, PhD, DVR, DipACVIM,
    MRCVS
Secretary and Director, NZVA
    Foundation for Continuing
    Education, Centre for
    Veterinary Education, Massey
    University, Palmerston North,
    New Zealand

Contributors

Kenneth Abrams
DVM, DipAVCO
Veterinary Ophthalmology Services, Inc., 42 Benefit
    Street, Warwick, Rhode Island, USA
Tel: 1 401 738 7337
Email: kabrams@mail.ids.net

T. James Anderson
BVM&S, MVM, PhD, DSAO, MRCVS
Research Fellow, Department of Veterinary Clinical
    Studies, University of Glasgow Veterinary School,
    Bearsden Road, Glasgow G16 1QH
Tel: 0141 330 5700
Fax: 0141 942 7215
Email: gvs07@udcf.gla.ac.uk

Jackie S. Barber
BVetMed, PhD, MRCVS
Department of Veterinary Parasitology, University of
    Liverpool, PO Box 147, Liverpool L69 3BX
Tel: 0151 7089393

Penney J. Barber
BMV&S, PhD, MRCVS
Research Fellow, Department of Veterinary Basic
    Sciences, Royal Veterinary College, University of
    London, Royal College Street, London NW1 0UT
Tel: 0171 468 5266
Fax: 0171 388 1027

Stephen Barr
BVSc, MVS, PhD, DipACVIM
Associate Professor of Medicine, Department of Clinical
    Sciences, College of Veterinary Medicine, Cornell
    University, Ithaca, New York
Tel: 1 607 253 3060
Email: scb6@cornell.edu

David Bennett
BSc, BVetMed, PhD, DSAO, MRCVS
Professor of Small Animal Studies, Department of Small
    Animal Studies, University of Glasgow, Veterinary
    School, Bearsden Road, Glasgow G16 1QH
Tel: 0141 330 5700
Fax: 0141 942 7215
Email: d.bennett@vet.gla.ac.uk

Malcolm Bennett
BVSc, PhD, MRCVS
Senior Lecturer, Department of Veterinary Pathology and
    Centre for Comparative Infectious Diseases, The
    University of Liverpool, Leahurst, Chester High Road,
    Neston, South Wirral L64 7TE
Tel: 0151 794 6015
Fax: 0151 794 6005
Email: m.bennett@liverpool.ac.uk

Laura Blackwood
BVMS, MVM, CertVR, MRCVS
Research Scholar, Department of Veterinary Pathology,
    University of Glasgow Veterinary School, Bearsden
    Road, Glasgow G61 1QH
Tel: 0141 330 5700
Fax: 0141 330 5602
Email: 8536541b@udcf.gla.ac.uk

Ross Bond
BVMS, PhD, DVD, MRCVS, DipECVD
Lecturer, Department of Veterinary Basic Sciences, Royal
    Veterinary College, University of London, Royal
    College Street, London NW1 0UT
Tel: 0171 468 5266
Fax: 0171 388 1027

H. Bourhy
DVM, PhD
Centre National de Référence pour la Rage, Institut
    Pasteur de Paris, 25, Rue du Docteur Roux, F-75724
    Paris cedex 15, France
Tel: 33 1 456 88785
Fax: 33 1 406 13020
Email: hbourhy@pasteur.fr

Bernard Brochier
DVM, PhD
Institut de Santé Publique–Louis Pasteur, 642, Rue
    Engeland, B-1180 Bruxelles, Belgium
Tel: 32 2 373 3256
Fax: 32 2 373 3174
Email: bbrochie@ben.vub.ac.be

Scott Brown
VMD, PhD, DipACVIM
Professor, Physiology and Pharmacology, College of
    Veterinary Medicine, University of Georgia, Athens,
    GA 30602, USA
Tel: 1 706 542 5857
Fax: 1 706 542 3015
Email: brown.s@calc.vet.uga.edu

Stuart D. Carter
BSc, PhD, FIMLS
Senior Lecturer, Departments of Veterinary Clinical
    Science and Veterinary Pathology, University of
    Liverpool, PO Box 147, Liverpool L69 3BX
Tel: 0151 794 4206
Fax: 0151 794 4219
Email: scarter@liverpool.ac.uk

Malcolm Cobb
MAVetMB, PhD, DVC, MRCVS
Leo Animal Health, Longwick Road, Princes Risborough,
    Buckinghamshire HP27 9RR
Tel: 01844 347333
Fax: 01844 272832

Brendan Corcoran
MVB, PhD, MRCVS
Lecturer, Department of Clinical Studies, Royal (Dick)
    School of Veterinary Studies, The University of
    Edinburgh, Small Animal Clinic, Edinburgh EH9 1QH
Tel: 0131 650 6061
Fax: 0131 650 6577

Andrew R. Coughlan
BVSc, CertSAO, CertVA, PhD, FRCVS
Animal Medical Centre, 511 Wilbraham Road, Chorlton,
    Manchester M21 0UB
Tel: 0161 881 3329
Fax: 0161 861 8553

Cathy F. Curtis
BVetMed, DVD, MRCVS
Dermatology Referral Service, 7 Chadwell, Ware,
    Hertfordshire SG12 9JX
Tel: 01920 484525
Fax: 01920 484525
Email: c.curtis@btinternet.com

Michael J. Day
BSc, BVMS (Hons), PhD, MASM, DipECVP, MRCPath,
    FRCVS
Senior Lecturer, Department of Clinical Sciences,
    University of Bristol Veterinary School, Langford
Bristol BS18 7DU
Tel: 0117 928 9427
Fax: 01934 853145
Email: m.j.day@bris.ac.uk

Robert DeNovo, Jr
DVM, MS, DipACVIM
Associate Professor, College of Veterinary Medicine,
    University of Tennessee, PO Box 1071, Knoxville, TN
    37901, USA
Tel: 1 423 974 8387
Fax: 1 423 974 5554
Email: rdenovo@ukt.edu

Jane M. Dobson
MA, DVetMed, MRCVS
Lecturer, Department of Clinical Veterinary Medicine,
    University of Cambridge, Madingley Road, Cambridge
    CB3 0ES
Tel: 01223 337600
Fax: 01223 337610
Email: jmd1000@cam.ac.uk

Hans Klaus Dreier
DVetMed
Millöckergasse 2, A-2500 Baden, Austria
Tel: 43 2252 86212
Fax: 43 2252 47710
Email: hans-klaus.dreier@telecom.at

John K. Dunn
BVM&S, MSc, DipECVIM, DSAM, MRCVS
Lecturer, Department of Clinical Veterinary Medicine,
    University of Cambridge, Madingley Road, Cambridge
    CB3 0ES
Tel: 01223 337600
Fax: 01223 337610

Katie Dunn
MAVetMB, CertSAM, MRCVS
Resident, Department of Clinical Veterinary Medicine,
    University of Cambridge, Madingley Road, Cambridge
    CB3 0ES
Tel: 01223 337600
Fax: 01223 337610

Jonathan Elliott
MAVetMB, PhD, CertSAC, MRCVS
Lecturer, Department of Veterinary Basic Sciences, Royal
    Veterinary College, University of London, Royal
    College Street, London NW1 0UT
Tel: 0171 468 5266
Fax: 0171 388 1027
Email: jelliott@rvc.ac.uk

Clive M. Elwood
MAVetMB, PhD, DipACVIM, DipECVIM, MRCVS
Lecturer, Department of Small Animal Medicine and
    Surgery, Royal Veterinary College, Hawkshead Lane,
    North Mymms, Hatfield, Herts AL9 7TA
Tel: 01707 666333
Fax: 01707 652090
Email: celwood@rvc.ac.uk

Margaret A. Fisher
BVetMed, CIBiol, MIBiol, MRCVS
Brentknoll Veterinary Centre, 152 Bath Road, Worcester
    WR5 3EP
Tel: 01905 355938
Fax: 01905 353902

Frederic P. Gaschen
DVM, DipACVIM
Assistant Professor, Klinik fur Kleine Haustiere,
    University of Berne, Laegnggrass-str.128, Bern,
    Switzerland
Tel: 41 31 631 2294
Fax: 41 31 631 2541

Caitlin C. Goodwin
MS
Veterinary Ophthalmology Services, Inc., 42 Benefit
    Street, Warwick, RI 02886, USA
Tel: 1 401 738 7338
E-mail: goodrice@ix.netcom.com

Neil T. Gorman
BVSc, PhD, FRCVS, DipACVIM (Oncology)
Vice President R&D, Mars Petcare Europe, Mill Street,
    Melton Mowbray LE13 1BB
Tel: 01664 416400
Fax: 01664 416696
E-mail: Neil.T.Gorman@btinternet

Craig E. Greene
DVM, MS, DipACVIM
Professor, Department of Small Animal Medicine, College
    of Veterinary Medicine, University of Georgia,
    Veterinary Medical Teaching Hospital, University of
    Georgia, Athens, Georgia, USA
Tel: 1 706 542 3221
Email: greene.c@calc.vet.uga.edu

Susan P. Gregory
BVetMed, PhD, DVR, DSAS, MRCVS
Lecturer, Department of Small Animal Medicine and
    Surgery, Royal Veterinary College, Hawkshead Lane,
    North Mymms, Hatfield, Herts AL9 7TA
Tel: 01707 666333

Edward J. Hall
MAVetMB, PhD, MRCVS
Lecturer, Department of Clinical Sciences, University of
    Bristol Veterinary School, Langford, Bristol BS18 7DU
Tel: 0117 928 9427
Fax: 01934 853145
Email: dred.hall@bris.ac.uk

C. Anthony Hart
BSc, MB, BS, PhD, FRCPath, FRCPCH
Professor and Head of Department, Department of
    Medical Microbiology and Centre for Comparative
    Infectious Diseases, University of Liverpool, PO Box
    147, Liverpool L69 3BX
Tel: 0151 7064380
Fax: 0151 7065805
Email: c.a.hart@liverpool.ac.uk

Richard Harvey
BVetMed, CIBiol, MIBiol, DVD, DipECVD, MRCVS
The Veterinary Centre, 207 Daventry Road, Coventry CV3
    5HH
Tel: 01203 717640
Fax: 01203 506008
Email: r.harvey@pop3.demon.co.uk

Herman A. W. Hazewinkel
DVM, PhD, DipRNVA, DipECVS
Professor, Department of Clinical Sciences of Companion
    Animals, Faculty of Veterinary Medicine, Utrecht
    University, PO Box 80.154, NL-3508 TD Utrecht, The
    Netherlands
Tel: 31 30 253 9411
Fax: 31 30 251 8126
Email: h.a.w.hazewinkel@ukg.dgk.ruu.nl

Julie I. Henfrey
BVM&S, Cert SAD, MRCVS
Sheriffs Highway Veterinary Hospital, 94 Sheriffs
    Highway, Low Fell, Gateshead NE9 5SD
Tel: 0191 487 7319

Dominique Heripret
Dr Vétérinaire, DipECVD
Porte D'Orleans, 43 Avenue Aristide-Briand, 94110
    Arcueil, France
Tel: 33 1 49 858300
Fax: 33 1 49 858301

Michael Herrtage
MA, BVSc, DVR, DVD, DSAM, MRCVS, DipECVDI,
    DipECVIM
Lecturer, Department of Clinical Veterinary Medicine,
    University of Cambridge, Madingley Road, Cambridge
    CB3 0ES
Tel: 01223 337600
Fax: 01223 337610
Email: mh10001@cam.ac.uk

Peter B. Hill
BVSc, PhD, CertSAD, MRCVS
Lecturer, Department of Clinical Studies, Royal (Dick)
    School of Veterinary Studies, The University of
    Edinburgh, Small Animal Clinic, Edinburgh EH9 1QH
Tel: 0131 650 6061
Fax: 0131 650 6577

Andrew Hopkins
BVSc, MVM, DipACVIM (Neurology), DipECVN
North Florida Neurology, 1015 SE Lake Lane, Keystone
    Heights, FL 32656
Tel: 1 904 269 7070

Christine C. Jenkins
DVM, DipACVIM
Technical Director, Department of Technical Services,
    Pfizer Animal Health, 812 Springdale, Exton, PA 19341,
    USA
Tel: 1 610 363 3411
Fax: 1 610 363 3286

Lennart Jönsson
DVM, PhD
Professor, Department of Pathology, Swedish University
    of Agricultural Sciences, Uppsala, Sweden

Peter P. Kintzer
DVM, DipACVIM
Laboratory Animal Medicine and Small Animal Medicine,
    Tufts University, 200 Westboro Road, North Grafton,
    MA 01536, USA
Tel: 1 508 839 5302
Fax: 1 508 839 7980

Peter Lees
CBE, BPharm, PhD, CBiol, FIBiol, Dr hc (Gent), Hon
    Assoc RCVS
Professor and Vice-Principal, Department of Veterinary
    Basic Sciences, Royal Veterinary College, University of
    London, Royal College Street, London NW1 0UT
Tel: 0171 468 5266
Fax: 0171 388 1027
Email: jelliott@rvc.ac.uk

Virginia Luis Fuentes
MAVetMB, PhD, DVC, MRCVS
Assistant Professor, College of Veterinary Medicine,
    Veterinary Medical Teaching Hospital, Clydesdale Hall,
    University of Missouri-Columbia, Columbia, MO
    65211, USA
Tel: 1 573 882 7821
Fax: 1 573 884 5444

Andrew Mackin
BSc, BVMS, MVS, DVSc, DSAM, FACVSc, DACVIM,
    MRCVS
WALTHAM Lecturer in Internal Medicine and Clinical
    Nutrition, Department of Veterinary Clinical Studies,
    Royal (Dick) School of Veterinary Studies, University
    of Edinburgh, Summerhall, Edinburgh EH9 1QH
Tel: 0131 650 6064
Fax: 0131 650 6577
Email: andrew.mackin@ed.ac.uk

Jill E. Maddison
BVSc, Dip Vet Clin Stud, PhD, FAVSc
Senior Lecturer, Department of Pharmacology, The
    University of Sydney, Sydney, NSW 2006, Australia
Tel: 61 2 9351 2315
Fax: 61 2 9566 2564
Email: jillm@pharmacol.usyd.edu.au

Ian S. Mason
BVetMed, PhD, MRCVS, CertSAD, DipECVD
2 Kempton Court, Kempton Avenue, Sunbury-on-
    Thames, Middlesex TW16 5PA
Tel: 01932 770769
Fax: 01932 779701
Email: ian_mason@msn.com

Christopher May
MRCVS
Grove Veterinary Hospital, Hibbert Street, New Mills,
    Stockport, Cheshire SK12 3JJ
Tel: 01663 745294
Fax: 01663 763419

Irene McCandlish
BVMS, PhD, MRCVS
Senior Histopathologist, Grange Laboratories, Grange
    House, Sandbeck Way, Wetherby,
West Yorkshire LS22 5JU
Tel: 01937 581649

Nicholas J. Millichamp
BVetMed, BSc, PhD, DVOpthal, DipACVO, MRCVS
Associate Professor, Department of Small Animal
    Medicine and Surgery, College of Veterinary Medicine,
    TX 77843, USA
Tel: 1 409 845 2351
Fax: 1 409 845 6978
Email: njm@cvm.tamu.edu

Joanna S. Morris
BSc, BVSc, PhD, FRCVS
Research Fellow, Department of Clinical Veterinary
    Medicine, University of Cambridge, Madingley Road,
    Cambridge CB3 0ES
Tel: 01223 337600
Fax: 01223 337610

David E. Noakes
BVetMed, PhD, FRCVS
Professor, Department of Large Animal Medicine and
    Surgery, Royal Veterinary College, Hawkshead Lane,
    North Mymms, Hatfield, Herts AL9 7TA
Tel: 01707 666333

Andrea Nolan
MVB, PhD, DVA, MRCVS
Senior Lecturer, Department of Veterinary Pharmacology,
    University of Glasgow Veterinary School, Bearsden
    Road, Glasgow G16 1QH
Tel: 0141 330 5700
Fax: 0141 942 7215

Paul-Pierre Pastoret
DVM, PhD, DHC
Professor, Department of Immunology–Vaccinology,
    Faculty of Veterinary Medicine, University of Liege,
    Sart Tilman, B-4000 Liege, Belgium
Tel: 32 4 366 4060
Fax: 32 4 366 4061
Email: pastoret@stat.fmv.ulg.ac.be

Mark E. Peterson
DVM, DipACVIM
Head of Division of Endocrinology, Department of
    Medicine, Animal Medical Center, 510 East 62nd
    Street, NY 10021, USA
Tel: 1 212 838 8100
Fax: 1 212 486 1699
Email: mark1311@AOL.COM

Simon Petersen-Jones
DVetMed, PhD, DVO, MRCVS
Department of Small Animal Clinical Sciences, College of
    Veterinary Medicine, Michigan State University, East
    Lansing, MI 48824-1314, USA

Peter Renwick
MAVetMB, DVOphthal, MRCVS
Willows Referral Service, 78 Tanworth Lane, Shirley,
    Solihull B90 4DF
Tel: 0121 745 1354
Fax: 0121 745 9340
Email: prenwick@aol.com

Jill Sackman
DVM, PhD, DipAVCS
Principal Scientist, Ethicon Endo-Surgery Inc., 4545
    Greek Road, Cincinnati, OH 45242, USA

J. Catherine R. Scott-Moncrieff
MS, MAVetMB, DipACVIM, DSAM, MRCVS
Associate Professor, Department of Veterinary Clinical
    Sciences, Purdue University, West Layfayette, Indiana,
    IN 47907-1248, USA
Tel: 1 317 494 1107
Fax: 1 317 496 1108
Email: scottmon@vet.purdue.edu

David F. Senior
BVSc, DipACVIM
Professor, Veterinary Clinical Sciences, School of
    Veterinary Medicine, Louisiana State University, Baton
    Rouge, LA 70803-9610, USA
Tel: 1 504 346 3108
Fax: 1 504 346 3295
Email: dsenior@vt8200.vetmed.lsu.edu

Ewa Sevelius
DVM, PhD
Specialist in Small Animal Disease, Chief of Staff, Small
    Animal Clinic, Animal Hospital of Helsingborg,
    Sweden

Nicholas J. Sharp
BVetMed, PhD, MVM, DipACVIM (Neurology),
    MRCVS
Associate Professor, College of Veterinary Medicine,
    North Carolina State University, 4700 Hillsborough
    Street, Raleigh, NC 27606, USA
Tel: 1 919 829 4233
Fax: 1 919 829 4336
Email: nick_sharp@ncsu.edu

David H. Shearer
BVetMed, CertSAD, PhD, MRVCS
Veterinary Dermatology Referral, 44 Meadowland Road,
    Henbury, Bristol BS10 7PW
Tel: 01179 837495
Email: shearer@dermatology.u-net.com

Kenneth W. Simpson
BVM&S, PhD, DipACVIM, MRCVS
Assistant Professor, Department of Clinical Sciences,
    College of Veterinary Medicine, Cornell University,
    Ithaca, NY 14853-6401, USA
Tel: 1 607 253 3570
Fax: 1 607 253 3055
Email: kws5@cornell.edu

Richard A. Squires
BVSc, PhD, DVR, DipACVIM, MRCVS
Secretary and Director, NZVA Foundation for Continuing
    Education, Centre for Veterinary Education, Massey
    University, Palmerston North, New Zealand
Tel: 64 6 350 5227
Fax: 64 6 350 5659
Email: r.a.squires@massey.ac.nz

Martin Sullivan
BVMS, PhD, DVR, MRCVS
Senior Lecturer, Department of Small Animal Studies,
    University of Glasgow Veterinary School, Bearsden
    Road, Glasgow G16 1QH
Tel: 0141 330 5700
Fax: 0141 942 7215

Joe Taboada
BS, DVM, DipACVIM
Associate Professor, Veterinary Clinical Sciences, School
    of Veterinary Medicine, Louisiana State University,
    Baton Rouge, LA 70803-9610, USA
Tel: 1 504 346 3108
Fax: 1 504 346 3295
Email: taboada@vt8200.vetmed.lsu.edu

Bryn J. Tennant
BVSc, PhD, CertVR, MRCVS
Veterinary Investigation Officer, Veterinary Services, Bush
    Estate, Penicuik, Midlothian EH26 0QE
Tel: 0131 445 5544

Hal Thompson
BVMS, PhD, MRCVS
Senior Lecturer, Department of Veterinary Pathology,
    University of Glasgow Veterinary School, Bearsden
    Road, Glasgow G16 1QH
Tel: 0141 330 5700
Fax: 0141 942 7215

Andrew G. Torrance
MAVetMB, PhD, DipACVIM, DipECVIM, MRCVS
Director, Bloxham Laboratories, George Street,
    Teignmouth, Devon TQ14 8AH
Tel: 01626 778844
Fax: 01626 779570

Sandy J. Trees
BVM&S, PhD, MRCVS
Professor, Department of Veterinary Parasitology,
    University of Liverpool, PO Box 147, Liverpool L69
    3BX
Tel: 0151 7089393
Email: trees@liverpool.ac.uk

Laurence Trepanier
DVM, PhD, DipAVCM
Assistant Professor, Department of Medical Sciences,
    School of Veterinary Medicine, University of
    Wisconsin-Madison, 2015 Linden drive West, Madison,
    WI 53706 1102, USA

Elizabeth J. Villiers
BVSc, CertSAM, CertVR MRCVS
Chesterford Cytology Service, Hills Cottage, Carmen
    Street, Great Chesterford, Saffron Walden, Essex CB10
    1NR
Tel: 01799 531904

Margaret W. Vroom
DVM
Boxtelsebaan 6
5061 VD Oidsterwijk
The Netherlands

Robert J. Washabau
VMD, PhD, DipACVIM
Associate Professor, School of Veterinary Medicine,
    University of Pennsylvania, 3900 Delancey Street,
    Philadelphia, PA 19104-6010, USA
Tel: 1 215 897 3395
Fax: 1 215 573 6050
Email: washabau@vet.upenn.edu

A. David J. Watson
BVSc, PhD, FACVSc, FFAAVPT, FRCVS
Associate Professor, Department of Veterinary Clinical
    Studies, Faculty of Veterinary Science, The University
    of Sydney, Sydney, NSW, Australia
Tel: 61 2 692 222
Fax: 61 2 566 2564

Alexander H. Werner
VMD, DipACVD
Valley Veterinary Speciality Services, 13125 Ventura Blvd,
    Studio City, CA 91604, USA
Tel: 1 800 781 VVSS
Fax: 1 818 981 6935

Zerai Woldehiwet
DVM, PhD, MRCVS
Lecturer, Department of Veterinary Pathology, University
    of Liverpool, Leahurst, Chester High Road, Neston,
    South Wirral L64 7TE
Tel: 0151 7946113
Fax: 0151 7946005
Email: zerai@liverpool.ac.uk

Preface to the Fourth Edition

The previous edition of this text was published eight years ago; the intervening years have seen a sustained expansion in the knowledge and understanding of the pathophysiology of the medical diseases that affect the dog. This has been complemented by significantly improved methods to diagnose and manage these diseases. The fourth edition of this textbook has been designed to reflect these many advances and has necessitated a radically different approach from the previous edition. Even with these changes it has not been possible to cover every disease in detail but this is a consequence of the volumes of clinical research. I hope that the logical approach to the management of clinical disease compensates for any omissions that there may be. There are fourteen sections, each with an editor to co-ordinate the chapters in that section. The number of authors contributing to this edition has expanded from twenty-nine to seventy-eight.

The first three sections have not been present in previous editions. Section 1 covers the principles of therapeutics and sets the platform for many of the following sections. It was felt important to separate this out as a section in order to give it the due prominence that the subject deserves. The key facts on infectious diseases of the dog are covered in the second section but there was insufficient space here to discuss the many exciting developments in bacteriology, virology and parasitology. As a result, the reader is referred to other texts which deal with the detail of these subjects.

Diagnostic laboratory investigations have become an integral part of the evaluation of the many presenting problems that face the small animal clinician. The sections on system-based diseases contain the relevant laboratory investigations and interpretation. There is the potential to misinterpret clinical laboratory data and Section 3 discusses some of the pitfalls that can occur and I hope that readers will find this section helpful in avoiding these pitfalls.

Sections 4–13 are system based and provide a logical guide to the diagnosis and management of diseases. The chapters within each section have been structured in a way to help the reader find the information they need clearly and easily. Each section has been written to give both concise reviews of the subject and a logical approach to the management of the clinical problems. A significant number of tables. flow diagrams and illustrations have been included to assist the clinician in accessing key clinical information. Section 14 gives a guide to the management of poisons in the dog.

I am delighted that this edition joins the impressive array of publications that has been produced by the BSAVA and hope that it will continue to be a reference text for use in clinical practice at all levels.

Neil T. Gorman
March 1998

Acknowledgements

This has been one of the most challenging projects I have had and am greatly indebted to the section editors who have worked with me on this project. They have given freely of their time and been prepared to be contacted at all times from all corners of the world. There have been many challenges since the inception of the project and fortunately, between us, we have been able to overcome these and ensure that the book is completed as planned. The authors of chapters have worked with their section editor to produce a co-ordinated view and have been under great pressure to deliver their work on time.

There are many other individuals who have given permission to use their material and who have given their advice, to whom I am grateful. Great credit is due to John Fuller who, as ever, has prepared illustrations in the text with meticulous care and creativity.

I am indebted to Richard Miles and Robert Dyer from Blackwell Science for their interest, enthusiasm and support in the production of the book. Finally, I would like to thank those who have supported me and in their own individual way helped me complete this book.

Section 1

Therapeutics

Edited by Jonathan Elliott

Chapter 1

Good Prescribing Practice

L. Trepanier and J. Elliott

INTRODUCTION

Practising veterinary surgeons should ensure that drugs are used in a safe and effective way by:

- complying with the legislation concerning medicines;
- recognising their potential hazards to themselves and their staff and understanding how to avoid these;
- considering the many factors that can interact with the chosen therapeutic agent and influence the outcome of therapy;
- considering the use of therapeutic drug monitoring, where appropriate, to assist in successful drug therapy.

This chapter considers all of these issues.

LEGAL ASPECTS OF MEDICINES AND PRESCRIBING

The legislation that governs the storage, handling, use and supply of medicines in veterinary practice includes:

- The Medicines Act 1968 and the Medicines (Restrictions on the Administration of Veterinary Medicinal Products) Regulations, 1994
- The Misuse of Drugs Act 1971 and The Misuse of Drugs Regulations 1985
- The Health and Safety at Work Act 1974 and The Control of Substances Hazardous to Health Regulations 1988.

The Medicines Act 1968

The Government ensures the quality, safety and efficacy of medicines for human and animal use by a system of marketing authorisations (formerly termed 'product licences'). Manufacturers and wholesale dealers of medicinal products require *manufacturer's* and *wholesale dealer's authorisations* respectively. An exemption to this law is that veterinary surgeons do not require a marketing authorisation to prepare a medicinal product themselves (or to request another veterinary surgeon to prepare such a product for them) for a particular animal under their care. The veterinary surgeon is only allowed to stock a very limited supply of a medicine prepared in this way (2.5 kg of solid and 5 litres of liquid). It is not permissible for vaccines (other than autogenous vaccines) to be prepared in this way.

Use of Unlicensed Products in Veterinary Medicine

The recent introduction of the Medicines (Restrictions on the Administration of Veterinary Medicinal Products) Regulations, 1994 has effectively made the British Veterinary Association's code of practice for the prescription of medicinal products by veterinary surgeons now a legal requirement. In dogs, the order in which the use of medicinal products should be considered is:

(1) a product which has a veterinary marketing authorisation for the dog and for the condition to be treated;
(2) one which is authorised for another condition or another veterinary species;
(3) if no veterinary licensed alternative exists, products authorised for human use may be used;
(4) special products made by the veterinary surgeon or by a pharmacist for the veterinary surgeon, which have

no marketing authorisation, should only be used if a veterinary or human authorised product does not already exist.

Guidance has been issued by the Veterinary Medicine Directorate which seems to allow the canine practitioner more flexibility in the use of unlicensed products for the management of his/her patients than these regulations would initially suggest. For example, if the age or concomitant disease state of the dog mean that the practitioner considers that the authorised product is unsuitable in this individual case, he or she may conclude that the authorised product does not exist and so prescribe an unlicensed product.

Legal Categories of Medicines

When granting a marketing authorisation for a drug the licensing body places the medicine into one of three main categories which are listed below in order of decreasing strictness of controls over their supply to the public.

- Prescription only medicines (POMs) including controlled drugs (CD)
- Pharmacy only medicines (P) including merchants' list (PML)
- General sales list medicines (GSL)

Table 1.1 Legal categorisation of medicinal products.

Legal category	Subcategory	Definition	Examples
Prescription only medicines (POM)	Controlled drugs	A subcategory of POM where the regulations for supply and storage are even more stringent than general POM medicines	Morphine (S2) Phenobarbitone (S3)

	General POM drugs	Can only be prescribed and dispensed by a veterinary surgeon or dispensed by a pharmacist against a prescription written and signed by a veterinary surgeon	Many veterinary medicines such as:
			    Antibacterial drugs
			    Vaccines
			    Any drug intended for parenteral
			        administration.

Pharmacy only medicines (P)	General P medicines	Any drug in this category may be sold over the counter by a registered pharmacist to the general public. A veterinary surgeon may supply drugs in this category for the treatment of animals under his/her care	Most P medicines are human products (e.g. famotidine) Veterinary example: Dermisol™
	Pharmacist Merchants' list (PML)	Drugs in this sub-category in addition to the general regulations described for P medicines may also be sold by agricultural merchants registered with the Royal Pharmaceutical Society to persons whose business involves animals (e.g. farmers)	Large animal anthelmintics Ectoparasiticides
	Saddlers' list (PML)	Saddlers who are registered with the Royal Pharmaceutical Society may sell certain anthelmintics to horse owners	Anthelmintics for horses
General sale list (GSL)	–	Medicinal products where the hazard to health or the need to take special precautions is sufficiently small that they can be sold without a prescription by pet shops or merchants who are not subject to special regulation. A number of veterinary products are GSL only when produced for external use or, when formulated for oral administration a maximum strength which may be sold is stipulated	Piperazine citrate Permethrin flea spray Pipronyl butoxide

More detailed information of these categories and their subdivisions is given in Table 1.1. In summary, the only category of medicine that can be sold direct to the public by a veterinary practice without the owner having consulted with a veterinary surgeon are GSL products. For all other categories of drugs, the animals for which they are intended should be under the care of a veterinary surgeon.

Storage, Dispensing and Labelling of Medicines

Storage
The manufacturer's recommendations should be carefully followed for each medicine in terms of storage temperature, sensitivity of the compound to light and humidity. Other important considerations are:

- Medicines should be stored in an area that is not accessible to the general public.
- Well designed shelves are essential to allow easy access to the drugs required reducing the possibility of breakage, spillage or misplacement of stock.

Box 1.1 Recommended containers for medicines.

Container	Medicine
Coloured flute bottles	Medicines for external application, e.g. shampoos, soaps, lotions. Enemas, eye and ear medications should be similarly dispensed if not already packaged in a suitable plastic container.
Plain glass bottles	Oral liquid medicines
Wide-mouthed jars	Creams, dusting powders, granules
Paper board cartons/ Wallets	Sachets, manufacturers' strip or blister packed medicines.
Airtight glass, plastic or metal containers (preferably child proof)*	All solid oral medicines (tablets or capsules)

* Discretion can be exercised with child-proof containers. Some aged and infirm clients may request plain screw top containers.

- A work surface should be provided which can be easily cleaned.
- Adequate refrigeration space should be available.

Effective stock control will save time and money ensuring that old stock is used before new so that medicines in stock do not exceed their expiry date and that the pharmacy does not run out of a particular medication.

Dispensing and Labelling
The containers recommended by the Council of the Royal Pharmaceutical Society for the dispensing of medicines from bulk packs are shown in Box 1.1. Note that paper envelopes and plastic bags are unacceptable forms of container.

The Medicines Act and the Medicine Labelling Regulations state the legal requirements for labelling of dispensed medicines. These regulations apply whether the medicines are dispensed in the manufacturer's original container or dispensed from bulk into smaller packages. Labels should be legible and indelible (written in biro or felt pen *not* washable ink or pencil). Printed labels can be generated by computers used in modern practices. A specimen label shown below indicates essential information which has to be provided by law and optional (but desirable) information to put on a label.

Essential   For Animal Treatment Only   Owner's name, pet identification and address   Date   Name & address of veterinary surgeon   Keep out of the reach of children
Optional   Quantity and strength of drug   Instructions for dosing

If the medication is for external use the words 'For external use only' should appear on the label. In addition, any safety precautions the owners should take when handling the drug should be added.

The Misuse of Drugs Act 1971 and The Misuse of Drugs Regulations 1985

This legislation controls the production, supply, possession, storage and dispensing of drugs where the potential of abuse by man exists. These drugs are a special category of POM products, the controlled drugs (CD), of which there are five schedules which are listed below with the drugs included in each schedule:

- *Schedule 1* (S1) – addictive drugs such as cannabis and hallucinogens mescaline and LSD.
- *Schedule 2* (S2) – the opiate analgesics morphine, etorphine, fentanyl and pethidine plus cocaine and amphetamine.
- *Schedule 3* (S3) – the barbiturates pentobarbitone and phenobarbitone plus the opiate analgesics, buprenorphine and pentazocine.
- *Schedule 4* (S4) – benzodiazepines such as diazepam and chlordiazepoxide.
- *Schedule 5* (S5) – certain preparations of cocaine, codeine and morphine that contain less than a specified amount of the drug. Examples: Codeine cough linctus, kaolin and morphine antidiarrhoeal suspension.

A veterinary surgeon does not have any general authority to possess or supply drugs from Schedule 1. Some of the other controlled drugs are subject to more stringent regulations than general POM medications as detailed below:

- *Purchase* of S2 and S3 drugs requires a written requisition to a wholesaler, manufacturer or pharmacist which includes the veterinary surgeon's signature, their name and address and profession, the purpose for which the drug is required and the total quantity of the drug required. If a messenger is sent to collect the drug, written authority has to be given by the veterinary surgeon for the messenger to receive the drug on their behalf.
- *Storage*: S2 drugs and buprenorphine (from S3) must be kept in a locked cupboard that is attached to a wall. The veterinary surgeon is responsible for the key to such a cupboard which should only be opened with his or her authority.
- *Records*: A bound register of all transactions involving S2 drugs must be kept. Details of purchases of S2 drugs and their outgoings (drugs given to animals on the practice premises or dispensed to an owner to give to their animal) should be recorded in separate parts of the register with a section for each individual drug in both parts of the register (i.e. the records for pethidine should be separated from those for morphine). Such registers for controlled drugs are available commercially. In addition, any S2 drug which is no longer required by the veterinary practice can only be disposed of in the presence of a Home Office Inspector. A record has to be made in the register which the Inspector is required to sign.
- *Special prescription requirements for controlled drugs*

apply to those drugs in S2 and S3. An example of a prescription is given below:

Mr J. Simmons, MA, Vet MB MRCVS
50, High Street, Comberton, Cambridge CB4 1RL
Tel: 01223 849623

25th September 1995

Mr J. R. Howe's dog 'Ludwig'
23, The Green,
Barton, Cambridge.

Rx
Tablets Pethidine 50 mg
Send 20 (ten)

Label: Give half a tablet twice a day for 5 days

For Animal Treatment Only

This animal is under my care

No repeats

The format is the same for any drug that the veterinary surgeon would like a pharmacist to dispense to one of his/her clients. In the case of S2 and S3 drugs, the name and address of the client, the date and the quantity (in numbers and words) and strength of the preparation should be written in the veterinary surgeon's own handwriting.

The Health and Safety at Work Act 1974 and The Control of Substances Hazardous to Health (COSHH) Regulations 1988

When common sense is used and a few general ground rules followed, the medicines used in most veterinary practices present a relatively small hazard to the health of employees. All data sheets of authorised medicines will discuss any hazards the medicine might pose to the person dispensing and administering the drug. Each veterinary practice should also have produced a COSHH assessment for the substances (including drugs) that personnel working in the practice come into contact with on a daily basis. If these safety measures are followed any risk will be reduced to the absolute minimum.

Drugs can get into the body by accident and have systemic effects in the operator in a number of ways:

(1) *Absorption across the skin* occurs particularly with lipophilic drugs such as:

- prostaglandins (luteolytic agents),
- insecticides,
- nitrovasodilators,
- compounds containing the solvent DMSO (dimethyl sulphoxide) which aids penetration of substances which are dissolved in it across the skin (e.g. the corticosteroid, flumethasone).

When handling such substances or when handling any substance when you have cuts or abrasions on your hands, gloves should be worn to prevent absorption across the skin. Washing hands after handling any medicine and rinsing splashes of liquid medicines from the skin as soon as they occur are good practices to follow.

(2) *Absorption across mucous membranes*: The conjunctiva nasal and oral mucous membranes are sites that drugs may reach if aerosols from liquid formulations or dust from powders containing the drug are formed, which can be accidentally sprayed into the eyes or mouth. Aerosols are formed most often when reconstituting lyophylised drugs for injection and when expelling air bubbles from a syringe. They can be avoided by:
- not over-pressurising the contents of vials when adding diluents,

- keeping the needle cover on the needle when expelling air bubbles from syringes,
- allowing trained personnel only to reconstitute cytotoxic drugs in designated areas (see Chapter 5).

Should accidental contamination of the eyes, nose or mouth occur, flush the area with copious amounts of water in the first instance and then seek appropriate help.

(3) *Accidental ingestion* of drugs can occur through aerosols or dust as described above or through contaminated food being eaten. Food and drink must not be consumed or stored in areas where drugs are being handled, including areas where topical sprays (e.g. flea sprays) are applied to animals. Smoking should also be prohibited form these areas.

(4) *Inhalation* of volatile substances such as gaseous anaesthetics, dust from powders and droplets from aerosols may cause irritation of the respiratory tract or the drugs can be absorbed and cause systemic effects. Hazards from inhalation can be minimised by:
- the use of an adequate scavenging circuit attached to the anaesthetic circuit,
- providing good ventilation of the operating room,

Table 1.2 Potentially hazardous drugs used in canine practice.

Hazardous drug	Comments
Etorphine	Highly toxic following accidental injection or exposure of skin or mucous membranes
Halothane	Repeated inhalation may damage the liver and has been incriminated in increasing the risk of miscarriages
Cytotoxic drugs	Many are mutagenic, carcinogenic and teratogenic
Prostaglandins	May cause asthma attacks, have serious effects on the cardiovascular system and cause uterine contractions. Should not be handled by asthmatics or women of child bearing age. (See British Veterinary Association code of practice for use of prostaglandins in cattle and pigs)
Antimicrobials Griseofulvin,	Teratogenic and should not be handled by women of child bearing age. Protective clothing, impervious gloves and a dust mask should be worn when handling the powdered form and adding this to feed
Penicillins and cephalosporins	May cause hypersensitivity on exposure in operators who are allergic to these drugs. The reaction can range from mild skin rash to swelling of the eyes, lips and face with difficulty breathing, symptoms which would require immediate medical attention. You should not handle drugs in these two families if you have a history of allergy to them
Chloramphenicol	Can cause a fatal aplastic anaemia in man, a reaction which is not related to the dose received and occurs in a very small number of people exposed to the drug when prescribed for them by doctors. Nevertheless, it is wise to avoid unnecessary exposure to this drug by taking the precautions mentioned above, including avoiding direct contact of the drug with the skin

- wearing dust masks and eye protection when dispensing powders from bulk packs,
- using insecticidal sprays in well ventilated areas only.

(5) *Accidental injection* is the final way in which drugs may get into the body. This risk may be minimised by keeping all needles covered until the injection is made and disposing of used needles in a safe way immediately after use. The quantity of drug that enters the body following penetration of the skin with a needle is very small. Oil based vaccines can, however, produce very severe reactions. Some drugs, such as etorphine, are extremely toxic to man such that even these minute quantities are hazardous.

Hazardous Drugs Used in Veterinary Practice

The groups of drugs mentioned in Table 1.2 carry special risks and so are worthy of note. It is important to realise that whilst some drugs may produce acute effects on the operator which are obvious shortly after exposure, other drugs can have cumulative effects, when exposure to small quantities occurs over a long period of time, which can be just as detrimental. For this reason it is good practice to keep exposure to all drugs handled to an absolute minimum by following the ground rules mentioned above.

As can be seen from the above discussion, hazards are greatest from drugs that are formulated in a liquid or powder form where aerosols, accidental injection or dust can lead to significant exposure of the operator. Many capsules and tablets can be safely handled with minimal or no contact with the drug, provided they are not broken or ground up to release the contents in a powdered form. For some tablets it is still good practice to wear gloves when handling them (e.g. cyclophosphamide, mitotane and griseofulvin). The use of a triangular metal or plastic tablet counter facilitates the counting of tablets and reduces any contact between the operator and the tablets to a minimum.

DRUG INTERACTIONS

A drug interaction occurs whenever there is a change in the action of one drug resulting from the following (Griffiths 1988; Wright 1992):

- adverse storage conditions,
- administration of other drugs,
- concurrent food intake.

Drug interactions may:

- produce a favourable effect (e.g. probenecid prolongs the duration of action of penicillin),
- be clinically insignificant,
- lead to an adverse outcome (toxicity or therapeutic failure).

A large number of adverse drug interactions have been reported in the human literature – only those reactions which have been shown to occur, or are likely to occur, in canine patients will be included here.

Unfavourable drug interactions can occur at any time from the moment a drug is chosen from the pharmacy shelf to the time the patient eliminates the drug or its metabolites from the body (see Table 1.3).

Problems Before Administration

Improperly stored drugs may oxidise, hydrolyse, or otherwise decompose to less active by-products. Outdated drugs are likely to have lost potency. A drug's expiration date indicates the date before which at least 90% of the labelled compound is stable and active, as guaranteed by the manufacturer. Routine use of outdated drugs is likely to lead to therapeutic failure, as there is no way to determine the appropriate dose for a patient since the concentration of active drug is no longer known.

Some drugs can become more toxic with prolonged storage, e.g. breakdown products of tetracyclines which form with prolonged exposure to heat, moisture, or acidic conditions, are nephrotoxic. The administration of outdated tetracyclines has been associated with renal tubular damage in dogs (Riond & Riviere 1989).

Table 1.3 Possible mechanisms of drug interactions.

Interactions before drug administration
- Reactions of a drug with its storage environment
- Interactions between drugs in the syringe, infusion line or specially prepared formulation

Pharmacokinetic interactions (drug–drug or drug–food)
- Absorption
- Distribution
- Metabolism
- Elimination

Pharmacodynamic interactions (drug–drug; additive, synergistic or antagonistic)
- Drugs with common receptor sites
- Drugs with actions on the same physiologic system

Table 1.4 Drugs that are incompatible for co-infusion.

Drug	Incompatible with
Ampicillin	Dextrose Gentamicin
Atropine	Diazepam
Calcium gluconate	Cephalothin Methylprednisolone sodium succinate
Cephalothin	Gentamicin Phenobarbitone Metoclopramide
Cimetidine	Cephazolin Pentobarbitone
Diazepam	Potassium chloride (40 mEq/l) Ranitidine Glycopyrrolate Heparin B complex with vitamin C
Frusemide	Gentamicin Metoclopramide
Glycopyrrolate	Pentobarbitone Diazepam Heparin
Heparin	Aminoglycosides Tetracyclines
Pentobarbitone	Phenytoin Sodium bicarbonate Cimetidine Ranitidine
Sodium bicarbonate	Adrenaline Dopamine Soluble insulin

From Paul 1982; Reilly & Isaacs 1983; Trissel 1990.

Problems during Administration

A large number of drugs are incompatible when combined before administration (see Table 1.4). Physical incompatibility can be detected by:

- change in colour
- increase in turbidity
- formation of precipitates

when two or more drugs are combined (Trissel 1990). Loss of activity of one or both drugs can occur without visible changes. Drugs with multiple incompatibilities include sodium bicarbonate, calcium gluconate, diazepam, heparin, ampicillin, gentamicin, and B complex vitamin solutions (Reilly & Isaacs 1983; Trissel 1990). Routine flushing of catheters with non-heparinised saline between drug boluses will avoid such interactions within infusion lines and it is best not to co-administer drugs in the same syringe.

Some drugs adsorb to fluid administration sets and become unavailable for delivery, e.g. insulin

- rapidly adsorbs to both glass and plastic;
- from 20% to 80% of a given infused dose may therefore never reach the patient (Trissel 1990);
- if the insulin infusion rate is individualised for each patient this is not a problem;
- over-dosing will occur if the infusion dose is later used as a starting dose for subcutaneous insulin administration.

Diazepam:

- adsorbs to plastic but not glass;
- for diazepam infusions in epileptic dogs, doses can be standardised by flushing the administration set with the fluid containing diazepam for 20–30 min before the calculated dose is administered to the patient.

Any drug that is supplied in an amber vial or bottle can be assumed to be photosensitive and may decompose with prolonged exposure to light (see Table 1.5 for examples). Most of these drugs, however, are reasonably stable in room light for short-term administration. If administering these drugs by prolonged infusion, infusion sets should be covered with foil (Griffiths 1988).

Pharmacokinetic Interactions

Interactions Affecting Absorption

Although there are many interactions that affect drug absorption, only a few of these are clinically significant in humans. The most common interactions affecting absorption involve:

Table 1.5 Stability of photosensitive drugs in room light.

Diazepam	at least 4 h
Amphotericin B	8–24 h
Metoclopramide	up to 24 h
Dopamine	36 h

From Trissel 1990.

- changes in gastric pH;
- the formation of drug complexes.

Gastric pH determines the ionisation state, and thus the ease of dissolution, of weakly acidic and weakly basic drugs. For example, drugs that raise gastric pH, such as antacids and H_2 blockers, markedly decrease the absorption of ketoconazole, which requires an acid environment for optimal dissolution and absorption. Insoluble drug complexes form between a number of drugs and:

- multivalent cations;
- sucralfate;
- adsorbents found in antidiarrhoeals.

To avoid such interactions it is important to establish what over-the-counter preparations are being administered by the owner. Important examples of such interactions are presented in Table 1.6.

Occasionally drugs will actually increase the absorption of other compounds. In some humans, digoxin is partially metabolised by gut flora before its absorption. Antibiotics such as erythromycin decrease the bacterial breakdown of digoxin in these patients and have led to toxicity at standard digoxin doses. The stool softener dioctyl sodium sulpho-

Table 1.6 Drug combinations which lead to altered absorption.

Drug	Absorption reduced when given with
Aspirin	Charcoal
Ciprofloxacin and erythromycin	Sucralfate Aluminium hydroxide Calcium, magnesium, iron, zinc
Digoxin	Antacids Neomycin Kaolin–pectin
Ketoconazole	Antacids, H_2 blockers
Lincomycin	Kaolin–pectin
Phenobarbitone and phenytoin	Charcoal
Tetracyclines	Antacids Sucralfate Calcium, magnesium, iron, zinc, Bismuth, kaolin–pectin Sodium bicarbonate

From Welling 1984.

succinate (DSS) can also increase the risk of digoxin toxicity by increasing the solubility and absorption of digoxin (Reilly & Isaacs 1983).

Most veterinarians tend to overlook the effect of food on drug absorption and efficacy. In general, the absorption of solid drug forms such as tablets and capsules is influenced more by the presence of food than is the absorption of suspensions and elixirs (Welling 1984). Table 1.7 lists important examples of drugs that should be given on an empty stomach. The effect of food on the absorption of antibiotics is further discussed in Chapter 4, Table 4.8. Lipophilic drugs may require some emulsification from bile salts for optimal absorption, and are best given with a fatty meal (Welling 1984; Griffiths 1988). For example, the systemic availability of mitotane is nearly 20 times greater when given to fed dogs compared with fasted dogs (Watson *et al.* 1987). Drugs formulated as esters are sometimes better absorbed with a fatty meal because dietary fat triggers the release of pancreatic esterases, which free the parent drug for absorption (e.g. chloramphenicol palmitate suspension in cats; Watson 1979).

Finally, drugs which affect gastric emptying (e.g. metoclopramide) can alter the rate of absorption of co-administered compounds. For most drugs, however, a moderate change in the rate, but not the extent, of absorption is not clinically significant. One exception is for drugs with low therapeutic indices, for which very rapid absorption and high peak serum concentrations would be dangerous. Metoclopramide should be avoided in the initial treatment of cases with paracetamol (acetaminophen) or ethanol toxicity, since it can enhance intestinal delivery and absorption of these intoxicants before gastric lavage can be performed (Welling 1984).

Distribution and Plasma Protein Binding

Many drugs exhibit some degree of binding to albumin and other plasma proteins. Protein binding:

- is reversible (i.e. protein-bound drugs are in a state of dynamic equilibrium between bound drug and free drug);
- increases drug solubility and provides a drug reservoir in the plasma;
- only free drug is able to cross biological membranes and exert its pharmacological effects.

Drugs that are protein-bound may be displaced by other compounds with higher affinities for protein binding sites resulting in increased free drug levels. For highly protein bound drugs (greater than 80–90%) which have low margins of safety, this displacement can lead to toxicity from the displaced drug.

Better absorbed on empty stomach	Feeding has little effect on extent of absorption*	Absorption (extent and/or rate) is enhanced by giving with food
Ampicillin	Amoxycillin	Chloramphenicol palmitate
Aspirin†	Digoxin	Diazepam
Captopril	Hydralazine	Griseofulvin
Ketoconazole	Prednisolone	Mitotane
Levothyroxine		Propranolol
Lincomycin		Spironolactone
Penicillin		Vitamin K_1
Tetracycline		
Theophylline		

Table 1.7 Effect of food on drug absorption.

* Rate of absorption may be slowed.
† Aspirin may cause less irritation if given with food.
From Welling 1984; Griffiths 1988.

Highly protein bound drugs susceptible to these interactions in humans are presented in Table 1.8, where examples of significant interactions are detailed. These interactions may or may not extrapolate to dogs, since there may be considerable species differences in the degree of protein binding for a given drug, and few drugs have been evaluated directly in dogs. Until more information is available in dogs, however, some caution is advisable. For example, because non-steroidal anti-inflammatory drugs increase the risk of bleeding in human patients treated with warfarin and other anticoagulants, these compounds should ideally be avoided in dogs with suspected warfarin toxicity.

Drugs may also compete for tissue binding sites, resulting in displacement and toxicity with certain drug combinations. This appears to be one of the mechanisms by which quinidine predictably increases serum digoxin concentrations. In dogs given digoxin chronically, the introduction of quinidine therapy results in increased serum digoxin levels, vomiting, and anorexia (DeRick & Belpaire 1981). Interestingly, the risk of digoxin-induced arrhythmias does not appear to be enhanced in these dogs, possibly due to the anti-arrhythmic effect of quinidine (Wilkerson & Beck 1987). Because of potential adverse gastrointestinal effects, however, veterinary cardiologists recommend that the combination of digoxin and quinidine be avoided in dogs, or, if both drugs are necessary, that the dose of digoxin be reduced by 50% when quinidine is added, with close monitoring for signs of digoxin toxicity.

Altered Hepatic Biotransformation

Many drugs, especially highly lipophilic compounds, require enzymatic biotransformation in the liver and other organs to decrease their pharmacological activity and/or enhance their water solubility for excretion in bile or urine.

- Individual cytochrome P450 enzymes in the liver have varied substrate specificities.
- Each may biotransform a number of drugs with markedly different chemical structures.
- Two drugs administered to the same patient, may compete for an enzyme such that the metabolism of one of the drugs is inhibited.
- Toxicity may result from higher serum concentrations of the unmetabolised drug.
- Cimetidine binds to the haem portion of a number of P450 enzymes and inhibits the metabolism of quite a few drugs – a significant number of adverse drug interactions are recognised with cimetidine in humans (see Table 1.9).
- Chloramphenicol binds irreversibly to cytochrome P450 enzymes and also inhibits the metabolism of many drugs in humans (see Table 1.9).

In dogs, chloramphenicol administration has been associated with:

- phenytoin toxicity (Sanders *et al.* 1979);
- profound sedation in canine epileptic patients when used in combination with primidone (Campbell 1983) or phenobarbitone;
- prolonged duration of barbiturate anaesthesia in dogs, an effect which lasts more than 3 weeks after a single intramuscular dose of 50 mg/kg of chloramphenicol sodium succinate (Teske & Carter 1971);
- recovery from chloramphenicol inhibition is dependent on synthesis of new liver enzymes rather than on

% plasma protein bound	Drug examples	Potential Interactions of importance
100–98	Acidic drugs	
	Phenylbutazone	Sulphonamides displace glipizide
	Sulphasalazine	causing hypoglycaemia
	Ibuprofen	(trimethoprim also inhibits glipizide
	Glipizide	metabolism)
	Basic drugs	Benet & Williams (1990)
	Diazepam	
98–95	Acidic drugs	
	Cloxacillin	Warfarin is displaced by many drugs
	Frusemide	including sulphonamides, NSAIDs
	Sulphadimethoxine	(which also inhibit platelet function)
	Warfarin	
95–85	Acidic drugs	
	Phenytoin	Drugs of the same chemical nature
	Digitoxin	(acidic or basic) tend to compete
		with each other most avidly.
		However, displacement is not
		always predictable
	Basic drugs	
	Clindamycin	
	Hydralazine	
	Propranolol	
	Quinidine	

Table 1.8 Drug plasma protein binding – examples of significant interactions from human medicine.

NSAIDs, non-steroidal anti-inflammatory drugs.

the clearance of chloramphenicol from the body, due to its irreversible mode of inhibition.

Other clinically useful drugs which have the side effect of being potent inhibitors of various families of cytochrome P450 enzymes are listed in Table 1.9. The data are taken from human medicine as canine studies are lacking. Until comparative data are available in dogs, it would be good prescribing practice to proceed with caution or avoid the combinations commented on in Table 1.9, where significant and potentially dangerous interactions are possible.

Drugs may also act as hepatic enzyme inducers by increasing the synthesis of one or more isoforms of cytochrome P450 enzymes. The classical example is phenobarbitone, which increases the liver content of a number of P450 enzymes, including those which metabolise phenobarbitone itself. This explains the:

- decrease in the elimination half-life of phenobarbitone observed with chronic dosing in dogs (Ravis *et al.* 1989);

- increased clearance of lignocaine (Esquivel *et al.* 1978) and possibly digoxin (Breznock 1975) in dogs receiving phenobarbitone;
- higher doses of mitotane required to treat Cushingoid dogs which are on phenobarbitone (Kintzer & Peterson 1991).

Phenytoin is another potent inducer of cytochrome P450 enzymes whose very short elimination half-life in dogs is further shortened by chronic therapy (Frey 1989). Co-administration of phenytoin and phenobarbitone has been shown experimentally to lower serum phenobarbitone concentrations in dogs (Frey *et al.* 1968). Table 1.10 lists the important interactions which result from enzyme induction. The additional drugs mentioned are again taken from human studies and canine studies are lacking.

Competition for Renal Elimination

Compared with the liver, the kidney is a much less common site for drug interactions. Drugs or their metabolites that reach the kidney may undergo:

Table 1.9 P450 enzyme inhibitors.

Enzyme Inhibitor	Drugs whose metabolism is inhibited	Comments and references	Relevance to canine medicine
Chloramphenicol	Barbiturates Phenytoin Oral hypoglycaemics Oral anticoagulants	Irreversible inhibitor Sande & Mandell 1990	Chloramphenicol leads to profound sedation when given to epileptics on primidone or phenobarbitone
Cimetidine	Diazepam Metronidazole Lignocaine Quinidine Phenytoin Propranolol Theophylline Warfarin	Most notable interaction in man is with theophylline Griffin *et al.* 1984 Somogyi & Muirhead 1987	Other H_2 blockers (ranitidine and famotidine) lack this effect at therapeutic dosages – best to use these in dogs receiving multiple drugs
Ciprofloxacin	Theophylline and other methylxanthines	Polk 1989	Enrofloxacin is metabolised to ciprofloxacin – should probably avoid enrofloxacin plus theophylline combinations in dogs
Erythromycin	Terfenadine (antihistamine) Theophylline Warfarin	Metabolite forms a stable intermediate complex with the enzyme – inhibition is prolonged Life-threatening arrhythmias have occurred in humans on erythromycin and terfenadine (Simons & Simons 1994)	Avoid combining erythromycin and new anti-histamines (e.g. in treating skin disease); avoid erythromycin in patients exposed to warfarin. Use with caution in combination with methylxanthines
Ketoconazole	Cyclosporin Terfenadine Warfarin	As for erythromycin, life-threatening arrhythmias may occur with terfenadine and ketoconazole	–
Metronidazole Phenylbutazone	Warfarin Phenytoin Warfarin	– – –	– – –

From Stockley 1991; Scott & Nierenberg 1992; and references cited in text.

- simple glomerular filtration,
- filtration and active tubular secretion,
- filtration and tubular reabsorption.

Although changes in protein binding will alter the amount of free drug available for glomerular filtration, drugs do not compete directly for glomerular filtration. Organic acids or bases have separate transport mechanisms for renal tubular secretion. Since tubular secretion is an active, saturable process, two acidic or two basic drugs may compete for secretion. For example, cimetidine and procainamide (both weak bases) compete for tubular secretion and cimetidine reduces the renal clearance of procainamide in humans leading to toxic serum procainamide concentrations in some patients given this combination (Somogyi & Muirhead 1987). This interaction has not been evaluated in dogs.

Passive renal tubular reabsorption of drugs is pH dependent, since urine pH will alter the ionisation state, and thus the lipid solubility, of drugs in the tubular lumen.

Table 1.10 P450 enzyme inducers.

Enzyme inducer	Enhances the metabolism of:*
Phenobarbitone (primidone will have the same effects)	corticosteroids *digoxin*† *griseofulvin* *lignocaine* *mitotane* (possibly) *phenobarbitone* *phenytoin* propranolol quinidine theophylline verapamil
Phenytoin	diazepam diazoxide fludrocortisone glucocorticoids *phenobarbitone* *phenytoin* theophylline thyroid hormones
Rifampicin	diazepam digoxin† doxycycline ketoconazole quinidine theophylline

* Drugs listed in italics are those for which there is evidence of induced metabolism in the dog. The remainder are extrapolated from human medicine.
† Although digoxin is primarily excreted by the kidneys, it may undergo some hepatic metabolism in dogs. In man, rifampicin increases serum digoxin levels in patients with renal failure.
From Stockley 1991, and references cited in text.

- Weak acids, (negatively charged at alkaline pH), are more readily eliminated (less likely to be reabsorbed) in alkaline urine.
- For intoxications by weak acids (e.g. barbiturates and aspirin) – use sodium bicarbonate to alkalinise the urine and hasten drug elimination (Rall 1990; Insel 1990).
- Weak bases, (e.g. amphetamines and quinidine) are non-ionised at alkaline pH and are eliminated more slowly in patients with alkaline urine.
- Co-administration of antacids or sodium bicarbonate with weak bases will delay the clearance of these drugs in humans.

(See Chapter 4 for further information on the effect of urine pH on the concentration of antibiotics in urine.)

Urine pH may also affect the solubility, and thus the toxicity, of renally excreted drugs such as sulphadiazine and other sulphonamides (weak acids). This means:

- they are poorly soluble in acid urine;
- they form crystals at low urine pH (sulphadiazine) which can lead to renal tubular damage in dogs and other species;
- urinary acidifiers such as ammonium chloride should be avoided in patients receiving sulphonamides, particularly sulphadiazine (Reilly & Isaacs 1983).

Pharmacodynamic Interactions

Pharmacological Antagonism

Many drug combinations, by virtue of their common sites of action, have antagonistic effects which may lead to loss of efficacy of one or both compounds. Most of these interactions can be predicted from a basic knowledge of the drugs' mechanisms of action, but other antagonistic interactions may be less obvious. For example, frusemide appears to mediate its diuretic and renal vasodilatory effects via the synthesis of renal prostaglandins (Hinchcliff & Muir 1991). Non-steroidal anti-inflammatory drugs which block prostaglandin synthesis, such as indomethacin, have been shown to blunt the diuretic response to frusemide in both humans and dogs, an effect which is enhanced by concurrent sodium restriction (Herchulez *et al.* 1989). Accordingly, these anti-inflammatory drugs should be avoided in dogs with congestive heart failure who are dependent on frusemide for the control of pulmonary oedema, particularly those dogs that are also on salt restricted diets.

Pharmacological Synergism

Other drug combinations lead to additive or synergistic toxicities which may or may not be evident from each drug's mechanism of action. For example:

(1) Acepromazine:
   - is a mild inhibitor of serum cholinesterase,
   - should not be used to treat excitation associated with organophosphate or carbamate intoxication, since it may worsen the cholinergic signs of intoxication from these insecticides (Reilly & Isaacs 1983).
(2) Aminoglycoside antibiotics:
   - also inhibit acetylcholine release and acetylcholine binding at the neuromuscular junction, and can cause neuromuscular blockade;

- large doses of these antibiotics, particularly when used for peritoneal lavage, have led to paralysis and respiratory arrest in human patients (Sande & Mandell 1990);
- the risk of paralysis is higher in those patients under general anaesthesia or with pre-existing neuromuscular weakness such as myasthenia gravis;
- this interaction has also been observed in dogs (Adams & Bingham 1971);
- these drugs are a poor antibiotic choice for canine patients who are sedated or anaesthetised, or who have pre-existing neuromuscular disease.

INFLUENCE OF PATIENT'S AGE AND DISEASE ON DRUG DISPOSITION

Neonates

Surprisingly, detailed descriptions of drug disposition in neonates and children are sparse in the human literature, despite the obvious need for accurate dosing information in these small patients (Snodgrass 1992). It is known that neonates have markedly different and rapidly changing physiology which alters drug handling in several important ways, which are presented in Table 1.11.

These differences increase the risk of toxicity from drugs with low therapeutic indices which rely on biotransformation or urinary excretion for elimination and demand a different dosing strategy in some, but not all cases. For example:

(1) Theophylline:
- has a larger volume of distribution but delayed elimination in one week old beagles compared with adults (Alberola et al. 1993);
- the optimal dose calculated for puppies (12 mg/kg b.i.d.) is slightly larger but less frequent than that reported for mature dogs (9 mg/kg q.i.d.);
- this information may be clinically useful, for example, in the treatment of smoke inhalation in puppies.
(2) Digoxin:
- disposition is surprisingly similar between 2-week-old and adult dogs;
- the recommended digoxin dose for puppies is the same as that for adults (Button & Gross 1980).

Because pharmacokinetic information is not available for many drugs in young dogs, the best course of action is to:

- avoid unnecessary drug therapy in these young patients;
- use drugs with large therapeutic indices whenever possible;
- where possible, use appropriate formulations of drugs for the patient's size to allow accurate dosing.

Table 1.11 Physiological differences between neonates and adults which influence drug handling.

Physiological difference of neonates compared to adults	Effect on drug handling	Comments and references
Decreased gastrointestinal motility Underdeveloped gut flora Immature mucosal enzymes	Lead to decreased absorption of some drugs	DeBacker (1985)
Increased total body water	Polar drugs have a larger volume of distribution (lower plasma concentration)	Short & Clarke (1984)
Immature liver metabolic capacity (glucuronyl and glutathione transferases and some cytochrome P450 enzymes)	Less efficient biotransformation of some drugs	Puppies are deficient at birth – these enzymes rapidly increase in the first 3–8 weeks of life (Kawalek & El Said 1990)
Decreased glomerular filtration rate, decreased renal tubular function	Less effective renal clearance of drugs	Deficiencies are present in puppies for the first 8 weeks of life (Horster & Valtin 1971)

Immature patients are at greater risk for certain drug reactions because of the increased susceptibility of some developing tissues to toxicity. For example:

- Tetracycline compounds cause tooth discoloration in puppies because of the deposition of drug in newly formed enamel and dentine; for this reason, tetracyclines should not be administered to patients with immature dentition.
- Enrofloxacin has been associated with degenerative cartilage lesions in the weight-bearing joints of growing dogs and is therefore contraindicated in any skeletally immature dog, which may preclude the use of this drug in some dogs (e.g. giant breeds) as old as 18 months.

Geriatrics

In humans, the risk of adverse drug reactions is increased in older patients (Vestal *et al.* 1992), owing to smaller body size, poor nutritional status, the presence of multiple disease processes, altered compliance and age-related changes in physiology and organ function (Montamat *et al.* 1989). Although the rate of decline in organ function can vary considerably among elderly individuals (Vestal *et al.* 1992), those factors which may lead to higher drug concentrations and therefore toxicity (drugs with low therapeutic indices) in elderly patients are:

- a decline in renal function – the most consistent change in older humans (Montamat *et al.* 1989), which is also evident in older dogs;
- sub-clinical decreases in glomerular filtration rate (GFR) are sufficient to increase the risk of toxicity from some renally excreted drugs such as:
  o gentamicin,
  o digoxin,
  o procainamide (Montamat *et al.* 1989);
- decreased lean muscle mass;
- decreased total body water leads to higher plasma drug concentrations from polar drugs such as cimetidine in humans (Vestal *et al.* 1992);
- small decreases in serum albumin concentrations and decreased binding affinity of some drugs for albumin cause:
  o minor effects overall in older humans,
  o appear to be involved in the higher incidence of side effects from non-steroidal anti-inflammatory compounds in these patients (Wallace & Verbeeck 1987);
- decreased liver mass and diminished liver blood flow (Vestal 1989) leads to reduced clearance of some cardiovascular drugs, such as propranolol and hydralazine.

Because the disposition of most drugs has not been evaluated in geriatric dogs, these patients should be monitored carefully when treated with drugs characterised by low therapeutic indices.

Congestive Heart Failure

Patients with congestive heart failure are susceptible to drug toxicity for several reasons. Many cardiac drugs have low therapeutic indices, cardiac patients are frequently treated with multiple drugs which interact (see Table 1.12), and drug disposition is altered when cardiac output is decreased. In congestive failure, blood is shunted from skeletal muscle and viscera to the brain and heart (Benowitz & Meister 1983). This can increase delivery of digoxin to the central nervous system and myocardium and result in side effects such as vomiting, anorexia, and arrhythmias. Pre-renal azotaemia resulting from cardiac failure merits a dose reduction of a number of cardiac drugs, including digoxin, procainamide and enalapril.

Poor visceral blood flow and gut oedema in heart failure impairs the absorption of some orally administered drugs in humans, such as frusemide, quinidine, and procainamide (Benet *et al.* 1976). Hepatic congestion and impaired cardiac output can affect drug metabolism, since cytochrome P450 enzymes require oxygen for catalytic activity (Benowitz & Meister 1983).

Hepatic Failure

Surprisingly, acute hepatic failure does not significantly affect the metabolism of most drugs, so that drug dose adjustments are usually not necessary for acute liver disease. Although inter-individual differences are considerable, drug metabolising capacity is reduced in most humans with chronic end-stage liver disease. For example, cirrhosis in man leads to:

- Shunting and decreased hepatic blood flow causing decreased clearance of drugs such as:
  o propranolol,
  o codeine,
  o hydralazine.
  [It is recommended that the oral dose of these drugs be reduced as much as 5 to 10 fold in human cirrhotic patients (Somogyi & Rolan 1986)]
- Decreased cytochrome P450 metabolism of some compounds, such as:
  o chloramphenicol,
  o metronidazole,
  o diazepam.

Table 1.12 Drug interactions in cardiovascular therapeutics.

Drugs interacting	Mechanism of interaction	Result of interaction
Pharmacodynamic interactions:		
Digoxin, propranolol and calcium channel blockers	All slow conduction through the AV node	Excessive reduction in heart rate and cardiac output
Vasodilators and diuretics	Both classes of drug may reduce cardiac pre-load	Excessive pre-load reduction resulting in hypotension and pre-renal azotaemia
Potassium sparing diuretics and ACE inhibitors	Both classes reduce potassium excretion	Hyperkalaemia could result
Loop diuretics and digoxin	Hypokalaemia and hypomagnesaemia enhances digoxin inhibition of the sodium pump	Increased digoxin toxicity
Potassium losing diuretics and anti-dysrhythmic agents	Hypokalaemia reduces the efficacy of anti-dysrhythmic agents and increases risk of pro-arrhythmic action Hypomagnesaemia is pro-arrhythmogenic	Failure of anti-arrhythmic therapy Increased toxicity of anti-arrhythmic drugs (particularly Classes Ia and III)
Pharmacokinetic interactions:		
Propranolol and lignocaine	Propranolol reduces hepatic blood flow and lignocaine clearance is dependent on hepatic blood flow	Increased blood levels of lignocaine
Quinidine and digoxin	Quinidine displaces digoxin from skeletal muscle binding sites	Increased blood levels of digoxin
Verapamil or diltiazem and digoxin	Verapamil and diltiazem reduce renal clearance of digoxin	Increased blood levels of digoxin

[These drugs should therefore be avoided in liver failure or used at 25–50% of standard doses with careful monitoring (Somogyi & Rolan 1986).]
- Hypoalbuminaemia and decreased protein binding affinity (McClean & Morgan 1991) may cause increased free drug concentrations of highly protein bound drugs such as:
  ○ phenylbutazone,
  ○ diazepam.
- The presence of ascites makes it difficult to dose drugs accurately:
  ○ can lead to an overestimation of body weight and overdosage of lipophilic drugs which do not distribute to ascites fluid;
  ○ polar drugs such as gentamicin do equilibrate with ascites fluid, leading to decreased serum drug concentrations and prolonged elimination rates (Somogyi & Rolan 1986).

Liver failure is also associated with enhanced sensitivity to central nervous system depressants. Opioids, benzodiazepines, acepromazine, and barbiturates may cause marked sedation in these patients due to an altered blood brain barrier and/or altered cerebral function (McClean & Morgan 1991). Patients with liver failure also have elevated serum aldosterone levels, and because of this are particularly prone to hypokalaemia following frusemide administration (Somogyi & Rolan 1986). Those drugs which are potentially hepatotoxic and which should be avoided in the liver failure patient are listed in Table 1.13.

Renal Failure

Drug pharmacokinetic changes associated with renal failure include decreased protein binding of acidic drugs, some alterations in hepatic drug metabolism, and, of course, decreased renal clearance of drugs due to decreased glomerular filtration rate (GFR), diminished active tubular secretion, and altered drug reabsorption (Aronson *et al.* 1986). Once the glomerular filtration rate is reduced to 30–40% of normal, elimination of renally cleared drugs becomes significantly impaired and drug dose adjustment becomes necessary (Riviere & Davis 1984) (see Table 1.14). This is particularly important for drugs with small therapeutic indices and even the dosages of relatively safe drugs,

Table 1.13 Potentially hepatotoxic drugs to avoid in liver failure patients.

Thiacetarsamide	Ketoconazole
Phenobarbitone	Anabolic steroids
Phenytoin	Halothane
Primidone	Tetracycline

Table 1.14 Drugs that merit dose adjustment in renal failure.

Penicillins
Cephalosporins
Sulphonamides
Digoxin
Cimetidine
Cyclophosphamide

Box 1.2 Fixed interval / reduced dose method.

The drug is given at the same frequency but the dose is divided by the patient's abnormal serum creatinine concentration* (Riviere 1981).

Example:
- serum creatinine of 2.5 mg/dl
- usual dose of cimetidine from 5 mg/kg t.i.d.
- adjusted dose of cimetidine 2 mg/kg t.i.d.

This method:
- results in less variability in serum drug concentrations over time
- avoids sub-therapeutic trough concentrations or excessively high peak concentrations
- can be used for many drugs, but is especially appropriate for bacteriostatic antibiotics and drugs with low therapeutic indices

* For these calculations, serum creatinine concentrations are measured in mg/dl. To convert from µmol/l to mg/dl divide by 88.4.

Box 1.3 Fixed dose / increased interval method.

The drug is given at the same dose but the dosing interval is extended by multiplying by the serum creatinine.

Example:
- serum creatinine of 3.0 mg/dl
- usual dose of gentamicin 3 mg/kg every 8 h
- adjusted dose 3 mg/kg every 24 h

This method:
- allows serum drug concentrations to fluctuate more widely
- for some drugs (e.g. aminoglycosides), low trough serum drug concentrations decrease the risk of toxicity (Riviere 1984).

Table 1.15 Drugs that should be avoided in renal failure.

Dose dependent nephrotoxins
   Aminoglycosides
   Oxytetracycline
   Thiacetarsamide
   Amphotericin B
   Cisplatin

Catabolic drugs
   Corticosteroids
   Tetracyclines

Drugs which reduce renal blood flow in hypotensive states
   Non-steroidal anti-inflammatory drugs
   Angiotensin converting enzyme inhibitors

such as penicillins, should be adjusted, since this reduces cost and may reduce toxicity.

There are two simple methods for dose adjustment of renally cleared drugs in azotaemic patients. These are shown in Boxes 1.2 and 1.3.

If the serum creatinine concentration exceeds 4.0 mg/dl, renal function is unstable (as in acute renal failure), or the patient has abnormally reduced muscle mass, the serum creatinine correlates poorly with GFR (Riviere 1984) and the above methods become inaccurate for dose adjustment.

Other drugs should be avoided altogether in azotaemic patients unless their use is absolutely necessary (see Table 1.15). These include:

- dose-dependent nephrotoxins which may further accelerate nephron loss,

- catabolic drugs which can increase blood urea nitrogen levels and increase the acid and nitrogen load on the kidney,
- non-steroidal anti-inflammatory drugs may worsen gastric ulceration and can acutely reduce renal blood flow.

THERAPEUTIC DRUG MONITORING

For many drugs, their therapeutic effects and predictable adverse toxic effects are directly related to the drug plasma concentration. The concept of monitoring the effect of drugs by measuring their plasma concentrations at known time intervals after dosing is logical as it would provide the clinician with an objective and individualised assessment of drug therapy.

It is important to recognise that there are a number of situations where measurement of the plasma concentration of the parent drug compound will not accurately predict therapeutic success. These are summarised in Table 1.16.

In many cases in canine practice, the safety margin for drug therapy is such that subjective monitoring of response to drug therapy is acceptable. In other situations, monitoring of the response to drug therapy and toxicity can be assessed objectively by looking at a marker of the effect of the drug. Common examples of such monitoring are shown in Table 1.17.

Measurement of drug plasma concentration is important in a number of circumstances for drugs which have:

- narrow therapeutic indices (e.g. anticonvulsants, anti-arrhythmics, cardiac glycosides and other cardiac drugs, anti-cancer drugs, anticoagulants, aminoglycoside antibiotics, methylxanthines);
- toxic effects which may be irreversible once clinically detectable;
- therapeutic or toxic effects which may take prolonged dosing to be recognised;
- effects against diseases with intermittent, unpredictable clinical signs making subjective assessment of response to therapy difficult.

Table 1.18 presents examples of drugs used in canine practice where measurement of plasma concentration of drugs may prove beneficial and recommends the target therapeutic range and the timing of blood samples in relation to the duration of therapy and the time of the last dose.

Table 1.16 Examples of drugs where measurement of the plasma concentration may not accurately predict therapeutic efficacy or drug toxicity.

Mechanism/explanation	Drug examples
Many bactericidal antibiotics have a post-antibiotic effect – their effect on infective organisms outlasts their presence in the body	Fluoroquinolones, aminoglycosides
Drug concentration at the site of action is much higher than that found in plasma:	
e.g. Concentrated in urine	Many antibiotics, e.g. penicillins
Bind tightly to target tissue and are slowly released (bound drug acts as a reservoir)	Non-steroidal anti-inflammatory drugs
Drug binds irreversibly to target receptor or enzyme, forms a covalent complex and rate of recovery from drug effect depends on rate of production of new protein (receptor or enzyme)	Phenoxybenzamine (α-receptor) Aspirin (cyclo-oxygenase) Omeprazole (proton pump)
The parent drug is not the active agent – active metabolites are formed (by the liver)	Enalapril (enalaprilat) Primidone (phenobarbitone and phenylethylmalonamide)
Type B adverse reactions: • not related to the drug's pharmacological effect • not dose related	Drug hypersensitivity (allergy) (penicillin, potentiated sulphas) Genetic idiosyncrasy (ivermectin in Collie dogs)

Drug	Objective test of drug action or toxicity
Insulin	Blood or urine glucose Plasma fructosamine, glycosylated haemoglobin to assess long-term therapy
Mitotane	Blood cortisol concentrations pre- and post-ACTH administration, plasma [Na] and [K]
Fludrocortisone	Plasma [Na] and [K]
Anti-hypertensive/vasodilator drugs (e.g. hydralazine)	Measurement of systemic arterial blood pressure
Anti-coagulant drugs (warfarin or heparin)	Serial measurement of OSPT (warfarin) or APTT (heparin)
Vitamin K therapy	OSPT measurement
Calcitriol, alphacalcidiol or dihydrotachysterol	Plasma calcium concentration Plasma parathyroid concentration (in management of CRF)

Table 1.17 Monitoring of response to drug therapy by objective markers of drug action.

ACTH, adrenocorticotrophin; APTT, activated partial thromboplastin time; CRF, chronic renal failure; OSPT, one stage prothrombin time.

Some important principles should be recognised when adopting this type of therapeutic drug monitoring for canine patients:

- Steady state drug kinetics will not be achieved until the drug has been administered for five half lives.
- Therapeutic ranges suggested for these drugs are often extrapolated from human medicine and are guides – toxic effects and therapeutic failure are possible with drug concentrations within the therapeutic range.
- Therapeutic success may be possible with drug concentrations below the suggested therapeutic range in individual patients.

In many cases, the therapeutic ranges quoted in Table 1.18 are derived from experimental studies; no large-scale well designed clinical studies using diseased animals have been undertaken to test their validity. Therapeutic drug monitoring allows the clinician to become aware of pharmacokinetic peculiarities of individual animals which may underlie lack of efficacy or enhanced toxicity and to tailor dose rates to the individual patient. Only by measuring the plasma levels of such drugs in our clinical cases will our knowledge of clinical pharmacology improve and so contribute to the success of therapeutics in veterinary practice. It should also be recognised, however, that variability in response to drug therapy may also occur for pharmacody-

Box 1.4 General recommendations for safe and effective therapy (adapted from Wright 1992)

(1) Elicit a careful and thorough drug history, including the concurrent administration of non-prescription medications.
(2) Learn about the mechanisms of action and mode of elimination of commonly prescribed drugs.
(3) Resist the urge to prescribe unnecessary drugs.
(4) Use careful clinical monitoring in patients with organ failure.
(5) Use caution when prescribing drugs with low therapeutic indices, use therapeutic drug monitoring in difficult cases.
(6) Always keep drug–drug interactions in mind when poor efficacy or toxic side effects are seen.

namic reasons such as reduced tissue density of receptors (down-regulation), predominance of a different receptor sub-type or the presence of endogenous physiological antagonist mediators reducing the effects of the administered drug.

Table 1.18 Recommendations for therapeutic drug monitoring in veterinary practice.

Drug	Elimination half-life	Duration of therapy before sampling	Timing of sampling in relation to dosing	Suggested therapeutic range
Phenobarbitone	50–70 h	10–14 days	Before next dose (trough level) 3–4 h after dosing (peak level)*	20–40 µg/ml
Digoxin	20–30 h	5–10 days	12 h after dosing (trough level) Avoid sampling within 8 h of dosing – long distributive phase may lead to assumption of toxic levels	1–2.5 ng/ml
Lignocaine	45 min	Daily monitoring with frequent changes in dosage if necessary	During an infusion to determine steady state concentrations	1.5–6.0 µg/ml Seizures occur at a mean concentration of 8.2 µg/ml
Procainamide	2–3 h	Wait at least 2 dose intervals after a change in dosage		10–15 µg/ml
Gentamicin	1–2 h	Monitor three times a week in patients at risk of toxicity	Peak concentrations 30 min after i.v. dosing (90 min after i.m. or s.c. doses) Trough concentrations just prior to next dose	5–12 µg/ml peak for efficacy (NB Marked post-antibiotic effect) <1.0 µg/ml trough to avoid toxicity
L-thyroxine	12–16 h	7 days (often wait 4–8 weeks to assess clinical response as well)	4–8 h after dosing	Use laboratory reference range – T_3 may be normal despite high T_4 If anti-thyroid antibodies are present these may interfere with assays

* Measure peak levels if suspect toxicity and trough levels if investigating lack of efficacy.

REFERENCES

Adams, H.R. & Bingham, G.A. (1971) Respiratory arrest associated with dihydrostreptomycin. *Journal of the American Veterinary Medical Association*, **159**, 179–180.

Alberola, J., Perez, Y. & Arboix, M. (1993) Theophylline kinetics in dog neonates. *Journal of Veterinary Pharmacology and Therapeutics*, **16**, 103–105.

Aronson, A.L., Bai, S.A., Riviere, J.E. & Aucoin, D.P. (1986) Effects of disease states on drug binding to serum proteins. In: *Comparative Veterinary Pharmacology, Toxicology, and Therapy*, (eds A. van Miert, M.G. Bogaert & M. Debackere), pp. 407–414. MTP Press, Lancaster.

Benet, L.Z., Greither, A. & Meister, W. (1976) Gastrointestinal absorption of drugs in patients with cardiac failure. In: *The Effect of Disease States on Drug Pharmacokinetics*, (ed. L.Z. Benet), pp. 33–50. American Pharmaceutical Association, Washington DC.

Benet, L.Z. & Williams, R.L. (1990) Design and optimization of dosage regimens; pharmacokinetic data. In: *Goodman and Gilman's The Pharmacologic Basis of Therapeutics*, (eds A.G. Gilman, T.W. Rall, A.S. Nies & P. Taylor), 8th edn. pp. 1650–1715. Pergamon Press, New York.

Benowitz, N.L. & Meister, W. (1983) Pharmacokinetics in patients with cardiac failure. In: *Handbook of Clinical Pharmacokinetics*, (eds M. Gibaldi & L. Prescott), pp. 182–200. ADIS Health Science Press, New York.

Breznock, E.M. (1975) Effects of phenobarbital on digitoxin and digoxin elimination in the dog. *American Journal of Veterinary Research*, **36**, 371–373.

Button, C. & Gross, D.R. (1980) A pharmacokinetic basis for the administration of digoxin to puppies. *Journal of Veterinary Pharmacology and Therapeutics*, **3**, 209–215.

Campbell, C.L. (1983) Primidone intoxication associated with concurrent use of chloramphenicol. *Journal of the American Veterinary Medical Association*, **182**, 992–993.

DeBacker, P. (1985) Comparative neonatal pharmacokinetics. In: *Comparative Veterinary Pharmacology, Toxicology, and Therapy*, (eds A. van Miert, M.G. Bogaert & M. Debackere), pp. 161–171. MTP Press, Lancaster.

DeRick, A. & Belpaire, F. (1981) Digoxin-quinidine interaction in the dog. *Journal of Veterinary Pharmacology and Therapeutics*, **4**, 215–218.

Esquivel, M., Blaschke, T.F., Snidow, G.H. & Meffin, P.J. (1978) Effect of phenobarbitone on the disposition of lignocaine and warfarin in the dog. *Journal of Pharmacy and Pharmacology*, **30**, 804–805.

Frey, H-H. (1989) Anticonvulsant drugs used in the treatment of epilepsy. *Problems in Veterinary Medicine*, **1**, 558–577.

Frey, H-H., Kampmann, E. & Nielsen, C.K. (1968) Study on combined treatment with phenobarbital and diphenylhydantoin. *Acta Pharmacologica et Toxicologica*, **26**, 284–292.

Griffin, J.W., May, J.R. & DiPiro, J.T. (1984) Drug interactions: theory versus practice. *American Journal of Medicine*, **77**(Suppl. 5B), 85–89.

Griffiths, J.P. (1988) Drug interactions. *Veterinary Clinics of North America: Small Animal Practice*, **18**, 1243–1265.

Herchulez, A., Derenne, F., Deger, F., *et al.* (1989) Interaction between nonsteroidal anti-inflammatory drugs and loop diuretics: modulation by sodium balance. *Journal of Pharmacology and Experimental Therapeutics*, **248**, 1175–1181.

Hinchcliff, K.W. & Muir, W.W. (1991) Pharmacology of furosemide in the horse: a review. *Journal of Veterinary Internal Medicine*, **5**, 211–218.

Horster, M. & Valtin, H. (1971) Postnatal development of renal function: micropuncture and clearance studies in the dog. *Journal of Clinical Investigation*, **50**, 779–795.

Insel, P.A. (1990) Analgesic-antipyretics and anti-inflammatory agents. In: *Goodman and Gilman's The Pharmacologic Basis of Therapeutics*, (eds A.G. Gilman, T.W. Rall, A.S. Nies & P. Taylor), 8th edn. pp. 638–681. Pergamon Press, New York.

Kawalek, J.C. & El Said, K.R.M. (1990) Maturational development of drug-metabolizing enzymes in dogs. *American Journal of Veterinary Research*, **51**, 1742–1745.

Kintzer, P.P. & Peterson, M.E. (1991) Mitotane (o,p'-DDD) treatment of 200 dogs with pituitary-dependent hyperadrenocorticism. *Journal of Veterinary Internal Medicine*, **5**, 182–190.

McLean, A.J. & Morgan, D.J. (1991) Clinical pharmacokinetics in patients with liver disease. *Clinical Pharmacokinetics*, **21**, 42–69.

Montamat, S.C., Cusack, B.J. & Vestal, R.E. (1989) Management of drug therapy in the elderly. *New England Journal of Medicine*, **321**, 303–309.

Paul, J.W. (1982) Drug interactions. *Modern Veterinary Practice*, **63**, 780–785

Polk, R.E. (1989) Drug–drug interactions with ciprofloxacin and other fluoroquinolones. *American Journal of Medicine*, **87**(Suppl. 5A), 76S–81S.

Rall, T.W. (1990) Hypnotics and sedatives. In: *Goodman and Gilman's The Pharmacologic Basis of Therapeutics*, (eds A.G. Gilman, T.W. Rall, A.S. Nies & P. Taylor), 8th edn. pp. 345–382. Pergamon Press, New York.

Ravis, W.R., Pedersoli, W.M. & Wike, J.S. (1989) Pharmacokinetics of phenobarbital in dogs given multiple doses. *American Journal of Veterinary Research*, **50**, 1343–1347.

Reilly, P.E.B. & Isaacs, J.P. (1983) Adverse drug interactions of importance in veterinary practice. *Veterinary Record*, **112**, 29–33.

Riond, J-L. & Riviere, J.E. (1989) Effects of tetracyclines on the kidney in cattle and dogs. *Journal of the American Veterinary Medical Association*, **195**, 995–997.

Riviere, J.E. (1981) Dosage of antimicrobial drugs in patients with renal insufficiency. *Journal of the American Veterinary Medical Association*, **178**, 70–72.

Riviere, J.E. (1984) Calculation of dosage regimens of antimicrobial drugs in animals with renal and hepatic dysfunction. *Journal of the American Veterinary Medical Association*, **185**, 1094–1096.

Riviere, J.E. & Davis, L.E. (1984) Renal handling of drugs in renal failure. In: *Canine Nephrology*, (ed. K.E. Bovee), pp. 643–685. Harwal Publ. Co., Philadelphia.

Sande, M.A. & Mandell, G.L. (1990) Antimicrobial agents. In: *Goodman and Gilman's The Pharmacologic Basis of Therapeutics*, (eds A.G. Gilman, T.W. Rall, A.S. Nies & P. Taylor), 8th edn. pp. 1098–1145. Pergamon Press, New York.

Sanders, K., Yeary, R.A., Fenner, W.R. & Powers, J.D. (1979) Interaction of phenytoin with chloramphenicol or pentobarbital in the dog. *Journal of the American Veterinary Medical Association*, **175**, 177–180.

Scott, G. & Nierenberg, D. (1992) Drug interactions. In: *Melmon & Morrelli's Clinical Pharmacology: Basic Principles in Therapeutics*, (eds K.L. Melmon, H.F. Morrelli, B.B. Hoffman & D.W. Nierenberg), 3rd edn. pp. 1073–1083. McGraw Hill, New York.

Short, C.R. & Clarke, C.R. (1984) Calculation of dosage regimens of antimicrobial drugs for the neonatal patient. *Journal of the American Veterinary Medical Association*, **185**, 1088–1093.

Simons, F.E. & Simons, K.J. (1994) The pharmacology and use of H_1-receptor-antagonist drugs. *New England Journal of Medicine*, **330**, 1663–1669.

Snodgrass, W.R. (1992) Drugs in special patient groups: neonates and children. In: *Melmon & Morrelli's Clinical Pharmacology:*

Basic Principles in Therapeutics, (eds K.L. Melmon, H.F. Morrelli, B.B. Hoffman & D.W. Nierenberg), 3rd edn. pp. 826–850. McGraw Hill, New York.

Somogyi, A. & Rolan, P. (1986) Drug disposition and dosing in hepatic disease. *Medical Journal of Australia*, **145**, 284–289.

Somogyi, A. & Muirhead, M. (1987) Pharmacokinetic interactions of cimetidine 1987. *Clinical Pharmacokinetics*, **12**, 321–366.

Stockley, I.H. (1991) *Drug Interactions*, 2nd edn. Blackwell Science, Oxford.

Teske, R.H. & Carter, G.G. (1971) Effect of chloramphenicol on pentobarbital-induced anesthesia in dogs. *Journal of the American Veterinary Medical Association*, **159**, 777–780.

Trissel, L.A. (1990) *Handbook on Injectable Drugs*, 6th edn. American Society of Hospital Pharmacists, Bethesda, MD.

Vestal, R.E. (1989) Ageing and determinants of hepatic drug clearance. *Hepatology*, **2**, 331–334.

Vestal, R.E., Montamat, S.C. Nielson, C.P. (1992) Drugs in special patient groups: the elderly. In: *Melmon & Morrelli's Clinical Pharmacology: Basic Principles in Therapeutics*, (eds K.L. Melmon, H.F. Morrelli, B.B. Hoffman & D.W. Nierenberg), 3rd edn. pp. 851–874. McGraw Hill, New York.

Wallace, S.M. & Verbeeck, R.K. (1987) Plasma protein binding of drugs in the elderly. *Clinical Pharmacokinetics*, **12**, 41–72.

Watson, A.D.J. (1979) Effect of ingesta on systemic availability of chloramphenicol from two oral preparations in cats. *Journal of Veterinary Pharmacology and Therapeutics*, **2**, 117–121.

Watson, A.D.J., Rijnberk, A. & Moolenaar, A.J. (1987) Systemic availability of o,p'-DDD in normal dogs, fasted and fed, and in dogs with hyperadrenocorticism. *Research in Veterinary Science*, **43**, 160–165.

Welling, P.G. (1984) Interactions affecting drug absorption. *Clinical Pharmacokinetics*, **9**, 404–434.

Wilkerson, R.D. & Beck, B.L. (1987) Increase in serum digoxin concentration produced by quinidine does not increase the potential for digoxin-induced ventricular arrhythmias in dogs. *Journal of Pharmacology and Experimental Therapeutics*, **240**, 548–553.

Wright, J.M. (1992) Drug interactions. In: *Melmon & Morrelli's Clinical Pharmacology: Basic Principles in Therapeutics*, (eds K.L. Melmon, H.F. Morrelli, B.B. Hoffman & D.W. Nierenberg), 3rd edn. pp. 1012–1021. McGraw Hill, New York.

Chapter 2

Decision Making in Fluid Therapy

J. Sackman

INTRODUCTION

Management of fluid and electrolyte abnormalities is a fundamental aspect of clinical medicine. In health, fluid balance is maintained by oral intake and renal, gastrointestinal and insensible losses. Fluid administration is an important supportive therapeutic measure in critically ill patients. Before the initiation of fluid therapy, identification of the disease process involved will help in formulating an appropriate plan. The first questions that a clinician should ask when deciding if fluid therapy is indicated are:

- Is the patient dehydrated?
- Are there significant electrolyte disturbances?
- Are there serious acid–base changes present?
- Are there ongoing fluid losses, such as vomiting that must be accounted for?

Once the decision to institute fluid therapy has been made, the following questions should be addressed:

- By what route should the fluids be given?
- What volume of fluid needs to be administered?
- What type of fluid should be used?
- How fast should the fluids be given?
- What supplements should be added to the standard fluid?
- How will hydration status be monitored?

STRUCTURE AND FUNCTION

Body Fluid Compartments

Total body water (TBW) represents 60% of body weight in adult animals. Two-thirds of TBW is located within the cell (intracellular) and one-third is located extracellularly. Extracellular fluid (ECF) is further divided into interstitial fluid (75% ECF) and intravascular fluid (25% ECF).

Fluid Electrolyte Concentration

Intracellular fluid volume is maintained primarily by the osmotic forces generated by the intracellular cations, potassium and magnesium. The principal extracellular ions are sodium, chloride, and bicarbonate. Sodium and potassium gradients are maintained by the membrane sodium–potassium ATPase pump. Variations in extracellular sodium concentration can have dramatic effects on cell hydration. In cases of pure water loss, such as with water deprivation, hypernatraemia occurs which can lead to net water movement from the cell to the extracellular space resulting in cell dehydration.

Regulation of Fluid Balance

The kidneys are responsible for the normal regulation of extracellular water and osmotic balance. Increases in plasma osmolality stimulates the release of antidiuretic hormone (ADH) from the pituitary. In turn, ADH causes increased water reabsorption from the collecting tubules in the kidney.

While osmoregulation occurs primarily through the release of ADH, volume regulation occurs primarily through baroreceptors in the cardiopulmonary circulation and kidneys. Decreases in blood volume detected by the renal baroreceptors leads to activation of renin–angiotensin system (RAS). Activation of RAS leads to aldosterone release and secondarily to increased renal sodium reabsorption and potassium loss. Mechanisms which defend the body against fluid volume overload are less well characterised. Stretch of the right atrium triggers the release of atrial natriuretic peptide from myocardial cells which enhances sodium and water excretion by the kidney.

Maintenance Fluid Requirements

Normal sources of water are those consumed directly or in food and that produced in the body through metabolism. Maintenance requirements are defined as the volume of fluid or electrolytes that is required on a daily basis to keep TBW and electrolyte content normal. In a healthy animal, water input equals water loss.

Daily water loss occurs by evaporation from the respiratory tract, from faeces, and from urine. The volume of fluid required for maintenance is calculated from two components:

- Insensible loss (loss not readily measurable from evaporation and faeces); estimated at 22 ml/kg per day.
- Sensible loss (readily measured such as urine production); estimated at 22–44 ml/kg per day.

Maintainence fluid volume is calculated by adding sensible and insensible water losses.

- Maintenance volume required for cats and small dogs is 66 ml/kg per day.
- Maintenance volume required for large dogs is 44 ml/kg per day.
- If intravenous fluid therapy is given for greater than 24 hours, daily electrolyte loss must be addressed by making sure that fluids contain 1 mEq/kg per day of sodium, potassium and chloride.*

* The dose of ions used is expressed in terms of electrical charge or milliequivalents

APPROACH TO THE PATIENT WITH FLUID LOSS

Assessment of the Patient Requiring Fluid Therapy

History

The first step in formulating a fluid therapy plan is to assess the degree of dehydration and electrolyte loss present in the patient. Historical information about the animal's disease and route of fluid loss will help in deciding on the type of electrolyte and acid–base changes present. The length of time over which fluid loss has occurred, an estimate of the magnitude of loss and information about water and food consumption can be obtained from the owners. Assessments about the source of fluid loss, such as gastrointestinal, urinary or traumatic (haemorrhage) are also helpful.

Technically, dehydration refers to loss of pure water from the body. In the clinical setting, most water loss is accompanied by electrolyte loss. Dehydration can occur following decreased intake due to water deprivation but, more commonly, results from increased loss of fluids in addition to reduced intake. Increased fluid loss can result from:

- polyuria (common)
- vomiting and diarrhoea (common)
- fever, panting
- large burn wounds
- excessive salivation
- haemorrhage.

Physical Examination

The use of physical examination to detect the degree of dehydration is helpful, but somewhat limited in sensitivity. Dehydration is not detected by clinical examination until at least 5% of body water has been lost. *Hydration status* is estimated by evaluating *skin turgor* or pliability, the *moistness of mucous membranes*, the *position of the eyes* in the orbit, *heart rate*, the character of *peripheral pulses*, *capillary refill time*, and *jugular venous distension*. Table 2.1 presents the significance of changes in these parameters and how they relate to the hydration status of the animal. Skin turgor is dependent upon subcutaneous fat and elastin as well as fluid content. Obese animals, because of subcutaneous fat, may appear well hydrated even if they are not. Likewise, emaciated and older animals may appear less hydrated than they are because of the loss of skin elastin and fat.

Table 2.1 Initial database of patients requiring fluid therapy.

History Include information on water and food intake, gastrointestinal losses, urine output, exposure to heat, trauma, hemorrhage, excessive panting, fever and diuretic use.

Physical examination findings

<5% dehydration	=	not detectable
5–6% dehydration	=	subtle loss of skin turgor
7–8% dehydration	=	delay in skin returning to normal position; prolonged capillary refill; tacky mucous membranes, eyes may be sunken in orbit.
10–12% dehydration	=	tented skin; prolonged capillary refill; eyes sunken in orbit; dry mucous membranes; signs of shock (tachycardia, weak peripheral pulses, collapse of peripheral veins)
12–15% dehydration	=	shock; collapse; death imminent
Determine body weight		Acute decrease in body weight may be due to fluid loss (1 kg = 1000 ml fluid)
Special procedures		Place indwelling urinary catheter to monitor urine output.
		Place jugular catheter and measure central venous pressure (CVP). CVP is a measure of right atrial pressure and intravascular blood volume.

Laboratory findings

Packed cell volume (PCV) and total plasma protein (TPP)

↑ PCV & TPP	intravascular dehydration
↑ PCV & normal or ↓ TPP	dehydration with hypoproteinaemia, splenic contraction (haemorrhage), polycythaemia
normal PCV & ↑ TPP	anaemia with dehydration, normal hydration & hyperproteinaemia
↓ PCV & ↑ TPP	anaemia with dehydration anaemia with hyperproteinaemia
↓ PCV & normal TPP	anaemia with normal hydration
normal PCV & TPP	acute blood loss normal hydration dehydration with anaemia and hypoproteinaemia
↓ PCV & ↓ TPP	blood loss anaemia & hypoproteinaemia overhydration

Urinalysis – dehydrated animals will have a reduced urine output if renal function is normal.
Urine specific gravity – elevated specific gravity (>1.030) represents a normal kidney response to dehydration.
Dilute urine in the face of dehydration suggests the kidney as a possible cause of fluid loss.

Serum biochemistries – electrolytes	K^+, Na^+
	Electrolytes will help determine the cause of fluid loss and the degree of replacement needed.
Blood urea nitrogen (BUN)	Elevated levels along with high urine specific gravity indicate a non-renal cause of dehydration. Elevated BUN and a urine specific gravity of <1.024 indicates that the kidney may be a source of the dehydration.
Bicarbonate or total CO_2	Will help evaluate metabolic status of the patient and determine type of replacement fluid necessary.

Initial Patient Database

- History and physical examination
- Laboratory tests.

Laboratory tests are helpful in establishing the nature and degree of fluid imbalance as well as monitoring the success of treatment. Tests to be included are: *packed cell volume* (PCV), *total plasma protein* (TPP), *urine specific gravity*, *blood urea nitrogen* (BUN), serum *potassium* and *sodium* and *total CO₂* (or bicarbonate). Other tests which may be indicated, but less available include *blood gases*, and *serum and urine osmolality*. Table 2.1 summarises the value of each test and significance of abnormal findings.

Replacement (Dehydration) Fluid Requirements

In patients requiring intravenous fluid therapy, three categories of fluid loss must be taken into consideration. These include losses related to normal body maintenance, ongoing losses resulting from the animal's underlying disease, and any existing deficits with which the animal presents. As indicated above, all patients will have normal fluid requirements generated from sensible and insensible fluid loss; these maintenance volumes must be added to any calculated fluid replacement volumes. Dehydration exists when TBW is less than normal. In the clinical situation, fluid loss is generally also associated with electrolyte loss.

The initial assesment of hydration by the clinician determines the volume of fluid needed to replace the hydration deficit. The *volume* of fluid to be replaced is then calculated based upon the estimated percentage dehydration and the patient's present body weight:

- % dehydration × weight (kg) = litres of fluid to be replaced

Along with replacement of the animal's fluid deficit, the clinician must add the maintainence fluid requirement as well as replacement of ongoing losses. The volume of ongoing losses is generally estimated. Blood loss during surgical procedures can be estimated and 3 ml of crystalloid solution is administered for each millilitre of blood lost. Total volume of fluid to be given to a patient is the result of adding rehydration volume to maintenance and ongoing losses:

- Rehydration = % dehydration × weight (kg)

$$= \underline{\hspace{2cm}} \text{litres}$$
$$+$$

- Maintenance requirements of
22–44 ml/kg per day = $\underline{\hspace{2cm}}$ litres
$$+$$
- Ongoing losses, estimated or measured
$$= \underline{\hspace{2cm}} \text{litres}$$

Determining the Type of Fluid to Give

Fluids available for treatment can be divided into several categories (Table 2.2):

- hypotonic solutions,
- hypertonic solutions,
- replacement electrolyte solutions,
- maintainance electrolyte solutions,
- colloids (plasma volume expanders) (see Table 2.3).

The choice of fluid should be based upon both the degree and nature of fluid loss. In some circumstances, the exact fluid required to treat a particular patient may not be available in a commercial preparation but can be formulated by mixing different preparations in the appropriate proportions and/or supplementing with concentrated additives (see Table 2.4).

Classification of Fluids

Fluids may be classified based upon their composition or use.

(1) *Osmolality*. Fluids may be categorised based upon the relationship of their osmolality compared with normal serum osmolarity of 300 mOsm/l. The osmolality of solutions is predominantly determined by their glucose and sodium content.
   - *Hypotonic fluids* have an osmolality of less than normal serum. An example is 5% dextrose in water (see Table 2.2).
   - *Hypertonic fluids* have an osmolality greater than serum. Use of these fluids has been advocated for volume replacement in patients with hypovolaemic and endotoxic shock. Small volumes of hypertonic saline produce immediate increases in cardiac output, arterial blood pressure, and peripheral perfusion. Haemodynamic improvement is believed to be secondary to a fluid shift from the interstitial and intracellular area to the intravascular component. Hypertonic fluids also have a direct positive inotropic effect on the heart. Administration of hypertonic (3–15%) saline

Table 2.2 Categorisation and composition of commercially available crystalloid fluids (concentrations in mmol/l unless stated).

Fluid category	Examples	Na	K	Cl	Ca/Mg	Glucose (g/l)	Buffer*	Osmolality (mOsm/l)	pH	Comments
1. Hypotonic	5% dextrose	0	0	0	0/0	50	0	252	4.0	ECF diluent (hypertonic dehydration)
2. Hypertonic	7.0% NaCl	1196	0	1196	0/0	0	0	2392	5.0	Increase intravascular volume (shock)
3. Replacement	Lactated Ringer's	131	5	111	1.5/0	0	23 (L)	272	6.5	Isotonic repair of ECF
	Plain Ringer's	147	4	156	2.25/0	0	0	310	5.0	Isotonic repair of ECF – acidifying
	0.9% NaCl	154	–	154	0/0	0	0	308	5.0	Isotonic repair of ECF but acidifying
Equivalent solutions†	Plasma-Lyte 148™ (water)	140	5	98	0/1.5	0	27(A) 23(G)	296	5.5–7.0	Human licensed product available in the UK
	Normosol R™	140	5	98	0/1.5	0	27(A) 23(G)	296	5.5–7.0	Licensed product available in USA
Potassium enriched	Darrow's solution	121	35	103	0/0	0	53(L)	312		Formulated for potassium replacement, not suitable for initial volume replacement
4. Maintenance	0.18% saline in glucose	31	0	31	0/0	43	0	300		Lacks potassium and bicarbonate precursor required for daily maintenance
	Plasma-Lyte M™ (dextrose 5%)	40	16	40	2.5/1.5	50	12(A) 12(L)	376	5.5	Human licensed product – provides daily fluid and electrolyte requirements for animals maintained nil by mouth
Plasma composition	Normal dog	145	4	105	2.5/1.5	1	25(B)	290	7.4	Values quoted are approx. mid-normal range values

ECF, extracellular fluid.
* Buffers use: A, Acetate; B, bicarbonate; G; gluconate; L, lactate.
† These solutions are replacement solutions but their composition more closely resembles that of plasma.

results in haemodynamic improvement in the dog for 2 h. By adding colloidal solutions (dextran 70) to hypertonic saline, the beneficial haemodynamic effects may be prolonged. Hypertonic saline resuscitation should always be followed by crystalloid fluid administration.

- *Isotonic fluids* have an osmolality near that of serum. Most crystalloid solutions (both replacement and maintenance solutions) fall into this category. Examples: lactated Ringer's solution and 0.9% sodium chloride.

(2) *Colloidal solutions* are large molecular weight substances that are restricted to the plasma compartment.

Colloids are generally administered to patients in shock and those with severe hypoalbuminaemia (albumin <20 g/l). Plasma proteins are colloids that are important in maintaining normal plasma oncotic pressure. Dextrans and hetastarch are high molecular weight substances which act much like plasma proteins in maintaining intravascular oncotic pressure (see Table 2.3).

Fresh (fresh frozen) plasma is a colloidal fluid administered to patients with hypoproteinaemia (<40 g/l plasma protein or 20 g/l albumin) or coagulopathy. Separated plasma frozen within 6 h of collection is called fresh frozen plasma (FFP). FFP is a source of coagulation factors, von Willebrand's factor, complement, fibrinolytic proteins, albumin, and immunoglobulins. FFP is generally not used as a resuscitation fluid.

(3) *Crystalloid solutions* (Table 2.2) contain ionised substances capable of passing a semipermeable membrane and are used for water and electrolyte supplementation and for intravascular volume expansion. Unlike colloids, crystalloid solutions distribute to sites outside of the intravascular compartment. Because of this, three times the volume of crystalloid must be given (compared with colloid) for effective plasma expansion. Crystalloid solutions may be classified as maintenance or replacement solutions.

- *Replacement fluids* are generally polyelectrolyte solutions to replace extracellular fluid volume deficits. The ideal replacement fluid, therefore has an electrolyte composition close to that of extracellular fluid, particularly with respect to its sodium ion concentration. Supplementation of replacement fluids may be required to correct acid–base imbalance or potassium deficits.

- *Maintenance fluids* are electrolyte solutions that are lower in sodium than replacement fluids and are often hypotonic. They are formulated to maintain homeostasis by replacing insensible fluid and electrolytes lost, when animals are not taking fluids orally. Examples of maintenance fluids include 0.18% sodium chloride in 4.5% dextrose. Such a preparation requires supplementation with potassium (up to 30 mmol/l) to satisfy maintenance requirements.

Table 2.3 Colloidal solutions (plasma volume expanders).

Preparation	Dosage	Use	Comments
Hetastarch – a synthetic hydroxy-ethyl starch, mol.wt 450 000 (6% in 0.9% NaCl)	Up to 20 ml/kg per day (can be given in one hour if severe hypovolaemia)	Correction of hypovolaemia, particularly in cases of hypoalbuminaemia	• Produces less hypersensitivity reaction than dextran 70 • Administration of hetastarch expands the plasma volume by twice the volume given • 40% of the volume increase persisting for 24–36 h • Causes elevated amylase values
Dextran 70 (linear polysaccharide molecule of average mol.wt 70 000) (6% in 0.9% NaCl or in 5% dextrose)	4–6 ml/kg per hour Up to 20 ml/kg per 24 h	Correction of hypovolaemia, particularly in cases of hypoalbuminaemia	• The larger the particle size of dextran the longer the dwell time in the circulation • Dextran 70 expands the plasma volume by twice the volume given • Less than 30% of the volume is retained in the circulation after 6 h • Both dextran 40 and 70 have been associated with anaphylactic reactions in 0.1% of dogs. • Dextrans prolong clotting times and decrease platelet function although this does not appear to be clinically significant
Gelatins of bovine origin, suitably treated to reduce their antigenicity e.g. Polygeline – average mol.wt 35 000 (3.5% in a polyionic solution – Haemaccel)	Equal to the estimated volume of blood lost (5 ml/kg can be given over 15 min to resuscitate an animal)	Correction of hypovolaemia, particularly in cases associated with hypoalbuminaemia	• Licensed veterinary product in the UK. • Smaller molecular weight than dextran 70 or hetastarch – expand the blood volume less effectively than dextran or hetastarch • 50% of the infused volume remains in the circulation after 4 h

SELECTING THE APPROPRIATE FLUID

(1) Collect initial physical examination, historical and laboratory data.

(2) Is the patient severely dehydrated or showing signs of shock?
- Consider rapid volume expansion with hypertonic saline, hypertonic saline and dextrans, or crystalloid solution (0.9% NaCl or lactated Ringer's solution). If there is active haemorrhage or the animal is hypernatraemic, volume expansion with hypertonic saline is contraindicated.

(3) Is the patient mildly dehydrated?
- Consider a balanced electrolyte solution.

(4) Does the patient have electrolyte abnormalities?
- *Hypokalaemia* (serum K+ < 3.0 mmol/l). Supplement fluids with KCl (see Table 2.4). The rate of administration should not exceed 0.5 mEq/kg per hour. Fluids used to maintain an animal should contain enough KCl to ensure daily losses of potassium (1 mEq/kg per day) are met, even if serum potassium concentration is in the normal range.
- *Hyperkalaemia* (serum K+ > 6.0 mmol/l). Give 0.9% NaCl or 0.45% NaCl and 2.5% dextrose. Begin ECG to evaluate for arrhythmias. If hyperkalaemia is causing life-threatening arrhythmias, emergency treatment to protect the heart may be necessary (see Chapter 62, Table 62.9). If there are no serious arrhythmias and the dog is producing adequate volumes of urine, therapy with potassium free fluids should correct the hyperkalaemia.
- *Hyponatraemia* (serum Na+ < 130 mmol/l). Give 0.9% NaCl. Does the patient have hypoadrenocorticism or has it been on diuretics?
- *Hypernatremia* (serum Na+ > 170 mmol/l) can be caused by pure water loss or hypotonic fluid loss or gain of sodium. Use a sodium free fluid such as 5% dextrose in water. The water deficit must be replaced slowly over 48–72 h with serial monitoring of the serum sodium concentration to avoid the development of cerebral oedema. Consider use of natriuretic diuretics (frusemide) to enhance sodium loss if initial cause was iatrogenic gain of sodium.
- *Hypocalcemia* (total serum Ca2+ < 2.0 mmol/l). Supplement fluids with calcium gluconate for symptomatic hypocalcemia (see Table 2.4).
- *Hypercalcemia* (total serum Ca2+ > 3.0 mmol/l). Diagnosis of the underlying cause of hypercalcaemia is most important in the successful management of this condition (see Chapter 35). Many hypercalcaemic animals will present in a dehydrated state due to excessive losses of fluid (renal, vomitus) and lack of fluid intake due to inappetance. Replacement of the calculated fluid deficit over 4–6 h, followed by continued fluid administration is warranted since mild volume expansion promotes calcium ion excretion. The most appropriate fluid is 0.9% NaCl which promotes renal excretion of calcium ions. Careful monitoring is required to ensure urine output is maintained and volume overload does not occur.

(5) Does the patient have metabolic acidosis (serum $HCO_3 < 12$ mmol/l; pH < 7.15)?
- If the patient has metabolic acidosis, supplement fluids with sodium bicarbonate (see Table 2.4). Total CO_2 (mmol/l) may be used in place of serum bicarbonate value for calculating the amount of alkali needed. Calculate the bicarbonate deficit by subtracting the patient's bicarbonate value from the normal value of 24 mmol/l. The deficit is then used in the following calculation:

HCO_3 deficit $\times 0.3 \times$ body weight in kg = missing mmol bicarbonate

Replacement bicarbonate should be administered slowly over several hours. Alternatively, a quarter of the calculated dose may be given i.v. slowly, followed by adding the remaining amount to the fluids for 24-h infusion. The acid–base status of the animal should be reassessed at regular intervals during the 24-h period and the dose rate adjusted according to the response to treatment. Do not add sodium bicarbonate to fluids that contain calcium as a calcium precipitate may occur.

- Without access to total CO_2 or blood gas analysis, sodium bicarbonate may be given if metabolic acidosis is suspected based upon history and clinical signs although this is much less reliable.
  - For *mild* metabolic acidosis, give 3 mEq/kg bicarbonate in fluids over 24 h.
  - For *moderate* metabolic acidosis, give 6 mEq/kg bicarbonate in fluids over 24 hours.
  - For *severe* metabolic acidosis, give 9 mEq/kg bicarbonate in fluids over 24 hours.
- In emergency situations that require immediate bicarbonate administration, 1–2 mEq/kg of sodium bicarbonate may be administered i.v. as a slow bolus injection.
- *Caution*: Overtreatment or rapid treatment of acidosis can result in alkalosis, paradoxical cere-

Table 2.4   Concentrated fluid additives.

Additive	Dosage	Route	Frequency	Use and monitoring
Potassium chloride available in various concentrations – the strong solution (15% or 2 mEq/ml) is most suitable for addition to fluids (mix thoroughly after addition)	Total infusion rate of potassium should not exceed 0.5 mEq/kg per hour	Intravenous	Continuous infusion at a slow rate	Correction of potassium deficit. Monitor plasma potassium concentration every 4–6 h. Monitor ECG for signs of hyperkalaemia
Calcium gluconate (10% solution contains 9.3 mg of Ca/ml) Calcium borogluconate (20% solution contains 15.2 mg Ca/ml)	5–15 mg of calcium per kg 5–15 mg Ca/kg per hour if signs of hypocalcaemia return and an infusion is required	Slowly i.v. Calcium gluconate or borogluconate salts can be given subcutaneously	Once (may be necessary to repeat bolus dose or set up infusion if signs of hypocalcaemia return). Avoid adding calcium salts to fluids containing bicarbonate or bicarbonate precursors)	Treatment of hypocalcaemic tetany Emergency treatment of hyperkalaemia Monitor ECG when giving calcium i.v. – stop if bradycardia occurs or QT interval shortens
Sodium bicarbonate (8.4% solution contains 1mEq/ml)	1–2 mEq/kg (empirical dose – see text for further details)	i.v. slowly	Once	Emergency treatment of hyperkalaemia monitor ECG and plasma [K+]
	Body weight (kg) $\times$ 0.3 $\times$ HCO$_3$ deficit (calculated dose – see text for further details)	Continuous i.v. infusion	Give 25% of dose i.v. slowly and add the remainder to the next 24 h of fluids	Correction of severe metabolic acidosis – monitor acid-base status every 6 h.
Dextrose (50%)	Add 20 ml of 50% dextrose per litre of fluid to raise the fluid glucose concentration by 1% Intravenous bolus dose of 1–2 ml per 10 kg body weight (usually diluted to a 10% solution) may be required in an emergency	i.v. (bolus and infusion)	As required to maintain plasma glucose	Treatment of hypoglycaemia

brospinal fluid (CSF) acidosis, ionised hypocalcaemia (increased binding of calcium to albumin),
and seizures.

(6) Is the patient hypoglycaemic?
   ● Investigate the cause of the hypoglycaemia.
   ● Fluids may be supplemented with 50% dextrose
     to vary the percentage of dextrose in the final
     solution which may be necessary to maintain the
     patient's blood glucose concentration (see Table
     2.4). Solutions that are less than 10% dextrose are
     not adequate sources of calories for anorexic
     patients.

(7) Is the patient severely anaemic (PCV < 0.151/l)?
   ● Give whole blood or packed red cell transfusion.

(8) Is the patient severely hypoproteinaemic (total protein
     <35 g/l)?
   ● Consider giving colloidal fluid such as fresh or
     fresh frozen plasma, hetastarch or dextrans.

(9) Should vitamins be added to parenteral fluids?
   ● Water soluble vitamins may be added to replenish
     urinary losses, especially in patients with renal
     failure. Thiamine deficiency, in particular, may be
     a clinical concern.

DETERMINING THE ROUTE OF FLUID ADMINISTRATION

The rate and route of fluid administration are dependent
upon the severity and nature of the patient's clinical
disease. Oral administration is useful in patients to maintain hydration and nutrition if vomiting and diarrhoea are
not present. Forced fluid therapy may be given through
nasogastric or percutaneously placed gastric tubes.

Subcutaneous Fluid Administration

Subcutaneous fluids are commonly administered to small
animal patients with minimal dehydration. The volume of
fluid that may be administered subcutaneously is limited by
the animal's skin elasticity. Absorption of fluids is often
unreliable, especially in conditions where peripheral perfusion is impaired, such as shock and severe dehydration.
Never rely on this route of fluid administration for critically
ill patients.

● Use intravenous fluids for critically ill patients and for
  those requiring accurate delivery of fluid volumes.
● Subcutaneous fluids are good for rehydration of minimally dehydrated patients.

● Administer isotonic or slightly hypotonic fluids if they
  are to be given subcutaneously.
● *Do not* administer 5% dextrose and water subcutaneously. Delayed absorption occurs with a resulting
  pocket of non-absorbed fluid.

Intravenous Fluid Administration

Critically ill patients require fluids that are administered
intravenously. Fluids given in this manner may be either
hypotonic, hypertonic or isotonic. Rapid volume re-
expansion is readily accomplished via the intravenous
route.

● The jugular and cephalic veins are most commonly
  used for intravenous catheter placement. The lateral
  saphenous and femoral veins may also be used. The use
  of the jugular vein has the advantages of being suitable
  for a large bore catheter, allowing measurement of
  central venous pressure (CVP) and enabling the administration of large volumes of fluid rapidly.
● Peripheral vein catheters are easy to place but they are
  frequently difficult to maintain and fluid flow is highly
  dependent on limb position.

Intraperitoneal Fluid Administration

Sterile isotonic fluids may be administered via this route
when a vein can not be catheterised. Severely anaemic
puppies may be tranfused by this route.

Intra-osseous Fluid Administration

Blood, isotonic and hypertonic fluids may be safely administered by this route. The femur, tibia or humerus is
catheterised with a large bore bone-marrow needle and
fluids are administered directly into the marrow cavity.
This route provides rapid vascular access and resuscitation
when a peripheral vein can not be catheterised and is particularly useful for this purpose in neonates.

Intravenous Catheter Placement and Care

Intravenous catheters should always be placed aseptically
and the catheter site covered with a gauze swab and antimicrobial ointment and bandaged. Catheter complications
include thrombophlebitis, bacteriaemia and bacterial
endocarditis.

- To minimise catheter complications, place aseptically and do not allow it to remain in any single vein for more than 72 h.
- Keep the catheter site clean and bandaged.
- Monitor the patient for leucocytosis and fever which may be related to the catheter.
- When the catheter is not in use, flush with heparinised saline to prevent thrombosis (0.9% NaCl with 5 units of heparin per ml).

DECIDING ON RATE OF FLUID INFUSION

The rate of fluid loss and clinical disease are critical in determining the rate of fluid administration. Dogs suffering from hypovolaemic shock secondary to sudden severe blood loss should have immediate rapid intravenous fluids administered to restore intravascular volume.

- In case of *hypovolaemic shock*, without concurrent cardiovascular disease, intravenous isotonic fluids should be administered at 90 ml/kg per hour (equal to one blood volume).
- In shock, hypertonic fluids, such as 7.0% NaCl or 7.0% NaCl and dextran-70, may be administered intravenously at 5 ml/kg slowly as a bolus over 5–10 min. The hypertonic solutions should be followed with an intravenous infusion of isotonic fluids at 20 ml/kg per hour for several hours.
- Patients with mild volume depletion require less aggressive fluid therapy. Generally, the fluid deficit can be replaced within 6–8 h with maintenance and contempory losses being distributed evenly throughout the day.

In cases where intravenous fluids can not be monitored 24 h per day, the 24-h fluid requirement may be given while someone is available to watch the infusion and the catheter heparinised until further use. After severe dehydration has been corrected, additional fluids may be given subcutaneously until the intravenous line can be started again the next day.

Setting the Administration Rate

Intravenous fluid administration sets are available as macro-drip sets (15 or 20 drops/ml) and micro-drip sets (60 drops/ml). Patient size and volume to be delivered determine the choice of administration set. Infusion pumps provide an accurate way to administer fluids, particularly in small volumes.

Once the fluid rate has been set, the infusion rate should be monitored hourly and the rate of administration adjusted to ensure the correct volume is given. Marking the fluid bag using adhesive tape will facilitate this process.

MONITORING THE SUCCESS OF FLUID THERAPY

The efficacy of fluid therapy should be monitored frequently and adjustments made based on the patient's response.

- Measure urine output during rapid infusion of large volumes of fluid. Urine output is a good guide to organ perfusion. In animals with persistent oliguria, rapid infusion of fluids can be dangerous; monitor for over-hydration by measuring central venous pressure (CVP) and auscultating lungs for pulmonary oedema.
- In severely shocked animals, serial measurement of arterial blood pressure by indirect means will facilitate assessment of response to aggressive fluid therapy. The

---

Example: 25 kg dog, 10% dehydrated		
Fluid deficit:	25 × 0.10	= 2.5 l
Maintenance requirement	22 ml/kg per day × 25	= 0.55 l/24 h
Total fluid requirement		= 3.05 l over 24 h
Rate of administration per hour	3050/24	= 127 ml/h
Using a macro giving set (20 drops/ml)	(127/60) × 20	= 42 drops/min or 1.5 drops/s

Box 2.1   Calculation of volume and rate of fluid administration.

aim should be to raise mean arterial pressure above 70 mmHg.
- Perform a thorough physical examination daily to evaluate rehydration. Evaluate mucous membrane moisture, skin turgor, capillary refill time, quality and rate of peripheral pulses, ongoing fluid loss due to vomiting, diarrhoea and polyuria.
- Daily body weight evaluation is important during fluid therapy. An acute gain or loss of 1 kg is equivalent to 1000 ml of body water.
- Monitor both PCV and total plasma protein (TPP) serially during fluid therapy – a decrease of both PCV and TPP is suggestive of rehydration.
- In animals with cardiovascular or renal disease, monitoring CVP is very useful. CVP should be monitored with a jugular catheter, the tip of which must be placed at the level of the right atrium. Normal values read on a manometer (filled with crystalloid fluid) run from 0 to 10 cmH$_2$O. Trends in CVP values are most important. Increasing values indicate that the cardiovascular system is incapable of handling the fluid load being administered and adjustments should be made.
- Serum electrolyte and blood gas values should be closely monitored in animals with electrolyte abnormalities and acid–base disturbances or those who are on fluid therapy for extended periods of time.

Handling Overhydration

Overhydration generally occurs in patients with underlying cardiovascular or renal disease who are unable to handle large volumes of fluids.

- Signs of overhydration include the accumulation of subcutaneous fluid leading to an oedematous feel to the skin, pulmonary oedema with tachypnoea and venous distension.
- Correction of overhydration is often difficult if there is an underlying disease. Stop all fluid infusions and give i.v. frusemide at 2–4 mg/kg. A second dose of 4–8 mg/kg may be given in 15 min if no diuresis occurs. Treat any underlying renal or cardiovascular disease.

TRANSFUSIONS

Blood cell transfusions are indicated in situations where low red cell mass severely compromises oxygen carrying capacity.

- Criteria for determining whether a blood transfusion is indicated include: haemorrhagic shock following volume replacement with crystalloid fluids; anaemia in dogs with a PCV < 0.151/l or less than 0.201/l if the animal is undergoing anaesthesia.

Canine Blood Groups

The dog has at least 13 different blood groups named dog erythrocyte antigens (DEA). The ideal canine blood donors are negative for DEA 1.1, 1.2 and 7 and are called universal donors. These three blood groups are the most important because:

- DEA 1.1 and 1.2 are the most potent stimulators of isoantibody production and transfusion of incompatible blood of these types can result in haemolytic reactions.
- Pre-formed antibodies to DEA 1.1 and 1.2 are rare and transfusion reactions generally do not occur unless the patient has been previously transfused with an incompatible blood group.
- Approximately 50% of dogs have naturally occurring isoantibodies to DEA 7.
- The clinical significance of isoantibodies to DEA 7 is uncertain – experimentally they have been shown to result in delayed destruction of transfused red cells (after 4–5 days) during the first transfusion.
- Compatible red cells survive for 80–100 days using blood stored for 2 weeks in acid citrate dextrose or 3 weeks in citrate phosphate dextrose adenine.

Blood Donors

To minimise the risk of disease transmission, full routine haematological examination of the blood donor should be performed before transfusion, if time permits. Canine blood donors should be:

- at least 25 kg in weight and have a PCV of at least 0.401/l,
- fully vaccinated,
- negative for *Ehrlichia canis*, *Babesia canis*, *Haemobartonella canis* and for microfilaria of *Dirofilaria immitis*,
- serologically negative for *Brucella canis*.

Cross Matching

A full cross match consists of major and minor parts. The major component is the cross matching of the donor cells to the recipient serum. Incompatibility is seen as either agglutination or haemolysis. The major cross match should always be compatible. The minor component is frequently not important. The main reasons for cross matching are to prevent transfusion reactions in previously sensitised patients. Because cross matching does not evaluate the compatibility of white blood cells and platelets, transfusion reactions can still occur in patients with compatible cross matches. In emergency situations, where crossmatching is not available and the patient has not received prior transfusions, a non-crossmatched transfusion can be performed. At worst, a first incompatible transfusion will result in delayed destruction of transfused cells and will sensitise the animal to subsequent transfusion of cells of the same blood group.

Collection and Storage of Blood Products

The following guidelines should be followed:

- Collect from a jugular vein using aseptic techniques (up to 20 ml/kg may be taken every 2–3 weeks from any one donor).
- Collect into commercially available plastic collection bag containing either:
  ○ citrate phosphate dextrose adenine – red cells remain viable for 4 weeks if stored at 4°C.
  ○ acid citrate dextrose – red cells remain viable for 3 weeks if stored at 4°C.
- Gently agitate during collection to ensure thorough mixing with anticoagulant.

Component Therapy

After blood has been collected into combined anticoagulant and preservative solutions, it may be separated into the different blood products. Blood products available include:

- fresh and stored whole blood,
- packed red cells,
- platelet rich plasma,
- fresh frozen plasma,
- frozen plasma,
- cryoprecipitate.

Deciding on Which Component to Use

(1) Whole blood – stored whole blood supplies red cells for oxygen delivery and plasma components for oncotic pressure, fibrinogen and stable clotting factors. Platelets and labile clotting factors (V, VIII,

von Willebrand's factor) are not preserved in stored whole blood. Fresh whole blood (stored for less than 12 hours) supplies platelets and all coagulation factors in addition to red cells and plasma proteins.
  - One unit of whole blood is equal to 450 ml.
  - Indications for whole blood transfusion include anaemia (stored), haemostatic abnormalities (fresh), and thrombocytopenia (fresh).
(2) Packed red cells are obtained following centrifugation of whole blood. Packed cells have less anticoagulant and less volume than whole blood.
  - One unit of packed cells contains approximately 250 ml. A typical haematocrit is 0.60–0.70 l/l. Packed cells can be added to fresh frozen plasma from the same donor to reconstitute a unit of whole blood with coagulation factors.
  - Use in patients with severe anaemia.
(3) Platelet rich plasma – is prepared by selective centrifugation of fresh whole blood and is an alternative low volume means of treating thrombocytopenic patients.
(4) Fresh frozen plasma (FFP) – plasma which has been separated from fresh whole blood and frozen within 6 h of collection. Rapid freezing protects labile coagulation factors. FFP is a good source of coagulation components, complements and oncotic proteins. One unit contains 200–250 ml.
  - Storage time is 1 year at −70°C (3 months at −20°C).
  - Used in cases of coagulopathy, von Willebrand's disease and hypoproteinaemia.
(5) If the time to separation and freezing exceeds 6 h, the product is called frozen plasma and is used as a source of oncotic proteins.

Guidelines for Blood Product Administration

- In dogs with anaemia, 2 ml of whole blood per kilogram will raise the PCV by 1% when the PCV of the donor blood is 0.40 l/l. If packed cells are used, 1 ml/kg will raise the PCV by 1%.
- The following equation can be used to determine the volume of blood required:

$$\text{volume of donor blood} = \text{BW recipient}\,(\text{kg}) \times 90 \times \frac{\text{desired PCV} - \text{recipient's PCV}}{\text{donors PCV}}$$

- A post transfusion PCV of 0.25–0.30 l/l is the goal in anaemic dogs.

- Rule of thumb dose rates for whole blood are:
  - Hypovolaemic animal: 13–22 ml/kg per hour
  - Normovolaemic   1–5 ml/kg per hour – do
    animal: not exceed 4 ml/kg
                           per hour if cardiac
                           insufficiency recognised
- Fresh frozen plasma should be administered at 10 ml/kg. This volume may be repeated until bleeding is controlled in animals with coagulopathies.
- Blood products are most commonly given slowly intravenously.
- Stored whole blood or packed cells should be warmed to body temperature and gently agitated before administration. Fresh frozen plasma should be slowly warmed to 37°C prior to use.
- Blood products are dripped through commercially available blood infusion sets with a nylon mesh filter (40 μm) capable of trapping microemboli and platelet aggregates.
- Do not infuse crystalloid solutions containing calcium through the same intravenous line as blood. Calcium containing solutions inhibit the anticoagulant resulting in the formation of micro-emboli.
- Do not infuse hypotonic crystalloid solutions through the same intravenous line as blood – these may cause red cell swelling and lysis.
- Prior administration of an antihistamine or glucocorticoid could be used to minimise the risk of a transfusion reaction.

Complications of Blood Transfusions

Immunological Reactions

(1) Haemolysis occurs secondary to infusion of blood to a patient that has previously been sensitised to a blood antigen (particularly DEA 1.1. and 1.2). In dogs that have not received a previous blood transfusion, uncrossmatched blood is very unlikely to lead to acute haemolysis but delayed red cell destruction can occur. Signs of acute haemolysis include:
- restlessness, fever (can also be caused by sepsis), vomiting, muscle tremors, tachycardia;
- haemoglobinaemia, haemoglobinuria and jaundice;
- may progress to disseminated intravascular coagulation or acute renal failure if transfusion not stopped;
- delayed haemolysis is more common than acute reactions and the animal is usually asymptomatic but may show an unexplained fall in PCV 10 to 21 days post-transfusion.

Action which should be taken in an acute haemolytic reaction:
- stop the transfusion immediately;
- give intravenous crystalloid fluids to support the circulation;
- administer an antihistamine (e.g. diphenhydramine 0.5 mg/kg i.v.) and/or glucocorticoids (e.g. hydrocortisone sodium succinate or methylprednisolone sodium succinate i.v.).

(2) Responses to foreign antigens on platelets and white cells can occur if antibodies are present in the donor or recipient's plasma. Mild allergic reactions can also occur to foreign proteins in the donor plasma. Signs include:
- fever,
- urticaria.

Action which should be taken:
- slow the rate of transfusion,
- administer antihistamines.

Non-Immunological Reactions to Transfusions

(1) Bacterial contamination of blood products may cause septicaemia and fever which to begin with may appear clinically similar to a transfusion reaction. To avoid this:
- stored blood which develops a brownish black tinge should be discarded;
- administer the entire bag within 24 h of warming or discard – do not warm and rechill blood.

(2) Circulatory overload may result. Signs include:
- vomiting,
- coughing, tachycardia, dyspnoea, cyanosis.

(3) Citrate intoxication can occur if large volumes of blood are transfused quickly or the animal has poor liver function. Signs are those of hypocalcaemia as citrate chelates calcium.

(4) Pulmonary microthromboembolism can occur if blood is administered without a filter.

(5) Iron overload is theoretically possible with repeated transfusions but is rare.

FLUID THERAPY IN SHOCK AND SEPSIS

Shock is a clinical syndrome that occurs when tissues are inadequately perfused secondary to cardiovascular collapse and/or increased tissue metabolic demand. When cardiac output fails to meet the demands of tissue metabolism, the patient is said to be in shock. Hypotension alone is not equivalent to shock.

Classification of Shock

Shock is classified into two broad categories:

- decreased circulating blood volume which is sub-divided into:
  - hypovolaemic
  - septic
  - neurogenic
- decreased cardiac function (cardiogenic shock).

Aggressive fluid therapy is only appropriate for the first broad category.

Hypovolaemic shock may be secondary to haemorrhage, fluid loss into the gastrointestinal tract (caused by obstruction) or severe dehydration. Clinical signs include pale and cool mucous membranes, slow capillary refill time, tachycardia and oliguria.

Septic shock is defined as clinical evidence of infection and a systemic response to that infection including tachycardia, hyperthermia and leucocytosis. Any pathogenic organism is capable of causing septic shock, however, Gram-negative rods are most commonly involved. Clinical signs include tachycardia, tachypnoea, slow capillary refill time (CRT), muddy coloured mucous membranes and hypotension. Initially, septic shock may present as a hyperdynamic state with high cardiac output and hypermetabolism. As septic shock progresses, the patient enters a hypodynamic state characterised by low cardiac output, peripheral vasoconstriction, oliguria and hypotension.

MANAGEMENT OF SHOCK

The underlying cause of the shock should be determined if possible. Perform a rapid physical examination and then proceed to the following steps:

- Place a large bore i.v. catheter in the jugular vein if possible. If jugular catheterisation is not possible, place catheters in both cephalic veins to enable large volumes of fluid to be administered.
- Begin administration of lactated Ringer's solution (or 0.9% sodium chloride) at 90 ml/kg in the first 15–20 min. Watch for signs of pulmonary oedema. Up to 200 ml/kg of fluids may be required to improve circulatory status. The fluid rate is adjusted based on the response

Box 2.2   Setting up constant infusions.

Example: Dosage (μg/kg per minute) × BW (kg)
= mg of drug added to 250 ml fluid
Administer at 1 drop/ 4 s from a biurette
giving set (60 drops per ml)

to therapy. Continual monitoring is necessary if such rapid rates of fluid administration are employed.
- An alternative to balanced electrolyte resuscitation is a combination of hypertonic saline (7.2%) and dextran 70 at 3–5 ml/kg slowly administered as a bolus over 5 min. Further doses of 2 ml/kg may be given up to a maximum total dose of 10 ml/kg. After hypertonic saline administration, the patient is maintained on isotonic replacement fluids at a rate of 10–20 ml/kg per hour until stable. Contraindications for hypertonic saline include: hypernatraemia, renal failure, cardiac failure and thrombocytopenia.
- Corticosteroids may suppress the systemic inflammatory response associated with shock. Water soluble drugs such as dexamthasone sodium phosphate (1–2 mg/kg i.v.) or prednisolone sodium succinate (10–20 mg/kg i.v.) may be given early in shock.
- Broad-spectrum antibiotics are indicated in most forms of severe septic shock. The cephalosporins or penicillins combined with the quinolones have excellent broad-spectrum of activity in the critical patient.
- Patients suffering from severe or prolonged shock (especially septic shock), are at risk for decreased myocardial function. In these patients, consider giving a positive inotropic drug. The most commonly used drugs in this category are dopamine (2–10 μg/kg per minute) and dobutamine (2–15 μg/kg per minute) both by continuous i.v. infusion.

CLINICAL EXAMPLES

Case 1

Signalment:	2-year-old male mixed breed dog (25 kg)
Presenting complaint:	Diarrhoea
History:	Bloody, liquid diarrhoea for 5 days, profound weight loss for 10 days
Physical examination:	10% dehydrated and depressed – no other abnormalities noted

Laboratory finding:	Sodium	115 mmol/l
	Potassium	3.5 mmol/l
	Chloride	80 mmol/l
	Total protein	65 g/l
	PCV	0.50 l/l
	BUN	39.3 mmol/l
	USG	1.030

Interpretation: Hypokalaemia, hyponatraemia, pre-renal azotaemia secondary to gastrointestinal fluid loss.

Treatment: Replacement fluid volume required:
$0.1 \times 25 = 2.5$ l

Maintenance fluid requirements for 24 h:
$44 \times 25 = 1100$ ml

A balanced electrolyte solution was adminsitered at 166 ml/h to correct 80% of the fluid deficit within 12 h. The fluid rate was then reduced to 130 ml/h to correct the remaining deficit and provide maintenance requirements. On the second day of fluid therapy, 20 mEq of KCl were added per litre of fluids.

Case 2

Signalment: 5-year-old female Labrador Retriever (25 kg)

Presenting complaint: Lethargy, anorexia and severe anaemia

History: Anorexia and lethargy for 1 week

Physical examination: Weak, lethargic, pale mucous membranes

Laboratory finding:	Sodium	147 mmol/l
	Potassium	4.5 mmol/l
	Chloride	110 mmol/l
	Total protein	42 g/l
	Albumin	10 g/l
	PCV	0.15 l/l
	BUN	7.9 mmol/l
	Faecal floatation	Severe hookworm infestation

Interpretation: Anaemia and hypoalbuminaemia secondary to chronic blood loss due to severe hookworm infestation.

Treatment: The dog was transfused with 700 ml of fresh whole blood to provide red cells and plasma protein. The dog's PCV after transfusion was 0.22 l/l. A course of pyrantel palmoate was prescribed to treat the hookworm infestation.

FURTHER READING

Authement, J.M. (1992) Blood transfusion therapy. In: *Fluid Therapy in Small Animal Practice*, (ed. S.P. DiBartola), pp. 371–383. W.B. Saunders, Philadelphia.

Authement, J.M. & Wolfshiemer, K.J. (1987) Canine blood component therapy: product preparation, storage and administration. *Journal of the American Animal Hospital Association*, **23**, 483–490.

Chew, D.J. (1994) Fluid therapy for dogs and cats. In: *Saunder's Manual of Small Animal Practice*, (eds. S.J. Birchard & R.G. Sherding), pp. 64–76. W.B. Saunders, Philadelphia.

Chew, D.J., Kohn, C.W. & DiBartola, S.P. (1982) Disorders of fluid balance and fluid therapy. In: *Quick Reference to Veterinary Medicine*, (ed. W.R. Fenner), pp. 465–480. J.B. Lippincott, Philadelphia.

DiBartola, S.P. (1992) Introduction to fluid therapy. In: *Fluid Therapy in Small Animal Practice*, (ed. S.P. DiBartola), pp. 321–340. W.B. Saunders, Philadelphia.

Kristensen, A.T. & Feldman, B.F. (1995) Blood banking and transfusion medicine. In: *Textbook of Small Animal Internal Medicine*, (eds S.J. Ettinger & E.C. Feldman), pp. 347–360. W.B. Saunders, Philadelphia.

Matrakos, P. & Meakins, J.L. (1994) Shock: causes and management of circulatory collapse. In: *Essentials of Surgery*, (eds D.C. Sabiston & H.K. Lyerly), 2nd edn. pp. 24–35. W.B. Saunders, Philadelphia.

Muir, W.W. (1990) Small volume resuscitation using hypertonic saline. *Cornell Veterinarian*, **80**, 7–12.

Senior, D.F. (1995) Fluid therapy, electrolytes and acid base control. In: *Textbook of Small Animal Internal Medicine*, (eds. S.J. Ettinger & E.C. Feldman), pp. 294–311. W.B. Saunders, Philadelphia.

Schertel, E.R. & Tobias, T.A. (1992) Hypertonic fluid therapy. In: *Fluid Therapy in Small Animal Practice*, (ed. S.P. DiBartola), pp. 471–485. W.B. Saunders, Philadelphia.

Chapter 3

Nutritional Support of the Critically Ill Patient

A. G. Torrance

INTRODUCTION

Most critical patients have an increased requirement for nutrients but a reduced nutrient intake due to lack of appetite or inability to eat. The resulting protein–energy malnutrition damages the immune system, impairs healing, depresses vital organ function and affects the chances of recovery. The objective of nutritional support is to avert protein–energy malnutrition by providing a formula of fuels and other nutrients in proportions that can be used by the patient with maximal efficiency and to deliver this formula with minimal discomfort.

THE NUTRITIONAL STATUS OF CRITICALLY ILL DOGS

Most of the available information on the effects of critical illness upon the nutritional status of dogs has been extrapolated from human patients and laboratory animal models of trauma and sepsis. It is assumed that:

- The response of dogs to critical disease is similar to that of other divergent species.
- The metabolic response of dogs to different critical disease processes is also similar to other species.

Clearly this is a gross oversimplification and until appropriate studies are performed the success of nutritional intervention in dogs with critical disease will depend upon close monitoring of the patient's response to an essentially arbitrary nutritional regimen.

When a normal dog is starved there is a decrease in metabolic rate coupled with an increase in fat oxidation and a reduction in protein catabolism. The effects of these changes are to conserve the function of the remaining tissue mass and to consume fat stores slowly.

When an animal is subjected to stresses such as trauma, sepsis or burns:

- In the initial shock phase there is often a reduction in metabolic rate.
- Once intravascular volume and tissue perfusion are restored, this is rapidly superceded by a hypermetabolic state which:
  - is characterised by increased oxygen consumption and energy expenditure and depends upon the severity of injury;
  - probably represents an attempt by the body to provide adequate glucose to optimise the host defences and wound repair at the privileged site of injury.
- Increased secretion of counter-regulatory hormones, glucagon, catecholamines, cortisol and growth hormone antagonise the effects of insulin and induce:
  - hyperglycaemia;
  - degradation of tissue protein to provide substrate for gluconeogenesis;
  - increased fat oxidation;
  - increased glucose oxidation but oxidation is less efficient and the overall contribution of glucose to energy expenditure is reduced;
  - rapid depletion of glycogen stores.
- The increase in metabolic rate is sustained by fat oxidation with continuing glucose wastage.

Stress Starvation

In 'simple starvation' fat oxidation is accompanied by ketogenesis and reduced protein degradation. When starvation and hypermetabolism occur at the same time (stress-starvation) protein degradation for gluconeogenesis is not suppressed and may accelerate. There are no protein stores in the body and substrates for gluconeogenesis are obtained at the expense of tissue structure and function such that:

- Breakdown of peripheral muscle sustains the patient for a while before more vital functions are affected.
- Organ systems which depend upon rapid cell turnover, such as the gut and the immune system, are very vulnerable.
- Gut-associated lymphoid tissue becomes depleted and there is a reduction in IgA secretion.
- The combination of depressed immune function and failure of the gastrointestinal mucosal barrier has grave consequences for the patient:
  ○ bacterial translocation from the gut lumen through the compromised mucosa into the portal blood increases;
  ○ reticuloendothelial system in the liver is also impaired and thus more bacteria and toxins of gut origin find their way into the systemic circulation leading to sepsis and endotoxaemia.
- Protein–energy malnutrition can be a major contributing factor in multiple organ failure and ultimately in the patient's demise.

Patients suffering from stress-starvation are relatively intolerant of glucose and use it inefficiently as an energy source. The hypermetabolic state is supported primarily by fat oxidation and protein breakdown. Fat and protein are therefore particularly important energy sources for the critical patient and should be emphasised when formulating diets for the critical care of dogs.

Despite this superficial understanding of the physiology of stress-starvation, there are no purely objective methods for determining the nutritional status of dogs in critical care. The consequence of this is that nutritional support is guided by a series of estimates based upon the maintenance energy requirements of groups of normal dogs multiplied by disease factors. Such estimates are wildly inaccurate (20–110%) when applied to the individual critical patient. Until simple, non-invasive methods for tracking nutritional status are developed, the provision of nutritional support is essentially arbitrary and the clinician is reliant upon close monitoring of the patient to determine the success or failure of the nutritional support measures.

Assessment of Nutritional Status in Critically Ill Dogs

The flow chart (Fig. 3.1) summarises the approach to assessment of nutritional status. Current methods for the objective assessment of nutritional status and the identifi-

cation of protein–energy malnutrition in canine patients are unsophisticated. The most useful information probably comes from careful history-taking and physical examination by an experienced veterinary surgeon.

The ideal objective index of nutritional status is a simple biochemical or physical measurement which is:

- sensitive and specific for protein–energy malnutrition,
- responds to nutritional repletion,
- an accurate indicator of nutritional complications.

Such an index does not exist in the human field and is a very distant goal in veterinary medicine. Unsuccessful candidates for this role have included albumin, prealbumin, transferrin, fibronectin, retinol binding protein and reduced peripheral lymphocyte counts. Most of these indices have proven too non-specific or insensitive in humans.

Albumin and peripheral lymphocyte counts are frequently measured in veterinary patients and have some role to play in the assessment of nutritional status but only as subsidiary indices to history and physical examination (Box 3.1).

Similar criticism can be applied to peripheral lymphocyte counts which are frequently altered by factors such as corticosteroid therapy that are unrelated to nutritional status. Methods for applying calorimetry and nitrogen balance studies to dogs in critical care and further nutritional markers such as insulin-like growth factor 1 (IGF1) and growth factor binding proteins are currently under investigation. In human patients, anthropometric measurements such as weight/height and triceps skinfold thickness can be used as objective indices of nutritional status. Development of similar measurements validated for each breed of dog would be a work of spectacular dedication but

Box 3.1 Plasma albumin as an indicator of nutritional status.

- Hypoalbuminaemia (<20 g/l) is:
  ○ a poor prognostic index in dogs undergoing surgical procedures,
  ○ an insensitive and non-specific marker of protein-energy malnutrition.
- Serum albumin only decreases late in starvation.
- Processes other than starvation, such as protein-losing enteropathy and nephropathy, frequently cause a precipitous drop in serum albumin in dogs with critical illness which may not reflect their overall nutritional status.

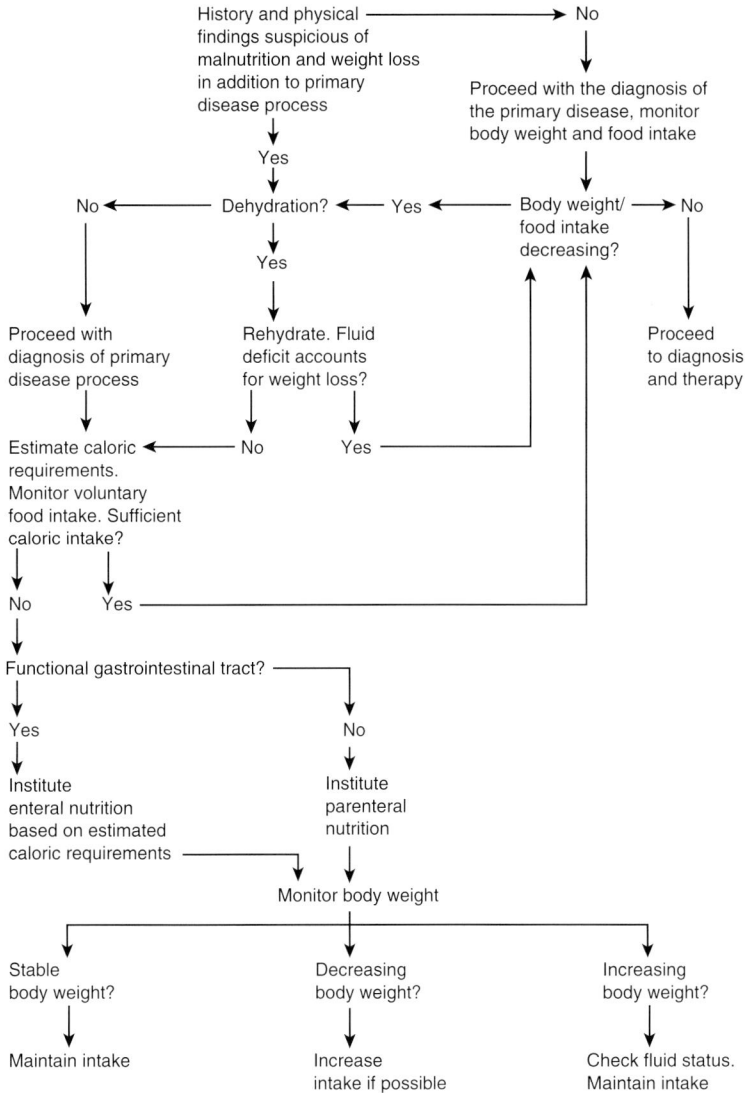

Fig. 3.1 Flow chart for the assessment of nutritional status in critically ill dogs

doubtful practicality. Such measurements could, however, be developed for cats.

Experienced veterinary surgeons are able to recognise the physical signs of protein–energy malnutrition in dogs. Dedicated owners are also very aware of loss of weight or condition in their pets. Generalised muscle loss in sick animals is usually due to protein–energy malnutrition unless there is a generalised myopathy or peripheral neuropathy. The combination of poor coat quality and generalised muscle loss often marks protein–energy malnutrition. Bilateral temporal atrophy is frequently the most readily appreciable sign of generalised muscle loss especially in breeds with thick coats. Acute weight loss is often due to dehydration and the actual loss of tissue mass can only be appreciated once the fluid deficit has been corrected. Weight gain in critical patients is often due to water retention rather than the acquisition of tissue. The importance of serial monitoring of body weight in the critical patient cannot be overemphasised. Each measurement must be interpreted carefully in the light of changes in the primary disease process, the nutritional status and the fluid status.

- Loss of 10% of hydrated body mass is an indication for nutritional support.
- Severely decreased food intake or complete anorexia for more than 5 days is an indication for nutritional support.

Overfeeding is a potential complication of nutritional support and may result in liver dysfunction due to fat or glycogen infiltration, aggravated glucose intolerance, azotaemia, increased energy expenditure and oxygen demand. In critical care, weight gain is generally not the goal of nutritional support as this might lead to oversupplementation of protein and energy in animals whose organs of excretion are compromised. Prevention of weight loss is the more realistic goal.

CALCULATION OF NUTRITIONAL REQUIREMENTS

The nutritional needs of a dog in critical care can be estimated using a simple equation for the maintenance energy requirement (MER) based upon body weight. The MER is an estimate of the energy required for maintenance of that animal during health, including provision for a modest amount of physical activity. The MER is then multiplied by disease factors for different disease processes which estimate, in a crude way, the additional metabolic requirement imposed by the disease process. In some cases, the caloric requirement is actually less than MER because of the lack of physical activity imposed during cage rest (Box 3.2).

These equations assume that the principal determinant of the quantity of food required is the energy (caloric) requirement of the patient. This assumption is reasonable only if the food source is balanced for energy, protein and other nutrients. It is advisable to use the commercially-available critical care diets designed specifically for dogs, rather than diets designed for use in humans, to ensure that the diet is appropriately balanced. Critical disease processes such as renal and hepatic failure impose additional nutritional demands which must be factored into the food requirement. For example the protein restriction needed in renal failure must be estimated and the energy intake maintained by addition of non-protein energy sources. In such cases monitoring blood urea and creatinine

Box 3.2 Calculation of energy requirements.

MER (kcals/day) = $125 \times$ [body weight(kg)]$^{0.75}$

Illness energy requirement (IER) = MER $\times$ Illness factors

Illness factors:
0.5–0.9 – hospitalisation
1.0–1.2 – minor surgery/trauma
1.2–1.5 – major surgery/trauma
1.5–2.0 – sepsis, neoplasia, burns, head trauma.

Quantity of food to feed = IER/caloric density of food.

Box 3.3 Calculation of quantities of nutrients for parenteral feeding.

- Maintenance protein requirement = 4 g/kg
- Dogs with extraordinary protein loss (burns, sepsis, neoplasia, trauma, surgery) protein requirement = 6 g/kg
- Dogs with renal or hepatic failure protein requirement = 1.5 g/kg
- Calories from 20% lipid emulsion (2 kcal/ml) usually make up 40–60% IER in parenteral nutrition
- Calories from 50% dextrose (1.7 kcal/ml) usually make up the remaining 40–60% IER

concentrations may be helpful in establishing the ideal protein and energy content of nutritional support.

In parenteral nutrition, the quantities of fat (20% lipid emulsion), carbohydrate (50% dextrose) and protein (amino acid solution) are calculated individually based on the IER and standardised protein requirements for adult dogs (see Box 3.3).

ROUTE OF ADMINISTRATION OF NUTRITION

Nutritional support can be provided via:

- intravenous infusion (parenteral),
- the gastrointestinal tract (enteral).

The enteral route is usually selected unless:

- the gut is non-functional,
- there is a specific contraindication such as intractable vomiting due to pancreatitis.

Parenteral Nutrition

This route of administration is required for a limited number of patients requiring nutritional support and most patients can be managed using the enteral route. Enteral nutrition is preferred because parenteral nutrition:

- is less physiological;
- is technically more demanding and requires:
  o prolonged maintenance of a central venous catheter,
  o continuous infusion controlled by an infusion pump,
  o strict asepsis in the preparation of an appropriate mixture to infuse;
- has less margin for error in estimating nutrient requirements – metabolic complications include:
  o hyperglycaemia which may cause osmotic diuresis and dehydration,
  o electrolyte abnormalities (hypochloraemia, hypokalaemia and hyperkalaemia),
  o acid–base disturbances, particularly metabolic alkalosis;
- carries a greater risk of sepsis (catheter or solution related).

For these reasons, parenteral nutrition should only be administered to those few cases where it is specifically indicated. Such cases would be best managed in specialist institutions where sophisticated critical care facilities and staff dedicated to the care of a small number of patients are available. For a detailed review of total parenteral nutrition see Lippert and Buffington (1992).

Enteral Nutrition

Methods for Administering Enteral Nutrition

Voluntary food intake is to be encouraged but most critical patients are either anorexic or dysphagic and unable to meet their nutritional needs without support. Numerous methods have been described to enhance voluntary intake and they include use of:

- favourite flavours;
- warming and wetting food;

- foods with strong odours and appealing textures;
- baby foods which are often very appetising to dogs but should not be used exclusively because they have an inappropriate balance of nutrients;
- careful coaxing by an individual dedicated to each patient – this is probably the most effective method for enhancing voluntary intake but is time-consuming and labour intensive;
- forced feeding which is not recommended in the critical patient because of the risks of increasing patient stress and of aspiration.

In many critical patients, the only way to control food intake completely and ensure that the patient has the best chance of recovery is to use a tube-feeding method. Numerous methods have been described – those currently recommended are listed in Box 3.4. The enterostomy tube has relatively few indications but may be an alternative to total parenteral nutrition in patients with pancreatitis and gastric causes of vomiting.

The advantages and disadvantages of these methods of enteral feeding are summarised in Table 3.1.

Naso-Oesophageal Tubes

Tube Placement Method
The following technique is recommended:

- Local anaesthetic drops are instilled into the right or left nostril.
- A 5–10 Fr long PVC or silicone infant feeding tube is then measured against the patient to extend from the external nares to the seventh rib-space.
- The lubricated tube is inserted into the nostril:
  o directed ventrally and medially into the ventral meatus,
  o entry into the ventral meatus may be facilitated by pushing the external nares dorsally once the tube is in contact with the nasal septum.
- The tube is advanced towards the pharynx and into the oesophagus until the marker tape is positioned against the external nares.
- Check the tube is correctly sited:

Box 3.4   Tube-feeding methods.

- naso-oesophageal
- oesophagostomy
- gastrostomy
- enterostomy

Method	Advantages	Disadvantages
Naso-oesophageal	Non-invasive No general anaesthetic required Easy to place	Mechanical interference by patient Short-term nutrition only Liquid diets only Tube regurgitation No use in oesophageal dysfunction Elizabethan collar often required
Oesophagostomy	Less mechanical interference Longer term nutrition possible	General anaesthesia needed More invasive
Gastrostomy	Use in oesophageal dysfunction Long-term support liquid/semi-solid diets No mechanical interference Dogs can exercise	General anaesthesia needed Invasive, rare but significant complications Not for short-term nutrition
Enterostomy	Use in pancreatitis	Invasive General anaesthesia Limited indications Osmotic diarrhoea

Table 3.1 The advantages and disadvantages of the different methods for administering enteral nutrition.

- o inject a small volume of saline down the tube to induce a cough should the tube have entered the trachea instead of the oesophagus,
  - o injecting 5–10 ml of air and auscultating the stomach for borborygmus.
- When satisfied that the tube is in the correct position, fix in place:
  - o suture or glue with fast acting adhesive to the external nares,
  - o tape butterflies are then used to secure the tube with sutures or glue up the middle of the nose and between the eyes to the top of the head,
  - o an Elizabethan collar may be necessary to prevent the patient interfering with the tube.

Use and Maintenance of the Tube

Naso–oesophageal tubes have a narrow bore and completely liquid diets should be used. Commercial liquid enteral diets are suitable.

- Diets can be administered:
  - o by continuous infusion,
  - o in intermittent boluses (more commonly).
- For bolus use check the position of the tube before each bolus of food is administered.

Complications of Naso-Oesophageal Tubes

These are rare but include:

- rhinitis,
- epistaxis,
- reflux or vomiting,
- tube or diet aspiration,
- oesophagitis with stricture formation.

The most common problems with these tubes are mechanical and include loss of positioning within the oesophagus and blockage with food.

Contraindications of Naso-Oesophageal Tubes

These include:

- unconscious patients,
- disease or dysfunction of:

○ nares,
○ larynx,
○ swallowing reflex,
○ oesophagus or stomach.

Termination of the tube in the oesophagus and not the stomach reduces the risk of reflux oesophagitis.

Oesophagostomy Tubes

Tube Placement Methods
Two techniques for placing oesophagostomy tubes have been described and used effectively with few significant complications (Crowe 1990).

The Percutaneous Technique
- Anaesthetise the patient.
- Insert curved foreceps into the oesophagus through the mouth.
- Turn the tips of the forceps and open slightly to locate the site for catheter insertion.
- Use a through-the-needle intravenous catheter (16–20 G).
- Insert the needle through the skin until it punctures the lumen of the oesophagus.
- Thread the catheter through the needle and advance towards the stomach.
- Check correct placement of the catheter by injecting air and auscultating the stomach.
- Fix the catheter to the skin using sutures and a light dressing.

The Cut-Down Technique
- Anaesthetise the patient.
- Place curved forceps with fine tips in the oesophagus through the mouth.
- Turn the tip of the forceps outwards to locate the site for incision.
- Make a small subcutaneous stab incision.
- Force the tip of the forceps through the oesophageal wall and out of the incision.
- Use a 5–12 Fr red rubber catheter or infant feeding tube.
- Grasp the end of the feeding tube with the forceps and pull through the oesophagus into the mouth.
- Bend the end of the tube back, reinsert it into the mouth and advance it down the oesophagus.
- Check the location of the catheter by auscultation of injected air.
- Fix the tube to the skin of the neck with sutures and a light dressing.

Use and Maintenance of the Oesophagostomy Tube
Suitable diets and daily management of the tube is similar to the naso–oesophageal tube.

Complications Oesophagostomy Tubes
- The only recorded problem of managing these tubes in a clinical trial involving 50 dogs and cats was infection at the entry site of the tube through the skin.
- Removal of these tubes is simple and scar tissue rapidly closes the stoma.

Contraindications of Oesophagostomy Tubes
These include:

- unconscious patients,
- laryngeal/swallowing dysfunction,
- oesophageal dysfunction or reflux,
- vomiting.

Percutaneous Gastrostomy Tubes

Tube Placement
Percutaneous gastrostomy tubes can be placed endoscopically or blindly using the ELD Gastrostomy Tube Applicator or a stomach tube. All methods require general anaesthesia.

Choice and Preparation of Tube

- Purpose-made human gastrostomy tubes are too expensive – tubes for small animals are made from alternative cheaper materials.
- Mushroom tipped urological catheters (16–20 Fr Bard Urological Catheter) are useful for this purpose and can be prepared as follows:
  ○ remove the small nipple on the mushroom tip,
  ○ cut a short length of the tube (3 cm) from the end and divided into 2 pieces of equal length,
  ○ make a small incision through the centre of each piece,
  ○ thread one of the pieces down the tube until it lies flush with the mushroom tip. (This acts as the internal anchor and the second piece will subsequently be used on the external side of the abdominal wall to lock the tube in place.) (See Fig. 3.2)

Endoscopic Tube Placement

- Two operators are required.
- Place the patient in right lateral recumbency.

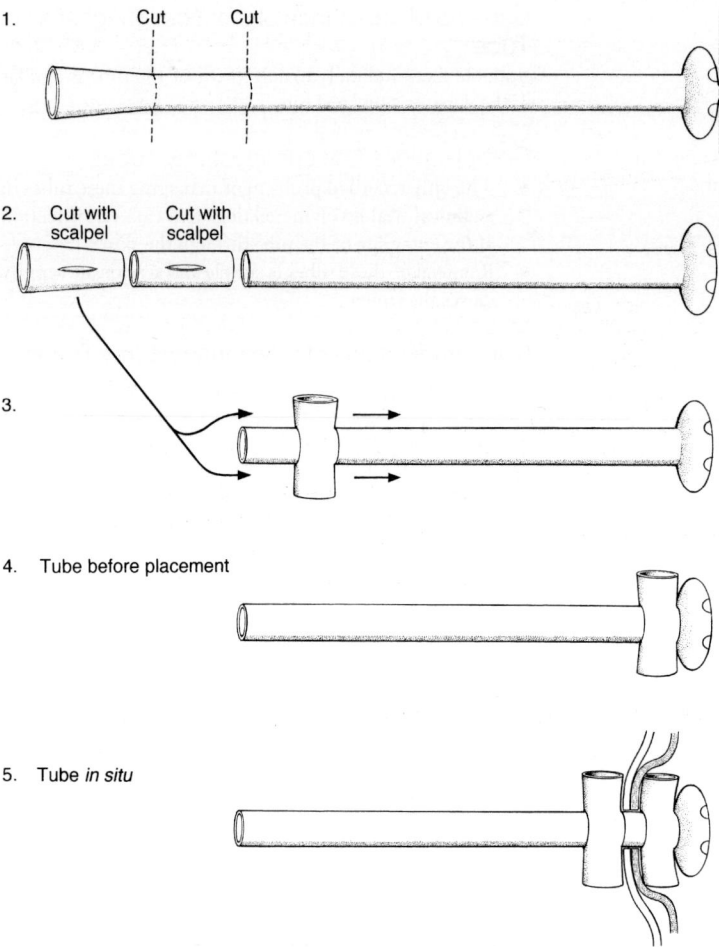

1.   Cut   Cut

2.   Cut with   Cut with
      scalpel   scalpel

3.

4.   Tube before placement

5.   Tube *in situ*

Fig. 3.2   Conversion of a
mushroom–tipped urological catheter
into a gastronomy tube (see text for a
description of each step).

- Clip an area behind the left costal arch and prepare aseptically.
- Pass the endoscope into the stomach.
- Inflate the stomach and transilluminate the left abdominal wall to ensure that the spleen is not trapped between the gastric and abdominal walls.
- The assistant depresses the abdominal wall with a finger and this is visualised with the endoscope.
- The finger is moved until a suitable insertion point is identified with the endoscope.
- Push a 16 or 18 G, over-the-needle catheter firmly through the body wall and into the gastric lumen.
- Remove the stylet and insert 3 metric monofilament nylon suture through the catheter into the stomach lumen.
- Catch the end of the suture with the endoscope biopsy foreceps.
- Withdraw the endoscope slowly from the stomach.

- Feed the suture from outside the abdominal wall until it is drawn out through the mouth.
- The catheter is then threaded off the suture which enters the abdomen behind the costal arch, passes into the gastric lumen, up the oesophagus and out of the mouth.
- Thread a hard plastic pipette tip onto the suture exiting the mouth with the sharp tip towards the patient (see Fig. 3.3).
- Pass the suture through the end of the tube with a needle and secure carefully with multiple knot ties (see Fig. 3.4).
- Draw the end of the tube into the pipette tip.
- Gently retract the suture emerging from behind the costal arch drawing the tube down the oesophagus and into the stomach.
- The second operator follows the tube down the oesophagus with the endoscope.

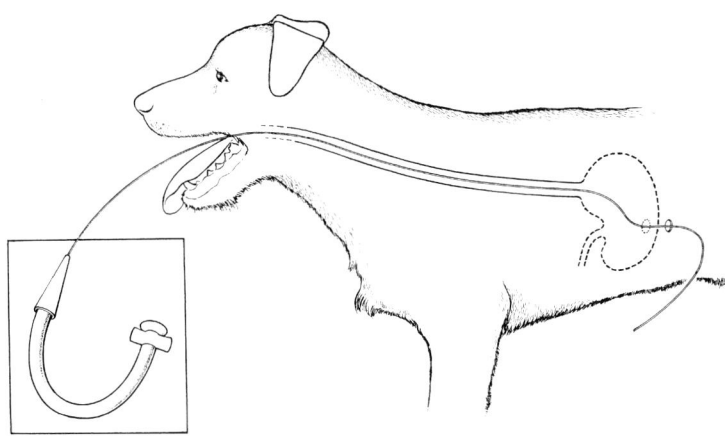

Fig. 3.3 Diagram showing how a gastronomy tube may be placed (see text for a description).

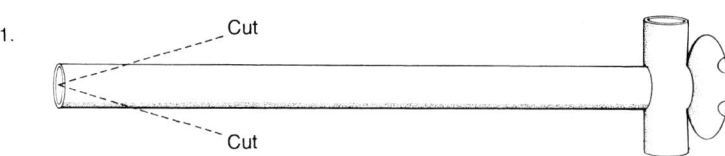

Fig. 3.4 Modification of a gastronomy tube to allow its percutaneous placement (see text for a description of each step).

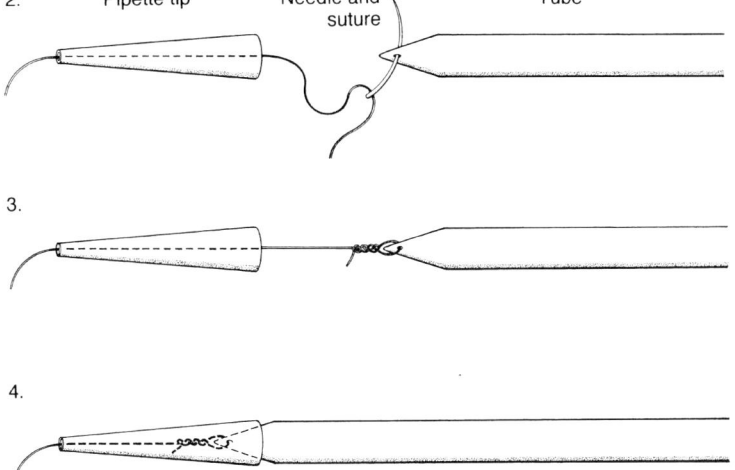

- Carefully enlarge the exit point of the suture with a scalpel blade until the sharp end of the pipette tip appears through the abdominal wall.
- As soon as it appears grasp it with a haemostat to take the pressure off the suture and further enlarge the exit point with a scalpel blade until the tube can be gently pulled out.
- Pull the tube out until the mushroom tip and anchor piece fit snuggly against the gastric mucosa.

- Thread the second rubber locking piece down the tube to secure it against the body wall.
- The second rubber locking piece should not be placed too tightly against the abdominal wall because the exit wound will swell during the healing period.
- Cap and secure the end of the tube against the body wall with a tape butterfly and a suture.
- Use a light bandage to hold the tube against the abdominal wall and to prevent patient interference.

Placement Using the ELD Gastrostomy Tube Applicator. This is quite a simple instrument for blind percutaneous placement of gastrostomy tubes. It comes in two sizes, one for cats and small dogs, and another for larger dogs. The instrument consists of a curved aluminium stomach tube with a sharp internal steel stylet operated by a spring-loaded plunger. The technique invloved is:

- Place the anaesthetised patient in right lateral recumbency.
- Pass the instrument through the mouth and into the stomach.
- Hold the handle of the instrument with the spring-loaded plunger in the left hand and use the curvature to push the end of the instrument against the gastric wall on the left side.
- Locate the end of the instrument with the right hand and isolate it between the fingers to ensure that the spleen is not trapped between the gastric and body walls.
- Depress the plunger and the sharp stylet appears through the abdominal wall.
- Tie a monofilament nylon suture through a hole in the end of the stylet.
- Retract the stylet (using the spring) into the instrument.
- Withdraw the instrument from the gastric lumen feeding the suture through the body wall until it extends from behind the costal arch, through the stomach and oesophagus and out of the mouth.
- From this point the tube placement is the same as that described above although the snug fit of the inner anchor and mushroom tip of the feeding tube against the gastric mucosa cannot be confirmed endoscopically.

This technique was evaluated recently in 15 cats and was found to be safe, rapid and effective and indicated when endoscopic or surgical gastrostomy is not feasible (Marks *et al.* 1994).

Another blind gastrostomy technique has been described which requires no special equipment at all (Fulton and Denis 1992). A lubricated vinyl tube is passed through the mouth into the stomach until the gastric end is seen to displace the abdominal wall. The tube is then grasped through the abdominal wall and manoeuvred so that the open end of the tube is pushed against the abdominal wall 2–3 cm caudal to the end of the left 13th rib. A small skin incision is made over the lumen of the tube and a 14–16 G over-the-needle catheter introduced. The location of the catheter within the end of the tube is verified by waggling the needle and feeling the the sides of the tube. The stylet is then removed and a guide-wire made from a banjo string is introduced and pushed up the lumen of the tube until it emerges at the mouth end of the tube. Monofilamant nylon

suture is attached to the wire outside the abdominal wall and pulled through into the stomach lumen, up the oesophagus and out of the mouth. From this point onwards the procedure is the same as the method described above. Limitations to this technique include all those for the endoscopic method with the addition of obesity. The method has been assessed in six dogs and 14 cats and found to be as successful as the endoscopic method.

Use and Maintenance of Gastrostomy Tubes
- Feeding through the tube is usually delayed for 24 h after placement.
- Start at one-third of the daily requirement in 6–8 feeds/day.
- Increase to the full daily requirement over 2–3 days.
- Flush the tube carefully after each feeding and if it becomes blocked relieve the obstruction using:
  - warm water,
  - pancreatic enzyme solution, or
  - cola.
- Record the quantity of flush solution that has entered the stomach.
- The volume of liquid diet given in each bolus should be judged for each individual patient but should not exceed 50 ml/kg per feed.
- Percutaneous gastrostomy tubes should be left in position for at least 5 days before removal to ensure that sufficient adhesions have developed between the stomach and the body wall.
- Gastrostomy tubes are removed by:
  - pulling the tube tight against the abdominal wall and then cutting it cleanly with scissors or a scalpel,
  - the mushroom tip and inner anchor are passed in faeces and the stoma closes rapidly with scar tissue.

Complications of Gastrostomy Tubes
These are very rare but include:

- splenic laceration,
- mild gastric haemorrhage,
- pneumoperitoneum,
- vomiting,
- aspiration pneumonia,
- inadequate gastric emptying,
- tube migration,
- infection of the stoma.

Animals with oesophageal dysfunction have a relatively high incidence of aspiration pneumonia associated with gastrostomy tube feeding.

Contraindications for Gastrostomy Tube Placement
These include:

- nutritional support anticipated for less than 5–7 days,
- intractable vomiting,
- severe gastric or intestinal dysfunction,
- pancreatitis,
- ascites.

Enterostomy Tubes

These tubes may be useful in animals with moderate gastric or oesophageal dysfunction where gastric emptying is impaired and there is a likelihood of aspiration pneumonia. Percutaneous enterostomy tubes are unlikely to have application in pancreatitis or inflammatory conditions of the stomach because of the necessity for placing a gastrostomy tube first (see below). Dogs with pancreatitis that require long-term nutritional support may benefit from a surgically placed jejunostomy tube, although there is still some pancreatic secretion associated with feeding. Total parenteral nutrition is not associated with significant pancreatic secretion and is therefore the preferred method if the infusion can be maintained in the long term. Specific indications based upon clinical application have not been reported yet.

Tube Placement Methods

Enterostomy tubes can be placed:

- by passing them through a percutaneous gastrostomy tube and guiding the end of the tube through the pylorus with the endoscope;
- surgically (jejunostomy tubes), often placed following major procedures on the stomach.

Use and Maintenance of Enterostomy Tubes

- Feeding through enterostomy tubes has to be controlled carefully to avoid osmotic overload and diarrhoea.
- Continuous low volume infusion of liquid enteral diet is the preferred method.

Complications of Enterostomy Tubes

These have not been carefully analysed because the tubes are used quite infrequently in canine practice.

Complications of Percutaneous Enterostomy Tubes

- all the complications mentioned above for percutaneous endoscopic gastrostomy (PEG) tubes,
- tube migration back through the pylorus,
- tube knotting or kinking distal to the pylorus making removal complicated,
- osmotic overload and diarrhoea.

Complications of Surgically Placed Jejunostomy Tubes

- leakage of gut contents into peritoneal cavity due to failure of surgical technique,
- osmotic overload and diarrhoea.

Contraindications for Enterostomy Tubes

- severe intestinal dysfunction,
- partial intestinal obstruction distal to the tube,
- ascites,
- nutritional support anticipated for less than 5–7 days.

ENTERAL DIETS FOR CRITICAL CARE

The ideal diet for critical care should:

- be highly palatable,
- be readily digestible,
- have high energy density to ensure sufficient energy is acquired from a small food intake,
- be liquid or semi-solid to facilitate tube feeding.

Fuel sources in the diet must be tailored to the patient's requirements. In most cases this means:

- provding a relatively high percentage of energy as protein and fat rather than carbohydrate;
- currently available critical care diets for dogs have:
  - ○ 20–25% kcal of protein,
  - ○ 50–55% kcal of fat,
  - ○ 25–26% kcal of carbohydrate;
- the diet should contain adequate quantities of trace minerals and vitamins – specific nutrients that are particularly important to the dog in critical care include glutamine, arginine and zinc.

(1) Glutamine
- is the major substrate for increased gluconeogenesis in stressed dogs;
- although not normally considered to be an essential amino acid, becomes conditionally essential in dogs suffering from stress-starvation;
- is an important fuel for rapidly dividing cells and deficiency leads to gut mucosal atrophy and compromise of the mucosal barrier to bacterial translocation;
- is too labile to be included in parenteral nutrition solutions and this may be the cause of the gut

atrophy seen in animals receiving total parenteral
nutrition;
- is supplemented in many of the available enteral
  diets;
- in high doses has a trophic effect on the gut
  mucosa.
(2) Arginine
- is an essential amino acid in dogs and deficiency
  can lead to failure of the urea cycle and
  hyperammonaemia;
- is deficient in standard human enteral diets which
  may cause hyperammonaemia in canine patients;
- has also been shown to improve the survival time
  of patients with sepsis by an immunostimulatory
  effect.
(3) Zinc
- plays an important role in protein and nucleic acid
  metabolism and promotes wound healing;
- deficiency for 1 week in animals with an enterotomy was associated with reduced collagen
  synthesis within the wound and hypoalbuminaemia.

This suggests that trace elements should be provided even
when only short-term nutritional support is anticipated.
Critical care diets suitable for tube feeding include Canine
Instant Concentration Diet (Waltham), A/D (Hills), and
Reanimyl (Virbac).

CASE EXAMPLES

Case 1

Signalment: Male cross bred dog, aged 14 years.

History: This dog had a long-term history of mild
dysuria which had never been investigated. He was
receiving a drug containing corticosteroids to control
arthritic pain. Five days before presentation the dog
became lethargic and less interested in food than normal
and appeared to be in pain when getting up. This progressed over the next few days to reluctance to move and
finally recumbency.

Medical investigation: On presentation the dog was collapsed with a temperature of 40.2°C, pulse 150/min and
respiratory rate 60/min. The mucous membranes were
brick red with rapid capillary refill and the prostate was
enlarged and painful. Haematology and biochemistry
revealed mild non-regenerative anaemia, degenerative left
shift and toxicity, mild azotaemia and mild non-specific

liver enzyme elevations. Urinalysis revealed concentrated
urine with a urinary tract infection with haemolytic
Escherichia coli. Thoracic and abdominal X-rays showed
microcardia and gross prostatic enlargement. Prostatic
ultrasound revealed a symmetrically enlarged prostate with
multiple fluid-filled cavities. Prostatic aspiration under
ultrasound guidance yielded an inflammatory fluid containing multiple bacterial rods.

Diagnosis: Septic shock with prerenal azotaemia secondary to severe prostatitis.

Treatment: Intravenous fluid therapy (Hartmann's) and
broad-spectrum, bactericidal antibiotics.

Nutrition: The body weight on presentation was 25 kg
and on a previous visit for vaccination the dog had weighed
30 kg. The estimate of dehydration was 8% and after fluid
replacement for 12 h the weight was 27.1 kg. The estimated
loss of lean body mass was 2.9 kg (=9.6%), coupled with a
highly catabolic process (sepsis) and anticipated stress-
starvation. The dog was recumbent and anorexic.
Nutritional support was indicated and an enteral tube
feeding method was ideal. A naso-oesophageal tube was
placed in the conscious dog and secured in position with
fast acting adhesive. A liquid critical care diet was selected.

On day two of hospitalisation, one-third of the amount
calculated in Box 3.5 was mixed into a liquid slurry with
water and administered at a constant rate through the tube
over a 24-h period. There were no adverse reactions to the
food and the dog remained recumbent and disinterested
and there were no mechanical problems with interference
with the tube. On day three of hospitalisation two-thirds of
the calculated requirement was administered. On day four
the full amount was given and the dog began to show signs
of improvement but still did not appear to resent the tube.

Box 3.5   Calculations of dietary requirements for Case 1.

Calculations: Daily MER = $125 \times [30]^{0.75} = 125 \times$
12.8 = 1600 kcals
The illness factor was 1.8 for a
markedly catabolic process
Daily IER = 1600 × 1.8 = 2880 kcals
The caloric density of the diet was
437 kcal/100 g dry matter
Therefore 2880/437 = 6.59 × 100 =
659 g of dry diet were required to
mix into a liquid slurry for
administration through the
tube/day.

By day six the dog was taking the liquid food voluntarily and the tube was removed. At no stage did the dog interfere with the tube and no Elizabethan collar was required to protect the tube. At the time of discharge the dog's weight was 27.5 kg. The dog made a complete recovery and was castrated to prevent recurrence one month after the first presentation. At that time the body weight was 30.5 kg.

Case 2

Signalment: Male Irish Setter aged 4 years.

History: Fourteen days before the current presentation this dog had undergone emergency surgery for a complete urinary obstruction due to oxalate uroliths. Recovery from surgery had been marred by the fact that the dog seemed unable to hold down food despite being hungry. The dog regurgitated unchanged food within minutes of ingestion.

Medical investigation: On physical examination the dog was not dehydrated but appeared very thin. The body weight was 28.5 kg and at the time of the emergency anaesthetic had been 33 kg. Allowing for 1 kg of water in the distended bladder the normal body weight was probably 32 kg. This gave an estimated loss of body mass of 10.9%. Biochemistry, haematology and urinalysis were essentially normal. A plain thoracic radiograph showed megaoesophagus. Endoscopic oesophagoscopy confirmed megaoesophagus but also revealed an oesophageal stricture just cranial to the gastro-oesophageal sphincter. There was patchy oesophagitis throughout the length of the oesophagus. The diagnosis was oesophageal stricture due to reflux oesophagitis which had occurred during emergency anaesthesia and surgery 14 days before.

Therapy: Complete oesophageal rest was required with a series of anaesthetics for blunt dilation of the stricture. Nutritional support was needed during the prolonged period of oesophageal rest. Gastrostomy tube feeding was elected and the tube was placed endoscopically. Fortunately the stricture was not so severe that the endoscope and the stomach tube could not pass. A liquid critical care diet was selected.

In this case gastro-oesophageal reflux was to be avoided at all costs and consequently the diet was administered in multiple very small boluses (7–10), through the tube per day. Urine output and hydration status were monitored closely and the liquid diet was found to provide adequate fluid intake in addition to nutrition. The dog was offered small quantities of water by mouth but was kept off any other oral intake. The quantity of diet fed was increased in

Box 3.6   Calculations of dietary requirements for Case 2.

Calculations: Daily MER = $125 \times [32]^{0.75} = 125 \times$ $13.45 = 1681$ kcals

The illness factor was 1.2 for a catabolic state with hospitalisation and reduced exercise.

Daily IER = $1681 \times 1.2 = 2018$ kcals

The caloric density of the diet was 437 kcal/100 g dry matter

Therefore $2018/437 = 4.6 \times 100 = 460$ g of dry diet were required to mix into a liquid slurry for administration through the tube/day.

the same way as the previous case over the first 3 days and then adjusted according to body weight. In this case weight gain to replace that lost during the period of regurgitation was a goal and the food intake was increased after 1 week because the weight was remaining stable. Thereafter the body weight began to increase slowly. The tube was left in place for 8 weeks and the dog returned home after a few days and was tube fed by the owners. Repeated blunt dilation of the stricture resulted in improvement but never complete reversal. The oesophagitis resolved and after 8 weeks of tube feeding the dog resumed oral intake. He remained on a liquid slurry fed from height and was stable on this regimen.

REFERENCES

Crowe, D.T. (1990) Nutritional support of the hospitalised patient: an introduction to tube feeding. *Compendium on Continuing Education for the Practicing Veterinarian*, **12**, 1711–1720.

Fulton, R.B. & Dennis, J.S. (1992) Blind percutaneous placement of a gastrostomy tube for nutritional support in dogs and cats. *Journal of the American Veterinary Medical Association*, **201**, 697–700.

Lippert, A.C. & Buffington, C.A.T. (1992) Parenteral nutrition. In: *Fluid Therapy in Small Animal Practice*, (ed. S.P. DiBartola), pp. 384–418. W.B. Saunders, Philadelphia.

Marks, S.L., Rishniw, M., Henry, C.J. & Kanaly, S.T. (1994) Blind percutaneous gastrostomy: a new technique. *Proceedings of the 12th Annual Veterinary Medical Forum of the American College of Veterinary Internal Medicine*, No. 31, p. 150.

FURTHER READING

Hill, R.C. (1994) Critical care nutrition. In: *The Waltham Book of Clinical Nutrition of the Dog and Cat,* (eds J.M. Wills and K.W. Simpson), pp. 39–61. Pergamon, Oxford.

Lippert, A.C. & Armstrong, P.J. (1989) Parenteral nutritional support. In: *Current Veterinary Therapy X,* (eds R.W. Kirk & J.D. Bonagura), pp. 25–30. W.B. Saunders, Philadelphia.

APPENDIX 1

Work Sheet for Calculating Daily Nutritional Requirements for Both Enteral and Parenteral Nutrition

1. Maintenance Energy Requirement (MER)
    $= 125 \times [\text{body weight(kg)}]^{0.75}$
    =......... kcal/day.
2. Illness Energy Requirement (IER)
    $= 0.5$–2.0 (depending upon the disease) $\times$ MER
    IER =..... $\times$ MER = ... kcal/day
3. Quantity of balanced enteral nutrition to give per day =
    IER/caloric density of food =..... g/day

4. Protein requirements (parenteral nutrition):
    = 4 g/kg adult dogs
    = 6 g/kg in dogs with extraordinary protein loss
    = 1.5 g/kg in dogs with renal or hepatic failure
    Protein requirements = ...g/day
5. Volumes of nutrient solutions required:
    (a) 8.5% Amino acid solution = 85 mg protein/ml
         To supply .... g of Protein need .... ml
    (b) 20% lipid solution = 2 kcal/ml
         To supply 40–60% IER (...... kcal)
         need .... ml
    (c) 50% dextrose solution = 1.7 kcal/ml
         To supply 40–60% IER (...... kcal)
         need .... ml
         (use half this volume on the first day and increase to full volume on the second day if no glucosuria)
6. Total volume of TPN solution = ... ml
    Administer at .... ml/h (4 ml/kg per hour)
7. Electrolyte requirements:
    Dependent upon patient status and products selected (mixed with amino acids)
8. Vitamin requirements: administer 0.5 mg/kg body weight s.c. vitamin K on the first day and weekly.
    Add 3 ml/10 kg/day of multivitamins to the total parenteral nutrition solution.

Chapter 4

Rational Use of Antibacterial Drugs

A. D. J. Watson, J. Elliott and J. E. Maddison

ASSESSING THE PATIENT

Is a Bacterial Infection Present?

A prime requirement when deciding whether antibacterial chemotherapy is indicated is an accurate clinical assessment. Learning and experience contribute importantly to this process, with valuable clues provided by recognition of previously observed patterns or syndromes, the gross appearance of any visible lesions, and the presence or absence of pyrexia and leucocytosis. However, several pitfalls await the unwary:

(1) *Inflammatory lesions* can also be caused by:
   - irritant chemicals,
   - trauma,
   - neoplasms,
   - allergies and other immune-mediated processes,
   - other non-bacterial infectious agents.
(2) *Pyrexia* can also occur with:
   - various other pathological processes, such as:
     - viral, fungal or rickettsial infections,
     - neoplasms,
     - drug reactions,
     - immune-mediated diseases,
     - other non-septic inflammatory conditions;
   - or certain physiological states, including:
     - excitement,
     - exercise,
     - high ambient temperature and humidity.
(3) *Leucocytosis* may be encountered also in patients with:
   - viral or fungal infections,
   - immune-mediated disorders,
   - tissue necrosis,
   - neoplasia,
   - regenerative anaemia,
   - excitement,
   - stress or glucocorticoid administration.

The prudent clinician will use all relevant items from the history, physical examination and any available laboratory data to decide, first, whether bacterial infection is likely and, second, whether systemic antibacterial drug therapy is warranted. A conservative approach to prescribing is advocated for several reasons:

- *Antibacterial drugs are not antipyretic agents.* They should not be used to treat pyrexia *per se*. If antipyretic treatment is required, administration of aspirin or a related compound is more appropriate.
- *Antibacterial drugs are not suitable placebos.* While placebo therapy may have some value in veterinary medicine (to placate an over-anxious owner for example) other products are more suited for this purpose, because antibacterials have the potential to disrupt the patient's normal flora and encourage development of drug resistance.
- *Inappropriate use can create a false sense of security.* This may delay appropriate investigation and more satisfactory therapy.
- *Administration of unnecessary drugs will increase costs and risks of toxicosis.* Neither of these can be regarded as a satisfactory outcome of therapy.

Determining the Site and Type of Infection

In most patients, it is not difficult to identify the site of a bacterial infection. Locations commonly involved in dogs are skin, lower urinary tract and the respiratory system. Although gastrointestinal diseases are prevalent in dogs, antibacterial therapy is not warranted in most cases.

In a minority of patients with signs suggesting an infectious disease the site of infection is not readily apparent. Detailed investigation may then be required to locate the lesion(s), assisted where necessary by radiography, ultrasonography, fine needle aspiration biopsy and cytology,

Table 4.1 Antibacterial drug selection for canine infections.

Site of infection	Diagnosis	Common organisms (less common in brackets)	Suggested drug for common organisms	Alternative drugs or comments
Cardiovascular system	Endocarditis*, septicaemia*	Various aerobic[†] or anaerobic organisms	Gentamicin plus a beta-lactam[‡]	Fluoroquinolone plus beta-lactam[‡]
Eye	Conjunctivitis	*Staphylococcus, Streptococcus, Escherichia, Proteus*	Topical neomycin, polymyxin, bacitracin	Topical chloramphenicol, gentamicin
Gastrointestinal tract	Cholecystitis, cholangitis	*Escherichia*, anaerobes	Amoxycillin clavulanate	Chloramphenicol
	Periodontitis, gingivitis and ulcerative stomatitis	Anaerobic and aerobic[†] bacteria	Penicillin G or V, clindamycin (teeth cleaning required)	Amoxycillin[§], metronidazole, spiramycin plus metronidazole
	Peritonitis (intestinal spillage)	*Escherichia, Enterococcus*, anaerobes	Beta-lactam[‡] plus gentamicin (Surgical management required)	Fluoroquinolone plus beta-lactam[§], cefoxitin
	Small intestine bacterial overgrowth	*Escherichia, Enterococcus, Staphylococcus, Clostridium*	Amoxycillin[§]	Amoxycillin-clavulanate, metronidazole, tylosin
Nervous system	Meningitis[a]	*Staphylococcus* (*Pasteurella, Actinomyces, Nocardia*)	Amoxycillin-clavulanate	Chloramphenicol, potentiated-sulpha[¶], fluoroquinolone
Respiratory system	Infectious tracheobronchitis[‖]	*Bordetella*, viruses (*Mycoplasma*)	Potentiated sulpha[¶]	Tetracycline
	Bacterial pneumonia*, aspiration pneumonia*	Single or mixed infection, various Gram-positive and negative aerobic[†] or anaerobic bacteria	Amoxycillin-clavulanate	Potentiated sulpha[¶] / Beta-lactam[‡] plus an aminoglycoside if very severe
	Pyothorax*, purulent pleuritis*	Commonly mixed infection: anaerobes, *Nocardia, Pasteurella, Staphylococcus*	Amoxycillin-clavulanate (Drainage of chest cavity most important)	Clindamycin, chloramphenicol, (sulpha with or without potentiator[¶] if Nocardia suspected)
Skeletal system	Discospondylitis	*Staphylococcus* (*Streptococcus, Brucella, Aspergillus*)	Amoxycillin-clavulanate	Cloxacillin**, lincosamide, cephalosporin
	Osteomyelitis*	*Staphylococcus* alone, or with other aerobic or anaerobic bacteria	Amoxycillin-clavulanate	Cloxacillin**, lincosamides, cephalosporin, fluoroquinolones (for *Pseudomonas*)
	Septic arthritis*	*Staphylococcus, Streptococcus* (other aerobic[†] or anaerobic bacteria)	Amoxycillin-clavulanate	Cephalexin

Table 4.1 (*Continued*)

Site of infection	Diagnosis	Common organisms (less common in brackets)	Suggested drug for common organisms	Alternative drugs or comments
Skin and soft tissue	Anal sac inflammation, abscessation	*Escherichia, Enterococcus* (*Clostridium, Proteus*)	Amoxycillin-clavulanate	Cephalexin
	Bite wounds, traumatic and contaminated wounds	*Staphylococcus, Streptococcus, Pasteurella*, anaerobes	Amoxycillin-clavulanate	Cephalexin
	Otitis externa	*Staphylococcus, Pseudomonas, Proteus*	Topical aminoglycoside	Topical polymyxin, chloramphenicol
		Malassezia	Topical nystatin	Topical thiabendazole, miconazole
	Otitis media, otitis interna*	*Staphylococcus, Streptococcus, Pseudomonas, Proteus*	Fluoroquinolone or chloramphenicol	Amoxycillin-clavulanate
	Pyoderma, pustular dermatitis	*Staphylococcus*, (secondary: *Escherichia, Proteus, Pseudomonas*)	Amoxycillin-clavulanate	Cloxacillin**, cephalexin, macrolide
Urogenital system	Lower urinary tract infection (see Chapter 67) If recurrent UTI always culture*	*Escherichia, Staphylococcus, Streptococcus, Proteus*, (*Klebsiella, Pseudomonas, Enterobacter*)	Amoxycillin§ (see Chapter 67 if pathogen known)	Potentiated sulpha¶, fluoroquinolones, amoxycillin-clavulanate
	Mastitis	*Escherichia, Staphylococcus, Streptococcus*	Macrolide or lincosamide (if Gram positive) chloramphenicol	Potentiated sulpha¶ amoxycillin-clavulanate
	Prostatitis	*Escherichia*, also *Staphylococcus, Klebsiella*, (*Proteus, Pseudomonas, Streptococcus*)	Potentiated sulpha¶ macrolide or lincosamide (if Gram positive)	Fluoroquinolone, chloramphenicol
	Pyelonephritis*	As for lower UTI but especially: *Escherichia, Proteus, Staphylococcus*	Amoxycillin-clavulanate	Fluoroquinolone, potentiated sulpha¶
	Pyometra* (metritis)	*Escherichia, Staphylococcus, Streptococcus*, anaerobes	Amoxycillin-clavulanate	Amoxycillin§ plus aminoglycoside

* Culture and susceptibility testing is advisable.
† 'Aerobic' includes facultative anaerobic organisms, 'anaerobic' indicates obligate anaerobic bacteria.
‡ Beta-lactam, e.g. cephalexin, amoxycillin or amoxycillin-clavulanate.
§ Also ampicillin.
¶ Trimethoprim, baquiloprim or ormetoprim as potentiators of sulphas (e.g. sulphadiazine or sulphadimethoxine).
‖ This infection is usually self-limiting unless animal immunocompromised.
** Also oxacillin, flucloxacillin.

microbial culture of body fluids, haematology, biochemistry or urinalysis.

Once the suspected site of infection has been identified, information about the type of bacteria involved may be sought in several ways:

- *Clinical experience.* In the absence of more specific information, the identity of the likely pathogen(s) may be surmised by considering the clinical diagnosis (or known site of infection) and the bacteria most frequently implicated therein.
- *Examination of smears of exudates or aspirates* from the infected site. These can be stained by Giemsa or Diff-Quik for cytology and Gram stain for bacterial classification.
- In vitro *culture of material from the infected location.* This usually provides more detailed information about the organism(s) present but may be unavailable or not feasible due to the added costs and ensuing delays.

Clinical experience (the deductive or best-guess approach), is used widely by veterinarians and seems satisfactory for many routine or less serious infections (Table 4.1). It can also be used as an initial step in patients with serious or life-threatening infections while awaiting results of microbiological investigations, with the option of changing to more appropriate medication once laboratory data become available

Identifying the Pathogen – Sample Collection and Handling

Direct Microscopic Examination

Microscopic examination of smears of exudates or aspirates from the infected site can assist diagnosis and therapy. The presence of a purulent inflammatory response (many neutrophils) suggests bacterial infection. Bacteria are readily apparent in smears when the number present exceeds 10^4–10^5/ml (Jones 1990). Examination of CSF or blood is often unrewarding because fewer bacteria are usually found in these fluids. Assessment of Gram-stained smears may indicate whether a single or mixed bacterial population is present (Table 4.2), and can facilitate selection of drugs likely to be effective.

Microbial Culture

Microbial culture and susceptibility testing may be unnecessary for routine infections that are not life-threatening. However, they can be very helpful whenever maximum antibacterial efficacy is desired and in conditions which are:

Table 4.2 Microscopic appearance of bacteria in clinical specimens.

Morphology and Gram-staining reaction	Possible microorganisms
Gram-positive cocci	*Staphylococcus, Streptococcus*, anaerobic cocci
Gram-positive rods with endospores	*Clostridium*
Gram-positive branching filaments, may show beading	*Actinomyces, Nocardia*
Gram-negative rods	Coliforms, *Pseudomonas, Pasteurella, Bordetella*, anaerobic rods

Jones (1990).

- serious (life-threatening),
- recurrent,
- poorly responsive.

Samples for culture should be taken:

- from the site of infection using aseptic technique, with a minimum of contamination from adjacent tissues or secretions;
- early in the course of disease because, with progression of the lesion and tissue necrosis, offending microbes may die or be overgrown by other bacteria (Jones 1990);
- before antimicrobial therapy commences if feasible – otherwise, sampling should be delayed as long as possible after the last dose was given, provided this does not endanger the patient. If antimicrobials are concentrated at the specimen site, as with urine, a delay of 48 h is suggested (Jones 1990).

Ideally, several millilitres or grams of material should be obtained for the laboratory. Tissue scrapings, biopsy material, fluid or surgically removed tissue may be preferable to swabs, particularly if anaerobic infections are suspected (Jones 1990). If lesions are present at several sites, multiple specimens should be submitted.

When sending samples to the laboratory (Jones 1990):

- place unfixed tissue samples in a sealed sterile container to prevent contamination and desiccation;
- submit tissue or fluid samples that have been aspirated using a sterile syringe and needle, in the syringe, after expelling residual air and capping the syringe;

- place swabs in transport medium or a humidified chamber for transport to avoid dessication;
- refrigerate samples if delivery to the laboratory will be delayed;
- consult the laboratory before undertaking special procedures or if uncertain about appropriate sample collection and handling.

PLANNING THE TREATMENT REGIMEN

Drug Selection

Any of the selection methods used, whether based on susceptibility testing, smear examination or deduction, might indicate a number of drugs that are likely to be effective against the pathogen. Several factors should be considered in choosing from these alternatives:

(1) *The width of antibacterial spectrum* (Table 4.3).
- Drugs that are more selective are generally to be preferred as they are less likely to disrupt the normal microflora.
- Habitual reliance on broad-spectrum antimicrobial agents merely because of the width of their spectra indicates a low standard of diagnosis on the part of the clinician and risks the selection of resistance genes in the bacterial population which may be tranferable to pathogens.
- In Table 4.3, 'Indication' is used to represent the clinically useful range of activity of the drug and does not correspond to the conventional antibacterial drug 'spectrum', e.g. aminoglycosides are active against various Gram-positive non-anaerobic pathogens but would not usually be used against them because more satisfactory agents are generally available. The same comment applies to cephalosporin groups two, three and four and cephamycins.

(2) *Bactericidal versus bacteriostatic activity* (Table 4.3).

Table 4.3 Actions of and indications for drugs used systemically against becterial pathogens.

Drug group and Action	Individual drugs	Aerobes and facultative anaerobes			Obligate anaerobes	Additional uses and comments
		Staphylococci producing β-lactamase	Other Gram-positive organisms	Gram-negative organisms		
Aminoglycosides *bactericidal*	Amikacin*, (dihydro) streptomycin, gentamicin, kanamycin, spectinomycin, tobramycin*			+++		Streptomycin is used against mycobacteria and *Leptospira* Plasmid mediated resistance is common
Beta-lactams						
1. Penicillins *bactericidal*	Amoxycillin, ampicillin		+++	+++	+++†	
	Amoxycillin–clavulanate	+++	+++	+++	+++	
	Carbenicillin			+++*		
	Cloxacillin, flucloxacillin, oxacillin	+++				
	Penicillin G (benzylpenicillin)		+++		+++†	
	Penicillin V (phenoxymethylpenicillin)		+++		+++†	
	Piperacillin			+++	+++	
	Ticarcillin, ticarcillin-clavulanate			+++*		
2. Cephalosporins, Cephamycins *bactericidal*	Oral cephalosporins – cephalexin	+++	+++	+++	+++†	
	Parenteral group I – cephazolin	+++	+++	+++	+++†	
	group II – cefotaxime			+++		
	group III – cefoperazone			+++*		
	group IV – cefoxitin				+++	
Fluoroquinolones *bactericidal*	Enrofloxacin, marbofloxacin	+++		+++		Active against *Brucella, Mycoplasma* and rickettsiae
Lincosamides *bacteriostatic*	Clindamycin, lincomycin	‡	+++		+++§	Active against *Mycoplasma*

Table 4.3   (*Continued*).

Drug group and Action	Individual drugs	Aerobes and facultative anaerobes			Obligate anaerobes	Additional uses and comments
		Staphylococci producing β-lactamase	Other Gram-positive organisms	Gram-negative organisms		
Macrolides *bacteriostatic*	Erythromycin, spiramycin tylosin	+++	+++			Erythromycin – drug of choice for *Campylobacter* enteritis. Tylosin is active against *Mycoplasma* & *Chlamydia*
Potentiated Sulphonamides *bactericidal*	Baquiloprim plus sulphadimethoxine. Trimethoprim plus sulphadiazine or sulphadoxine	‡	+++	+++	¶	Pyrimethamine is potentiator against toxoplasma
Sulphonamides alone‖ *bacteriostatic*	Sulphadiazine, sulphadimethoxine, sulphadoxine etc.		+++	+++		Drug of choice for *Nocardia*. Active against protozoa and *Chlamydia*
Tetracyclines *bacteriostatic*	Chlortetracycline, doxycycline, minocycline, oxytetracycline tetracycline		+++	+++		Active vs *Borellia* rickettsiae, protozoa, chlamydia and mycoplasma
Miscellaneous *bacteriostatic*	Chloramphenicol, florfenicol	+++	+++	+++	+++	Active against rickettsiae & *Chlamydia*
bactericidal	Metronidazole				+++	Active against anaerobic protozoa
	Rifampicin	+++				Resistance develops rapidly

+++ Denotes the clinical indication for the drug or group of drugs and may not correspond to the conventional antibacterial drug spectrum.

* Used principally against *Pseudomonas*.

† Activity against *Bacteroides fragilis* may be poor.

‡ Could be effective but resistant strains are common in some hospitals.

§ Clindamycin especially.

¶ Good activity *in vitro* but *in vivo* activity may be hindered by substances in necrotic tissue.

‖ Sulphonamides are now mostly given with potentiators.

- Bactericidal drugs are often favoured because they may be more effective when host defences are impaired.
- There may be little difference in efficacy between bactericidal and bacteriostatic drugs when treating non-critical infections in otherwise healthy patients.
- The division into bactericidal and bacteriostatic groups is based on *in vitro* activity. The distinction is not absolute and may vary with drug concentration and bacterial species.

(3) *Distribution*. The selected drug must reach the site of infection at adequate concentrations to kill or inhibit the growth of bacteria following administration by the chosen route of administration (see below).

(4) *Cost*. The cost of some drugs (newer β-lactams and aminoglycosides; fluoroquinolones, clindamycin) may preclude their use, especially in large dogs. It may then be necessary to choose a cheaper alternative despite possibly lower efficacy.

(5) *Toxicity*. Most of the antibacterial drugs in common

use are relatively safe when correct dosages are employed. However, one should be aware of potential adverse effects of any drug used.

(6) *Intercurrent disease.* The presence of kidney or liver disease may increase toxic risks with some drugs, either because they damage these organs or because impaired excretion or metabolism allows the drug or its metabolites to accumulate to toxic levels (Tables 4.4 and 4.5).

(7) *Pregnant or neonatal patients.* Particular care may be necessary in these patients because of known or suspected adverse effects (Table 4.6).

Route of Administration

Usually there is a choice of routes, although some drugs (such as aminoglycosides) must be given parenterally if systemic therapy is desired. Table 4.7 lists drugs which are absorbed following oral administration, those which are not but which are stable in the gastrointestinal tract so could be given orally to treat a gastrointestinal infection and those whose oral bioavailability is poor because of instability in the gastrointestinal tract.

Other factors influencing route selection include the disease being treated, likely treatment duration, the patient's temperament and owner's capability.

Topical Administration

● This route is valuable for disorders of eye and ear, and some skin or gut infections.
● High drug concentration may be achieved locally using this route.
● Some drugs too toxic for routine systemic administration (polymyxins, bacitracin, neomycin) can be useful topically.

Oral Administration

● This route is adequate in most infections and is usually preferable for home treatment.
● Some owners find it easier to administer drugs orally with food.
● Potential adverse effects of ingesta on systemic drug availability should be considered, especially with penicillins, erythromycin products and most tetracyclines (Table 4.8).

Table 4.4 Systemic antibacterials in dogs with renal failure.

Category	Drugs or drug groups
Probably safe	Chloramphenicol
	Clindamycin
	Doxycycline
	Macrolides
	Penicillins (including clavulanate)*
Consider dosage adjustment in moderate or severe failure†	Cephalosporins (most)
	Fluoroquinolones
	Lincomycin
	Sulphonamides
	Sulphonamide–trimethoprim
Hazardous, avoid Accumulation of drug or its metabolites can increase side effects or non-renal toxicity	Nalidixic acid
	Nitrofurantoin
	Tetracycline‡ (except doxycycline)
Nephrotoxic, avoid Drug may exacerbate renal damage	Aminoglycoside
	Polymyxins

Watson (1994).
* Sodium or potassium salts of these agents may cause electrolyte abnormalities.
† See Chapter 1 for discussion of adjustment of dose in renal failure.
‡ There are some reports of nephrotoxicity of tetracyclines which are probably due to impurities in out-dated or improperly stored products.

Table 4.5   Systemic antibacterials in dogs with liver failure.

Category	Drugs or drug groups
Probably safe Drugs not known to be hepatotoxic and unlikely to accumulate to toxic levels in liver disease	Aminoglycosides Cephalosporins Penicillins
Caution advised Drugs metabolised by the liver that *might* accumulate to toxic levels in hepatopathy	Chloramphenicol Lincosamides Macrolides Metronidazole Sulphonamides Tetracyclines
Potentially toxic Drugs that may cause hepatic injury	Chlortetracycline Erythromycin estolate Rifampicin Sulphonamide- trimethoprim

Watson (1994).
There is little information on the effects of liver failure on antibacterial drug therapy. These warnings might constitute relative rather than absolute contraindications. Some antimicrobial drugs can affect metabolism of other drugs by the liver (e.g. chloramphenicol, erythromycin and rifampicin; see Chapter 1).

Table 4.6   Systemic antibacterials in pregnancy and neonates.

Category	Drugs of durg groups
Probably safe Studies have shown safety in dogs and cats, or there are no reported adverse effects in women or laboratory animals	Cephalosporins Erythromycin (not estolate form) Lincosamides (data lacking in neonates) Penicillins (including clavulanate)
Safe with caution Some risk may have been identified in laboratory animals, but the drugs either appear safe in dogs and cats or are safe if not give near parturition or to neonates	Nitrofurantoin Sulphonamides (avoid long acting forms) Sulphonamide–trimetoprim Tylosin (no data available)
Potential risk Risk identified in women, laboratory animals or dogs and cats. Avoid these agents in neonates and use cautiously if lacking alternatives in pregnancy	Aminoglycosides Chloramphenicol Metronidazole
Contraindicated Drugs shown to cause congenital malformation, embryotoxicity or neonatal lesions	Fluoroquinolones Nalidixic acid Rifampicin Tetracyclines

Watson (1994).

Table 4.7 Suitability of antibacterial drugs for oral administration.

Good/fair absorption – oral route suitable for systemic infections*	Poor absorption but oral route suitable for gut infections	Poor absorption and unsuitable for gut infections (unstable)
Aminopenicillins (ampicillin, amoxycillin)	Aminoglycosides	Carbenicillin
Baquiloprim	Bacitracin	Cephalosporins (parenteral groups 1 to 4)
Cephalosporins (oral group)	Polymixins	Methicillin
Chloramphenicol	Sulphonamides (N^1 & N^4 substituted e.g. succinylsulphathiazole)	Penicillin G (benzylpenicillin)
Clavulanate		Piperacillin
Florphenicol		Ticarcillin
Fluoroquinolones		
Isoxazoyl penicillins (cloxacillin, oxacillin, flucloxacillin)		
Lincosamides (clindamycin, lincomycin)		
Macrolides (erythromycin, spiramycin, tylosin)		
Metronidazole		
Penicillin V (phenoxymethylpenicillin)		
Rifampicin		
Sulphonamides (N^1 substituted – most)		
Tetracyclines		
Trimethoprim		

* Oral bioavailability may be affected by the presence of food (see Table 4.8 and Chapter 1).

Table 4.8 Suggested administration of oral antibacterlal drugs in dogs in relation to feeding.

Category	Drugs or drug groups
Better when fasting Drug absorption may be impaired by ingesta. Fasting means no food for at least 1–2 h before and 1–2 h after dosing	Cephalosporins Erythromycin (free base) Erythromycin stearate Lincomycin Most penicillins Most sulphonamides Most tetracyclines*
Better with food Drug availability is improved, or gastrointestinal upsets are reduced, by ingesta	Doxycycline† Erythromycin estolate Erythromycin ethylsuccinate Metronidazole* Minocycline Nitrofurantoin*
No restriction needed	Chloramphenicol Erythromycin coated formulations Fluoroquinolones

Watson (1994). Data from human studies except penicillins and chloramphenicol.
* Avoid milk and other foods rich in calcium ions in particular.
† Food may reduce gut irritation without hindering absorption importantly.

Parenteral Administration

- This route is not routinely advantageous, but can be useful for fractious, unconscious or vomiting patients, or those with painful mouths.
- Intramuscular or subcutaneous administration may be equally satisfactory.
- Intravenous route gives the highest peak plasma concentrations if given as a bolus injection.
- Intravenous dosing should be considered if maximum plasma drug concentrations are desired immediately after dosing, e.g. life-threatening infections, shocked or hypotensive patients where poor tissue perfusion may impede drug absorption after administration by other routes.

Dose and Frequency of Administration

Dosing regimens for commonly used antibacterial drugs are suggested in Table 4.9. The ideal regimen will vary with the case, depending on:

- susceptibility of the pathogen to the chosen antibacterial under conditions found at the site of infection *in vivo*;
- penetration of the drug to the site of infection which is influenced by:
  - ○ physicochemical characteristics of the chosen drug,

Table 4.9 Suggested dosage regimes for antibacterial drugs in dogs.

Drug	Route	Dose
*Aminoglycosides**		
Amikacin	i.v., i,m., s.c.	10 mg/kg t.i.d.
Gentamicin	i.v., i.m., s.c.	2–4 mg/kg t.i.d.
Neomycin	p.o.	10 mg/kg q.i.d.
Streptomycin	p.o.	20 mg/kg q.i.d.
	i.m., s.c.	10 mg/kg b.i.d.
Tobramycin	i.v., i.m., s.c.	1–2 mg/kg t.i.d.
Beta lactams		
1. Cephalosporins		
Oral		
Cefadroxil	p.o.	20 mg/kg b.i.d.–t.i.d.
Cephalexin	p.o.	20–30 mg/kg b.i.d.–t.i.d.
Parenteral Group I		
Cephazolin	i.v., i.m., s.c.	20–30 mg/kg t.i.d.–q.i.d.
Cephapirin	i.v., i.m., s.c.	10–30 mg/kg t.i.d.–q.i.d.
Parenteral Group II		
Cefamandole	i.v., i.m., s.c.	15–30 mg/kg t.i.d.
Cefotaxime	i.v., i.m., s.c.	20–50 mg/kg b.i.d.–t.i.d.
Parenteral Group III		
Cefoperazone	i.v., i.m., s.c.	30 mg/kg t.i.d.–q.i.d.
Parenteral Group IV		
Cefoxitin	i.v., i.m., s.c.	20–40 mg/kg t.i.d.–q.i.d.
2. Penicillins		
Amoxycillin	p.o., i.v., i.m., s.c.	10–20 mg/kg b.i.d.–t.i.d.
Amoxycillin– clavulanate	p.o., i.m., s.c.	12.5–25 mg/kg b.i.d.–t.i.d.
Carbenicillin	i.v., i.m., s.c.	50 mg/kg t.i.d.–q.i.d.
Cloxacillin	p.o.	30 mg/kg t.i.d.
Dicloxacillin	p.o.	50 mg/kg t.i.d.
Methicillin	i.v., i.m.	25–50 mg/kg q.i.d.
Oxacillin	p.o.	30 mg/kg t.i.d.
Penicillin G, Na, K	i.v., i.m., s.c.	20 000–40 000 U/kg t.i.d.–q.i.d.

Table 4.9 (*Continued*).

Drug	Route	Dose
Penicillin G, procaine	i.m., s.c.	20 000 U/kg s.i.d.–b.i.d.
Penicillin G, benzathine	i.m.	40 000 U/kg every 3–5 days
Penicillin V	p.o.	10 mg/kg t.i.d.
Ticarcillin	i.v., i.m., s.c.	50–75 mg/kg t.i.d.–q.i.d.
Fluoroquinolones†		
Ciprofloxacin	p.o.	5–15 mg/kg b.i.d.
Enrofloxacin	p.o., i.m., s.c.	2.5–10 mg/kg b.i.d.
Marbofloxacin	p.o.	2 mg/kg s.i.d.
Norfloxacin	p.o.	5–20 mg/kg b.i.d.
Lincosamides		
Clindamycin	p.o., i.v., i.m., s.c.	5–10 mg/kg b.i.d.–t.i.d.
Lincomycin	p.o.	10–20 mg/kg b.i.d.–t.i.d.
	i.v., i.m.	10 mg/kg b.i.d.
Macrolides		
Erythromycin	p.o.	10–20 mg/kg b.i.d.–t.i.d.
Tylosin	p.o.	10 mg/kg t.i.d.
	i.v., i.m.	5–10 mg/kg b.i.d.
Potentiated sulphonamides		
Sulphadiazine-trimethoprim	p.o., i.v., i.m., s.c.	30 mg/kg s.i.d.–b.i.d.
Sulphadimethoxine-baquiloprim	s.c.	12 mg/kg s.i.d. or 30 mg/kg every 48 h
	p.o.	30 mg/kg every 48 h
Tetracyclines		
Chlortetracycline	p.o.	20 mg/kg t.i.d.
Doxycycline	p.o., i.v.	5–10 mg/kg b.i.d.
Minocycline	p.o.	5–15 mg/kg b.i.d.
Oxytetracycline	p.o.	20 mg/kg t.i.d.
	i.v., i.m.	10 mg/kg b.i.d.
Tetracycline	p.o.	20 mg/kg t.i.d.
	i.v., i.m.	10 mg/kg b.i.d.
Miscellaneous		
Chloramphenicol	p.o., i.v., i.m., s.c.	50 mg/kg t.i.d.
Metronidazole	p.o.	10–20 mg/kg b.i.d.–t.i.d.
Rifampicin	p.o.	10–20 mg/kg b.i.d. (max. 600 mg daily)

* Recent studies suggest administration of the total parenteral daily dose in one bolus rather than as split doses may reduce toxic potential without compromising efficacy.
† Use lower end of dosage ranges for urinary infections, higher end for soft tissue infections or osteomyelitis.

○   blood flow to the infected area,
○   tissue barriers to diffusion of the drug;
● immunocompetence of the patient.

Each of these factors affect the outcome of an antimicrobial treatment as outlined below. Demonstration of therapeutic efficacy ultimately depends on large clinical trials conducted for specific infections under carefully monitored circumstances. Such data are lacking in most areas of canine medicine and many recommended dose rates remain empirical. Nevertheless, considerations relating minimum inhibitory concentration (MIC) data to the pharmacokinetics of the drugs should help in making logical choices of antibacterial drugs and appropriate dosages.

For example, smaller doses may suffice in lower urinary tract infections using drugs excreted in high concentration in urine (see below), but larger or more frequent doses may be required for relatively resistant pathogens or infections in areas where drug penetration is poor (e.g. central nervous system, prostate gland, bronchial secretions).

Bacterial Susceptibility

Various factors need to be considered in drug susceptibility testing:

● The MIC is the drug concentration that must be attained at the infection site to inhibit bacteria. In general bacteria that are resistant to a drug *in vitro* will be resistant *in vivo*.
● If a bacterium is susceptible *in vitro* the drug may be effective *in vivo* depending on other factors.

It would seem logical to aim for drug concentrations at the site of infection which exceed the MIC value of the drug for the target bacterium. Indeed, in assessing data from pharmaceutical companies applying for product authorisations, the rule of thumb for antibacterial products is that efficacy claims should be supported by demonstration that:

● The peak plasma concentration of the drug exceeds twice the MIC value for the causative organism involved (MIC data from recent field isolates).
● The plasma concentration of the drug is maintained above the MIC value for at least half of the proposed inter-dosing interval.

These guide-lines seem logical and are most applicable to bacteriostatic drugs and for infections in sites where drugs have no difficulty penetrating. The following points show the limitations of this approach:

● *In vivo* susceptibility of bacteria does not always correlate well with *in vitro* susceptibility data because of:
   ○   host factors (innate and specific immune responses),
   ○   environmental factors at the site of infection (see below).
● Frequency of dosing required may be less than suggested by these rules for antibacterials that demonstrate a marked post-antibiotic effect (some bactericidal drugs such as aminoglycosides and fluoroquinolones).
● Drugs may concentrate in some sites to give concentrations higher than found in plasma, whereas at other sites penetration of drugs may be poor, giving much lower concentrations than found in plasma (see below).

Distribution to the Site of Infection (Pharmacokinetic Phase)
(see Tables 4.10 and 4.11)

To be effective an antimicrobial agent must be distributed to the site of infection in adequate concentration and come into contact with the pathogen. The drug plasma concentration reflects the concentration in extracellular fluid of bone and soft tissues, as the unbound portion of the drug in the plasma crosses most tissue capillaries by diffusing between the endothelial cells. A high degree of plasma protein binding may limit the distribution to tissues, particularly to sites which are difficult to penetrate (e.g. brain) or which have a low blood flow. The following factors should be considered:

(1) High peak plasma concentrations, as after following i.v. administration, generally aid tissue penetration
(2) The brain is a 'special tissue' as the junctions between capillary endothelial cells are tight and 'glial feet' abut against the capillary endothelium. Only very lipophilic drugs cross the normal blood brain barrier effectively (chloramphenicol, fluoroquinolones, potentiated sulphonamides) and therefore enter cerebrospinal fluid and brain tissue.
(3) Penetration of drugs into transcellular fluids depends on their lipid solubility and the barrier caused by the epithelial/mesothelial lining the compartment. Transcellular fluids include: CSF, ocular fluids, prostatic fluid, milk, bronchial secretions, bile and intestinal secretions, peritoneal, pleural and joint fluid.

(4) The ion trapping effect of differing pH in transcellular fluid will affect the distribution of weak acids and weak bases across epithelial membranes:
- lipophilic weak bases will tend to accumulate in fluids with pH less than plasma;
- lipophilic weak acids will tend to accumulate in fluids with pH greater than plasma.

(5) Urine is a special transcellular fluid because:
- all unbound drugs are freely filtered into the glomerular filtrate;
- the lipophilicity of the drug determines whether the drug is reabsorbed or remains in the urine;
- renal tubular epithelium has transport processes that secrete some acidic and basic drugs into the urine;
- these factors can lead to some drugs which are filtered, not reabsorbed and actively secreted reaching very high drug concentrations in urine (e.g. penicillins).

(6) Bile is also a special transcellular fluid – some drugs can be secreted unchanged into bile and undergo enterohepatic re-circulation (e.g. tetracyclines).

(7) Penetration of drugs into cells is also governed by these physicochemical properties (lipophilicity needs to be sufficient to cross plasma membranes and ion trapping can occur within cells, where the pH is lower than extracellular fluid). Intracellular bacteria, e.g. *Salmonella*, *Brucella*, *Listeria*, will not be affected by antimicrobial agents that remain in the extracellular space.

(8) Tissues with poor blood supply (e.g. connective tissue, heart valves and devitalised tissue) attain poor tissue concentrations of antibiotics. Where possible, devitalised tissue should be surgically removed so that it does not act as a nidus for infection.

Many studies on tissue penetration of antibacterial drugs are carried out in healthy animals, and for many drugs we understand little about the influence of disease on drug disposition. Factors that restrict access of drugs to the infected site include abscess formation, pus and oedema

Table 4.10 Antibacterial drugs – physicochemical properties and effects on tissue distribution.

Polar (hydrophilic) drugs of low lipophilicity		Drugs of moderate to high lipophilicity			Highly lipophilic molecules with low ionisation
Acids	Bases	Weak acids	Weak bases	Amphoteric	

Beta lactams
Penicillins
  Aminopenicillins
  Carbenicillin
  Isoxazolypenicillinl*
  Penicillin G and V
  Piperacillin
  Ticarcillin
Cephalosporins (all
  groups)
Beta lactamase
  inhibitors
  Clavulanate
	Polymyxins
	Polymyxin B
	Polymyxin E (colistin)
	Aminoglycosides
	Amikacin
	Dihydrostreptomycin
	Gentamicin
	Kanamycin
	Neomycin
	Streptomycin
	Tobramycin
	Spectinomycin
		Sulphonamides
		Sulphadiazine
		Sulphadimethoxine
		Sulphadoxine
		Sulphafurazole
		Sulphamethazine
		Sulphamethoxazole
		Sulphathiazole
			Diaminopyrimidines
			Baquiloprim
			Ormetoprim
			Trimethoprim
			Lincosamides
			Clindamycin
			Lincomycin
			Macrolides
			Erythromycin
			Spiramycin
			Tylosin
				Tetracyclines
				Chlortetracycline
				Oxytetracycline
				Tetracycline
					Fluoroquinolones
					Enrofloxacin
					Marbofloxacin
					Lipophilic tetracyclines
					Minocycline
					Doxycycline
					Miscellaneous drugs
					Chloramphenicol
					Florphenicol
					Metronidazole
					Rifampicin

These drugs:		These drugs:			These drugs:
Do not readily penetrate 'natural body barriers' so that effective concentrations in CSF, milk and other transcellular fluids will not always be achieved. Adequate concentrations may be achieved in joints, pleural and peritoneal fluids where the barrier to penetration is less (Penetration may be assisted by acute inflammation)		Cross cellular barriers more readily than polar molecules so enter transcellular fluids to a greater extent. Weak bases will be ion trapped (concentrated) in fluids which are more acidic than plasma, e.g. • prostatic fluid • milk • intracellular fluid if lipophilic enough to penetrate (e.g. erythromycin). Penetration into CSF and ocular fluids is affected by plasma protein binding as well as lipophilicity – sulphonamides and diaminopyrimidines penetrate effectively whereas macrolides, lincosamides and tetracyclines do not			Cross cellular barriers very readily. Penetrate into difficult transcellular fluids such as prostatic fluid and bronchial secretions. All penetrate into intracellular fluids. All penetrate into CSF except tetracyclines and rifampicin

* Cloxacillin, oxacillin and flucloxacillin are highly plasma protein bound (>95%) in the dog – higher dose rates are required than in man.

fluid. An infectious process usually adversely affects the distribution of a drug *in vivo*. An exception is meningitis which reduces the barrier between blood and CSF and allows drugs that normally cannot penetrate the barrier to gain access to the CSF.

Table 4.10 summarises the physicochemical properties of the commonly used antibacterial drugs and the effects these have on their tissue distribution within the body. Table 4.11 summarises the modes of elimination of drugs from the body indicating which are excreted in active forms in urine and bile.

Favourable Environmental Conditions (Pharmacodynamic Phase)

As well as hindering the access of antimicrobial agents to the site of infection the inflammatory process can create an unfavourable environment for antimicrobial drug action such as:

(1) *Unfavourable conditions* may slow growth of bacteria thus rendering them less susceptible to antimicrobials

Table 4.11   Excretion of antibacterial durgs in urine and bile.

Urinary excretion*			Biliary Excretion of Unchanged Drug
Hepatic metabolism important for elimination of drug	Urinary excretion of the unchanged drug is the important route of elimination		
Filtration plus good/fair reabsorption	Filtration plus little/no reabsorption	Filtration plus active secretion in proximal convoluted tubule	Secreted in bile and generally undergo enterohepatic circulation
Chloramphenicol Florphenicol	Aminoglycosides	Cephalosporins (most) Fluoroquinolones	Cefoperazone Chloramphenicol† Fluoroquinolones
Diaminopyrimidines (esp. in alkaline urine), e.g.	Polymyxins	Penicillins (all groups)	Lincosamides Macrolides
Baquiloprim Ormetoprim Trimethoprim	Tetracyclines Chlortetracycline Oxytetracycline Tetracycline	Sulphonamides (short) acting drugs), e.g. Sulphadiazine	Rifampicin Tetracyclines (except minocycline)
Lincosamides Macrolides (esp. in alkaline urine)		Sulphadimidine Sulphafurazole Sulphamethoxazole Sulphathiazole	
Metronidazole Sulphonamides (esp. in acidic urine), e.g. Sulphadimethoxine Sulphadoxine Tetracyclines, e.g. Doxycycline Minocycline			

* Mean 8-h urinary concentrations of antibacterial drugs used to treat urinary tract infections are given in Chapter 67. Even drugs which are reabsorbed following filtration may still reach urinary concentrations adequate to treat urinary tract infections (e.g. trimethoprim and baquiloprim)
† Glucuronides of chloramphenicol can be hydrolised in the gut and the active drug absorbed from the intestine

that act by inhibiting cell wall synthesis. Bacteria must be actively multiplying for these drugs (e.g. penicillins, cephalosporins) to be effective.

(2) *Accumulation of purulent material* may bind or inactivate the drug. For example, sulphonamides and aminoglycosides can be substantially bound by pus and unable to contact the bacteria to exert an antibacterial effect.

(3) *Lowered pH and oxygen tension* can also hinder the activity of various antimicrobial agents. For example the lethal action of penicillins depends on autolytic enzyme activity in bacteria which is impaired in low pH conditions. Low pH also hinders substantially the activity of aminoglycosides, erythromycin and fluoroquinolones.

(4) A *foreign body* at an infected site reduces the likelihood of effective antimicrobial therapy. In attempting to phagocytose and destroy the foreign body, phagocytes degranulate and are depleted of intracellular bactericidal substances. Thus they become relatively inefficient in killing bacterial pathogens.

These factors highlight the importance of creating an environment conducive to wound healing and antibacterial action by removing foreign bodies and providing surgical drainage and wound cleansing.

ASSESSMENT AND DURATION OF THERAPY

In acute infections, it is usually evident within 2 or 3 days whether treatment is having the desired effect. An inadequate response should prompt re-evaluation of the diagnosis and treatment. If underdosing or poor tissue penetration is suspected, increased dosage of the same drug might be appropriate. Otherwise, selection of a different drug is warranted. For the majority of uncomplicated, acute infections in dogs, treatment for 4 or 5 days, up to a week, seems adequate.

With chronic infections, it may take longer to determine whether treatment is being effective and prolonged administration is usually required. This can be explained by the existing tissue damage, impaired blood supply and compromised local immunity. Treatment for 4–6 weeks or more is generally required when bacterial infections are chronic. Similarly prolonged treatment is also advised for pyoderma, prostatitis, pyelonephritis, recurrent lower urinary tract infections, septic arthritis, osteomyelitis, septicaemia, pneumonia and bacterial endocarditis.

ADJUNCTIVE TREATMENTS

Many bacterial infections are not cured by systemic antibacterial drug therapy alone and require additional specific or supportive measures:

- *Fluid therapy* may be crucial to correct acid–base imbalances and dehydration and maintain the patient while antibacterial therapy is undertaken.
- *Surgery* may be needed to remove necrotic tissue, calculi or foreign material or to establish drainage from the site.
- *Fever* is common in more severe infections and may benefit the patient by inhibiting proliferation of pathogens (Davis 1985).
  - Antipyretic treatment is usually not warranted and may obscure the natural course of the disease or the response to antibacterial treatment.
  - Sustained hyperthermia exceeding 41°C can be detrimental and warrants intervention (cool baths, cool water enemas) to quickly reduce body temperature to safe levels (Davis 1985).
- *Glucocorticoid administration* is potentially deleterious in animals with sepsis because it may suppress the host's defences and mask signs of infection but:
  - A shorter acting glucocorticoid (such as prednisolone) for a few days can help by suppressing an acute inflammatory response that is causing pain or discomfort and provoking self-trauma.
  - If glucocorticoid is introduced along with antibacterial therapy, then a bactericidal drug should be selected because bacteriostatic drugs are more dependent on the patient's defence mechanisms to control the infection.

ENHANCING THERAPEUTIC COMPLIANCE

Studies have shown that a substantial proportion of human patients comply poorly with drug therapies prescribed by physicians. Limited observations suggest non-compliance is also prevalent in veterinary medicine: in two canine studies, only 27% of owners gave the prescribed number of doses during short-term antibiotic treatment (Bomzon 1978, Barter 1994). Underdosing and dosing at suboptimum intervals were common problems, but overdosing also occurred (Barter 1994).

Undesirable consequences of poor compliance include:

- inadequate response to treatment,
- increased costs,
- creation of doubts in the mind of the client about the effectiveness of both the drug and the clinician.

Potential difficulties with compliance should be addressed by scheduling administration to suit the owners' routines where possible, deciding with the owners the dosage form they can best manage, demonstrating its use, and providing clear verbal and written instructions. Human studies have shown that the risk of missed doses increases with treatment complexity. Accordingly, if no therapeutic difference exists between several alternative treatments, the one with the least complex regimen should be chosen. Likewise, additional medications of questionable value are best avoided, because complicated treatment schedules could reduce the owners' ability to comply with the regimens recommended for the more important drugs.

PROPHYLACTIC ANTIBACTERIAL USE

(1) Prophylactic antimicrobial drugs are not indicated for routine, clean surgery where no inflammation is present, the gastrointestinal or respiratory systems have not been invaded, and aseptic technique is maintained.
(2) Prophylactic use of antibacterials is indicated for:
    - complicated orthopaedic surgery where the time required may be prolonged;
    - dental procedures with associated bleeding;
    - patients with leucopenia, where the consequences of sepsis would be disastrous and potentially irreversible or life threatening;
    - contaminated surgery.
(3) For antibacterial chemoprophylaxis drugs should be administered before the procedure so that adequate concentrations are present *in vivo* at the time of surgery – for best effect the drug must be present in the wound when contamination occurs:
    - appropriate doses, given by i.v. at the time of anaesthetic induction or i.m. injection, 60 min beforehand, should give optimum concentrations;
    - repeated doses may be necessary if surgery is prolonged (every 3 h for β-lactam drugs).
(4) The likely contaminating pathogens should be considered when selecting the appropriate drug for prophylaxis.
(5) The advantages of chemoprophylaxis are lost if administration is commenced more than 3 h after contamination.

ADVERSE EFFECTS OF ANTIBACTERIAL DRUGS

The goal of antimicrobial therapy is to assist elimination of infectious organisms without toxicity to the host. However, like all drugs, antimicrobial agents are not without toxicity and may cause:

- selection or promotion of antimicrobial resistance,
- hypersensitivity reactions,
- direct tissue or organ toxicity,
- toxic interactions with other drugs,
- interference with the protective effect of normal host microflora,
- tissue necrosis at injection sites,
- impairment of host immune or defence mechanisms.

Selection or Promotion of Resistance

Although many previously fatal bacterial infections can now be successfully treated with antimicrobial drugs, widespread use of these agents has resulted in emergence of drug-resistant pathogens and increasing costs as new drugs are developed against resistant bacteria.

(1) Antimicrobial agents do not cause bacteria to become resistant but their use selects for resistant populations. Genes coding for resistance have been identified in bacterial cultures established before antimicrobial agents were available.
(2) Various mechanisms produce antimicrobial resistance, the most important involving R (resistance) plasmids. R plasmids are cytoplasmic genetic elements that can transfer antimicrobial resistance to susceptible bacteria. Transmissible resistance can occur between species and may produce resistance to unrelated antimicrobial agents.
(3) *Acquired resistance is not a problem in all bacterial species.* For example, Gram-positive bacteria, with the exception of staphylococci, are often unable to acquire R plasmids, whereas resistance is an increasing problem in many Gram-negative pathogens such as Enterobacteriaceae, *Pasteurella*, *Bordetella* and *Haemophilus*. The intestine is the major site of transfer of antimicrobial resistance.
(4) Nosocomial infections (acquired during hospitalisation) by resistant bacteria.
    - These are an emerging problem in veterinary hospitals, although they are not as prevalent as currently experienced in human hospitals.

- *Klebsiella*, *Escherichia*, *Proteus* and *Pseudomonas* have been associated most frequently with nosocomial infections.
- Predisposing factors include age (young or old), severity of disease, duration of hospitalisation, use of invasive support systems, defective immune responses and previous use of antibacterial agents.

(5) Disturbance of the normal gut flora
- Antibacterials with the greatest potential to suppress endogenous flora that normally keep pathogenic enteric bacteria in check are:
  - aminopenicillins,
  - chloramphenicol,
  - lincosamides and macrolides,
  - tetracyclines.
- Antibacterials that do not generally have this effect:
  - most parenteral cephalosporins,
  - aminoglycosides,
  - parenterally administered narrow spectrum penicillins.
- Antibacterials with the least effect on normal gut flora are:
  - fluoroquinolones,
  - sulphonamides and sulphonamides with potentiators.

Hypersensitivity

Hypersensitivity reactions to antibacterials are reported less often in veterinary medicine than in human patients where they constitute 6–10% of all drug reactions.

- Hypersensitivity reactions depend on the combination of antigen and antibody and are:
  - usually not dose related,
  - cannot be anticipated, although atopic individuals reportedly are at greater risk.
- Hypersensitivity reactions have been reported most frequently in veterinary patients with penicillins, cephalosporins and sulphonamides.
- *Doberman Pinschers* appear to have increased risk of sulphonamide hypersensitivity, possibly due to delayed sulphonamide metabolism. Other breed susceptibilities have not been reported.
- The probability of an anaphylactoid reaction is increased if penicillin preparations containing methylcellulose as a stabiliser are used.
- To induce an allergic response:
  - the drug molecule must be able to form covalent bonds with macromolecules such as proteins;

  - bonding with the protein carrier enables reaction with T lymphocytes and macrophages;
  - the reactive moiety is usually a drug metabolite, for example the penicilloyl moiety of penicillins and the sulphonamide metabolite, hydroxylamine.

Drug hypersensitivity may manifest in different ways.

- Acute anaphylaxis
  - associated with IgE and mast cell degranulation,
  - characterised by one or more of the following signs: hypotension, bronchospasm, angioedema, urticaria, erythema, pruritus, pharyngeal and/or laryngeal oedema, vomiting and colic.
- Immune complex deposition in tissues and activation of complement leading to:
  - lymph node enlargement,
  - neuropathy,
  - vasculitis,
  - glomerulonephritis,
  - polyarthritis,
  - urticaria,
  - fever.
- Haematological perturbations
  - haemolytic anaemia,
  - thrombocytopenia,
  - agranulocytosis (rarely).
- Cutaneous reactions may be caused by immune complex deposition or delayed hypersensitivity.

Allergy to antimicrobial agents can only occur if there has been previous exposure to the drug or a related substance (this includes earlier doses in the current regimen). However, certain anaphylactoid substances present in formulations may not require previous exposure to elicit a reaction. A hypersensitivity reaction will probably recur every time the drug or related substance is administered. It is often difficult in practice to demonstrate that re-exposure will induce a reaction (and hence prove that drug allergy exists) because of concerns that this will endanger or discomfort the patient. Treatment of drug hypersensitivity involves discontinuation of the drug and treatment with adrenaline, antihistamine, corticosteroid and intravenous fluids as necessary.

Direct Tissue or Organ Toxicity

Renal

Aminoglycosides

Aminoglycosides (except (dihydro)streptomycin) may cause renal toxicity in dogs and their use must be closely monitored to avoid toxic effects. Neomycin is too nephrotoxic for use by systemic administration.

- Renal toxicity may be enhanced by:
  - concurrent administration of diuretics,
  - dehydration from other causes that deplete extracellular fluid and may raise circulating drug concentrations,
  - pre-existing renal dysfunction (subclinical renal failure),
  - fever, acidosis and sepsis.
- Nephrotoxicity is correlated with the degree of tubular reabsorption of the aminoglycoside and the degree to which phospholipid metabolism in proximal renal tubular cells is inhibited. Therefore, of the systemically administered aminoglycosides, gentamicin has the greatest potential to cause nephrotoxicity. Amikacin and tobramycin are less likely to be nephrotoxic.

Polymyxins
- Azotaemia, proteinuria, haematuria and tubular casts formation can occur with systemic administration of polymyxins.
- Damage may progress after withdrawal of therapy.
- Systemic use is best avoided if safer alternatives are available.

Sulphonamides
- Crystalluria, haematuria and urinary tract obstruction can occur as a result of concentration of sulphonamides in renal tubules, particularly at acid pH.
- It is important to ensure that animals receiving sulphonamides are well hydrated and not receiving urinary acidifiers.

Tetracyclines
- When given intravenously tetracyclines have been reported to cause renal tubular damage in several species if:
  - large doses are given,
  - the animal is dehydrated, debilitated or stressed,
  - degraded tetracyclines are administered.
- With the exception of doxycycline and minocycline, tetracyclines should be avoided in patients with renal disease.

Hepatotoxicity

Hepatic toxicity induced by antibacterials is not common. Hepatocellular damage has been reported in domestic animals with chloramphenicol, tetracyclines, lincomycin and novobiocin.

- Parenteral administration of *tetracyclines* has been reported to cause acute hepatotoxicity in pregnant bitches.
- Chloramphenicol, erythromycin, enrofloxacin and metronidazole may inhibit liver enzyme activity and interact with other drugs in this way (see Chapter 1, Table 1.9).
- Rifampicin is a potent liver enzyme inducer and may cause significant drug interactions (see Chapter 1, Table 1.10).

Gastrointestinal Toxicity

The major cause of gastrointestinal dysfunction following use of antimicrobial drugs involves disturbance of normal enteric flora (see above). Adverse effects may also occur for the following reasons:

- Diarrhoea may occur after oral administration of many antibacterials because of:
  - interference with gut motility (chloramphenicol),
  - impaired absorption of nutrients (neomycin, kanamycin).
- Nausea and vomiting may occur occasionally with antibacterial treatment.
  - common with erythromycin (affects smooth muscle activity),
  - also reported with metronidazole and tetracycline.
- Vomiting may occur if crystalline penicillin is given rapidly intravenously.
- Nitrofuran derivatives may cause anorexia, vomiting, diarrhoea and gastrointestinal bleeding.

Neurotoxicity (Including Neuromuscular Blockade)

Aminoglycosides
- *Ototoxicity*, affecting both vestibular and auditory function, may be caused.
- Potential for ototoxicity is increased by concurrent administration of frusemide.
- Also occasionally neuromuscular blockade is caused, usually in association with anaesthesia or administration of other neuromuscular blocking agents. Patients with myasthenia gravis are particularly susceptible.

Lincosamides
- Neuromuscular blockade due to inhibition of acetylcholine release may be seen after rapid intravenous dosing, particularly if given whilst animal is anaesthetised.

Metronidazole

- Chronic treatment at relatively high doses has caused seizures, weakness and disorientation in dogs.

Penicillin

- High doses of benzylpenicillin given intravenously can cause neurological disturbances in dogs.
- Inadvertent administration of procaine penicillin G by the intravenous route can cause CNS excitability and seizures due to procaine toxicity.

Polymyxins

These drugs are safe when used topically but systemic administration may cause:

- peripheral neuropathy (blurred vision, loss of sensory function),
- blockade of neuromuscular transmission,
- polymyxin E (colistin) is less toxic than polymyxin B.

Musculoskeletal System Toxicity

- The *fluoroquinolones* cause erosion of articular cartilage in young animals.
- Intra-articular injection of some antimicrobial preparations can cause moderate to severe synovitis. This arises because of the strength of solution, its pH or the solubilising agent. The same preparations are irritant to muscle and other tissues when injected and so cause pain. These include:
  - cephalosporins (most),
  - erythromycin,
  - metronidazole,
  - polymyxins (sulphates but not sulphonates),
  - sulphonamides (sodium salts),
  - tetracyclines.
- *Tetracyclines* are deposited in growing teeth and bones and will cause *tooth discoloration* if used in young animals during development of permanent teeth. *Bony hypoplasia* is also a serious concern with use of these drugs in young animals.

Haematopoietic and Cardiovascular Toxicity

Apart from immune-mediated hypersensitivity reactions, few haematological side effects have been reported with antibacterial use in veterinary medicine.

- *Chloramphenicol* can inhibit erythropoiesis in most species in a dose dependent and reversible manner.

Chloramphenicol-induced idiosyncratic fatal aplastic anaemia that occurs in humans has not been reported in domestic animals.

- *Sulphaquinoxaline* can cause haemorrhagic diathesis in dogs due to suppression of bacterial synthesis of vitamin K.
- Bone marrow suppression has been reported associated with *sulphonamide* administration.

A number of antibacterial drugs can cause severe cardiovascular depression if administered quickly by the intravenous route. Hypotension resulting from effects of high concentrations of the drugs on the heart and vasculature are presumed to be the cause. Examples include:

- aminoglycosides,
- chloramphenicol,
- lincosamides,
- tetracycline.

Skin

The major dermatological manifestations of adverse reactions to antibacterial drugs concern hypersensitivity reactions such as ulcerative dermatitis associated with immune complex deposition. Penicillins are most frequently incriminated. Photosensitisation may occur with sulphonamide or tetracycline therapy.

Eye

Keratoconjunctivitis sicca (dry eye) may occur with prolonged use of some sulphonamides including sulphadiazine. It is probably most commonly associated with sulphasalazine because this drug is used for long-term treatment of colitis.

REFERENCES

Barter, L.C. (1994) *Aspects of small animal therapeutics*. BSc(Vet) thesis, The University of Sydney.

Bomzon, L. (1978) Short-term antimicrobial therapy – a pilot compliance study using ampicillin in dogs. *Journal of Small Animal Practice*, **19**, 697–700.

Davis, L.E. (1985) General care of the patient. In: *Handbook of Small Animal Therapeutics*, (ed. L.E. Davis), pp. 1–19. Churchill Livingstone, New York.

Jones, R.L. (1990) Laboratory diagnosis of bacterial infections. In:

Infectious Diseases of the Dog and Cat, (ed. C.E. Greene), pp. 453–460. Saunders, Philadelphia.

Watson, A.D.J. (1994) Appropriate use of antimicrobial drugs in dogs and cats. In: *Antimicrobial Prescribing Guidelines for Veterinarians*, (ed. B.S. Cooper), pp. 55–81. Postgraduate Foundation, The University of Sydney.

Ferguson, D.C. and Lappin, M.R. (1992) Antimicrobial therapy. In: *Small Animal Medical Therapeutics*, (eds M.D. Lorenz, L.M. Cornelius & D.C. Ferguson), pp. 457–478. Lippincott, Philadelphia.

Prescott, J.F. and Baggot, J.D. (1993) *Antimicrobial Therapy in Veterinary Medicine*, 2nd edn. Iowa State University Press, Ames.

FURTHER READING

Cooper, B.S. (1994) *Antimicrobial Prescribing Guidelines for Veterinarians*. Postgraduate Foundation, The University of Sydney.

Chapter 5

Cytotoxic and Immunosuppressive Drugs

J. M. Dobson

CYTOTOXIC DRUGS

Cancer is a common disease in dogs, the diagnosis and treatment of which is assuming increasing importance in clinical veterinary practice. The modern veterinary approach to treatment of cancer owes a great deal to the human experience, indeed all the cytotoxic drugs discussed in the following chapter have been developed and licensed for use in human cancer therapy. Although anti-cancer chemotherapy is a relatively recent development, there is now considerable veterinary experience in the use of cytotoxic drugs, and a large volume of published literature exists to support the use of these drugs in selected tumours in the dog. Chemotherapy is not a panacea for cancer however, and the actions of cytotoxics are not selective for neoplastic cells. Potentially life-threatening damage to normal tissues is an almost invariable consequence of their use. Great care is needed when prescribing these drugs and they should never be used empirically.

BASIC PRINCIPLES

The use of cytotoxic drugs in cancer treatment requires a basic understanding of:

- tumour biology,
- pharmacology of cytotoxic drugs.

Tumour Biology

The majority of naturally occurring cancers arise from the neoplastic transformation of a single precursor or stem cell.

The growth characteristics of a tumour are summarised in Fig. 5.1. In the early stages of development most tumours grow rapidly, but the growth rate tends to slow towards a plateau phase as the tumour reaches larger proportions.

The major tumour-related factors that determine the success of chemotherapy are:

- tumour doubling time/growth fraction,
- tumour cell heterogeneity,
- drug resistance.

Tumour/Mass Doubling Time

The time it takes for a tumour to double in size is a function of:

- *growth fraction*: the number of actively dividing cells within the tumour, i.e. those in G_1, S, G_2 or M stages of the cell cycle (Fig. 5.2);
- *cell cycle time*: the time it takes for the dividing cells to complete the cyclical process of cell division;
- *cell loss factor*: the number of tumour cells being lost through cell death.

The mass doubling time of most human tumours at the time of diagnosis is in the order of weeks to months, but detailed studies show the mass doubling time for sub-populations of well nourished cells within such tumours to be approximately 1–5 days. This discrepancy is explained by estimates that suggest that up to 90–95% of tumour cells are fated to die through 'starvation' as a result of impoverished tumour blood supply.

The *growth fraction* is the single most important factor governing tumour response to chemotherapy because most cytotoxic drugs are only active against dividing cells. The *mitotic index* or *mitotic count*, which refers to the percentage of mitoses (M phase cells) visible in tumour sections by

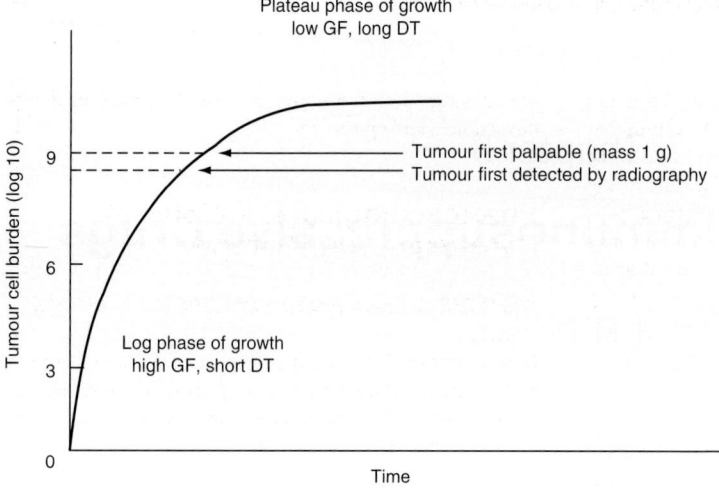

Fig. 5.1 Growth characteristics of a tumour. A tumour cannot be detected by palpation or radiography until it reaches approximately 1 cm in diameter or 0.5–1 g in weight, by which time it has undergone approximately 30 doublings and contains in the order of 10^8–10^9 cells.

During the early stages of tumour growth a high proportion of tumour cells are actively dividing, i.e. the growth fraction (GF) is high and the doubling time (DT) short, but, by the time most solid tumours can be detected clinically, only a small proportion of the cells are dividing, i.e. the growth fraction is low (and doubling time long).

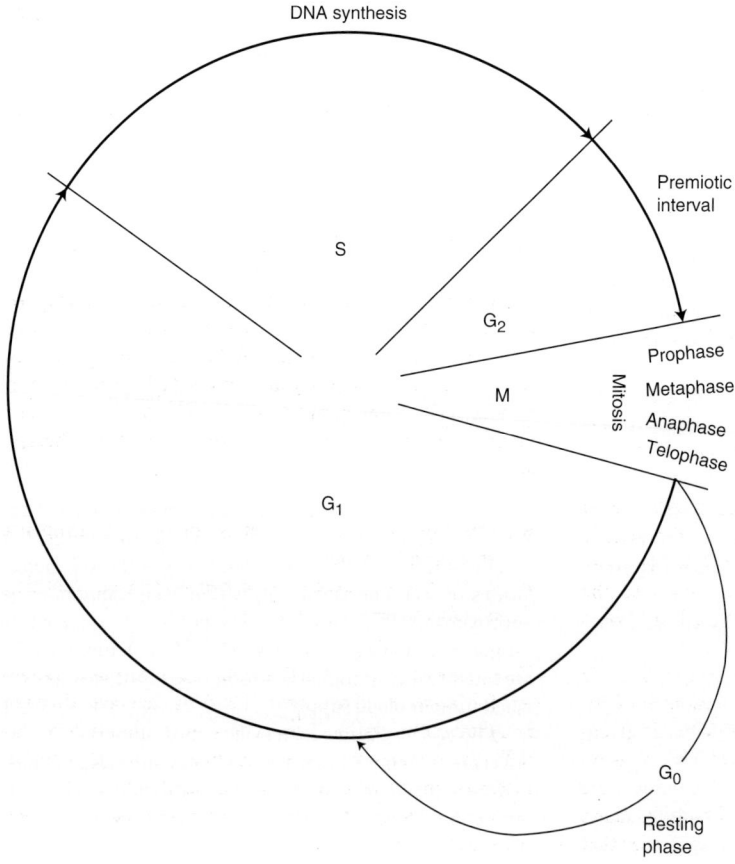

Fig. 5.2 The cell cycle. Cell division is a cyclical process with cells progressing through a series of well defined stages of mitosis (M), growth (G_1), synthesis of DNA (S) and further growth (G_2) including preparation of the mitotic spindle. Cells which are not actively dividing enter the 'G_0' or resting phase and may re-enter the cycle in response to a number of stimuli.

Cells may be more or less sensitive to different drugs or to radiation at different stages of the cell cycle. Resting cells are relatively resistant to the actions of radiation and cytotoxic drugs and therefore form an important reservoir of cells from which the tumour may repopulate.

light microscopy, is a useful indicator of the growth fraction of an individual tumour, but is distinct from the GF in that the latter includes all dividing cells and not just those in the M phase. The fraction of viable, resting (G_0) cells in the tumour is also important because these cells form a 'protected' reservoir of cells from which the tumour may repopulate and thus these cells govern the ultimate outcome of treatment.

Tumour Cell Heterogeneity

The original homogeneity of the tumour does not persist through the later stages of tumour growth. Cancer cells continually modify their properties through small mutations occurring during cell division. Hence, although the cells in the tumour mass may share some features of the original precursor cell, they are heterogeneous in many properties including biochemical, morphological and drug-response characteristics.

Drug Resistance

Drug resistance describes the ability of a tumour cell to survive the actions of an anti-cancer drug when administered at a dose which would normally be expected to cause cell damage and death. Certain tumours are refractory to the actions of cytotoxic drugs from the outset. This may result from the growth kinetics of the tumour being inappropriate for the use of drugs, for example a slowly growing fibrosarcoma, but some rapidly growing tumours may also fail to respond to therapy and in such cases it is concluded that the cell type of the tumour is *intrinsically* resistant to the actions of cytotoxic drugs. This is the case with many carcinomas and melanomas.

Tumour cells may also *acquire* drug resistance, as exemplified by the clinical situation in which a previously drug-responsive tumour regrows and is no longer sensitive to further treatment with the same agent.

Intrinsic and acquired drug resistance is considered to arise through mutations occurring due to the genetic instability of a tumour. Many clinically applicable resistance mechanisms have been identified for most of the commonly used cytotoxic drugs, as detailed in Boxes 5.1–5.6.

Tumour cells can acquire resistance to drugs which are outwith the drug groups used to treat the tumour initially. Multi-drug resistance (MDR) is associated with a P-glyco-protein membrane transport mechanism which acts as an export pump for certain cytotoxic drugs. This reduces the intracellular concentration of the drug and thereby allows the tumour cell to survive exposure to the drug. Drugs that

are substrates for the pump include the vinca alkaloids, doxorubicin and epirubicin.

Pharmacological Principles of Cytotoxic Drug Therapy

Mechanisms of Action of Cytotoxic Drugs

Most cytotoxic drugs act upon the processes of cell growth and division. Agents are commonly divided into six classes on the basis of their characteristic sites or modes of action, anti-tumour activity and toxicity.

- alkylating agents – interfere with replication of DNA
- anti-metabolites – prevent the synthesis of DNA and RNA
- anti-tumour (cytotoxic) antibiotics – interefere with replication of DNA
- vinca alkaloids – antimitotic agents which cause metaphase arrest
- hormones – corticosteroids and sex hormones and their antagonists
- miscellaneous – several drugs do not fit into the above categories

These agents and their actions are detailed in Boxes 5.1–5.6.

Normal Tissue Toxicity ('Side Effects')

Cytotoxic drugs are most effective against growing or dividing cells but these actions are not selective for tumour cells and normal tissue toxicity follows a similar pattern to that of tumours: organs containing a high proportion of dividing cells are most susceptible to drug-induced toxicity. Hence the most common 'side effects' of chemotherapy are:

- *bone marrow* toxicity – myelosuppression, neutropenia and thrombocytopenia;
- *gastrointestinal* toxicity – anorexia, nausea, vomiting and diarrhoea.

Fortunately, these normal tissues have a tremendous capacity for recovery from cytotoxic drug damage through recruitment of resting stem cells. Hence, although potentially life-threatening, these toxic effects are usually quickly reversible on discontinuation of treatment.

Some cytotoxic agents have other toxic actions which are less reversible:

Box 5.1 Alkylating agents.

Mechanism of action: substitute alkyl radicals ($R—CH_2—CH_3$) for hydrogen atoms in the DNA molecule. Alkylation of nucleotide bases causes breaks, cross-linkages and abnormal base pairing in DNA, all of which interfere with replication of DNA and transcription of RNA. These actions are not cell cycle specific.

Mechanisms of resistance: defective transport mechanisms, intracellular inactivation of the drug and / or increased DNA repair.

Main tumour activities: variable, see below.

Major toxicities: myelosuppression is the major side effect of alkylating agents. They also affect the GIT and can cause anorexia, vomiting and diarrhoea. May affect gametogenesis and cause alopecia or thinning of the coat in some breeds of dog.

Individual agents	Indications	Toxicity
Nitrogen mustard derivatives		
Cyclophosphamide	Lymphoproliferative disorders Myeloproliferative disorders Multiple myeloma (certain sarcomas/carcinomas in combination protocols) Immunosuppression	Myelosuppression Gastrointestinal (V & D) *Urologic – haemorrhagic cystitis* Alopecia or thinning of coat
Chlorambucil	Chronic lymphocytic leukaemia Multiple myeloma Lymphoma (maintenance) (polycythaemia vera) (immunosuppression)	Myelosuppression – mild
Melphalan	Multiple myeloma Lymphoproliferative disorders (certain carcinomas & sarcomas in combination protocols)	Myelosuppression – may be delayed Gastrointestinal (V & D)
Ethenamine derivatives		
Thiotepa (triethylenethiophosphoramide)	Instillation in body cavities for malignant pleural or peritoneal effusions Bladder instillation for transitional cell carcinoma of bladder (not widely used)	Myelosuppression (even following local instillation)
Alkyl sulphonates		
Busulphan	Chronic granulocytic leukaemia Polycythaemia vera	Myelosuppression (pulmonary fibrosis – rare) (endocrinological disorders – rare) (ocular, lens changes – rare)
Triazine derivatives		
Dacarbazine (imidazole carboxamide) (in addition to alkylating actions, also inhibits DNA & protein synthesis)	Lymphoma (combination protocols) (?malignant melanoma)	Gastrointestinal: anorexia nausea & vomiting Myelosuppression (hepatotoxicity) (alopecia) Irritant – perivascular reactions
Nitrosureas Lipophilic agents, pass into CSF		
Carmustine	Brain tumours (malignant glioma) (carcinoma, gastric/colorectal, hepatoma, LPD in humans)	Myelosuppression – cumulative, delayed onset marrow stem cell toxicity (pulmonary fibrosis)
Lomustine	Brain tumours (carcinoma, brochogenic/colorectal, Hodgkin's disease in humans)	Myelosuppression – cumulative, delayed onset Gastrointestinal – nausea, vomiting stomatitis Alopecia Neurological reactions

Box 5.2   Anti-metabolites.

Mechanism of action: structural analogues of metabolites required for purine and/or pyrimidine synthesis. They interfere with DNA and RNA synthesis by enzyme inhibition or by causing synthesis of non-functional molecules. Anti-metabolites are cell cycle specific, acting during the 'S' phase of the cell cycle.

Mechanisms of resistance: deactivation by intracellular enzymes, defective transport – reduced uptake, use of alternative metabolic pathways.

Main tumour activities: variable, see below.

Major toxicities: myelosuppression, gastrointestinal (anorexia, vomiting and diarrhoea). Renal and neurological toxicities are features of individual drugs (see below).

Individual agents	Indications	Toxicity

Antifolates
  Methotrexate
	Lymphoproliferative diseases
	Transmissible venereal tumour
	  (sertoli cell tumour) (soft tissue
	  sarcoma and osteosarcoma)
		Myelosuppression
		Gastrointestinal – can be severe in
		  the dog
		Renal tubular necrosis – with high
		  dose regimens

Pyrimidine analogues
  5-Fluorouracil
	(mammary, gastrointestinal, hepatic
	  & pulmonary carcinoma)
	Topical – basal cell and squamous
	  cell carcinomas of the skin
		Myelosuppression
		Gastrointestinal
		Neurotoxicity-cerebellar ataxia and
		  seizures

Cytarabine (cytosine arabinoside, Ara-C)	Lymphoproliferative disease Myeloproliferative disease Acute myelogenous leukaemia Acute lymphoblastic leukaemia	Myelosuppression Gastrointestinal

Purine analogues
  6-Mercaptopurine
	Lymphoproliferative &
	  myeloproliferative diseases
		Myelosuppression
		  (Gastrointestinal – rare)

6-Thioguanine	Lymphoproliferative &
	  myeloproliferative diseases
		Myelosuppression
		  (Gastrointestinal – rare)

Azathioprine	Immunosuppression	Myelosuppression (hepatic toxicity reported in humans)

- cyclophosphamide – haemorrhagic cystitis,
- doxorubicin – cardiomyopathy (see later),
- cisplatin – nephrotoxicity.

The Theoretical Basis for Cytotoxic Drug Administration

The objective of cancer treatment is to reduce the tumour cell population to zero.

Tumour Cell Kill

One of the most important basic principles of anti-cancer chemotherapy is described by the 'fractional cell kill hypothesis' which suggests that a given dose of a cytotoxic drug kills a fixed percentage of the total tumour population as opposed to a set number of tumour cells (Skipper *et al.* 1964). Although some assumptions upon which this hypothesis is based are not entirely accurate in naturally occurring tumours, it does establish the following practical principles for the use of cytotoxic drugs:

Box 5.3   Antitumour antibiotics.

Antitumour antibiotics are a group of compounds derived mainly from soil fungi which have inhibitory actions on the growth of tumour cells. This group contains some of the most potent, broad-spectrum anticancer agents identified to date.

Mechanism of action: form stable complexes with DNA by intercalation, thus inhibiting DNA synthesis and transcription. These actions are not cell cycle specific.

Mechanisms of resistance: decrease in membrane binding and uptake, inactivation by intracellular enzymes, multiple drug resistance.

Main tumour activities: broad-spectrum of antitumour activity, see below.

Major toxicities: myelosuppression is the major side effect of antitumour antibiotics (with the exception of bleomycin). They also cause a dose related gastrointestinal toxicity with anorexia, vomiting and diarrhoea. Diverse range of selective toxicities of individual members of group – see below.

Individual agents	Indications	Toxicity
Actinomycin D (dactinomycin)	Lymphoproliferative disorders (vet. experience limited)	Myelosuppression Gastrointestinal
Bleomycin	Lymphoproliferative disorders (carcinomas)	Minimal myelosuppression Hypersensitivity reactions Pulmonary fibrosis Gastrointestinal
Doxorubicin (Adriamycin)	Lymphoproliferative & myeloproliferative diseases Soft tissue & osteogenic sarcoma (carcinoma)	Vesicant* Myelosuppression Gastrointestinal *Cardiac (acute and chronic)* Alopecia Hypersensitivity reactions
Epirubicin	Lymphoproliferative & myeloproliferative diseases Soft tissue & osteogenic sarcoma (carcinoma)	Vesicant Myelosuppression Gastrointestinal Cardiac (acute and chronic – less than doxorubicin) Alopecia Hypersensitivity reactions
Mitozantrone	Lymphoproliferative diseases ? soft tissue sarcoma (human – advanced breast cancer)	Myelosuppression Gastrointestinal Cardiac (acute and chronic – less than doxorubicin)

* Extremely severe local tissue toxicity resulting in serious damage if injected perivascularly

- Cytotoxic drugs should always be used at the highest possible dose to effect the highest possible fractional kill.
- Even a highly effective drug acting upon a highly sensitive tumour cell population is unlikely to eradicate the tumour cell population in a single dose.
- Chemotherapy should be instituted when the tumour burden is at its lowest, i.e. when the tumour is first detected or, in the treatment of micrometastases, immediately following surgical removal of the primary tumour.
- Chemotherapy is unlikely to be effective if used as a last resort for the treatment of extensive and advanced disease.

Box 5.4   Vinca alkaloids.

Plant alkaloids extracted from the periwinkle *Vinca rosea*.

Mechanism of action: bind specifically to microtubular proteins (tubulin) and inhibit the formation of the mitotic spindle, thus blocking mitosis and causing a metaphase arrest. These actions are cell cycle specific, acting during the M phase. (May have other, less well documented cytotxic effects including enzyme inhibition.)

Mechanisms of resistance: reduced efficiency of binding to tubulin, multiple drug resistance.

Main tumour activities: variable, see below.

Major toxicities: vesicant, neurological complications documented in humans. Vincristine is not myelosuppressive.

Individual agents	Indications	Toxicity
Vincristine	Lymphoproliferative & myeloproliferative diseases ?Mast cell tumours Transmissible venereal tumour (thrombocytopenia)	Vesicant – perivascular reactions Peripheral & autonomic neuropathies Alopecia – mild
Vinblastine	Lymphoproliferative diseases (mammary & testicular carcinomas)	Myelosuppression Vesicant – perivascular reactions Neurological Gastrointestinal

---

Box 5.5   Hormones.

CORTICOSTEROIDS

Widely used in the management of cancer for both therapy and palliation.

Mechanism of action: anti-inflammatory/immunosuppressive actions, lympholytic, suppress mitosis in lymphocytes and cause redistribution of circulating lymphocytes.

Agents	Indications	Toxicity
Prednisolone	Lymphoproliferative & myeloproliferative diseases Mast cell tumours Brain tumours Management of complications of neoplasia Palliation of advanced neoplastic disease Immune-mediated disease	Pancreatitis Diarrhoea Hyperadrenocorticism

SEX HORMONES & ANTAGONISTS

Hormonal manipulation has a major role in the management of human breast, endometrial and prostatic cancer. In veterinary oncology, although sex hormones play a role in the development and progression of a number of comparable tumours, the value of hormonal manipulation in the management of these tumours has not been established.

Box 5.6A　Miscellaneous agents.

L-Asparaginase – Crisantaspase	L-asparaginase is an enzyme which hydrolyses asparagine. Although most normal mammalian tissues synthesise asparagine in amounts sufficient for protein synthesis, lymphoid tumours do not have this ability.

Indications
Lymphoproliferative disease
  (mast cell tumour)

Toxicity
Hypersenstivity reactions
Gastrointestinal
Haemorrhagic pancreatitis has been reported in the dog

Hydroxyurea　Inhibits DNA synthesis. Acts by inhibiting the enzyme ribonucleoside diphosphate reductase. This enzyme acts at a critical and rate limiting step in the biosynthesis of DNA. This action is cell cycle specific (S phase)

Indications
Polycythaemia rubra vera
Chronic granulocytic leukaemia

Toxicity
Myelosuppression

Mitotane　*o,p'*DDD is a derivative of the chlorinated hydrocarbon insecticides. It causes destruction of the zona fasiculata and reticularis of the adrenal cortex, through actions on the cytochrome P_{450} dependent enzymes in adrenocortical cells.

Indications
Hyperadrenocorticism

Toxicity
Nausea, vomiting
Hypoadrenocorticism
Neurotoxicity (occasionally)

Box 5.6B　Platinum co-ordination compounds.

Mechanism of action: inhibit protein synthesis by the formation of both inter- and intra-cross links in the strands of DNA. The N7 atom of guanine is particularly reactive and platinum cross-links between adjacent guanines on the same DNA strand are most readily demonstrated. These agents also react with other nucleophiles such as the sulphydryl groups of proteins and these reactions may produce some of the toxic effects.

Mechanisms of resistance: ? decreased drug uptake and increased DNA repair.

Main tumour activities: broad spectrum of activity against solid tumours, see below.

Major toxicities: severe toxicity has limited veterinary use: myelosuppression is a minor side effect. Gastrointestinal tract toxicity is common, direct actions on the chemoreceptor trigger zone can cause acute and severe vomiting. Nephrotoxicity is the main concern.

Individual agents	Indications	Toxicity
Cisplatin	Osteogenic and soft tissue sarcoma Carcinomas	Nephrotoxic – acute proximal tubular necrosis Gastrointestinal – vomiting (myelosuppression)
Carboplatin	Osteogenic and soft tissue sarcoma Carcinomas	Myelosuppression Nephrotoxic – less than cisplatin Nausea & vomiting – less than cisplatin

Clinical Application of Cytotoxic Drugs

The clinical application of cytotoxic drugs depends on:

- the objective of treatment, i.e. whether the intent is cure, long-term remission or short-term palliation,
- the phase of treatment.

It is difficult to achieve a complete cure through the short-term use of chemotherapy. Even the most chemosensitive human tumours usually require 3–6 months of aggressive chemotherapy to effect a cure or prolonged remission. Several different phases of treatment can be described according to the extent and response of the disease as outlined in Fig. 5.3.

Induction Therapy

The aim of induction therapy is to reduce the number of tumour cells to a minimal level. This usually involves an intensive course of treatment administered over a defined period of time. Certain chemoresponsive tumours, for example lymphomas, often show a remarkable response following one or two courses of chemotherapy. Clinically this may be seen as a complete regression of the tumour

and remission of any associated signs. A *clinical remission* is not synonymous with *cure* and unless treatment is continued there will be a rapid expansion of the residual tumour mass resulting in a 'relapse' or clinical recurrence of the disease.

Maintenance Therapy

Where clinical remissions can be achieved through the use of intensive treatment schedules, a less aggressive treatment may then be adopted to maintain this remission.

Rescue Therapy

In clinical practice, anti-cancer drugs do not always achieve the desired effect in terms of tumour response and duration of response. In some cases the tumour may not respond to the initial therapy, in others, the initial response appears to be good but the tumour eventually recurs despite continued treatment; this is usually the result of tumour drug resistance. The aim of rescue therapy is to establish a further remission of the tumour and this usually involves recourse to more aggressive therapy, preferably with agents to which the tumour has not been exposed. Drugs that have similar mechanisms of action, or similar chemistry, are likely to share resistance mechanisms.

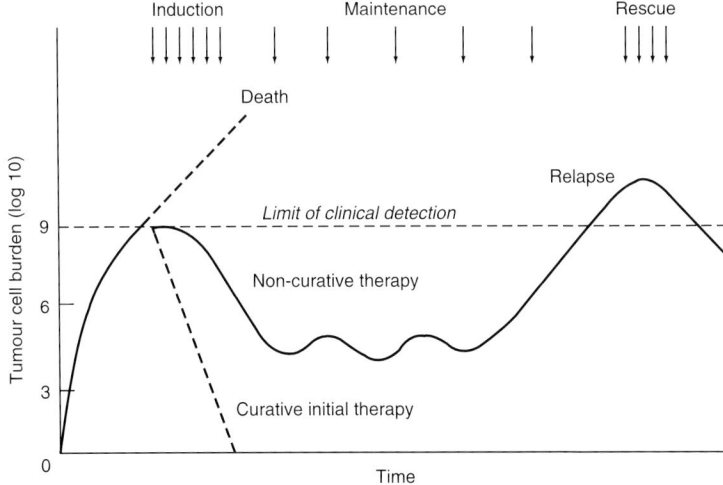

Fig. 5.3 Phases and outcome of cytotoxic treatment. Conceptual summary of tumour growth and tumour burden during phases of cytotoxic treatment. Without treatment tumour progression and death are a certain outcome. The initial intensive induction therapy often results in a clinical remission of the tumour, initial therapy is rarely curative.

The residual (sub-clinical) tumour mass eventually becomes resistant during the maintenance phase of treatment resulting in tumour regrowth or relapse. Rescue therapy may be attempted at this stage but, as a result of drug resistance, the tumour is rarely as responsive to rescue treatment as it was to the initial induction treatment.

Single Agent Versus Combination Therapy

In most circumstances, a combination of cytotoxic agents has proved to be more effective in cancer therapy than the use of a single agent. By treating a tumour with a combination of agents which employ different mechanisms of action and have different spectra of normal tissue toxicity, the overall response can be enhanced often without an increase in toxicity. Most combination drug protocols are designed according to these criteria. Examples are provided in Chapter 35 on lymphoproliferative and myeloproliferative disease.

Dosage and Timing of Treatments

Timing

It is more beneficial to administer a cytotoxic drug in 'pulse doses', allowing the normal tissues to recover between treatments than to use continuous therapy where the normal tissues are constantly exposed to the drug and unable to repair or repopulate.

The interval between treatments has to be carefully timed:

- The time interval should be long enough to allow for recovery of the normal tissues without expansion of the residual tumour population.
- If the time interval is too short, cumulative toxicity will occur resulting in leucopenia and thrombocytopenia, vomiting and diarrhoea.
- If the time interval is too long the tumour will repopulate and the benefit of the preceding treatment will have been lost.
- For most cytotoxic agents maximum bone marrow suppression occurs at about day 7–10 following treatment with recovery by day 21. Hence 3-week cycles of treatment are commonly employed in clinical practice.

Dosage

As a general rule the dosages of cytotoxics used in human therapy are not appropriate in the dog because the severe toxicities resulting from such treatment cannot be managed on a routine basis in veterinary medicine. Dosages recommended for animals are invariably a compromise between efficacy and toxicity. As recommended doses vary according to the circumstances of treatment, dose rates are not provided in this Chapter but may be found in later sections on individual conditions where chemotherapy is recommended.

Dose Rate Calculation

Doses of cytotoxic drugs are usually calculated as a function of body surface area (in m²) rather than body weight

Box 5.7   Calculation of surface area.

$$\text{Surface area} = \frac{K \times \text{body weight (kg)}^{0.66}}{10^4}$$

K = 10.1 for dogs and 10.0 for cats.
(see Appendix 1 for canine body weight – surface area conversion chart)

Table 5.1   Modification of drug dosage based on clinicopathological findings of organ dysfunction.

Hepatic dysfunction	Renal dysfunction
Doxorubicin	Methotrexate
Vincristine	Cisplatin
Vinblastine	Bleomycin
	Hydroxyurea
	Cyclophosphamide*
	Thiotepa

* Cyclophosphamide is inactive *in vitro* and requires activation *in vivo* by hepatic metabolism to produce cytotoxic metabolites. The value of administration of cyclophosphamide in cases of severe hepatic dysfunction must be given careful consideration.

because the blood supply to the organs responsible for detoxification and excretion (liver and kidneys) is more closely related to surface area than body weight. Body weight is used to calculate surface area by the formula shown in Box 5.7.

Consideration should be given to the presence of significant renal or hepatic dysfunction when calculating dose rates of cytotoxic drugs. Dosages should be reduced in proportion with the degree of organ dysfunction (see Table 5.1 and Chapter 1 for further discussion).

INDICATIONS FOR CHEMOTHERAPY IN VETERINARY MEDICINE

The main indication for chemotherapy in veterinary cancer medicine is in the treatment of systemic or disseminated malignant disease. In practice there are broadly two categories of disease where the value of chemotherapy has been established in the dog:

- in the treatment of lymphoproliferative and myeloproliferative diseases which are generally systemic in nature;

- as an adjunct to surgical and/or radiation treatment of the primary malignant tumours with a high risk of distant metastatic disease, e.g. osteosarcoma, haemangiosarcoma.

Detailed consideration of the role of chemotherapy in the management of lymphoproliferative and myeloproliferative disorders are the subject of Chapter 35. The following basic considerations apply to the use of cytotoxic drugs in any clinical circumstance.

Patient Selection and Evaluation

The diagnostic evaluation of the patient is of great importance in the management of cancer. The basic requirements of this evaluation are listed in Table 5.2, these include:

Histopathological Diagnosis

- A diagnosis of tumour type and grade before embarking upon therapy is essential.
- Only when the nature of the disease is known can the most effective therapy be prescribed.

- Histological examination of needle, incisional or excisional biopsy samples is the most accurate method of cancer diagnosis.

Clinical Staging

- Successful treatment depends upon eradication of all tumour stem cells.
- This can only be achieved if the extent of the disease is fully appreciated.
- The initial evaluation of the cancer patient should determine:
  - the local extent of a tumour,
  - the possibility of lymphatic or haematogenous metastasis.

Evaluation of Tumour Related Complications and Concurrent Disease

- Tumours may be associated with a number of medical complications:

Table 5.2 Techniques for the diagnostic evaluation of the cancer patient.

Aim	Technique
Achieve definitive diagnosis	*Incisional or excisional biopsy* of lesion: to allow histopathological examination of representative tissue from the tumour

Clinical staging
  T: Primary tumour
  N: Lymph nodes (local & regional)
  M: Distant metastases
	Physical examination of primary site, local and regional lymph nodes
	Radiography of primary tumour site, if adjacent to bone; for assessment of deep lymph nodes (e.g. sublumbar, mediastinal). Right and left lateral, inflated thoracic films essential for assessment of pulmonary metastases
	Ultrasonography for assessment of liver, spleen and kidneys
	Cytological (histological) evaluation of any suspicious lesions or lymphadenopathy

Evaluate tumour related concurrent disease	*Haematology*: full haematological assessment of red cells, white cell and platelets
	Biochemical screen: including
	  urea, creatinine – renal function
	  alkaline phosphatase, ALT, AST, GGT, bile salts – liver function
	  electrolytes – especially calcium
	  protein (albumen : globulin ratio)
	  glucose

Establish base-line parameters	*Haematology*: white cell (neutrophil) and platelet counts *Liver & renal* function *Cardiac*: ECG and ultrasound assessment of cardiac muscle fractional shortening

ALT, alanine aminotransferase; AST, aspartate aminotransferase; GGT, gamma glutamyl transferase.

Table 5.3 Haematological response to cytotoxic drugs.

Drug	Major element suppressed	Degree of suppression	Nadir (days)	Recovery (days)	Comments
Alkylating agents					
Busulphan	G	Severe*	Delayed	Several weeks	Does not spare stem cells, hence severe effects which are prolonged
Chlorambucil	G & L	Moderate	21	42–56	Less myelosuppressive than other agents of this group. Onset delayed but recovery rapid
Melphalan	G & P	Mild/moderate	10	21	Recovery can be slow sometimes
Cyclophosphamide	G	Moderate	14	18–21	Significant myelosuppression is more common with i.v. high dose therapy (250 mg/m²) than low dose oral therapy (50 mg/m² every other day)
Carmustine/lomustine (nitroureas)	G	Severe	Delayed	Several weeks	Does not spare stem cells, hence severe effects which are prolonged
Antimetabolites					
Cytarabine (Cytosine arabinoside)	G & P	Moderate to severe	10	21	More myelosuppressive but also more efficacious if given as an infusion over 24 h rather than as daily dosages
5-Fluorouracil	G	Mild/moderate	10	21	
Methotrexate	G & P	Mild	10	14	
Antitumour antibiotics					
Doxorubicin	G & P	Moderate	14	21	Thrombocytopenia can be marked. Other antitumour antibiotics have similar effects
Vinca alkaloids					
Vinblastine	G & P	Mod/severe	10	21	
Vincristine	G	None	–	–	
Platinum dye products					
Cisplatin	G & P	Mild/moderate	6–7 and 15	21–28	May induce biphasic myelosuppression. Can cause significant thrombocytopenia
Carboplatin	G & P	Moderate	14	21–28	More likely to cause thrombocytopenia than cisplatin

G, granulocytes; P, platelets; L, lymphocytes.
* All the doses used for the treatment of chronic granulocytic leukaemia/polycythemia do not usually cause severe myelosuppression.

○ some are life-threatening and require emergency management,
○ others, while not being immediately life-threatening, may affect the animal's ability to tolerate future treatment and influence the prognosis.

● Many animals presenting with cancer are elderly and may have concurrent cardiac, renal or hepatic dysfunction. The presence of these and/or other problems may also influence the prognosis and affect the patient's tolerance of treatment.

Establish Base Line Parameters for Monitoring Patient

- *Haematology* – as most cytotoxic drugs are myelosuppressive it is essential to establish base-line haematological values, especially total white blood cell and neutrophil counts from which treatment related toxicity can be assessed.
- *Biochemistry* – renal and hepatic function are particularly important in cytotoxic chemotherapy. Impaired metabolism or excretion of these drugs will enhance the likelihood of toxicity occurring at dose rates usually employed.

COMPLICATIONS OF CHEMOTHERAPY

Complications of chemotherapy can be life threatening and may require emergency treatment. It is important that the animal is monitored regularly for any signs of toxicity. In this way potential problems can often be detected at an early stage and remedial action taken. Complications of chemotherapy can arise at any time during therapy; they include:

- myelosuppression leading to infection,
- gastrointestinal toxicity,
- hypersensitivity/anaphylaxis,
- phlebitis.

Myelosuppression and Infection

The vast majority of the chemotherapeutic drugs used to treat neoplastic conditions in animals are myelosuppressive. The most notable *exceptions* are:

- vincristine sulphate,
- L-asparaginase.

Myelosuppression is the main dose-limiting factor in veterinary chemotherapy. Rapidly dividing haemopoietic precursor cells are susceptible to cytotoxic drugs and thus cell production is diminished. The red cells, granulocytes and platelets in the circulation at the time of administration are unaffected but replacement of these cells as they are removed from the circulation may be inadequate. If no cells at all were produced then granulocytes would disappear within about a week, platelets within 2 weeks and erythrocytes would vanish after 4 months. The actual haematological response to cytotoxic drugs used in veterinary practice is summarised in Table 5.3.

The clinically significant effects of myelosuppression are:

- *neutropenia* (neutrophil count of less than $2 \times 10^9/1$) leads to a significant risk of overwhelming infection/sepsis;
- *thrombocytopenia* (a platelet count of less than $70 \times 10^9/1$) rarely severe enough to cause bleeding.

Anaemia is rarely clinically significant and is often indistinguishable from anaemia associated with the neoplasm itself.

Haematological monitoring is *vital* in all cases receiving potentially myelosuppressive drugs.

Treatment of Neutropenic Patients

This depends on the neutrophil count and clinical presentation. Recommendations for adjustment of dose rates of chemotherapy according to the neutrophil count are presented in Table 5.4.

Neutropenia predisposes the cancer patient to infection.

Table 5.4 Management of chemotherapy according to neutrophil counts.

Neutrophil count ($10^9/1$)	Degree of myelosuppression	Chemotherapy adjustment required
>3.0 Normal	Not significant	Use recommended dose rates of myelosuppressive drugs (no adjustment necessary)
2.0–3.0	Significant	Reduce dose of myelosuppressive cytotoxics by 50%
1.0–2.0	Serious	Stop all myelosuppressive cytotoxics
<1.0	Severe, life threatening	Stop all cytotoxics, administer broad-spectrum bactericidal antibiotics

Infectious organisms may gain entry to the body through the respiratory, urogenital or gastrointestinal tracts, or through disruption of normal barriers (e.g. skin and mucosa) by the tumour or indwelling catheters. Absorption of enteric bacteria through damaged intestinal mucosa is the most common source of infection in animal cancer patients and *Escherichia coli* and *Klebsiella pneumoniae* are two of the most common pathogenic organisms. Identification or detection of sepsis can be difficult in the neutropenic patient because the inflammatory response is altered by the neutropenia. Pyrexia is the most consistent sign of sepsis.

Pyrexic Neutropenic Patients

These patients represent a medical emergency, and must be provided with intensive medical support and treated aggressively with antibiotics. Blood and swabs of suspicious lesions should be submitted for culture and sensitivity testing but before identification of the causative organism, the following steps should be taken:

- all cytotoxic drugs except corticosteroids should be discontinued immediately;
- supportive therapy: intravenous fluids, electrolytes, glucose as indicated;
- bactericidal antibiotics: cephalosporins plus gentamicin, or fluoroquinolones (can alter later based on sensitivity) (enrofloxacin is often used in preference to gentamicin due to the nephrotoxicity of the latter agent);
- 5–7 days of trimethoprim plus sulphonamide (TMP : S) combination therapy after clinical recovery and restoration of neutrophil numbers.

Asymptomatic, Afebrile Neutropenic Animals

These patients should be treated with:

- potentiated sulphonamide drug combinations (baquiloprim or trimethoprim plus sulphonamide),
- discontinuation of the offending drug until neutrophil numbers recover.

Although potentiated sulphonamides are broad-spectrum antibacterials, they spare many of the normal gut flora probably because of the high concentrations of thymidine which are present in the intestinal fluid resulting from desquammated enterocytes and dead bacteria. Thymidnine antagonises the antibacterial effect of potentiated sulphonamides. This is advantageous as these bacteria are involved in local defence in the intestines. Potentiated sulphonamides also have broad-spectrum bactericidal activity (see Chapter 4).

Anorexia, Vomiting and Gastrointestinal Toxicity

Many cytotoxic drugs have adverse effects on the gastrointestinal tract either as a direct result of the action of the drug on the oral, gastric and intestinal epithelium or as a result of non-specific myelosuppression. Death and desquamation of alimentary epithelium usually occurs 5–10 days following administration of the drug and leads to stomatitis, vomiting and mucoid or haemorrhagic diarrhoea. In the majority of cases such problems are self-limiting and the animal recovers spontaneously as the normal alimentary epithelium regenerates. Some drugs induce nausea and vomiting by stimulation of the chemoreceptor trigger zone, these include cisplatin and doxorubicin.

Treatment is symptomatic:

- Intravenous fluid therapy should be given in cases where the vomiting/diarrhoea is severe or prolonged.
- Anti-emetics are useful in the prevention or control of drug-induced vomiting:
  ○ metaclopramide,
  ○ 5-HT$_3$-receptor antagonists (e.g. ondansteron) have proved most successful in human medicine although can have disturbing side effects.
- Mucosal injury can also predispose to systemic infection and parenteral antibiotics may be indicated, as discussed above.

Hypersensitivity/Anaphylaxis

Hypersensitivity reactions to cytotoxic drugs are rare but have been reported in dogs in association with:

- L-asparaginase,
- doxorubicin,
- cisplatin,
- cytarabine.

Most cytotoxic drug hypersenstivities are immune-mediated reactions but some drugs (e.g. doxorubicin) can displace histamine from mast cells directly and other agents may activate the alternative complement pathway.

Prevention

- The route of administration can affect the incidence of hypersensitivity reactions. L-asparaginase may produce anaphylaxis in up to 30% of dogs when administered intravenously, for this reason it is recommended that the drug should always be given by the intramuscular route.

- Pre-treatment with diphenhydramine (2–4 mg/kg i.m 30–60 min before administration of the cytotoxic drug) can reduce the frequency of some drug reactions and this is usually recommended before infusion of doxorubicin.

Treatment

In the event of a hypersensitivity reaction:

- stop administration of the drug immediately,
- treat with intravenous fluids, soluble corticosteroids, adrenaline or antihistamines as appropriate for the severity of the reaction.

The animal should not be treated with the same agent again.

Phlebitis and Tissue Necrosis

The following cytotoxic drugs are intensely irritant and can cause severe local tissue necrosis after perivascular injection or extravasation from the intravenous injection site:

- vinca alkaloids – vincristine and vinblastine: extravasation will cause local erythema, irritation and possible slough;
- antitumour . antibiotics – doxorubicin, epirubicin: extravasation can cause severe progressive tissue necrosis.

Prevention

- Adequate restraint of the patient.
- Use of an intravenous catheter for administration of the drug. The latter should be flushed with saline before and after administration of the agent.

Treatment

In the event of perivascular leakage:

- Aspirate affected area immediately and flush with physiological saline to try and remove as much of the agent as possible and to dilute any residual drug.
- Soluble corticosteroids (e.g. dexamethasone) may help stabilise cell membranes.
- Cold compresses may also help reduce the inflammatory response (but see below).

Specific recommendations:

- Doxorubicin:
  ○ locally administered sodium biocarbonate (8.4% solution) is recommended,
  ○ preclinical studies show a reductant, DHH3 may be valuable (Averbuch *et al.* 1986);
- Vincristine: manufacturer's recommend local infiltration of hyaluronidase with the application of heat to disperse the drug.

Specific Drug Associated Toxicity

Cyclophosphamide: Haemorrhagic Cystitis

Metabolites of cyclophosphamide (in particular acrolein) are excreted in the urine and have an irritant action on the bladder mucosa, resulting in an acute inflammation, often accompanied by profuse bleeding. This sterile haemorrhagic cystitis can occur at any time during cyclophosphamide therapy but is more common following administration of high doses or after long-term, continuous low-dose therapy. In some cases the cystitis resolves following withdrawal of treatment but, in severe cases, resolution can take considerable time. There is no specific treatment for cyclophosphamide-induced haemorrhagic cystitis. It is therefore important to try and minimise the risk of this problem by:

- administration of the drug in the early morning;
- ensuring a good fluid intake;
- encouraging frequent emptying of the bladder;
- the urine of dogs receiving cyclophosphamide should be checked regularly for blood and protein to help detect the problem in its early stages;
- the drug mesna (Uromitexan™) is used prophylactically in some human cancer patients receiving high dose cyclophosphamide, however, there is little experience of its use in dogs.

Doxorubicin (& related drugs): Cardiotoxicity

Doxorubicin can cause acute and chronic cardiac toxicity through actions on myocardial calcium metabolism. The rate of infusion can influence this cardiac toxicity and it is recommended that the drug is administered as an infusion over at least 15 min.

Acute Changes
- Tachycardia and arrhythmias may occur on administration of the drug:

○ pulse rate and character should be monitored throughout administration and immediately afterwards,

○ if problems occur the infusion should be stopped or slowed.

• During treatment, ECG changes such as sinus tachycardia, T-wave flattening, S-T segment depression and arrhythmias are often noted.

Chronic Changes

• Cumulative, dose-related damage to the myocardium leads in some (but not all) cases to an irreversible cardiomyopathy.

• All dogs should have thoracic radiographs, an ECG and ultrasound assessment of ventricular fractional shortening before treatment.

• There is no absolute dose at which cardiomyopathy occurs in all dogs – there is tremendous variation between patients.

• The total dose of the drug administered should be limited to $240\,mg/m^2$, as it is above this level at which cardiomyopathies usually occur.

Cisplatin (Carboplatin): Nephrotoxicity

Platinum co-ordination compounds accumulate in renal tubular epithelial cells where they block oxidative phosphorylation leading to acute proximal tubular necrosis. The drug may also affect renal blood flow. In order to minimise these effects cisplatin must be administered with intensive fluid diuresis:

• pre-hydration – intravenous saline (0.9%) at rate of $25\,ml/kg$ per hour for 3 h;

• cisplatin – given as a slow intravenous infusion over 15 min;

• diuresis – intravenous saline (0.9%) continued at $15\,ml/kg$ per hour for 3 h;
[NB These represent significant fluid loads administered over a short period of time. Careful assessment of cardiac and renal function should be undertaken before treatment to ensure the animal can withstand such fluid loading. The animal should also be monitored during treatment to ensure urine production is matching fluid input.]

• mannitol – may be used to assist diuresis;

• frusemide – may be administered if urine production is not adequate;

• an anti-emetic, e.g. chlorpromazine or metoclopramide should be given after the cisplatin to control nausea and vomiting.

IMMUNOSUPPRESSIVE DRUGS

Modification of the immune response by pharmacological agents and antibodies is an important and developing area in both human and veterinary medicine. The primary function of the immune system is to process antigen and protect the body from invasion by foreign agencies. The activation and the control of the immune system is dependent on a series of complex cellular and molecular interactions. Self-recognition is an essential feature of the immune response. In human medicine there has been great impetus to develop drugs which modulate the immune response to prevent graft rejection following organ transplant. Organ transplant is of less relevance in veterinary practice, but 'auto-immune' diseases resulting from altered and abnormal responses to auto-antigens are recognised and immunosuppressive agents may be used to modulate the aberrant immune response in these diseases. Immune-mediated diseases of the skin, blood and joints are well characterised in the dog and are discussed in the relevant chapters of this book. As more is known about disease processes affecting other organs there is increasing evidence that the immune system may also play a role in the aetiology of certain gastrointestinal, renal, hepatic, endocrinological, neuromuscular and ocular disease conditions.

CATEGORIES OF IMMUNOSUPPRESSIVE AGENTS

A number of different classes of drug may be used for immunosuppression:

• corticosteroids,

• cytotoxic immunosuppressives: cyclophosphamide, azathioprine,

• cyclosporin,

• danazol.

Corticosteroids (see also Chapter 6)

Corticosteroids are the most widely used agents in veterinary medicine for the management of immune-mediated conditions. Although they are often described as potent immunosuppressants, technically the immunosuppressive activity of corticosteroids in terms of suppressing primary or secondary antibody responses is poor. They are, however, very potent anti-inflammatory agents and many of their beneficial effects in the management of immune-mediated diseases stem largely from their ability to reduce the inflammatory component of the immune response and to antagonise cell-mediated immunity. Actions of corticosteroids are summarised in Chapter 6.

Corticosteroids with an intermediate duration of effect, for example prednisolone, are generally preferred for immunosuppressive therapy. This allows dosing regimes to be used that cause minimal suppression of the hypothalamic–pituitary–adrenal axis. Newer, more potent corticosteroids appear to offer little advantage over prednisolone and are more expensive.

Cytotoxic Immunosuppressants

Many cytotoxic drugs cause immunosuppression through their cytotoxic actions on the production of myeloid and lymphoid cells. However, as a result of their toxicity, relatively few cytotoxic drugs are used routinely in the management of non-neoplastic conditions. The ideal cytotoxic immunosuppressant is a drug that has potent immunosuppressive activity but minimal or at least, readily reversible toxicity.

Cytotoxic immunosuppressants used in veterinary practice are:

- azathioprine,
- cyclophosphamide (and other alkylating agents) acts by inhibiting the synthesis of DNA, thereby preventing proliferation of stimulated T and B lymphocytes and preventing both the production of autoantibodies and the clonal expansion of activated T cells,
- vincristine (actions – see below).

Azathioprine

- It is the cytotoxic drug of first choice to use for immunosuppression.
- It is a prodrug, which is metabolised in the body to 6-mercaptopurine, this results in a slow release of the drug in the tissues which may explain its superior immunosuppressive activity.
- It can be administered orally at doses of 2.0 mg/kg (approximately 50 mg/m^2) daily or on alternate days.

Cyclophosphamide

Cyclophosphamide is a very potent and effective immunosuppressive agent, but is less popular than azathioprine for maintenance of long-term immunosuppression because of the risk of toxicity:

- drug-induced haemorrhagic cystitis,
- myelosuppression.

Cyclophosphamide is recommended by some authors in the treatment of dogs with immune-mediated haemolytic anaemia (IMHA) showing evidence of autoagglutination or acute intravascular haemolysis. The management of IMHA is discussed in Chapter 33.

The alkylating agents melphalan and chlorambucil may also be used for immunosuppression.

Vincristine

Vincristine has a useful role in the management of immune-mediated thrombocytopenia partly because of immunosuppressive actions but also by virtue of its special ability to cause thrombocytosis by stimulating the shedding of platelets from megakaryocytes. The value of this action obviously depends on the presence of maturing platelet and functional megakaryocytes within the bone marrow. This may not be the case if the thrombocytopenia is secondary to lymphoproliferative or myeloproliferative disease.

Cyclosporin

Cyclosporin is a fungal metabolite (produced by *Tolypocladium inflatum*). Cyclosporin is a potent immunosuppressant, the discovery of which seems set to revolutionise immunosuppressive therapy. Cyclosporin was developed for use in human transplant patients to prevent allograft rejection and this is still its major licensed application in human medicine.

Mode of Action

Cyclosporin specifically inhibits helper T cell activation by inhibiting the production of cytokines (interleukin 2) by T cells and by blocking the response of T cells to cytokines (IL-1 & IL-2).

Toxicity

- Cyclosporin is the first potent immunosuppressant to act specifically on T cells (and T cell-B–cell interactions) without causing bone marrow suppression.

- Although neutropenia is not a problem, the T cell suppression can predispose patients to development of bacterial, fungal and protozoal infections.
- Increased incidence of viral-related tumours including forms of lymphoma has also been reported in human patients receiving long-term immunosuppressive therapy.
- In humans cyclosporin is markedly nephrotoxic and this is the main factor limiting its use – nephrotoxicity appears to be less of a problem in the dog.
- Adverse effects reported with the use of cyclosporin in dogs include gastrointestinal irritation and gingival hypertrophy (Gregory 1995).

Clinical Application

Cyclosporin has been used to treat a variety of immune-mediated conditions in dogs including auto-immune haemolytic anaemia and immune-mediated thrombocytopenia and is currently under investigation for control of inflammatory bowel disease, ulcerative colitis and some inflammatory dermatoses such as sebaceous adenitis. Its only authorised application in the dog is ophthalmic: as topical agent for application to the eye in treatment of chronic superficial keratitis.

Danazol

Danazol is a synthetic 'attenuated' androgen which, in human medicine, is given by mouth primarily in the treatment of endometriosis, other uterine disorders and benign breast conditions. In veterinary medicine, danazol has been used in treatment of immune-mediated throbocytopenia and haemolytic anaemia (Bloom *et al*. 1989; Holloway *et al*. 1990; Stewart and Feldman 1993).

Mode of Action

The immunosuppressive actions of danazol are thought to arise through:

- a reduction in the number of immunoglobulin (Fc) receptors on the surface of macrophages,
- a decrease in the amount of antibody on the surface of target cells.

Toxicity

In humans, adverse effects are mainly androgenic although effects on carbohydrate metabolism, the liver, the skin and emotional status are also reported. Large scale clinical trials concerning the long-term use of danazol have not been reported in the dog. In small studies, use of danazol for up to 6 months has not, to date resulted in hepatopathy, but androgenic effects including increased muscle mass and decreased hair production have been reported.

Clinical Application

In veterinary medicine, danazol has been used in conjunction with corticosteroids (and cytotoxic immunosuppressants) in the treatment of immune-mediated thrombocytopenia and haemolytic anaemia. In these conditions, danazol may be beneficial in cases refractory to more conventional treatment or allow earlier reduction of corticosteroid dosage. There is a wide dose range of 4–10 mg/kg b.i.d. or t.i.d. The onset of action may be slow (2–3 weeks) and so the dose of prednisolone or other drugs should not be reduced immediately.

CLINICAL APPLICATION OF IMMUNOSUPPRESSIVE DRUGS

As with anti-cancer chemotherapy, the objectives of immunosuppressive therapy can be divided into two phases: *induction* of remission and *maintenance*. Corticosteroids are usually the drug of first choice but opinions vary on whether corticosteroids should be used alone or combined with other immunosuppressants for induction treatment. The most common reason for treatment failure or relapse of the condition is too rapid a reduction in the level of treatment. Most cases require at least 4 weeks of induction treatment, then providing a satisfactory response has been achieved, doses and frequency of treatment can be gradually reduced to a maintenance level (see Chapter 6). Further discussion on the clinical application of immunosuppressive agents is provided in relevant chapters of this book.

SAFETY OF HANDLING CYTOTOXIC/ IMMUNOSUPPRESSIVE DRUGS

The general principles of safe handling of medicines are discussed in Chapter 1. Many cytotoxic drugs are carcinogenic and mutagenic, some are also teratogenic and as such represent a special hazard to personnel. Many cytotoxic drugs are also extremely irritant and produce harmful local effects after direct contact with the skin or eyes. The following are guide-lines to the precautions which should be taken to reduce the exposure of personnel to cytotoxic drugs. Detailed local rules and practices should be established for the safe handling of cytotoxic drugs at places where they are used.

Cytotoxic drugs should not be handled by pregnant staff.

Cytotoxic drugs are commonly available in two forms:

- tablets or capsules for oral administration,
- powder or solutions for injection.

Tablets/Capsules

- Tablets should never be broken or crushed and capsules should not be opened.
- Disposable latex gloves should be worn when handling any tablet which does not have an inert barrier coat.
- Where tablets are provided in individual wrappers, they should always be dispensed in this form.
- In addition to the statutory requirements for the labelling of medicinal products, all containers used for dispensing cytotoxic drugs must be child-proof and carry a clear warning to keep out of the reach of children. Containers should also be clearly labelled with the name of the agent.
- Staff and owners should receive clear instructions on the administration of tablets. Disposable plastic or latex gloves should always be worn when administering these tablets because the protective barrier may break down on contact with saliva.
- Always wash hands after handling of any drug.
- Excess or unwanted drugs should be disposed of by incineration in a chemical incinerator.

Injectable Solutions

The main risk for exposure to personnel arises during the preparation and administration of injectable cytotoxics, many of which are presented as freeze-dried material or powder, requiring reconstitution with a diluent. Potential dangers in the handling and manipulation of these products are:

- the creation of aerosols during preparation/reconstitution of the solution, and

- accidental spillage of solutions either on to work surfaces or body surfaces (skin, mucous membranes, eyes).

Reconstitution

- The drug should only be reconstituted by trained personnel.
- Reconstitution of the drug should only be performed in a designated area, free from draughts, and well away from thoroughfares and food.
- Techniques should be used to prevent high pressure being generated within the vials and minimise the risk of creating aerosols. When excess air is expelled from a filled syringe it should be exhausted into a pad and not straight into the atmosphere.
- Adequate protective clothing should be worn. This varies according to the agent. The minimum requirement should be:
  - latex gloves,
  - a gown with long sleeves to protect the skin,
  - a protective visor or goggles to protect the eyes,
  - a surgical mask to provide some protection against splashes to the face.
- Some cytotoxic drugs, e.g. doxorubicin, should only be reconstituted in a protective, vertical-flow, biological safety cabinet .

Drug Administration

- Luer lock fittings should be used in preference to push connections on syringes, tubing and giving sets.
- All animal patients must be adequately restrained by trained staff (who should also wear protective clothing). Fractious or lively animals may need to be sedated.

Waste Disposal

- Adequate care and preparation should be taken for the disposal of items (syringes, needles etc.) used to reconstitute and administer cytotoxic drugs.
- 'Sharps' should be placed in an impenetrable container specified for the purpose and sent for incineration.
- Solid waste (e.g. contaminated equipment, absorbent paper etc.) should be placed in double sealed polythene bags and incinerated.

In the event of spillage the following actions should be taken:

- Personal protective equipment should be put on.
- The spilt material should be mopped up with disposable absorbent towels (these should be damp if the spilt material is in powder form). The towels should be disposed of as above.
- Contaminated surfaces should be washed with plenty of water.

Individual products vary with regard to irritancy and potential carcinogenic, mutagenic and teratogenic hazard. Data sheets and Health Hazard sheets should be consulted before use of any such agent.

REFERENCES

Averbuch, S.D., Gandiano, G., Koda, T.H., *et al.* (1986) Doxorubicin-induced skin necrosis in the swine model: protection with a novel radical dimer. *Journal of Clinical Oncology*, **4**, 88–94.

Bloom, J.C., Meunier, L.D., Thiem, P.A. & Sellers, T.S. (1989) Use of danazol for treatment of corticosteroid resistant immune-mediated thrombocytopenia in a dog. *Journal of the American Veterinary Medical Association*, **194**, 76–78.

Gregory, C.R. (1995) Cyclosporin. *Waltham Focus*, **5** (1), 29–31.

Holloway, S.A., Meyer, D.J. & Mannella, C. (1990) Prednisolone and danazol for treatment of immune-mediated anaemia, thrombocytopenia and ineffective erythroid regeneration in a dog. *Journal of the American Veterinary Medical Association*, **197**, 1045–1048.

Skipper H.E., Schabel F.M. & Wilcox W.S. (1964) Experimental evaluation of potential anticancer agents XIII: on the criteria and kinetics associated with 'curability' of experimental leukaemia. *Cancer Chemotherapy Reports*, **35**, 1.

Stewart, A.F. & Feldman, B.F. (1993) Immunemediated haemolytic anaemia. Part II. Clinical entity, diagnosis and treatment theory. *Compendium on Continuing Education for the Practicing Veterinarian*, **15**, 1479–1490.

FURTHER READING

Calabresi, P. & Chabner, B.A. (1996) Chemotherapy of neoplastic diseases. Section X. In: *Goodman and Gilman's The Pharmacological Basis of Therapeutics*, (eds J. Hardman, A. Goodman Gilman & L.E. Lambird), 9th edn. pp. 1225–1232. McGraw-Hill, New York.

Carter, S.K. (1987) Principles of cancer chemotherapy. In: *Veterinary Cancer Medicine*, (eds G.H. Theilen & B.R. Madewell), 2nd edn. pp. 167–182. Lea & Febiger, Philadelphia.

Chabner, B.A. & Collins, J.M. (eds) (1990) *Cancer Chemotherapy*. J.B. Lippincott, Philadelphia.

Chabner, B.A., Allegra, C.J., Curt, G.A. & Calabresi, P. (1996) Antineoplastic agents. In: *Goodman and Gilman's The Pharmacological Basis of Therapeutics*, (eds J. Hardman, A. Goodman Gilman & L.E. Lambrid), 9th edn. pp. 1233–1287. McGraw-Hill, New York.

Couto, C.G. (1990) Clinical management of the cancer patient. *Veterinary Clinics of North America, Small Animal Practice*, **20**, 4.

Dobson, J.M. & Gorman, N.T. (1993) *Cancer Chemotherapy in Small Animal Practice*. Blackwell Science, Oxford.

Gorman, N.T. (1986) The use of cytotoxic drugs in the management of neoplasia. In: *Contemporary Issues in Small Animal Practice, Vol 6. Oncology*, (ed. N.T. Gorman), pp. 121–146. Churchill Livingstone, New York.

Gorman, N.T. (1991) Chemotherapy. In: *Manual of Small Animal Oncology*, (ed. R.A.S. White), pp. 127–159. BSAVA Publications, Cheltenham.

Hahn, K.A. & Richardson, R.C. (1995) *Cancer Chemotherapy. A Veterinary Handbook*. Williams & Wilkins, Baltimore.

Hefland, S.C. (1990) Principles and applications of chemotherapy. *Veterinary Clinics of North America, Small Animal Practice*, **20**, 987–1013.

Ogilvie, G.K. (1996) Chemotherapy. In: *Small Animal Clinical Oncology*, (eds S.J. Withrow & E.G. MacEwan), 2nd edn. pp. 70–86. W.B. Saunders, Philadelphia.

Safety

COSHH Regulations (1988) *General Approved Code of Practice for the Control of Substances Hazardous to Health and Approved Code of Practice for the Control of Carcinogenic Substances*. HMSO, London.

HSE (1983) *Guidance Notes MS21 from the Health and Safety Executive*. 1983 Precautions for the safe handling of cytotoxic drugs. HMSO, London.

Hitchings, C.R. (1983) Working Party Report. Guidelines for the handling of cytotoxic drugs. *Pharmaceutical Journal*, 26 February, 230.

Swanson, L. (1988) Potential hazards associated with low dose exposure to anti-neoplastic agents. *Compendium on Continuing Education for the Practicing Veterinarian*, **10**, 293–300.

APPENDIX 1

Body Weight: Surface Area Conversion for Dogs

kg	m²	kg	m²
0.5	0.06	26.0	0.88
1.0	0.10	27.0	0.90
2.0	0.15	28.0	0.92
3.0	0.20	29.0	0.94
4.0	0.25	30.0	0.96
5.0	0.29	31.0	0.99
6.0	0.33	32.0	1.01
7.0	0.36	33.0	1.03
8.0	0.40	34.0	1.05
9.0	0.43	35.0	1.07
10.0	0.46	36.0	1.09
11.0	0.49	37.0	1.11
12.0	0.52	38.0	1.13
13.0	0.55	39.0	1.15
14.0	0.58	40.0	1.17
15.0	0.60	41.0	1.19
16.0	0.63	42.0	1.21
17.0	0.66	43.0	1.23
18.0	0.69	44.0	1.25
19.0	0.71	45.0	1.26
20.0	0.74	46.0	1.28
21.0	0.76	47.0	1.30
22.0	0.78	48.0	1.32
23.0	0.81	49.0	1.34
24.0	0.83	50.0	1.36
25.0	0.85		

Chapter 6

Corticosteroids

A. Nolan

INTRODUCTION

Corticosteroids are among the most commonly used anti-inflammatory drugs. Their therapeutic potential and diversity of action are almost as great as their scope for misuse. Endogenous corticosteroids are synthesised from cholesterol in the adrenal cortex and are released under the influence of adrenocorticotrophic hormone (ACTH). Historically, the corticosteroids may be classified into two groups:

- mineralocorticoids which exert their effects on electrolyte homeostasis,
- glucocorticoids which are both anti-inflammatory and gluconeogenic.

However, this division is not clear-cut and many corticosteroids have relative activity on all three systems. In general, the desired therapeutic effect with the corticosteroids is anti-inflammatory. Thus, the glucocorticoids or their synthetic analogues are the most widely used by the clinician. Unfortunately, it has not proved possible to separate the anti-inflammatory actions of these drugs and their metabolic effects. The adrenal cortex is essential for life, both in maintenance of homeostasis and in response to 'stress', and removal of this portion of the gland will result in death unless corticosteroid hormone replacement therapy is given. The adrenal cortex also secretes androgens, oestrogen and progesterone.

HYPOTHALAMIC–PITUITARY–ADRENAL GLAND AXIS

- Cortisol synthesis and secretion is stimulated by ACTH released from the pituitary gland.

- ACTH secretion is regulated by corticotrophin releasing factor (CRF).
- CRF is released from the hypothalamus and its secretion is influenced by neuronal inputs to the hypothalamus.

Feedback control of this system occurs at two levels (see Fig. 6.1):

- circulating levels of cortisol (hydrocortisone) the endogenous corticosteroid in the dog, inhibit ACTH release from the pituitary,
- cortisol and ACTH also inhibit the secretion of CRF.

This inhibitory feedback mechanism is important clinically because exogenously administered corticosteroid analogues will have a similar suppressive effect on adrenal glucocorticoid production (known as hypothalamic–pituitary–adrenal (HPA) suppression) which, if prolonged, may lead to adrenal cortical atrophy (ACTH is trophic for the adrenal gland cortex).

Production of aldosterone, the endogenous mineralocorticoid, is mainly independent of ACTH stimulation, rather it is under the control of renin and angiotensin. Aldosterone increases sodium retention and enhances potassium excretion.

PHARMACOLOGY OF CORTICOSTEROIDS

Relative Glucocorticoid to Mineralocorticoid Activity

All the corticosteroids have a basic structure, a 4-ring 21-carbon steroid nucleus (a pregnane nucleus, Fig. 6.2). Substitutions made to this molecule alter the therapeutic

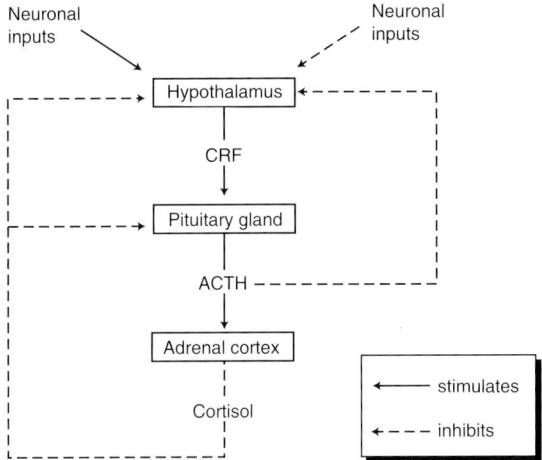

Fig. 6.1 The hypothalmic – pituitary – adrenal axis

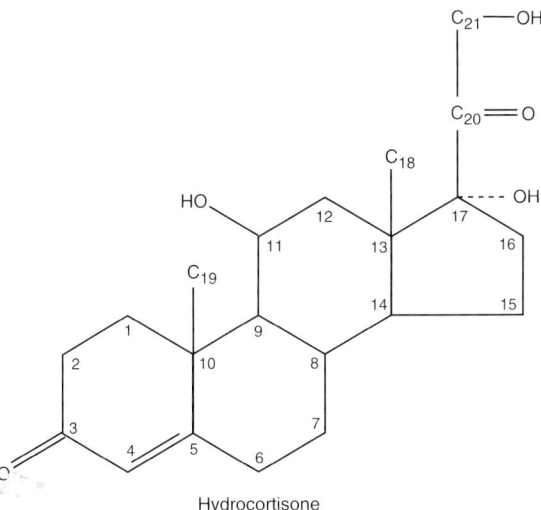

Fig. 6.2 The steroid nucleus

properties of the drug and consequently, glucocorticoids have been synthesised which have, relative to cortisol, increased anti-inflammatory potency but reduced mineralocorticoid effect, e.g. dexamethasone (Table 6.1). The duration of biological effect of these compounds also varies and the figures quoted in Table 6.1 apply following administration of preparations that are rapidly absorbed from their site of administration (see below).

Prednisone and cortisone require enzymic conversion in the liver before they are active, being converted to prednisolone and hydrocortisone respectively. For this reason, prednisolone may be used in preference to prednisone in animals with severe liver disease who require corticosteroid therapy, although the degree of hepatic pathology would have to be severe to restrict metabolism.

Pharmacokinetics of Corticosteroids

Routes of Administration

Topical Application

- Common route for treatment of inflammatory conditions of the skin, eyes and ears.
- Results in high drug concentrations achieved locally at the site of application while reducing the risk of side effects.
- If the animal licks the sites of application, the drug concentration at the site will be reduced and systemic side effects can occur following oral absorption.
- Betamethasone-17-valerate and beclomethasone dipropionate are only poorly absorbed from the gut but have high local activity.
- Drugs may be absorbed from skin in sufficient concentrations to induce HPA suppression, particularly where the preparation is being applied frequently for a long period, e.g. greater than 1 week.

Oral and Parenteral Administration

Most corticosteroids are well absorbed if given orally and are generally administered by this route to dogs and cats on medium or long-term therapy. Parenteral therapy is generally used to initiate a course of short-term therapy although depot preparations with long duration of action are available (see below).

Absorption

Glucocorticoids may be formulated in a number of ways which will confer therapeutically desirable characteristics. They are free alcohols and so they are presented esterified to various compounds which vary in their water solubility and hence their rate of absorption following intramuscular injection (see Table 6.2). Esters are not active themselves and are converted back to the parent compound after absorption. The preparations available for clinical use are shown in Table 6.2. Formulations given by the oral route are usually the free steroid or the acetate ester, which is

Table 6.1 Properties of available glucocorticoid drugs.

Compound	Relative glucocorticoid activity	Relative mineralocorticoid activity	Duration of biological effect (h)	Additional comments and availability of products for veterinary use
Hydrocortisone	1	1	8–12	Identical to natural hormone (cortisol). Parenteral and oral preps are all human products
Cortisone	0.8	0.8	8–12	Metabolised to cortisol to be activated. No authorised veterinary products
Prednisolone	5	0.8	12–36	Oral forms authorised for veterinary use, parenteral forms are human products
Prednisone	4	0.8	12–36	Metabolised to prednisolone. No authorised veterinary products
Methylprednisolone	5	Minimal	12–36	Both oral and parenteral preps are authorised for veterinary use
Triamcinolone	5*	None	24–48	Only long acting parenteral prep is authorised for veterinary use. Oral forms are human products.
Dexamethasone	30	Minimal	36–72	Both oral and parenteral preps are authorised for veterinary use
Betamethasone	30	Negligible	36–72	Both oral and parenteral preps are authorised for veterinary use

* Some authors suggest triamcinolone is 30 times more potent than hydrocortisone.

rapidly hydrolysed in the gut, and the drug is rapidly and effectively absorbed from the gastrointestinal tract.

Metabolism and Excretion

Glucocorticoids are metabolised primarily in the liver where they are reduced and conjugated with glucuronic acid, and are then excreted in the urine. Drugs that enhance hepatic enzyme activity such as phenobarbitone and phenytoin, may increase the metabolism of glucocorticoids (see Chapter 1).

Mechanism of Action and Effects of Corticosteroids

Cellular Mechanism of Action of Corticosteroids

Glucocorticoids exert their effects on cellular metabolism through the interaction with specific hormone receptors located intracellularly. They cross the cell membrane by diffusion and bind to steroid specific cytoplasmic receptor molecules to form a complex which is subsequently translocated into the nucleus where it binds to discrete elements of DNA. These complexes stimulate cell DNA to induce the transcription of specific mRNAs which result in new protein synthesis. There are believed to be 10 to 100 steroid responsive genes in each cell. One example of a new protein produced is lipocortin (more correctly, a family of proteins), which appears to be a specific inhibitor of phospholipase A_2. Inhibition of this enzyme, which catalyses the release of arachidonic acid from cell membranes (see Chapter 7, Fig. 7.1), may be responsible for mediating the anti-inflammatory effects of the glucocorticoids, although this is not the sole mechanism by which glucocorticoids induce their anti-inflammatory effect. As well as switching on the expression of genes, glucocorticoids can also turn off gene expression and therefore inhibit production of proteins, for example, the cyclo-oxygenase 2 enzyme, important in the generation of prostaglandins in inflammation.

Table 6.2 Formulations of glucocorticoid preparations for injection.

Preparation	Duration of action following i.m. injection*	Examples (authorised veterinary products unless stated)
Short acting		
Free steroid alcohols solubilised in a suitable vehicle (polyethylene glycol)	12–72 h (rapid onset of action)	Dexamethasone
Soluble esters sodium succinate sodium phosphate	12–72 h (onset of action within mins)	Betamethasone Dexamethasone Hydrocortisone† Methylprednisolone
Intermediate acting Insoluble esters		
acetate diproprionate isonicotinate phenylproprionate undecanoate	2–4 weeks (slow onset of action) Some products are co-formulated with soluble esters to give rapid onset of action	Betamethasone Dexamethasone Methylprednisolone Triamcinolone
Long acting Very insoluble esters		
acetonide pivalate	>4 weeks (very slow onset of action)	Triamcinolone Dexamethasone

* Approximate guide only, also depends on the vehicle in which the drug is formulated and dose given.
† Only available in human authorised products.

Systemic Actions of Corticosteroids

Metabolic Effects of Glucocorticoids

The corticosteroids have a wide range of physiological actions, particularly influencing carbohydrate, protein and fat metabolism.

Carbohydrate Metabolism. Glucocorticoids are physiological antagonists to insulin in the body, tending to raise blood glucose concentration and cause insulin resistance. Their effects are:

- inhibition of glucose uptake into cells;
- increased formation of glucose from lactate and amino acids (gluconeogenesis);
- simulation of glycogen synthesis by the liver, possibly as a result of increased insulin secretion in response to hyperglycaemia;
- where hyperglycaemia does develop, it aggravates and may even trigger the development of diabetes mellitus.

Protein Metabolism. Glucocorticoids have a general inhibitory effect on cellular protein synthesis and increase the rate of protein breakdown, particularly in muscle. The prolonged conversion of amino acids into glucose by gluconeogenesis accounts for the catabolic effect on proteins and is responsible for reduced growth in young animals on long-term therapy, and decreased wound healing after surgery or injury.

Fat Metabolism. The glucocorticoids promote redistribution of body fat. In the dog, fat is deposited in the lumbar region. Overall, gluconeogenesis favours fat metabolism.

Mineral Metabolism. Glucocorticoids have several actions that result in negative calcium balance and hypercalciuria:

- decrease calcium absorption from the intestine;
- increase calcium excretion by the kidney (reduce tubular absorption);
- increase secretion of parathyroid hormone;
- inhibit osteoblast and stimulate osteoclast activities, mobilising calcium and phosphate from bone;
- block the vitamin D_3 induced synthesis of osteocalcin.

Prolonged treatment with glucocorticoids can lead to osteoporosis particularly in young growing animals. There is a concurrent catabolic effect on bone matrix which is particularly severe in highly trabecular bone such as the vertebrae and ribs.

Water and Electrolyte Balance. An effect of glucocorticoids which is often evident when these drugs are used clinically is an increase in urine production and consequently an increase in thirst. These drugs affect renal concentrating mechanisms by:

- inhibiting the secretion of antidiuretic hormone (ADH);
- reducing the responsiveness of the kidney to the effects of ADH.

Most of the synthetic glucocorticoids do have some affinity for mineralocorticoid receptors and thus enhance potassium excretion and reduce sodium excretion by the kidney to a degree.

Anti-Inflammatory and Immunosuppressive Actions of Glucocorticoids

The most important clinical effect of glucocorticoid therapy is on inflammation and the anti-inflammatory effects are complex. Glucocorticoids suppress:

- early (acute) inflammatory process – i.e. dilation of capillaries, oedema formation and migration of polymorphs;
- later stages of inflammation – i.e. proliferation of fibroblasts and deposition of collagen (repair of tissue damage).

It is important to recognise that both stages of inflammation are affected and that as well as suppressing the heat, pain and swelling of inflammation glucocorticoids also:

- reduce the amount of scar tissue formed after injury;
- decrease the strength and increase the possibility of wound breakdown;
- slow healing.

Glucocorticoids inhibit many humoral and cellular elements of the inflammatory response. For example:

- Humoral responses – glucocorticoids inhibit the formation of:
  - prostaglandins,
  - leukotrienes,
  - platelet activating factor,
  - cytokines (e.g. interleukins),
  - complement components.
- Cellular responses – glucocorticoids inhibit:
  - migration of neutrophils and macrophages into

tissues, preventing their adherence to vascular endothelium,
  - ability of phagocytes to generate oxygen free radicals,
  - ability of macrophages to kill organisms they phagocytose,
  - clonal expansion of T and B lymphocytes,
  - activity of fibroblasts reducing fibrosis and wound healing.

Glucocorticoids reduce the numbers of circulating lymphocytes (in particular T lymphocytes), eosinophils, monocytes and basophils and therefore suppress cell-mediated immunity (see Chapter 5). They reduce the migration of lymphocytes and monocytes to inflammatory sites and reduce granulocyte adhesion to vascular endothelium in response to inflammatory stimuli. Although this may be a clinical asset in the prevention of graft rejection and in the treatment of auto-immune disease, it suppresses the resistance of animals to parasitic, bacterial and viral infections. The numbers of circulating neutrophils increase following glucocorticoid administration because:

- the survival time for neutrophils is increased,
- the margination pool of neutrophils is reduced (more are circulating),
- the release of mature neutrophils from bone marrow is accelerated.

In theory, glucocorticoids could potentially reduce the immunogenic response to vaccination, however, studies in dogs treated with prednisone indicated that the dogs responded well to vaccination. However, immunosuppression will depend on the dose and type of glucocorticoid used and consequently, it is not recommended to vaccinate animals receiving glucocorticoids or within 4 weeks of such therapy.

Other Desirable Effects of Glucocorticoids

Glucocorticoids have an antitumour effect, distinct from their anti-inflammatory action and are used in the management of malignant haematological neoplasia.

Some steroids possess sedative properties, the best known of which is probably alphaxalone/alphadolone (a progesterone derivative) and it may be that the glucocorticoids affect CNS function. This might explain the sense of well-being or euphoria experienced in humans treated with glucocorticoids and the dramatic if temporary improvement often observed in sick animals after treatment. Reports of anxiety and aggression in humans undergoing treatment with corticosteroids have been documented and similar observations of aggressive behaviour have been made anecdotally in dogs undergoing high dose glucocorticoid therapy.

Mineralocorticoid Effects

Corticosteroids with mineralocorticoid activity, which include all of them to some degree but particularly hydrocortisone, cortisone, 11-deoxycorticosterone and fludrocortisone, act on the distal tubule of the kidney, mimicking the effect of the natural hormone, aldosterone, to promote retention of sodium and water and excretion of hydrogen and potassium ions.

PRINCIPLES OF CORTICOSTEROID THERAPY

It is imperative to remember that treatment with the corticosteroids is purely palliative except where there is a primary adrenal cortical insufficiency. Before treating an animal with corticosteroids, certain questions should be addressed:

- How serious is the underlying disease?
- How long will therapy be required?
- Does the animal have a pre-existing condition that will predispose it to side effects?

For most therapeutic purposes, a compound with minimal mineralocorticoid activity is preferred, in order to minimise side effects unless using corticosteroids as replacement therapy for adrenal insufficiency where hydrocortisone may be appropriate in the acute crisis, providing both glucocorticoid and mineralocorticoid effects in a preparation which can be given intravenously (see below for further detail).

The more potent and long-acting compounds are associated with greater risk of toxicity. Thus, dexamethasone, betamethasone and triamcinolone are associated with more severe side effects than shorter acting, less potent compounds such as prednisolone.

Clinical Indications for Glucocorticoid Therapy

Glucocorticoid drugs are indicated for the following problems in small animal veterinary medicine:

- replacement therapy in hypoadrenocorticism;
- diagnostic testing for hyperadrenocorticism;
- suppression of acute inflammation where the inflammatory response may cause serious damage to the tissues;

- suppression of chronic inflammatory disease where the underlying cause cannot be addressed or ascertained;
- management of immune-mediated disease;
- treatment of hypercalcaemia once the underlying cause has been identified;
- as part of a cytotoxic drug therapy protocol for malignant lymphoma, multiple myeloma and mast cell tumours;
- treatment of central nervous system oedema (neoplasia and trauma);
- treatment of circulatory shock (endotoxaemic shock in particular).

Although in many of the above situations glucocorticoids are being used as palliative rather than curative therapy, their use is of great value in the control of these diseases and in some cases they can be life-saving. The indications have been listed in approximate order of the dose of glucocorticoid generally required in each case, which may vary from one individual animal to the next.

Selection of Appropriate Drug and Formulation

In deciding which drug and which formulation should be used it is necessary to consider the following:

- Is the duration of therapy likely to be short term or long term?
- Is an immediate onset of action necessary?
- Is additional mineralocorticoid action desirable or undesirable?
- What is the most practical route of administration for the animal concerned?

Short-Term Therapy

Acute conditions which benefit from short-term glucocorticoid treatment may only require one dose. The most appropriate choice in these situations would be the drugs with the long duration of action (betamethasone and dexamethasone) administered in a formulation which gives a rapid onset of action (soluble esters or the free steroid), usually by intravenous injection as most of the indications for short-term therapy require an immediate onset of effect. Orally administered drugs will be rapidly absorbed and should produce their effects as rapidly as intramuscular or subcutaneous injections of soluble formulations. Indications for short-term therapy include:

- anaphylactic reactions;
- circulatory shock (particularly endotoxaemic shock);

- CNS trauma or oedema of other causes (e.g. neoplasia);
- prevention of post-surgical oedema (e.g. following airway surgery);
- emergency management of severe hypercalcaemia;
- management of acute moist dermatitis (hot spots).

In general, with short-term usage of glucocorticoids, the adverse effects discussed below are not considered to be a problem.

Long-Term Glucocorticoid Therapy

With long-term therapy adverse effects of glucocorticoids are a major consideration. These can be predicted from the actions of glucocorticoids discussed above and in the choice of agent and its formulation for long-term therapy we are primarily concerned with limiting adverse effects. The practicalities of long-term dosing mean that either the oral route or topical administration are chosen.

The principles that are followed in the situations where long-term glucocorticoid therapy is necessary are:

- once the condition you are treating is brought under control, find the lowest possible effective dose of glucocorticoid;
- administer this dose with the longest possible inter-dosing interval;
- consider other additional treatments which may lower the dose of glucocorticoid necessary;
- re-evaluate the animal on a regular basis to detect complications of therapy or concomitant disease which may lead to failure of therapy.

The most suitable glucocorticoid drugs for long-term therapy are those with an intermediate duration of biological effect (e.g. prednisolone). If these drugs can be used on an every-other-day basis, the long-term complications which can occur with glucocorticoid therapy tend to be much less severe. In theory, dosing every 48 h with a drug whose biological effect lasts a maximum of 36 h leaves the body at least 12 h between each dose to recover from the effects of the drug. This is particularly true of the effects of HPA axis suppression which can lead to severe adrenal cortical atrophy with long-term continuous glucocorticoid dosing. This scheme works because glucocorticoids tend to have a longer anti-inflammatory effect than HPA inhibitory effect. HPA axis suppression has been documented with administration of topical preparations containing glucocorticoids.

Time of dosing of glucocorticoids is often recommended such that it coincides with the peak of cortisol and ACTH secretion. In man there is a definite diurnal rhythm for cortisol secretion and glucocorticoids are recommended to be given in the morning to minimise HPA axis suppression. Currently, it is recommended that dogs are dosed in the morning and cats in the evening to minimise HPA axis suppression although the scientific validity of this suggestion is open to question.

Dose Rates and Dosing Regimes

The dose of glucocorticoid required to treat a particular problem will depend on the nature of the problem. In most inflammatory and immune-mediated diseases, where long-term treatment is necessary, an induction dose will be required for a variable period of time to bring the disease under control, followed by a reduction in dose in an attempt to find the dose rate which keeps the disease under control without giving unacceptable adverse effects (see below).

Dosing Regimens

Each animal should be treated as an individual and dose rates given below should be considered as guide-lines only. Any animal that has received glucocorticoid therapy for more than 24 h should have the dose of glucocorticoid it is receiving gradually reduced rather than abruptly stopped to prevent glucocorticoid withdrawal syndrome due to HPA axis suppression. The severity of HPA axis suppression increases with the duration of therapy and the dose used. Recommendations for dose reduction in inflammatory and immune-mediated diseases are discussed below.

In order that the adverse effects of glucocorticoids should be avoided or minimised with chronic therapy, the lowest dose of oral prednisolone which will control the disease process should be established as soon as possible. Again, only guide-lines can be suggested and individual patients should be managed according to their response.

Anti-Inflammatory Therapy

In general terms, most inflammatory diseases can be brought under control after 5–7 days of treatment at an induction dose rate, but this may depend on the chronicity of the disease. With anti-inflammatory doses, the first stage is to reduce the frequency of dosing. In some very pruritic dogs, the anti-inflammatory effect of prednisolone has been found to wane by the end of the non-treatment day. In these animals, it is possible to start therapy on a daily basis and gradually reduce the dose one day, while increasing it the next, thus converting to an alternate day regimen. Three points should be taken into consideration with alternate day therapy:

- The daily dose must be doubled.
- It must be given as a single dose every alternate day.
- The drug chosen must have an intermediate duration of action – prednisone, prednisolone or methylprednisolone, which suppress the adrenal gland for less than 36 h (as discussed above).

If control is not achieved with prednisolone, it may be worth trying another glucocorticoid provided the animal has been fully evaluated for any factors that would complicate the response to steroid therapy. It should be appreciated that every-other-day therapy with dexamethasone, betamethasone or triamcinolone will still produce significant HPA axis suppression and other adverse effects with long-term administration. Moving to every third day therapy with these drugs is not usually possible without losing control of the problem.

A further step which may be taken to reduce the risk of adrenal hypofunction either after daily or alternate day therapy, is to reduce the dose gradually before terminating treatment. This is done over a period of months in human medicine and allows the adrenal glands time to recover.

Immunosuppressive Therapy

When using prednisolone for immunosuppressive therapy, the same principles as discussed for anti-inflammatory therapy should be followed. The time scale over which the dose can be reduced is usually longer, however, with 10–28 days of dosing at the induction dose rate being required to bring the disease under control. It may be necessary to use other immunosuppressive drugs at this stage to help control refractory cases and reduce the dose of glucocorticoid required (see Chapter 5). Frequent monitoring for signs of recurrence of the disease under treatment should be undertaken as the dose is reduced.

Specific Conditions Requiring Glucocorticoid Therapy (Table 6.3)

Table 6.3 gives examples of inflammatory disorders and suggests dose rates, formulations and routes of administration of corticosteroid which might be used to treat them. These are guide-lines only. Further comments concerning some of these conditions are given in the text below.

Inflammatory Conditions of the Eye and Skin

Corticosteroids are indicated in acute conditions where the inflammatory response is more damaging than the underlying condition, e.g. iritis, uveitis, severe keratoconjunctivitis where the animal may inflict further trauma upon itself by rubbing. However, where there is corneal ulceration, corticosteroids are contraindicated because they delay healing and predispose to perforation of the cornea. In animals suffering from chronic allergic skin conditions or otitis, they give symptomatic relief and by breaking the itch–scratch cycle, they reduce further self-inflicted trauma. In all inflammatory conditions, they should be used in combination with appropriate therapy for the underlying cause and corticosteroids should be withdrawn gradually from the therapeutic regime as early as possible.

Respiratory Distress

Glucocorticoids have been used in many conditions involving respiratory distress. Inflammatory respiratory tract conditions are generally treated with anti-inflammatory doses of prednisolone but higher doses (2–4 mg/kg) may be necessary depending on the condition being treated (e.g. pulmonary infiltrative eosinophilia) and the response achieved. It is however evident that where a pneumonia is caused by infectious agents, the long-term benefit of corticosteroid therapy is limited and may even be detrimental. Where corticosteroids are used in conjunction with antimicrobial drugs to control the inflammatory process associated with bacterial infection, bactericidal antimicrobial drugs are recommended. Antimicrobial drugs that are bacteriostatic (e.g. oxytetracycline, lincomycin, erythromycin) rely on the host's immune system to eliminate the bacteria and theoretically would be less effective if given in conjunction with glucocorticoids.

Management of Circulatory Shock

Two acute clinical syndromes which may respond to corticosteroid therapy are those of shock and cerebral oedema. In both these conditions, large doses of the short-acting soluble steroids, particularly the succinate esters, should be given intravenously. The evidence supporting the therapeutic efficacy of corticosteroid therapy for shock is still sketchy, since most studies pretreat animals before the induction of haemorrhagic or endotoxic shock. The reason for their 'claimed' success in the treatment of shock is not completely clear, but probably reflects improved circulation in small blood vessels which prevents tissue anoxia and the onset of irreversible shock. It is generally agreed that if corticosteroids are to be used, they are most beneficial if given early and in large doses. Dose rates of 15–30 mg/kg methylprednisolone sodium succinate or 5–10 mg/kg dexamethasone sodium phosphate have been recommended in the dog. Methylprednisolone is given as an infusion over 30 min and has a more rapid onset of action, while

Table 6.3   Recommendations for dose rates of glucocorticoids.

Therapeutic aim	Examples of disease states*	Preferred preparation and initial dose	Additional comments
Glucocorticoid replacement therapy	Addison's disease Glucocorticoid withdrawal syndrome	Prednisolone (oral) 0.2 mg/kg per 24 h As above	Used in maintenance phase of the disease, particularly if animal is to encounter stress. In emergency crisis dose as for shock
Anti-inflammatory therapy	Atopic/flea allergic dermatitis	Prednisolone (oral) 0.5–1.0 mg/kg per 24 h	These are standard anti-inflammatory doses for dogs. Reduce dose after 5 to 7 days (see text)
	Chronic/allergic bronchitis	As above	Inflammatory bowel diseases in dogs are generally treated with immunosuppressive doses
Immunosuppression	Immune mediated: anaemia thrombocytopenia polyarthritis skin disease	Prednisolone (oral) 2–4 mg/kg per 24 h	These are standard immunosuppressive doses Reduce dose after 10–28 days according to response (see text)
Cancer chemotherapy	Malignant lymphoma Multiple myeloma Mast cell tumour	Consult individual chemotherapy protocols	Use as part of a chemotherapy protocol – if used alone, glucocorticoids can induce multiple drug resistance in cancer cells
CNS oedema	Brain trauma or neoplasia leading to acute problems	Dexamethasone (soluble prep i.v.) 2 mg/kg per 6 h	Use for 24 h then reduce dose and switch to oral prednisolone if still required
	Spinal cord trauma	Methylprednisolone sodium succinate – 30 mg/kg i.v. per 6 h	Use for 24 h and then stop
Management of shock	Acute trauma and haemorrhage	Dexamethasone (soluble preparation) 5 mg/kg i.v. once	Use of glucocorticoids in shock is controversial. Experimentally, the beneficial effects come from pre-treatment of animals, particularly in endotoxaemic models of shock
	Endotoxaemic shock	Prednisolone sodium succinate 15 mg/kg i.v. once	

* These examples are illustrative and not meant to be an exhaustive list – consult texts on individual disease states for more detailed information.

dexamethasone is given i.v. over 2–3 min and has a more prolonged effect. The action of corticosteroids via lipocortin to prevent the generation of the eicosanoids may also be useful. However, this will take some time to occur, perhaps up to 30 min, since cells generate lipocortin *de novo*. The action of the non-steroidal anti-inflammatory drugs on eicosanoid (prostanoid and thromboxane) production is likely to be quicker and these drugs have proved useful in the management of endotoxic shock (see Chapter 7).

Treatment of Cerebral Oedema

The use of glucocorticoids is well established in the management of cerebral oedema and cerebral reperfusion injury after cardiovascular resuscitation. Large doses of glucocorticoids have been recommended in the management of cerebral oedema. Intravenous doses of 5–10 mg/kg methylprednisolone and 1–3 mg/kg dexamethasone have been recommended and may be repeated every 6 h for up to 48 h, although lower doses of dexamethasone have been reported to be successful. Clearly animals in a shocked state must receive fluid therapy, and ancillary therapy is generally appropriate (i.e. frusemide etc). Methylprednisolone and dexamethasone similarly appear to have beneficial effects in high doses (30 mg/kg and 2 mg/kg respectively) in the therapy of post-resuscitation cerebral ischaemia. They have inhibitory effects on lipid peroxidation which reduce the amount of tissue-damaging oxygen free radicals formed. Moreover, they help to increase cerebral perfusion following a period of hypoperfusion. Methylprednisolone sodium succinate (25–30 mg/kg, i.v. followed by 12.5 mg/kg i.v. 2 and 4 h later and 2.5 mg/kg per hour by i.v. infusion from 6 to 42 h) has been recommended for animals with moderate to severe head injuries and in a shocked state.

Management of Joint Disease

Corticosteroids have been used for the treatment of osteoarthritic conditions and in some cases are considered to be useful. This is certainly the case in animals that are unable to tolerate non-steroidal anti-inflammatory drugs or where there is a significant inflammatory component to the disease. However, since they have osteoporotic side effects, although these effects are not commonly observed in dogs, long-term therapy is ill advised. Local administration by intra-articular injection is rarely indicated, particularly for weight bearing joints, where high concentrations of corticosteroids are achieved locally and predispose to cystic degeneration of bone matrix and cartilage erosions. At low doses, corticosteroids may be useful in the early stages of degenerative joint disease in delaying the osteophyte production and inhibiting degradative enzyme production.

Management of Haematological Neoplasia

Glucocorticoids are used as part of a combination therapeutic regime in the management of malignant haematological neoplasia both for their anti-tumour activity and in the management of the secondary complications of malignant disease such as hypercalcaemia, thrombocytopenia and haemolytic anaemia. Prednisone and prednisolone are the most commonly used drugs and have the advantage over most other cancer chemotherapeutic agents that they do not induce myelosuppression, although there is a risk of iatrogeneic hyperadrenocorticism. Glucocorticoids also have a role in the management of solid neoplasms. Although the mass may not be directly affected, the inflammatory process surrounding the mass is often controlled by glucocorticoid administration.

Management of Hypoadrenocorticism

Emergency therapy of dogs with Addison's disease can be carried out with hydrocortisone sodium succinate, given intravenously by infusion along with fluid therapy until a good response is observed. Doses up to 0.625 mg/kg per hour have been recommended. However, administration of hydrocortisone will interfere with the ACTH stimulation test. For this reason, dexamethasone is sometimes recommended for the emergency treatment of an Addisonian crisis. Most cases of Addison's disease respond well to chronic replacement therapy with fludrocortisone acetate, a synthetic oral mineralocorticoid, alone and do not require glucocorticoid supplementation on a regular basis. However, prednisolone tablets should be readily available to the owner (0.2 mg/kg daily) where the dog may be undergoing any form of stress. These animals should be pretreated with glucocorticoids before stressful veterinary interventions such as anaesthesia and surgery (see Chapter 59).

UNDESIRABLE EFFECTS OF CORTICOSTEROID THERAPY

Toxicity to corticosteroids is probably much more common than is appreciated and has increased in incidence since the longer lasting depot preparations became available. Two main syndromes occur:

- *iatrogenic Cushing's syndrome*, associated with long-term high dosage administration;
- *adrenal insufficiency* associated with the sudden withdrawal of corticosteroid after prolonged therapy.

Iatrogenic Cushing's Syndrome

Iatrogenic Cushing's syndrome has the same clinical features as natural Cushing's disease reflecting excessive corticosteroid levels leading to:

- muscle wasting,
- skin atrophy and hair loss,
- osteoporosis,
- polyuria and polydipsia (interference with the action of antidiuretic hormone).

The risk of inducing Cushing's syndrome is reduced by administering minimal doses of steroid for long-term

Therapeutics

Table 6.4 Some adverse effects of glucocorticoids leading to specific concerns over their use.

Organ/system	Adverse effect	Comments
Cardiovascular	Hypertension	Tendency to cause sodium retention varies with the preparation chosen. Should avoid glucocorticoids in states where this may contribute to the disease process e.g.
	(sodium and water retention and vascular effects)	• Cardiac disease where salt and water retention may precipitate signs of congestion • Chronic renal disease, animals are unable to excrete excess salt and water and tend to be hypertensive and hypokalaemic (esp. cats) • Some forms of liver disease where hyperaldosteronism is already a complicating factor in the disease, leading to oedema formation and hypokalaemia
Endocrine	Insulin antagonism	Glucocorticoids antagonise the effects of insulin on peripheral tissues – subclinical diabetics may become overtly diabetic and clinical diabetics will require more insulin for control
Eyes	Raise intra-ocular pressure	Glucocorticoids do raise intra-ocular pressure with long-term use but may be helpful in the acute phase of some forms of glaucoma where there is also an anterior uveitis present.
	Delay corneal healing	Glucocorticoids are contraindicated in ulcerative keratitis as they delay corneal healing and potentiate infectious agents
Gastrointestinal	Ulceration of gastrointestinal tract	Slow the rate of turn over of enterocytes and inhibit production of cytoprotective prostaglandins. May potentiate the ulcerogenic effects of non-steroidal anti-inflammatory drugs
	Perforation of gastrointestinal tract	Trauma to the spinal cord may predispose to gastrointestinal tract ulceration severe enough to cause colonic perforation. Dogs undergoing spinal surgery are particularly susceptible to this problem
	Pancreatitis	Although controversial, it has been suggested that glucocorticoids can be one of the trigger factors for acute pancreatitis and as such should be avoided in dogs with a history of this problem
	Hepatopathy	Glucocorticoids cause accumulation of glycogen in hepatocytes and also lead to organelle damage with prolonged high dose therapy. Some forms of liver disease with active inflammatory pathology will respond to glucocorticoids, in others glucocorticoids will be detrimental, particularly where there is hepatic encephalopathy (catabolic effects) or ascites (sodium retaining effects).
Musculoskeletal	Arthropathy	There are clear indications for steroid use in inflammatory arthritides but in degenerative joint disease their use is controversial. They inhibit cartilage synthesis, may accelerate its destruction and reduce its proteoglycan content, particularly after multiple intra-articular injections. Their use in degenerative joint disease is reserved for refractory cases to provide symptomatic relief after other treatment has failed
	Osteoporosis	Osteoporosis and vertebral compression fractures occur in man. Less of a problem in dogs and cats but would expect bone healing to be slow and metabolic bone disease to be potentiated in conditions such as renal failure
Nervous system	Behaviour changes	These are not well documented in veterinary medicine. High dose glucocorticoid therapy can cause increased anxiety and aggression in some patients. Anecdotal reports would suggest the same is true of dogs
Reproductive system	Infertility, birth defects and abortion	Glucocorticoids are not recommended for use during pregnancy because of these potential adverse effects

therapy and instituting alternate day therapy wherever possible with glucocorticoids of intermediate duration of action such as prednisolone.

Adrenal Insufficiency After Corticosteroid Withdrawal

Excessive use of glucocorticoids also induces adrenal gland hypofunction and atrophy as a consequence of suppression of the HPA axis by negative feedback. Abrupt termination of prolonged therapy leaves the animal with a poorly functioning adrenal cortex which is unable to respond to stress and may lead to an Addisonian type crisis with vomiting, diarrhoea, lethargy, weakness, hypoglycaemia leading to shock and if no therapy is initiated, ultimately death. This is exacerbated if the animal is stressed. In order to avoid adrenal atrophy, an alternate day dosing regime discussed above has been developed. This regimen allows the adrenal gland to recover on the following day, during which there is no exogenous steroid administration, and thus no negative feedback on the gland.

Other Undesirable Actions

These are shown in Table 6.4.

In summary, the adverse effects of glucocorticoids are best avoided by:

- using the lowest dose of glucocorticoid that is necessary, dosing on an alternate day basis with oral prednisolone if possible;
- monitoring animals on glucocorticoids carefully, not merely increasing the dose when the owner reports that signs of the disease have re-appeared, but examining the animal carefully for new problems which may require different therapy;
- recognising concomitant diseases which will be exacerbated by glucocorticoids and deciding on the risk–benefit of glucocorticoid therapy;

- managing withdrawal of glucocorticoid therapy carefully to avoid iatrogenic hypoadrenocorticism.

FURTHER READING

Behrend, E.N. & Greco, D.S. (1995) Clinical applications of glucocorticoid therapy in nonendocrine disease. In: *Current Veterinary Therapy XII (Small Animal Practice)*, (ed. J.D. Bonagura), pp. 406–413. W.B. Saunders, Philadelphia.

van den Broek, A.H.M. & Stafford, W.L. (1992) Epidermal and hepatic glucocorticoid receptors in dogs and cats. *Research in Veterinary Science*, **52**, 312–315.

Ferguson, E.A. (1993) Glucocorticoids – use and abuse. *Manual of Small Animal Dermatology*, (eds P.H. Locke, R.G. Harvey & I.S. Mason), pp. 233–243. BSAVA Publications, Cheltenham.

Keen, P.M. (1984) Uses and abuses of corticosteroids. In: *Veterinary Annual*, (eds C.G.S. Grunsell, F.W.G. Hill & M.E. Raw), 27th edn. pp. 45–62. Scientechnica, Bristol.

Moore, G.E., Mahaffey, E.A. & Hoenig, M. (1992) Hematologic and serum biochemical effects of long term administration of anti-inflammatory doses of prednisone to dogs. *American Journal of Veterinary Research*, **53**, 1033–1037.

Roberts, S.M., Lavach, J.D., Macy, D.W. & Severin, G.A. (1984) Effect of ophthalmic prednisolone acetate on the canine adrenal gland and hepatic function. *American Journal of Veterinary Research*, **45**, 1711–1714.

Rutgers, H.C., Batt, R.M., Valliant, C. & Riley, J.E. (1995) Subcellular pathologic features of glucocorticoid induced hepatopathy in dogs. *American Journal of Veterinary Research*, **56**, 898–907.

Scott, D.W. (1995) Rational use of glucocorticoids in dermatology. In: *Current Veterinary Therapy XII (Small Animal Practice)*, (ed. J.D. Bonagura), pp. 573–581. W.B. Saunders, Philadelphia.

Zenoble, R.D. & Kemppainen, R.J. (1987) Adrenocortical suppression by topically applied corticosteroids in healthy dogs. *Journal of American Veterinary Medical Association*, **191**, 685–688.

Chapter 7

Non-steroidal Anti-inflammatory Drugs

P. Lees

MECHANISMS AND MEDIATORS OF INFLAMMATION

Acute or chronic inflammation is the fundamental process that underlies many pathophysiological and pathological conditions of mammals. It occurs as the response to noxious stimuli and is one of the most complex and finely regulated responses of living organisms.

Noxious stimuli may be physical, chemical or biological and the latter may damage tissues as a consequence of immunological and microbiological agents or through the actions of a range of endoparasites and ectoparasites. The distinction between these classes of stimuli is of course in some degree artificial, since biological and physical as well as chemical stimuli ultimately mediate their effects through released chemicals, inflammatory mediators.

Inflammatory Processes

The purpose of the inflammatory response is to mobilise the body's defence mechanisms against the noxious stimulus, remove it from the site of invasion and repair damage to the tissues, thus restoring them to normal function. Acute inflammatory processes facilitate the movement of phagocytic cells to the area of the stimulus and direct the microcirculation of tissue fluid from the affected area towards the local lymph node, where a specific immunological response against the invading stimulus will be mounted. Acute inflammation is followed by repair of tissue damage when the invading stimulus has been successfully removed or by chronic inflammation should the stimulus persist. These processes are considered in more detail below.

Acute Inflammation

The cardinal signs of acute inflammation which have been recognised for centuries are:

- heat,
- redness,
- pain,
- swelling,
- loss or disturbance of tissue function.

The microcirculatory events underlying the cardinal signs are:

- arteriolar dilation,
- increased capillary and small vein permeability,
- leucocyte migration to the extravascular space,

all of which lead to the formation of cell-rich oedema fluid. The first mediator of inflammation to be identified was histamine, described in the 1920s as the cause of the now classical Lewis triple response in the skin – a central red area, a surrounding flare and the subsequent weal in the central area of damage. Table 7.1 gives examples of some mediators believed to be important in the process of inflammation.

Resolution of the Inflammatory Response and Chronic Inflammation

Much is now known of the identity and roles of mediators of acute inflammation, whereas much less is known about mediators in chronic inflammatory states. It is, however, crucial to note that the desirable and common outcome of the inflammatory process is removal of the noxious stimulus and restoration of normal tissue function by repair processes. Mediators thought to be important in the repair

Table 7.1   Some mediators that are important in the inflammatory process.

Mediator	Mechanism of production	Contribution to the inflammatory process
Mediators derived from plasma		

1. Complement
    C3a
    C3b
    C5a
	Activation of complement by the alternative pathway or the enzymic splitting of C3 by plasmin and fibrin	C3a – releases histamine from mast cells.
		C3b – facilitates phagocytosis ('opsonin')
		C5a – releases histamine from mast cells, increases permeability of postcapillary venules, attracts white blood cells ('chemotaxin') and activates these cells

2. Kinin system Bradykinin	Formed by the breakdown of kininogen (plasma α-globulin)	Vasodilation (endothelium dependent) Increased vascular permeability Stimulation of pain nerve endings (nociceptive receptors of sensory nerves)
Mediators derived from cells		
1. Histamine	Secreted by mast cells	Arteriolar dilation (direct effect and via the axon reflex caused by stimulation of sensory nerves) – also contracts non-vascular smooth muscle (e.g. to cause bronchoconstriction) Increased vascular permeability (post-capillary venules) Itching (stimulation of sensory nerves) Inhibits functions of most leucocytes but enhances activity of eosinophils

2. Neuropeptides/tachykinins
    Calcitonin gene related peptide (CGRP)
    Tachykinins – substance P (SP)
    Vasoactive intestinal peptide (VIP)
	Synthesised and stored in nerve fibre terminals and released on neuronal stimulation	CGRP and VIP – arteriolar dilation
		SP – increased postcapillary venule permeability
		SP – activation of neutrophils and eosinophils
		SP – releases histamine from mast cells

3. Prostanoids	Generated *de novo* from arachidonic acid (released from membrane phospholipid) by the action of cyclooxygenase (COX) (see Fig. 7.1)	PGE_2, PGI_2 and PGD_2 are potent vasodilators in their own right and are synergistic with other inflammatory mediators PGE_2, PGI_2 and PGD_2 do not affect vascular permeability directly but by their arteriolar dilator action potentiate the actions of bradykinin and histamine PGE_2, PGI_2 and PGD_2 sensitise afferent C fibres to the actions of bradykinin and histamine (hyperalgesia) PGE_2 is implicated in the production of fever, mediating the effects of interleukin 1 on the hypothalamus
4. Leukotrienes	Generated *de novo* from arachidonic acid (released from membrane phospholipid) by the action of 5-lipoxygenase (5-LO; see Fig. 7.1)	LTB_4 causes adherence, chemotaxis and activation of neutrophils, eosinophils and monocytes, increases cytokine production by lymphocytes and macrophages and induces arteriolar vasodilation LTC_4, LTD_4 and LTE_4 increase postcapillary venule permeability, induce contraction of bronchial smooth muscle and increase bronchial mucus secretion LTE_4 activates eosinophils

Table 7.1 (*Continued*).

Mediator	Mechanism of production	Contribution to the inflammatory process
5. Platelet activating factor (PAF)	Generated *de novo* from action of phospholipase A_2 which releases lysoPAF (and arachidonic acid), which is acetylated to form PAF	Vasodilation Increased postvenular permeability Chemoattractant for neutrophils and macrophages Spasmogen for bronchial and gastrointestinal smooth muscle Sensitises pain nerve endings (hyperalgesic effect)
6. Nitric oxide	A free radical gas, generated *de novo* by activated macrophages which express the inducible form of nitric oxide synthase when stimulated by cytokines	Vasodilation Involved in macrophage mediated cell killing processes Possible role in cartilage matrix turnover
7. Neutral proteases and oxygen free radicals	Released by neutrophils when they are activated to secrete their products or form toxic oxygen radicals within tissue fluids	Neutral proteases and oxygen free radicals should not normally be released from the neutrophil. Under some circumstances their release into the tissues occurs inappropriately and results in tissue damage during inflammation
8. Cytokines Interleukins (1–10) Tumour necrosis factor Interferon-γ Transforming growth factor β Platelet derived growth factors β-chemokines	Peptides produced by macrophages and lymphocytes predominantly but also other cell types. Synthesised *de novo* on cell activation	Cytokines form a complex network of mediators, the functions of which are not yet fully understood. They are responsible for activating inflammatory cells, transmitting signals between lymphocytes and phagocytic cells and thus co-ordinating innate responses to foreign stimuli with specific immune responses. IL-1 is an endogenous pyrogen, causing swelling, leucocyte adherence and the breakdown of proteoglycans in cartilage. Some of cytokines initiate tissue healing processes which repair damage to the tissues, while others limit the spread of viral infections

processes include the cytokines, platelet derived growth factor, transforming growth factor and various fibroblast growth factors. If the inflammatory stimulus persists (e.g. persistent infections, allergic conditions where exposure to the allergen cannot be prevented, chronic autoimmune conditions), the processes of tissue destruction and local proliferation of cells and connective tissue proceed together to produce chronic inflammation. Cell types involved in chronic inflammatory reactions are typically mononuclear with greatly increased activity of fibroblasts and angiogenesis (growth of new blood vessels) occurring.

PHARMACOLOGY OF NON-STEROIDAL ANTI-INFLAMMATORY DRUGS

Clinically the use of anti-inflammatory drugs may be justified and even essential for the relief of inflammatory pain or the suppression of persistent or overwhelming (even life-threatening) responses. However, the clinician should recognise the basic protective nature of inflammation and the potential for inhibiting the final, reparative stages. Such inhibition is, for example, characteristic of steroids but not of NSAIDs.

Of fundamental importance to the inflammatory process and to the actions of NSAIDs is the arachidonic acid cascade (Fig. 7.1). Arachidonic acid is a 20-carbon unsaturated fatty acid component of cell membrane phospholipid where it exists in esterified form. Inflammatory stimuli cause the release of endogenous peptides, called lipocortins, which activate phospholipase A_2, an enzyme which de-esterifies arachidonic acid. The free acid serves as a substrate for both cyclo-oxygenase (COX) and 5-lipoxygenase (5-LO) enzymes. By further enzyme action these pathways lead, respectively, to prostanoids (PGE$_2$, PGI$_2$, PGD$_2$ and TxA$_2$) and leukotrienes (LTB$_4$, LTC$_4$, LTD$_4$ and LTE$_4$). Both sub-groups of eicosanoids are inflammatory mediators (Table 7.1). As discussed later, the principal mechanism of action of NSAIDs is inhibition of COX. They thereby blunt both the pain and microvascular components of the inflammatory response, although experimental animal studies suggest that higher doses are generally required to inhibit oedema formation than to produce analgesia.

Box 7.1 Summary of the inflammatory process.

- Inflammation is the integrated manifestation of an intricate network of tissues, systems, cells and mediators involving endocrine, paracrine, autocrine and neural components.
- Inflammatory mediators include cytokines, eicosanoids, other lipid mediators such as platelet activating factor, adhesion molecules, nitric oxide, leucocytic and tissue derived enzymes, oxygen free radicals and components of the complement cascade (see Table 7.1).
- The identity of many mediators and systems contributing to the inflammatory response is now established, but there is little doubt that other mediators remain to be discovered by future researches, particularly those of importance in chronic inflammation.
- The cell types involved and the temporal sequence in which mediators are released as well as the manner in which they interact to inhibit or enhance the effects of other mediators will undoubtedly provide a basis for future advances in our understanding of inflammatory mechanisms.

Development of NSAIDs

Salicylic acid, as the sodium salt, was the first synthetic NSAID to be used clinically and this was followed by the introduction of acetylsalicylic acid (aspirin) in 1897. Phenylbutazone was introduced into human and veterinary therapeutics in the 1950s. Since these early developments, there has been a great expansion in the number of compounds synthesised and introduced into human therapy, and several compounds are now authorised for use in canine therapeutics.

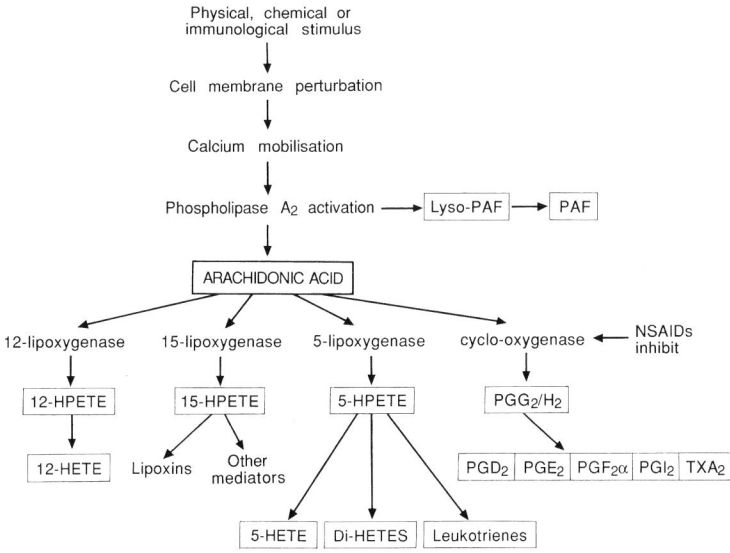

Fig. 7.1 Arachidonic acid cascade illustrating production of inflammatory mediators, indicating site of action of NSAIDs as inflammatory mediators.

Classification of NSAIDs

NSAIDs are classified on the basis of chemical structure into two principal groups: carboxylic acids (R-COOH) and enolic acids (R-OH). Both groups are further divided into several sub-groups on the basis of detailed chemical structures (Table 7.2).

The 2-arylpropionic acid group of NSAIDs (profens) are of particular interest since three compounds (carprofen, ketoprofen and vedaprofen) have been developed relatively recently for canine use. They are characterised by the presence of a centre of asymmetry and are therefore chiral compounds. They are marketed as racemic (50:50) mixtures of the two optical isomers. Several profens undergo a unique type of metabolic chiral inversion, which normally is unidirectional with the (R)-enantiomer being converted into the (S)-enantiomer. However, a few instances of (S)- to (R) inversion have been reported, for example 2-phenylpropionic acid and oxindanac. Bioinversion of profens can take place in several organs and tissues (kidney, liver, lung, fat and muscle) but the liver is the major organ involved. The (S)-enantiomers of profens are widely regarded as the active enantiomers, when the effect considered is inhibition of COX. The potency ratio is strongly in favour of the (S)-enantiomer. In in vitro studies, values of 1:100 or greater are common. However, results from in vivo studies are less conclusive and there are reports suggesting equal potency of the enantiomers in vivo. In most cases this is due to chiral inversion of $R(-)$ to $S(+)$ profens.

Mechanisms and Sites of Action

The actions of NSAIDs have been attributed, following the classical studies of Vane (1971) and Smith and Willis (1971), to their capacity to inhibit prostaglandin (PG) endoperoxide synthase (cyclo-oxygenase; COX). However, several additional mechanisms of action have been proposed (Table 7.3) and, in recent years, the existence of two isoforms of COX has been a major discovery.

Cyclo-oxygenase-1 (COX-1)

COX is a membrane bound haemoprotein and glycoprotein, present in the endoplasmic reticulum of prostanoid-forming cells. It both cyclises arachidonic acid and adds a 15-hydroperoxy group to form PGG_2. It is constitutively expressed as COX-1 in most tissues and blood platelets. COX-1 is involved in cellular 'housekeeping' functions, such as regulating vascular homeostasis, gastroprotection, renoprotection and co-ordination of the actions of circulating hormones.

Table 7.2 Chemical classification of NSAIDS.

Carboxylic acids (R—COOH)	Enolic acids (R—COH)
Salicylates	Pyrazolones
Sodium salicylate‡	Phenylbutazone*
Acetylsalicylic acid*	Oxyphenbutazone§
Quinolines	Dipyrone†
Cinchophen*	Isopyrin (ramifenazone)†
Propionic acids	Oxicams
Carprofen*	Meloxicam*
Ketoprofen*	Piroxicam
Vedaprofen*	Tenoxicam
Naproxen	
Ibuprofen	
Flurbiprofen	
Oxindanac	
Anthranilic acids	
Flunixin*	
Tolfenamic acid*	
Clonixin	
Meclofenamic acid†	
Mefenamic acid	
Indolines	
Indomethacin	

* Drugs licensed for canine use.
† Drugs licensed for veterinary but not canine use.
‡ Also a metabolite of acetylsalicylic acid.
§ Also a metabolite of phenylbutazone.

Table 7.3 NSAIDs: mechanisms of action.

Inhibition of cyclo-oxygenase in the arachidonic acid cascade

In addition some drugs:
- inhibit 5-lipoxygenase in the arachidonic acid cascade,
- inhibit actions of eicosanoids on their receptors,
- inhibit actions of bradykinin,
- inhibit release of lysosomal and non-lysosomal tissue degrading enzymes,
- modulate release/secretion of cytokines, e.g. IL-1,
- inhibit neutrophil chemotaxis,
- inhibit neutrophil activation preventing:
  - release of enzymes, e.g. β-glucuronidase,
  - release of free radicals, e.g. superoxide,
- modulate synthesis of nitric oxide,
- inhibit signal transduction mechanisms.

Cyclo-oxygenase-2 (COX-2)

COX-2 is an inducible isoform of the enzyme, encoded by a different gene from COX-1. COX-2 shares 62% of the amino acid sequence of the constitutive enzyme. Its biosynthesis is stimulated by serum, growth factors, some cytokines and lipopolysaccharides. COX-2 is also induced by mitogens and mediators of inflammation and its expression is inhibited by glucocorticoids (which do not inhibit COX-1). COX-2 produces the prostanoids involved in inflammation. There is therefore considerable current interest in the development of specific COX-2 inhibitors (see below).

Non-COX Mechanisms of Action

Several other actions of NSAIDs, independent of COX inhibition, have been described. For example, some modify the oxidative burst induced by a range of stimuli in neutrophils. They may also inhibit β-glucuronidase release (a marker of neutrophil activation) from neutrophils and from synoviocytes. A disruptive action of NSAIDs on molecular interactions within the cell plasmalemma and an interruption of signal transduction at guanosine triphosphate (GTP) binding protein or G protein levels have also been proposed as possible mechanisms of action.

Some fenamate NSAIDs inhibit not only the synthesis of inflammatory prostanoids but also their actions on prostanoid receptors while other NSAIDs of several groups inhibit 5-LO to block the synthesis of leukotrienes *in vitro*, although this action has not generally been demonstrated with clinical dose rates *in vivo*. In addition to their peripheral actions at sites of inflammation, it has been reported that salicylates injected into the lateral cerebral ventricle can inhibit peripheral inflammation in rats, and that this action is not due to systemic penetration of the drug. Moreover, the centrally mediated (spinal) analgesic effect of NSAIDs has also recently been better defined. The several non-COX actions of NSAIDs described are not shared by all drugs, even within the same chemical sub-group and the extent to which they contribute to therapeutic effects is not known. Carprofen is possibly unique amongst NSAIDs used commonly in canine medicine, in that therapeutic dose rates in the dog do not inhibit either COX-1 or COX-2 and its mechanism of action is unknown.

Pharmacokinetics of NSAIDs

The important pharmacokinetic properties of NSAIDs are summarised in Table 7.4.

Absorption

In general NSAIDs are well absorbed after intramuscular, subcutaneous and oral administration in the dog; values for bioavailability approaching 100% have been reported for orally administered flunixin and ketoprofen in dogs. Because NSAIDs are weak acids (pK_a = 3.0–5.5), absorption from the canine stomach is facilitated by diffusion (ionic) trapping from acidic gastric juice, the pH of which may be as low as 1.0 (Fig. 7.2). Although conditions in the small intestine are less favourable (less acidic) for absorption, the surface area is much greater, so that efficient absorption continues, since the non-ionised forms of most NSAIDs are lipophilic.

Distribution

Most NSAIDs are highly bound to plasma protein (in most cases binding is in excess of 95% and sometimes greater than 99%; see Chapter 1). High protein binding limits passage from plasma into interstitial fluid. Hence, the volume of distribution is, in general, low and values of 0.3 l/kg or less are common. However, a high volume of

Table 7.4 General pharmacokinetic properties of NSAIDs.

Property	Consequence
Marked species variation in elimination half-life	Cannot transpose pharmacokinetic data between species Dosage schedules must be established separately for each species
High degree (>99%) of binding to plasma proteins	Low volume of distribution (Vdarea, Vdss) Tendency to accumulate at sites of inflammation
Well absorbed from intramuscular and subcutaneous injection sites	Bioavailability approaches 100%
Well absorbed from gastrointestinal tract	Absorption from stomach favoured by diffusion trapping as a consequence of acid pH; bioavailability generally exceeds 80%

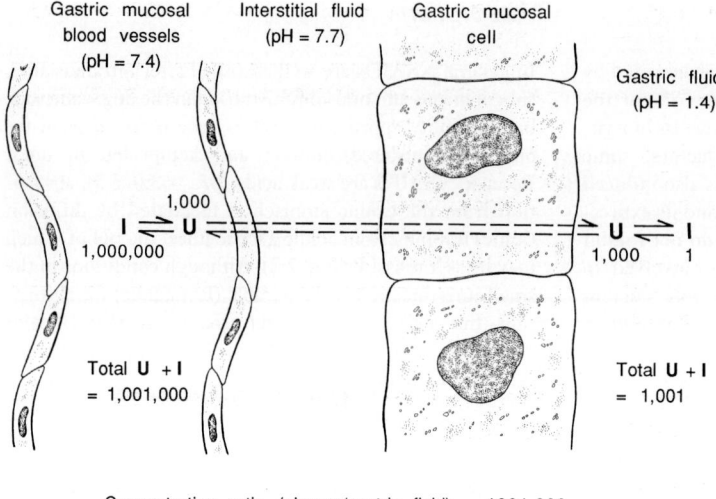

Gastric mucosal   Interstitial fluid   Gastric mucosal
blood vessels   (pH = 7.7)   cell
(pH = 7.4)

Gastric fluid
(pH = 1.4)

1,000
I ⇌ U ══════════════════ U ⇌ I
1,000,000   1,000   1

Total **U** + **I**   Total **U** + **I**
= 1,001,000   = 1,001

Concentration ratio (plasma/gastric fluid) = $\dfrac{1001,000}{1,001}$

= 1,000 : 1

Fig 7.2   Facilitation of absorption of NSAIDs from an acidic medium (gastric juice) into the circulation by diffusion (ionic) trapping (U = unionised; I = ionised).

distribution has been reported for tolfenamic acid in dogs. The reason for this is not clear but it could be a consequence of the presence of an enterohepatic circulation, as established for indomethacin in the dog.

For the clinician, an advantage of the high degree of plasma protein binding of NSAIDs is the resulting accumulation in inflammatory exudate. Since exudate is rich in extravasated plasma protein, the attachment of NSAIDs to this protein will facilitate penetration into and persistence at the desired site of action. This is reflected in a slower rate of elimination of drugs from this fluid compared with their rate of elimination from plasma. The ready penetration into and persistence in exudate is a likely explanation for the maintained efficacy of these drugs when plasma concentrations have decreased to low levels. It is also a likely explanation of the fact that NSAIDs with relatively short half-lives in the dog (e.g. flunixin, ketoprofen, tolfenamic acid, phenylbutazone) are usually clinically effective with once daily dosing schedules. However, an additional factor determining duration of effect is the negative hysteresis (delay in onset of action) reported for NSAIDs; experimental studies have shown that the time of maximal inhibition of PGE_2 in inflammatory exudate occurs some time after peak drug concentrations occur.

Elimination

Since all commonly used NSAIDs are weak acids, their elimination by the kidney will depend on urine pH. Ionic (diffusion) trapping in urine pH will favour excretion in herbivorous species (horses and ruminants) in which urinary pH is alkaline relative to omnivores and carnivores (dogs and cats) in which species urine is generally acid. In the dog urine pH can be as low as 4.5. The acidic urine of the dog suppresses ionisation and the unionised moiety, being lipid soluble, will be readily absorbed into peritubular capillaries. In addition, the high degree of plasma protein binding of NSAIDs will greatly limit their penetration into glomerular ultrafiltrate in the first instance. Together, these two factors (protein binding and acidic urine) combine to ensure that only small fractions of the administered dose of most NSAIDs are excreted in unchanged form in canine urine. Although relatively little published data are available, it is likely that most NSAIDs are eliminated by hepatic biotransformation to less active (or inactive) metabolites. Some drugs, including aspirin and phenylbutazone, on the other hand, are converted to active metabolites (salicylate and oxyphenbutazone, respectively). In the case of aspirin the initial de-acetylation is, in part, spontaneous, so that the parent compound has a half-life of several minutes only. It is believed that salicylate accounts for most of the analgesic and anti-inflammatory properties of aspirin, whereas aspirin itself provides the anti-thrombotic actions (see page 116). The elimination half-life of NSAIDs varies considerably between drugs and also between species. Half-life values for NSAIDs in the dog are reported in Table 7.5.

Table 7.5 Elimination half-life of NSAIDs in the dog.

Drug	Half-life (h)
Aspirin	0.2
Carprofen*	8–12
Flunixin	3.7
Indomethacin	0.3
Ketoprofen*	3–5
Meloxicam	12–36
Naproxen	35–74†
Phenylbutazone	2.6–6.0‡
Piroxicam	48
Salicylate	8.6
Tolfenamic acid	2.3
Vedaprofen*	13–17

* Administered as racemic (50 : 50) mixtures; half-life values differ for the component enantiomers, the $R(-)$ enantiomers having greater values for carprofen and vedaprofen and the $S(+)$ enantiomer half-life being longer for ketoprofen.
† Breed dependent (shorter in Beagles than mongrels).
‡ Dose-dependent kinetics: elimination half-life increases with administered dose.

TOXICITY OF NON-STEROIDAL ANTI-INFLAMMATORY DRUGS

For most drugs toxic effects are a direct consequence of their mechanism of action as therapeutic agents, and NSAIDs are no exception. Prostaglandins are pleiotropic compounds, whose capacity for synthesis in the body is widespread. They are associated with a wide range of physiological functions, in addition to their role as inflammatory mediators, and inhibition of these functions is the primary basis of NSAID toxicity.

The clinically most important side-effects of NSAIDs in animals are exerted on the gastrointestinal tract. Other major target organs are the kidney, liver, central nervous system and leucocytes (see Table 7.6). The ready availability and extensive use of three NSAIDs, aspirin, paracetamol and ibuprofen, on general sale in human medicine has led to a widespread belief that NSAIDs as a group possess a relatively wide safety margin. This belief is as unwarranted in canine as it is in human medicine.

Table 7.6 Undesirable properties (possible side-effects) of NSAIDs.

- Gastrointestinal irritation leading to emesis and possibly ulceration
- Renotoxicity
- Hepatotoxicity
- Blood dyscrasias
- Inhibition of haemostatic mechanisms
- Delayed parturition

Gastrointestinal Irritation and Ulceration

In early reports the toxicity of NSAIDs on the gastrointestinal tract (irritation possibly leading to ulceration) was attributed to their local/topical actions, leading to increased back diffusion of luminal hydrogen ions into the mucosal tissue. However, the toxic actions of NSAIDs on the gastrointestinal tract occur not only after oral but also after parenteral administration, suggesting that toxicity is not a consequence solely of their topical actions. Early studies demonstrated that ulcerogenic doses of indomethacin reduced prostaglandin (PG) concentrations in the gastric mucosa. In subsequent studies dose-related inhibition of gastric mucosal PG generation, following both oral and parenteral administration of several NSAIDs, has been reported. Since PGs act as local hormones to increase gastric mucosal blood flow, inhibition of this action by NSAIDs is likely to cause ischaemia and thereby contribute to the ulcerogenic action. A further local hormonal role of PGs is the formation of mucus and bicarbonate secretions to provide the viscous alkaline lining barrier which normally limits or prevents back diffusion of acid to mucosal cells. Removal or reduction of this protective mechanism will also contribute to the ulcerogenicity of NSAIDs. In addition, NSAIDs reduce the rate of mitosis at the edge of ulcer sites, creating a futile cycle that prevents healing of the ulcer.

A major role for neutrophils in the development of NSAID-induced gastrointestinal tract toxicity has been suggested, since NSAID administration has been shown to increase the number of leucocytes (mainly neutrophils) adhering to the local vascular endothelium. Moreover, the use of monoclonal antibodies to prevent leucocyte adhesion to the local vascular endothelium impairs the severity of NSAID-induced gastropathy and the gastropathy is also markedly reduced in neutropenic animals. Wallace has proposed that NSAID-induced leucocyte adherence to the vascular endothelium can contribute to mucosal injury in two ways:

(1) If adherence is accompanied by activation of neutrophils this may lead to the release of oxygen derived free radicals and proteases.
(2) Neutrophil adherence could lead to capillary obstruction, resulting in a reduction in gastric mucosal blood flow and hypoxia.

A further hypothesis advanced to explain NSAID-induced gastropathy involves the vasodilator free radical gas, nitric oxide (NO). Suppression of the gastric damage produced by a range of NSAIDs when they are converted to nitroxybutyl- (nitroso-) esters has been reported. The nitroso group acts as a NO donor *in vivo*. The increased leucocyte adherence elicited by NSAIDs does not occur with the nitroso derivatives. In addition, the released NO may, through its vasodilator action, directly increase gastric mucosal blood flow thereby inhibiting NSAID-induced ischaemic hypoxia. Whatever the mechanism of the gastro-protection produced by NO-conjugated NSAIDs, these compounds hold out promise as novel therapeutic agents, although more work is required to confirm and extend existing data on their efficacy and safety.

A second novel means of limiting or preventing NSAID-induced gastrointestinal tract mucosal injury is by co-administration with a cytoprotective E-type prostaglandin. For example, misoprostol, a stable derivative of PGE_1, has been developed as a combination product with diclofenac for use in man. Significant inhibition by misoprostol of the gastric ulceration induced in dogs by aspirin and flunixin has been demonstrated, although to date authorised products for veterinary use containing misoprostol have not been developed.

Renotoxicity

Adverse effects of NSAIDs on the kidney generally do not occur in healthy animals with free access to water, implying that PGs do not have a crucial role in kidney physiology. *However*, inhibition of COX by NSAIDs in:

- sodium depleted animals with decreased renal blood flow and glomerular filtration rate;
- hypovolaemic subjects;
- animals with systemic hypotension;

can precipitate acute renal failure.

Under the conditions listed above, activation of the sympathetic nervous system and of the renin–angiotensin system in the kidney occurs, the latter ensuring that glomerular filtration rate is maintained in the face of reduced renal perfusion pressure. Angiotensin II is a potent vasoconstrictor which may reduce nutrient blood flow in the kidney, particularly to the renal medulla. Local produc-

tion of two vasodilators, PGI_2 in the glomerulus and PGE_2 in the medulla, counteract the vasoconstrictor actions of angiotensin II and noradrenaline, protecting renal tissue from ischaemic damage under these conditions. Blockade of the renoprotective action exerted by increased intrarenal release of PGs in these pathophysiological conditions has been postulated to explain occasional reports of acute renal failure with normal (even single) doses of flunixin in the dog. If the PG inhibition theory is correct, it follows that most other NSAIDs which are potent inhibitors of COX may also cause renal failure in the above pathophysiological circumstances.

Other Potential Adverse Effects

Hepatic dysfunction is uncommon in animals receiving NSAIDs. However, hepatic toxicity has been associated with the use of phenylbutazone in elderly human patients and aged horses, possibly because of prolongation of half-life of the drug in older subjects. In the dog, phenylbutazone administration has been linked to blood dyscrasias but whether this is a dose-related phenomenon or an idiosyncratic reaction is unclear. As far as is known, blood dyscrasias do not occur to other NSAIDs, administered at clinical dose rates to the dog.

Table 7.7 Factors potentially enhancing or predisposing towards NSAID toxicity.

Impairment of drug biotransformation and/or excretory pathways (hepatic and renal disease) leading to raised plasma and tissue concentrations
Administration to dogs with gastrointestinal inflammation or ulceration
Too high and/or too frequent dosing
Concomitant administration of two (or more) NSAIDs at maximum recommended dosage rates
Administration of NSAIDs together with:

- corticosteroids
- agents which compete with NSAIDs for binding to plasma proteins

Administration to neonates *and* elderly dogs at high dose rates
Administration to hypotensive, hypovolaemic, dehydrated and sodium depleted patients or subjects with pathological cardiovascular conditions
Administration with renotoxic anaesthetics, e.g. methoxyflurane

Enhancement or Predisposition Towards NSAID Toxicity

Table 7.7 summarises those factors which could enhance the potential adverse effects of NSAIDs and indicates conditions and circumstances in which particular care is warranted in using NSAIDs.

CLINICAL APPLICATIONS OF NSAIDS

NSAIDs are widely and increasingly used in canine medicine. Their therapeutic properties are summarised in Table 7.8.

The potential advantages of choosing an NSAID for therapy in canine practice over alternative drugs are presented in Table 7.9.

Therapy for Musculoskeletal Conditions

In dogs the most common use of NSAIDs is in the treatment of musculoskeletal conditions. In particular, they are used in older dogs with various arthropathies notably osteoarthritis. The principal objective of NSAID therapy is suppression or abolition of pain (analgesic effect). A second objective in some patients is inhibition of swelling of components of the locomotor system (muscle, synovial and capsular membranes, etc.) (anti-inflammatory or anti-oedematous action). Canine musculoskeletal conditions which are successfully treated, though rarely completely controlled, by NSAIDs include traumatic arthritis, degenerative joint disease, tendinitis and myositis.

Currently there is controversy and uncertainty as to whether NSAIDs, in providing undoubted benefit through their analgesic actions, affect the progression of cartilage degeneration in dogs with osteoarthritis. Both *in vitro* and *in vivo* studies have shown that some NSAIDs, including aspirin, accelerate cartilage loss, while others seem to have no effect and some have even been shown to enhance the rate of cartilage matrix (proteoglycan) synthesis by chondrocytes or cartilage explants in tissue culture. This has been demonstrated *in vitro* for piroxicam and carprofen and, while this might provide the basis for a chondroprotective action *in vivo*, it must be emphasised that:

- some of these data have been generated in laboratory animal species;
- confirmation of reduction of cartilage erosion in canine patients with osteoarthritis is lacking.

The effect on cartilage matrix homeostasis of increasing joint mobility and usage, which the analgesic action of NSAIDs facilitates, is also uncertain. It is possible that increased loading of the joint might lead to an enhanced rate of erosion but a degree of loading is an essential stimulus to normal cartilage turnover. Experimentally, total joint immobility leads to marked thinning of articular cartilage. In the light of these uncertainties, the judicious use of NSAIDs in patients with osteoarthritis is both justified and recommended.

Table 7.8 Therapeutic properties/uses of NSAIDs.

Action	Effects achieved
Analgesic	Suppression of inflammatory pain
Anti-inflammatory	Reduction of swelling and/or leucocyte infiltration
Antipyretic	Suppression of raised body temperature in patients with fever
Anti-endotoxaemic	Suppression of cardiovascular and systemic effects of lipopolysaccharide
Anti-thrombotic (aspirin*)	Inhibition of platelet function in haemostasis
Anti-cancer	Possible future use of drugs inhibiting COX-2
Chondroprotection	Reduced cartilage breakdown through prevention of cartilage matrix (proteoglycan) loss†

* Aspirin (unlike other NSAIDs) inhibits platelet cyclo-oxygenase (COX-1) irreversibly and therefore permanently (for the lifespan of the platelet).
† A property of a minority of NSAIDs; significance for chondroprotection *in vivo* unclear.

Table 7.9 Advantages of NSAIDs in canine medicine.

Possess analgesic, anti-inflammatory, antipyretic and anti-endotoxaemic properties
Available in a range of formulations for oral and parenteral dosing
Unlike other classes of analgesic, produce no CNS depression with clinical dose rates
Unlike corticosteroids not immunosuppressant
Usually well tolerated at clinical dose rates
Tend to accumulate at sites of acute inflammation
Provide pharmacological effects for 12–24 h (or longer) permitting once daily dosing for short or long term use

Therapy of Acutely Painful Conditions

There is increasing use of NSAIDs to control acute pain arising from accident-induced trauma, from surgical pain and in some medical conditions, examples of which are presented in Table 7.10.

Comparative trials have indicated that, in controlling postoperative pain, NSAIDs may be as potent as recommended doses of opioids such as papaveretum, while being longer acting and free from the central nervous depressant side-effects of opioids. There is now considerable interest in pre-emptive analgesia, that is the administration of analgesic drugs as part of the premedication protocol or during anaesthesia, (pre- and peri-operatively, respectively), not only to improve surgical conditions but also in anticipation of the need to control pain postoperatively. It has been shown that postoperative analgesic dose requirements are significantly reduced when pre-emptive analgesia has been provided. For NSAIDs there is the added reason for pre-emptive analgesia that, if administration of the drug is delayed until consciousness has returned, the delay between administration and onset of action and the further delay between achievement of peak levels in plasma and the attainment of maximal response may lead to failure to control pain in the early postoperative period.

Against the use of NSAIDs before recovery from anaesthesia has occurred is the rare but potentially lethal possibility of inducing acute renal failure. As mentioned earlier, if a dog is dehydrated before anaesthesia and/or there is significant blood loss during anaesthesia and/or the actions of anaesthetics and ancillary agents (such as halothone and acepromazine) produce significant hypotension, intrarenal PG release will protect renal blood flow. In these circumstances, normal doses of NSAIDs may adversely affect renal function. Of the drugs with marketing authorisations for canine use, carprofen may be the drug of choice for pre- or peri-operative use. Carprofen is a 'prostaglandin-sparing' NSAID, clinical dose rates do not significantly inhibit either COX-1 or COX-2, its mechanism of action being unknown. It seems likely that carprofen will not inhibit the renal PG pathway at recommended dose rates in the dog. A specific interaction has been described for flunixin and the renotoxic inhalational anaesthetic, methoxyflurane; co-administration of these drugs in the dog produces acute renal failure.

Recommended dosages of NSAIDs for canine use are given in Table 7.11.

Antithrombotic Actions of NSAIDs

All NSAIDs can potentially inhibit haemostatic mechanisms by blocking COX-1 in platelets; this enzyme releases the pro-aggregatory eicosanoid, thromboxane A_2 (TxA_2). However, at clinical dose rates most NSAIDs do not impair clotting mechanisms or prolong bleeding time. This may be due to the fact that COX-1 blockade of TxA_2 production by platelets is balanced by inhibition of COX-1 in endothelial cells, resulting in blockade of release of the anti-aggregatory eicosanoid PGI_2. The action of aspirin on haemostatic mechanisms among commercially available NSAIDs is unique. It acetylates COX-1 covalently and therefore irreversibly, so that it is inhibited for the life-span of the platelet. This makes aspirin the NSAID of choice as an anti-thrombotic agent. However, it is more likely than other NSAIDs to cause or exacerbate haemorrhage at high dose rates.

FUTURE DEVELOPMENTS IN ANTI-INFLAMMATORY THERAPY

The increasing recognition by both veterinarians and pet owners that dogs feel and probably also suffer pain as does man will stimulate both the introduction of more drugs of the NSAID class and the increased usage of existing agents. Novel means of administering these agents can also be anticipated; products containing NSAIDs in formulations applied topically for transcutaneous absorption are available for use in man. Local application to achieve a localised action and thereby minimise the toxic side-effects of NSAIDs will be a logical development in canine therapeutics.

Several new classes of anti-inflammatory and analgesic agents are currently under development. Their use in the dog can be anticipated on the grounds that:

Table 7.10 Medical and surgical conditions which cause severe pain and for which use of NSAIDs might be considered.

Surgical conditions causing severe pain	Medical conditions causing severe pain
Aural surgery	Otitis externa
Anal surgery	Pancreatitis
Orthopaedic surgery	Bone tumours
Upper abdominal surgery	Disc lesions
Oral surgery	Various ophthalmic conditions
	Acute moist dermatitis

Table 7.11 Formulations and recommended dosages of NSAIDs for canine use.

Product	Active ingredients	Formulation	Route of administration	Dosage
Rheumatine™ Aspirin (non-proprietary)	Acetylsalicylic acid	Tablets	p.o.	10–25 mg/kg up to 3 times daily. Thromboembolic disorders up to 75 mg every 3 days
Zenecarp™	(RS)-Carprofen	Tablets	p.o.	2–4 mg/kg daily in divided doses for 7 days then 2 mg/kg once daily
Zenecarp™	(RS)-Carprofen	Injection	s.c. or i.v. injection	4 mg/kg
Finadyne™	Flunixin	Tablets	p.o.	1 mg/kg daily for up to 3 days (repeat once weekly if necessary)
		Injection	s.c.	1 mg/kg daily for up to 3 days
			i.v. (slow)	In endotoxic shock 1 mg/kg up to twice daily for a maximum of 3 doses
Ketofen™	Ketoprofen	Tablets	p.o.	1 mg/kg once daily for up to 5 days
		Injection	s.c., i.m. or i.v.	2 mg/kg once daily for up to 3 days
Metacam™	Meloxicam	Suspension	p.o.	0.2 mg/kg once daily for 7 days then 0.1 mg/kg daily
Naprosyn™ Naproxen (not licensed for canine use)	Naproxen	Suspension tablets	p.o.	Initial dose 5 mg/kg then 2 mg/kg once daily
Companazone™ Phenogel™ Phenycare™ Phenylbutazone	Phenylbutazone	Tablets	p.o.	2–20 mg/kg daily in divided doses up to 7 days, then reduce to lowest effective dose
Feldene™ Piroxicam (not licensed for canine use)	Piroxicam	Tablets capsules	p.o.	0.3 mg/kg on alternate days
Tolfedine™	Tolfenamic acid	Tablets	p.o.	4 mg/kg once daily
		Injection	s.c. or i.m.	4 mg/kg to be repeated once only after 24 h if required
PLT™	Cinchophen (200 mg) + prednisolone (1 mg)	Tablets	p.o.	0.5 to 2 tablets twice daily reducing to lowest effective dose
Buscopan™ compositum	Dipyrone (500 mg) + hyoscine (4 mg)	Injection	i.m. or i.v.	1.0–2.5 ml

Table 7.12   New classes of analgesic/anti-inflammatory drugs and drug combinations.

Drug class or combination	Examples	Potential advantages/uses
NSAID – prostaglandin analogue combinations	Aspirin + misoprostol; Flunixin + misoprostol	Retention of therapeutic properties with reduction of side-effects e.g. gastrointestinal tract irritation of NSAIDs
Nitroso-NSAIDs	Nitrosoketoprofen Nitrosoaspirin	Retention of therapeutic properties with reduction of side-effects e.g. gastrointestinal tract irritation of NSAIDs
Prostaglandin sparing NSAIDs	Carprofen	Possess anti-inflammatory and analgesic properties but less likely to cause gastrointestinal tract irritation and other side-effects
NSAIDs inhibiting cytokine (e.g. IL-1) release	IX 207-887	Possibly wider spectrum of activity with fewer side-effects
Specific COX-2 inhibitors	Nimesulide SC58125 DuP697 L-745,337	Avoidance of most NSAID side-effects through very weak inhibition of COX-1
5-LO inhibitors	BAY Y1015 Lofrin	Inhibition of LT synthesis; of potential value in canine allergic skin and airway diseases and arthritides
Phosphodiesterase IV (PDE IV) inhibitors	Rolipram Ro20-1724 RP73401 CDP840	Increase intracellular levels of cyclic-AMP at sites of inflammation to provide anti-inflammatory effects

- some will retain the desirable therapeutic actions of NSAIDs but possess fewer and/or less serious side-effects;
- some will possess novel modes of action and may therefore be therapeutically superior to NSAIDs or possess fewer side-effects or extend the range of therapeutic indications.

Some of these compounds are listed in Table 7.12.

FURTHER READING

Cunningham, F.M. & Lees, P. (1994) Advances in anti-inflammatory therapy. *British Veterinary Journal*, **150**, 115–134.

Lees, P., May, S.A. & McKellar, Q.A. (1991) Pharmacology and therapeutics of non-steroidal anti-inflammatory drugs. 1. Dog and cat in general pharmacology. *Journal of Small Animal Practice*, **32**, 183–193.

Lewis, A.J. & Furst, D.E. (eds) (1994) *Non-Steroidal Anti-Inflammatory Drugs. Mechanisms and Clinical Uses*, 2nd edn. Marcel Dekker, New York.

McKellar, Q.A., Lees, P. & Getinby, G. (1994) Pharmacodynamics of tolfenamic acid in dogs. Evaluation of dose response relationships. *European Journal of Pharmacology*, **253**, 191–200.

McKellar, Q.A., May, S.A. & Lees, P. (1991) Pharmacology and therapeutics of non-steroidal anti-inflammatory drugs in the dog and cat. 2. Individual agents. *Journal of Small Animal Practice*, **32**, 225–235.

McMillan, R. & Williams, T. (eds) (1995) World Congress on Inflammation, Abstracts. *Inflammation Research*, **44** (Suppl. 33), 5221–5299.

Smith, J.B. & Willis, A.L. (1971) Aspirin selectivity inhibits prostaglandin production in human platelets. *Nature*, **231**, 235–237.

Trevethick, M.A., Clayton, N.M., Strong, P. & Harman, I.W. (1993) Do infiltrating neutrophils contribute to the pathogenesis of indomethacin induced ulceration of the rat gastric antrum? *Gut*, **34**, 156–160.

Vane, J.R. (1971) Inhibition of prostaglandin synthesis as a mechanism of action for aspirin-like drugs. *Nature*, **231**, 232–235.

Vane, J., Botting, J. & Botting, R. (eds) (1996) *Improved Non-Steroidal Anti-Inflammatory Drugs. Cox-2 Enzyme Inhibitors*. Kluwer, Dordrecht, and William Harvey Press, London.

Wright, V. (1995) Decisions on non-steroidal anti-inflammatory prescribing. *British Journal of Rheumatology*, **34** (Suppl. 1), 1–31.

Section 2

Infectious Diseases

Edited by Malcolm Bennett

INTRODUCTORY COMMENTS

This section aims to cover the essential features of the main specific infectious diseases in dogs. Some other microbial diseases, where the aetiology is more complex than a single infectious agent, will be found elsewhere in the book (e.g. pyometra, page 772, enteric bacterial overgrowth page 501, bacterial skin infections pages 861 and 878). The following is not intended to be a comprehensive microbiology, parasitology or infectious diseases text, but rather to cover the clinical signs and those aspects of the aetiology and patho-genesis of use to the clinician in making a diagnosis and prognosis. For more detailed information the reader is referred to more specialist books and reviews. To avoid cluttering the text, we have also opted for a list of further reading at the end of the section rather than cited references.

The bias of the section is heavily towards those infections most likely to be encountered in Europe, but we have included brief accounts of some of the infectious diseases encountered elsewhere not least because they may be seen in imported dogs. We have also included brief chapters on canine zoonoses, where the infectious agent often causes no disease in the dog, and on the general principles of vaccination and possible causes of vaccine failures.

Chapter 8

Infectious Gastroenteritis

B. J. Tennant

The purpose of this section is to give an overview of the clinical features, diagnosis and control of infectious gastrointestinal disease. There are many causes of acute gastroenteritis, and the precise aetiology is often not defined because of similarities in presenting signs and the interaction of different factors. Treatment is often non-specific, and the clinical management of diseases of the gastrointestinal tract is covered in detail in Section 6.

VIRAL GASTROENTERITIS

The major viral causes of viral gastroenteritis are listed in Table 8.1

CANINE PARVOVIRUS INFECTION

See Chapter 9.

CANINE DISTEMPER

See Chapter 11.

CANINE CORONAVIRAL ENTERITIS (CCV)

Aetiology

Found world-wide, with seroprevalence rates up to 54% in family dogs and 100% in kennel populations. All ages and breeds are susceptible to infection, although younger dogs (6–12 weeks old) appear more susceptible to disease.

After ingestion, CCV infects mucosal epithelial cells overlying the upper two-thirds of small intestinal villi, causing epithelial loss and villus atrophy; crypt cells are unaffected. Colonic and alveolar epithelium, and mesenteric lymph nodes may also be infected. Viral shedding persists for ≥16 days post-infection and virus neutralising antibodies are detected by day 5. Virus may be isolated from dogs with or without diarrhoea.

Clinical Features

CCV infection is predominantly associated with mild or subclinical disease with low mortality rates. The following are the salient features of the disease:

- Incubation period varies from 1 to 7 days.
- Mild, often watery diarrhoea.
- Occasionally, vomiting, depression and anorexia.
- Haemorrhagic diarrhoea, pyrexia and leucopenia are *not* features of CCV infection; but may reflect concomitant infections.
- Spontaneous recovery occurs over 7–10 days, although diarrhoea may persist for several weeks.
- CCV infection of tissues other than the small intestine does not appear to be associated with disease.

Distended intestinal loops and enlarged oedematous mesenteric lymph nodes may be noted post-mortem.

Table 8.1   Viral causes of gastroenteritis.

Canine parvovirus-1 (CPV-1)
Canine parvovirus-2 (CPV-2)
Canine distemper virus (CDV)
Canine rotavirus (CRV)
Canine coronavirus
Reovirus
Calicivirus

Histologically, atrophy and fusion of intestinal villi, deepening of crypts and increased cellularity of the lamina propria may be seen.

Diagnosis

As clinical signs are mild and dogs respond well to symptomatic treatment, confirmation of the diagnosis is not usually attempted. Demonstration of virus particles by electron microscopy or virus isolation is suggestive for a coronaviral enteritis. Viral particles are easily disrupted during prolonged storage, so fresh faecal samples must be submitted immediately for isolation. A rising antibody titre may allow the diagnosis to be made retrospectively.

Treatment, Prognosis and Control

Dietary modification and oral rehydration are all that are usually required. Motility modifiers may be of use when diarrhoea is severe. Young dogs under 12 weeks old may require more intensive supportive therapy. The prognosis is good for a complete recovery. Prevention of CCV disease may be achieved using killed systemic CCV vaccines, available in the USA and certain parts of Europe, but although safe, their efficacy is doubtful. Newer live systemic vaccines are also available and may provide better protection against both disease and virus shedding.

CANINE ROTAVIRUS (CRV)
Aetiology

CRV infection is widespread, with a seroprevalence of 62–84% in Europe. Dogs over 6 months of age appear to be resistant to infection. In neonates, the virus colonises the epithelium on the upper half of the villi in jejunum and ileum causing mild or moderate villous atrophy; crypt cells

are unaffected. The incubation period ranges from 1 to 7 days.

Clinical Features

A mild watery to mucoid self-limiting diarrhoea can develop in puppies ≤4 weeks old, causing significant fluid losses. Supportive fluid therapy is required in such cases. Death due to CRV infection is rare. Diagnosis can be confirmed by the detection of viral particles in faeces by electron microscopy, virus isolation, or polyacrylamide gel electrophoresis. The prognosis for recovery is good. Clinical disease is more likely in overcrowded conditions, particularly where hygiene is poor. There is no vaccine available.

OTHER VIRUSES

Reoviruses have been found in faecal samples from dogs with and without diarrhoea. Their significance is unknown. Caliciviruses have been detected in diarrhoea samples from dogs, although their significance is not yet clear. There are some reports of the possible transmission of the virus from dogs to man. Other viruses have been identified in canine faeces, including a paramyxovirus, a herpesvirus related to felid herpesvirus-1, astroviruses, 'small round viruses' and various enteroviruses (including coxsackie and polio viruses). The clinical significance of these viruses is unknown.

BACTERIAL GASTROENTERITIS

Some of the major bacterial causes of gastroenteritis are listed in Table 8.2.

Table 8.2   Bacteria associated with gastroenteritis.

Campylobacters
Salmonellae
Clostridia
Enterococcus durans
Escherichia coli
Yersinia enterocolitica
Aeromonas hydrophilia
Plesiomonas shigelloides

CAMPYLOBACTEROSIS

Aetiology

Campylobacter spp. can be isolated from symptomatic and asymptomatic dogs at similar frequencies, suggesting that the organisms are not primary pathogens. *C. jejuni* is the commonest species identified and is more likely to be isolated from:

- animals with diarrhoea,
- young animals,
- stressed animals,
- overcrowded animals with poor hygiene,
- animals with other enteric pathogens.

Thus campylobacters may be synergistic or opportunistic in their mechanisms of disease. *C. jejuni* is a potential zoonosis, although the significance of dogs as a source for human infection is unclear.

Clinical Features and Diagnosis

The more common presenting sign is watery or mucoid diarrhoea, this can occasionally be haemorrhagic. Pyrexia, depression, vomiting and anorexia are rare. *Campylobacter* spp. may be detected by dark-field or phase-contrast microscopy. The use of Gram-stain on faecal or colonic smears for early presumptive diagnosis has been reported. As *C. jejuni* are microaerophilic, samples should be placed in anaerobic transport medium, stored at 4°C and processed at the earliest opportunity.

Treatment and Control

The disease is usually self-limiting and rarely systemic, although chronic diarrhoea may develop in some patients. Therapy may not affect the clinical outcome, but may reduce the duration of bacterial shedding. *C. jejuni* is usually sensitive to erythromycin, but the choice of antibacterial therapy should be based on *in vitro* testing. The prognosis for recovery is good. There is no vaccine available but the risk of disease can be minimised by the reduction of the environmental burden with good hygiene.

SALMONELLOSIS

Aetiology

Salmonella spp. are obtained through contact with infected animals or ingestion of contaminated food. Salmonellae may be intermittently isolated from faecal samples over prolonged periods, and from the colon and mesenteric lymph nodes of asymptomatically infected dogs, suggesting a high prevalence of carrier animals; these animals pose a risk to man and other animals. Risk of disease depends upon the bacterial strain, competition from established flora, age of the host, host defence factors and the presence of other pathogens.

Clinical Features and Diagnosis

Salmonella spp. uncommonly cause clinical disease in the dog. The organism may be responsible for:

- acute and chronic diarrhoea of a variable nature; or
- septicaemia, characterised by anorexia, pyrexia, vomiting, diarrhoea, severe depression and death, particularly in neonates and geriatric patients or following a severe gastroenteritis.

Culture of the bacteria from faeces or blood is required for a definitive diagnosis.

Treatment and Control

Patients with septicaemia require:

- Prompt systemic antibacterial therapy (as determined by *in vitro* sensitivity testing). Appropriate antibacterials include fluoroquinolones, potentiated sulphonamides and chloramphenicol.
- An essential part of therapy is intravenous fluid management, full details of which are covered in Chapter 2, page 24. The prognosis is guarded in animals with septicaemia.

For patients with diarrhoea only:

- Antibacterials are of limited value and may promote a carrier status.
- Supportive therapy may be required.
- Dietary modification using highly digestible diets is often helpful.
- The prognosis is good in animals with diarrhoea.

Following the resolution of clinical signs, culture of further samples is recommended to ensure that the animal is not continuing to shed salmonellae. Individuals in contact with infected animals should wear protective clothing and disinfection of the contaminated environment with phenolic compounds or 1:32 Chlorox (sodium hypochlorite) solution should be performed.

CLOSTRIDIAL DISEASES

Aetiology and Clinical Features

Clostridium spp. may be isolated from asymptomatic dogs, but *C. perfringens* and *C. difficile* may cause severe disease in some dogs. *C. perfringens* can be associated with either acute haemorrhagic diarrhoea, or chronic mucoid, large bowel diarrhoea. The disease associated with *C. difficile* is poorly characterised, but the organism may be responsible for severe depression, vomiting and gastroenteritis

Diagnosis

Diagnosis of clostridial diseases is difficult. It may be attempted by demonstration of:

- large numbers of *C. perfringens* bacteria in faecal cultures,
- large numbers of spore forming bacteria in faecal smears,
- *C. perfringens*/*C. difficile* toxin in faecal samples.

Treatment

Antibacterials active against anaerobic bacteria (e.g. amoxycillin, chloramphenicol, clindamycin, tetracycline, tylosin, metronidazole) are useful. Prolonged, sometimes indefinite treatment, may be required. Metronidazole is the preferred antibacterial for *C. difficile*. Where *C. perfringens* causes large bowel diarrhoea, feeding a high fibre diet may resolve the problem by altering the colonic microenvironment.

MISCELLANEOUS BACTERIAL INFECTIONS

Aetiology

Yersinia enterocolitica, *Aeromonas hydrophilia* and *Plesiomonas shigelloides* have been reported to cause acute

and chronic gastroenteritis in dogs, particularly puppies, although *Y. enterocolitica* is more commonly found in pigs and the soil. Several strains of *Escherichia coli* are known to cause severe gastroenteritis in man, but although *Enterococcus durans* and enterotoxigenic *Escherichia coli* have been isolated from puppies with acute diarrhoea, their significance as primary pathogens in dogs is unclear. Recently, colonisation of the stomach by *Helicobacter pylori* has been linked with the development of gastric and duodenal ulcers and gastric carcinoma in man. Gastric *Helicobacter*-like organisms (HLOs) have been described in the dog in association with glandular degeneration, accumulation of lymphocytes and neutrophils, mucosal oedema and lymphocytoplasmic infiltrates. It has not yet been shown whether these bacteria are the cause of such changes.

Clinical Features

Small bowel diarrhoea of variable nature may be associated with any of these organisms other than *Helicobacter*-like organisms. *Y. enterocolitica* may cause colitis whereas *Helicobacter*-like organisms may cause gastritis. All these bacteria may be cultured from faeces; *Y. enterocolitica* requires enriched media. For HLOs, however, isolation should be attempted from gastric biopsy samples.

Treatment

Supportive and appropriate antibacterial therapy (as determined by *in vitro* sensitivity tests) are required. *Y. enterocolitica* is often sensitive to tetracyclines and HLOs to erythromycin. Treatment should be continued for at least 3 days beyond the resolution of signs. Protective clothing must be worn by in-contact people. The prognosis is generally good, although these organisms, in particular *Escherichia coli* and *Enterococcus durans*, may cause death if untreated.

ALIMENTARY TRACT PARASITIC INFECTIONS

Aetiology

Several endoparasites may be associated with gastroenteritis in the dog (Table 8.3).

- The whipworm (*Trichuris vulpis*) is most commonly found in kennels or where dogs are exercised on grass runs. Adults burrow into the colonic and caecal

Table 8.3 Alimentary tract endoparasites.

Roundworms	Tapeworms	Hookworms	Whipworm
Toxocara canis *Toxascaris leonina*	*Dipylidium caninum* Echinococcosis *Taenia* spp.	*Uncinaria stenocephala* *Ancylostoma* spp.	*Trichuris vulpis*

Table 8.4 Clinical features of endoparasites.

Trichuris vulpis	Roundworms	Tapeworms	Hookworms	Coccidia	*Giardia*
Haematochezia Protein-losing enteropathy Diarrhoea, sometimes severe enough to cause hyponatraemia and hyperkalaemia	Poor growth, poor hair coat Poor weight gain A 'pot-bellied' appearance Diarrhoea Intestinal or, very rarely, biliary obstruction	Anal irritation is the commonest sign Heavy infestations may cause intestinal obstruction, or mild diarrhoea *Taenia stenocephala* is generally considered to be non-pathogenic	Tropical hookworms cause severe anaemias May see skin lesions	Often clinically insignificant Where dogs are exposed to large numbers of oocysts, a mild to severe, often haemorrhagic, diarrhoea may develop; blood loss may be marked	May be responsible for a mild to severe diarrhoea. This may be persistent, intermittent or self-limiting The nature of the diarrhoea varies from 'cowpat'-like to mucoid. Melena is not usually a feature Chronic diarrhoea can be associated with weight loss

mucosa, causing inflammation, bleeding and protein loss.

- Roundworms (*Toxocara canis* and *Toxascaris leonina*) are obtained by ingestion of ova directly, via paratenic hosts or transplacentally (*Toxocara canis*). Adults are found in the small intestine. Larvae of *T. canis* migrate through other tissues.
- Dogs are infested with tapeworms when they consume infected intermediate hosts, e.g. fleas and lice for *D. caninum* or wild animals for most *Taenia* spp.
- *Ancylostoma* spp. (warmer climates) and *Uncinaria* spp. (colder climates) infest dogs primarily through ingestion of ova, although transmammary or percutaneous infestation by larvae may occur. Adults are found predominantly in the small intestine.
- Following ingestion of *Isospora* and *Sarcocystis* spp., oocysts invade the intestinal mucosa destroying epithelial cells.
- *Giardia* colonises the small intestine. Giardial cysts are quite resistant to environmental factors and persist for

long periods in the environment, particularly in damp conditions.

Clinical Features

The clinical features of endoparasites are shown in Table 8.4.

Diagnosis

Ova of roundworms, hookworms, *Echinococcus* spp. (eggs of other tapeworms are not usually detected as they are confined to the segments) and whipworms, coccidial oocysts and giardial oocysts may be observed using faecal flotation techniques; multiple sampling is required for whipworms, coccidia and *Giardia*. Coccidial oocysts should not be confused with those of *Giardia* spp. Transplacental migration of roundworms may result in neonatal disease before ova

are produced. Adult worms may be observed endoscopically and tapeworm segments can be seen in faeces.
Giardiosis is particularly difficult to diagnose. Motile
trophozoites may occasionally be found in fresh faeces,
while duodenal cytology and washes can be used to demonstrate the organism.

Treatment and Prognosis

Various anthelmintics available to treat intestinal parasite
infestations are listed in Table 50.14, page 503.

- Pyrantel and piperazine are safe for use in young
  animals infested with roundworms.
- Fenbendazole (50 mg/kg per 24 h) from day 40 of gestation until 2 weeks postpartum reduces the somatic
  roundworm and hookworm burden in bitches and
  reduces transplacental and transmammary migration
  respectively.
- Newborn pups may be treated with fenbendazole 100
  mg/kg p.o. for 3 days to provide a 90% kill of prenatally
  acquired larvae.
- Praziquantel is effective against all tapeworm species
  and is preferred to other drugs (niclosamide and

bunamidine). Control of flea and lice infestations is
required to prevent re-infestations.
- Coccidiosis can be controlled with sulphonamide
  drugs, administered for 3 weeks. Hygiene should be
  improved to reduce exposure to oocysts.
- Metronidazole and furazolidone are effective anti-
  giardial drugs. Where recurrence of infection occurs,
  re-infection or drug resistance must be considered.
  Prolonged therapy may be required in some cases.

The prognosis for recovery from most intestinal parasite infestations is good, although severely stunted puppies
may not attain their adult size.

MISCELLANEOUS CAUSES OF INFECTIOUS GASTROENTERITIS

Histoplasma capsulatum is a fungal agent that may affect the
gastrointestinal tract causing diarrhoea and weight loss.

Prototheca zopfii and *P. wickerhamii* are algae that may
cause colitis. See page 165.

Chapter 9

Canine Parvovirus Infection

I. McCandlish

Virology

There are three distinct canine parvoviruses, the non-pathogenic canine adeno-associated virus, canine parvovirus 1 (CPV-1), also known as canine minute virus, and canine parvovirus 2 (CPV-2) the cause of canine parvovirus enteritis. CPV-1 can be isolated from canine faeces and appears to be widespread in the dog population but is of uncertain and apparently limited pathogencity.

Canine parvovirus 2 emerged in the late 1970s probably in Europe and rapidly spread globally within the next few years. It is a small, extremely resistant virus which may have arisen by mutation from the parvovirus of cats or another carnivore. Further antigenic divergence took place in the early 1980s and the original CPV-2 has largely been replaced by either CPV-2a or CPV-2b. These newer strains differ from the original in certain epitopes defined by monoclonal antibodies but the main neutralising epitopes are still shared so that vaccines based on the original CPV-2 will protect dogs from challenge with CPV-2, CVP-2a or CPV-2b.

Epidemiology

- CPV-2 is the most important virus infection of dogs in Britain. Its success is based on its ability to survive in the environment, up to a year under favourable conditions, and the vast amount of virus excreted from an infected dog.
- Active shedding of virus probably lasts no more than 2 weeks but during that time many thousands of millions of virus particles are excreted. CPV-2 will replicate only in dividing cells and this is the reason for its tropism for lymphoid tissues, the myocardium of puppies less than 3 weeks of age and the epithelial cells of the intestinal crypts of dogs of all ages.
- Since 1981 CPV-2 infection has been endemic in most countries where dogs are kept.

- Most of the adult dog population has now encountered the infection naturally or has been vaccinated against it.
- Transmission is by the faecal–oral route and indirect transmission can be as important as direct contact. In the mid 1980s some 10% of puppies presented for primary vaccination at 12 weeks of age in Britain had already encountered the infection. CPV-2 is now, and will continue to be, predominately an infection of young dogs which have lost their maternal immunity but which have not yet acquired active immunity. More cases of CPV enteritis are seen in the months of August and September as the spring born puppies come of age.
- Most breeding bitches are now solidly immune and provide protection for their puppies *in utero* and via the colostrum for the first few weeks when CPV-2 infection could result in myocarditis.
- Myocarditis is now extremely rare and occurs almost exclusively in the pups of individual, non-immune pet bitches which come into contact with infection at or about the time of birth. One of the most likely ways in which this may arise is the pet bitch which has difficulty in whelping and is brought to a veterinary surgery for a caesarean.

CPV enteritis is the main form of CPV-2 infection. It occurs most commonly in puppies between the ages of 5 and 16 weeks and in this age of dog can usually be linked to the breeding kennel or point of sale. Infection is also common in older unvaccinated pups up to 12 months of age. This type of dog is most frequently found in the shifting urban population and forms the bulk of the strays which pass through rescue centres. Occasional cases still occur in adult or aged animals, usually those which have never been vaccinated and have led very isolated lives until for some reason, e.g. boarding, they encounter infection.

Pathogenesis

- Following oral infection the initial site of viral replication is the thymus (from 1 day post-infection), rapidly followed by other lymphoid tissues. Viral replication in these organs results in lymphocytolysis and depletion. Lysis of infected lymphoid cells results in a lymphopenia and a cell free plasma viraemia (at 3 and 4 days post-infection) which permits localisation of virus to the mitotically active proliferative zones of the intestinal epithelia (from 4–5 days post-infection).
- Destruction of intestinal crypt proliferative cells results in excretion of virus in the faeces and with damage to the intestinal structure the first signs of enteric disease follow shortly.
- The incubation period of CPV enteritis, which is the base mark for many disputes, is 7 days plus or minus 2. It is known however, that low levels of maternal antibody may delay this sequence so that range should be widened to between 5 and 11 days. There is rapid development of the humoral immune response (from 5 days post-infection) and as serum antibody rises so virus is eliminated from the body.

Most of the stages of CPV infection described above, i.e. replication in lymphoid tissue, plasma viraemia, localisation to intestine, virus excretion and antibody response, always take place in the non-immune susceptible host. However the degree of viral damage to the intestinal architecture varies widely, apparently depending on the intestinal crypt mitotic rate at the time of viral localisation. If the mitotic rate is high, extensive damage and severe disease will result: if the rate is low, only limited viral replication with minor pathology and only asymptomatic viral excretion will result.

- Of the many factors that affect intestinal crypt mitotic rate, age, change in diet and the nature of the intestinal flora are probably the most important.
- Clinically significant CPV enteritis is rare in healthy adult dogs and is also unusual in puppies less than 4 weeks of age. In both, the crypt mitotic rate is slow whereas clinical disease is most common in young recently weaned pups with changing diet and variations in intestinal flora.
- The difference between infection and disease is one of the most difficult concepts for lay people to understand. It is not surprising that those breeders who have nine perfectly healthy pups at home find it hard to accept that the tenth puppy which they have just sold and which has died of CPV enteritis within a few days of sale acquired the infection on their premises. An antibody screen of the healthy puppies would confirm that they too have been infected.

The pathogenesis of CPV-2 myocarditis follows a similar pattern. Oral infection of neonate pups results in the same initial phase of lymphocytolysis and viraemia as in older animals but virus localises to the myocardium where, at this time, mitotic activity is prominent. CPV then appears to persist in the heart muscle and by 3–4 weeks of age a non-suppurative myocarditis is developing. Depending on the severity and extent of the myocarditis affected pups may die rapidly in acute heart failure usually between 4 and 6 weeks of age, or may gradually develop more sub-acute heart failure at anything up to 1 year or more.

Clinical Features

CPV Enteritis

'Dull the first day, vomiting on the second, diarrhoea on the third and dead or better on the fourth' neatly sums the clinical features of CPV enteritis. There is a wide range in severity of clinical signs from the peracute dysenteric animal which collapses and dies within 24 h to the protracted case which, with treatment, may linger on for weeks. Sudden onset depression and anorexia is the first sign. Vomiting occurs early in the course of disease and can be severe and persistent. The vomitus is clear and mucoid and can be missed as it mingles with the hair. A nasal discharge and mild conjunctivitis may complicate the picture and raise suspicions of early distemper infection particularly in younger pups. In the older pups between 6 and 16 months of age the constant vomiting and the impression of foreign body which may be created by the enlarged mesenteric lymph nodes can lead to surgical intervention. Diarrhoea which follows within 24 h of vomiting quickly confirms that mistake. The faeces are usually profuse and fluid and flecks or streaks of blood may be present. The faeces can vary from simply soft or pasty to grossly dysenteric. Dehydration and weight loss are often profound and can develop extremely rapidly when there is repeated vomiting and severe diarrhoea. Severely affected dogs, particularly pups may become moribund very quickly. All breeds can be affected but there is a strong clinical impression that the course of disease is faster and decline more severe in Rottweilers and Dobermans.

The rectal temperature is variable (28.5–40°C). Marked pyrexia is uncommon and the temperature may be subnormal in moribund dogs. There is usually a lymphopenia early in the infection but reduction in total leucocyte count (with neutropenia as well as lymphopenia) is seen only in cases with severe enteric lesions. The reserve pool of neutrophils is lost through the damaged gut mucosa. A leucocytosis will develop during the recovery phase.

The course of the disease is usually short and in severe

cases without the institution of fluid therapy death may occur within 24 h. In many animals recovery is surprisingly rapid but in a proportion of cases prolonged therapy is required. Once recovered there should be no lasting side effects but occasional cases of osteoporosis have been reported in larger breeds of puppies. It is not clear if these cases are related to direct viral damage or as seems more likely an imbalance of meat in the diet as the owner attempts to rebuild the puppies' condition.

CPV Myocarditis

CPV myocarditis is, as has been explained, now very rare. It is a litter problem and something like 70% of the pups will die in heart failure by 8 weeks of age. The surviving pups in affected litters will also have some degree of heart pathology and die in the subsequent months or even years later of heart failure. Sudden death is first seen in young pups about 4 weeks of age following a period of stress or excitement such as feeding or play. Apparently healthy pups collapse and die within minutes. Pale mucosae, cold extremities and terminal convulsions have been noted. These cases are usually described by the breeder as they are rarely seen by a veterinary surgeon. He or she will then be asked to examine what appears to be a perfectly normal litter and auscultation will be unremarkable. The worst fears will now be confirmed if other pups start to die in the next few weeks and microscopic examination of their heart muscle confirms CPV myocarditis. By 8–12 weeks some of the survivors may present in subacute heart failure with tachynoea, dyspnoea and tachycardia with ascites and hepatomegaly.

The prognosis in clinical cases is hopeless. It is impossible to regard litter mates as normal animals and the breeder should be advised of the possibility of their death in heart failure at a later stage. Many responsible breeders opt for euthanasia.

Diagnosis

- CPV myocarditis is confirmed by histological examination of the myocardium.
- Sudden onset of severe vomiting and diarrhoea with dehydration in pups between 5 weeks and 1 year is at the moment very likely to be due to CPV enteritis.
- The similarity of some early cases to upper intestinal obstruction has been mentioned and particularly in older animals it can be difficult to differentiate between peracute dysenteric cases of CPV and classical canine haemorrhagic gastroenteritis.
- In milder cases it can be impossible on purely clinical grounds to differentiate between CPV-2 infection and

other causes of diarrhoea/vomiting, e.g. dietary upset, other viruses, bacteria.

CPV-2 can be isolated from faeces and its natural resistance means that there is no problem with transportation of samples to the laboratory. The simplest and cheapest method to screen for CPV-2 is to use either the haemagglutinin assay or an enzyme-linked immunosorbent assay (ELISA) test. The haemagglutin assay depends on the ability of CPV-2 to agglutinate pig erythrocytes. However non-specific agglutinins are often present in faeces and the test must be carefully controlled. The peak period of excretion is early in the infection and in dogs which have been ill for 2 or 3 days the excretion of free virus drops below detectable levels. The ELISA tests which are quick and simple to use in practice are excellent and specific but again the virus has to be present. Antibody develops rapidly in CPV-2 infection and dogs which have been ill for a few days will have reached their peak antibody titre. In clinically affected animals it is essential that both faeces and serum are submitted for confirmation of diagnosis.

- In fatal cases of CPV enteritis histopathology of the intestines and lymph nodes is the most reliable method of confirmation. At post-mortem examination the carcass is thin and dehydrated.
- There is usually intestinal congestion which may be mild or severe although in young pups the intestine may appear blanched. Typically the intestines feel thickened or inelastic and the serosal surface has a roughened granular appearance.
- The mucosa at first glance may seem unremarkable and novice pathologists are often surprised at the lack of congestion or haemorrhage. Closer inspection will reveal that the surface is denuded and floccules of mucosal debris can be noted in the fluid, blood-tinged content. The stomach usually contains grey, mucoid fluid and the spleen will be mottled. The mesenteric lymph nodes will be enlarged and oedematous. There will be thymic atrophy in puppies.

The extent and severity of the pathology may vary along the length of the intestine and three samples should be taken for confirmation of diagnosis from the duodenum, jejunum and ileum. CPV-2 infection is confirmed by the characteristic changes which include sloughing and necrosis of villi, and dilation of the crypts. Inclusion bodies are more difficult to find in dogs with CPV-2 infection compared with cats with feline infectious enteritis.

Treatment and Management

Treatment of CPV enteritis is fluids, more fluids and even more fluids. Details of fluid therapy are covered in Chapter

2. In brief the author recommends intravenous lactated Ringer's solution as the fluid of choice to compensate for the electrolyte imbalance along with fluid loss. In dysenteric animals in circulating collapse whole blood or plasma volume expanders may be used in preference to simple electrolyte. Short duration corticosteroid therapy may also be useful to reverse circulatory collapse. Supportive antibiotic therapy is advisable because bacterial invasion of the damaged intestinal mucosa is common.

Special problems of prophylaxis and control of CPV enteritis arise in large breeding kennels, puppy farms, dog rescue shelters and pet shops where there is a continuous turnover of susceptible pups. Each successive generation of pups picks up the virus and excretes a great deal more thus increasing the burden of challenge presented to the next generation. The resistance of CPV-2 to physical and chemical agents combined with the varied and often *ad hoc* construction of many kennels, wooden buildings, grass or gravel runs etc., results in a heavily contaminated environment which is impossible to disinfect. Outbreaks and individual cases of CPV enteritis occur on a regular basis in such places and disease can be difficult to control even with blanket vaccination.

In such situations, the adult breeding stock will be immune and high antibody titres are often present. It might be expected that pups born from such bitches would inherit maternal protection which would last till 12 or even 16 weeks of age, indeed some do, and therefore take them beyond the age when they are most susceptible to disease. However in such premises disease or death often occur in puppies at or about 6–10 weeks of age. A number of factors contribute to this paradox. First in such large kennels management at whelping may be poor; the puppies may not receive or may not absorb the correct amount of colostral antibody which might be expected. Second, and more importantly, the burden of CPV-2 challenge to which the puppies are subjected is immense and such a weight of infection will break through maternal protection 2 or even 4 weeks before a vaccine would immunise.

Management of CPV enteritis in kennels is obviously difficult. There is no point in repeated vaccination of the breeding stock; they are already solidly immune with antibody titres which will not be significantly increased by vaccination. Equally there is little point in early vaccination of the pups; their maternal antibody, though insufficient to resist challenge will be sufficient to prevent response to vaccination. Since the problem lies in the heavy and continuous environmental challenge to the pups by CPV-2, this is where attempts at control must first be directed. In some kennels it is possible to manage the problem by removal (or sale) of pups to a clean environment at an early age before their antibody levels fall sufficiently for them to be susceptible to disease. If this is not possible then rotation of the puppy area within the kennel should be considered.

An initial reduction of environmental challenge can be achieved by thorough cleansing of the kennel particularly the area used as puppy accommodation. This is most easily achieved by depopulating the kennels of pups even if in breeding establishments or shops, this means stopping breeding or sales for a short period. CPV-2 is resistant to many commonly used disinfectants. Only formalin and sodium hypochlorite (bleach) have high activity against CPV-2 and both of these are rapidly inactivated by organic material. Consequently thorough cleaning with removal of all organic debris is a prerequisite for effective disinfection. Thorough cleaning with lots of water will substantially reduce the burden of infection by simple dilution. Although bleach and formalin are cheap they are both unpleasant to handle with destructive side effects on skin and fabrics. A newer range of disinfectants based on glutaraldehyde are now available which are pleasant, effective and safe to use but relatively expensive. Sprays containing these products should be mandatory in each veterinary surgery to clean tables between consultations.

Subsequent management practices should be such as to minimise repeated build-up of infection and transfer of infection, e.g. litters or groups of pups should be batched and kennels cleared between batches. Nevertheless there is a tendency for infection to build up with recurrence of disease at peak breeding periods. For breeders keeping replacement stock the control programme should be combined with a suitable vaccination schedule based if necessary on analysis of the antibody status of the bitches. Modified live CPV-2 vaccine is best in these difficult situations as it provides rapid protection and is more capable of dealing with low levels of maternal antibody than the inactivated products.

Owners who have lost an individual pup from CPV enteritis are frequently worried about the risk to any new pups they might acquire. It is impracticable to talk to such owners about formalin fumigation or bleach disinfection or to give a definite time limit before acquiring a new dog. The most reasoned advice would be to wait for a reasonable period of say 4–6 weeks during which time the area of the house contaminated by the previous dog is cleaned. Time, with dilution, is the important factor in the equation. The next pup acquired should, if at all possible, be an older pup which has already been vaccinated or a dog which has been shown to be immune by antibody testing. The best pup of course would be a surviving littermate who has acquired natural immunity but given the drama and tragedy of the initial loss this substitute is rarely acceptable.

Chapter 10

Infectious Canine Hepatitis

H. Thompson

Aetiology

Canine adenovirus type 1 (CAV-1) is responsible for the generalised disease known as infectious canine hepatitis (ICH) or Rubarth's disease. This acute infection is the most dramatic manifestation of the encounter between this virus and a susceptible dog.

Epidemiology

Infectious canine hepatitis is not common and although it has been claimed that serological evidence of CAV-1 infection in unvaccinated dogs is widespread this has not been assessed in Britain for many years. Infection spreads by direct and indirect contact with virus in urine, faeces or saliva. Faecal and salivary excretion is short lived but urinary shed from individual animals may persist for up to 9 months.

- Most cases of ICH occur in individual dogs less than 6 months old.
- In a litter of 10 infected puppies fatalities rarely exceed 3 or 4.
- Infection can persist in larger kennels such as commercial Beagle colonies.
- The red fox is susceptible to ICH and maybe reservoir of infection.

Adenoviruses are moderately stable in the environment and may persist in moist conditions for up to 10 days in sawdust. Steam heat, aldehyde, phenol and hypochlorite will destroy the virus.

Pathogenesis

- Infection by the oral route leads to multiplication of virus in tonsils, Peyer's patches and lymph nodes.

- Lymphadenitis at 3 days post-infection is followed by anaemia, lymphopaenia and further viral multiplication in endothelial cells and hepatocytes.
- Antibody is detectable by 5 days post-infection and the critical collision of virus versus host defence determines the outcome of infection.
- In most dogs the defences win, the illness is short or undetected and the dog returns to normality.
- ICH is the catastrophic consequence of viral success or excess.

Initial periacinar necrosis in the liver becomes widespread causing acute hepatic failure and jaundice etc. Widespread haemorrhages are also common due primarily to endothelial damage with a superimposed consumptive coagulopathy. This bleeding tendency is exacerbated by failing liver function with decreased production of clotting factors. At this stage viral damage is also apparent in the intestine, the renal glomeruli, the eye and the salivary glands.

- Corneal oedema (blue-eye) is a common sequel in dogs recovering from ICH (about 20% are affected).
- Viral induced lysis of viral and corneal endothelial cells is followed by the deposition of immune complexes with complement fixation which develops 10–15 days after infection. This leads to a leakage of fluid into the corneal oedema. One or both eyes may be affected.
- Blue-eye may occur as a clinical syndrome in its own right.
- Some recovered dogs will excrete the virus for many months.

Virus will persist in the renal epithelia even though antibody is present and the infected cells are surrounded by macrophages, lymphocytes and plasma cells. These dogs have no compromise of renal function and the foci form only small white nodules in the renal cortex.

Clinical Features

- Mild forms of the infection present as slight malaise, partial anorexia and transient elevation of rectal temperature. The dog invariably recovers and the diagnosis of CAV-1 infection might go unsuspected unless a serological test was carried out or blue eye develops a week or so later.
- Infectious canine hepatitis is a peracute or acute illness. Some animals die suddenly without previous signs. Dogs with ICH are profoundly dull, anorexic and pyrexic (up to 41°C (106°F)) with enlarged lymph nodes and swollen red tonsils. Vomiting occurs initially and scanty blood tinged diarrhoea may develop. Palpation of the anterior abdomen usually elicits pain and hepatomegaly may be detected. The dog is in shock with pale mucosae and widespread petechiation visible in the mucosae or skin. Terminal seizures or coma finally result from CNS haemorrhage and hepatic encephalopathy. Most cases die before showing jaundice but this can be intense if the dog survives for a few days.
- Sudden blue-eye maybe the only indication of CAV-1 infection in some dogs.
- The dog that persistently excretes the virus in the urine may never have shown any clinical illness.

Diagnosis

Definitive diagnosis of infectious canine hepatitis is on the isolation of CAV-1. Virus can be isolated from tonsillar swabs from acutely ill dogs but this will be increasingly difficult as the dogs move into the recovery phase. The detection of carrier animals by culture of urine is possible but not particularly practical given that the excretion will be in low amounts and intermittent.

A rise in circulating antibody to CAV-1 can also give confirmation of the diagnosis, but paired serum samples at intervals of 2 weeks apart are rarely available and in most cases only a single sample in the recovery phase is obtained. Following recent infection the serum neutralisation titre to CAV-1 will be generally much higher than that seen after vaccination, and there will be a significant difference in the titre measured to CAV-1 compared with that obtained if CAV-2 is used in a similar neutralisation test. The differential test is of particular value when dogs already have a history of vaccination.

Histological examination of the liver and lymph nodes for viral inclusions and cell necrosis is the easiest means of confirmation in fatal cases. The liver is usually swollen and mottled with strands of fibrin between the lobes. The lymph nodes are bright red and oedematous. Oedema of the gall bladder is a classical feature but is not present in every case. Many cases of ICH are mistaken clinically for CPV enteritis. Fortunately in cases of CPV infection there are characteristic changes of intestinal epithelial cell necrosis that are readily apparent in fixed intestinal samples which have been submitted to a laboratory.

Treatment and Control

- Mild cases of CAV-1 infection will respond with the minimal of treatments.
- Severe cases of ICH require aggressive fluid therapy to counteract shock and specific treatment to deal with the hyperammoniaemia and hypoglycaemia of liver failure. Dogs with coagulation problems may require whole blood.
- Corneal oedema will resolve uneventfully in the vast majority of cases but a check for glaucoma may be warranted in some susceptible breeds.
- Live vaccines containing CAV-2 are very effective; vacines based on CAV-1 are rarely used nowadays and were associated with vaccine-induced blue eye.

Chapter 11

Canine Distemper

H. Thompson

Aetiology

- Canine distemper virus (CDV) is a morbillivirus, and as such belongs to a group which includes human measles, cattle rinderpest and the recently discovered phocine (seal) and piniped (dolphin) viruses.
- It is a large virus and a very delicate structure with a lipid coat.
- It is quickly inactivated by sunlight and is susceptible to most disinfectants including detergents.
- There is one antigenic form of the virus, although within that form there are strains which vary in virulence and in particular in neurotropism.

Epidemiology

CDV is commonly spread by aerosol exposure and the virus is present in respiratory exudates from infected dogs during the 2 or 3 weeks and possibly longer. As the virus is extremely labile, spread of infection occurs by dog-to-dog contact or by aerosol spread over a short distance. The pattern of infection in canine populations depends on the numbers and density of that population and the availability and use of vaccination. Before vaccination the disease was endemic in urban areas where a large number of dogs lived in relatively close contact. Most cases occurred between 3 and 6 months of age as pups that lost maternal derived antibody started to encounter the infection. The majority of dogs that survived to adulthood were immune. In isolated canine communities the pattern was different as there would be insufficient numbers of new susceptible dogs to sustain the infection. Outbreaks of CDV in these situations would appear as mini-epidemics and all ages of animals would be affected. Dogs would either die or become immune, and the infection would die out only to return in a few years time.

The emergence of effective vaccines, which became widely available in Britain in the 1950s, added a socio-economic dimension to this basic pattern. Distemper largely disappeared from the more affluent parts of towns and cities as dogs in these areas were vaccinated and kept under better control. Pockets of infection remained in the poorer areas and in particular in the larger estates which sprang up on the edges of all major cities. In smaller towns and rural areas the use of vaccine prevented dramatic epidemics but the seasonal pattern of the disease still remained. In holiday towns, distemper would be seen in unvaccinated dogs a few weeks or months following the annual influx of visitors and their pets. Between the mid 1950s and the early 1970s the incidence of distemper in the charity clinics serving the poorer areas of Glasgow did not change. Within the last 10 years that has changed dramatically and classical cases of distemper are now uncommon. This dramatic fall in the number of cases of distemper reflects the better control of dog numbers in the city but, more importantly, the vaccination of all new animals at local animal shelters. A similar picture has emerged in other parts of the country and one can now say that CDV is uncommon. Many veterinary surgeons in small animal practice in Britain will not have diagnosed a case of distemper in the last 5 years. The infection has not disappeared however. A reservoir of unvaccinated dogs still remain and the complex movements of susceptible puppies within the pet trade means that isolated cases of canine distemper can and do occur in unexpected situations.

Pathogenesis

- Virus inhaled as aerosol droplets is taken up by respiratory and oropharyngeal macrophages and spreads to the lymph nodes, spleen and thymus. It multiplies in these sites before spreading to epithelial and nervous tissues.
- The critical period is 8–10 days after infection when the contest between the virus and the immune system is decided. If the immune system wins, as it must do in

the majority of cases, the virus is eliminated and the dog is left with a strong cellular and humoral immunity. If viral multiplication is unchecked then the lymphoid system is overwhelmed and the virus spreads to the epithelia causing classical catarrhal distemper with respiratory, alimentary and oculonasal signs.

- This happens about 2 or 3 weeks after infection, and the immune response in these dogs will be greatly depressed. By this time the virus has also spread to the nervous system and the skin and hyperkeratosis (hard pad) and nervous signs first appear about 4–5 weeks post-infection.
- Some dogs develop a partial immune response which may eliminate the virus from the epithelia but is unable to prevent, although it may delay, the onset of nervous signs and hard pad.

The wide variation in the severity of the signs of CDV infection is further complicated by differences in virulence of strains and the fact that the situation in which some puppies contract distemper are also those situations in which other agents such as *Bordetella bronchiseptica* abound. Variation in genetically determined susceptibility of the dog must also be an important factor but little hard scientific evidence is available on this issue.

Clinical Features

- The onset of clinical distemper is insidious and the variation in speed of onset and the range of clinical signs often take the owner and their veterinary surgeon by surprise. The realisation that the disease is distemper comes with the failure to halt the progression of what at first would seem a minor problem.
- Dullness, anorexia and pyrexia (39.4°C to 40°C (103° to 104°F)) may herald the start of illness, and the end of illness, as many dogs must recover at this stage.
- Vomiting can be an early sign. Diarrhoea, however, is more common. The diarrhoeic faeces are mostly yellow and can be spotted with blood. Although the diarrhoea is not life threatening it will prove difficult to treat.
- A cough is almost invariably present and at first is soft in character but becomes harsh and is often accompanied by the expectoration of mucus. Some cases show hyperpnoea or tachypnoea if pneumonic.
- Early in the disease, the nose becomes dry, and beads of serous fluid will often form at each nostril. This gradually becomes purulent and sneezing is common. The skin rhinarium becomes thickened, fissured and may even ulcerate. Congestion of the conjunctivae is common. A purulent discharge will form at the inner canthus and if unchecked will become adherent to the cornea and the eyelids. During this initial period which

may last 2 or even 3 weeks the rectal temperature will fluctuate but more often than not will hover around (39.4°C (103°F)).

- Definite palpable foot pad hyperkeratosis (hard pad) is detectable in about one-third of clinical cases at or after the third week of illness. At first the pads may be tender, then they become smooth and shiny and on compression from side to side a decided edge is palpable. As the disease progresses the pad becomes very thickened and 'wooden'.

Fits, chorea and paralysis may occur separately or in combination. About 50% of cases of catarrhal distemper are likely to develop fits. Classical epileptic fits develop around the fourth to eighth week of illness. Before that time dogs may go through a phase of restlessness and whining and whimpering which may continue night and day. Sudden bouts of apparent apprehension which cause the dog to run around wildly with yelping have also been observed. Chorea, a clonic spasm of a muscle or muscle group, is a classical sign of distemper. It commonly affects the head or limbs. It is caused by regular, rhythmic twitch of the muscle group and is quite distinct from shivering. Chorea tends to be permanent and continuous even when the animal is sleeping. A dog may sometimes attack an area which has a chorea twitch and make an indolent wound at this site.

In severe cases complete paralysis of the hind limbs may develop, with loss of control of defecation and urination. Less affected animals may just show inco-ordination of gait, staggering or dragging the hind limbs so that the anterior surface of the toenails become worn.

Diagnosis

Confirmation of CDV diagnosis in the living dog is difficult because laboratory tests can be unrevealing and expensive.

- Virus isolation is difficult and usually impractical from a distance given the labile nature of this virus. The most reliable isolation method is direct culture of alveolar lavage fluid which would only be possible in exceptional circumstances.
- Detection of inclusions in smears of conjunctival or tonsillar epithelial is often advocated but requires an experienced observer. Examination of cells from urinary deposits gives a cleaner preparation but still requires experience, and even then false negatives will be common.
- Detection of rising levels of antibody to CDV either by neutralisation or ELISA will allow definite diagnosis but is most useful when a number of dogs are involved. Interpretation of serological results from individual

dogs is difficult. At the time the sample is taken the level may well have reached its peak which, in the case of severely ill dogs that are immunosuppressed, will be low. Dogs with very high titres to CDV have usually recovered from the infection.

- Detection of antibody to CDV in cerebrospinal fluid is diagnostic since it is produced locally and indicates viral infection within the brain. It is always best to compare the level with that present in the serum and to check an additional antigen, say CPV-2 to make sure that the CSF sample has not been contaminated with blood.
- If the dog is to be destroyed a wide range of tissues will be available and portions of lymph nodes, spleen, lung, bladder and brain (including hind brain) should be placed in formal–saline before dispatch to the laboratory. Virus isolation is only possible if direct or immediate access to the laboratory is possible.

Management and Prognosis

Treatment for CDV is symptomatic and many owners will request euthanasia for their dog once nervous signs appear. The dogs must be kept warm, dry, comfortable with regular cleaning of discharges from the eyes and nose. Antibiotics should be given to control secondary infection. Antisera may be used but it appears of little value. Phenobarbitone can be used to control the fits, and chorea or occasional seizures are often well tolerated by both owners and dogs. The owner should be warned that the course of the illness will be protracted and that hindlimb paralysis may develop.

Chapter 12

Kennel Cough

I. McCandlish

Aetiology

Kennel cough (infectious tracheobronchitis or contagious respiratory disease) can be caused by several infectious agents either alone or in combination (Table 12.1).

Epidemiology

Kennel cough is a disease syndrome that follows mixing of dogs and circulation of any pathogens that are present. Infection occurs mainly by direct contact and short distance aerosol transmission. Indirect contact by fomites, on feed bowls for example, is possible but less important. Ideal conditions for spread occur in several circumstances:

- boarding kennels,
- dog shows, training clubs, race meetings,
- veterinary hospitals or waiting rooms.

Disease often peaks in late summer towards the end of the holiday season. Cases do occur in individual pets with no obvious kennel or group contact. Enzootic disease with coughing in successive litters of pups may prove a problem in large breeding kennels or puppy trading premises with a high or continuous throughput of animals.

Pathogenesis

Infection occurs by inhalation for all agents with direct infection of epithelia.

- *Bordetella bronchiseptica*
  - colonisation of respiratory epithelial cilia
  - acute rhinitis and tracheobronchitis
  - cough from 3–4 days after infection for up to 10 days

  - bacteria persist in airways for up to 3 months
  - local immunity of short duration (18–24 months)
- CPIV
  - multiplication in nasophayngeal and tracheo-bronchial epithelia
  - mild rhinitis and tracheobronchitis
  - slight cough by *7 days post-infection* lasts only a few days
  - viral excretion usually stopped by *14 days post-infection*
  - local immunity of short duration (12–18 months)
- *B. bronchiseptica*
  - CPIV – dual infection results in more severe synergism and longer lasting disease.
- CAV-1 & CAV-2
  - Aerosol infection causes necrotising bronchiolitis. Respiratory disease can occur in pups with low maternal antibody that protects against systemic infectious canine hepatitis (ICH). High circulating antibody from systemic vaccines protects against respiratory disease.

Severe disease with pneumonia due either to the agents of kennel cough or secondary bacterial infection is most likely in young pups, immunocompromised animals or dogs with cardiac or other respiratory diseases, e.g. tracheal collapse. A few dogs that suffer repeated episodes of kennel cough may develop chronic bronchial disease.

Clinical Features

- Coughing is the main, and often only clinical sign. Typically harsh, dry and hacking, it is readily induced by excitement, exercise or tracheal palpation. Moist, more obviously productive cough is less common. Coughing may last only 2–3 days, typically resolves within 2 weeks and exceptionally persists for over 3 weeks. In severe cases, bouts of paroxysmal cough end

Table 12.1 Some causes of kennel cough.

Bordetella bronchiseptica	Commonly isolated, produces typical disease experimentally
Canine parainfluenza virus (CPIV)	Commonly isolated, produces mild disease experimentally
Canine adenovirus (CAV-1 & CAV2)	Less common, most frequent in, unvaccinated pups, produces significant disease experimentally
Canine herpesvirus (CHV)	Uncommon, produces mild/inapparent disease
Reoviruses	Uncommon, produce mild/inapparent disease
Mycoplasmas	May complicate other infections
Canine distemper (CDV)	May occur in similar situations to kennel cough and must be distinguished from it

in retching that may be interpreted as vomiting by inexperienced owners. Recently fed dogs do rarely regurgitate food during paroxysms.

- Respiratory rate is usually normal although pups with CAV-induced disease may be markedly tachypnoeic and hyperpnoeic. Lung sounds may be harsh and there may be some increase in adventitious sounds.
- Sneezing and serous to mucoid, rarely mucopurulent, nasal discharges occur occasionally.
- Tonsillar enlargement and cranial or cervical lymphodenopathy is often present.
- Typical cases are bright and non-pyrexic. Depression, fever, anorexia and markedly abnormal lung sounds indicate supervening pneumonia.

Diagnosis

The typical clinical syndrome in individual cases or kennel outbreaks is easily recognised without need of ancillary tests or laboratory back-up. Specific aetiological diagnosis is time consuming, expensive and often unrewarding, and can probably only be justified in severe kennel outbreaks or if there is a question of litigation.

- *Bordetella bronchiseptica* can be difficult to isolate from naso-pharyngeal swabs. Tracheal aspirates or swabs may be more useful.
- Nasopharyngeal swabs in transport medium for viral isolation are best collected from early, not established cases.
- Since most viral transport media contain antibacterials, separate samples are needed for bacterial and viral culture.
- Demonstration of rising antibody titres on paired sera may confirm infection with specific agents. Single samples are unhelpful since antibody is widespread. Animals with good local antibody responses may not show a classical rising serum antibody response.
- Fatal cases in young pups necessitate post-mortem

examination. Samples of lung and trachea should be taken for histopathology in 10% formalin. Deep tracheobronchial swabs for bacterial and viral culture should be collected aseptically.

Treatment and Management

Most cases of kennel cough recover uneventfully without treatment in 2–3 weeks. Antibacterials are indicated in individuals with evidence of pneumonia or risk of transmission of bordetellosis to more susceptible animals.

- Trimethoprim–sulphonamide, oxytetracycline, ampicillin and cephalexin are usually effective against *Bordetella bronchiseptica in vitro*. Maximal doses should be given for up to 10 days.
- Aerosolisation with gentamicin or kanamycin can reduce *Bordetella* burdens in airways but is impractical in most circumstances.

Methods of ameliorating severe or paroxysmal coughing vary from a variety of drugs (although efficacy studies for these are lacking) to management factors.

- Short acting glucocorticoids and antitussives are considered by many to be effective. These are contraindicated in dogs with pneumonia, immunosuppression or very moist productive coughs.
- Bronchodilators may ease wheezing coughs where there is a suspicion of bronchospasm.
- Unnecessary excitement should be avoided and exercise restricted. Racing and working dogs should not resume normal training or activity until they have recovered fully.
- Shoulder harnesses may prevent stimulation of coughing by pressure from collars.

Control within kennels depends not only on use of vaccines but also on good kennel design, management and hygiene.

- Vaccines against *Bordetella bronchiseptica* and CPIV may reduce the likelihood of kennel cough but cannot be guaranteed to prevent it.
- Vaccines should ideally be administered 1–2 weeks before anticipated challenge.
- Small kennel blocks with good ventilation are preferable to large units with common, poorly ventilated airspaces.
- Kennels should be used on a rota system to prevent mixing new occupants with long-stay residents and to allow periodic depopulation, cleaning and disinfection.
- Food and water bowls and other moveable equipment should be thoroughly cleaned and disinfected.
- Disinfectants recommended for CPIV will also be effective against the agents of kennel cough.

Chapter 13

Canine Filaroidiasis

I. McCandlish

Aetiology

Filaroides (*Oslerus*) *osleri* is a nematode parasite, occurring world-wide, that causes nodular parasitic tracheobronchitis. The life cycle is direct. Adult female worms embedded in nodules concentrated around the predilection site of the carina extrude embryonated eggs in the trachaobronchial lumen. Eggs of hatched larvae are coughed up or swallowed. Larvae in sputum or faeces are immediately infective and if ingested by a susceptible dog migrate through the intestine to the lungs and mature in nodules at the carina. The pre-patent period is 10–18 weeks and adult parasites can remain *in situ* for many months. *F. hirthi* is a related parasite that causes low grade chronic parasitic pneumonia, mainly in laboratory Beagles.

Epidemiology

Infection is uncommon overall. Association with particular kennels, in which many dogs infected, often gives a local breed prediction. Pups of infected bitches, exposed to heavy infection, are most likely to show clinical signs but since these seldom occur before 4–8 months of age, cases often present in individual pet dogs. Most cases are seen in dogs less than 2 years of age but older animals can be affected.

Clinical Signs

Many infections are asymptomatic. Chronic coughing or wheezing occurs over several months. Coughing spasms may produce white or blood tinged sputum. Hyperpnoea, dyspnoea and exercise intolerance develops in cases with severe airway narrowing. Such dogs become distressed or cyanotic on forced exercise. Affected dogs are bright and maintain body condition except in the severest infestations. Auscultation ranges from normal to harsh respiration or increased adventitious sounds in severe cases.

Diagnosis

- Radiography may reveal an irregular tracheal outline or distinct nodules around the carina.
- Bronchoscopy will show distinct pale 2–5 mm nodules protruding into the trachaobronchial lumen. The tails of female worms may stick out from the nodules. Biopsy of nodules will show the parasites. Thin walled larvated eggs or larvae with distinctly kinked tails are readily seen in bronchoscopic brushings, tracheal mucus aspirates or sputum. Faecal examination is less rewarding.

Treatment and Control

Thiabendozole (32 mg/kg b.i.d. for 3 weeks), levamisole (7–5 mg/kg daily for 30 days) and albendazole (25 mg/kg b.i.d. for 5 days) have been used with variable success. Ivermectin has been suggested more recently but there is no published data available. Small fibrous nodules or scars may be left even after elimination of the parasite.

Cases in individual pets should be traced to the kennel of origin, although control within kennels may be difficult. Infected bitches excreting larvae should not be used for breeding. Strict faecal disposal may reduce environmental contamination.

Chapter 14

Aspergillosis and Penicillinosis

N. J. Sharp

Aetiology

Nasal aspergillosis and penicillinosis cause destructive rhinitis and sinusitis. *Aspergillus* spp. cause the majority of cases; *Penicillium* spp. are much less common. All ages and breeds are susceptible with the exception of brachycephalic dogs.

Most dogs have no predisposing factors to explain how these ubiquitous saprophytic fungi become pathogenic. *Aspergillus* spp. secrete haemolytic and necrotising toxins which cause extensive turbinate necrosis by local vascular injury. Hyphae may erode through the nasal bones, into periorbital soft tissues, or into the brain.

Clinical Signs

The three *clinical hallmarks* of infection are:

- chronic, profuse, sanguinopurulent nasal discharge,
- ulceration of the external nares,
- nasal or facial pain.

The incidence of clinical features is shown in Table 14.1.

Diagnosis

It is recommended that the dog be positive for at least *two* of the following four criteria before treatment for fungal disease is considered:

Radiology

- A dorsoventral image of the nasal chamber is made using a piece of non-screen film inside the dog's mouth.
- Turbinate destruction with an overall increase in radio-

lucency is seen in aspergillosis due to replacement of turbinates with air.
- In neoplasia the turbinate destruction is associated with an overall increase in radiopacity due to soft tissue invasion.

Rhinoscopy

Rhinoscopy is very useful due to the large air space created by destructive rhinitis. Fungal colonies appear as greenish-white plaques. These should be sampled for culture or cytological examination.

Mycology

Fungal hyphae can be demonstrated by either direct culture of plaques, cytological examination of discharge, or histopathological evaluation of turbinate tissue. Culture of nasal discharge is not recommended; even if *Aspergillus* spp. or *Penicillium* spp. grow the result is impossible to interpret. These organisms can be cultured from swabs of the nasal chamber in 40% of both normal dogs and those with nasal neoplasia.

Serology

Enzyme-linked immunoabsorbent assays (ELISA) and agar gel double diffusion (AGDD) are both very useful tests, but about 15% of normal dogs may be seropositive in the absence of infection.

Several features differentiate this condition from nasal neoplasia:

- The discharge is profuse and purulent; in neoplasia it tends to be serous and intermittent.
- Nasal pain or ulceration are uncommon in neoplasia.

Table 14.1 Incidence of clinical features.

Clinical feature	% Affected
Profuse nasal discharge	>90
Nasal pain	>80
Ulceration of external nares	>70
Sanguinopurulent discharge	>70
Epistaxis	>60
Sinusitis	>60

Treatment

- The systemic antifungals are not so highly active against *Aspergillus* spp. or *Penicillium* spp. and so tend to be effective in only 50–70% of cases. Itraconazole is the most effective.
- Topical enilconazole or topical clotrimazole will cure about 90% of dogs with nasal aspergillosis and penicillinosis.
- Surgery is used solely to insert tubes into the frontal sinuses and nasal chambers for drug irrigation. Recently it has been shown that tubes are just as effective when inserted through the nostrils. Rhinotomy and turbinectomy are not recommended as they often result in permanent nasal discharge despite elimination of fungus.
- Dogs with extranasal soft tissue involvement should receive combination topical and systemic therapy.
- The best indication of treatment success is the resolution of sanguinous discharge, nasal pain and ulceration. In such cases the long-term prognosis is excellent.

Chapter 15

Canine Leptospirosis

M. Bennett

Aetiology

Dogs can become infected with several serovars of *Leptospira interrogans* but those most often isolated are *icteroheamorrhagiae*, *canicola* and *grippotyphosa*. The source of infection in dogs is usually direct or indirect contact with rodents rather than other dogs, but may be bite wounds, infected meat and even placental transfer. A combination of good hygiene and vaccination means that canine leptospirosis is not commonly reported in many areas. Affected dogs are usually non-vaccinated with a history of swimming in stagnant or slow-moving water.

Pathogenesis and Clinical Signs

Leptospires usually enter through mucous membranes or broken skin, and replication occurs in the blood, renal tubules and liver. The course of the disease depends on the dose and serovar of leptospire, and on the age of dog and degree of immunity – pre-existing high antibody titres lead to elimination of the organism, and moderate antibody titres to mild or asymptomatic infection with apparent recovery within 2–3 weeks. After recovery from acute or subacute leptospirosis, chronic renal failure or hepatitis may develop. Full-blown, peracute clinical disease is generally seen only in unvaccinated dogs or vaccinated dogs infected with a serovar not included in the vaccine, e.g. *L. interrogans grippotyphosa*.

Most infections, however, are chronic rather than acute or subacute, with rather more vague clinical signs such as pyrexia of unknown origin, or progressive, chronic renal or hepatic failure. Infected dogs may excrete leptospires in urine for months or even years. Clinical signs of acute leptospirosis are shown in Table 15.1.

Diagnosis

- Diagnosis is often based on clinical signs and history (environment and lack of vaccination), supported by haematology (leucocytosis, thrombocytopenia) and blood biochemistry (urea and creatinine levels raised, elevated liver enzymes and bilirubin).
- Serology is expensive and can be difficult to interpret.
- Isolation from urine and blood is difficult as leptospires

Table 15.1 Clinical signs of acute leptospirosis.

Peracute disease due to massive leptospiraemia	Sub-acute disease
Pyrexia	Fever
Shivering	Anorexia
Muscle tenderness	Vomiting
Vomiting	Dehydration
Dehydration	May be reluctant to move owing to abdominal pain
Shock	Jaundice
Death	Mucous membranes congested possibly with petechial haemorrhage
	Progressive loss of renal function (oligouria and anuria)

do not survive long and need special transport media. The organism can also sometimes be seen in urine by dark-ground microscopy, but a negative result does not rule out leptospirosis.

- Leptospires can also be detected by immunofluorescence in liver or kidney sections snap frozen in liquid nitrogen then sent frozen to the laboratory.

Treatment and Control

Antibiotic Therapy

Penicillin G (25 mg/kg i.v. or i.m. b.i.d.) or ampicillin (10 mg/kg i.v., i.m. or s.c. b.i.d., or 10–20 mg/kg p.o. t.i.d.) for 2 weeks to control bacteraemia.

Dihydrostreptomycin (15 mg/kg, i.m. or s.c. b.i.d.) for 2 weeks to eliminate renal infection. *Only use streptomycin once renal function has returned to normal.*

Supportive therapy, including rehydration, blood transfusion if necessary, and possible use of diuretics or even peritoneal dialysis in persistently oligouric animals. Appropriate nutritional management of chronic renal failure is useful.

Control

Control is mainly by vaccination with killed *L. interrogans icterohaemorrhagiae* and *canicola* and avoidance of known contaminated environments.

Chapter 16

Canine Rabies

P.-P. Pastoret, B. Brochier and H. Bourhy

Key Features of the Aetiology and Epidemiology

- Rabies virus is a member of the genus *Lyssavirus* in the family Rhabdoviridae. Lyssaviruses comprise six known species; *Lyssavirus*-1 is responsible for the present European fox rabies epizootic.
- Rabies is present in all continents except Australasia and Antarctica, although several countries, because of geographical barriers, are presently free of infection, e.g. UK, Eire, Iceland, Spain and Portugal.
- Rabies virus does not survive for long outside the body. It is maintained either by serial infection in wildlife ('sylvatic rabies') or by cycles of infection in domestic dogs ('urban rabies').
- Biological variants of the virus species exist, each adapted to different hosts. The strain prevalent in Western Europe is adapted to the red fox (*Vulpes vulpes*) and far less well to the dog – 10^5 times more virus is required to infect dogs than foxes, and dogs are rare excretors of this virus.
- The Western European virus probably originated at the Russian–Polish border in dogs and became adapted to foxes. The epizootic advanced 20–60 km each year, although recently this seems to have stopped, possibly due to variation in virus strain or the ecology of transmission.
- Although the red fox is the vector and reservoir of the disease, humans are mainly at risk from affected domestic animals such as cattle and cats.
- Apart from terrestrial rabies, another European epizootic of rabies exists in insectivorous bats, caused by other species of *Lyssavirus*.

Pathogenesis and Pathology

- Rabies virus is mainly transmitted by biting. The virus multiplies locally within myocytes and moves up the axons of associated nerves to the CNS to produce encephalitis.
- The susceptibility of animals to rabies virus varies enormously, depending on the
  - host species, its immune status and age,
  - virus dose and strain (biotype).
- In dogs, the incubation period is very variable, usually 10 days to 4 months, but possibly up to of 10 months. This variability depends largely on:
  - the site and severity of the bite,
  - the dose and strain of the virus.
- In foxes the incubation period depends mainly on the dose of virus and varies from 10 to 41 days.
- Dogs may excrete virus in saliva for up to 14 (but generally only 3) days, and foxes for 29 days, before the onset of disease.
- The incubation period is characterised by silent progression of infection without any detectable antibody response. Thus there is no serological test for if an animal is infected.
- Rabies is usually fatal. But rare recovery of dogs has been described with silent excretion of rabies virus by apparently healthy animals.
- Gross pathological findings are minimal: possibly
  - emaciation,
  - evidence of self-trauma,
  - foreign bodies in the gut (through pica).
- Neurons may contain intracytoplasmic inclusions (Negri bodies). These are pathognomonic for rabies. Although found in most cases, their absence does not exclude rabies, and diagnosis usually relies on a combination of a fluorescent antibody test on brain smears, and virus isolation in mice and cell cultures.

Clinical Signs

In Dogs

Prodromal Stage

Most cases commence with a change of temperament, and often a rise in body temperature. Saliva may contain large amounts of virus, so dogs in known infected areas which show sudden changes in temperament should be handled cautiously.

Furious Form

In about 25% of rabid dogs (depending on the virus strain), the disease gradually develops into a phase of hyperexcitation, characterised by:

- Restlessness and irritability – snapping at restraints and imaginary objects.
- Possible depraved appetite – chew and swallow stones, wood, carpet or straw.
- Spells of hyperexcitation may be short and infrequent, but may last 5 h and recur after periods when the dog may be friendly.
- If free to wander, rabid dogs may travel 25 miles or more.

Generalized signs of paresis gradually develop – weakness of legs and tail, difficulty in swallowing, and drooping jaw and eyelids. 'Hydrophobia' does not apply to dogs as it does to man. May die during convulsive seizures, but usually the paralysis progresses and animals die in coma.

Dumb Form

This is the most common form of the disease seen in dogs, and may be more difficult to diagnose; prodromal and furious phases can be either absent or transient.

- Progressive paralysis of all muscles.
- Jaw and eyelids droop, the eyes tend to squint.
- Conjunctival congestion is usually marked.
- May drool from the jaws.
- Dogs with dumb rabies can and will bite if provoked.

Not all dogs have typical dumb or furious rabies. A variety of other nervous signs may be observed. The bark may become high pitched and hysterical. Sexual aberration may be seen. The duration of the disease from the first noted clinical signs until death is usually less than 7 days but rarely may extend to 10 days.

In Foxes

- Clinical disease lasts 3–5 days.

- The furious form is relatively rare.
- Most foxes become apathetic and develop paralysis.
- Thus rabid foxes do not usually wander far from their original territory – this may explain why the front of a fox rabies epizootic progresses slowly.

Diagnosis and Action to be Taken with Suspected Cases

In the UK, where rabies is not enzootic, most veterinary surgeons are inexperienced in dealing with the disease. Nevertheless, because of the public health risk, a diagnosis of rabies should always be considered in dogs with signs of neurological disease. Advice can be sought from the local Divisional Veterinary Officer (DVO).

- Suspect cases must be detained in isolation on the premises on which they have been examined, and the local DVO of the Ministry of Agriculture, Fisheries and Food or Department of Agriculture, Northern Ireland must be notified immediately.
- The veterinary surgeon and any other handler should carry out a thorough personal disinfection with soap or detergent and water, and any contaminated clothing should be changed.
- If anyone is bitten or scratched, it is imperative to wash and flush the wound immediately with soap or detergent (not both, as soap inhibits quaternary ammonium compounds) and water, then water alone, followed by application of 40–71% alcohol, tincture or aqueous solutions of iodine, or 0.1% quaternary ammonium compounds (e.g. cetrimide).
- No further animals should enter the consulting room until the case is diagnosed as negative, or the premises satisfactorily cleansed and disinfected under the supervision of the Ministry veterinary officer.
- The names and addresses of any contacts (e.g. those in the waiting room) should be recorded.
- The veterinary officer will inform the medical officer for environmental health of any necessary further action.
- If the animal dies or is killed, the head and neck should be removed by an MAFF veterinary officer and transported fresh and intact to an appropriate diagnostic laboratory (in the UK, the Central Veterinary Laboratory, Weybridge). It should be packed in a sealed container, held at a low temperature, but not frozen.

Prevention and Control

Human Exposure

Veterinarians and others exposed to an increased risk of infection should be protected by preventive vaccination. Human post-exposure treatment requires several vaccinations, together with an injection of specific immunoglobulin if the exposure was severe. Only preventive vaccination is generally carried out in animals, although in some countries post-exposure vaccination may be allowed if they have previously been vaccinated. Attenuated vaccines, widely used in the past, still have residual pathogenicity for some species, and cases of vaccine-induced rabies occasionally occur. Humans exposed to attenuated veterinary vaccines are treated in the same way as after wild-type virus exposure. Recently, safe and potent inactivated vaccines have been developed for veterinary use, and these have now largely superseded attenuated vaccines.

Rabies Control in the UK

Control measures in Britain presently rely on 6 months quarantine in approved premises for all mammals, except farm-stock and horses which are subject to other controls. All animals entering quarantine are vaccinated with an approved, inactivated rabies vaccine, and dogs must also be vaccinated against distemper. Vaccination other than in quarantine or for export is not allowed in the UK. Commercially traded dogs from EC states no longer undergo quarantine, but must come from approved premises, be vaccinated, tested positive for antibody and be permanently identified with a microchip transponder.

Control Measures in Countries Where Rabies is Endemic

Apart from measures aimed at wildlife control, the incidence of the disease in dogs may be reduced by the elimination of strays, licensing, restricting movement and by vaccination. Several vaccines are available for use in dogs (e.g. for USA, see vaccines listed under the Compendium of Animal Rabies Control, 1990). In dogs, primary vaccination is generally not recommended before 3 months of age, followed by a booster 1 year later; thereafter annual or triennial boosters are commended, depending on the vaccine. At least 1 month should be allowed for the development of immunity.

Control of Rabies in Wildlife

Fox rabies is still present in most of continental Western Europe, and the destruction of foxes does not prevent the spread of the epizootic as the fox population rapidly recovers and rabies then recurs. Most recent research on the control of fox rabies has concentrated on the development of methods of vaccination of foxes, notably with a recombinant vaccinia-rabies vaccine in baits. This approach seems very promising, and many areas in mainland Europe are now free from rabies as a result of this.

Chapter 17

Infections of Reproduction and Neonates

C. E. Greene

CANINE HERPESVIRUS INFECTION

Aetiology

Canine herpesvirus (CHV) causes systemic and fatal infection of neonatal and prenatal pups, and a localised respiratory and genital infection of adult dogs. The virus is endemic in dog populations and resides as a inhabitant of the mucosa of the nasopharynx, upper respiratory tract and external genitalia. Infection may spread between adult animals by respiratory or venereal means. Recrudescence and shedding may accompany periods of stress or immunosuppression. Newborn puppies may acquire infection from the genital tract of their dam. *In utero* transmission can occur from subclinical viraemia in susceptible dams.

Pathogenesis

After oronasal exposure, CHV infects the upper respiratory epithelium and in susceptible hosts spreads by viraemia throughout the body into the mononuclear phagocyte system and parenchymal organs. The amount of maternal immunity acquired and body temperature appear to be important factors in determining resistance to the systemic spread of the virus. Temperature regulation of the newborn pup is insufficient until 3 weeks of age so that chilled pups during the first week of life are highly susceptible.

Puppies nursing immune, recovered bitches do not develop clinical illness because of maternal immunity passed in colostrum.

Clinical Signs

There are no signs of illness in bitches that have puppies die of CHV infection. The pups can die at any stage of gesta-

tion with the earliest losses manifest by abortion of dead or mummified fetuses and later infection by abortion or birth of stillborn pups. In neonatally acquired infections, the signs are usually seen between 1 to 3 weeks of age. Puppies develop a fatal illness first manifest by loss of interest in nursing, passing of soft faeces and persistent crying, restlessness and shivering. A serous to mucopurulent or haemorrhagic nasal discharge may be apparent. Petechial haemorrhages may be found on mucous membranes. Discomfort is noticeable on abdominal palpation and papules or vesicles and subcutaneous oedema of the ventral abdominal and inguinal region may be noted. Vesicles are sometimes apparent on the genital and oral mucosae. Puppies develop neurologic dysfunction manifest by opisthotonus and seizures just before death which usually occurs after 24–48 h of illness.

Slightly older puppies may develop upper respiratory tract disease, similar to mild kennel cough.

Diagnosis

The diagnosis of canine herpesvirus infection is usually suspected from the clinical history and physical examination. The pathological changes are usually pathognomonic with multifocal haemorrhagic and necrotic foci throughout parenchymal organs especially the kidney. Viral isolation can be made from culture of many parenchymal tissues of dead neonates. In adult animals, the virus is only temporarily shed from the respiratory and genital mucosae for 2–3 weeks after infection but may re-shed following stress or immunosuppression. Culturing and testing to eliminate infection is not accurate or effective in screening dogs for infection. As a result, the disease in neonates is best prevented by husbandry measures.

Treatment of affected litters is often unsuccessful because puppies die suddenly. Mortality in remaining unaffected or subclinically infected littermates can be reduced by warming their body temperatures to 38.5 to 39.5°C. In addition parenteral administration of hyperimmune sera from recovered bitches may offer some protection from dissemination of virus early in the course of infection. The sporadic nature of the disease and difficulty of producing solid immunity to herpesvirus makes the development of a vaccine unlikely. The prognosis for bitches having infected litters is good because the immunity they develop protects against infection of subsequent litters.

BRUCELLOSIS

Canine brucellosis is caused by a small Gram-negative bacterium (*Brucella canis*) that infects dogs and causes reproductive disorders including infertility and abortion. The organism is acquired by mucosal contact. The highest numbers of infecting organisms are shed in the semen and vaginal discharges and less in urine. Once they gain entry into the body, these organisms are phagocytised by mononuclear phagocytes where they are transported to lymphatic and genital tract tissues where they multiply. A cell-associated bacteraemia can last for many months. Serum antibody titres increase in an attempt of the body to eliminate this persistent intracellular organism.

Clinical Signs

Lymphadenomegaly may be the only manifestation noted in mature dogs, and systemic manifestations of the bacteraemia are rare. Overt clinical disease seen in bitches in late gestation is abortion of pups in the last trimester. Pups are usually aborted partially autolysed and abortion is accompanied by a greenish-black vaginal discharge that can last up to 6 weeks. Infertility, and birth of stillborn puppies can also be noted.

Male dogs show more overt reproductive abnormalities than females. Males develop scrotal swelling from epididymal enlargement and from irritation produced by licking the painful area. Secondary scrotal dermatitis and pyoderma from skin microflora is common.

Dogs may also develop non-reproductive abnormalities from localisation of the blood-borne organisms in various tissues. Lameness, paresis and pain has resulted from osteomyelitis or discospondylitis. Ataxia, hyperaesthesia and cranial nerve dysfunction has been observed with meningoencephalomyelitis. Recurrent anterior uveitis or panophthalmitis has been observed with ocular localisation.

Diagnosis

The diagnosis of brucellosis is usually confirmed by serological testing although definitive incrimination can be made by culture of the organism from blood or tissues. Clinical laboratory abnormalities include: hyperglobulinaemia in many cases; pleocytosis with meningitis; and semen abnormalities in male dogs with epididymitis. Haemoglobin-free specimens should be used for serological tests because false-positive reactions can occur in agglutination assays. Some bacteria are antigenically cross-reactive with *B. canis* producing false-positive reactions in the rapid slide agglutination test (RSAT) and tube agglutination tests (TAT). Mercaptoethanol is used in the screening test, the RSAT, to improve the specificity by removing nonspecific IgM agglutinins. TAT is usually done after the RSAT to quantify serum antibodies. Titres of 50 to 100 are considered suspicious of infection while dogs with 200 or greater are usually bacteraemic. The agar gel immunodiffusion test (AGID), the final serological means of confirmation, is more sensitive and specific when both the somatic and cytoplasmic antigens respectively, are used. The AGID test is performed by a limited number of laboratories but is indicated to resolve discrepant serologic results or to determine if infection may still be present when agglutination tests have become negative after treatment. Blood culture is also used to confirm suspicious titre results or if serological tests are not available. Blood cultures are more time consuming and require special media.

Treatment

Therapy for canine brucellosis is difficult because of the intracellular location of the bacterium. The infection appears to be controlled by several antibiotics but the bacteraemia may reoccur weeks to months after treatment is discontinued, and the organism may be cultured from treated and apparently recovered animals at necropsy. Bitches have been known to clear their infection after treatment although the risk of transmitting a potentially inapparent infection to offspring is never completely eliminated. Male dogs become sterile and aspermic as a result of infection, and therefore treatment of reproductively intact dogs is not advised. Although infected pets are a potential source of zoonotic infection, those that are neutered are of less risk. Antimicrobials that have been effective *in vivo* in treating canine brucellosis are the lipid-soluble tetracyclines (minocycline and doxycycline), aminoglycosides (dihydrostreptomycin, gentamicin), trimethoprim–sulfonamides, and the fluoroquinolones. The most effective regimen that has been evaluated under scrutiny for its effectiveness is high dose minocycline or doxycycline (12.5

mg/kg given orally b.i.d.) for 2 weeks accompanied by gentamicin (2 mg/kg given i.m. or s.c., b.i.d.) for 1 week. Localised infections in isolated tissues such as the intervertebral disc or eye require repeated or longer term therapy.

Preventative measures are most important in avoiding brucellosis in a breeding kennel. Carrier dogs maintain infection and so all animals entering the facility should be screened serologically. Any found positive should be removed from the facility, even if they are neutered, treated, and are kept as pets.

STREPTOCOCCAL INFECTIONS

Beta-haemolytic group G streptococci are normal inhabitants of the skin and mucosal surfaces of dogs yet the veterinary literature contains numerous reports of infection with these organisms including metritis, vaginitis, infertility, abortion and neonatal death. Isolation of these organisms from dying puppies may therefore involve more than simple variation in virulence between isolates. Streptococci are acquired from the bitch during whelping and they may gain entrance by the umbilical vein and can spread into the liver and eventually to the systemic circulation. The neonatal puppy may initially become contaminated at birth; however, it is stress of uncleanliness, improper umbilical disinfection and improper nursing which allow the infection to overwhelm host defences. Puppies may show clinical illness during the first few weeks of life, or they may develop delayed manifestations of systemic infection with embolic localisation of infection in such areas as the joints with manifestations of fever and polyarthritis. Diagnosis of beta-haemolytic streptococcal infection can be achieved by culturing the organism from tissues or body fluids involved with suppurative infection. Streptococcal infections are very susceptible to penicillin and its derivatives. Solitary abscesses should be surgically drained with addition of systemic antimicrobial therapy.

Chapter 18

Canine Papillomas

M. Bennett

Clinical Signs

Canine papillomavirus is a common cause of oral papillomas in puppies world-wide. Cutaneous papillomas and warts in older dogs may also be caused by a papilloma virus, but, if so, the virus appears to be different from, and not so readily transmissible as, that of puppies.

The papillomas are:

- initially smooth pale, or pink, papules,
- which later develop into larger, irregular, cauliflower-like lesions,
- usually limited to the buccal mucosa and tongue,
- occasionally on the conjunctivae and rarely the oesophagus and skin around the nose and mouth.

The lesions are benign and self-limiting, and puppies usually recover in 1–5 months. However, large papillomas can sometimes interfere with eating, or may be associated with halitosis or mild oral haemorrhage.

Diagnosis

Generally made from the clinical signs, but can be confirmed by histopathology, especially immunocytochemistry. Like most papillomaviruses, canine papillomavirus cannot be grown in cell culture.

Treatment and Control

Usually unnecessary, but if the tumours are causing discomfort, obstruction or persist, surgical removal may be indicated. Care must be taken not to spread lesions by inoculation of infective material into fresh sites during surgery. The value of autogenous vaccines in affected animals is debatable. Commercial, or specially-produced autogenous vaccines are available in some areas, but are only recommended for use during outbreaks in kennels with large numbers of dogs.

Chapter 19

Tetanus

B. J. Tennant

Aetiology

The cause of tetanus is *Clostridium tetani. Cl. tetani* spores persist in the environment for prolonged periods of time. Contamination of a deep wound or an area of tissue damage with these spores may result in their conversion to a vegetative form with the consequent production of a neurotoxin, neurospasmin. This toxin ascends peripheral nerves to the spinal cord where it blocks the release of neurotransmitter from inhibitory interneurons. Release of extensor muscles from inhibition results in increased involuntary activity ranging from tremors to opisthotonus.

Clinical Signs

Clinical signs (Table 19.1) may develop from 5 to 20 days after wound infection.

Diagnosis

Cl. tetani infection is diagnosed primarily on the basis of clinical signs and a history of wounding, although on occasion no wound is found. Isolation of the organism from wounds is difficult and is not necessary for the diagnosis.

Treatment

Cl. tetani infections should be treated immediately with:

- Wound debridement. *Cl. tetani* is an anaerobic bacteria, thus physically opening and draining wounds limits further growth of the bacteria.
- Antibiotics. Penicillin G (25 mg/kg i.v. every 4–6 h, i.m. every 12 h) or metronidazole (10 mg/kg i.v., s.c. or 30 mg/kg p.o. every 12 h) are suitable drugs. Intravenous administration is indicated initially. They should be adminstered for 2 weeks or until clinical signs resolve.
- Neutralisation of the toxin. The administration of tetanus antitoxin intravenously or locally just proximal to the wound site in dogs with localised tetanus has been recommended. As it does not penetrate the CNS, its efficacy is doubtful once clinical signs are established. There is a risk of anaphylactic reactions, thus, a test dose should be injected intradermally 30 min before administration of the treatment dose. If no wheal develops, antitoxin may be administered. The dose is not repeated as therapeutic blood levels persist for 7–10 days after one injection.
- Rest. Affected dogs should be housed in a quiet, dark environment to minimise CNS stimulation.

Table 19.1 Clinical signs of tetanus.

Mild or early tetanus	Severely affected animals
A stiff gait	Hyperaesthesia
Erect ears	Muscle spasms
An elevated tail	Recumbency
Contraction of facial muscles	Extensor rigidity of all four legs and opisthotonus
Signs are often most pronounced in areas adjacent to where the toxin is produced.	Seizures (rare)
	Faecal and urinary retention

- Muscle spasms may be controlled with diazepam (0.5–2 mg/kg i.v., p.o. p.r.n.) and chlorpromazine (0.5 mg/kg i.v. every 8 h) or acepromazine (0.1–0.2 mg/kg i.m. every 6 h), or methocarbamol (220 mg/kg i.v. slowly p.r.n. or 45 mg/kg p.o. every 8 h). Seizures can be controlled with pentobarbitone (5–15 mg/kg i.v. to effect).
- Supportive care. Intravenous fluid therapy and nutritional support are used as required. Urinary and faecal retention are managed by repeated catheterisation and enemas when necessary.

Prognosis

Clinical signs begin to resolve within 1 week, but may persist for up to 4 weeks. If signs progress rapidly, the prognosis is poor with many severely affected dogs dying within 5 days from respiratory failure.

Chapter 20

Tuberculosis

M. Bennett

Aetiology

Tuberculosis in dogs is usually caused by *Mycobacterium tuberculosis*, less commonly by *M. bovis*, or, very rarely, by *M. avium-intracellulare* complex. In addition, various other mycobacteria may be involved in chronic wounds and abscesses.

Epidemiology

Tuberculosis is an uncommon disease of dogs. *M. tuberculosis* and *M. bovis* infections are generally contracted from humans, although cattle and wild mammals might be an alternative source of infection in some areas. *M. avium* is a saprophyte found in soil and water, and a rare opportunist pathogen of animals and man. Generally tuberculosis is acquired by the respiratory or oral route and infection is often subclinical.

Clinical Signs

These are summarised in Table 20.1.

Diagnosis

Usually based on a combination of history and the demonstration of acid-fast organisms in biopsies or smears of exudates. Isolation may be possible on special media, but can be a lengthy process. Radiography may reveal large granulomas in the respiratory tract. Skin tests give inconsistent results in dogs, although intradermal BCG (Bacille Calmette–Guérin vaccine, 0.1–0.2 ml in the inner surface of the pinna) is said to give more consistent results than purified protein derivative (PPD). A hard swelling between 48 and 72 h of injection is taken as positive; erythema alone is taken to be negative. Very often, the diagnosis is made at necropsy.

Table 20.1 Clinical features of tuberculosis.

Respiratory infection	Intestinal infection
Retching	Chronic weight loss and wasting
Non-productive cough	Anaemia and diarrhoea due to malabsorption
Dysphagia or hypersalivation	Palpably enlarged mesenteric lymph nodes
Chronic ulceration of the oropharynx, tonsils and draining lymph nodes	Anorexia
Bronchopneumonia	Infection may spread to plurae or abdominal organs
Anorexia	Generalised lymphadenopathy, or skin lesions.
Wasting	Infection may spread to plurae or abdominal organs
Infection may spread to plurae or abdominal organs	
Generalised lymphadenopathy, or skin lesions	

Treatment

Successful treatment of dogs experimentally infected with
M. tuberculosis has been reported with rifampicin, isoniazid
and streptomycin for 23 months. However, as bacteriological cure is rare, euthanasia is often recommended on public
health grounds.

Atypical Mycobacterial Infections

Occasionally, various saprophytic *Mycobacteria* including
M. fortuitum–M. chelonei complex, *M. smegmatis*, *M. xenopi*
and *M. phlei* have been isolated from superficial or, rarely,
deeper, persistent abscesses and ulcerative or granulomatous lesions of dogs.

Treatment is by surgical removal/drainage combined
with antibiotics. Gentamicin (2 mg/kg i.m. or s.c. b.i.d.) or
potentiated sulphonamides (10–15 mg/kg p.o. b.i.d.), are
sometimes useful as the usual anti-tuberculous antibiotics
are often ineffective.

Chapter 21

Lyme Disease

S. D. Carter

Epidemiology and Aetiology

Lyme disease is a multisystemic disorder arising from infection with the spirochaete, *Borrelia burgdorferi* and was first described by Willi Burgdorfer in children with sudden onset polyarthritis and erythematous skin rash in Lyme, Connecticut, USA in 1975. Although parasitism with *B. burgdorferi* (borreliosis) occurs in many domesticated mammalian species, it only regularly causes clinical syndromes resembling Lyme disease in some; and only the dog appears to be affected as seriously as man, with canine cases reported in both the USA and Europe. *B. burgdorferi* is epizootic and transmitted primarily by ixodid ticks, which in the USA are *Ixodes dammini* or *I. pacificus* and in Europe is *I. ricinus*. These ticks were originally associated with deer and sheep but now are known to be carried by many small rodents, which are probably the main reservoir hosts. All stages of the tick (larva, nymph and adult) can be effective vectors, although the nymph is most often implicated. Tick larvae or nymphs become infected when they take a blood meal from a reservoir host, many of which are persistently infected. The organisms are transmitted in salivary secretions during feeding and are secondarily transmitted to other mammals including man, cats, horses and dogs.

Pathogenesis

Not all infected animals, particularly the primary hosts, show clinical signs of infection. In animals showing clinical signs, infection with *B. burgdorferi* has been shown in all tissues in which there are pathological changes. The infection is spread through both the blood and the lymphatics. Organisms are rare in infected tissues but may be detected by sensitive molecular biology techniques. Most pathology is caused by the host's inflammatory response, primarily as a result of activation of phagocytes. The immune response which develops during infection is not adequate to eradicate the organism, even though it is only slow growing. In dogs, lesions are seen primarily in joints. The typical erythematous skin rash seen in man is not seen in the dog.

Clinical Features

Predominantly acute or subacute.
Common signs in the dog:

- lameness,
- fever,
- anorexia,
- lethargy,
- lymphadenopathy.

In lame dogs, one or more joints may be involved: the joints are swollen, hot and painful.

Other clinical signs which may be seen include carditis, glomerulonephritis and neurological signs (behavioural changes, aggression, seizures).

Investigations

Clinical examination for joint disease, neurological defects, carditis, pyrexia. Serology for *B. burgdorferi* infection (interpret with caution). Analysis of synovial fluid from affected joints shows cytological changes consistent with an inflammatory arthropathy, usually of low grade. Radiographs of affected joints may be normal, or show only soft tissue swelling in the joints. Dogs with Lyme disease most commonly present with acute, migratory monoarthritis or pauciarthritis; true polyarthritis is rare. Episodes of lameness typically last only a few days and there is often an associated pyrexia and lymphadenopathy.

Table 21.1   Criteria for diagnosis of canine Lyme disease.

(1)   A history of potential exposure to *B. burgdorferi* and ixodid ticks.
(2)   Seasonal incidence: associated with peaks in tick activity, particularly the nymph or adult stages which are more likely to transmit *B. burgdorferi*.
(3)   Appropriate clinical signs: including fever, malaise, lethargy, inappetence, lymphadenopathy, lameness, carditis (heart block), neurological signs and, possibly, glomerulonephritis.
(4)   Laboratory/radiological support for the diagnosis: in cases of Lyme arthritis this should include radiographic evidence of a synovial effusion and synovial fluid analysis consistent with synovitis.
(5)   Positive serological test for *B. burgdorferi*. Many asymptomatic animals are positive for anti-*Borrelia* antibodies.
(6)   Response to antibiotic therapy.
(7)   Identification of *B. burgdorferi* in blood, urine, synovial fluid, CSF or other tissues.
(8)   Culture of *B. burgdorferi* from blood, urine, synovial fluid, CSF, or other tissues.
(9)   Exclusion of other possible causes of similar clinical signs: including traumatic arthritis, osteoarthritis and the immune mediated polyarthritides.

Diagnosis

A diagnosis of Lyme disease is difficult to establish with certainty. Lameness is a common clinical presentation in dogs as a result of injuries to the foot pads, trauma, osteoarthritis or many other diseases of bones and joints. Serological testing is of value although subclinical infections can occur and the antibodies to *B. burgdorferi* may cross react with other spirochaetes or bacteria. The mere presence of a positive serum anti-*Borrelia* antibody in a dog with lameness is insufficient evidence on which to base a diagnosis of Lyme disease. Furthermore, *B. burgdorferi* is notoriously difficult to culture from clinical cases. The study of Lyme disease in dogs is hampered by these diagnostic difficulties and by the lack of an early marker of clinical disease. The typical skin rash occurring in early Lyme disease of man is not seen in dogs and the stages of clinical disease are less well defined than they are in man. Diagnosis of Lyme disease in dogs presently relies on the expertise of the clinician and the support of laboratory aids, particularly serology.

A diagnosis of Lyme disease in dogs should satisfy criteria 1, 3, 4, 5 and 9 in Table 21.1. Criterion 6 should subsequently be satisfied in almost all cases. Ideally, criteria 7 and 8 should also be satisfied, but this may be difficult as the organism is difficult to culture and may only be present in very low numbers. Even in low numbers, the organism can be detected by polymerase chain reaction or *in situ* hybridisation, but these techniques are not in common use for routine Lyme diagnosis at present.

Treatment and Control

Once a diagnosis has been reached, antibiotics should be used as early as possible. Most antibiotics are effective and should be used for as long as 3–4 weeks. If there is no response within 10 days, the antibiotic should be changed. Prophylactic use on tick bitten dogs is not recommended. Vaccination with components of *B. burgdorferi* is now commercially available in some countries, although not in the UK.

Prognosis

Chronic infection is rare. Antibiotic therapy, particularly given early is usually effective and usually results in falling antibody titres.

Chapter 22

Tularaemia

S. Barr

Aetiology and Epidemiology

Caused by the zoonotic bacterium *Francisella tularensis*, a small, pleomorphic, Gram-negative, non-spore forming bacillus. Two biotypes:

- Type A (ferments glycerol and highly virulent to rabbits) occurs only in North America and produces classic disease in human beings.
- Type B (does not ferment glycerol and is less virulent to rabbits) occurs throughout the Northern Hemisphere, has low virulence for human beings, and is more commonly associated with rodents and waterborne infections.

Various tick species (the 'dog tick' *Dermacentor variabilis*, the 'wood tick' *Dermacentor andersoni*, the 'Lone-Star tick' *Amblyomma americanum*, and the 'Pacific Coast tick' *Dermacentor occidentalis*), and the deerfly, *Chrysops discalis*, are primary vectors for dogs and cats. Trans-stadial and transovarial passage occurs in ticks. Dogs and cats can become infected by tick or fly bites, ingestion of contaminated water or infected mammals. *Francisella tularensis* can survive up to 4 months in water, mud, or decaying carcasses.

Pathogenesis and Clinical Features

Dogs are considered resistant to tularaemia although puppies are more susceptible than older dogs. From the site of inoculation, the bacterium spreads through the regional lymphatics to disseminate by blood. Experimentally, 48 h after ingestion of infected material, dogs develop fevers and mucopurulent ocular-nasal discharge lasting for 5 days. Intradermal challenge produces fever, pustules at the inoculation site, and regional lymphadenopathy. Intramuscular or subcutaneous challenge produces draining abscesses at the site, regional lymphadenopathy, septicemia with high fever and high mortality. Naturally acquired cases are rare. After exposure, dogs develop a low-grade fever, anorexia, listlessness, sudden death, and occasionally uveitis.

Diagnosis

Direct or indirect fluorescent antibody tests on biopsied or aspirated material (especially lymph nodes or bone marrow) is the most expedient method of diagnosis. Culture of *F. tularensis* requires special sample handling, special media (blood–glucose–cysteine agar), and takes 24–48 h to grow. Some laboratories will not attempt culture because of the high risk of laboratory-acquired disease.

Management and Prognosis

There are no reports on the efficacy of antimicrobial therapy for canine tularaemia. Few naturally infected cats and dogs have been reported to survive infection.

- Streptomycin (15–20 mg/kg per day) is the drug of choice in man.
- Gentamicin (5 mg/kg per day) is an acceptable alternative.
- Tetracycline and chloramphenicol are alternatives but are associated with relapses.

Chapter 23

Canine Rickettsiosis

Z. Woldehiwet

Aetiology and Pathogenesis

Rickettsiae are obligately intracellular Gram-negative bacteria requiring host cells for their metabolism. Most of those pathogenic to dogs belong to the tribe Ehrlichieae, e.g. *Ehrlichia canis*, the cause of canine ehrlichiosis and tropical canine pancytopenia, *E. platys*, the cause of infectious cyclic thrombocytopenia, and *Neorickettsia helmintheca* and *N. elokominica*, which cause salmon poisoning disease and Elokomin fluke liver fever. Other rickettsiae which may cause disease in dogs include *Rickettsia rickettsii*, the cause of Rocky Mountain spotted fever; *Rickettsia conorii*, the cause of boutonneuse or tick bite fever; *Haemobartonella canis*, which usually causes no disease but may cause anaemia and jaundice; and *Coxiella burnetii*, which causes Q-fever in man, cattle and cats but non-clinical infections in dogs. After entry through a tick bite or other route, the organisms gain access to their target tissues through phagocytosis or endocytosis. The mechanisms of leukopenia and thrombocytopenia are not clearly established but are thought to be related to the sequestration of infected cells. The other pathological changes such as anaemia and hyperglobulinaemia (haemobartonellosis, canine ehrlichiosis) could be due to misdirected immune responses.

Epidemiology

With the exception of *C. burnetii* and *Neorickettsia*, all the agents are transmitted by ticks. The former does not require any intermediate hosts while the latter requires a trematode, snails and fish as intermediary hosts before infecting dogs. The geographical distributions (Table 23.1) of the diseases caused by these agents is therefore determined by the distribution of their vectors. For example, coxiellosis which is not dependent on a biological vector is present world-wide while the ehrlichial agents are found wherever their ticks are found.

Clinical Features

The different rickettsial infections have some common clinical and haematological features, including fever, depression, anorexia, lethargy, anaemia and various degrees of leukopenia (summarised in Table 23.2). Canine ehrlichiosis may be acute, chronic or subclinical. Acute ehrlichiosis lasts for 2–4 weeks and may be followed by complete recovery or sub-clinical infection lasting up to 4–5 years. Tropical canine pancytopenia is a severe and chronic sequel of subclinical infection. Clinical cases of acute and chronic ehrlichiosis may be difficult to differentiate and are often complicated by other infections including babesiosis, haemobartonellosis and other infections.

Dual infections with two or more rickettsial agents (e.g. *E. canis*, *E. platys* and/or *H. canis*) may occur.

Diagnosis

Ehrlichial infections should be suspected in endemic areas when the common clinical signs of anorexia, depression, fever, anaemia and haemorrhages are seen in association with recent exposure to ticks. Diagnosis can be confirmed on haematology, isolation and immunological detection.

Haematology and Clinical Chemistry

- Blood or lymph node smears for presence of rickettsiae
  - within infected mononuclear cells (*E. canis*, *Neorickettsia* spp.),
  - within neutrophils (*E. canis*),
  - within blood platelets (*E. platys*),
  - or on the surface of erythrocytes (*H. canis*).
- Leukopenia/lymphopenia, decreased PCV, increased bleeding time and sometimes positive Coombs' test.
- Hyperglobulinaemia and hypoalbuminaemia in acute and chronic ehrlichiosis.

Table 23.1 Geographic distribution of rickettsial agents causing disease in dogs.

Agent	Disease	Target cells	Transmission	Geographic distribution
Coxiella burnetii	Coxiellosis Q-fever	Reticuloendothelial cells	Birth fluid, milk, dust	World-wide
Ehrlichia canis	Ehrlichiosis Tropical pancytopenia	Mononuclear cells, macrophages	*Rhipicephalus sanguineus*	N. & S. America, Africa, Asia, S. Europe
Ehrlichia platys	Infectious anaemia	Patelets	Ticks?	N. America S. Europe
Haemobartonella canis	Haemobartonellosis	Erythrocytes	Arthropods?	World-wide
Neorickettsia helmintheca	Salmon poisoning disease	Lymphoid system	Infected salmonid fish	USA and Canada (Pacific Coast)
Neorickettsia elokominica	Elokomin fluke liver fever	Macrophages		
Rickettsia conorii	Boutonneuse or tick bite fever	Epithelial cells	Ticks	Africa, S. Europe
Rickettsia rickettsii	Rocky Mountain spotted fever	Vascular endothelium	*Dermacentor* spp.	The Americas

Table 23.2 The main clinical and haematological features of canine rickettsiosis.

Disease	Prepatent period	Clinical signs	Haematology
Canine ehrlichiosis (acute) (*E. canis*)	8–20 days	Fever (41–41.5°C), oedema, depression, weight loss, anaemia	Reduced PCV, increased sedimentaion and bleeding time, thrombocytopenia, leukopenia
Tropical canine pancytopenia	As above	Fever (longer duration), anaemia, corneal opacity, petechiation, oedema, death	Reduced PCV, pancytopenia, hyperglobulinaemia
Infectious cyclic thrombocytopenia (*E. platys*)	3–20 days	Fever (39.4–40.3°C), anaemia	Thrombocytopenia, low PCV, leukopenia
Salmon poisoning disease (SPD) (*N. helmintheca*)	5–7 days	Fever (40–42°C), anorexia, weight loss, diarrhoea, vomiting, thirst, anaemia	Mild leukopenia, thrombocytopenia, lymphopenia
Elokomin fluke liver fever (EFF) (*N. elokominica*)	5–12 days		Mild leukopenia, thrombocytopenia
Rock Mountain spotted fever (RMSF) (*R. rickettsii*)	2–3 days?	Fever (≥38°C), anorexia, depression, Petechiae, epistaxis, lymphadonopathy, subcutaneous oedema	
Haemobartonellosis (*H. canis*)	2–21 days	Anaemia (moderate or mild), icterus, splenomegaly	Low PCV (20%)

- Elevated alkaline phophatase and alanine transaminase in chronic ehrlichiosis and Rocky Mountain spotted fever (RMSF), with hypoalbuminaemia in RMSF.

Immunology and Isolation in Culture

- Demonstration of antigens in tissues or antibody in sera.
- In monocytic/macrophage cells (*E. canis*, *Neorickettsia* spp.).
- Embryonated fowl eggs (*C. burnetii*, *R. rickettsii*). N.B. both are serious human pathogens and must be handled in designated laboratories.

Other Investigations

- Polymerase chain reaction (PCR) or DNA-hybridisation.
- Trematode eggs in dog faeces for salmon poisoning disease/Elokomin fluke liver fever.

Treatment

Many cases will require hospitalisaion and symptomatic therapy for severe emesis and diarrhoea. In those cases where severe anaemia develops blood transfusions are required.

Antibiotic Therapy

- Oxytetracycline/tetracycline hydrochloride, 22 mg/kg t.i.d. for 1 week (SPD/EFF and RMSF), 2 weeks (for haemobartonellosis) or 3–4 weeks (for ehrlichiosis and infectious cyclic thrombocytopenia).
- Doxycyline 5–10 mg/kg, b.i.d. for 2 weeks, or imido-carb dipropionate 5 mg/kg once weekly for 2–3 weeks for ehrlichiosis.
- Chloramphenicol, 22–50 mg/kg t.i.d. for 1–3 weeks for most rickettsiae.
- Praziquantel, 10–30 mg/kg to eliminate trematodes in SPD/EFF.

Chapter 24

Deep Mycoses

S. Barr

The following diseases are discussed in this chapter:

- Blastomycosis
- Histoplasmosis
- Cryptococcus
- Coccidiomycosis
- Sporotrichosis
- Rhinosporidosis
- Candidiasis
- Trichosporosis.

BLASTOMYCOSIS

Aetiology and Epidemiology

Caused by *Blastomyces dermatitidis*, a dimorphic fungus which grows in tissues as a yeast. The organism is a soil saprophyte, endemic world-wide but particularly on the eastern seaboard, Great Lakes region, and Mississippi, Ohio, and St Lawrence river valleys of the USA. Transmission from dog to dog or man is remote although reported.

Pathogenesis and Clinical Features

Three forms of disease are identified: primary pulmonary disease after inhalation of spores; disseminated disease after spread from a pulmonary infection; and local cutaneous disease after inoculation of spores into the skin. Inhaled spores deposited within alveolae are phagocytosed by macrophages, where they multiply. Yeast rupture out of macrophages and continue to divide within the lungs promoting a considerable inflammatory response. The immune response may limit the infection to the lungs and local lymph nodes, or dissemination by the lymphatic and haematogenous routes to other organs (skin, eyes, CNS,

heart, joints etc.) may occur. Localised pulmonary forms may go unrecognised or exhibit anorexia, weight loss, fever, cough, and occasionally dyspnoea. Disseminated forms present with signs of systemic disease (fever and more than one organ system involved) often including pulmonary involvement (non-productive cough, dyspnoea). Cutaneous (fistulous tracts in nodular lesions, generalised lymphadenopathy) and ocular (uveitis, glaucoma, retinal detachment) disease occur in nearly half of disseminated cases. Osseous involvement (single osteolytic lesions with periosteal reactions of a long bone) resulting in lameness and sinus tracts occur in up to 25% of cases. Urogenital and central nervous system involvement are less common.

Diagnosis

- Non-regenerative anaemia is common in chronic disease. Leukocytosis with a left shift, monocytosis and lymphopenia is usually present. Hypercalcaemia is occasionally seen.
- Pulmonary radiographs often reveal generalised, diffuse, miliary nodular interstitial pattern with mediastinal and tracheobronchial lymphadenopathy. Osseous lesions are usually confined to the epiphyseal region of one long bone especially below the stifle and elbow.
- Finding yeast in stained aspirates (lymph nodes, lungs, ocular) or impressions (fistulous discharges, transtracheal washes, CSF, urine, pleural fluid) yields a definitive diagnosis in most animals.
- Culture isolation is not often advised because of the ease of identifying organisms on cytology or histopathology, and the high risk of human laboratory infection from the mycelial phase.
- Serology (agar gel immunodiffusion and counter immunoelectrophoresis) is highly sensitive and specific.

Table 24.1 Recommended drugs for the treatment of deep mycoses.

Systemic drug	Dosage (mg/kg per day)	Route	Interval	Duration (months)
Amphotericin B	0.5	i.v.	3 times weekly	Up to total dose of 4 mg
Ketoconazole	10–30	p.o.	every 12 h	4–6
Itraconazole	10	p.o.	every 24 h	4–6
Fluconazole	5–10	p.o.	every 12–24 h	4–6
Na iodide (20%)	44	p.o.	every 8 h	1 after cure

Drugs Used in Treatments

● Amphotericin B with or without ketoconazole or itraconazole (see Table 24.1).

HISTOPLASMOSIS

Aetiology and Epidemiology

Caused by *Histoplasma capsulatum*, a dimorphic fungus which grows in tissues as a yeast. The organism is a soil saprophyte preferring soils rich in bird and bat faeces. Endemic world-wide but disease mainly seen in the Mississippi, Ohio, and Missouri river valleys of USA.

Pathogenesis and Clinical Features

Pulmonary histoplasmosis is acquired by inhalation of spores into alveoli where they multiply as yeast, spread to local lymph nodes, and are disseminated. Gastrointestinal histoplasmosis without pulmonary disease suggests that the gastrointestinal tract may be also a primary site of infection. Dogs frequently develop gastrointestinal dysfunction (weight loss, large bowel diarrhoea eventually also involving small bowel with watery loose stools and protein-losing enteropathy) sometimes including hepatomegaly, splenomegaly, icterus and ascites. Pulmonary involvement may be manifested by cough, dyspnoea, and abnormal lung sounds.

Diagnosis

● Normocytic, normochromic, non-regenerative anaemia is common. Leukocytosis with a left shift, monocytosis and lymphopenia is usually present, although leukopenia may be present. *Histoplasma*

organisms may be seen in blood monocytes or neutrophils, especially on buffy coat smears or bone marrow aspirates. Serum chemistry profiles reflect organ dysfunction (liver, kidney) or protein-losing enteropathy.
● Pulmonary radiographs often reveal generalised, diffuse, miliary nodular interstitial pattern. Hilar lymphadenopathy is often prominent in dogs. Osseous lesions are rare.
● Intracellular organisms (2–4 μm round bodies) are numerous in aspirates of lymph nodes, lungs, or rectal scrapings. Culture is not often advised because of the ease of identifying organisms on cytology or histopathology, and the high risk of human laboratory infection from the mycelial phase. Intradermal skin tests and serology are often falsely negative in dogs and cats.

Drugs Used in Treatments

● Amphotericin B with or without ketoconazole or itraconazole (see Table 24.1).

CRYPTOCOCCOSIS

Aetiology and Epidemiology

Caused by the saprophytic budding yeast, *Cryptococcus neoformans*. It is found world-wide.

Pathogenesis and Clinical Features

Primary portal of entry is the respiratory tract but the CNS is the most common site of infection resulting in granulomatous meningoencephalitis; ocular lesions are also common. Skin lesions are less common; involvement of the lungs, bone, lymph nodes, kidneys, heart, spleen, nasal cavity have been reported.

Diagnosis

Aspirate cytology of nasal lesions and skin masses usually reveals numerous capsulated organisms. A latex cryptococcal antigen test to detect capsular antigen in serum, CSF, urine, or aqueous is sensitive. Antigen levels parallel the severity of infection and can be used to monitor treatment efficacy.

Drugs Used in Treatments

- Itraconazole, ketoconazole, and rarely, amphotericin B (see Table 24.1).

COCCIDIOMYCOSIS

Aetiology and Epidemiology

Caused the soil-borne fungus, *Coccidioides immitis*, found in dry desert-like areas of southwestern United States. Infection occurs by inhalation of airborne arthrospores. In tissues, *Coccidioides* forms large (20–100 μm) spherules that release endospores.

Clinical Signs

Fever, cough, dyspnoea are common due to acute and chronic granulomatous pneumonia and tracheobronchial lymphadenopathy. In contrast to some of the other deep mycoses coccidioides rarely dissemination to affect multiple tissues. It is more common for the infection to be subclinical.

Diagnosis

- Serology is fairly reliable.
- Thoracic radiographs are similar to histoplasmosis.
- Definitive diagnosis depends on identifying spherules in affected tissues or culturing in Sabouraud's medium.

Treatment

- Ketoconazole or itraconazole for 8 to 12 months (see Table 24.1).

SPOROTRICHOSIS

Aetiology and Epidemiology

Caused by the dimorphic fungus, *Sporothrix schenckii*, which has a world-wide distribution. Infection is usually as a result of inoculation into the skin by thorns or plant material.

Clinical Signs

- The cutaneous form consists of dermal or subcutaneous nodules which may ulcerate to form crusts.
- The cutaneolymphatic form usually develops nodules on the distal aspect of a single limb with lymphadenopathy and draining sinuses from the lymph tissue.
- The disseminated form may arise after autoinfection from localised cutaneous forms, dissemination via lymphatics, and involvement of internal organs.

Definitive Diagnosis

- Depends on demonstrating the organism (pleomorphic round or oval yeast) in exudates or in aspirates from lesions (difficult as numbers of organisms are low), or on histological sections of lesion.
- Direct immunofluorescent test on biopsied tissue and culture may aid a diagnosis.

Treatment

- Inorganic iodides, ketoconazole, and itraconazole for 2 months (see Table 24.1).

RHINOSPORIDIOSIS

Clinical Features, Diagnosis and Treatment

Caused by the fungal agent *Rhinosporidium seeberi*, which is endemic in India, Sri Lanka, and Argentina but occurs sporadically in other areas of the world. The major clinical finding is a unilateral polypoid single mass in the anterior nares resulting in sneezing, epistaxis, and stertorous breathing. Definitive diagnosis depends on demonstrating the organism (100–400 µm nucleated sporangia) in exudates, or in aspirates or histological sections of lesions. Treatment is the surgical removal of the mass.

CANDIDIASIS

Aetiology and Epidemiology

Caused by the dimorphic fungus *Candida* spp. The yeast phase is a commensal inhabitant of the alimentary, upper respiratory, and genital mucosa of mammals. Infection is initiated by local proliferation in wounds or on mucosal surfaces before dissemination which may occur if the cell-mediated immune system (especially neutrophil function) is compromised. Embolic colonisation of multiple sites results in microabscess formation.

Clinical Signs

- Localised candidiasis is characterised by non-healing ulcers of the oral, gastrointestinal, and genitourinary mucosa in immunocompromised animals.
- Systemic candidiasis is usually widespread resulting in multiple organ involvement usually including erythematous to haemorrhagic skin lesions which eventually ulcerate.

Diagnosis

Culture of organisms from specific sites (such as aseptically collected urine samples, deep biopsies of skin lesions) are needed to rule out normal inhabitants of the skin. Histology may be needed to confirm deep infections.

Treatment

Localised lesions are best treated with local application of nystatin, gentian violet (1:10000), miconazole creams. Ketoconazole and itraconazole are indicated for systemic infections (see Table 24.1).

TRICHOSPOROSIS

Aetiology and Epidemiology

Caused by the saprophytic yeast like fungus *Trichosporon* spp. The organism has a world-wide distribution, and causes rare infections in cats.

Clinical Signs

Mixed suppurative and granulomatous inflammation of the mucosal and submucosal or subcutaneous tissues, lymphadenopathy, and one cat developed cystitis.

Diagnosis

Diagnosis relies on demonstrating intracellular yeast in exudates or aspirates from lesions. Biopsy or culture of deep tissue can confirm infection instead of a skin commensal.

Treatment

Ketoconazole and itraconazole until resolved (see Table 24.1).

Chapter 25

Protothecosis

J. Taboada

Aetiology

Prototheccosis is a rare multisystemic disease of dogs caused by unicellular saprophytic organisms of the genus *Prototheca*. Two *Prototheca* species, *P. zopfii* and *P. wickerhamii*, are reported to cause disease. *Prototheca* species are morphologically similar to *Chlorella* species of green algae but lack chlorophyl. Using nucleic acid sequence comparison of primarily small subunit (ss) rRNA, *Prototheca* species are classified as protistan organisms in the same phylogenetic branch of blue-green algae. The organisms are closely related to the oomycotic organism, *Pythium insidiosum*, that causes cutaneous and gastrointestinal pythiosis (phycomycosis) in dogs.

Epidemiology

Prototheca has caused disease in dogs, cats, humans, other mammals, fish, and reptiles. The first cases of canine protothecosis were reported in 1969. Since that time 22 cases have been reported in the veterinary literature. While in most species, protothecosis is characterised by localised cutaneous infection, the disease in dogs is generally systemic in nature. Most affected dogs are female (14 of 18 in one study). There is no age predilection (range 2 to 10 years) but a disproportionate number of cases have occurred in Collies (6 of 22) suggesting a breed predisposition.

Pathogenesis

Prototheca infections are not transmissible from one dog to another. Dogs are more likely to encounter the organisms in water, soil, or food contaminated with raw or treated sewage, animal wastes, or other organic matter. Only rare exposures to *Prototheca* organisms will result in disease. Immunocompromised states such as defective cell-mediated immunity or neutrophil function may be important predisposing factors in dogs that do become infected. The most likely portal of entry for *Prototheca* is the gastrointestinal tract, especially the colon. From this site the organisms likely spread via the blood and local lymphatics to mesenteric lymph nodes and other tissues such as the eyes, central nervous system, heart, kidneys, liver, pancreas, lungs, thyroid, skeletal muscle, peripheral lymph nodes, spleen, cochlea, aorta, and skin. While any organ system can become involved, clinical signs are usually attributable to granulomatous inflammation of the colon, eyes, and central nervous system. *Prototheca* can cause localised infection of the skin or nasal cavity without systemic involvement but this form of the disease is less common.

Clinical Features

Systemic Disease

Most dogs with protothecosis will be presented to a veterinarian for debilitating disease that has been ongoing for months. Signs will vary significantly depending on the tissues involved. Bloody diarrhoea or blood containing faeces and posterior-segment ocular disease characterised by exudative retinal detachment, chorioretinitis, retinal haemorrhage, and vitreal clouding are the most common presenting clinical signs. Sudden blindness may result in an acute presentation and sudden death caused by myocarditis has been reported.

The most typical clinical features of canine protothecosis are:

- diarrhoea (usually hemorrhagic) with weight loss and debility,
- blindness (caused by exudative retinal detachment or panuveitis with chorioretinitis and retinal hemorrhage),

- central nervous system signs (with may include depression, ataxia, head tilt, circling, paresis, deafness, and cranial nerve deficits).

Less common clinical features include:

- lymphadenopathy,
- nodular skin disease,
- polyuria/haematuria,
- otitis externa,
- rhinitis/sinusitis,
- neuromuscular weakness,
- mucocutaneous disease.

Localised Disease

Nodular skin disease, ulcerated mucocutaneous disease, and nasal disease is occasionally seen in dogs without evidence of systemic involvement. Localised disease may be more commonly associated with *P. wickerhamii* infection than that with *P. zopfii*.

Diagnosis

Non-specific abnormalities associated with multisystemic disease and chronic inflammation may be noted on the complete blood count and chemistry profile. Protein increases and neutrophilic or mononuclear cell pleocytosis may be noted on CSF analysis. Definitive diagnosis of protothecosis is dependent on demonstration of organisms which are readily apparent in samples taken from affected tissues. Specific tests that may yield organisms are listed in Table 25.1.

Prototheca organisms can be identified as oval to spherical basophilic organisms ranging in diameter from 1.5 to 20 μm with a thick (0.05 μm) slightly birefringent capsule. Cells reproduce by endosporulation and may contain two to 20 endospores (also termed daughter cells). The organisms stain variably with haematoxylin and eosin stain and Giemsa-based stains but stain well with fungal stains such as Gridley's, Gomori's methenamine-silver or periodic acid-Schiff (PAS). *Prototheca* grows well on cycloheximide-free Sabouraud's medium. *P. zopfii* can be differentiated from *P. wickerhamii* by culture and immunofluorescent antibody techniques.

Management

Few dogs with protothecosis have been successfully treated. Ketoconazole, itraconazole and amphotericin B have all been used with limited success in management of systemic disease. Cutaneous and nasal disease may be more responsive to therapy than systemic disease. Focal cutaneous lesions should be surgically excised. Widespread cutaneous disease may respond to ketoconazole or itraconazole. Localised nasal infections may respond to topical clotrimazole or enilconazole administration. Immunostimulants have been used together with systemic antifungal therapy in people and one reported dog with protothecosis but their role in the management of *Prototheca* infections remains to be defined.

Table 25.1 Specific antemortem tests that may yield organisms for culture, cytological, or histological identification.

Vitreal or subretinal aspirate manifestations.	This is the most useful diagnostic test in dogs with ocular manifestations Samples can be submitted for both fungal culture and cytology
Biopsy of nodular or ulcerated lesions	Small white to tan nodular lesions are usually composed of a mass of organisms with minimal lymphoplasmacytic inflammation. Occasionally severe granulomatous inflammation may be noted
Rectal scrapings (occasionally faecal samples will yield organisms)	For cytology and fungal culture

Fine needle aspirate of:
  lymph nodes
  liver
  spleen
	For cytology and fungal culture

Swabs or impression smears from ulcerated skin lesions or nasal discharge	For cytology and fungal culture
Urinalysis	Sediment examination occasionally demonstrates organisms
Blood cultures	Must be subcultured on to fungal media

Chapter 26

Neosporosis and Toxoplasmosis

J. S. Barber and A. J. Trees

OVERVIEW OF AETIOLOGY

The protozoan parasites causing toxoplasmosis and neosporosis in dogs (*Toxoplasma gondii* and *Neospora caninum* respectively) are almost identical morphologically, although they can be distinguished antigenically. The two disease syndromes are also very similar, and it is probable that before the identification of *Neospora caninum* in the 1980s, many cases of toxoplasmosis were, in fact, neosporosis.

NEOSPOROSIS

Aetiology

Neosporosis was first described in a litter of Boxer puppies from Norway in 1984, but the parasite was not fully described and named until 1988 in the USA. Cases have since been reported from many parts of the world including Europe, Australia, Japan and South Africa. Retrospective studies have shown that *N. caninum* was occurring in canine tissues at least as long ago as the 1950s. *Neospora* spp. are also pathogenic in cattle, causing abortion, and have been found naturally infecting sheep, goats and an equine fetus, but not cats. The life cycle of this parasite is incompletely understood – tachyzoites are found most commonly in muscle and nerve tissue, but may occur in almost any organ; bradyzoites within tissue cysts have been reported only within CNS and eye; sexual stages have not yet been described.

Clinical Signs

Neosporosis usually manifests as a neurological problem, most typically presenting as a hindlimb ataxia/paresis in puppies from a few weeks of age onwards. Proprioceptive deficits and loss of patellar reflex is common, although pain perception is usually retained. Initially dogs remain bright and eat normally, but as the condition progresses they become quiet, depressed and some become incontinent. Pain may be detected in some dogs, particularly over the quadriceps or lumbar spine. The condition often progresses to paraplegia, with or without a rigid hyperextension of one or both hindlimbs, followed by forelimb weakness, dysphagia and dyspnoea. The onset is usually acute, with rapid deterioration, but in some cases may be milder and more chronic, with anecdotal reports of spontaneous recovery in a few pups.

Mature dogs may also develop similar signs, and other neurological presentations may occur, such as hemiparesis, forelimb ataxia, head tilt, cranial nerve deficits and/or behavioural changes. Non-neurological presentations include sudden collapse, due to myocarditis, and dermatitis.

Diagnostic Tests

Serology

Serum indirect fluorescent antibody test (IFAT) titres of ≥ 50 are considered specific for infection by *N. caninum*, although dogs with very high anti-*Toxoplasma* titres may also produce a very low titre against *Neospora* owing to partial cross-reactivity. Clinical cases usually have titres ≥ 800. Some clinically normal dogs are seropositive (around 10% of pet dogs in the UK) but almost all have low (≤ 800) titres.

Haematology and Serum Biochemistry

Routine blood tests are not particularly useful in diagnosis neosporosis, although many dogs have increased liver enzyme levels, and, in cases involving myositis, very high creatine kinase levels.

CSF Examination

CSF cell counts and protein estimation are variable in cases of neosporosis, but antibody detection may be useful (titres are generally lower than serum levels) and tachyzoites have been occasionally identified in the cell sediment. Antigen detection methods may prove useful in the future.

Imaging Techniques (e.g. Radiography, Myelography)

Useful for confirming/repudiating differential diagnoses.

EMG/Nerve Conduction Studies

Often reveal abnormalities, but varied results as neosporosis is generally a multifocal disease.

Biopsy

Muscle and nerve biopsies may reveal typical inflammatory lesions and the presence of tachyzoites, which can be differentiated from toxoplasmosis by immunoperoxidase staining. This is the most assured way of diagnosing neosporosis in the live animal.

Differential Diagnosis

- Trauma.
- Orthopaedic problems, e.g. 'wobblers', disc disease, hip dysplasia, cruciate rupture.
- Inherited neurological problems, e.g. progressive axonopathy in Boxers.
- Other infections, e.g. toxoplasmosis, distemper, tetanus, rabies.
- Metabolic conditions, e.g. porto-systemic shunts.

Treatment

The following drugs are recommended:

- clindamycin, 20–50 mg/kg daily, divided into 2 or 3 doses;
- potentiated sulphonamides, 30 mg/kg daily, divided

into 2 doses; given in combination with pyrimethamine (human anti-malarial drug) at 1 mg/kg once daily.

Pyrimethamine may also be used to supplement clindamycin therapy. In addition, corticosteroids at anti-inflammatory doses, can be a beneficial adjunct to anti-protozoal therapy. Initial improvement in clinical condition may be rapid, but often treatment must be continued for many weeks. Appropriate supportive therapy, including physiotherapy, should be given.

Prognosis

Although many dogs that are diagnosed as having neosporosis are euthanased, early treatment can result in many dogs making a full or functional recovery.

Pathology

There are often no gross lesions post-mortem. Histology typically reveals multifocal areas of mononuclear cell infiltration with necrosis, most usually in muscle and CNS, but can occur in most organs. Tachyzoites, or, in CNS, tissue cysts may be identified, and confirmed as *N. caninum* by immunoperoxidase staining.

Routes of Infection

N. caninum is transmitted from subclinically infected bitches transplacentally to their puppies. The number infected in each litter ranges from none to all, and several subsequent litters may contain infected pups. Most of these congenitally infected pups will not develop signs of neosporosis. Epidemiological studies suggest that around 10% of the pet dog population are seropositive. Evidence is now accumulating that post-natal infection also occurs.

TOXOPLASMOSIS

Aetiology

The first fatal case of canine toxoplasmosis was described in Italy in 1910, since when numerous cases of toxoplasmosis have been reported world-wide. Dogs may become infected by eating tissue cysts in raw or undercooked animal tissue, by ingesting oocysts (shed by cats) contaminating the environment, or, rarely, congenitally. Most infections remain subclinical; clinical signs are usually associated with immunosuppression, e.g. concurrent canine distemper infection, and are mostly seen in young dogs.

Clinical Signs

- Neuromuscular, e.g. ataxia, limb paralysis, tremors, seizures, stupor. May have a chronic course.
- Generalised – intermittent fever, pneumonia, anaemia, diarrhoea and vomiting. Involvement of the eye is apparently uncommon.

Diagnostic Tests

Serology

Several types of test are available to detect (mainly IgG) antibodies to *T. gondii*. But remember that most infections do not give rise to clinical signs, and acute cases may not have developed IgG antibodies. Distemper titres, indicating concurrent canine distemper virus infection, may be useful.

Tachyzoites

May be identified in CSF/broncho-alveolar lavage sediment and/or biopsy samples.

Differential Diagnosis and Treatment

As for neosporosis.

Chapter 27

Miscellaneous Protozoal Diseases

S. Barr

LEISHMANIASIS

Aetiology and Epidemiology

Caused by the zoonotic protozoan *Leishmania* spp.

Leishmania species have been classified traditionally based on geographic distribution (Old vs. New World) and clinical presentations (cutaneous vs. visceral) in people. However infections in dogs are invariably systemic. Most reports in dogs in the Old World (usually caused by *L. donovani infantum*) have been from around the Mediterranean basin, Portugal, with sporadic autochthonous cases reported in northern France, Switzerland, and the Netherlands. In the New World (usually caused by *L. donovani* complex, but also *L. braziliensis*) areas of South and Central American are endemic, with extension into Mexico. Cases in dogs (Oklahoma and Ohio) and cats (Texas) have been reported in the United States. Sandfly vectors become infected by ingesting parasitised macrophages (amastigotes) while feeding from an infected host. In the vector, amastigotes multiply, transform into a flagellate (promastigotes), and are injected back into the skin of a host. Promastigotes transform into amastigotes.

Pathogenesis and Clinical Features

After infection, amastigotes enter macrophages in the skin, spread throughout the body to infect most organs. Clinical signs may develop from 1 month to several years post-infection. Normal immune regulation is impaired with B lymphocyte proliferation (with excessive immunoglobulin production), and disturbed T lymphocyte regulation. The resulting circulating immune complex formation and deposition in such organs (glomerulus of kidneys, vessel walls of joints) can lead to renal failure (a main cause of death in dogs), polyarthritis, and bleeding tendencies. Other contributing factors to haemorrhagic diathesis can include

hyperglobulinaemia, uremic interference with platelet function, thrombocytopenia (due to splenic pooling, autoantibodies, immune complex formation), and disseminated intravascular coagulation. Dogs invariably develop cutaneous lesions. Initially, hyperkeratosis, depigmentation of the muzzle and foot pads, scaling of the nose, around the eyes, ears, and even diffuse alopecia are prominent signs. Mucocutaneous ulcers and small intradermal nodules are seen in some dogs. Muscle atrophy with weight loss are often the first signs of visceral involvement. Ocular disease (usually eyelid and conjunctival involvement) is common and may be the only signs present in the course of the disease. Terminally, many dogs die from renal failure but are often severely debilitated from hepatic, splenic, and bone marrow parasitosis.

Diagnosis

- Clinical laboratory abnormalities usually include hyperglobulinaemia, hypoalbuminaemia, and elevated liver specific enzymes. Thrombocytopenia and azotaemia are seen in about 50% of dogs.
- Identification of intracellular amastigotes in lymph node or bone marrow aspirates stained with Giemsa.
- Culture of aspirates in Novy–MacNeal–Nicolle or Schneiders' Drosophila medium plus 10% fetal bovine serum.
- Serology (using many different technologies to detect anti-leishmanial antibodies). A positive titre should indicate current infection but most tests have a poor sensitivity and specificity.

Management and Prognosis

Treatment is less effective in dogs than in man. As the organism is never eliminated, recurrence of signs is the norm. Meglumine antimonate (100 mg/kg) or sodium stibogluconate (50 mg/kg) given i.v. or s.c. once daily for 4 weeks have given the best results in dogs. Relapses are common requiring another round of therapy. Allopurinol (15 mg/kg, p.o., b.i.d. for 8 weeks) has been effective in man and shows promise in dogs. Prognosis is dependent on renal function before treatment, being very poor if renal insufficiency is present.

HEPATOZOONOSIS
Aetiology and Epidemiology

Caused by the coccidian protozoan *Hepatozoon canis*. Infects dogs (and cats but of little clinical significance) throughout Africa, southern Europe, Asia, Pacific Islands, Middle East, and Texas Gulf Coast in the United States. Tick vectors, *Rhipicephalus sanguineus*, become infected by ingesting gametocyte-containing monocytes and neutrophils in blood. Transmission to the host occurs when the vector is ingested. Wild Canidae and Felidae serve as reservoir hosts.

Pathogenesis and Clinical Features

After ingestion of infected ticks, sporozoites penetrate intestinal epithelium, set up cycles of schizogony first in mononuclear phagocytes and endothelial cells, then disseminate to skeletal muscle, myocardium, lungs, liver, spleen lymph nodes and skin to develop microschizonts (cyst-like structures). Released micromerozoites will infect blood monocytes and neutrophils to develop into gametocytes which are infective to tick vectors.

Dogs typically present with intermittent fever, weight loss, lumbar and hind limb pain, and oculonasal discharge. The signs tend to be intermittent with sometimes months between bouts, although spontaneous remission of signs have been reported.

Diagnosis

Major clinical laboratory abnormalities usually include a marked leukocytosis (up to 200 000 cells/µl) consisting mainly of a marked mature neutrophilia, monocytosis, and lymphocytosis. Radiographs characteristically reveal periosteal bone proliferation at the insertions and origins of skeletal muscles mainly on vertebrae, pelvis, mandible, and long bones. Identification is confirmed by intracellular gametocytes within neutrophils or macrophages in blood smears (Romanowsky's stain), or smears of the buffy coat or splenic aspirates. Muscle biopsy can reveal microschizonts.

Management and Prognosis

No effective treatment has been reported. Palliative treatment with non-steroidal anti-inflammatory drugs can make dogs more comfortable. Prognosis is unpredictable as remission or full recovery is possible in even severely debilitated animals.

BABESIOSIS
Aetiology and Epidemiology

Caused by the tick-borne intracellular erythrocytic piroplasm *Babesia* spp.

Several *Babesia* species infect dogs and cats. *B. canis* and *B. gibsoni* are the main species affecting dogs (*B. vogeli* less rarely) and some wild Canidae, and have world wide distribution. Babesiosis is considered one of the most important infectious diseases of dogs in South Africa. Ixodid tick vectors become infected by ingesting parasitised erythrocytes from a host. *Babesia* spp. are introduced into a host by a tick bite. The parasites only parasitise erythrocytes in the host.

Pathogenesis and Clinical Features

Clinical signs, due almost entirely as a consequence of parasitosis of erythrocytes, are related to speed of destruction of the parasitised erythrocytes. Young dogs are more susceptible to clinical disease than older dogs. Species and strain of parasite will also determine disease severity; for example, infection with *B. gibsoni* produces more severe disease than *B. canis* in the United States, and isolates of *B. canis* in the United States are less pathogenic than *B. canis* from South Africa.

Three main syndromes account for the main clinical entities:

- *Hyperacute*. Hypotensive shock, hypoxia with extensive tissue damage occurring as a result of massive intravascular erythrolysis.
- *Acute*. Haemolytic anaemia associated with anorexia, lethargy, vomiting, haematuria, icterus can be noted. Thrombocytopenia, splenomegaly, and occasionally lymphadenopathy can occur. Animals that recover from acute disease are usually chronic carries.
- *Chronic* disease of intermittent fever and weight loss can occur. A wide variety of vague clinical signs have also been reported but may be associated with other concurrent infections (*Ehrlichia canis*).

Diagnosis

Haematological abnormalities are dependent on disease severity and therefore, the strain of the parasite involved. For example, *B. canis* isolated in South Africa (SA) produces a more severe but less responsive anaemia than seen in France or the Philippines (which probably have the same parasite strain). Neutrophilia and monocytosis are higher in SA. Generally, a regenerative anaemia and thrombocytopenia are the major clinical laboratory abnormalities. Serum chemistry abnormalities are variable and are determined by dehydration, shock, metabolic acidosis, erythrocyte destruction (haemoglobinaemia/uria, bilirubinuria).

Definitive diagnosis is made by identifying organisms on a Giemsa-stained blood smear. Large (2.5 × 5.0 m) piriform intraerythrocytic bodies usually in pairs is typical of *B. canis*; smaller (1 × 3 m) single organisms is typical of *B. gibsoni*. Organisms are rarely evident in chronically infected animals, and the numbers of organisms does not necessarily indicate the severity of disease.

An indirect fluorescent antibody test may help detect chronic infections in dogs with subpatent parasitaemias. False negative results can occur in dogs under 6 months of age.

Management and Prognosis

- Diminazene aceturate (3.5 mg/kg, i.m., once) is the drug of choice in uncomplicated cases. Due to its hypotensive and anticholinergic effects it should be avoided in complicated cases.
- Phenamidine isethionate (15 mg/kg, s.c., twice, 24 h apart) is similar to diminazene but side effects (vomiting, histamine release, severe tissue reactions) occur more frequently.
- Imidocarb dipropionate (6 mg/kg, s.c. or i.m., once) can produce transient salivation, diarrhoea, dyspnoea immediately after injection (effects can be controlled by atropine at 0.05 mg/kg).
- Trypan blue (10 mg/kg, i.v. as a 1% solution, once) is the drug of choice in compromised babesiosis patients as it has few side effects. However, it does not eliminate infection with parasites (and clinical signs in some) reappearing 9 to 12 days post-treatment.
- Primaquine phosphate (0.5 mg/kg, i.m. or p.o., every 3 days for 3 treatments) is the only effective drug against *B. felis* of cats.
- Supportive therapy of whole blood transfusion for severe anaemia, fluids and glucocorticoids for the treatment of shock when indicated.
- Vaccination, as being developed in Europe and South

Africa, may be an effective means of decreasing the incidence of disease.

AMERICAN TRYPANOSOMIASIS

Aetiology and Epidemiology

Caused by the haemoflagellate protozoan parasite *Trypanosoma cruzi*. Trypanosomiasis (Chagas' disease) is endemic in dogs in many parts of South and Central America, and Mexico. Hunting breeds of dogs from Texas, Louisiana, Oklahoma, Florida, North Carolina, and Virginia have been diagnosed with the disease. Infected vectors (Reduviidae) and reservoir hosts (opossums, raccoons, skunks, armadillos) have been found from Maryland to California. Dogs may become infected when infected faeces from a vector contaminates a vector bite wound or mucous membrane, dogs eat infected vectors or contaminated meat of reservoir hosts, or by blood transfusion, congenitally, or via milk.

Pathogenesis and Clinical Features

Once the parasites (trypomastigotes) enter the bloodstream, they enter the cytoplasms of multiple tissues (mainly myocardium and brain) to multiply. Parasitaemias reach a peak approximately 2 weeks post-infection which coincides with rupture of trypomastigotes out of cells causing severe destruction and inflammation of the organ (myocarditis) producing clinical signs of acute disease. If dogs survive the acute phase, parasitaemias drop as immunity against the organism increases, and there is a prolonged asymptomatic period (8–24 months). During this asymptomatic period, the myocardium degenerates eventually leading to dilated cardiomyopathy and ventricular arrhythmias which are eventually fatal.

Clinical signs of acute disease include depression, generalised lymphadenopathy, first or second degree heart block, signs of right and left cardiac insufficiency. Multifocal neurological disease not unlike distemper may be apparent. Chronic disease is characterised by initially right-sided heart failure followed by biventricular failure and ventricular arrhythmias.

Diagnosis

Haematological and serum chemistry abnormalities are non-specific. During acute disease, trypomastigotes (15 × 20 μm) can be identified in the blood, on buffy coat smears, or lymph node aspirates and biopsy. After 3 weeks post-infection, serology is reliable. Parasitaemias are subpatent but the organism may be cultured from a large volume of blood in Liver Infusion Tryptose medium.

Management and Prognosis

Nifurtimox (2–7 mg/kg, p.o., q.i.d. a day for 5 months) and benznidazole (5 mg/kg, p.o., once daily for 2 months) decrease parasitaemias in man but with severe side effects and unknown efficacy in dogs. Allopurinol is under investigation in man. Some newer inhibitors of sterol biosynthesis show considerable efficacy in mice.

ENCEPHALITOZOONOSIS
Aetiolgy and Epidemiology

Caused by the microsporidian protozoan, *Encephalitozoon cuniculi*. Widespread throughout the world infecting sporadically dogs and cats, both domestic and wild, and rabbits. Canine encephalitozoonosis is primarily a kennel problem of highest incidence in South Africa and in farm-reared blue fox cubs in Nordic countries. Animals are thought to become infected by oral or nasal route following contact with infected urine, ingestion of infected mammals, or transplacentally.

Pathogenesis and Clinical Features

The parasite becomes intracellular in renal tubular epithelial cells, tissue macrophages, endothelial cells, and less frequently glial cells, myocytes, and hepatocytes. Stunted growth and unthriftiness are seen in pups a few weeks postpartum with several in a litter affected. As more organs become involved, there is progression of clinical signs referable to central nervous system and renal involvement.

Diagnosis

A normocytic, normochromic anaemia is a consistent finding. Azotaemia may be present. Spores may be readily identified in the urine (Gram or Ziehl–Neelsen stain). A positive indirect fluorescent antibody test is indicative of active infection.

Management and Prognosis

No specific treatment is known but prophylaxis is based on improving environmental hygiene.

Chapter 28

Heartworm Disease

S. Barr

Aetiology and Epidemiology

Caused by the filarial worm, *Dirofilaria immitis*. Important disease in parts of Europe, Australia, certain states of the United States (Southeastern, Atlantic coast, and Midwestern) and Japan. Cats and ferrets are also susceptible to infection, but prevalence is much lower than in dogs. Microfilaria (L1, about 315 μm long) are discharged from adult females (about 28 cm long) into the bloodstream where they can survive for up to 3 years. Development to L3 (infective stage) occurs over approximately 2 weeks after ingestion by mosquito vectors. The L3 and L4 migrate in the connective tissues for about 4 months. After the last molt, immature adults migrate to the pulmonary arteries and right heart. Microfilaria appear in circulation 6–7 months after infection.

Pathogenesis and Clinical Features

The most clinically significant physiological burden on the host is impedance of pulmonary artery blood flow by adult worms, and the development of endarteritis, obstructive fibrosis, and thromboembolism to the pulmonary vascular bed. The result of these inflammatory and obstructive lesions are pulmonary hypertension leading eventually to right sided heart failure. Immune complexes associated with microfilaria can produce glomerulonephritis.

Caval syndrome may develop when a large number of adults occupy not only the pulmonary arteries but the right atrium, caudal and cranial vena cava, and even hepatic veins.

Using clinical, radiographic, and laboratory examinations, heartworm-infected dogs can be classified into 1 of 3 classes:

- *Class 1*: Asymptomatic.
- *Class 2*: Exercise intolerance with occasional cough; moderate ventricular, main pulmonary artery, and caudal lobar artery enlargements (radiology); mild anaemia (haemogram).
- *Class 3*: Cardiac cachexia ± signs of right sided cardiac insufficiency (ascites), constant fatigue, persistent cough, dyspnoea, perhaps occasional haemoptysis; right atrial and ventricular enlargements, deformity and enlarged lobar arteries, diffuse pulmonary densities (thromboembolism), enlarged main pulmonary artery (radiology), anaemia (PCV < 20%). Dogs with caval syndrome (with haemoglobinuria and thrombocytopenia) enter Class 3 after surgical removal of worms.

Diagnosis

Based on identifying microfilaria in peripheral blood and/or a positive adult antigen test in dogs with clinical or radiographic findings consistent with infection.

Characteristic radiographic findings in dogs include enlarged and tortuous lobar pulmonary arteries, increased prominence of the main pulmonary artery, perivascular parenchymal pattern, right ventricular enlargement. In cats, caudal lobar pulmonary artery enlargement is the most common finding. Echocardiography to identify adults is best used to confirm caval syndrome (when adults are present in the right atrium or ventricle) as identifying parasites in pulmonary arteries is unreliable.

Microfilaria may be found on a blood smear (if counts are high) but a concentration technique (modified Knott's test, filter test) will increase sensitivity. Microfilaria of *D. immitis* should be differentiated from those of the non-pathogenic filarids of dogs (*Dipetalonema reconditum* and *Dip. repens*) based on morphology.

Diagnosis of occult infections (adults present but amicrofilaraemic) relies on adult antigen tests coupled with clinical signs and radiographic evidence of infection. In cases with a positive antigen test but no clinical or radiographic signs, the antigen test should be repeated using a test from a different manufacturer. Antigen tests are the tests of choice in dogs receiving chronic preventative therapy with ivermectin, milbemycin, or moxidectin as these drugs will produce occult infections after 6–8 months in microfilaraemic dogs.

Management and Prognosis

Adulticides

- Thiacetarsamide sodium (2.2 mg/kg, i.v., b.i.d. for 2 days) has low efficacy (especially to female worms), is hepatotoxic and mildly nephrotoxic, and produces severe tissue necrosis if injected perivascularly. Treatment should be delayed a month if dogs show signs of toxicity during the treatment course. Class 3 dogs have increased mortality from thromboembolic complications post-treatment.
- Melarsomine dihydrochloride (2.5 mg/kg, i.m., twice at 24-h intervals) has high efficacy (100% male, 96% female worms), low toxicity, and lower incidence of thromboembolic complications than seen in thiacetarsamide treatment. Class 3 dogs can be successfully treated with a single injection monthly for 3 months, or

a single 2.5 mg/kg injection followed 1 month later by 2.5 mg/kg, given twice, 24 h apart.

Microfilaricide

- Dogs with microfilaraemias 30 days post-adulticide therapy should receive ivermectin (50 μg/kg, p.o. once) or milbemycin oxime (0.5 mg/kg, p.o. once). These doses can be used safely in Collies. A shock-like reaction (especially if the microfilaraemia is high) due to rapid microfilaria kill may develop in any breed of dog within 6 h of treatment and should be treated with shock doses of i.v. fluids and glucocorticoids.

Preventative

- Diethylcarbamazine (3.0 mg/kg daily) has been superseded as the main preventative by the very effective and more convenient macrocyclic lactone compounds including ivermectin (6 μg/kg monthly), milbemycin (0.5 mg/kg monthly), and moxidectin (3 μg/kg monthly). Ivermectin (24 μg/kg monthly) is an effective preventative in the cat.

Chapter 29

Canine Zoonoses

M. Bennett and C. A. Hart

INTRODUCTION

Although dogs and man have lived together generally to their mutual benefit for thousands of years, there is no doubt that the potential for transmission of diseases as diverse as rabies and flea infestation from dogs to man has put a strain on this relationship from time to time. This is not intended to be an exhaustive account of all the possible canine zoonoses, but rather will concentrate on those not covered elsewhere in this book (often because they cause no disease in dogs) or which have been the subject of recent medical (and potentially owner) comment.

Zoonoses can be defined as infections transmissible between vertebrate animals and man, a definition which excludes many other important mechanisms by which dogs contribute to human ill health (e.g. allergy, accidents, environmental contamination and fear). It is also important to remember that the susceptibility of both man and dogs to an infectious agent does not necessarily mean that transmission occurs between the two.

VIRUS ZOONOSES

- *Rabies*: see page 144.
- *Canine distemper virus* (CDV) has been suggested as a possible cause of Paget's disease, an abnormality of growth plate development, in man, but suggestions that CDV might be involved in multiple sclerosis have been largely disproven.
- *Canine calicivirus* infection has been reported associated with diarrhoea in both dogs and people.
- *Lymphochoriomeningitis virus* is found in wild rodents and only rarely transmitted to man. After experimental dog infection, dog-to-dog transmission occurred – but whether this has any epidemiological significance in the field is another matter.
- Dogs can also be experimentally infected with human strains of *rotavirus* and natural human–canine reassortants have been reported.
- *Reoviruses* are well known for being able to cross species, but, again, it is not known whether canine reoviruses are transmitted to man, especially as human reovirus infections are generally asymptomatic.
- *Enteroviruses*, particularly some *coxsackie viruses* and *polioviruses*, can naturally infect dogs, but dogs are thought unlikely to be sources of human infection.

BACTERIAL ZOONOSES

- *Bite wounds*: By far the most frequent and important canine zoonosis. *Pasteurella multocida* and, less frequently, *P. pneumomotropica* are found in the mouths of dogs and cats and *P. multocida* infection involved in >30% bite infections. *Capnocytophagia canimorsus* and *C. cynodegmi* (dysgonic fermenter type 2; DF-2, and DF-2-like) are also part of the normal oral flora of many animal species, although not man, and are transmitted to man via bites and scratches. In man, they are generally of low pathogenicity, although in the immunosuppressed infection can kill. *Eikenella corrodens* is found in gingival plaque of dogs and is commonly isolated from dog bites. Also frequently isolated from bites are *pseudomonads*, *actinobacilli*, *streptococci*, *staphylococci*, *corynebacteria* and a variety of *anaerobes*.
- *Escherichia coli*: pathogenic strains are generally host-specific, but can carry transferable genes encoding virulence or antibiotic resistance. Although enterotoxigenic and enterohaemorrhagic *E. coli* have been detected in dogs, there is no evidence of transmission to man or vice versa.

- *Salmonellosis*: most frequently *S. typhimurium*, but other species may be more common in a local outbreak. Prevalence varies; 1–5% of dogs excreting in most European surveys but in the USA up to 50% prevalence reported in normal young dogs ≤6 months old. Age is important; in one survey, only 5% adults excreting, but 25% of normal dogs ≤6 months. It is not known how often dogs are the source of human infection.

- *Campylobacteriosis*: several reports in the medical literature accuse dogs of being the source of human infection, and surveys suggest that about 24% of dogs excrete *Campylobacter* spp., mainly *C. jejuni*. But the significance of this to human health is unknown – common sources of infection are as likely as transmission from dog to man. See page 123. *C. upsalensis* is a more important pathogen, and infection of dogs and possible transmission to man has been reported.

- *Anaerobiospirillum* spp. – recently described spiral bacterium, isolated from the faeces of children with diarrhoea but not from normal human faeces. However, it is a normal finding in dog faeces, and transmission from a puppy to a baby has been reported.

- *Tuberculosis* – man-to-dog spread seems more common than dog-to-man. See page 153.

- *Leptospirosis* continues to be a problem in man, but dogs are rarely incriminated nowadays. Most human leptospirosis is associated with contaminated water (rats) or cattle, and those most at risk are farmers and water sports enthusiasts. See page 142.

- *Streptococci* – although fairly species-specific, group A streptococci, the most common serotype found in man, has been isolated from dogs, and associated with recurrent human infections within families. In addition, canine strains (generally group G) have been isolated from man.

- *Staphylococci*: there is little evidence of frequent transmission in the field. But non-phage-typable '*S. aureus*' isolates from humans are sometimes *S. intermedius*, and the possibility of zoonotic spread exists.

- *Rickettsias*: various rickettsias listed in Table 23.1 are infectious to man, but dog-to-human transmission is rare.

PROTOZOA

- *Giardiasis* is a cause diarrhoea in dogs and man, and dog-to-human transmission has been reported although a common source of infection, e.g. a contaminated water supply, is more often the case.

- *Cryptosporidiosis* is a common cause of diarrhoea in children, and sometimes also in adults. The disease is particularly severe in immunosuppressed individuals, and is a common infection in people with acquired immunodeficiency syndrome (AIDS). Infection in dogs is generally sub-clinical, and while dog-to-human infection is theoretically possible it has not been reported. Human infection associated with subclinical infection in a cat has been reported.

- *Leishmaniasis*: Dogs are an important reservoir of infection in the Mediterranean region, and via sand-flies, can be a source of human infection. Direct dog-to-man transmission is also possible, but very rare.

HELMINTHS

Toxocariasis

Causes visceral larva migrans in man. The prevalence of antibody in man is fairly high, but clinical disease, including retinal granuloma (which can be mistaken for retinoblastoma) is rare. Possibly also linked with asthma in children. Zoonotic risk arises from dogs shedding large numbers of *Toxocara canis* eggs (15 000 eggs /g in puppy faeces), and ability of eggs to remain infectious in soil for several years (≈10% soil samples in public parks contain viable eggs). The most important sources of *T. canis* eggs are puppies up to about 6 months old and pregnant and lactating bitches (both directly and as the source of puppy infection transplacentally and via milk). See page 125.

Echinococcus Granulosus Infection

Segments containing embryonated eggs are shed in faeces. Embryos can survive in the soil for ≤2 years, and are ingested by ruminant intermediate hosts or man. Cysts in sheep and horses rarely cause clinical signs. In man, however, pulmonary hydatids cause severe respiratory distress, and those in the liver grow to enormous size. Rupture of a cyst can cause anaphylactic shock and death. Treatment in man is generally surgical excision. (See also page 125.)

Others

Various other canine helminths, including some hookworms and *Dipylidium caninum*, can also rarely infect humans, generally causing abdominal pain.

ECTOPARASITES

- *Fleas*. See page 903. In addition to the dog fleas (*Ctenocephalides felis* and *C. canis*) transmissible to man, the human flea (*Pulex irritans*) can also be transmitted to and from dogs.

- *Ear mites*. Very rarely, *Otodectes cynotis* can be transmitted to man where it can cause superficial skin irritation or painful ear infestations.
- *Sarcoptic mange*. Although fairly host-specific, transmission to man can occur. See page 914.

Chapter 30

Vaccination

M. Bennett

ROUTINE VACCINATION PROGRAMMES

Which vaccines are given, and precisely when, varies between countries and according to local factors such as disease prevalence and husbandry system (for example, dogs living individually might require a different vaccination regime from those in a colony). Table 30.1 lists the vaccines generally available for use in the dog. This section describes the principles of routine canine vaccination, based on those vaccines available in the UK. More details of specific protocols may be found in individual sections on that infectious disease, but it is important to:

> ALWAYS READ THE MANUFACTURER'S RECOMENDATIONS, AND CONSULT WITH THE MANUFACTURER BEFORE DEVIATING FROM THEIR INSTRUCTIONS.

Vaccination in Puppies

- Aim is to provide active, vaccine-derived immunity as early as possible.
- But maternally derived antibody (MDA) may block effective vaccination in young animals (Fig. 30.1). For distemper, live measles vacines are sometimes used in an attempt to overcome MDA, although many modern live distemper vaccines are probably just as effective.
- Standard protocol is often therefore to vaccinate at 8 or 9 weeks and then repeat at 12 weeks old.
- In puppies over 12 weeks old, one dose of live vaccine may suffice – but two doses at least 2 weeks apart are usually recommended.

- Extra doses of vaccine, earlier and/or later than standard may be given, for example during an outbreak of disease.

Almost all MDA in puppies is derived from colostrum – transplacental MDA is negligible in dogs. Fig. 30.1 shows the decline in antibody titre (half-life approximately 10 days) over the first 14 weeks of life, and the dotted lines indicate how variation in initial titre between and within litters can affect how long MDA persists. The aim of vaccination is to provide protection against disease as soon as possible – but Fig. 30.1 demonstrates that:

- vaccination too early may be blocked by MDA, and
- because attenuated vaccine virus is less virulent than wild-type virus, there will often be a short period when vaccination will not be effective but the animal is susceptible to wild-type infection and disease.

Furthermore, through variation in antibody titre in bitches and in colostrum uptake by puppies, the optimum vaccination time will differ between individuals.

Vaccination of Adult Dogs

For many live vaccines, one dose may be all that is necessary to provide protection in an an adult dog, but two doses are usually recommended, and are particularly important for many killed vaccines.

Annual re-vaccination is recommended for most vaccines, although some (for example distemper) may need only be given every other year, while more frequent dosing may be advised for others (for example the intranasal *Bordetella bronchiseptica* kennel cough vaccine.) But see Box 30.1 on boosters.

Table 30.1 Dog vaccines available.

Vaccine	Type	Route*	See page
Canine distemper†	Live	s.c.	133
Canine parvovirus	Live or killed	s.c.	127
Infectious canine hepatitis‡	Live or killed	s.c.	131
Leptospirosis			
L. interrogans icterohaemorrhagiae and _L. interrogans canicola_	Killed	s.c.	142
Kennel cough			
Canine parainfluenza	Live	s.c.	136
Bordetella bronchiseptica	Live	i.n.	136
Canine coronavirus§	Killed/live	s.c.	121
Borreliosis§	Killed	s.c.	155
Rabies‖	Killed	s.c./i.m.	144

* s.c. = subcutaneous injection, i.n. = intranasal.
† Live measles virus is sometimes used to overcome maternally-derived antibody to distemper.
‡ Vaccine is canine adenovirus (CAV) type 2 which protects against both CAV-1 (hepatitis) and CAV-2 (laryngotracheitis).
§ Not available in the UK at time of writing.
‖ Not routinely used in UK. See p ••.

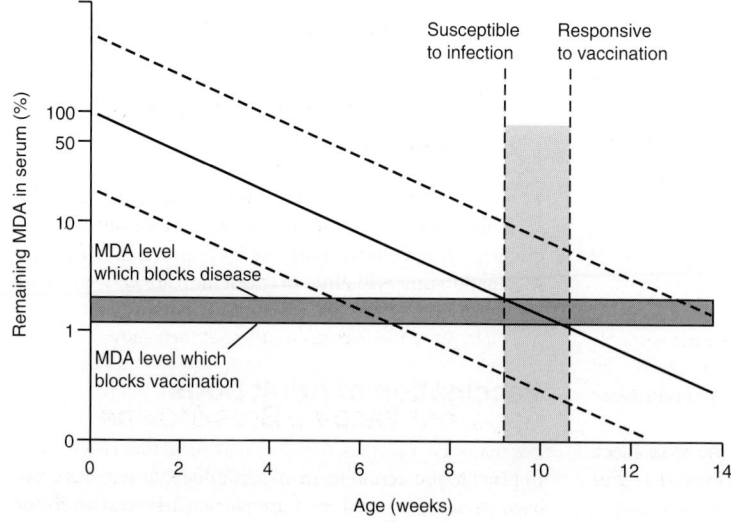

Fig. 30.1 The decline in serum levels of maternally derived antibody (MDA) in puppies.

Box 30.1   To boost or not to boost.

The need for annual booster vaccination of pets has recently been the subject of much debate, sometimes acrimonious, in both the veterinary and lay literature. For most canine vaccines, it is not known when the immunity derived from vaccination declines to non-protective levels, and therefore when revaccination is necessary. The reason for this lack of information largely reflects a combination of ethical considerations and the cost of keeping large numbers of experimental dogs over such long periods for challenge studies. Annual booster recommendations are therefore largely based on antibody studies (on the assumption that antibody level indicates protective immunity – not necessarily the case for all diseases) over 6–12 months after vaccination of young animals, and on a policy of playing-safe. Certainly, there are some studies which show increased disease in dogs in colonies in which routine booster vaccinations are not given. On the other hand, for live canine distemper vaccination, for example, there is experimental evidence to suggest that most adult dogs are protected for many years, if not life, by a single dose of live vaccine.

It can be argued that we expect more of our dog (and cat) vaccines than we do of most vaccines used in other species, since the owners of dogs generally wish to protect individual animals rather than the herd or population. The protection of 'most animals for many years' is not regarded as sufficient, and, in the absence of any hard evidence of untoward effects, annual boosters are therefore recommended.

However, there are also strong arguments to be made for review of present blanket vaccination policies and consideration of more flexible policies based on individual vaccines and particular circumstances. Probably the best advice is to follow the manufacturer's recommendations as routine, but to be willing to consider alternative protocols and take advice from the manufacturer whenever appropriate.

APPARENT VACCINE FAILURE

Apparent Vaccine Reactions

Defined as disease apparently caused by the vaccine. Apparent reactions usually occur within a week or so of vaccination, and while true reactions may be due to either the biological component (i.e. the virus or bacteria) or some other component of the vaccine (usually the adjuvant), many apparent reactions have other causes.

Apparent Biological Reactions

- *Incomplete attenuation* of virus or bacterial component. – Uncommon, but possible. Report suspected cases to the manufacturer and/or other appropriate body. Most often combined with:
- *Increased susceptibility* to infection with attenuated pathogen, e.g. a live vaccine given to a very young or immunosuppressed animal
- Vaccine given by incorrect route, e.g. a live systemic vaccine given orally.
- *Animal infected* and incubating disease at time of vaccination. As can be seen in Fig. 30.1, puppies and kittens are often vaccinated just when maternal antibody levels are declining and so the animal is most susceptible to infection. This is probably the single most common

reason for apparent biological reactions to vaccination at 8–12 weeks old.
- It is normal for some live vaccines to provoke *mild clinical signs*, e.g. injection of many live vaccines gives rise to mild systemic clinical signs such as depression, lethargy and inappetance, generally lasting only 24 h.

Apparent Reactions to Non-Biological Components of the Vaccine

These are usually due to an inappropriate response to the adjuvant or a particular adjuvant–antigen combination.

- Mild skin reactions at the site of subcutaneous injection – most common.
- Generalised hypersensitivity reactions – rare.

Apparent Vaccine Breakdowns

Defined as the development of the disease despite vaccination. Apparent breakdowns usually occur several weeks or more after vaccination, but within the period of immunity normally expected. Possible causes of apparent vaccine breakdown include:

- *Faulty (non-potent) vaccine* – uncommon, but possible. Report suspected cases to the manufacturer and/or other appropriate body.

- *Incorrect storage* of vaccine – a likely cause of non-potency. Do not use vaccines after their recommended use-by date, and always store them according to the manufacturer's instructions. Live vaccines, especially canine distemper virus vacines, are particularly liable to loss of potency if stored incorrectly.

- *Incorrect administration* of vaccine – usually the result of the injection of an inadequate dose of vaccine.

- *Inhibition of vaccination by maternally-derived antibody* – a very common cause of apparent vaccine failure in young animals. If the last vaccine dose is given before the puppy or kitten is 12 weeks old, or if the animal has particularly high MDA, vaccination may not provide active immunity and protection.

- *Animal already infected* – vaccination rarely prevents the development of disease in an already infected animal, or eliminates a carrier state. Another very common cause of apparent vaccine failure.

- *Intercurrent disease* or *immunosuppression* – either at the time of vaccination or later.

- *Infection with different organisms or strains* from those contained in the vaccine – before a clinical disease can be ascribed to vaccine breakdown, the causative organism(s) must be identified, e.g. not all cases of haemorrhagic gastroenteritis in dogs are caused by canine parvovirus.

- *Overwhelming infection* – if the challenge with the infective agent is great enough then a vaccinated dog may still develop the disease. The chance of such a high challenge under field conditions is low, but more likely in, e.g. puppy farms, with high population densities and inadequete hygiene.

FURTHER READING FOR SECTION 2

Allaker, R.P., Langlois, T. & Hardie, J.M. (1994) Prevalence of *Eikenella corrodens* and *Actinobacillus actinomycetemcomitans* in dental plaque of dogs. *Veterinary Record*, **134**, 519–520.

Alvar, J., Molina, R., San-Andres, M., *et al.* (1994) Canine leishmaniasis: Clinical, parasitological and entomological follow-up after chemotherapy. *Annals of Tropical Medicine and Parasitology*, **88**, 371–378.

Amela, C., Mendez, I., Torcal, J.M., *et al.* (1995) Epidemiology of canine leishmaniasis in the Madrid region, Spain. *European Journal of Epidemiology*, **11**, 157-161.

Barr, S.C. (1991) American trypanosomiasis in dogs. *Compendium on Continuing Education for the Practicing Veterinarian*, **13**, 745–755.

Barber, J.S. & Trees, A.J. (1996) Clinical aspects of 27 cases of neosporosis in dogs. *Veterinary Record*, **139**, 439–443.

Barton, C.L., Russo, E.A., Craig, T.M., *et al.* (1985) Canine hepatozoonosis: a retrospective study of 15 naturally occurring cases. *Journal of the American Animal Hospital Association*, **21**, 125–134.

Bauer, D. (1994) The capacity of dogs to serve as reservoirs for gastrointestinal disease in children. *Irish Medical Journal*, **87**, 184–185.

Barrs, V.R., Malik, R. & Love, D.N. (1995) Antimicrobial susceptibility of staphylococci isolated from various disease conditions in dogs – a further survey. *Australian Veterinary Practitioner*, **25**, 37–42.

Baumgartner, W., Boyce, R.W., Weisbrode, S.E., *et al.* (1995) Histologic and immunocytochemical characterization of canine distemper-associated metaphyseal bone lesions in young dogs following experimental infection. *Veterinary Pathology*, **32**, 702–709.

Bell, J.A., Sundberg, J.P., Ghim, S.J., *et al.* (1994) A formalin-inactivated vaccine protects against mucosal papillomavirus infection – a canine model. *Pathobiology*, **62**, 194–198.

Bell, S.C., *et al.* (1991) Canine distemper viral antigens and antibodies in dogs with rheumatoid arthritis. *Research in Veterinary Science*, **50**, 64.

Beynon, P.H. & Edney, A.T.B. (eds) (1995) *Rabies in a Changing World: Symposium of the Royal Society of Medicine and British Small Animal Veterinary Association.* British Small Animal Veterinary Association, Cheltenham.

Brochier, B., Kieny, M.P., Costy, F., *et al.* (1991) Large scale eradication of rabies using recombinant vaccinia-rabies vaccine. *Nature*, **354**, 520–522.

Chalmers, W.S.K. & Baxendale, W. (1994) A comparison of canine distemper vaccine and measles vaccine for the prevention of canine distemper in young puppies. *Veterinary Record*, **135**, 349–353.

Chomel, B.B., Jay, M.T., Smith, C.R., *et al.* (1994) Serological surveillance of plague in dogs and cats, California, 1979–91. *Comparative Immunology, Microbiology and Infectious Diseases*, **17**, 111.

Corboz, L., Ossent, P. & Gruber, H. (1993) Lokale und sytemische Infektionen mit Bakterien der Gruppe EF-4 bei Hundeen, Katzen und bei einem Dachs: Bakeriologische und Pathologisch-anatomische Befunde. *Schweizer Archiv fur Tierheilkunde*, **135**, 96–99.

Craig, T.M. (1990) Hepatozoonosis. In: *Infectious Disease of the Dog and Cat*, (ed. C.E. Greene), pp. 778–785. WB Saunders, Philadelphia.

Croese, J., Fairley, S., Loukas, A., *et al.* (1996) A distinctive aphthous ileitis linked to *Ancyclostoma caninum*. *Journal of Gastroenterology and Hepatology*, **11**, 524–531.

Delgado, S. & Carmenes, P. (1995) Canine seroprevalence of *Rickettsia conorii* infection (Mediterranean spotted fever) in Castilla-Y-Leon (Northwest Spain). *European Journal of Epidemiology*, **11**, 597–600.

Dubey, J.P. & Linsay, D.S. (1993) Neosporosis. *Parasitology Today*, **9**, 452–458.

Enderlin, G., Morales, L., Jacob, R.F., *et al.* (1994) Streptomycin and alternative agents for the treatment of tularemia: Review of the literature. *Clinical Infectious Diseases*, **19**, 42–47.

Faggi, E., Gargini, G., Pizzirani, C., *et al.* (1993) Cryptococcosis in domestic animals. *Mycoses*, **36**, 165–170.

Font, A., Roura, X., Fondevila, D., *et al.* (1996) Canine mucosal leishmaniasis. *Journal of the American Animal Hospital Association*, **32**, 131–137.

Gevrey, J. (1994) Encephalitozoonosis in domestic carnivores. *Recueil de Medecine Veterinaire de l'Ecole d'Alfort*, **169**, 477–481.

Gordon, M.T., Bell, S.C., Mee, A.P., *et al.* (1993) Prevalence of canine distemper antibodies in the pagetic population. *Journal of Medical Microbiology*, **40**, 313–317.

Greenwood, N.M., Chalmers, W.S.K., Baxendale, W., *et al.* (1995) Comparison of isolates of canine parvovirus by restriction enzyme analysis, and vaccine efficacy against field strains. *Veterinary Record*, **136**, 63.

Greenwood, N.M., Chalmers, W.S.K., Baxendale, W., *et al.* (1996) Comparison of isolates of canine parvovirus by monoclonal antibody and restriction enzyme analysis. *Veterinary Record*, **138**, 495–496.

Hermanns, W., Kregel, K., Breuer, W., *et al.* (1995) Helicobacter-like organisms: histopathological examination of gastric biopsies from dogs and cats. *Journal of Comparative Pathology*, **112**, 307–318.

Houston, D.M., Ribble, C.S. & Head, L.L. (1996) Risk factors associated with parvovirus enteritis in dogs – 283 cases (1982–1991). *Journal of the American Veterinary Medical Association*, **208**, 542–546.

King, A. & Turner, G.S. (1993) Rabies: a review. *Journal of Comparative Pathology*, **108**, 1–39.

Hoskins, J.D. (1991) Ehrlichial diseases of dogs: diagnosis and treatment. *Canine Practice*, **16**(3), 13–21.

Malik, R., Dilmacky, E., Martin, P., *et al.* (1995) Cryptococcosis in dogs – a retrospective study of 20 consecutive cases. *Journal of Medical and Veterinary Mycology*, **33**, 291–297.

Modiano, J.F., Getzy, D.M., Akol, K.G., *et al.* (1995) Retrovirus-like activity in an immunosuppressed dog – pathological and immunological findings. *Journal of Comparative Pathology*, **112**, 165–183.

Orloski, K.A. & Edison, M. (1995) *Yersinia pestis* infection in three dogs. *Journal of the American Veterinary Medical Association*, **207**, 316–318.

Pastoret, P.P., Boulanger, D. & Brochier, B. (1995) The rabies situation in Europe. In: *The Veterinary Annual*, Vol. 35, (eds M.-E. Raw & T.J. Parkinson), pp. 1–17. Blackwell Science, Oxford.

Patronek, G.J., Glickman, L.T., Johnson, R., *et al.* (1995) Canine distemper in pet dogs. 2: A case control study of risk factors during a suspected outbreak in Indiana. *Journal of the American Animal Association*, **31**, 230–235.

Proceedings of the Heartworm Symposium. (1992) Austin, Texas. American Heartworm Society, Batavia, USA. ISBN 1-878353-29-2.

Richardson, E.F. & Mathews, K.G. (1995) Distribution of topical agents in the frontal sinuses and nasal cavity of dogs: comparison between current protocols for treatment of nasal aspergillosis and a new, non-invasive technique. *Veterinary Surgery*, **24**, 476–483.

Rudmann, D.G., Coolman, B.R., Perez, C.M., *et al.* (1992) Evaluation of risk factors for blastomycosis in dogs: 857 cases (1980–1990). *Journal of the American Veterinary Medical Assoiation*, **201**, 1754–1759.

Schetters, T.P.M., Kleuskens, J.A.G.M., Scholtes, N.C., *et al.* (1994) Vaccination of dogs against *Babesia canis* infection using parasite antigens from culture supernatants with emphasis of clinical babesiosis. *Veterinary Parasitology*, **52**, 219–233.

Shif, I., Silberstein, I. & Mendelson, E. (1994) Evidence that human babies may become infected by animal rotaviruses. *Israel Journal of Medical Sciences*, **30**, 387–391.

Slappendel, R.J. (1988) Canine leishmaniasis. A review based on 95 cases in the Netherlands. *The Veterinary Quarterly*, **10**, 1–16.

Tennant, B.J., Gaskell, R.M., Jones, R.C., *et al.* (1993) Studies on the epizootiology of canine coronavirus. *Veterinary Record*, **132**, 7–11.

Tennant, B.J., Gaskell, R.M., Jones, R.C., *et al.* (1991) Prevalence of antibodies to four major canine viral diseases in dogs in a Liverpool hospital population. *Journal of Small Animal Practice*, **32**, 175–179.

Urbina, J.A., Payares, G., Molina, J., *et al.* (1996) Cure of short- and long term experimental Chaga's disease using D0870. *Science*, **273**, 969–971.

Watt, P.R., Robins, G.M., Galloway, A.M., *et al.* (1995) Disseminated opportunistic fungal disease in dogs – ten cases (1982–1990). *Journal of the American Veterinary Medical Association*, **207**, 67–70.

Yamane, I., Gardner, I.A., Ryan, C.P., *et al.* (1994) Serosurvey of *Babesia canis*, *Babesia gibsoni* and *Ehrlichia canis* in pound dogs in California, USA. *Preventive Veterinary Medicine*, **18**, 293–304.

Yamane, I., Thomford, J.W., Gardner, I.A., *et al.* (1993) Evaluation of the indirect fluorescent antibody test for diagnosis of *Babesia gibsoni* infections in dogs. *American Journal of Veterinary Research*, **54**, 1579–1584.

Woldehiwet, Z. & Ristic, M. (eds) (1993) *Rickettsial and Chlamydial Diseases of Domestic Animals*. Pergamon Press, Oxford, UK.

Section 3

Interpretation and Misinterpretation of Laboratory Data

Edited by Richard A. Squires

Chapter 31

Avoiding Misinterpretation of Clinical Laboratory Data

R. A. Squires

INTRODUCTION

Diagnostic reasoning is an intricate, error-prone process; the success of which depends entirely upon the collection and correct interpretation of accurate clinical information (Kassirer 1989; Barosi *et al.* 1993). To make a diagnosis, the small animal clinician should first:

- obtain and carefully consider the historical and physical examination findings,
- identify the clinical problems of the patient and list appropriate differential diagnoses, and
- perform necessary diagnostic tests (such as radiographs, blood work and urine analysis) to help rule in or rule out differential diagnoses.

At this stage the clinician then uses inferential reasoning to refine his or her understanding of the clinical problems of the patient. More specific diagnostic tests may be necessary to approach a diagnosis. A 'definitive' diagnosis can be deduced, once the clinical problems are understood with a sufficient degree of precision. The diagnosis should be precise enough to permit accurate prognostication and formulation of an optimal therapeutic plan (see Fig. 31.1).

Clinical laboratory data can help the clinician to reach a definitive diagnosis, by augmenting the historical and physical examination findings. Laboratory tests should certainly not be used to 'fish' blindly for a diagnosis. Ideally, laboratory tests should be done to confirm or deny differential diagnoses derived from the history and physical examination rather than to generate differential diagnoses *de novo*. This will help to reduce the frequency of diagnostic errors in several ways:

- Over-reliance on laboratory test results will be minimised.

- Naïve, uncritical acceptance of spurious or artifactual test results is less likely to occur.
- Relevant laboratory tests are more likely to be selected in the first place.
- Confusion arising from misinterpretation of irrelevant tests (which should not have been done in the first place) will be minimised.

This chapter will provide information to help clinicians avoid possible pitfalls in the interpretation of clinical laboratory data. Most of the information presented here will concern interpretation of routine haematological parameters, serum biochemical profiles and urine analyses. A few comments will be made concerning more specialised tests. It will be assumed that a careful history has been taken, a physical examination has been carried out, differential diagnoses have been considered, and specific clinical laboratory tests have been deemed appropriate to help pursue a diagnosis.

CONCEPTS OF NORMALITY AND ABNORMALITY

An 'abnormal' laboratory test result is generally defined as one that lies outside of the reference range (Farver 1989). The reference range is determined by analysis of random samples from a representative population of normal animals. 'Representative' is the key word here: it is very important that the population used to determine the reference range is truly representative of the patient under study. Differences in species, breed, age and sex must be taken into account, so that:

(1) It is entirely inappropriate to evaluate canine haematological and serum biochemical values using feline reference values.

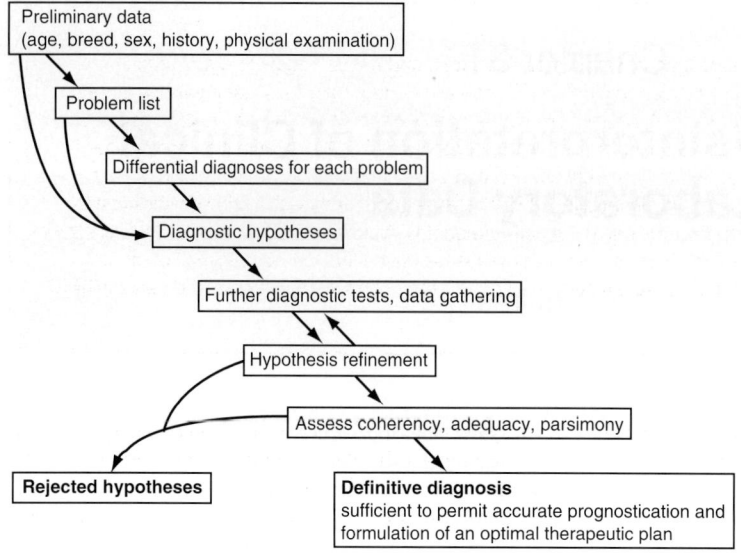

Fig. 31.1   The process of diagnostic reasoning.

(2) It should be recognised that laboratory values for healthy young puppies differ from those of healthy adult dogs.
(3) Each clinical laboratory should establish its own reference ranges for veterinary patients of varying species, age, breed and sex.
(4) Each laboratory should provide the most applicable reference range when reporting laboratory results for a particular patient.

Unfortunately most laboratories have established reference ranges only for adult dogs and cats of mixed breeds and sexes. It is the responsibility of the clinician to ensure that the provided reference range is truly representative of the patient under study. If it is not, the clinician must try to persuade the laboratory to develop a more suitable reference range, or may have to rely upon published reference ranges provided by other laboratories (Bounous *et al.* 1995; Jacobs *et al.* 1995).

Once samples from a suitable representative population of normal animals have been analysed, statistical methods are used to determine a reference range that usually includes about 95% of normal animals, assuming a normal distribution of the population. This means that for a particular analyte, about 2.5% of normal, healthy animals will have a value below the lower limit of the reference range and about 2.5% of normal, healthy animals will have a value above the upper limit of the reference range. Furthermore, consider a typical 15-test serum biochemical profile done on a normal, healthy animal. The probability that *all 15* results will be in the normal range is 0.95 raised to the power of 15 or 0.46. Therefore, more often than not,

a healthy animal will have at least one spurious abnormal value on a 15-test biochemical profile. This simple calculation highlights once again the danger of uncritical acceptance of abnormal laboratory test results, and demonstrates the need for interpretation of laboratory data in light of other, relevant clinical information.

A laboratory test result slightly above or below the limits of the reference range should be evaluated particularly critically: the patient may be an outlier in perfect health, or may be showing subtle evidence of mild or early disease. To help discriminate, the test result should be interpreted in light of the history and physical examination. If appropriate, the test can be repeated, or alternative tests that address the same diagnostic issue can be done.

INITIAL APPRAISAL OF CLINICAL LABORATORY DATA

Whenever an abnormal laboratory test result is obtained, the clinician should consider several questions to diminish the likelihood of misinterpretation:

- Does this result confirm diagnostic hypotheses generated from the history and physical examination, or is it quite unexpected (and therefore worthy of particularly sceptical scrutiny)?
- Is the magnitude of deviation from normal small, medium, or large?

Case example

A 14-year-old, female-spayed, Wire-haired Dachshund is presented for inappetance. Physical examination reveals mild dehydration, severe dental tartar and moderate gingivitis. Dental work under general anaesthesia is planned. Routine preanaesthetic blood work shows that the serum creatinine concentration is slightly above the upper end of the reference range. In view of this, the clinician should review the history and physical examination findings for evidence of polydipsia, polyuria, dehydration or abnormal urinary tract palpation findings. Urine specific gravity should be checked, to help determine if urine concentrating ability has been compromised. A urine dipstick test for proteinuria should be done as a first step towards ruling out glomerulopathy. A urine sediment examination will help to rule out urinary tract infection. These and other tests will help to assess the patient for the presence of renal disease and should be considered before detailed discussion with the owner concerning the risks and benefits of general anaesthesia.

- Although it is 'flagged' as abnormal, could the result be normal *for this particular patient*, given the species, breed, age and sex?
- Could the abnormal result be a consequence of suboptimal specimen collection or handling?
- Could the abnormal result be a consequence of artifact, or interfering substances in the specimen? (e.g. is there a comment on the report stating that haemolysis, lipaemia or hyperbilirubinaemia was present in a blood specimen?)
- What further steps (if any) are necessary to corroborate the abnormal finding and to approach a definitive diagnosis?

The information provided in the remainder of this chapter will show the pertinence of these questions and will help the clinician to answer these questions in future. The rest of the chapter is divided into sections dealing with patient factors, specimen factors and human factors that can contribute to misinterpretation of clinical laboratory data.

PATIENT FACTORS THAT CAN LEAD TO MISINTERPRETATION OF LABORATORY DATA

Species

Reference ranges for a multitude of clinical laboratory parameters have been established for dogs and cats (Jacobs *et al.* 1995). It is clear that there are important differences between the species. Canine reference ranges should not be used when evaluating feline laboratory data, and *vice versa*. Some veterinary clinical laboratories report feline patient results alongside canine reference ranges. Human clinical laboratories may report canine and feline patient results

alongside human reference ranges. If in doubt, the clinician should contact the clinical laboratory to ascertain that the correct reference range is being provided.

Important differences between canine and feline clinical laboratory parameters are provided in Table 31.1. Compared with cats, dogs have a higher blood haemoglobin concentration, a higher haematocrit and larger red blood cells. The upper limit of the normal feline lymphocyte count is higher than that of the dog.

A noteworthy difference between dogs and cats concerns the serum activity of alkaline phosphatase (ALP). ALP is a membrane-associated enzyme that is released into plasma from a variety of tissues. The two most important tissues, from a diagnostic point of view, are bone and hepatobiliary tissue. In dogs:

- Large amounts of ALP are produced by:
  - growing or diseased bone,
  - cholestastic liver disease,
  - glucocorticoid excess.
- Plasma activity of ALP is a non-specific indicator of hepatobiliary disease (Center *et al.* 1992) because:
  - the isoenzyme of ALP produced by the liver in response to cholestasis can also be induced by anticonvulsants and glucocorticoid drug therapy (Sanecki *et al.* 1990),
  - the canine liver produces a distinct glucocorticoid-induced isoenzyme of ALP in response to glucocorticoid therapy and a diverse variety of illnesses.

Thus drug therapy, cholestasis, and a variety of other illnesses associated with increased circulating endogenous glucocorticoids can all lead to a prompt, dramatic increase in canine serum ALP activity.

In contrast, in cats:

- A glucocorticoid-induced isoenzyme of ALP is not produced.
- ALP production does not increase dramatically in

Table 31.1 Differences between canine and feline clinical laboratory values.

Laboratory value	SI units	Feline	Canine	Species differences
Routine haematology*				
Haematocrit	l/l	0.24–0.45	0.37–0.55	Cats normally have a lower haematocrit and haemoglobin concentration than dogs
Haemoglobin	g/l	80–140	120–180	
Mean corpuscular volume	fl	40–55	66–77	Feline red blood cells are much smaller than those of most dogs
RBC morphology				Heinz bodies may be present on a proportion of the RBCs in normal feline blood. Heinz bodies are not typically seen on normal canine RBCs
White blood cell count	×10^9/l	5.5–19.5	6.0–17.0	Normal feline white blood cell counts may be a bit higher than those of dogs
Lymphocytes	×10^9/l	1.5–7.0	1.0–4.8	Normal feline lymphocyte counts can be higher than those of dogs
Serum biochemistry†				
Alanine aminotransferase	U/l	10–75	0–130	Normal feline ALT, ALP and bilirubin concentrations are lower than those of dogs. ALP is particularly important: modest elevations of ALP are much more significant in cats than in dogs
Alkaline phosphatase	U/l	0–90	0–200	
Total bilirubin	μmol/l	0–4	0–7	
Cholesterol	mmol/l	1.5–6.0	2.74–9.5	Cholesterol is usually lower in cats than in dogs
Creatine kinase	U/l	0–580	0–460	CK values can be variable in both species, but particularly in cats
Creatinine	μmol/l	75–180	55–145	The normal range for creatinine extends higher in cats than in dogs
Phosphorus	mmol/l	1.03–2.82	0.5–2.6	The normal ranges for phosphorus and urea extend lower in dogs than in cats
Urea	mmol/l	5.0–10.0	2.1–9.7	
Urine analysis				
Random specific gravity	–	1.001–1.070	1.001–1.060	Maximal urine concentrating ability in normal cats is greater than in normal dogs
Bilirubin	–	Negative	Positive or negative	Normal cats do not have bilirubin in their urine. Normal dogs of both sexes may have bilirubin present (males more than females), particularly in concentrated urine

* Reference values from Jain 1986.
† Reference values from Clinical Pathology Laboratory, Department of Pathology, Ontario Veterinary College; cited by Jacobs *et al.* 1995.
ALP, alkaline phosphatase; ALT, alanine aminotransferase; CK, creatine kinase; RBC, red blood cell.

response to cholestasis or drugs.
- The major ALP isoenzyme has a short plasma half-life (6 h) compared with that in dogs (about 70 h).
- A modest elevation in serum ALP activity is much more significant than in dogs, and is a more specific indicator of hepatobiliary disease (Center et al. 1986).

Another difference between dogs and cats of direct relevance here concerns urinary excretion of bilirubin. Normal cats do not excrete dipstick-detectable bilirubin in their urine, but dogs of both sexes may do so. In dogs, hyperbilirubinuria precedes hyperbilirubinaemia and clinical jaundice as cholestasis progresses. In cats with only modest elevation of serum ALP, the presence of hyperbilirubinuria may portend cholestatic disease. Other causes, such as haemolysis must, of course, be ruled out. Conversely, bilirubin is frequently detected in the urine of normal dogs. Absence of bilirubin from the urine of a dog with substantially elevated serum ALP activity should prompt the clinician to consider other causes for the enzyme elevation.

Age

Puppies differ from adult dogs in some haematological, serum biochemical and urine analysis findings (Jacobs et al. 1995). Important differences are shown in Table 31.2. Most of the important differences are caused by rapid skeletal growth and continuing postnatal maturation of the lymphatic and urinary systems and the bone marrow.

Breed

There are some recognised breed variations in reference values for canine laboratory tests. Most concern normal haematocrit, which varies substantially among canine breeds. It is very likely that further breed variations will be recognised as our profession's collective clinical experience grows. Table 31.3 lists various breeds and known breed-associated variations. Perhaps the most striking breed variation concerns the Akita. Typically, these Japanese working dogs have unusually small red blood cells (MCV 52–60 fl) compared with members of other canine breeds. In addition, they may have an unusually high ionic concentration of potassium in the cytoplasm of their erythrocytes. Consequently haemolysis caused at the time of venipuncture, or afterwards, can lead to pseudohyperkalaemia. This phenomenon, thought to be a consequence of retained sodium-potassium ATPase activity in Akita erythrocyte plasma membranes, can lead uninformed clinicians to misdiagnose hypoadrenocorticism, acute renal failure, or other disorders that are associated with hyperkalaemia.

Gender and Pregnancy

Little has been published recently concerning the effects of gender or neutering status on canine clinical laboratory data. Early studies of Beagles suggested that males have slightly higher blood haemoglobin concentration than females (Andersen and Gee 1958). More recent studies did not support the earlier findings (Robinson and Ziegler 1968). Any minor effects of gender or neutering status on routine haematology and serum biochemistry are not likely to lead to diagnostic errors. However, in the case of some specialised tests, errors can be made if the gender of the patient is not taken into account. Sex hormone assays must obviously be interpreted with the age, sex and neutering status of the patient borne in mind. In intact females, the stage of the oestrus cycle must also be considered. Less obviously, it has recently been shown that there are significant differences in the serum concentration of alpha-1-antitrypsin that depend upon gender and neutering status (Hughes et al. 1995). Among healthy dogs, the serum alpha-1-antitrypsin concentration was significantly higher in sexually intact females than in spayed females, sexually intact males and castrated males. Measurement of serum alpha-1-antitrypsin concentration may in future prove useful in the diagnosis of pulmonary emphysema, hepatic failure, pancreatitis and other disorders.

Pregnancy in dogs has been shown to be associated with a decline in haematocrit. In one study, the mean packed cell volume (PCV) of a group of Beagles decreased from 0.53 l/l before pregnancy to a nadir of 0.321 l/l at term (Andersen and Gee 1958). After parturition, the mean haematocrit increased, returning to normal by 9 weeks postpartum. Similar effects should be expected in other canine breeds. The anaemia is thought to be a consequence of fluid retention and increased plasma volume. Other expected effects of fluid retention, such as hypoalbuminaemia, are less well characterised in dogs.

Drugs

Numerous drugs can alter the results of routine haematology, serum biochemistry, urine analysis and more specialised laboratory tests (Burkhard and Meyer 1995). Such alterations may be a consequence of physiological effects of the drug, or may merely reflect interference with the methodology used in a particular test. Some of the altered results are caused by drug toxicity; others do not indicate detrimental effects in the patient, but may lead to misdiagnosis. Important examples of some of these drug effects are discussed below.

Table 31.2 The effects of age upon various canine clinical laboratory values.

Laboratory value	Age differences
Routine haematology	
Mean corpuscular volume	Puppies are born with large fetal erythrocytes. The MCV at birth is about 95–100 fl. Postnatal RBCs of smaller size replace fetal cells over the first few months of life
Packed cell volume	Puppies are born with a slightly higher packed cell volume and Hb concentration than adults. These parameters decline over the first month of postnatal life to below adult
Haemoglobin	values. This is because of destruction of fetal RBCs, rapid growth of the young animal and the low concentration of iron in mother's milk. From the beginning of the second
Red blood cell count	month of postnatal life, these parameters increase. Puppies take about a year to reach adult levels
White blood cell count	In general, the WBC count is high in young animals, declines with age and increases again late in life. Differences are mainly due to changes in lymphocyte and neutrophil numbers. Superimposed on this general trend, there are fluctuations in neutrophil and lymphocyte counts in the first 2 months of life
Serum biochemistry	
Calcium	Associated with active bone growth, serum calcium and phosphorus are higher in
Phosphorus	puppies than in adults. Phosphorus is usually more substantially elevated than calcium
Alkaline phosphatase	Puppies have two to three fold higher serum alkaline phosphatase than adults throughout the period of skeletal growth. This is a consequence of the bone isoenzyme. Levels are even more impressive (20- to 25-fold elevation over adult levels) during the first few days of postnatal life. This may be because of intestinal absorption of intact alkaline phosphatase from colostrum
Bilirubin	Slightly higher in very young puppies than in adults. It declines to the adult level by about two weeks of age
Creatinine	Somewhat lower in young animals than adults, because of relatively low muscle mass
Urea	Serum urea nitrogen concentration depends heavily on the length of the pre-sample fast and the protein content of food previously ingested. Making the rather artificial assumption of equal duration of fast, and identical food; urea would be somewhat lower in puppies than adult dogs
Total protein	Concentration is lower in young animals than in adults because of low albumin and globulin levels. Albumin concentration reaches an adult level by about two months of age. Globulin takes longer
Urine analysis	
Random specific gravity	On average, urine specific gravity will be lower in young animals than in adults. Puppies have immature renal tubular function. They are unable to concentrate or dilute urine to the same extent as adults
Dipstick findings	Glucosuria in the face of normal blood glucose concentration is a common incidental finding in young puppies. It usually disappears by 3 weeks of age, as renal tubular function matures.

MCV, mean corpuscular volume; Hb, haemoglobin; RBC, red blood cell; WBC, white blood cell.

Table 31.3 Known breed-related variations in clinical laboratory data of *normal dogs*.

Breed	Variation
Akita	Some have microcytic RBCs (typical MCV 55–65 fl), high RBC count, and normal PCV; some have high potassium concentration inside their RBCs, leading to pseudohyperkalaemia with haemolysis
Beagle, Boxer, Chihuahua, Dachshund, Greyhound	Higher RBC count, PCV and Hb values than most other breeds of dog
Dalmatian	Urate crystals are commonly observed on urine sediment examination. In other breeds, an equivalent number of crystals might indicate liver disease or a portosystemic vascular shunt
German Shepherd Dog	Higher RBC count, PCV and Hb values and eosinophils than most other breeds of dog
Cavalier King Charles Spaniel	Large size of platelets may lead to apparently low platelet count by automated techniques as a high proportion of the platelet population will be above the largest size recognised by the machine
Miniature Poodle	High RBC count, PCV and Hb; macrocytic RBCs in some individuals (MCV 80–100 fl in affected individuals)

MCV, mean corpuscular volume; Hb, haemoglobin; RBC, red blood cell; PCV, packed cell volume.

Glucocorticoids

Serum activities of some liver enzymes may be elevated in dogs that have recently received glucocorticoid medication, though the magnitude of the effect is unpredictable. The enzymes usually affected are ALP, gamma glutamyltransferase (γGT) and, to a lesser extent, alanine transaminase (ALT). Parenteral, oral and topical routes of glucocorticoid administration can all be associated with this effect (Moriello *et al.* 1988; Meyer *et al.* 1990; Ridgway and Moriello 1993). Therefore, the clinician should inquire about the use of topical medications when investigating a patient with raised liver enzymes. Increased serum activities of ALP (which may be dramatic) and γGT are in part due to glucocorticoid-induced *de novo* synthesis of these liver enzymes. Glucocorticoid-induced hepatocellular swelling and consequent cholestasis may also play a role. Elevation of serum ALT concentration is thought to be a consequence of increased hepatocellular membrane permeability and enzyme leakage secondary to hepatocellular swelling. A recent publication described in detail the biochemical and subcellular pathological features of glucocorticoid-induced hepatopathy in dogs (Rutgers *et al.* 1995).

An indistinguishable profile of liver enzyme elevations may be found in patients that have received glucocorticoid medication, patients with cholestasis (both intrahepatic and posthepatic) and patients with true hyperadrenocorticism (Cushing's syndrome). Therefore, when faced with elevated liver enzyme test results, it is essential to consider the possibility that administered glucocorticoid, rather than cholestasis or Cushing's syndrome is responsible for the result. The owner should be asked whether glucocorticoid has recently been administered *by any route*. Questions concerning aural, cutaneous and ophthalmic medications should not be forgotten.

Glucocorticoids have powerful effects on leukocyte trafficking and consequently affect the results of routine haematological tests. Shortly after an oral dose of prednisone, mature neutrophilia, lymphopenia and eosinopenia develop. Neutrophilia is a consequence of reduced margination and reduced egress of cells from the circulating pool. Fewer cells leave the circulation to traffic to sites of inflammation. Lymphopenia is thought to develop because some T-lymphocytes are redistributed to extravascular lymphoid tissues, such as lymph nodes, spleen and bone marrow. The mechanisms leading to eosinopenia in glucocorticoid-treated dogs are incompletely understood (Jain 1986). Glucocorticoids inhibit survival of human eosinophils *in vitro* (Wallen *et al.* 1991). In dogs, glucocorticoid administration can cause monocytosis. This is rather unusual; in several other species these drugs cause monocytopenia. Glucocorticoid-induced changes in the leukogram may be misinterpreted as evidence of severe infection. This can lead to unnecessary further laboratory tests and inappropriate, empirical antimicrobial therapy (see also Chapter 4).

Administered glucocorticoids tend to suppress the hypothalamic–pituitary–adrenal axis. As a consequence of suppressed adrenocorticotropin (ACTH) secretion, endogenous cortisol secretion is decreased. Over time, the adrenal cortices atrophy. If a test of adrenal function is done after several days of oral glucocorticoid administration; or several days after a patient has received an injection of long-lasting glucocorticoid medication; a false low result is likely to be obtained. The ACTH stimulation test (see Chapter 54) is one such adrenal function test that is substantially affected by administration of glucocorticoid medications. Although performance of this test after *known* glucocorticoid administration is not usually recommended, the ACTH stimulation test is an excellent means of distinguishing iatrogenic from true hyperadrenocorticism in a patient showing unexplained clinical signs of hypercortisolism. Plasma cortisol concentration in a patient that has recently been receiving exogenous glucocorticoid medication will usually be low and will fail to rise much in response to ACTH. In contrast, a patient with true hyperadrenocorticism will usually have an exaggerated increase in plasma cortisol concentration in response to ACTH.

To further complicate matters, some steroid medications (hydrocortisone, prednisone, prednisolone) interfere with the measurement of cortisol in assays used to test the hypothalamic–pituitary–adrenal axis. Hydrocortisone is identical to cortisol; and prednisone and prednisolone show significant cross reactivity with cortisol in radioimmunoassays leading to falsely elevated values. For this reason, such medications should be discontinued at least 24 h before blood is drawn for cortisol measurement. Another glucocorticoid (dexamethasone) does not interfere in cortisol assays and can therefore be used in tests of adrenal function, such as the low dose dexamethasone suppression test (LDDST). Dexamethasone can be given before or during an ACTH stimulation test without adversely affecting the test result. This knowledge can be helpful when dealing with a suspected Addisonian crisis (hypoadrenocortical crisis). It is not necessary to withhold potentially life-saving glucocorticoid therapy while carrying out this diagnostic test, so long as dexamethasone is used in preference to prednisolone, or other short-acting glucocorticoids.

Other effects of glucocorticoids upon clinical laboratory parameters include lowering of urine specific gravity and lowering of serum thyroxine concentration. The clinician should enquire about the use of glucocorticoids when investigating polydipsia and when dealing with patients with suspected hypothyroidism. The discussion above is summarised in Table 31.4.

Anticonvulsants

Phenobarbitone, phenytoin and primidone can increase serum liver enzyme activities. Enzyme induction and, to a lesser extent, hepatocellular swelling and secondary cholestasis are contributing factors. At conventional doses, these anticonvulsants cause less marked elevation of serum ALP and γGT activities than do glucocorticoids. These anticonvulsants may also lower serum thyroxine concentration, perhaps by increasing its metabolism and excre-

Table 31.4 Summary of the effects of glucocorticoids on clinical laboratory test results.

Effect	Consequence
Induction of *de novo* synthesis of ALP and γGT	↑ plasma activity of ALP and γGT
Hepatocellular swelling and cholestasis	↑ plasma activity of ALP and γGT
Increased hepatocellular membrane permeability	↑ ALT
Decreased margination and reduced egress of neutrophils from blood vessels	Neutrophilia
Redistribution of T lymphocytes to lymph nodes and bone marrow	Lymphopenia
Reduced survival of eosinophils	Eosinopenia
Reduced ACTH secretion as a consequence of negative feedback on the hypothalamus/pituitary, leading to adrenal gland atrophy.	Reduced responsiveness in the ACTH stimulation test
Cross reaction with cortisol in RIA (hydrocortisone, prednisolone and prednisone)	Falsely elevated resting and post-ACTH stimulation cortisol measurements
Reduced ADH secretion and diminished responsiveness of renal tubular cells to ADH, thus reducing urine concentrating ability	Lower urine specific gravity
Reduced capacity of thyroid hormone binding globulin to bind thyroxine	Lower serum thyroxine concentration

ALP, alkaline phosphatase; γGT, gamma glutamyl transferase; ALT, alanine transaminase; ACTH adrenocorticotropin; RIA, radioimmunoassay; ADH anti-diuretic hormone.

tion (Evinger and Nelson 1984). In addition, anticonvulsants reduce urine concentrating ability and glucose tolerance.

Potassium bromide, which has recently undergone renaissance as an anticonvulsant (Trepanier 1995) interferes with the measurement of serum chloride concentration. An artificially high result is obtained because bromide appears as chloride in commonly used assays. Bromide also interferes with the measurement of serum cholesterol concentration (Burkhard and Meyer 1995).

Nonsteroidal Anti-inflammatory Drugs (NSAIDs)

Patients receiving aspirin or paracetamol when blood is drawn for a serum chemistry profile may have an artificially low serum glucose concentration. Aspirin can cause gastrointestinal ulceration and haemorrhage. This is mild and clinically insignificant in most patients, but may be sufficient to cause a positive faecal occult blood test result due to subclinical gastric ulceration. In other patients, NSAID-induced gastrointestinal haemorrhage may be a severe problem. Clinical judgement must therefore be exercised when interpreting tests results for faecal blood in patients receiving NSAIDs.

NSAIDs have many other pathophysiological effects that may genuinely alter clinical laboratory data. Prolongation of bleeding time is routine with aspirin use; since the drug causes thrombocytopathia. This effect may be beneficial or detrimental to the patient, depending on clinical circumstances. Other potential adverse consequences of NSAID use include hepatocellular injury leading to increased serum ALT activity, and renal vasoconstriction with consequent azotaemia. These are more likely to develop if pre-existing liver or renal disease is present. Azotaemia is particularly likely to develop in hypovolaemic or hypotensive patients.

Antibiotics

Certain antibiotics can produce false positive results in tests for proteinuria. Penicillins, cephalosporins and sulfisoxazole affect the sulphosalicylic acid precipitation test. Those drugs which alkalinise urine can affect both dipsticks and the sulphosalicylic precipitation test (Burkhard and Meyer 1995). Potentiated sulphonamides have been reported to cause reversible, iatrogenic hypothyroidism when used at moderately high doses (Hall and Campbell 1995). However, no effect on thyroid function test results was noted when one product (trimethoprim–sulphadiazine, Tribrissen™) was used at the manufacturer's recommended dose (Panciera and Post 1992). Sulpha drugs can also raise serum

liver enzyme activities by enzyme induction, or by causing an idiosyncratic hepatopathy (Rowland *et al.* 1992). Beta-lactam antibiotics (penicillins and cephalosporins) may falsely elevate serum creatinine.

Other Drugs

Renally excreted radiographic contrast agents can falsely increase urine specific gravity and give a false positive 'dipstick' protein reaction. These agents may crystallise in acid urine, producing unusual urine sediment examination findings for several days after their use.

Reducing agents such as ascorbic acid (vitamin C) and aspirin falsely lower serum glucose concentration measured by the glucose oxidase method and can produce a false negative result for urine glucose when a reagent strip is used to test urine from a diabetic patient. Ascorbic acid can also falsely increase serum creatinine concentration and can falsely increase urine glucose measured by copper reduction methods.

Hydration and Nutritional Status

Dehydration increases the concentration of solutes and cellular elements in blood. Diagnostic errors can be made if dehydration is missed during physical examination and clinical laboratory data is evaluated uncritically. In animals with normal urine concentrating ability, dehydration is associated with high urine specific gravity. Elevated serum creatinine and urea nitrogen should always be interpreted in light of physical examination findings and urine specific gravity. In the presence of concentrated urine, azotaemia is most likely to be prerenal, rather than renal or postrenal in origin (see Chapter 62). Prerenal azotaemia is usually corrected promptly after rehydration is achieved. As a matter of routine, urine should be obtained *before* fluid therapy in dehydrated patients.

Hyperalbuminaemia is strong serum biochemical evidence of dehydration, because the only recognised cause of this particular abnormality is dehydration. Other possible findings in a dehydrated patient include:

- hyperglobulinaemia,
- increased serum electrolyte concentrations (hypernatraemia, hyperchloraemia, hyperphosphataemia, hyperkalaemia, hypercalcaemia),
- reduced total CO_2 (metabolic acidosis due to tissue hypoperfusion), and
- raised haematocrit.

Occasionally, significant anaemia and hypoproteinaemia may be masked by dehydration (see Chapter 1). The clinician should critically evaluate the packed cell volume and total plasma protein in light of the estimated hydration deficit in severely dehydrated animals. Does it seem likely that rehydration of the patient in question will unmask anaemia or hypoproteinaemia? If so, further monitoring steps and possible therapeutic interventions, such as the administration of a plasma expander or blood transfusion may be appropriate.

Fasting, or feeding of a protein-restricted diet can:

- lower the serum urea nitrogen (SUN) concentration,
- decrease the SUN:creatinine ratio (because serum creatinine concentration is relatively unaffected by fasting compared with SUN),
- reduce the maximal urine concentrating ability (because of low renal medullary urea concentration).

Feeding a high protein diet, or gastrointestinal haemorrhage has the opposite effect on SUN and urine concentrating ability of feeding a protein-restricted diet (Bartges and Osborne 1995).

Prolonged starvation or protein malnutrition can also lead to:

- hypoalbuminaemia,
- hypokalaemia,
- raised liver enzyme serum activities.

Eating a normal meal tends to raise the blood concentrations of:

- glucose,
- cholesterol,
- triglycerides,
- trypsin–like immunoreactivity (TLI),
- total bile acids,
- ammonia.

The effects of feeding on serum total bile acids and blood ammonia are well known, and are useful in diagnostic tests of liver function that may include preprandial and postprandial blood sampling. Serum TLI is also raised by feeding; in this case making difficult the diagnosis of exocrine pancreatic insufficiency. Blood for TLI measurement should therefore be drawn after a 12-h fast. The magnitude of glucose elevation after feeding is modest, and is unlikely to contribute to diagnostic errors. Patients with suspected borderline diabetes mellitus should be evaluated with serial blood glucose measurements, rather than a single measurement. The time of the most recent meal should be taken into consideration when evaluating blood glucose values. Postprandial hypertriglyceridaemia, on the other hand, can be substantial. Sufficient lipaemia may be present in a postprandial serum specimen to cause turbidity

and consequently to alter the results of several other laboratory tests. Lipaemia can also cause *in vitro* haemolysis, worsening the confusion (see the following section on specimen factors that can lead to misinterpretation of clinical laboratory data). Postprandial hypercholesterolaemia does not usually lead to diagnostic errors.

To avoid the confounding effects of lipaemia and other postprandial vagaries, it is best to obtain blood samples for most purposes after a 10–12 h fast.

Stress and Intercurrent Illness

Stress and illness produce physiological effects that may manifest in routine clinical laboratory data. These effects are summarised in Table 31.5.

The stress of venipuncture is sufficient to raise blood glucose concentration in many cats. This can occasionally hinder the diagnosis of borderline diabetes mellitus in this species. In stressed or ill dogs, the 'stress leukogram' (consisting of neutrophilia, lymphopenia, eosinopenia and monocytosis) is a familiar haematological finding that may be mistaken for evidence of inflammation. The 'stress leukogram' is thought to be a consequence of glucocorticoid and adrenalin release.

Stress and non-adrenal illnesses may raise plasma cortisol levels sufficiently to complicate adrenal function testing (Kaplan *et al.* 1995). Acute stress should not alter the results of an ACTH stimulation test, because in this test a pharmacological dose of ACTH is given to assess the maximum capacity of the adrenal glands to produce cortisol. In contrast, chronic stress might affect ACTH stimulation test results due to adrenal gland hypertrophy; this can lead to a false positive result. Stress can also lead to false positive results in the low dose dexamethasone suppression test (LDDST). As a general rule physical restraint and other stressful procedures should be avoided as much as possible during the course of adrenal function tests.

Hypoglycaemia is another potential cause of false positive results in these tests, because low blood glucose is a potent stimulus for glucocorticoid secretion. It is important to ascertain that patients (particularly those with diabetes mellitus) are not hypoglycaemic during the course of LDDSTs and ACTH stimulation tests. Stress- or illness-induced plasma cortisol elevation may also lead to increased serum ALP activity, because of steroid-induced isoenzyme synthesis. This combination of findings may lead the unwary clinician to misdiagnose hyperadrenocorticism. A patient with raised serum ALP activity and an adrenal function test result suggestive of hyperadrenocorticism should be evaluated critically. Does other clinical information (e.g. history, physical examination findings, imaging studies) support a diagnosis of hyperadrenocorticism? If

Table 31.5 Summary of the effects of stress on clinical laboratory data.

Clinical laboratory test	Effects of stress and intercurrent illness
Blood glucose	Hyperglycaemia may result from the acute stress of venipuncture in cats. This can occasionally hinder diagnosis of borderline diabetes mellitus
Leukogram and differential white blood cell count	Stressed or ill dogs often show the stress leukogram (neutrophilia, lymphopenia, eosinopenia and monocytosis) which may be mistaken for evidence of inflammation
Cortisol	Acute stress, physical restraint, stressful procedures and illness may raise plasma cortisol
Low dose dexamethasone suppression test (LDDST) Adrenocorticotropin (ACTH) stimulation test	• Chronic stress of non-adrenal illness may lead to adrenal gland hypertrophy and altered responsiveness of the hypothalamic–pituitary–adrenal axis. Under these circumstances, false positive results indicative of hyperadrenocorticism may be obtained in these diagnostic tests • Acute stress may result in failure to suppress in the LDDST. Excessive physical restraint and other stressful procedures should be avoided during this test • Hypoglycaemia is a potent stimulus for ACTH and therefore cortisol secretion. It is important to ensure that patients with diabetes mellitus are not hypoglycaemic during LDDST and ACTH stimulation tests
ALP	Chronic stress or illness may increase plasma cortisol concentration, leading to increased hepatic synthesis of the steroid-induced isoenzyme of ALP. Increased plasma activity of ALP may contribute to misdiagnosis of hyperadrenocorticism
T_4 and T_3	Various non-thyroidal illnesses can lower serum thyroid hormone concentrations leading to the potential for misdiagnosis of hypothyroidism. Measurement of free T_3 and T_4, measurement of TSH or performance of a TSH stimulation test can help the clinician to avoid this form of misdiagnosis

not, a false positive result is a distinct possibility in a patient with non-adrenal illness (Kaplan *et al.* 1995). Repetition of adrenal function testing, ultrasound imaging of the liver and adrenal glands, ACTH assay and test therapy with a non-adrenolytic drug (such as ketoconazole) can be used in combination to resolve this potential diagnostic dilemma (see Chapter 59). Ideally, repeat adrenal function testing should be done with minimal stress after any known non-adrenal illness has been successfully treated.

As stated previously, raised serum ALP activity may be a consequence of stress. Occasionally this finding will lead to misdiagnosis of cholestatic liver disease. To avoid this mistake, the clinician should assess the patient for evidence of cholestasis by other means. Abdominal ultrasound examination, preprandial and postprandial serum bile acid

quantitation, and assessment of bilirubin concentration in urine and blood can be used to help rule in or rule out cholestasis. Separation and quantitation of the various ALP isoenzymes that make up the total serum ALP activity is possible (Teske *et al.* 1986; 1989). This turns out to be of modest value when attempting to distinguish cholestasis from other causes of raised ALP. When the serum activity of the glucocorticoid-induced isoenzyme of ALP is markedly elevated (>2000 IU/l), or when it forms a substantial portion of total ALP (>90% of total ALP), a diagnosis of hyperadrenocorticism is highly likely (Solter *et al.* 1993). Although this does not rule out cholestasis absolutely, it may help the clinician who chooses to apply careful diagnostic parsimony to the patient with raised serum ALP.

Non-thyroidal illnesses can temporarily lower serum thyroid hormone concentrations, potentially leading to misdiagnosis of hypothyroidism (Tibaldi and Surks 1985; Chastain and Panciera 1995). These effects have been termed euthyroid sick syndrome. Thyroid hormones circulate in free and protein-bound forms. The free hormones are physiologically active. Total thyroid hormone concentrations are measured and reported by most clinical laboratories, although free thyroxine (T_4) can be measured accurately by equilibrium dialysis assay (Ferguson 1994). Illnesses leading to decreased binding protein concentration will be associated with decreased total thyroid hormone concentration, but normal free hormone concentration, euthyroidism being maintained. Other debilitating illnesses, such as congestive heart failure (Panciera and Refsal 1994), diabetic ketoacidosis, hyperadrenocorticism, hypoadrenocorticism, renal failure and severe liver disease may be associated with decreased circulating free and/or total thyroid hormone concentrations (Nelson et al. 1991). Thyroid hormone supplementation is not appropriate for patients with euthyroid sick syndrome. Most patients with euthyroid sick syndrome can be distinguished from patients with true hypothyroidism on the basis of a thyroid-stimulating hormone (TSH) response test. Serum or plasma TSH assay can also prove useful in making the distinction.

Some illnesses cause alterations in clinical laboratory data that, at first glance, seem paradoxical or indicative of completely different illnesses. For example, immune-mediated haemolytic anaemia (IMHA) is frequently associated with marked neutrophilic leukocytosis and a left shift (Weiser 1995). This so-called 'leukemoid response' is often misinterpreted as evidence of a serious infection or marrow neoplasia. If unaware of this possible feature of IMHA, the clinician may be inclined empirically to institute potent antibiotic therapy and to delay immunosuppressive therapy. This would be inappropriate, since the leukemoid response does not indicate an infectious process. Rather, it is thought to be a corollary of bone marrow hyperactivity consequent to haemolysis. In some cases, it may reflect an inflammatory underlying cause for the immune-mediated disease. The specific cytokines or other mechanism(s) responsible for the leukemoid response in canine IMHA have not yet been elucidated.

Neoplastic illnesses frequently cause potentially-confusing alterations in clinical laboratory data, termed paraneoplastic effects. Paraneoplastic effects are caused by humoral factors secreted by tumour cells. Secretion of such humoral factors is generally inappropriate, or unexpected, given the neoplastic tissue of origin (see Chapter 35). For example, hypercalcaemia is a routine finding in patients with apocrine gland adenocarcinoma of the anal sac. This particular form of paraneoplastic hypercalcaemia is caused by tumour secretion of parathyroid hormone-related peptide (PTHrP) (Weir et al. 1988; Rosol et al. 1990). Clinicians unaware of this disease association might fail to carry out (or repeat) a thorough rectal examination and might expend resources pursuing other causes of hypercalcaemia, such as lymphoma or multiple myeloma. Some further examples of potentially-confusing alterations in clinical laboratory data caused by neoplastic and non-neoplastic illnesses are shown in Table 31.6.

Table 31.6 Potentially confusing effects of selected disorders on clinical laboratory data.

Abnormal laboratory value	Increase/decrease	Usual disease associations	Potentially confusing associations
Routine haematology			
Mean corpuscular volume	Decrease	Blood loss anaemia	Portosystemic shunts may be associated with microcytosis or microcytic anaemia
Packed cell volume	Increase	Dehydration	Polycythaemia may be caused by renal tumours and some other expansile renal lesions because of increased renal erythropoietin production. Haematocrit may be higher than 70%, and may lead to seizures or other signs of blood hyperviscosity. Dehydration may be misdiagnosed if the physical examination findings and the total plasma protein are not taken into consideration
Haemoglobin concentration		Breed variation	
Red blood cell count		Exposure to high altitude	
		Chronic hypoxaemia	
		Polycythaemia rubra vera	
			Paraneoplastic erythrocytosis may also occasionally be caused by other tumours

Table 31.6 *Continued*

Abnormal laboratory value	Increase/ decrease	Usual disease associations	Potentially confusing associations
Neutrophil count	Increase	Infection Inflammation	Immune-mediated haemolytic anaemia frequently causes a marked neutrophilic leukocytosis with a left shift. The mechanism is incompletely understood. This 'leukemoid response' may be misinterpreted as evidence of infection, unnecessarily delaying immunosuppressive therapy Paraneoplastic neutrophilia is occasionally reported
Neutrophil count	Decrease	Toxic bone marrow suppression Primary bone marrow disorder	A severe inflammatory focus may cause transient neutropenia as polymorphonuclear leukocytes marginate and leave the circulation in large numbers. A 'degenerative left shift' with more young, band neutrophils than mature, segmented neutrophils in the peripheral blood may develop.
Platelet count	Increase	Acute blood loss Inflammation Primary (essential) thrombocytosis	Chronic gastrointestinal blood loss may cause marked thrombocytosis in addition to microcytic, hypochromic anaemia. The high platelet count can be a useful marker of chronic gastrointestinal bleeding, but can also lead to misdiagnosis of a primary bone marrow disorder.
Serum biochemistry Calcium	Increase	Skeletal immaturity Lymphoproliferative disorders Hypervitaminosis D	Apocrine adenocarcinomas of the anal sac are associated with hypercalcaemia in about 80% of cases. If careful rectal examination is not done, hypercalcaemia may be incorrectly attributed to lymphoma, myeloma or some other cause.
Glucose	Decrease	Artifact Neonatal and juvenile forms Insulinoma	Sepsis, leukaemia, large liver tumours, and other tumours are less well recognised causes of hypoglycaemia

SPECIMEN FACTORS THAT CAN LEAD TO MISINTERPRETATION OF LABORATORY DATA

Sample Collection and Handling

Venipuncture

In an ideal world, every blood sample would be obtained rapidly by uncomplicated venipuncture. In practice, problems with patient restraint, patient conformation and technical expertise often slow or disrupt the procedure. Difficulties encountered during or immediately after venipuncture often lead to unwanted blood coagulation, haemolysis and other problems:

- If there is a sufficient delay in collecting blood from the vein and transferring it to the anticoagulant blood tube, blood may begin to clot in the syringe or vacutainer.
- If blood is inadequately mixed with anticoagulant once it is collected, it will clot in the tube.
- If undetected, partial coagulation will lead to errors in routine haematological testing. In particular, platelet counts will be artificially low.
- Blood vessel walls may be punctured several times during difficult venipuncture. Damaged blood vessel wall components and tissue fluid may be aspirated into the syringe or vacutainer, accelerating clotting and compromising the results of coagulation and other tests.
- Haemolysis may result from use of excessive negative pressure while drawing blood, or from forcing blood through a small lumen needle into the blood tube. Haemolysis interferes with several haematogical and serum biochemical tests.
- If an insufficient volume of blood is obtained during difficult venipuncture and is then mixed with a relative excess of anticoagulant, artifactual alterations in erythrocyte indices will occur. For example, ethylenediaminetetracetic acid (EDTA) excess causes shrinkage of red blood cells, falsely lowering PCV and MCV, but raising mean corpuscular haemoglobin concentration (MCHC).
- If the vein is raised for an excessive period of time, the tourniquet effect may slightly alter the results of several haematological and biochemical tests (e.g. ammonia and lactate quantitation).

Cystocentesis

Potential technical problems with cystocentesis are comparable to those experienced with venipuncture. In most cases, urine samples intended for bacterial or fungal culture are ideally obtained by cystocentesis. This is because urine aspirated directly from the bladder, through surgically-prepared skin, is free of contaminating organisms. Urine obtained by catheter, or by free-catch, is contaminated to a lesser or greater extent (Lulich and Osborne 1995).

Technical difficulties experienced during attempted cystocentesis most commonly lead to failure to obtain a urine specimen. Sometimes a blood-contaminated specimen is obtained. Rarely in ascitic patients, the urine specimen may be contaminated with ascitic fluid, or ascitic fluid may be obtained instead of urine. Even more rarely, the colon is punctured and the specimen may be contaminated with faeces.

Factors that Complicate Cystocentesis Include

- Obesity of the patient – palpation or immobilisation of the bladder is more difficult in a grossly obese dog.
- Tenseness of the abdominal wall – nervous patients, or patients with abdominal pain may tense their abdominal muscles making palpation of the bladder difficult.
- Struggling of the patient – cystocentesis is best carried out on a well-restrained, relaxed patient.
- Degree of fullness of the bladder – cystocentesis is more difficult if the bladder is nearly empty. Patients with lower urinary tract disease are usually candidates for cystocentesis; unfortunately, their illness causes them to empty their bladder frequently. Sometimes, to permit cystocentesis, fluid therapy must be given to encourage filling of the bladder.
- Location of the bladder – cystocentesis is usually more difficult if the patient has an intrapelvic bladder or a retroflexed bladder in a perineal hernial sac.

Sample Handling and Storage

Once a specimen of blood or urine is collected it must be handled appropriately. This is more critical for some analyses than others.

Urine

- Urine intended for bacterial culture should be processed within 30 min or promptly refrigerated at 4°C. Failure to do this may permit bacterial replication in the urine specimen and may lead to misdiagnosis of urinary tract infection. This is more likely to happen if catheter-obtained or free-catch specimens are mishandled, because the number of bacteria is greater in specimens obtained by these routes. Refrigerated specimens may be stored for up to 6 h without a significant increase in bacterial numbers; however fastidious organisms may die during storage. Refrigeration of urine chemically preserved using a mixture of boric acid, glycerol and formate is an option if culture cannot be started within 6 h (Allen *et al.* 1987). Bacterial viability has been reported to be up to 72 h using this technique.

- Urine sediment examination is best carried out on fresh urine specimens. Cellular elements and tubular casts degenerate in stored specimens, particularly if urine is stored at room temperature. Crystals may form in refrigerated urine. Urine should be warmed to room temperature before analysis.

- Urine should not be exposed to fluorescent light for a long period of time before the reagent strip tests for urobilinogen and bilirubin are done. Bilirubin is rapidly oxidised to biliverdin and urobilinogen to urobilin upon exposure to ultraviolet light. The urine takes on a green colour and the strip tests may yield false negative results.

- Glucose present in infected urine that is not handled properly may be consumed by bacteria, leading to a false negative dipstick result.

Blood

After blood collection, serum or plasma should ideally be separated from blood cells within 20–30 min. This will prevent consumption of glucose by cells in the specimen and may reduce the amount of *in vitro* haemolysis. The specimen should then be stored either refrigerated at 4°C or frozen at −20°C until analysis. Most analytes in serum or plasma are stable in a refrigerator at 4°C for 24 h or more, however there are important exceptions. Handling of blood specimens intended for quantitation of glucose, ammonia, ionised calcium and blood gases requires special care because these analytes are particularly labile.

Storage of whole blood at room temperature leads to a decrease in blood glucose concentration of about 0.39 mmol/l per hour, or about 10% per hour (Leifer 1986). The rate of *in vitro* glucose consumption is dependent upon the number of cells per unit volume in the sample and may be more rapid in specimens from patients with polycythaemia, leukocytosis or thrombocytosis. If serum or plasma cannot be separated promptly from blood cells to avoid artifactual hypoglycaemia, blood can be collected into a sodium oxalate/fluoride tube. Sodium oxalate/fluoride is both an anticoagulant and a glucose preservative, oxalate binds the Ca^{2+} and anticoagulates. Certain enzymatic methods for glucose quantitation cannot be used with fluoride-containing specimens, because the enzyme used in the assay is 'poisoned' by fluoride. This applies to many of the commercially available 'sticks' for the determination of blood glucose. If in doubt, the clinician should contact the clinical laboratory to discuss methods for optimising blood glucose measurement.

Blood ammonia determination is sometimes useful in the diagnosis of severe liver disease, particularly if hepatic encephalopathy is present. Used in this setting, the test has high specificity but low sensitivity. Blood for ammonia determination is usually collected into heparinised tubes. For obvious reasons ammonium heparin tubes should not be used; lithium, sodium or potassium heparin tubes are suitable. After collection, blood should immediately be placed on ice and transported to the clinical laboratory. Plasma should be harvested in a precooled centrifuge and ideally the analysis should be carried out within an hour of blood collection. Storage of canine whole blood or plasma intended for ammonia quantification, even in a −20°C freezer, leads to erroneous results (Hitt and Jones 1986).

Blood ionised calcium measurement provides a more accurate assessment of calcium homeostasis than does serum total calcium because ionised calcium comprises the physiologically active fraction. Homeostatic mechanisms regulate blood ionised calcium concentration, not total calcium. An increasing number of veterinary clinical laboratories are offering to measure blood or serum ionised calcium. The astute clinician should be aware of some potential pitfalls when handling specimens for ionised calcium measurement.

- pH changes may occur after collection of a whole blood specimen and alter the ionised calcium concentration. Glycolysis (with consequent formation of lactic acid) causes a decrease in pH and a rise in the concentration of ionised calcium in the sample. Blood cells should therefore be separated from serum or plasma if the specimen cannot be promptly analysed. A study has shown that heparinised venous whole blood can be stored at 4°C for up to 3 h after collection without significant alteration in ionised calcium concentration (Szenci *et al.* 1994).

- The same study showed that serum and plasma can be collected and stored anaerobically at 4°C for much longer (up to 240 h) without significant alteration in ionised calcium concentration.

- Ionised calcium is substantially bound by all standard anticoagulants, including heparin. Therefore ionised calcium concentration is a little lower in plasma than in serum taken from the same patient at the same time. The assay is very sensitive to the concentration of anticoagulant used, therefore this should be standardised. Calcium-titrated heparin (S 4500 Heparin for ionised calcium analysis, Radiometer, Copenhagen) is the preferred anticoagulant, if plasma rather than serum is to be submitted to the laboratory. The use of serum to avoid these chelation problems is an acceptable alternative. The normal range for ionised calcium is much narrower than for total calcium, artifacts can take the estimated value outside the normal range and therefore greatly hinder diagnosis.

Specimens for blood gas analysis should be collected and transported to the laboratory anaerobically on ice. The rectal temperature of the patient and the blood haemoglobin concentration (or at least the PCV) should be measured at the time that the blood gas specimen is drawn. The laboratory needs to be informed of these values to permit correct measurement of blood gases.

Interfering Substances

Ideally, each veterinary clinical laboratory would be aware of the effects of commonly encountered interfering substances on their own laboratory test results and would provide the inquisitive clinician with detailed information concerning these interfering substances upon request. Simple graphs can be produced that show the effects of increasing amounts of lipid, bilirubin and haemoglobin upon test results (Glick *et al.* 1986). In practice, it can be quite difficult to get hold of such information, even from a university veterinary hospital. A useful, but less complete alternative is provided by some clinical laboratories. Test results from specimens that were found by the laboratory to contain interfering substances are 'rubber stamped' with a list of known effects of the interfering substance.

Lipaemia

Lipid droplets in canine plasma or serum may cause visible turbidity of what is normally a clear, straw-coloured fluid. Lesser degrees of lipaemia may be inapparent on examination of the specimen, or may cause a slight haze. Marked lipaemia of whole blood may give the specimen the appearance of a 'strawberry milk shake'. Lactescent plasma or serum is routinely encountered when postprandial blood specimens are centrifuged for analysis. If encountered in a true fasting specimen, lipaemia may be indicative of hypothyroidism, hyperadrenocorticism, pancreatitis, diabetes mellitus, or a primary hyperlipidaemia.

Effects of lipaemia include the following:

- The scattering of light caused by fat droplets affects certain laboratory tests that depend upon absorption or refraction of light.
- New analytical methods that employ dry reagent technology are less affected by lipaemia than are conventional wet chemical methods.
- Spectrophotometric and flame photometric determinations are affected, but ion selective electrodes are not.

Therefore, electrolyte measurements obtained by flame photometry (e.g. sodium and potassium) will be decreased; but values obtained using ion selective electrodes are unaffected.

- Refractometry is substantially affected, so that artificially high results for total plasma protein are obtained, compared with the results obtained using biochemical methods. Total plasma protein values obtained by refractometry of specimens from healthy, lipaemic animals may exceed 130 g/l.
- Serum bile acids (SBAs) are artificially elevated by lipaemia, which frequently causes problems in interpreting postprandial SBAs. A modest amount of food should be fed during the test. The objective is to provide sufficient food to cause emptying of the gall bladder and no more.

Lipaemia can enhance *in vitro* haemolysis. Therefore the interferences mentioned below in the section concerning haemolysis can be a consequence of both lipaemia and haemolysis.

Haemolysis

Lysis of erythrocytes *in vitro* causes interference with a number of clinical laboratory tests.

- PCV is decreased.
- The MCHC is increased as the machine measures all the haemoglobin in the sample and calculates MCHC from the red cell count.
- Spectrophotometric tests that depend upon transmission (or absorption) of light may be substantially affected, artificially elevating the values of:
  - ALT,
  - albumin,
  - total bilirubin,
  - calcium,
  - cholesterol,
  - glucose and
  - phosphate.
- Newer analytical systems are more resistant to this sort of interference.
- Canine erythrocytes are not particularly rich in potassium, so pseudohyperkalaemia is not a common sequel to *in vitro* haemolysis, except in specimens from Akitas.
- Erythrocytes are rich in lactate dehydrogenase (LDH) and aspartate aminotransferase (AST). Serum concentrations of these enzymes increase after haemolysis.

Hyperbilirubinaemia

Hyperbilirubinaemia may artificially increase the concentrations of albumin, cholesterol, glucose and total protein; depending on the biochemical methods used for the determination of each of these analytes. The concentration of serum creatinine may be artificially decreased if the Jaffé method is used for analysis.

Timing of Specimen Collection

Blood samples for certain purposes must be collected at specific times relative to feeding or administered medications. Examples include :

- postprandial SBAs (120 min after food);
- serum trypsin-like immunoreactivity (after a 12-h fast);
- ACTH stimulation test (before and 30–120 min after ACTH administration, depending upon the ACTH preparation used and the laboratory);
- serum T_4 for assessment of adequacy of thyroid medication (about 6 h post pill); and
- serum digoxin level (8–12 h post pill).

If specimens are inadvertently collected at an incorrect time, or if the clinician is unaware of the necessity for careful timing, diagnostic errors may be made.

HUMAN FACTORS THAT CAN LEAD TO MISINTERPRETATION OF LABORATORY DATA

Human beings have a natural proclivity to err; we tend to cut corners, jump to conclusions, and overlook things. Veterinarians are far from being immune to these tendencies. Yet despite the complexity of our work, development and maintenance of a habit of thoroughness can help considerably in the avoidance of diagnostic errors. In the approach to clinical laboratory data, it is useful to follow a set of guidelines, similar to the one offered here.

(1) First assess specimen quality. Look for comments concerning unwanted coagulation, lipaemia, haemolysis, or hyperbilirubinaemia. These can cause spurious, marked alterations in some parameters. If you are uncertain of the possible effects of an interfering substance, make enquiries of the clinical laboratory.

(2) Peruse the reported laboratory values and identify abnormal values. Classify the degree of abnormality of each as mild, moderate, or marked. This should go beyond simple numerical considerations. For some analytes (e.g. serum calcium or sodium) a small percentage increase is highly significant. For others (e.g. ALP) a 10-fold increase is not overwhelmingly impressive. When faced with an unfamiliar analyte, avoid errors concerning units of measurement by meticulous examination of results.

(3) Consider whether or not any of the abnormalities might be normal for the particular patient under study (e.g. anaemia of late pregnancy; puppy hypercalcaemia; raised serum ALP activity in a patient receiving glucocorticoid therapy).

(4) Consider whether inadequate patient preparation, or inappropriate timing of specimen collection might be responsible for an abnormal result (e.g. postprandial hypercholesterolaemia; failure to fast a patient before TLI quantitation; collection of blood for T_4 measurement at an inappropriate time post pill).

(5) Rank the problems identified from the clinical laboratory data in order of importance, taking into consideration both the degree of abnormality and the physiological relevance of the analyte. Consider possible hierarchical relationships among the problems. Group problems together loosely, in an interchangeable format. Consider differential diagnoses for individual problems, or for groups of problems.

(6) Decide what further investigations are required to rule in or rule out your differential diagnoses. Discuss the costs, risks and benefits of these investigations with the owner of the patient. If deemed appropriate, carry out the investigations needed to permit accurate prognostication and formulation of an optimal therapeutic plan.

REFERENCES

Allen, T.A., Jones, R.L. & Purvance, J. (1987) Microbiologic evaluation of canine urine: Direct microscopic examination and preservation of specimen quality for culture. *Journal of the American Veterinary Medical Association*, **190**, 1289–1291.

Andersen, A.C. & Gee, W. (1958) Normal blood values in the beagle. *Veterinary Medicine*, **53**, 135.

Barosi, G., Magnani, L. & Stefanelli, M. (1993) Medical diagnostic reasoning: Epistemological modeling as a strategy for design of computer-based consultation programs. *Theoretical Medicine*, **14**, 43–55.

Bartges, J.W. & Osborne, C.A. (1995) Influence of fasting and eating on laboratory values. In: *Kirk's Current Veterinary*

Therapy XII – Small Animal Practice, (ed. John D. Bonagura), pp. 20–23. W.B. Saunders Company, Philadelphia.

Bounous, D.I., Boudreaux, M.K. & Hoskins, J.D. (1995) The hematopoitic and lymphoid systems. In: *Veterinary Pediatrics – Dogs and Cats from Birth to Six Months*, (ed. Johnny D. Hoskins), 2nd edn. pp. 337–376. W.B. Saunders Company, Philadelphia.

Burkhard, M.J. & Meyer, D.J. (1995) Causes and effects of interference with clinical laboratory measurements and examinations. In: *Kirk's Current Veterinary Therapy XII – Small Animal Practice*, (ed. John D. Bonagura), pp. 14–20. W.B. Saunders Company, Philadelphia.

Center, S.A., Baldwin, B.H., Dillingham, S., Erb, H.N. & Tennant, B.C. (1986) Diagnostic value of serum gamma-glutamyl transferase and alkaline phosphatase activities in hepatobiliary disease in the cat. *Journal of the American Veterinary Medical Association*, **188**, 507–510.

Center, S.A., Slater, M.R., Manwarren, T. & Prymak, K. (1992) Diagnostic efficacy of serum alkaline phosphatase and gammaglutamyltransferase in dogs with histologically confirmed hepatobiliary disease: 270 cases (1980–1990). *Journal of the American Veterinary Medical Association,* **201**, 1258–1264.

Chastain, C.B. & Panciera, D.L. (1995) Hypothyroid diseases. In: *Textbook of Veterinary Internal Medicine*, (eds Stephen J. Ettinger & Edward C. Feldman), 4th edn. pp. 1487–1501. W.B. Saunders Company, Philadelphia.

Evinger, J.V. & Nelson, R.W. (1984) The clinical pharmacology of thyroid hormones in the dog. *Journal of the American Veterinary Medical Association*, **185**, 314.

Farver, T.B. (1989) Concepts of normality in clinical biochemistry. In: *Clinical Biochemistry of Domestic Animals*, (ed. Jiro J. Kaneko), 4th edn. pp. 1–20. Academic Press, London.

Ferguson, D.C. (1994) Update on diagnosis of canine hypothyroidism. *Veterinary Clinics of North America Small Animal Practice*, **24**, 515–539.

Glick, M.R., Ryder, K.W. & Jackson, S.A. (1986) Graphical comparisons of interferences in clinical chemistry instrumentation. *Clinical Chemistry*, **32**, 470–474.

Hall, J.A. & Campbell, K.L. (1995) The effect of potentiated sulfonamides on canine thyroid function. In: *Kirk's Current Veterinary Therapy XII – Small Animal Practice*, (ed. John D. Bonagura), pp. 595–597. W.B. Saunders Company, Philadelphia.

Hitt, M.E. & Jones, B.D. (1986) Effects of storage temperature and time on canine plasma ammonia concentrations. *American Journal of Veterinary Research*, **47**, 363–364.

Hughes, D., Elliott, D.A., Washabau, R.J. & Kueppers, F. (1995) Effects of age, sex, reproductive status, and hospitalization on serum alpha(1)-antitrypsin concentration in dogs. *American Journal of Veterinary Research*, **56**(5), 568–572.

Jacobs, R.M., Lumsden, J.H. & Vernau, W. (1995) Canine and feline reference values. In: *Kirk's Current Veterinary Therapy XII – Small Animal Practice*, (ed. John D. Bonagura), pp. 1395–1417. W.B. Saunders Company, Philadelphia.

Jain, N.C. (1986) The eosinophils. In: *Schalm's Veterinary Hematology*, (ed. Nemi C. Jain), 4th edn. pp. 731–755. Lea & Febiger, Philadelphia.

Kaplan, A.J., Peterson, M.E. & Kemppainen, R.J. (1995) Effects of disease on the results of diagnostic tests for use in detecting hyperadrenocorticism in dogs. *Journal of the American Veterinary Medical Association*, **207**, 445–451.

Kassirer, J.P. (1989) Diagnostic reasoning. *Annals of Internal Medicine*, **110**, 893–900.

Leifer, C.E. (1986) Hypoglycemia. In: *Kirk's Current Veterinary Therapy IX – Small Animal Practice*, (ed. Robert W. Kirk), pp. 982–987. W.B. Saunders Company, Philadelphia.

Lulich, J.P. & Osborne, C.A. (1995) Bacterial infections of the urinary tract. In: *Textbook of Veterinary Internal Medicine*, (eds Stephen J. Ettinger & Edward C. Feldman), 4th edn. pp. 1775–1788. W.B. Saunders Company, Philadelphia.

Meyer, D.J., Moriello, K.A., Feder, B.M., Fehrer-Sawyer, S.L. & Maxwell, A.K. (1990) Effect of otic medications on liver function test results in healthy dogs. *Journal of the American Veterinary Medical Association*, **196**, 743–744.

Moriello, K.A., Fehrer-Sawyer, S.L., Meyer, D.J. & Feder, B. (1988) Adrenocortical suppression associated with topical otic administration of glucocorticoids in dogs. *Journal of the American Veterinary Medical Association*, **193**, 329–331.

Nelson, R.W., Ihle, S.L., Feldman, E.C. & Bottoms, G.D. (1991) Serum free thyroxine concentration in healthy dogs, dogs with hypothyroidism, and euthyroid dogs with concurrent illness. *Journal of the American Veterinary Medical Association*, **198**, 1401–1407.

Panciera, D.L. & Post, K. (1992) Effect of oral administration of sulfadiazine and trimethoprim in combination on thyroid function in dogs. *Canadian Journal of Veterinary Research*, **56**, 349–352.

Panciera, D.L. & Refsal, K.R. (1994) Thyroid function in dogs with spontaneous and induced congestive heart failure. *Canadian Journal of Veterinary Research*, **58**, 157–162.

Ridgway, H.B. & Moriello, K.A. (1993) Iatrogenic Cushing's syndrome in a dog from owner's topical corticosteroid [letter]. *Archives of Dermatology*, **129**(3), 379.

Robinson, F.R. & Ziegler, R.F. (1968) Clinical laboratory values of beagle dogs. *Laboratory Animal Care*, **18**, 39–49.

Rosol, T.J., Capen, C.C., Danks, J.A., *et al.* (1990) Identification of parathyroid hormone-related protein in canine apocrine adenocarcinoma of the anal sac. *Veterinary Pathology*, **27**, 89–95.

Rowland, P.H., Center, S.A. & Dougherty, S.A. (1992) Presumptive trimethoprim-sulfadiazine-related hepatotoxicosis in a dog. *Journal of the American Veterinary Medical Association*, **200**, 348–350.

Rutgers, H.C., Batt, R.M., Vailant, C. & Riley, J.E. (1995) Subcellular pathologic features of glucocorticoid-induced hepatopathy in dogs. *American Journal of Veterinary Research*, **56**, 898–907.

Sanecki, R.K., Hoffmann, W.E., Dorner, J.L. & Kuhlenschmidt,

M.S. (1990) Purification and comparison of corticosteroid-induced and intestinal isoenzymes of alkaline phosphatase in dogs. *American Journal of Veterinary Research*, **51**, 1964–1968.

Solter, P.F., Hoffmann, W.E., Hungerford, L.L., Peterson, M.E. & Dorner, J.L. (1993) Assessment of corticosteroid-induced alkaline phosphatase isoenzyme as a screening test for hyperadrenocorticism in dogs. *Journal of the American Veterinary Medical Association*, **203**, 534–538.

Szenci, O., Besser, T.E., Stollar Z. & Brydl, E. (1994) Effect of storage time and temperature on canine ionised calcium concentration in blood, plasma and serum. *Journal of the American Animal Hospital Association*, **30**, 495–499.

Teske, E., Rothuizen, J., de Bruijne, J.J. & Mol, J.A. (1986) Separation and heat stability of the corticosteroid-induced and hepatic alkaline phosphatase isoenzymes in canine plasma. *Journal of Chromatography*, **369**, 349–356.

Teske, E., Rothuizen, J., de Bruijne, J.J. & Rijnberk, A. (1989) Corticosteroid-induced alkaline phosphatase isoenzyme in the diagnosis of canine hypercorticism. *Veterinary Record*, **125**, 12–14.

Tibaldi, J.M. & Surks, M.I. (1985) Effects of nonthyroidal illness on thyroid function. *Medical Clinics of North America*, **69**, 899–911.

Trepanier, L.A. (1995) Use of bromide as an anticonvulsant for dogs with epilepsy. [Review]. *Journal of the American Veterinary Medical Association*, **207**, 163–166.

Wallen, N., Kita, H., Weiler, D. & Gleich, G.J. (1991) Glucocorticoids inhibit cytokine-mediated eosinophil survival. *Journal of Immunology*, **147**(10), 3490–3495.

Weir, E.C., Burtis, W.J., Morris, C.A., Brady, T.G. & Insogna, K.L. (1988) Isolation of 16,000-dalton parathyroid hormone-like proteins from two animal tumors causing humoral hypercalcemia of malignancy. *Endocrinology*, **123**, 2744–2751.

Weiser, M.G. (1995) Erythrocyte responses and disorders. In: *Textbook of Veterinary Internal Medicine*, (eds Stephen J. Ettinger & Edward C. Feldman), 4th edn. pp. 1864–1891. W.B. Saunders Company, Philadelphia.

Section 4

Haematology, Oncology, Immunological Disease

Edited by Jane M. Dobson

Chapter 32

The Haematopoietic System: The Structure and Function of Bone Marrow

L. Blackwood and E. J. Villiers

INTRODUCTION

Haematopoiesis is the process by which blood cells are formed. *In utero*, erythropoiesis (the production of red blood cells) occurs firstly in the blood islands of the yolk sac. After the third week of gestation the liver becomes active in haematopoiesis and is the main source of erythrocytes until the marrow becomes the primary site of erythropoiesis in late gestation. In contrast, intra-uterine production of granulocytes and platelets occurs largely in the fetal bone marrow. In neonates and immature dogs, the marrow of all bones is actively involved in blood cell production. As maturity is reached, haematopoiesis becomes restricted to the flat bones (such as the sternum, ribs, pelvis and vertebrae) and the proximal ends of the marrow cavity of long bones (especially the humerus and femur). All blood cell types are produced within the marrow, but the peripheral lymphoid tissues also produce lymphocytes. The liver and spleen retain the capacity to produce blood cells in abnormal circumstances in later life: this is referred to as extramedullary haematopoiesis.

THE STRUCTURE OF BONE MARROW

There are two types of bone marrow:

- red marrow, which is haematopoietically active,
- yellow marrow, which does little other than store fat.

Yellow marrow is substituted for red as the animal matures,

except in selected sites (as above), but can be reactivated when demand for erythrocyte production increases. Red marrow comprises a mixed population of cells involved in haematopoiesis and a supportive connective tissue stroma. The stromal elements of the bone marrow consist of a variety of cell types (including fibroblasts, endothelial cells and macrophages) supported by a meshwork of collagen and reticular fibres. The microenvironment created by these cells supports blood cell production. Factors produced locally by stromal cells are involved in the control of haematopoiesis. The endothelial cells of the marrow form wide, thin walled sinusoids with a discontinuous basement membrane, and the cells themselves are modified to favour macromolecular transport. These sinusoids allow exchange between the plasma and the marrow stromal microenvironment. Maturing blood cells are thought to exit the marrow by squeezing through temporary 'migration pores' in the endothelium. Macrophages, involved in phagocytosis of debris, are found associated with the sinusoids. Adipocyte-like fat storing cells are also found in the stroma, even in red marrow.

The haematopoietic cells of the bone marrow can be divided into three groups:

- pluripotent stem cells,
- differentiating progenitor cells and
- fully functional mature blood cells.

The early, pluripotent stem cells are capable of self-renewal. As cells become more committed to a certain cell lineage, their ability to proliferate is reduced and eventually lost. Thus the marrow has a pyramidal structure, where one stem cell gives rise to many daughter cells. Fig. 32.1 shows a schematic representation of haematopoiesis, and Figs 32.2 and 32.3 show the pyramidal structure of the marrow.

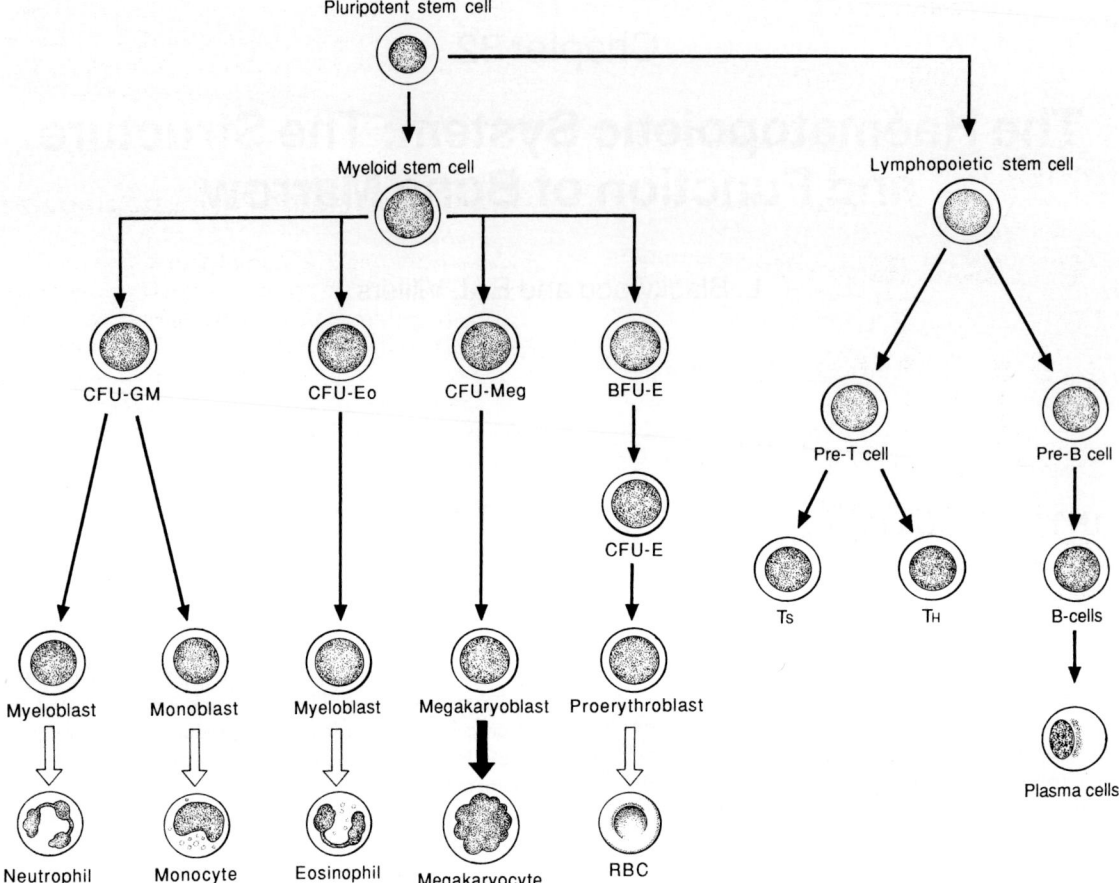

Fig. 32.1 A diagrammatic representation of haematopoiesis showing the differentiation of the various cell lineages.

THE FUNCTION OF BONE MARROW

Erythropoiesis

Erythrocytes are normally produced in the bone marrow. This development occurs in islets around central ('nurse') macrophages, which phagocytose debris (e.g. extruded nuclei, abnormal cells), store iron and contribute to local control of the microenvironment. Extramedullary haematopoiesis in the liver and spleen is stimulated only if the marrow is unable match the demand. It takes approximately 7 days for red cells to differentiate in the marrow, and they continue to mature for 24–48 h in the circulation or spleen. The average life span of red cells in the canine circulation is 110–120 days, and most effete red cells are phagocytosed by splenic macrophages.

During erythropoiesis, the pluripotent stem cell in the marrow is influenced by factors called 'burst promoting activity' (BPA) to form colonies of cells called 'erythroid burst forming units' (BFU-E). It has been hypothesised that BPA is the cytokine interleukin-3 produced by T lymphocytes. BFU-E differentiate into 'erythroid colony forming units' (CFU-E) in response to erythropoietin, stimulation by which also causes differentiation of CFU-E into the first recognisable erythroid precursor, the proerythroblast. This cell continues to differentiate through the early, intermediate and late normoblast stages to the reticulocyte and then the mature erythrocyte (Fig. 32.2). (British and American nomenclature for the erythroid series differ and are shown in Appendix 1.)

ERYTHROPOIESIS

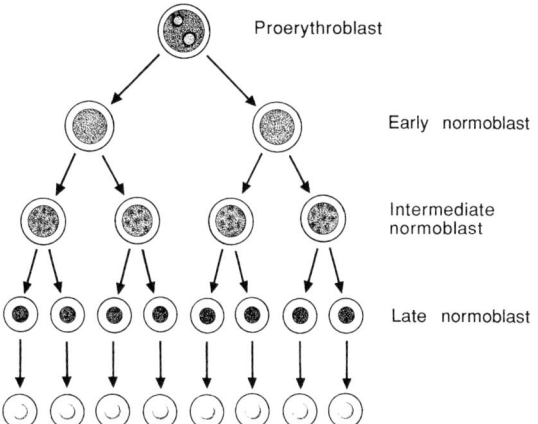

Fig. 32.2   A diagrammatic representation of erythrocyte differentiation from the first morphologically recognisable precursor, the proerythroblast, through to mature red cells. Note the pyramidal arrangement of cells, i.e. increasing numbers or progeny from a single proerythroblast.

The glycoprotein hormone erythropoietin is the main regulator of erythropoiesis and is produced by the kidney in response to lowered oxygen tension. Although the liver can produce erythropoietin in man, this is not the case in dogs.

Granulopoiesis and Lymphopoiesis

In contrast to erythropoiesis, where the role of erythropoietin is well understood, factors controlling granulopoiesis are less well defined. Although it is simpler to assume that lymphoid cells have a separate stem cell from the granulocyte/monocyte cell lines, the possibility of there being additional bipotent stem cells which can produce both myeloid and lymphoid progeny has not been ruled out.

CFU-C (so called because they were first described in 'colony forming units in culture') are the multipotent stem cells which have been shown to give rise to mixed colonies of cells. These stem cells are morphologically similar to small lymphocytes. In the presence of colony stimulating factor (CSF) these will grow and differentiate into cells of the granulocyte–monocyte lineages. CFU-GM (granulo-

GRANULOPOIESIS

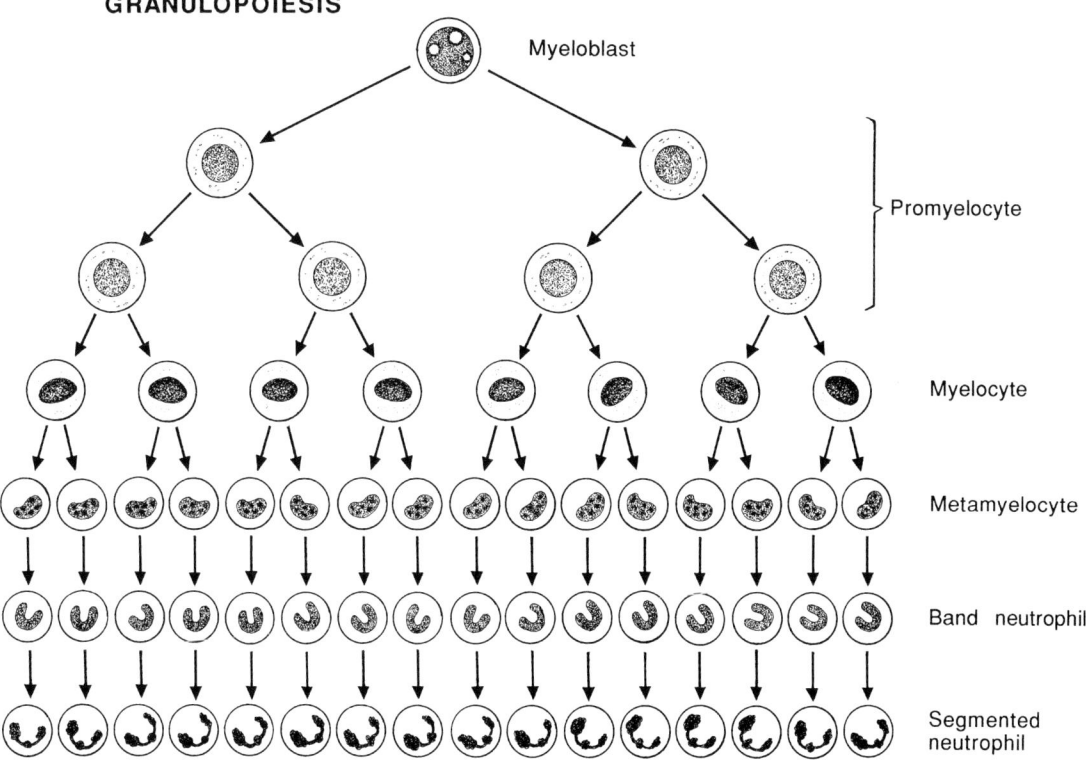

Fig. 32.3   A diagrammatic representation of neutrophil maturation from the first morphologically recognisable precursor, the myeloblast. The capacity to divide is lost at the metamyelocyte stage.

cyte–monocyte colony forming unit) has been identified as the particular CFU-C progenitor cell which gives rise to both granulocytes and monocytes.

Colony stimulating factor is not thought to be a single hormone, and there is probably a separate CSF for each cell lineage. Macrophages, monocytes, activated lymphocytes and endothelial cells all produce local factors which stimulate granulopoiesis including interleukin-3. Unless there is continued stimulation for granulocyte release (e.g. presence of endotoxins) then inhibitory substances from mature neutrophils and prostaglandin E from macrophages have a 'negative feedback' effect on granulopoiesis.

The first morphologically recognisable granulocyte is the myeloblast. These cells differentiate through progranulocyte, myelocyte, metamyelocyte and band forms to become mature granulocytes (Fig. 32.3). The capacity for cell division is lost at the metamyelocyte stage, by which time 16 to 32 myelocytes have arisen from each myeloblast.

Neutrophils

Within the marrow there is a maturation pool of neutrophils, consisting of metamyelocytes, band cells and segmented neutrophils. This pool acts as a reserve should there be a sudden demand for neutrophils, and contains approximately 5 days supply of cells. The marrow transit time for a neutrophil (time to enter the pool) is about 4 days. In contrast to red cells, the half-life of circulating neutrophils is only 6–14 h, and is shortened during acute infections as most of the neutrophils pass into the tissue pool. Approximately half the neutrophils in the total blood pool are circulating at any given time, while the remainder are adherent to the vascular endothelium (the circulating and marginal pools, respectively). There is no significant pool of neutrophils in the tissue (tissue pool) of normal animals. A diagrammatic representation of neutrophil distribution is shown in Fig. 32.4.

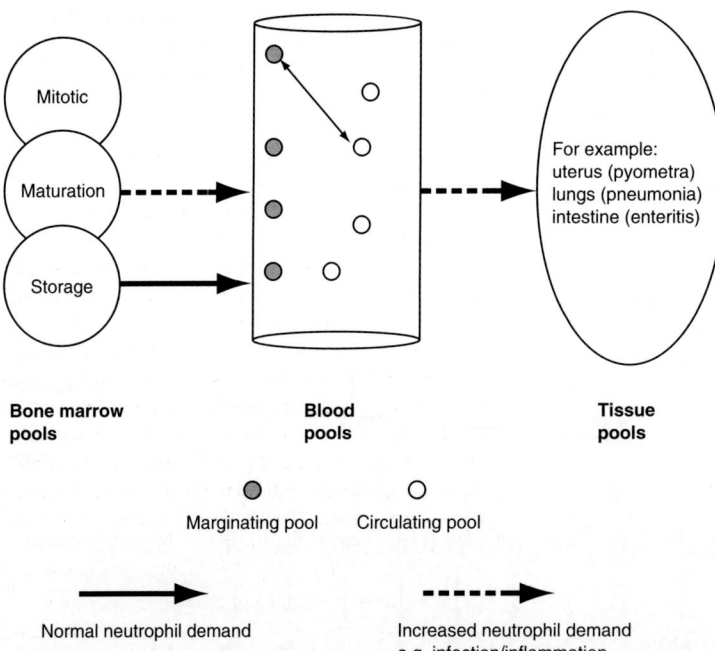

Fig. 32.4 Diagrammatic representation of neutrophil distribution within the body. In the normal animal, neutrophils are released from the storage pool to replace those lost from the bloodstream. When this storage pool is insufficient to meet demand, immature neutrophils are released from the maturation pool and a left shift results. The marginating pool consists of cells stuck to or rolling along small blood vessels, particularly in the spleen, lungs and splanchnic circulation. The neutrophil spends about 8 h in the blood before migrating into the tissue pool. In health there are very few neutrophils in the tissue pool.

Monocytes

Monocytes share a common precursor with neutrophils. They are produced from monoblasts with fewer maturation steps than granulocytes. Monocytes circulate in the blood for a variable period of hours to days. They then enter the tissues, where they mature into macrophages.

Eosinophils and Basophils

The progenitor cell for eosinophils is CFU-Eo. Division and differentiation occurs in response to stimulation by T lymphocytes and an undefined humoral factor. Basophils are thought to arise from CFU-C (the myeloid precursor) or a precursor derived from this cell, which is also thought to give rise to mast cells.

Lymphocytes

Lymphopoiesis occurs within the bone marrow and peripheral lymphoid tissue. The marrow stem cells can differentiate into either B or T cells. T cells arise in the thymus due to the influence of different microenvironmental factors. An equivalent to the avian bursa has not been identified in mammals and B cells are thought to arise in the marrow. These cells then migrate to the peripheral lymphoid tissues, where they can mature and proliferate, and develop into plasma cells, memory B cells and so on which respond to antigenic stimulation. Much of the lymphopoiesis in normal marrow is independent of antigenic stimulation, though a few B cells will undergo antigen-dependent development into plasma cells in the marrow. Populations of T lymphocytes regulate B cell function, and also are involved of the production of granulocytes and monocytes. Many of the lymphocytes in the blood are long-lived (months to years), recirculating T and B memory cells.

Megakaryopoiesis

Megakaryocyte colony-forming units (CFU-Meg) are the committed precursor cells derived from the pluripotent stem cells which give rise to platelets. These cells undergo nuclear division without accompanying cytoplasmic division, resulting in a multinucleate cell with copious cytoplasm: the megakaryocyte. During platelet production, megakaryocytes protrude cytoplasmic processes close to or into the marrow sinusoids. Thus platelets break off from these processes as the vesicles around small regions of cytoplasm unite. Platelets arise in the bone marrow but some may arise from megakaryocytes that become fixed in the pulmonary parenchyma.

THERAPEUTIC APPLICATION OF HAEMATOPOIETIC GROWTH FACTORS

Many of the growth factors required for the control of blood cell proliferation, differentiation and survival have been identified and produced *in vitro* using recombinant DNA technology. The therapeutic potential of these agents is vast.

(1) *Erythropoietin.* Human recombinant erythropoietin has been used in dogs with chronic renal failure to increase erythropoiesis, with some success. Unfortunately, dogs develop antibodies to this foreign glycoprotein which limit long-term use. Patients receiving the drug must be closely monitored, as adverse effects include systemic hypertension, iron deficiency, hyperkalaemia and polycythaemia (Ogilvie & Obradovich 1992) (see also Chapters 33 and 62).

(2) *Colony stimulating factors.* Human recombinant G-CSF and GM-CSF have been used experimentally in dogs, and have been shown to promote granulopoiesis, resulting in increased production of mature, functional neutrophils. There is some evidence that GM-CSF enhances the cell killing activity of the neutrophils produced, and this factor also has effects on other cell lines (but not erythroid and megakaryocytic cell lines). As with erythropoietin, dogs rapidly produce antibodies to human recombinant factors, so that the human recombinant proteins can only be used in the short term. However, this is all that would be required in many clinical situations. Results with recombinant canine factors have been encouraging: they have been shown to be of benefit in prevention of clinically significant neutropenia after chemotherapeutic drug administration (see Chapter 35), and to ameliorate cyclic haematopoiesis by preventing clinically significant neutropenia (Mischu *et al.* 1992). These factors could be used in the treatment of canine parvovirus, overwhelming sepsis, septic shock, and primary bone marrow disorders.

(3) *Interleukin-3.* Interleukin-3 is thought to support and promote the development of the pluripotent stem cell, and has effects on red cells and platelets as well as on granulocytic cells. Early work in man has shown that it takes several weeks for the beneficial effects of this drug to be apparent, but it has been successfully used in cases of myelodysplasia and aplastic anaemia (Morstyn & Sheridan 1993; Ogilvie 1993).

While the potential applications of haematopoietic growth factors in the clinical situation are wide reaching, these drugs are still in the early stages of development. The long-term effects of their use are unknown, for example whether it is possible that they might eventually produce bone marrow failure as a result of forced cell differentiation, whether they may compromise the killing of tumour cells by cytotoxic drugs, and even whether they could promote neoplastic transformation leading to leukaemia.

ASSESSMENT OF BONE MARROW

The bone marrow should be evaluated in conjunction with haematological assessment (see later). Indications for sampling the bone marrow include:

- unexplained cytopenias, e.g. non-regenerative anaemia, thrombocytopenia, neutropenia, pancytopenia;
- abnormal/immature lymphocytes or granulocytes in the peripheral blood;
- inexplicably high levels of any cell line;
- multicentric lymphoma;
- hyperproteinaemia (associated with monoclonal or polyclonal gammopathy);
- hypercalcaemia (of unknown origin);
- pyrexia of unknown origin.

Samples of bone marrow may be collected and evaluated in two ways:

- cytological examination of an aspirate,
- histological examination of a core biopsy.

Both techniques can be carried out under local anaesthesia and sedation, and although some animals may not require

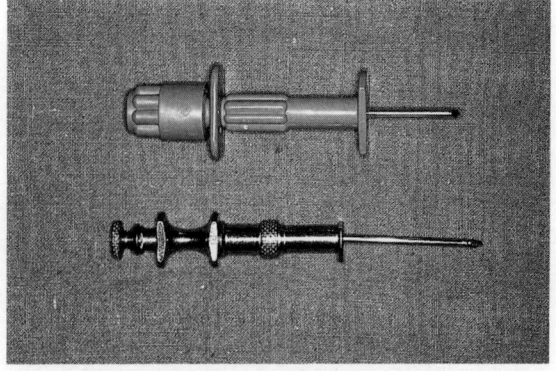

Fig. 32.5a   Specialised needles for bone marrow aspiration. There is a Klima needle (bottom) and a Jamshidi Disposable Modified Illinois Sternal Iliac Bone Marrow Aspiration Needle (Baxters Healthcare, Thetford, England).

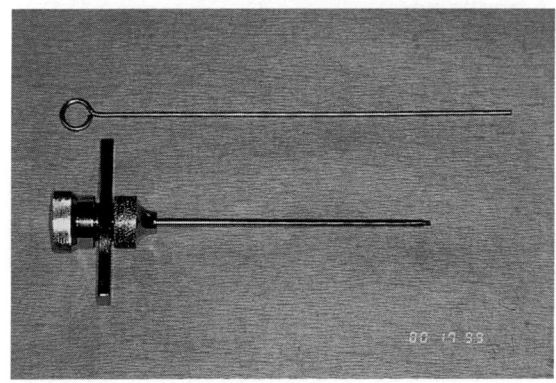

Fig. 32.5b   A Jamshidi needle for bone marrow core biopsy. The blunt ended probe (above) is used to push the harvested core in reverse direction from the tip to the hub, from which it is expelled.

Table 32.1   Examples of needles for bone marrow sampling.

	Gauge	Length
Aspiration needles		
Klima (reuseable) (Fig. 32.5a)	16 G or 18 G	20–80 mm
Disposable, e.g. Jamshidi Disposable sternal/iliac bone marrow aspiration needles (Baxters Healthcare, Thetford, England)	15 G or 18 G	48 mm or 38 mm
Biopsy needles		
Jamshidi	14 G or 18 G	95 mm

chemical restraint, local anaesthesia should always be used. Specialised needles incorporating an in-built central stylet are required for bone marrow sampling (Table 32.1 and Figs 32.5a and b).

Bone Marrow Aspirate

Collection of bone marrow aspirates is a relatively quick and simple technique (Box 32.1).

- To achieve satisfactory marrow aspirates, adequate personnel must be available to restrain the animal and assist in the rapid making of smears.
- In all but the smallest and most obese dogs the iliac crest is the site of choice for the bone marrow aspirate. The gluteal surface of the wing of the ileum, trochanteric fossa, the cranial aspect of the proximal humerus and the tibial crest are alternatives. If the trochanteric fossa is used it is the authors' preference to carry out this technique under general anaesthesia, due to the proximity of the sciatic nerve to the biopsy site and the absolute requirement for adequate restraint.

Failure to Aspirate Marrow

The most common reason for failure to aspirate marrow is the needle being positioned in cortical bone rather than within the marrow cavity:

- If the needle has not been advanced fully through the near cortex, the stylet should be re-inserted and the needle advanced further before further attempts to aspirate.

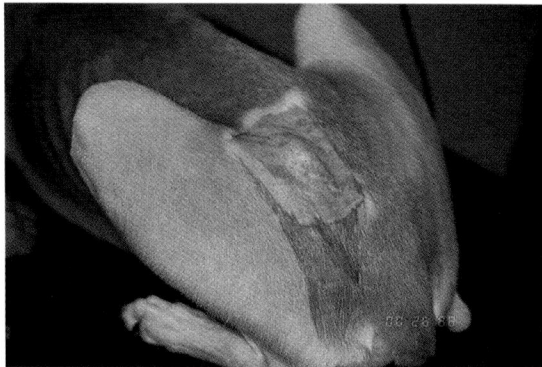

Fig. 32.6 A dog in sternal recumbency, positioned and prepared for marrow aspiration. Note the prominent iliac crest.

Box 32.1   Bone marrow aspiration technique.

- Pre-position several clean glass slides near vertically against, e.g. a sandbag on the bench. Further slides are needed to make smears.
- Place the dog in sternal recumbancy with the hind legs fully flexed and drawn close to the body. The iliac crest should now be readily palpable (Fig. 32.6).
- Clip, aseptically prepare and drape the area.
- Local anaesthesia: infiltrate the skin and subcutis, then advance the needle onto the periosteum (which should feel hard). 1–2 ml of lignocaine should be infiltrated into the periosteum (Fig. 32.7).
- Make a small stab incision in the skin over the iliac crest.
- Grasp the iliac crest, tensing the overlying skin and advance the Klima needle through the subcutis onto the bone of crest (Fig. 32.8).
- Advance the needle through the cortical bone by applying firm pressure, twisting back and forth. Keep the needle vertical or slightly ventromedial.
- Once through the cortex, the needle will be firmly lodged in the bone (moving the needle from side to side will move the dog from side to side).
- Remove the central stylet. Attatch a 20 ml syringe to the needle, and apply vigorous suction. The dog may show transient pain as the marrow is aspirated. 0.5–2 ml of bloody fluid (the marrow) should appear in the syringe. As soon as marrow appears release the negative pressure (excess pressure will result in haemodilution and cell damage) (Fig. 32.9).
- Remove the needle and syringe as one unit. Apply a drop of marrow to each slide. Marrow spicules remain on the slide whilst blood gravitates downwards (Fig. 32.10).
- Make the smears: a second slide is placed flat over the first slide at right angles, in doing so lightly crushing the marrow spiccules. The upper slide is drawn across the lower slide creating a smear on the underside of the upper slide (Fig. 32.11).
  Smears should be made rapidly before the sample clots (within about 30 s).
- The wound is closed with a single skin suture.

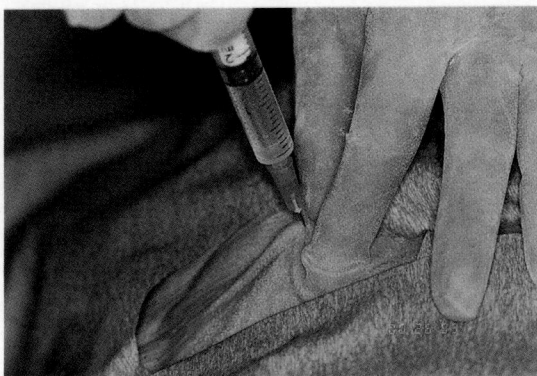

Fig. 32.7   Local anaesthetic is infiltrated into the skin and soft tissue over the iliac crest, and most importantly into the periosteum.

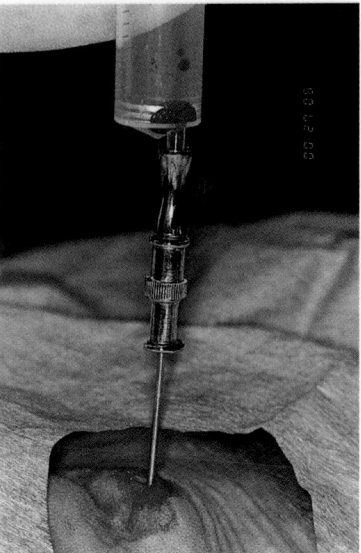

Fig. 32.9   Marrow is aspirated into the needle and bloody fluid appears in the syringe.

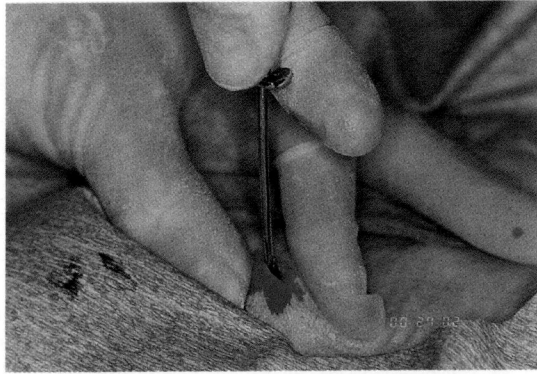

Fig. 32.8   The iliac crest is grasped between thumb and forefinger. Using the other hand, the Klima needle is firmly advanced into the cortical bone using a twisting motion.

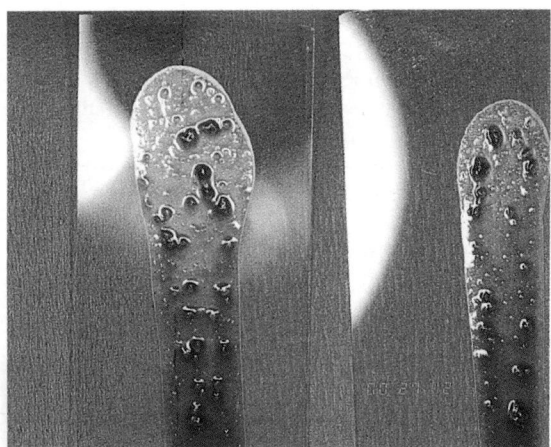

Fig. 32.10   The aspirated marrow and blood have been applied to a slide. Spicules of marrow can be seen stuck to the slide as the blood gravitates downwards.

- If it is suspected that the needle is lodged in the far cortex, then it should be gradually withdrawn until aspiration is successful.
- If aspiration remains unsuccessful, the needle should be withdrawn, the stylet replaced and a second attempt made in a different direction (e.g. obliquely into the wing of the ileum) or at an alternative site.

Repeated unsuccessful attempts, i.e. a 'dry' tap, may be due to myelofibrosis or packing out of the marrow by tumour infiltrate rather than poor technique. A core biopsy is indicated in these situations.

Processing the Smears

The smears are air dried and stained with May–Grünwald and Giemsa stains. In addition a Perls' Prussian blue stain should be carried out to evaluate iron stores. If smears are being sent to a laboratory they should be fixed in methyl alcohol for 3 min before dispatch.

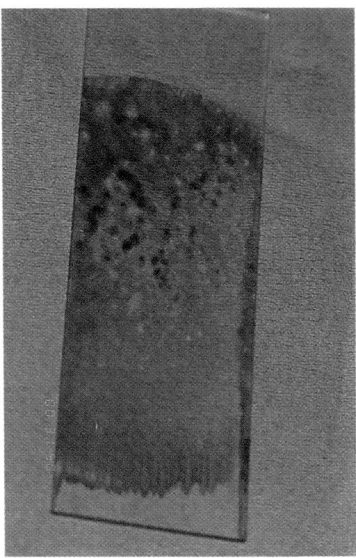

Fig. 32.11 A smear of the marrow aspirate, on which numerous spicules are evident.

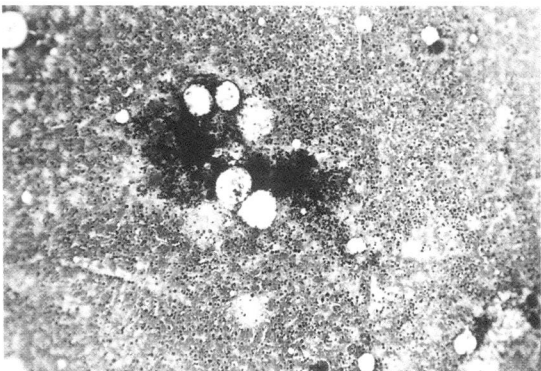

Fig. 32.12 A smear of a bone marrow aspirate, examined under low power. The dark staining densely cellular areas are spicules (or flecks) of marrow.

Interpretation of the Marrow Smears

Low Power

- Initially, the smear is scanned under low power to evaluate quality and cellularity of the sample. Marrow cells are present in clusters called spicules (Fig. 32.12). If no spicules are present, the aspirate is sub-optimal, and this makes accurate interpretation difficult or impossible.
- The number of megakaryocytes present should then be evaluated. These large multinucleate cells are seen within the flecks. There should be three or more megakaryocytes within a large fleck examined under low power.

Low and Then High Power

- The granulocytic or myeloid series is examined. Early granulocytes have pink granules within light blue cytoplasm. The maturation of the myeloblasts through to neutrophils should be orderly, that is there should be more bands and neutrophils than myeloblasts and promyelocytes (Fig. 32.13). An increase in the number of immature forms and decreased numbers of mature forms indicates a maturation arrest, or exhaustion of the storage pool.

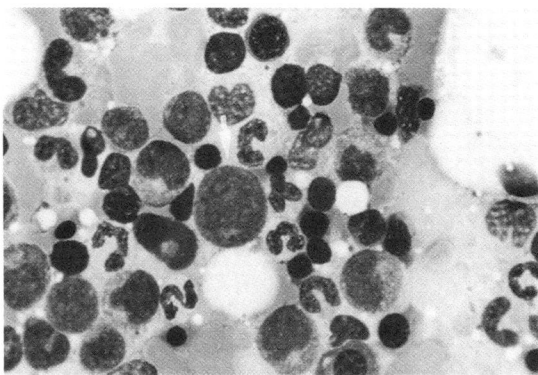

Fig. 32.13 In the centre of the field a promyelocyte (with basophilic cytoplasm and faint pinkish azurophilic granules). Myelocytes, metamyelocytes (which have a kidney bean shaped nucleus), band and mature segmented neutrophils are also seen.

- The erythroid series is examined next. Again the maturation of proerythroblasts through to late normoblasts should be orderly, with a higher proportion of intermediate and late normoblasts than proerythroblasts and early normoblasts (Fig. 32.14). In contrast to granulocyte precursors, proerythroblasts do not have pink cytoplasmic granules, but have deep blue agranular cytoplasm.
- The myeloid : erythroid ratio can be estimated subjectively. The normal value of this ratio is between 0.75 : 1 and 2 : 1.
- Up to 15% of cells present in normal marrow may be lymphoid, mostly small lymphocytes. Normal marrow

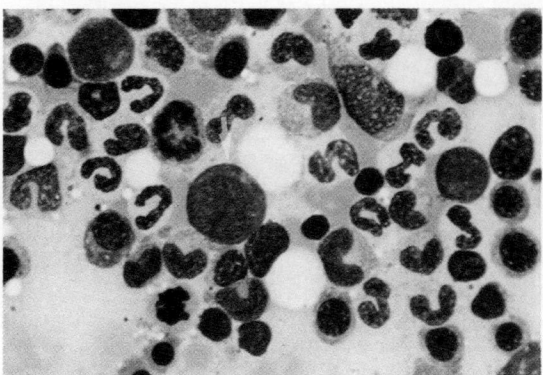

Fig. 32.14 In the centre of the field a proerythroblast with densely staining agranular blue cytoplasm is seen. In the bottom right, two early and an intermediate normoblast are seen. Just left of centre at the lower edge of the field is a late normoblast. Metamyelocytes and band neutrophils are seen throughout the field.

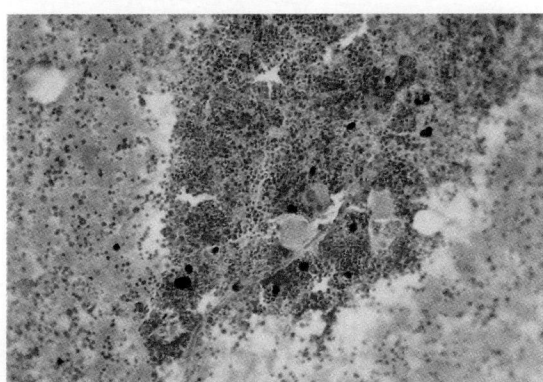

Fig. 32.15 Perls' stain, showing insoluble haemosiderin staining deep blue. This haemosiderin is seen within macrophages.

contains small numbers (no more than 2%) of plasma cells which are seen singly. Small numbers of macrophages are also present.
- Iron stores are best assessed on Prussian blue (Perls') stain (Fig. 32.15). Iron is stored as small soluble ferritin aggregates within developing erythroid cells and larger insoluble masses of haemosiderin within macrophages in flecks. Haemosiderin stains deep blue with Perls'.

Box 32.2   Bone marrow core biopsy technique.

- Position and prepare dog as for bone marrow aspirate, including local anaesthesia.
- Insert the Jamshidi needle through the cortex of the iliac crest as for aspirate.
- Remove the central stylet and advance the needle a further 1–2 cm into the marrow cavity.
- Rotate the needle vigorously in one direction to ensure the biopsy sample is sectioned at its base.
- Remove the needle.
- Use the blunt ended probe (not the stylet) to push the sample out of the top of the needle (the needle tapers slightly and pushing through the distal end may crush the sample).
- Close the skin wound with a single suture.

Bone Marrow Core Biopsy

In a core biopsy the architecture of the marrow is preserved, and the supporting stromal tissue within the marrow cavity can be evaluated as well as the haematopoietic cells. One disadvantage is the delay incurred by decalcification of the sample, which may take 5–7 days. However, before fixing the core in formalin, a smear can be made by rolling the core of marrow along a glass slide and this can be cytologically assessed in the interim.

The indications for a marrow core biopsy include:

- failure to harvest an aspirate,
- an aspirate of non-diagnostic quality,
- suspected myelofibrosis.

The technique for bone marrow core biopsy is outlined in Box 32.2.

CONDITIONS AFFECTING THE BONE MARROW

The bone marrow is the primary site of disease in many lymphoproliferative and myeloproliferative conditions but may also be affected to a greater or lesser extent by most disease states.

Primary conditions of the bone marrow include:

- neoplasia: lymphoproliferative and myeloproliferative diseases (Chapter 35),

- dysplasia: myelodysplastic syndromes (Chapter 33),
- myelofibrosis (which may be a primary condition of marrow fibroblasts, or secondary to another disease process) (Chapter 33),
- marrow necrosis (Chapter 33),
- autoimmune disease (with intramedullary destruction).

Marrow changes are also seen as a result of:

- infectious diseases,
- myelophthisis (metastasis of a tumour to the marrow),
- other neoplasms,
- autoimmune disease,
- myelotoxicoses/idiosyncratic drug reactions,
- cytotoxic drug administration.

With the exception of the effects of drugs and infectious diseases on marrow, these conditions are discussed in other chapters as indicated.

Bone Marrow Toxicoses

Myelotoxicoses may occur as a result of exposure to certain toxins, hormones and drugs. Drug toxicity takes two forms:

- Predictable toxicity occurs with drugs such as chemotherapeutic agents, which by their very nature act on dividing cells. The mechanisms of action and toxicities of cytotoxic drugs are fully discussed in Chapter 5 in the therapeutics section of this book. Haematological monitoring is *vital* in all cases receiving potentially myelosuppressive drugs.
- Idiosyncratic toxicity is seen in individual adverse reactions to other drugs.

Idiosyncratic Drug Reactions

Idiosyncratic reactions are individual adverse reactions to a drug which occur in only a small proportion of treated individuals. Many drugs have been reported to cause bone marrow toxicity on isolated occasions.

The proposed mechanisms of haematological toxicity include:

- direct drug induced myelotoxicity causing ultrastructural and microenvironmental changes in the marrow;
- suppression of progenitor cells (direct or indirect);
- immune-mediated destruction of blood cells which have been released into the circulation.

Oestrogen

The dog is very susceptible to oestrogen toxicity, although considerable individual variation exists. Toxicity associated with exogenous oestrogen administration can result from:

- overdosage,
- prolonged low level dosage, or
- idiosyncratically after dosage within the recommended range.

Oestradiol, which is widely used for misalliance, is especially toxic. As there are no methods to predict, prevent or effectively treat oestrogen toxicity the therapeutic use of oestrogen must be considered carefully, and alternative drugs used if at all possible.

Oestrogen toxicity is also seen as a paraneoplastic syndrome, most commonly in male dogs in association with testicular sertoli cell tumours which produce oestrogen. This syndrome is more likely where the tumours are extrascrotal (i.e. in cases of cryptorchidism.) Oestrogenic effects on the bone marrow have also been reported in cases of seminoma and, rarely, in association with interstitial cell tumours. Functional granulosa cell tumours (of ovary) can produce oestrogen toxicity in bitches.

Mechanism. The mechanism of oestrogen induced myelotoxicosis is unknown. Recent work suggests that oestrogen acts indirectly, inducing production of a factor which inhibits haematopoiesis rather than directly damaging marrow progenitor cells (Farris & Benjamin 1993). The thymus has been postulated as a source of the inhibitory factor.

Clinical Signs. In the early stages of oestrogen myelotoxicosis, there is a granulocytosis, manifest as a neutrophilia with left shift, and thrombocytopenia. Within 2–3 weeks, granulocytopenia, further thrombocytopenia and non-regenerative anaemia develop. The clinical signs reflect the haematological abnormalities.

- Petechial and ecchymotic haemorrhages, melaena, epistaxis and pallor occur because of thrombocytopenia. These signs often predominate and persist for many weeks.
- Pyrexia and sepsis occur secondary to neutropenia.
- Pallor, lethargy and collapse occur due to the anaemia.
- Non-specific signs include anorexia, inactivity, weight loss and weakness.

Male dogs with the paraneoplastic syndrome may also show feminisation, and prostatic abnormalities.

Diagnosis of Suspected Oestrogen Myelotoxicosis. Bone marrow aspirates from dogs affected by oestrogen myelotoxicosis show cellular hypoplasia, with a paucity of all cell lines. Fat and variable numbers of plasma cells, lymphocytes and mast cells are seen. If bone marrow is aspirated during the early phase of granulocytosis (first 2–3 weeks) then myeloid hyperplasia with reduced erythroid activity and low numbers of megakaryocytes may be seen.

Treatment. Treatment of patients with oestrogen myelotoxicosis is supportive, and can include:

- bactericidal antibiotic therapy;
- fresh blood transfusion, or platelet rich transfusion;
- prednisolone, androgens and anabolic steroids have also been used in an attempt to stimulate erythropoiesis, but have not been successful in halting disease progression;
- lithium carbonate therapy.

Lithium carbonate or lithium citrate therapy has been of some benefit in small number studies (Maddux & Shaw 1983; Hall 1992) but has not gained wide acceptance. Lithium is thought to stimulate division of pluripotent stem cells (by enhancement of production of colony stimulating activity) and thus facilitate marrow repopulation (Harker *et al.* 1977). Lithium has beneficial effects in increasing the numbers of neutrophils and platelets, but is of lesser benefit in stimulating red cell production. It is potentially nephrotoxic, serum levels of the drug are unpredictable and must be monitored carefully (optimal therapeutic serum lithium concentration in the dog is reported to be 0.5–1.8 mEq/l, Hall 1992). The drug has been used in humans to treat chemotherapy-induced myelosuppression and aplastic anaemias (Barrett *et al.* 1977; Lynam *et al.* 1980).

Prognosis. Recovery is heralded first by the presence of reticulocytes in the blood, then increasing white cell numbers and eventually platelet numbers. This recovery takes months. Unfortunately, most severely affected dogs do not recover from oestrogen myelotoxicosis.

Antimicrobial Agents

- *Chloramphenicol* causes a mild, dose dependent reversible myelosuppression in dogs, but irreversible aplastic changes as seen in humans have not been reported (Watson 1977). In reversible anaemia, chloramphenicol acts in part by causing defective haem synthesis.
- *Trimethoprim–sulphonamide* combinations have been linked with myelosuppression. As both drugs in this combined therapy block folate metabolism, long-term high dosage can result in anaemia. However, pancytopenia has also been reported (Weiss & Adams 1987; Weiss & Klausner 1990). This may be immune mediated.

- *Cephalosporins* have been also associated with experimentally induced marrow changes after prolonged high dose administration (Deldar *et al.* 1988), and there are reports of neutropenia occurring after therapeutic use (Latimer & Meyer 1989).

Non-Steroidal Anti-Inflammatory Agents

In humans, many non-steroidal anti-inflammatory drugs (NSAIDs) have been implicated in idiosyncratic drug induced myelotoxicosis.

- *Phenylbutazone* is the most frequently documented cause of NSAID induced bone marrow toxicity in the dog (Watson *et al.* 1980; Badame *et al.* 1984; Weiss & Klausner 1990). This myelotoxicosis is not dose dependent and can occur after relatively short courses. Severe pancytopenias or 'bicytopenias' develop, and bone marrow is hypocellular. Although some cases recover, fatalities are not uncommon.
- *Meclofenamic acid* has been suspected of causing bone marrow 'failure' after a prolonged course (Weiss & Klausner 1990).

Miscellaneous Drugs

- *Quinidine* is myelosuppressive in humans and has been reported to cause severe myeloid and erythroid hypoplasia in a dog (Weiss & Klausner 1990).
- *Organic arsenicals* such as thiacetarsamide are used to treat dirofilariasis and have been reported to cause marrow hypoplasia and pancytopenia (Watson 1979).

Lead

Lead becomes concentrated in the marrow where it has specific effects in cases of lead toxicosis. There may be erythroid hypoplasia, but erythroid hyperplasia is also recorded. Lead also causes damage to marrow sinusoids, and this may allow escape of nucleated red cells into the bloodstream. Thus nucleated red cells and reticulocytes are frequently, but not invariably, seen. Basophilic stippling of red cells may be seen in bone marrow or peripheral blood, but is not a consistent finding and is of questionable diagnostic value. Bone marrow evaluation shows an increase in erythroid elements. Other red cell changes include anisocytosis, polychromasia, poikilocytosis, target cells, and hypochromasia. There is a neutrophilia. The clinical picture is dominated by gastrointestinal (abdominal pain, anorexia) and/or neurological signs (convulsions, hysteria, ataxia) rather than those referable to the haematological abnormalities (Chapter 106, Poisons).

Bone Marrow Changes in Infectious Diseases

The marrow changes in infectious diseases generally reflect the demands placed upon the marrow as a result of the primary disease. For example, where there is acute bacterial infection and overwhelming sepsis, the marrow neutrophil maturation and storage pools may become exhausted, so that marrow aspirated at this time would give the appearance of a maturation arrest within the myeloid lineage, with many immature and few mature forms, possibly accompanied by erythroid hyperplasia. Conversely, in situations where the marrow is able to keep up with demand and recovery is occurring there may be myeloid hyperplasia.

THE HAEMOGRAM

A great deal of valuable information can be obtained by careful interpretation of the haemogram. Outlined below is the interpretation of the leukogram: red cell and platelet parameters are discussed in detail in Chapters 33, 34 & 36.

Neutrophils

Neutrophil Function

The neutrophil is a vital line of defence against various pathogens and can kill or inactivate bacteria, yeasts, fungi and parasites. It is able to eliminate infected or transformed cells, to amplify or modulate the immune response and is involved in the regulation of granulopoiesis.

Neutrophil Kinetics

The neutrophils in the body are distributed between the three pools previously described (Fig. 32.4).

Table 32.2 Normal leukocyte count ranges in the adult dog.

Cell type	Normal values ($\times 10^9$/l)
Total white cell count	6–17
Neutrophils	3–11.5
Monocytes	0.2–1.5
Lymphocytes	1–4.8
Eosinophils	0.1–1.3
Basophils	0–0.2

In the marrow:

- the mitotic pool (CFU-GM → myelocyte),
- the maturation pool (metamyelocytes and band cells),
- the storage pool (a 5-day supply of mature neutrophils stored in the marrow).

In the blood:

- the circulating pool,
- the marginating pool,
- (the tissue pool).

The leukogram gives information only about the circulating pool.

Interpretation of the Nutrophil Count

The neutrophil count is influenced by the rate of neutrophil production and release from the bone marrow, movement between the circulating and marginating pool, and the rate of entry to the tissue pool.

It is normal for young dogs to have neutrophil counts at the upper end of the normal range. Pups have high neutrophil counts at birth, which decline during nursing, but increase again on weaning to peak at 2–3 months of age. The counts decline to adult values by around 6 months of age.

Neutrophilia

NEUTROPHIL COUNT $> 11.5 \times 10^9$/l

The causes of neutrophilia are listed in Table 32.3.

Table 32.3 Causes of neutrophilia.

- Physiological response
- Stress/corticosteroid induced neutrophilia
- Acute inflammatory response
  - ○ bacterial infection (localised or generalised)
  - ○ immune-mediated disease, e.g. haemolytic anaemia
  - ○ polyarthritis
  - ○ neoplasia especially tumour necrosis
- Chronic granulocytic leukaemia
- Neutrophil dysfunction
  - ○ congenital
  - ○ acquired
- Paraneoplastic syndromes

Physiological Neutrophilia

Physiological neutrophilia results from acute emotional stress or fear, an effect more marked in the cat than the dog. Increased levels of adrenaline result in an increased rate of blood flow and in release of cAMP, both of which reduce marginating neutrophil adherence to the vessel endothelium. Thus neutrophils are 'washed' from the marginating pool to the circulating pool. A mild neutrophilia (up to $15 \times 10^9/l$) without a left shift results.

Stress/Steroid Induced Neutrophilia

This is part of the 'stress leukogram' characterised by neutrophilia (without a left shift), monocytosis, lymphopenia and eosinopenia. Neutrophilia results from a shift of cells from the marginating and storage pools into the circulating pool. In addition endothelial adherence is reduced which results in prolonged neutrophil circulating time. This contributes to the immunosuppressive effect of steroids. Concurrent lymphopenia results from steroid induced movement of cells from the circulation, then later lymphocytolysis. The stress response is seen as a result of exogenous steroid administration, hyperadrenocorticism and prolonged 'medical' stress.

Acute Inflammatory Response

This response is caused by:

- bacterial infection (most common cause),
- immune–mediated disease, e.g. haemolytic anaemia, polyarthropathies,
- neoplasia (especially tumour necrosis).

The acute inflammatory response is characterised by a neutrophilia (usually $20–30 \times 10^9/l$) with a left shift ($>1 \times 10^9/l$ bands). Increased numbers of cells are released from the marrow storage pool. There is an increased rate of myelopoiesis to meet the increased demand, but as the storage pool becomes depleted bands or metamyelocytes are released into the circulation and this is described as a left shift. This left shift may be either regenerative or degenerative.

- *A regenerative left shift* is characterised by an absolute increase in neutrophil numbers with immature cells in the circulation and is indicative of an adequate response.
- *A degenerative left shift* arises when the bone marrow is unable to make an adequate response. The storage pool becomes exhausted, neutropenia develops and the left shift persists. It is a poor prognostic indicator.

Severe localised or systemic bacterial infection results in *toxic changes* within the neutrophils. Within the marrow, there is defective neutrophil maturation at the level of the myeloblast. Toxic changes include:

- increased cytoplasmic basophilia,
- cytoplasmic vacuolation,
- Döhle bodies (round blue cytoplasmic structures),
- giant band cells.

The number of toxic neutrophils present closely follows the clinical signs. A fall in the number of toxic neutrophils present is an accurate prognostic indicator of recovery, and will occur before neutrophilia resolves.

Neutrophilia persists once the inflammatory response is established, and the left shift resolves with time. Thus the degree of neutrophilia and left shift depend to some extent on the time of sampling. A concurrent monocytosis is seen in chronic inflammation and is suggestive of tissue necrosis.

Pelger–Hüet Anomaly

An apparent left shift is seen in the inherited *Pelger–Hüet anomaly* which has been recorded in the Cocker Spaniel, Coonhound, Foxhound, Basenji and Boston Terrier (Schull & Powell 1978; Latimer *et al.* 1987). Defective nuclear segmentation results in lobar, band neutrophils which have condensed nuclear chromatin and mature cytoplasm. On the leukogram there is a persistent left shift with a normal white blood cell count. The neutrophils are functionally normal and the syndrome is usually an incidental finding. This condition has an hereditary basis.

Extreme Neutrophilia

Two types of extreme neutrophilia have been described:

- 'Leukaemoid reaction' – total white cell count greater than $75 \times 10^9/l$ with a severe left shift.
- 'Neutrophilic leukocytosis' – neutrophil count of greater than $100 \times 10^9/l$ with a mild left shift.

The causes of extreme neutrophilia include:

- severe localised pyogenic infections (e.g. pyometra),
- immune-mediated disease (especially haemolytic anaemia),
- chronic granulocytic leukaemia,
- diseases of neutrophil dysfunction with secondary infection,
- paraneoplastic disease: extreme neutrophilic leukocytosis has been reported in association with a case of renal carcinoma, and of metastatic fibrosarcoma (Chinn *et al.* 1985; Lappin & Latimer 1988; Latimer & Meyer 1989). This is thought to be due to the release of colony stimulating factors from the tumour.

Distinguishing these extreme neutrophilias from chronic granulocytic leukaemia can be difficult. The presence of toxic neutrophils is indicative of bacterial infection, and a leukaemoid reaction should be suspected. Chronic granulocytic leukaemia is characterised by excessive, uncontrolled production of neutrophils resulting in release of large numbers of mature neutrophils into the blood, and this diagnosis is supported by:

- concurrent mild to moderate anaemia or thrombocytopenia in some cases,
- splenomegaly (due to extramedullary haematopoiesis),
- positive staining using the alkaline phosphatase technique.

The neutrophils in granulocytic leukaemia may show variable staining with the alkaline phosphatase technique whereas neutrophils in health or inflammatory disease will not. (This cytochemical staining is not yet widely available but may have a place in distinguishing neoplasia from leukaemoid responses in the future.)

Diseases of Neutrophil Dysfunction

Congenital Neutrophil Dysfunction
Four congenital syndromes have been recognised:

- Canine granulocytopathy syndrome in Irish Setters (Renshaw *et al.* 1975; Renshaw & Davis 1979);
- complement deficiency in Brittany Spaniels (Winkelstein *et al.* 1981; Blum *et al.* 1985);
- neutrophil defect in Doberman Pinschers (Breitschwerdt *et al.* 1987);
- immunodeficiency in Weimaraners (Studdert *et al.* 1984);
- sporadic cases of immunodeficiency may occur in other breeds.

Clinically, these syndromes manifest as recurrent, prolonged infections commonly affecting the skin, respiratory system and gastrointestinal tract. Osteomyelitis, lymphadenopathy and subcutaneous abscesses may also be seen. There is a marked neutrophilia either with or without a left shift. There is generally a progressive non-responsiveness to antibiotic treatment with worsening recurrent episodes of infection until terminal illness. In Dobermans, there may be a partial neutrophil defect resulting in intermittent infection (commonly respiratory infection) with the dogs surviving for years with intermittent antibiotic treatment.

In vitro neutrophil function tests are available (e.g. at local hospitals), but a major limiting factor is the need for fresh cells – the tests should be performed within 2 h of blood collection. Neutrophil adhesion, migration, phagocytosis, oxygen metabolism and bacterial killing activity can be evaluated (Renshaw *et al.* 1977; Renshaw & Davis 1979; Gosset *et al.* 1983/1984).

Acquired Neutrophil Dysfunction
This is most commonly a consequence of:

- diabetes mellitus,
- neoplasia (thought to be due to the release of colony stimulating factors from the tumour: see above).

In diabetes mellitus, hyperglycaemia results in reduced neutrophil bacterial killing activity, due to impaired adherence, migration and phagocytosis. The degree of neutrophil adherence is inversely correlated with serum glucose level. Therefore hyperglycaemic diabetics frequently develop infections such as bacterial cystitis (which may be emphysematous due to gas forming organisms) as well as pyodermas, respiratory infections etc. Haematological evaluation reveals a high neutrophil count.

Neutropenia

NEUTROPHIL COUNT $< 3.0 \times 10^9/l$

Neutropenia (Table 32.4) may be caused by:

Overwhelming Demand
Neutropenia results when the demand for neutrophils outstrips the capacity of the marrow to produce them. This is seen in peracute bacterial infections, especially where there is Gram-negative sepsis, associated with conditions such as peritonitis, pyometra or aspiration pneumonia. A degenerative left shift with toxic neutrophils is seen.

Reduced Granulopoiesis
Reduced granulopoiesis may be associated with:

- aplastic anaemia (leading to pancytopenia),
- myeloproliferative and lymphoproliferative disease,

Table 32.4   Causes of neutropenia.

- Overwhelming demand
- Reduced granulopoiesis
- Ineffective granulopoiesis
- Cyclic haematopoiesis
- Immune-mediated neutropenia
- (Hereditary neutropenia of Border Collies)

- myelophthisis (neoplastic invasion of the bone marrow),
- infections such as canine parvovirus,
- cytotoxic drug related myelosuppression,
- idiosyncratic reactions to other drugs,
- endogenous and exogenous oestrogens may also cause reduced granulopoiesis as part of their myelotoxicosis. (See previous section.)

Ineffective Granulopoiesis

Ineffective granulopoiesis (i.e. an arrest in granulocytic maturation) may be seen in:

- myeloproliferative diseases (e.g. acute myeloid leukaemia),
- myelodysplastic diseases,
- cyclic haematopoiesis.

Cyclic Haematopoiesis

Cyclic haematopoiesis is an inherited (autosomal recessive) disease of Grey Collies (Jones *et al*. 1975a; Campbell 1985). There is a cyclic fluctuation in all types of circulating cells due to defective stem cell proliferation (Patt *et al*. 1973). The length of the cycle is the same for all cell types (12 days) although the cycles are asynchronous. The neutrophilic cycle is the most dramatic with a profound neutropenic episode (lasting 2–4 days) followed by a marked neutrophilia (up to $67 \times 10^9/l$). Affected animals are highly susceptible to infections with death usually occurring before 6 months of age. Lithium carbonate and endotoxins have been shown to stabilise neutrophil numbers to some extent although both of these agents have undesirable side effects (Hammond *et al*. 1982; Hammond *et al*. 1987). Canine colony stimulating factors (GM-CSF, G-CSF) have been shown to prevent significant neutropenia and associated clinical signs, but did not eliminate cycling completely (Mishu *et al*. 1992). Bone marrow allograft is curative (Dale & Graw 1974; Jones *et al*. 1975b).

Table 32.5   Monocytes.

Monocytes
   Normal adult monocyte count: $0.2–1.5 \times 10^9/l$

Monocytosis
- Acute trauma
- As part of stress leukogram
- Chronic inflammatory response secondary to: suppuration, necrosis, malignancy, internal haemorrhage, pyogranulomatous inflammation
- Immune-mediated disease
- Compensatory monocytosis secondary to neutropenia
- Haemolysis
- Monocytic or myelomonocytic leukaemia

Immune Mediated Neutropenia (IMN)

Although anti-neutrophil antibody tests for dogs are not routinely available, individual cases of neutropenia resolving following treatment with immunosuppressive doses of steroids have been reported, suggesting an immune-mediated aetiology (Maddison *et al*. 1982). On haematological evaluation, there is a profound neutropenia with a compensatory monocytosis, and there may be clumping of neutrophils suggesting autoagglutination. Bone marrow aspiration shows myeloid hyperplasia with granulopoiesis

Table 32.6   Lymphocytes.

Lymphocytes
   Normal adult lymphocyte count: $1–4.8 \times 10^9/l$
   Before 6 months of age pups may have lymphocyte counts at or beyond the high end of the normal range, the peak being around 6–8 weeks of age.

Lymphocytosis
Physiological:
- acute response to emotional stress, lymphocytes are mobilised from the rapidly accessible pool
Reactive:
- chronic infection
- transient post-vaccination phenomenon
Proliferative:
- leukaemia, ALL & CLL very high lymphocyte counts may be seen
- lymphoma, mild lymphocytosis may be seen unless marrow is involved where levels may be higher
(Hypoadrenocoricism – inconsistent)

Lymphopenia
Corticosteroids:
- endogenous (hyperadrenocorticism)
- exogenous
(due initially to a shift from the circulating pool to other body compartments, then lymphocytolysis) Increased utilisation, e.g. acute viral infection
Loss of lymphocytes:
- chylothorax, loss of lymphocytes into the pleural space
- lymphangiectasia
Decreased production due to:
- immunosuppressive drug therapy
- (myelophthesis)
- (radiation)
Obstruction of lymph flow due to:
- inflammation
- neoplasia

ALL, acute lymphoblastic leukaemia; CLL, chronic lymphocytic leukaemia.

to the level of the bands, but a severe depletion of mature neutrophils.

Hereditary Neutropenia in Border Collies

Hereditary neutropenia has been reported in families of Border Collies in Australia and New Zealand (Gething *et al.* 1995). This condition is thought to have an autosomal recessive inheritance. Affected animals usually present within the first 2–3 months of life, and are persisitently neutropenic. All cases reported to date have been euthanased because of intractable infection. Bone marrow evaluation shows myeloid hyperplasia, and an apparent 'shift to the right'. It is thought that the neutropenia is due to an inability of neutrophils to escape from the marrow into the blood (myelokathexis).

Table 32.7 Eosinophils.

Eosinophils
- Normal adult eosinophil count: 0.1–1.3 × 10^9/l
- Eosinophil distribution is thought to be similar to that of neutrophils with marrow storage and maturation pools, circulating and marginating pools and a tissue pool.

Eosinophilia
Parasitic infection
Inflammatory/hypersensitivity reactions:
- eosinophilic enteritis
- pulmonary infiltrate with eosinophils (PIE)
- eosinophilic myositis
- panosteitis
- allergic skin disease

(A local tissue eosinophilia may be present without a circulating eosinophilia)
Mast cell tumour (mast cells release chemotactants for eosinophils)
(Hypoadrenocorticism inconsistent)

Eosinopenia
Corticosteroids:
- endogenous (hyperadrenocorticism)
- exogenous administration

Sequestration of eosinophils into the marginating pool, reduction in release from storage pool and reduced production in the bone marrow
Acute infection

Table 32.8 Basophils.

Basophils
- Normal adult basophil count: 0–0.2 × 10^9/l

Basophilia
- Parasitic infections
- Hypersensitivity/inflammatory reactions

Lymphocytes, Monocytes, Eosinophils and Basophils

Abnormalities in numbers of other white blood cells may result from a variety of physiological and disease states as shown in Tables 32.5 to 32.8.

REFERENCES AND FURTHER READING

Structure and Function of Bone Marrow

Cormack, D.H. (1987). Myeloid tissue. In: *Ham's Histology*, (ed. D.H. Cormack), 9th edn. pp. 214–233. J.B. Lippincott, Philadelphia.

Greenberg, M.L., Atkins, H.L. & Schiffer, L.M. (1966). Erythropoietic and reticuloendothelial function in bone marrow in dogs. *Science*, **152**, 526–528.

Harvey, J.W. (1984). Canine bone marrow: normal haematopoeisis, biopsy techniques, and cell identification and evaluation. *Compendium on Continuing Education for the Practicing Veterinarian*, **6**, 909–925.

Latimer, K.S. & Meyer, D.J. (1989). Leukocytes in health and disease. In: *Textbook of Veterinary Internal Medicine*, Vol. 2, (ed. S.J. Ettinger), 3rd edn. pp. 2181–2224. W.B. Saunders, Philadelphia.

Quesenberry, P. & Levitt, L. (1979). Haematopoietic stem cells. (First of three parts) *New England Journal of Medicine*, **301**, 755–760.

Quesenberry, P. & Levitt, L. (1979). Haematopoietic stem cells. (Second of three parts) *New England Journal of Medicine*, **301**, 819–823.

Wickramasinghe, S.N. (1986). Normal haemopoiesis: cellular composition of normal bone marrow. In: *Systemic Pathology, Vol. 2: Blood and Bone Marrow*, (ed. S.N. Wickramasinghe), 3rd edn. pp. 41–72. Churchill Livingstone, London.

Colony-Stimulating Factors

Cowgill, L.D. (1989). Application of recombinant human erythropoietin in dogs and cats. In: *Current Veterinary Therapy X*

(*Small Animal Practice*), (eds R.W. Kirk & J.D. Bonagura), pp. 484–487. W.B. Saunders, Philadelphia.

Elmslie, R.E., Dow, S.W. & Ogilvie, G.K. (1991). Interleukins: biological properties and therapeutic potential. *Journal of Veterinary Internal Medicine*, 5, 283–293.

Giger, U. (1992). Erythropoietin and its clinical use. *Compendium on Continuing Education for the Practicing Veterinarian*, 14, 25–34.

Mischu, L., Callahan, G., Allebban, Z., *et al.* (1992). Effects of recombinant canine granulocyte colony-stimulating factor on white blood cell production in clinically normal and neutropenic dogs. *Journal of the American Veterinary Medical Association*, 12, 1957–1964.

Morstyn, G. & Sheridan, W.P. (1993). Haematopoietic growth factors in cancer. In: *Cancer Chemotherapy and Biological Response Modifiers, Annual 14*, (eds H.M. Pinedo, D.L. Long and B.A. Chabner), pp. 344–366. Elsevier, Amsterdam.

Ogilvie, G.K. (1993). Haematopoietic growth factors: tools for a revolution in veterinary oncology and haematology. *Compendium on Continuing Education for the Practicing Veterinarian, Small Animal Oncology*, 15, 851–854.

Ogilvie, G.K. & Obradovich, J.E. (1992). Haematopoietic growth factors: clinical use and implications. In: *Current Veterinary Therapy XI (Small Animal Practice)*, (eds R.W. Kirk & J.D. Bonagura), pp. 466–470. W.B. Saunders, Philadelphia.

Ogilvie, G.K., Obradovich, J.E., Cooper, M.F., *et al.* (1992). Use of recombinant canine granulocyte colony-stimulating factor to decrease myelosuppresson associated with administration of mitoxantrone in the dog. *Journal of Veterinary Internal Medicine*, 6, 44–48.

Queenberry, P.J. (1989). Treatment of marrow stem-cell disorder with granulocyte colony-stimulating factor. *New England Journal of Medicine*, 320, 1343–1345.

Bone Marrow Sampling and Examination

Dunn, J.K. (1992). Bone marrow aspiration and biospy in small animals: indications and techniques *Veterinary Annual*, 32, 107–118.

Grindem, C.B. (1989). Bone marrow biopsy and evaluation. *Veterinary Clinics of North America*, 19, 669–696.

Harvey, J.W. (1984). Canine bone marrow: normal haematopoeisis, biopsy techniques, and cell identification and evaluation. *Compendium on Continuing Education for the Practicing Veterinarian*, 6, 909–925.

Jain, N.C. (1993). Examination of the blood and bone marrow. In: *Essentials of Veterinary Haematology*, (ed. J.C. Jain), pp. 1–18. Lea & Febiger, Philadelphia.

Tyler, R.D. & Cowell, R.L. (1989). Bone marrow. In: *Diagnostic Cytology of the Dog and Cat*, (eds R.L. Cowell & R.D. Tyler), pp. 99–119. American Veterinary Publications, Santa Barbara.

Weiss, D.J. (1986). Histopathology of canine non-neoplastic bone marrow. *Veterinary Clinical Pathology*, 15, 7–11.

Oestrogen Myelotoxicosis

Bland-Van Den Berg, P., Bomzon, L. & Lurie, A. (1978). Oestrogen-induced bone marrow aplasia in a dog. *Journal of the South African Veterinary Association*, 49, 363–365.

Edwards, D.F. (1981). Bone marrow hypoplasia in a feminised dog with a sertoli cell tumour. *Journal of the American Veterinary Medical Association*, 178, 494–496.

Farris, G.M. & Benjamin, S.A. (1993). Inhibition of myelopoiesis by serum from dogs exposed to oestrogen. *American Journal of Veterinary Research*, 54, 1374–1379.

Gaunt, S.D. & Pierce, K.R. (1986). Effects of oestradiol on haematopoietic and marrow adherent cells of dogs. *American Journal of Veterinary Research*, 47, 906–909.

Hall, E.J. (1992). Use of lithium for the treatment of oestrogen-induced bone marrow hypoplasia in a dog. *Journal of the American Veterinary Medical Association*, 200, 814–816.

Legendre, A.M. (1976). Oestrogen-induced bone marrow hypoplasia in a dog. *Journal of the American Animal Hospital Association*, 12, 525–527.

Maddux, J.M. & Shaw, S.E. (1983). Possible beneficial effect of lithium therapy in a case of oestrogen-induced bone marrow hypoplasia in a dog: a case report. *Journal of the American Animal Hospital Association*, 19, 242–245.

McCandlish, I.A.P., Munro, C.D., Breeze, R.G. & Nash, A.S. (1979). Hormone producing ovarian tumours in the dog. *Veterinary Record*, 105, 9–11.

Sherding, R.G., Wilson, G.P. & Kociba, G.J. (1981). Bone marrow hypoplasia in eight dogs with sertoli cell tumour. *Journal of the American Veterinary Medical Association*, 178, 497–501.

Suess, R.P., Barr, S.C., Sacre, B.J. & French, T.W. (1992). Bone marrow hypoplasia in a feminised dog with an interstitial cell tumour. *Journal of the American Veterinary Medical Association*, 9, 1346–1348.

Lithium Therapy

Barrett, A.J., Hugh-Jones, K., Newton, K. & Watson, J.G. (1977). Lithium therapy in aplastic anaemia. *Lancet*, i, 202 (Letter).

Bille, P.E., Jensen, M.K., Jensen, J.P. & Poulsen, J.C. (1975). Studies on the haematologic and cytogenetic effect of lithium. *Acta Medica Scandinavica*, 198, 281–286.

Hall, E.J. (1992). Use of lithium for the treatment of oestrogen-induced bone marrow hypoplasia in a dog. *Journal of the American Veterinary Medical Association*, 200, 814–816.

Harker, W.G., Rothstein, G., Clarkson, D., Athens, J.W. & Macfarlane, J.L. (1977). Enhancement of colony-stimulating activity production by lithium. *Blood*, 49, 263–267.

Lynam, G.H., Williams, C.C. & Preston, D. (1980). The use of lithium carbonate to reduce infection and leukopenia during systemic chemotherapy. *New England Journal of Medicine*, **302**, 257–260.

Maddux, J.M. & Shaw, S.E. (1983). Possible beneficial effect of lithium therapy in a case of oestrogen-induced bone marrow hypoplasia in a dog: a case report. *Journal of the American Animal Hospital Asociation*, **19**, 242–245.

Non-cytotoxic Drug Associated Myelotoxicoses

Atwell, R.B., Thornton, J.R. & Odlum, J. (1981). Suspected drug-induced thrombocytopenia associated with levamisole therapy in a dog. *Australian Veterinary Journal*, **57**, 91–93.

Badame, F.G., Van Slyke, W. & Hayes, M.A. (1984). Reversible phenylbutazone-induced pancytopenia in a dog. *Canadian Veterinary Journal*, **25**, 269–270 (Letter).

Deldar, A., Lewis, H. & Weiss, L. (1988). Cephalosporin-induced change in the ultrastructure of canine bone marrow. *Veterinary Pathology*, **25**, 211–218.

Latimer, K.S. & Meyer, D.J. (1989). Leucocytes in health and disease. In: *Textbook of Veterinary Internal Medicine*, Vol. 2, (ed. S.J. Ettinger), 3rd edn. pp. 2181–2224. W.B. Saunders, Philadelphia.

Neiger, R.D. (1989). Arsenic poisoning. In: *Current Veterinary Therapy X (Small Animal Practice)*, (eds R.W. Kirk & J.D. Bonugura), pp. 159–161. W.B. Saunders, Philadelphia.

Watson, A.D.J. (1977). Chloramphenicol toxicity in dogs. *Research in Veterinary Science*, **23**, 66–69.

Watson, A.D.J. (1979). Bone marrow failure in a dog. *Journal of Small Animal Practice*, **20**, 681–690.

Watson, A.D.J., Wilson, J.T., Turner, D.M. & Culvenor, J.A. (1980). Phenylbutazone-induced blood dyscrasias suspected in three dogs. *Veterinary Record*, **107**, 239–241.

Weiss, D.J. & Adams, L.G. (1987). Aplastic anaemia associated with trimethoprim sulphadiazine and fenbendazole administration in a dog. *Journal of the American Veterinary Medical Association*, **9**, 1119–1120.

Weiss, D.J. & Klausner, J.S. (1990). Drug-associated aplastic anaemia in dogs: eight cases (1984–1988). *Journal of the American Veterinary Medical Association*, **196**, 472–475.

Other Myelotoxicoses

Bratton, G.R. & Kowalczyk, D.F. (1989). Lead poisoning. In: *Current Veterinary Therapy X (Small Animal Practice)*, (eds R.W. Kirk & J.D. Bonugura), pp. 152–159. W.B. Saunders and Company, Philadelphia.

Khanna, C., Boermans, H.J., Woods, P. & Ewing, R. (1992). Lead toxicosis and changes in the blood lead concentration of dogs exposed to dust containing high levels of lead. *Canadian Veterinary Journal*, **33**, 815–817.

Mitema, E.S., Oehme, F.W., Penumarthy, L. & Moore, W.E. (1980). Effect of chronic lead exposure on the canine bone marrow. *American Journal of Veterinary Research*, **41**, 682–685.

Infectious Diseases

Boosinger, T.R., Rebar, A.H., DeNicola, D.B. & Boon, G.D. (1982). Bone marrow alterations associated with canine parvoviral enteritis. *Veterinary Pathology*, **19**, 558–561.

Brunner, C.J. & Swang, L.J. (1985). Canine parvovirus investigation: effects on the immune system and factors that predispose to severe disease. *Compendium on Continuing Education for the Practicing Veterinarian*, **7**, 979–989.

Huxsoll, D.L., Hildebrandt, P.K., Nims, R.M. & Walker, J.S. (1970). Tropical canine pancytopenia. *Journal of the American Veterinary Medical Association*, **157**, 1627–1632.

Walker, J.S., Rundquist, J.D., Taylor, R., *et al.* (1970). Clinical and clinicopathological findings in tropical canine pancytopenia. *Journal of the American Veterinary Medical Association*, **157**, 43–55.

The Leukogram

Chinn, D.R., Myers, R.K. & Matthews, J.A. (1985). Neutrophilic leukocytosis associated with metastatic fibrosarcoma in a dog. *Journal of the American Veterinary Medical Association*, **186**, 806–809.

Jain, N.C. (1993). Interpretation of leukocyte parameters, In: *Essentials of Veterinary Haematology*, (ed. J.C. Jain), pp. 295–306. Leah & Febiger, Philadelphia.

Lappin, M.R. & Latimer, K.S. (1988). Haematuria and extreme neutrophilic leukocytosis in a dog with renal tubular carcinoma. *Journal of the American Veterinary Medical Association*, **192**, 1289–1292.

Latimer, K.S. & Meyer, D.J. (1989). Leukocytes in health and disease. In: *Textbook of Veterinary Internal Medicine*, Vol. 2, (ed. S.J. Ettinger), 3rd edn. pp. 2181–2224. W.B. Saunders Philadelphia.

Diseases of Neutrophil Dysfunction or Neutropenia

Blum, J.R., Cork, L.C. & Morris, J.M. (1985). The clinical manifestations of a genetically determined deficiency of the third component of complement in the dog. *Clinical Immunology and Immunopathology*, **34**, 304–315.

Breitschwerdt, E.B., Brown, T.T., Buysscher, E.V., *et al.* (1987). Rhinitis, pneumonia, and defective neutrophil function in the

Doberman Pinscher. *American Journal of Veterinary Research*, **48**, 1054–1061.

Campbell, K.L. (1985). Canine cyclic haematopoiesis. *Compendium on Continuing Education for the Practicing Veterinarian*, **7**, 57–62.

Couto, C.G. & Giger, U. (1985). Congenital and acquired neutrophil functional abnormalities in the dog. In: *Current Veterinary Therapy X (Small Animal Practice)*, (eds R.W. Kirk & J.D. Bonugura), pp. 521–525. W.B. Saunders Philadelphia.

Dale, D.C. & Graw, R.G. Jr. (1974). Transplantation of allogeneic bone marrow in canine cyclic neutropenia. *Science*, **199**, 83–84.

Gething, M.A., Allan, F.J., Jones, B.R., *et al.* (1995). Hereditary neutropenia in Border Collies. *British Small Animal Veterinary Association – Paper Synopses, Clinical Research Abstracts*, 216.

Gosset, K.A., MacWilliams, P.S., Enright, F.M. & Cleghorn, B. (1983/1984). *In vitro* function of canine neutrophils during experimental inflammatory disease. *Veterinary Immunology and Immunopathology*, **5**, 151–159.

Guilford, G. (1987). Primary immunodeficiency diseases of dogs and cats. *Compendium on Continuing Education for the Practicing Veterinarian*, **9**, 641–650.

Hammond, W.P., Adamson, J.W. & Dale, D.C. (1982). Canine cyclic haematopoiesis: the effect of endotoxin on erythropoiesis. *Journal of Haematology*, **50**, 283–294.

Hammond, W.P., Rodger, E.R. & Dale, D.C. (1987). Lithium augments GM-CSA generation in canine cyclic haematopoiesis. *Blood*, **69**, 117–123.

Jones, J.B., Lange, R.D. & Jones, E.S. (1975a). Cyclic haematopoiesis in a colony of dogs. *Journal of the American Animal Hospital Association*, **166**, 365–367.

Jones, J.B., Lange, R.D., Yang, T.J., Vodopick, H. & Jones, E.S. (1975b). Canine cyclic neutropenia platelet cycles after bone marrow transplantation. *Blood*, **45**, 213–219.

Latimer, K.S., Duncan, J.R. & Kircher, I.M. (1987). Nuclear segmentation, ultrastructure, and cytochemistry of blood cells from dogs with Pelger–Huet anomaly. *Journal of Comparative Pathology*, **97**, 61–72.

Maddison, J.E., Hoff, B.H. & Johnson, R.P. (1982). Steroid responsive neutropenia in a dog. *Journal of the American Animal Hospital Association*, **19**, 881–886.

Patt, H.M., Lund, J.E. & Maloney, M.A. (1973). Cyclic haematopoiesis in Grey Collie dogs: a stem cell problem. *Blood*, **42**, 873–884.

Renshaw, H.W. & Davis, W.C. (1979). Canine granulocytopathy syndrome: an inherited disorder of leukocyte function. *American Journal of Veterinary Pathology*, **95**, 731–744.

Renshaw, H.W., Chatburn, C., Bryan, G.M., Bartsch, R.C. & Davis, W.C. (1975). Canine granulocytopathy syndrome: neutrophil dysfunction in a dog with recurrent infections. *Journal of the American Veterinary Medical Association*, **166**, 443–447.

Renshaw, H.L., Davis, W.C. & Renshaw, S.J. (1977). Canine granulocytopathy syndrome: defective bactericidal capacity of neutrophils from a dog with recurrent infections. *Clinical Immunology and Immunopathology*, **8**, 385–395.

Yang, T.J., Jones, J.B., Jones, E.S. & Lange, R.D. (1974). Serum colony-stimulating activity of dogs with cyclic neutropenia. *Blood*, **44**, 41–48.

Schull, R.M. & Powell, D. (1979). Acquired hyposegmentation of granulocytes (pseudo-Pelger–Huet anomaly) in a dog. *Cornell Veterinarian*, **69**, 241–247.

Shelly, S.M. (1988). Causes of canine pancytopenia. *Compendium on Continuing Education for the Practicing Veterinarian*, **10**, 9–16.

Studdert, V.P., Phillips, W.A., Studdert, M.J. & Hosking, C.S. (1984). Recurrent and persistent infections in related Weimeraner dogs. *Australian Veterinary Journal*, **61**, 261–263.

Winkelstein, J.A., Cork, L.C., Griffin, D.E., Griffin, J.W., Adams, R.J. & Price, D.L. (1981). Genetically determined deficiency of the third component of complement in the dog. *Science*, **212**, 1169–1170.

APPENDIX 1

British and American Nomenclature for the Erythroid Series

British nomenclature	American nomenclature
Proerythroblast	Rubriblast
Early normoblast	Prorubricyte
Intermediate normoblast	Rubricyte: basophilic
	Rubricyte: polychromatophilic
Late normoblast	Metarubricyte
Reticulocyte	Reticulocyte
Erythrocyte	Erythrocyte

Chapter 33

Anaemia

J. K. Dunn

Anaemia can be defined as a decrease in the total red blood cell (RBC) count, haemoglobin (Hb) concentration and packed cell volume (PCV), taking into account variations for the age and breed of dog.

PATHOPHYSIOLOGY OF ANAEMIA

The main stimulus for increased erythropoiesis is tissue hypoxia via the renal production of erythropoietin. The bone marrow is the primary site of erythropoiesis, which is described in more detail in Chapter 32. Extramedullary haemopoiesis occurs in the spleen and liver in response to chronic hypoxia. The earliest recognisable erythroid precursor in the bone marrow is the proerythroblast which divides and differentiates through early, intermediate and late normoblast stages (Fig. 33.1) to become a reticulocyte. This maturation process takes approximately 5 days. Reticulocytes remain in the bone marrow for a further 2–3 days before their release into the circulation where they become mature erythrocytes. The average circulating lifespan of a red blood cell is approximately 110–120 days.

An absolute decrease in the number of circulating red cells may occur in three ways:

- haemorrhage;
- increased red cell destruction, usually associated with a decrease in red cell lifespan;
- inadequate production of red cells by the bone marrow either as a result of reduced proliferation of red cell precursors (hypoproliferative anaemias) or the defective synthesis of haemoglobin or nuclear chromatin (maturation defect anaemias).

DIAGNOSTIC APPROACH TO ANAEMIA

A logical diagnostic approach to anaemia is essential in order to provide an accurate prognosis and initiate appropriate therapy. The main objectives are as follows:

- Determine whether the anaemia is regenerative or non-regenerative on the basis of the reticulocyte count and red cell indices.
- Identify the pathophysiological mechanism and underlying cause responsible for the anaemia.

Anaemias due to haemorrhage or haemolysis are typically regenerative; hypoproliferative and maturation defect anaemias are non-regenerative (see section below on classification of anaemias).

History

The history of the animal may provide diagnostically useful indicators as to the nature of the disease. Important points are detailed in Table 33.1.

The *age, breed and sex* of an animal may provide several important diagnostic clues. Certain congenital (in most cases hereditary) and acquired bleeding disorders are more common in certain breeds, for example, von Willebrand's disease occurs most frequently in Dobermann Pinschers and German Shepherds; splenic haemangiosarcoma is relatively common in older German Shepherds and may result in intra-abdominal haemorrhage. Haemophilia A (classical haemophilia) is a sex-linked condition, occurring only in males. Severely affected animals may be expected to bleed

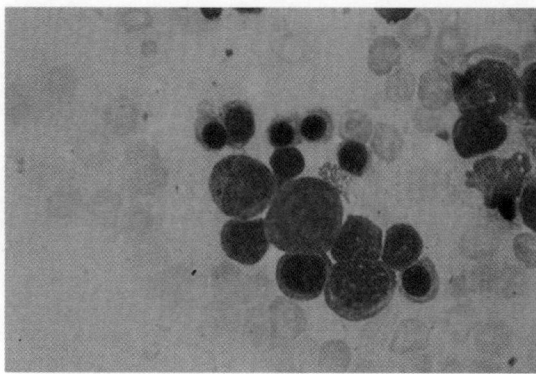

Fig. 33.1 Giemsa-stained bone marrow aspirate showing a large proerythroblast (centre) surrounded by intermediate and late normoblasts.

Table 33.1 Diagnostic approach to anaemia: history.

- Age, breed, sex
- Rate of onset: acute vs. chronic
- Trauma
- Exposure to toxic drugs or chemicals (non-steroidal anti-inflammatory drugs, anticoagulant rodenticides, oestrogens, cytotoxic agents, e.g. cyclophosphamide)
- External blood loss (epistaxis, haemoptysis, haematuria, melaena) or haemolysis (haemoglobinuria)
- Recent vaccination history
- Lived in or visited foreign countries
- Presence of other systemic signs (vomiting, diarrhoea, polydipsia, polyuria etc.)
- Signs of recurrent infection

at an early age. Some inborn errors of metabolism, for example deficiencies in certain red cell enzymes, although relatively rare, also have a higher incidence in certain breeds (e.g. red cell pyruvate kinase deficiency in Basenjis and phosphofructokinase deficiency in Springer Spaniels). Copper storage disease in Bedlington Terriers may cause hepatic necrosis and is occasionally associated with acute intravascular haemolysis. The age and breed of an animal and the effects of other non-disease states should also be taken into consideration when interpreting red cell parameters (see below).

Acute versus chronic onset. Clinical signs such as lethargy, anorexia and weight loss are present in most anaemic animals. The severity of these signs depends on the severity and rate of onset of the anaemia. A rapid onset of signs is more suggestive of acute haemorrhage or haemolysis. In

comparison, the majority of non-regenerative anaemias tend to be more insidious in onset and clinical signs are often not apparent until much later on in the course of the disease.

Consider the possibility of internal haemorrhage especially if there is a history of *trauma* or exposure to *toxic drugs or chemicals* (anticoagulant rodenticides, oestrogenic compounds, non-steroidal analgesics and cytotoxic agents). The owner should also be questioned regarding evidence of external blood loss; a history of epistaxis, haemoptysis, haematuria or haemoglobinuria, or melaena may indicate a more generalised bleeding tendency.

Check recent *vaccination history* and whether animal has *travelled or lived abroad*. Immune-mediated thrombocytopenia occasionally occurs as a sequel to modified live vaccination. Anaemia may be a feature of imported diseases such as ehrlichiosis, leishmaniasis and babesiosis.

In addition to the non-specific signs described above a history of vomiting, diarrhoea, polyuria or polydipsia, either alone or in combination, suggests the presence of an *underlying systemic disease* (for example chronic renal failure or hypoadrenocorticism).

Clinical Examination

Clinical examination of the patient should provide an indication of the severity of the disease and may provide clues as to the nature as detailed in Table 33.2.

Common clinical manifestations of anaemia include:

- lethargy,
- inappetance or anorexia,
- weakness,
- exercise intolerance,
- respiratory distress or occasionally collapse, and
- pallor of the mucous membranes.

These signs reflect the reduced oxygen carrying capacity of blood (hypoxaemia) and inadequate tissue oxygenation.

Other clinical signs are a consequence of haemodynamic alterations or various physiological compensatory mechanisms which become operative in the anaemic animal.

The severity of the clinical signs present depends on:

(1) Rate of onset and severity of the anaemia, i.e. acute or chronic. Signs of hypovolaemic shock predominate following acute blood loss (pale mucous membranes, weak, rapid femoral pulse, capillary refill time greater than 2s and tachycardia). An animal that becomes acutely anaemic either as a result of haemorrhage or haemolysis is more likely to show signs of respiratory embarrassment at rest. Tissue hypoxia and decreased

Table 33.2 Diagnostic aproach to anaemia: clinical examination.

- Signs of hypoxaemia and tissue hypoxia (lethargy, inappetence or anorexia, generalised weakness, exercise intolerance, dyspnoea, collapse, mucosal pallor)
- Tachycardia (acute) or heart rate normal (chronic); accentuated heart sounds; 'haemic' murmur
- Femoral pulse weak and rapid (acute) or sharp and bounding (chronic)
- Pyrexia (underlying infectious, inflammatory or immune-mediated disease, neoplasia, primary bone marrow disease resulting in neutropenia or immunosuppression)
- Icteric mucous membranes (primary liver disease or acute haemolysis)
- Ecchymotic or petechial haemorrhages (thrombocytopenia, functional platelet defect or vasculitis)
- Hepatomegaly or splenomegaly (extramedullary haemopoiesis, neoplasia or extravascular destruction of red blood cells and/or platelets)
- Lymphadenopathy (lymphoma, lymphoid or myeloid leukaemias, immune-mediated polyarthritis, systemic lupus erythematosus)
- Abdominal pain, abdominal masses or fluid
- Rectal examination to check for presence of melaena

blood viscosity result in a reflex tachycardia. With chronic anaemias or anaemias where blood loss occurs more slowly fluid moves from the tissues into the circulation to maintain circulatory volume. In these cases the heart rate is often within normal limits or only slightly increased, a bounding femoral pulse may be present and the dog may show respiratory signs only when exercised or excited.

Heart sounds may be accentuated and a low grade, mid-systolic 'haemic' murmur is often present with more severe anaemias (PCV < 0.15l/l). 'Haemic' murmurs are usually attributed to decreased blood viscosity and increased flow velocity and have a point of maximal intensity over the left cardiac apex. They usually disappear when the anaemia is corrected; failure to do so indicates concurrent cardiac pathology.

(2) The degree of physiological compensation. Older animals are less able to compensate for severe reductions in blood volume and the effects of tissue hypoxia because the reserve capacity of their cardiovascular and respiratory systems is compromised. Increased

cardiac workload in an animal with pre-existing heart disease may lead to cardiac decompensation and signs of congestive heart failure.

Clinical signs referrable to the underlying cause of the anaemia may also be present. For example, a history of vomiting, polydipsia and polyuria in an anaemic dog with uraemic breath and tongue ulcers is highly suggestive of chronic renal failure.

Pyrexia

Pyrexia may indicate the presence of an underlying infectious, inflammatory/immune-mediated or neoplastic disease process. The more common causes of fever in an anaemic animal include immune-mediated haemolytic anaemia (especially acute intravascular haemolysis resulting in release of red cell pyrogens) or immune-mediated thrombocytopenia. Primary bone marrow disorders (e.g. myeloproliferative and lymphoproliferative disease or true aplastic anaemia) in addition to causing anaemia may result in persistent neutropenia or more generalised suppression of B and/or T lymphocyte responses and predisposition to recurrent infection.

Icteric Mucous Membranes

The increased destruction of red cells may result in icteric mucous membranes (consider primary liver disease or acute intravascular haemolysis if jaundice is severe).

Ecchymotic or Petechial Haemorrhages

Check the gingivae, conjunctivae, sclera, external genitalia and skin, especially areas where the skin is thin and susceptible to trauma, e.g. inguinal region, for signs of haemorrhage. The most common cause of petechial and ecchymotic haemorrhages is thrombocytopenia (less common causes include platelet function defects and vasculitis). Retinal haemorrhages occasionally may be present in severely thrombocytopenic animals.

Hepatomegaly or Splenomegaly

Enlargement of the spleen and/or liver in an anaemic animal may be caused by extramedullary erythropoiesis, increased extravascular destruction of opsonised red cells or platelets, or neoplastic infiltration (e.g. lymphoproliferative or myeloproliferative disease).

Lymph Node Enlargement

Moderate to marked non-painful enlargement of all peripheral lymph nodes in an anaemic animal is highly suggestive of malignant lymphoma. A milder degree of generalised lymph node enlargement is often seen with systemic immune-mediated disorders such as polyarthritis or systemic lupus erythematosus or when lymph nodes are secondarily infiltrated with neoplastic cells from a primary bone marrow neoplasm, e.g. lymphoid or myeloid leukaemia. Cytological examination of a fine needle aspirate from an affected node may help to determine the cause of the lymphadenopathy.

Abdominal Pain or Abdominal Masses

The abdomen should be palpated for the presence of abnormal masses, fluid or pain. Splenic neoplasms, particularly haemangiosarcoma or lymphoma, occasionally rupture resulting in acute intra-abdominal haemorrhage.

Rectal Examination

A rectal examination should be performed to check for the presence of melaena.

LABORATORY INVESTIGATION OF ANAEMIA

The initial diagnostic plan for the investigation of anaemia should include the following:

- full routine haematological examination including reticulocyte and platelet counts;
- examination of a blood film for the presence of red cell parasites (*Haemobartonella* sp., *Babesia* sp.);
- a complete biochemical profile*;
- urine analysis;
- lateral radiographs of the thorax and abdomen to check for the presence of abnormal masses, organomegaly and bleeding into a body cavity.

*A complete biochemical screen at the Department of Clinical Veterinary Medicine, University of Cambridge, includes urea, creatinine, glucose, alanine aminotransferase (ALT), aspartate aminotransferase (AST), alkaline phosphatase (ALP), gamma-glutamyl transferase (GGT), creatinine phosphokinase (CPK), calcium, phosphate, sodium, potassium and chloride.

Based on the results of the above additional more specific tests may be indicated in order to define more accurately the cause of the anaemia. These include tests to detect the following:

- abnormalities in iron metabolism (see below),
- abnormalities in blood clotting (see Chapter 36),
- red cell antibodies (direct antiglobulin test),
- faecal occult blood,
- bone marrow aspiration or biopsy (see Chapter 32).

Tests to Detect Abnormalities in Iron Metabolism

Alterations in iron metabolism may be helpful in differentiating between the various causes of anaemia (particularly non-regenerative anaemia) (Table 33.3).

Serum Iron

Serum iron levels begin to fall only when the total body reserves of iron are virtually depleted and usually before anaemia develops.

Causes of *low serum iron* levels include:

- chronic haemorrhage (true iron deficiency),
- chronic inflammatory or neoplastic disease (anaemia of chronic disease),
- portosystemic shunts.

With chronic haemorrhage the stores of non-haem iron in the liver and bone marrow are depleted; with anaemia of chronic disease the stores of non-haem iron are typically normal or increased. The concentration of serum iron therefore on its own does not provide an estimate of total body iron reserves.

Increases in serum iron concentration occur with:

- chronic haemolysis,
- some cases of aplastic or hypoplastic anaemia,
- glucocorticoid administration (Harvey *et al.* 1987).

Normal values for serum iron in the dog are 101 ± 23 mg/dl (Smith 1989).

Total Iron Binding Capacity (TIBC)

- In dogs the normal TIBC is 334 ± 26 mg/dl (Smith 1989) and the TIBC does not change significantly with true iron deficiency.

Table 33.3 Interpretation of serum iron, total iron binding capacity (TIBC), percentage saturation of transferrin and ferritin assays in the dog.

Parameter	Chronic haemorrhage	Anaemia of chronic disease	Chronic haemolysis
Serum iron	Decreased	Decreased	Increased
TIBC	Usually no significant change	Decreased or low normal	Decreased?
% Transferrin saturation	Decreased	Decreased (or normal if TIBC and iron decrease in parallel)	Increased
Ferritin	Decreased	Increased	Increased

- Anaemia of chronic disease is associated with low or low normal TIBC.

Percentage Saturation of Transferrin

The percentage saturation of transferrin (serum iron/TIBC) may provide a more accurate indicator of an animal's iron status than either serum iron or TIBC alone. Alterations in the ratio are summarised in Table 33.3.

Serum Ferritin

Serum ferritin assays have recently been developed and validated for use in the dog although they are not yet routinely available (Weeks *et al.* 1989; Andrews *et al.* 1992). The concentration of ferritin correlates well with the concentration of non-haem iron in the liver and spleen and provides a reliable means of estimating total body iron reserves in dogs (Weeks *et al.* 1989). Serum ferritin concentrations in one recent study ranged from 80 to 800 ng/ml with a mean of 252 ng/ml (Andrews *et al.* 1992). Ferritin is an acute phase protein and any increase should be interpreted relative to the serum concentrations of other acute phase proteins such as ceruloplasmin or haptoglobin.

Bone Marrow Iron Stores

Bone marrow iron (haemosiderin) stores can be stained with Prussian blue (see Chapter 32) and may help differentiate true iron deficiency anaemia from the anaemia of chronic disease in which there is impaired release of iron from bone marrow reticuloendothelial stores.

INTERPRETATION OF HAEMATOLOGICAL RESULTS

Influence of Physiological and Other Non-Disease Variables on Red Cell Parameters

Consideration should be given to the following factors when interpreting red cell parameters.

Age of Animal

Puppies less than 3 weeks of age have a high PCV and mean cell volume (mean cell volume may be as high as 95 fl). At 2–3 months there is a marked decrease in these parameters as the fetal red cells are replaced by adult red cells. Thereafter the total red cell count, haemoglobin concentration, PCV and total plasma protein concentration remain low until 6–9 months of age. A PCV of 0.30–0.35 l/l is not unusual for a 3 month old pup.

Effects of Exercise

Athletic breeds such as Greyhounds or working Border Collies may have a higher PCV and MCV. Post-exercise increases have been documented in total RBC count, haemoglobin concentration and PCV (Feldman & Lassard 1992).

Breed

The total red cell count, haemoglobin concentration and PCV are increased in most adult Greyhounds (PCV 0.55–0.601/l); some Poodles also have a high PCV due to the presence of macrocytic erythrocytes. Many healthy Japanese Akitas have microcytic red cells without being anaemic (Squires 1993a).

Pregnancy

During pregnancy the red cell count, haemoglobin concentration and PCV decrease before returning to normal during lactation (Allard *et al.* 1989).

Causes of Artefactual Results

Poor sample collection and handling may also influence haematological results.

- Haemolysis occurs if blood is subjected to a delay in transit or exposed to a high environmental temperature. Haemolysis can lower the total red cell count, PCV and mean cell volume (MCV), and increase the total plasma protein concentration and mean cell haemoglobin concentration (MCHC).
- Excessive anticoagulant in an EDTA collection tube owing to inadequate filling with blood causes shrinkage of red cells and a decrease in the PCV which in turn affects the validity of the MCV and MCHC calculations.
- Gross lipaemia may increase the haemoglobin concentration.

- Platelet clumping in a blood sample may artificially lower the platelet count.

Total Plasma Protein Concentration

The total plasma protein (TPP) concentration should always be interpreted in association with the PCV. A low TPP concentration accompanied by a low PCV in an adult dog suggests ongoing or recent haemorrhage. Severe dehydration may increase both the PCV and TPP concentration and therefore may mask the true degree of anaemia.

Laboratory Classification of Anaemia

Anaemias may be classified on the basis of the red cell indices, i.e. mean corpuscular volume (MCV), mean corpuscular haemoglobin (MCH) and mean corpuscular haemoglobin concentration (MCHC) as follows:

- macrocytic and hypochromic,
- normocytic and normochromic,
- macrocytic and normochromic,
- microcytic and hypochromic.

Some of the more common causes of each of these types of anaemia are given in Table 33.4. Normal haematological values for the dog (Department of Clinical Veterinary Medicine, University of Cambridge) are given in Appendix 1.

A more helpful pathophysiological classification of anaemia takes into account the degree of bone marrow responsiveness. Anaemia can be classified as regenerative or

Table 33.4 Classification of anaemia based on red cell morphology.

Morphological classification	Possible aetiology
Macrocytic, hypochromic (increased MCV, decreased MCHC)	• Haemorrhage or haemolysis, i.e. regenerative anaemias
Normocytic, normochromic (normal MCV, normal MCHC)	• Following acute blood loss before erythroid regeneration occurs • Most non-regenerative anaemias caused by primary or secondary failure of erythropoiesis, i.e. hypoproliferative anaemias
Macrocytic, normochromic (increased MCV, normal MCHC)	• Myeloproliferative disease • Occasionally small intestinal malabsorption, neoplasia, liver disease and prolonged anorexia
Microcytic, hypochromic (decreased MCV, decreased MCHC)	• Iron deficiency anaemia due to chronic blood loss • Portosystemic shunts • Anaemia of chronic disease

MCV, mean cell volume; MCHC, mean cell haemoglobin concentration.

Table 33.5 Features of regenerative and non-regenerative anaemias.

Feature	Regenerative	Non-regenerative
Reticulocytosis i.e. >5% reticulocytes or evidence of polychromasia	Yes	No
Anisocytosis	Yes	No
Poikilocytosis	Yes	No
Normoblastosis	Yes	Possible in myeloproliferative disease or if damage to marrow stroma
Increased numbers of Howell–Jolly bodies	±	No
Reactive leukocytosis	Yes	No

non-regenerative based on the reticulocyte count. The major differentiating features of regenerative and non-regenerative anaemias are listed in Table 33.5.

REGENERATIVE ANAEMIAS

Regenerative anaemias are caused by either *haemorrhage* or *haemolysis*. A regenerative anaemia is characterised by the presence of increased numbers of large immature red cells with bluish/pink cytoplasm (polychromasia) and nucleated red blood cells (normoblasts) on a Giemsa-stained blood film (Figs 33.2 and 33.3). Evidence of polychromasia is a reliable indicator of increased erythropoiesis. The presence of increased numbers of large immature red cells results in marked anisocytosis, a variable degree of poikilocytosis and an increase in the MCV. Regenerative anaemias are therefore typically macrocytic and hypochromic and most are associated with a reactive neutrophilia with or without a variable left shift. Increased numbers of Howell–Jolly bodies may also be present in intensely regenerative anaemias. Howell–Jolly bodies are remnants of nuclear material which, on a Romanowsky-stained blood film, appear as single basophilic spherical structures within the red cell (Fig. 33.3).

Reticulocyte Counts

Reticulocytes on a blood film are demonstrated using a supravital stain such as new methylene blue. Small numbers of reticulocytes, usually less than 1%, are present in the blood of healthy dogs. Following an acute haemorrhagic or haemolytic episode reticulocytes do not appear in the circulation for up to 48–72 h, reaching maximal production by 7 days. The reticulocyte response may be classified as mild (1–4%), moderate (5–20%) or marked (>20%). The number of reticulocytes present generally correlates with the degree of erythropoietic activity.

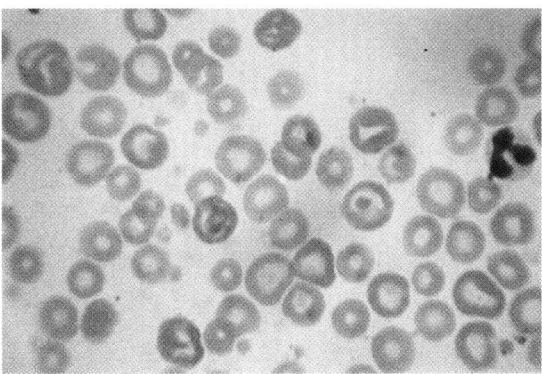

Fig. 33.2 Giemsa-stained blood film from a dog with an intensely regenerative anaemia. Note the marked anisocytosis and polychromasia. Some of the larger polychromatophilic cells have a target cell appearance.

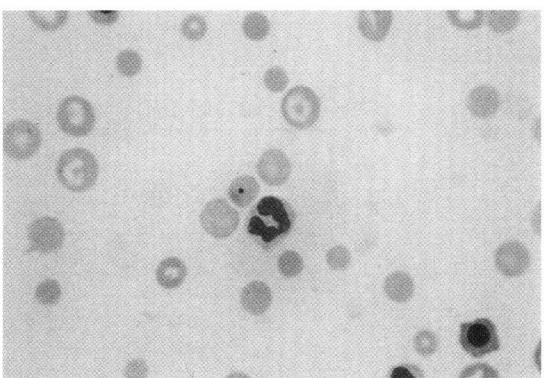

Fig. 33.3 Giemsa-stained blood film showing marked anisocytosis and evidence of polychromasia. The smaller dark-staining cells are spherocytes. A nucleated red blood cell (normoblast) is present at the bottom right of the picture. A red blood cell next to the neutrophil contains a Howell–Jolly body.

Reticulocyte Correction Factors

The younger, larger 'shift' reticulocytes released in response to haemorrhage or haemolysis have a longer maturation time and circulating half-life. The observed percentage of reticulocytes may therefore overestimate the degree of marrow responsiveness at any one time since it does not take into account variations in circulating red cell numbers and changes in reticulocyte maturation time.

- The *absolute reticulocyte count* corrects for variation in red cell number, i.e. the degree of anaemia.

$$\text{Absolute reticulocyte count } (\times10^9/\text{l}) =$$
$$\text{observed reticulocyte } (\%)$$
$$\times \text{ RBC count } (\times10^{12}/\text{l}) \times 10$$

An absolute reticulocyte count $> 60\times10^9/\text{l}$ is evidence of an erythroid response.

- The *corrected reticulocyte count* also corrects for variation in red cell number.

$$\text{Corrected reticulocyte count } (\%) =$$
$$\frac{\left(\text{observed reticulocyte count } (\%) \times \text{ measured PCV } (\text{l}/\text{l})\right)}{\text{average PCV for species } (0.45/\text{l})}$$

A corrected reticulocyte count greater than 1% is indicative of active erythropoiesis.

- The *reticulocyte production index* (RPI) takes into account the prolonged maturation time of younger reticulocytes.

$$\text{RPI} = \frac{\text{corrected reticulocyte count } (\%)}{\text{Maturation factor}}$$

Maturation factor (days)	PCV (l/l)
1.0	0.45
1.5	0.35
2.0	0.25
2.5	0.15

RPI < 1 indicates anaemia is non-regenerative;
RPI between 1 and 2 indicates eyrthropoietically active marrow;
RPI > 2 indicates accelerated erythropoiesis;
RPI > 3 is more consistent with haemolysis than haemorrhage.

Inappropriate Red Cell Response

An inappropriate red cell response is one in which the numbers of normoblasts exceed the numbers of reticulocytes present. Such a response may be an indicator of damage to the marrow stroma (e.g. myeloproliferative disease or myelodysplasia). A similar type of response is sometimes seen in dogs with lead poisoning or in response to chronic hypoxia (e.g. congestive heart failure).

Haemorrhage

Acute Haemorrhage

The PCV does not reflect the degree of blood loss for the first 12–24 h following an acute haemorrhagic episode. Initially the red cell parameters are within normal limits since red cells and plasma are lost in proportions similar to whole blood and splenic contraction may help offset any fall in PCV. The PCV and TPP concentration fall only when blood volume is expanded by movement of interstitial fluid into the vascular space. Since reticulocytes do not appear in the circulation for at least 48 h following blood loss, the anaemia initially appears normocytic, normochromic and non-regenerative. A neutrophilic leucocytosis and left shift are often present especially following haemorrhage into a body cavity. Platelet numbers also transiently increase and large granular 'shift' platelets are released into the circulation (Fig. 33.4). When haemorrhage into a body cavity occurs red cells may undergo a process of autotransfusion and re-enter the circulation. In doing so they become distorted and poikilocytes (acanthocytes) may be evident on the blood film. The PCV may take up to 2 weeks to return to normal following a single acute haemorrhagic episode.

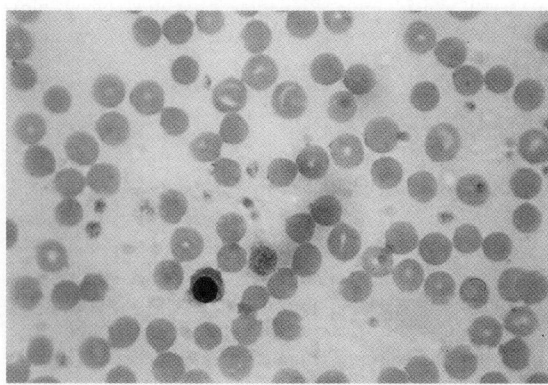

Fig. 33.4 Giemsa-stained blood film showing a large granular shift platelet next to a nucleated red blood cell.

Causes of acute haemorrhage include:

- trauma,
- surgery,
- bleeding gastrointestinal ulcers or tumours,
- renal or bladder neoplasia,
- idiopathic renal haematuria,
- congenital or acquired defects in haemostasis (haemophilia A, von Willebrand's disease, anticoagulant rodenticide toxicity, liver disease, thrombocytopenia, disseminated intravascular coagulation),
- rupture of vascular splenic tumours.

Chronic Haemorrhage

Chronic blood loss gradually leads to depletion of bone marrow iron stores and ultimately an iron deficient state. As iron stores become depleted the reticulocyte response diminishes and the red cells become progressively smaller until iron stores are virtually exhausted at which point the anaemia is typically microcytic, hypochromic and non-regenerative. Thrombocytosis is a relatively consistent feature of chronic haemorrhage. Chronic blood loss most commonly occurs via the urinary or gastrointestinal tracts (see causes for acute haemorrhage above) or less frequently as a result of severe flea or hookworm (*Ancylostoma caninum*) infections.

Haemolysis

Haemolytic anaemias can be classified as intrinsic or extrinsic.

(1) *Intrinsic haemolytic anaemias* are rare and are caused by an inherent metabolic defect in the red cell. Two examples are
   ○ Red cell pyruvate kinase deficiency in Basenjis (Searcy *et al.* 1979).
   ○ Red cell phosphofructokinase deficiency in Springer Spaniels (Giger *et al.* 1985a).
(2) *Extrinsic haemolytic anaemias* involve external factors such as red cell parasites, drugs or antibodies directed against the red cell membrane that render the red cells abnormal and more susceptible to phagocytosis by cells of the monocyte–phagocyte system. The net result is a reduction in red cell lifespan. Red cells are destroyed extravascularly in the liver, spleen or bone marrow, or intravascularly (or by a combination of both mechanisms). The major causes of extrinsic haemolytic anaemia are listed in Table 33.6.

Table 33.6   Causes of extrinsic haemolytic anaemia.

Immune-mediated disease
- Intravascular haemolysis; often via activation of complement attached to IgM antibody
- Extravascular haemolysis; frequently IgG antibodies directed against red cell membrane ± complement (C3) activation

Primary
   ○ Idiopathic immune-medicated haemolytic anaemia

Secondary
   ○ Associated with myeloproliferative or lymphoproliferative disease
   ○ Red cell parasites e.g. *Haemobartonella* sp., *Babesia* sp.
   ○ Drug-induced (e.g. trimethoprim–sulphadiazine, cephalosporins)
   ○ Neonatal isoerythrolysis
   ○ Incompatible blood transfusion
   ○ Manifestation of systemic lupus erythematosus

Oxidant damage to red cells
- Paracetamol toxicity resulting in Heinz body haemolytic anaemia
- Onion toxicity

Infectious agents
- Leptospirosis (*Leptospira icterohaemorrhagiae*)
- *Haemobartonella canis*
- *Babesia canis, B. gibsoni, B. vogeli*
- *Ehrlichia canis*

Miscellaneous
- Lead poisoning

Primary Immune-Mediated Haemolytic Anaemia

Most cases of haemolytic anaemia in the dog are immune-mediated involving the production of IgG or IgM antibodies (or both) directed against the red cell membrane. Most cases of primary or idiopathic immune-mediated haemolytic anaemia (IMHA) are probably autoimmune implying an aberrant antibody response against self-antigens on the surface of red cells. However since confirmation of true autoimmunity is rarely established the term immune-mediated is probably more appropriate and will be used in preference throughout this chapter.

The consequence of antibody attachment to red cells depends on the amount of antibody present, the antibody class and its ability to fix complement. Opsonised red cells are phagocytosed by splenic, hepatic and in some cases bone marrow macrophages. IgG antibodies are incomplete antibodies in that on their own they do not cause direct agglutination or cell lysis. Red cells coated with IgG antibodies alone therefore are more likely to be destroyed in the spleen since a much higher percentage of splenic macrophages possess receptors for the Fc portion of the IgG molecule (Stewart & Feldman 1993a). Activation of the complement cascade following attachment of the antibody to the red cell membrane makes the destructive process more effective since macrophages also possess CR1 and CR3 receptors. Macrophage receptors for the Fc portion of IgM are located primarily in the liver (only 20% in the spleen); IgM-mediated red cell destruction, in contrast, therefore tends to occur intravascularly (especially if complement is activated) or extravascularly in the liver (Stewart & Feldman 1993a). Pure complement-mediated lysis is uncommon.

Clinical and Clinicopathological Features of Immune-Mediated Haemolytic Anemia

Primary (idiopathic) IMHA has a higher incidence in females and Old English Sheepdogs, Irish Setters, Cocker Spaniels, Springer Spaniels, Poodles, Border Collies and, in the author's experience, Dobermann Pinschers appear to be over-represented (Dodds 1977; Klag *et al*. 1993). The higher incidence in certain breeds suggests genetic factors may induce failure of self-tolerance. A seasonal incidence has been recognised with most cases occurring in the spring (Stewart & Feldman 1993b) and an association with dioestrus has also occasionally been observed (J.K. Dunn, unpublished observations).

The rate of onset and severity of clinical signs vary according to the class and thermal dependency of antibody, the presence or absence of haemagglutination or haemolysis, and whether red cell destruction is occurring intravascularly or extravascularly.

Classification of Immune-Mediated Haemolytic Anaemia

Class 1 In-saline acting agglutinins
- In-saline acting agglutinins may be IgG or IgM. The red cells agglutinate on a glass slide and agglutination persists if blood is diluted with a drop of normal saline to the blood, differentiating it from rouleaux formation.
- Onset usually acute and prognosis guarded especially if IgM involved and haemolysis is occurring intravascularly.

Class 2 Intravascular haemolysins
- Usually IgM antibodies which fix complement resulting in acute intravascular haemolysis.
- Onset acute and prognosis extremely guarded.

Class 3 Incomplete warm acting antibodies
- Most common type of IMHA usually involving IgG antibodies.
- Antibody opsonises red blood but is unable to cause direct intravascular cell lysis or agglutination.
- Direct antiglobulin test (Coombs' test) required to detect their presence.
- Onset more insidious, disease follows a more chronic course and prognosis is generally more favourable.

Class 4 Cold haemagglutinins
- Rare form of IMHA.
- Active at 4°C and usually IgM antibodies.
- Red cells clump if cooled to 4°C (reverses if warmed to 37°C).

Class 5 Non-agglutinating, haemolytic cold antibodies
- Rare form of IMHA.
- Non-agglutinating IgG antibodies which require a direct antiglobulin test to detect.

The following clinical and clinicopathological findings may be seen with all types of IMHA:

- Pyrexia (may be intermitttent or sustained).
- Splenomegaly, hepatomegaly and mild generalised lymph node enlargement.
- Anaemia usually intensely regenerative and may be associated with a neutrophilic leucocytosis. Cases of suspected non-regenerative IMHA have been reported (Holloway *et al*. 1990; Cotter 1992; Klag *et al*. 1993; Scott-Moncrieff *et al*. 1995). In these cases antibodies may be directed against erythroid precursors resulting in ineffective erythropoiesis, characterised by a late maturation arrest of the erythroid series, and a delayed reticulocyte response (Stockham *et al*.1980; Jonas *et al*. 1987). Increased numbers of plasma cells and evidence of intramedullary destruction of red cells may be seen in some cases (Jonas *et al*. 1987; Holloway *et al*. 1990; Cotter 1992; Dunn *et al*. 1995).
- Concurrent thrombocytopenia is common in cases of IMHA.
- Liver enzymes (ALT and ALP) are often increased especially with acute haemolysis.

Clinical Signs Associated with Intravascular Haemolysis

- Onset of anaemia usually acute. More likely to be Class 1 or Class 2 IMHA.
- Haemoglobinaemia and haemoglobinuria occur if

plasma haptoglobin system (haptoglobin binds free haemoglobin) is saturated.

- Hyperbilirubinaemia may result in jaundice; greater than 90% of the total bilirubin present in plasma may be the free (unconjugated) form during the acute stage of the disease.
- Liver enzymes often increased as a result of hepatocellular hypoxia.
- Prolonged haemoglobinuria may lead to acute renal tubular necrosis.

Clinical Signs Associated with Extravascular Haemolysis

- Anaemia more insidious in onset and affected animals rarely jaundiced. Most frequently Class 3 IMHA.
- Splenomegaly more common.
- Spherocytes (Figs 33.3 and 33.5) may be noted on blood film. These small dark-staining erythrocytes lack central pallor and represent red cells which have been partially phagocytosed by splenic or hepatic macrophages. An absence of spherocytes should not be regarded as evidence that an animal does not have IMHA.
- Total plasma proteins, especially the globulin fraction, may be increased.

Miscellaneous Clinical Signs

- Class 4 IMHA is characterised by microthromboemboli formation resulting in erythema, swelling, ulceration and ischaemic necrosis of the extremities (feet, tail, ears and nose).
- Class 5 IMHA is extremely rare and manifests as intermittent haemoglobinuria in cold weather.

Complications

Pulmonary thromboembolism and disseminated intravascular coagulation (DIC) are important complications of IMHA which may be difficult to diagnose antemortem (Klein *et al.* 1989). The acute onset of dyspnoea in an animal with IMHA should raise suspicion of acute pulmonary thromboembolism. Arterial blood gases show hypoxaemia and normocapnoea. Coagulation tests are usually normal and thoracic radiography may reveal a pronounced interstitial pattern and evidence of mild pleural effusion (Klein *et al.* 1989). The clinical and clinicopathological features of DIC are described in Chapter 36.

Secondary Immune-Mediated Haemolytic Anaemia

- The production of anti-erythrocyte antibodies may occur in association with certain systemic infectious, inflammatory, neoplastic and other immune-mediated disorders for example:
  - ○ sub-acute bacterial endocarditis (Calvert 1982),
  - ○ lymphoproliferative or myeloproliferative disease,
  - ○ systemic lupus eythematosus (SLE),
  - ○ as a sequel to some viral infections, vaccination with modified live vaccines or as a result of an incompatible blood transfusion.
- Red cell parasites (*Haemobartonella canis* or *Babesia* sp.) cause intravascular and/or extravascular haemolysis by increasing red cell fragility. In addition to direct cell damage immune-mediated (antibody dependent) haemolysis may contribute to the anaemia seen with both these diseases.

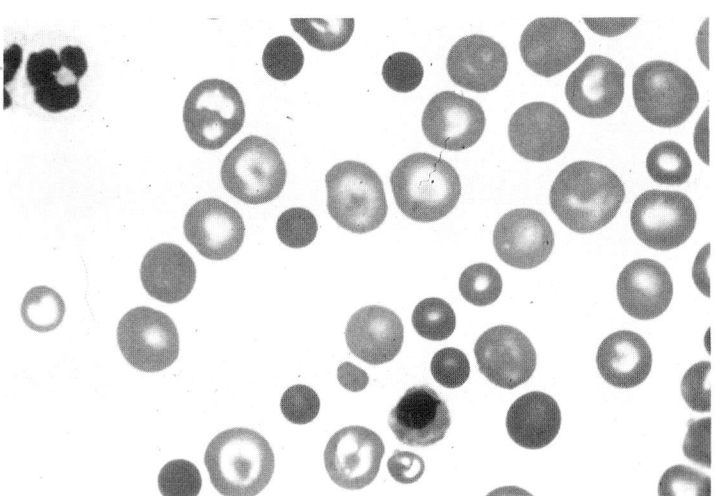

Fig. 33.5 Blood from a dog with auto-immune haemolytic anaemia. Many of the red cells are macrocytic and some appear as folded leptocytes. The small, dark-staining cells which lack central pallor are spherocytes; the nucleated red cell at the bottom right of the picture is a normoblast. Photo courtesy of Prof. N. T. Gorman.

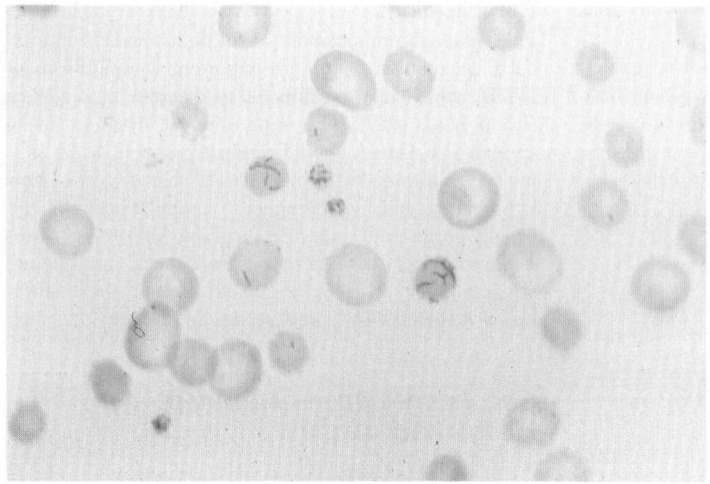

Fig. 33.6 Red blood cells parasitised with *Haemobartonella canis*. The organisms appear as blue, coccoid or rod-like bodies which extend in chains across the surface of the erythrocytes. Photo courtesy of Prof. N. T. Gorman.

Red Cell Parasites

Haemobartonellosis. Unlike haemobartonellosis in cats, *Haemobartonella canis* infections appear to be rare, occurring only in dogs that have previously been splenectomised. The anaemia is occasionally Coombs' positive. Diagnosis requires detection of small basophilic coccoid or coccobacillary rickettsial organisms on a blood film stained with Giemsa or acridine orange (Fig. 33.6).

Babesiosis. Canine babesiosis occurs sporadically in dogs in quarantine kennels. The disease does not occur spontaneously in the United Kingdom. The three species of babesia which can parasitise canine red cells are *B. canis*, *B. gibsoni* and *B. vogeli*. The intermediate host is the brown dog tick, *Rhipicephalus sanguineus*. Acute infection is characterised by intravascular and extravascular haemolysis. In some cases the anaemia is Coombs' positive. Animals that recover from acute infection may progress to a chronic carrier state. Chronically infected animals develop premunition and may show a recurrence of clinical signs following splenectomy or if subjected to a stressful stimulus, for example intercurrent disease. Diagnosis of babesiosis is made by examining a Giemsa-stained film of capillary blood for the presence of paired trophozoites in red blood cells (Fig. 33.7). An immunofluorescent test has been developed for detecting occult parasitaemia. Treatment with parasiticidal drugs such as imidocarb dipropionate or diminazene aceturate may clear the parasitaemia but often does not completely eliminate the infection.

Drug-Induced Haemolytic Anaemia

Drug-induced haemolytic anaemia occurs when antibodies are produced against a cell-bound drug (hapten) or against

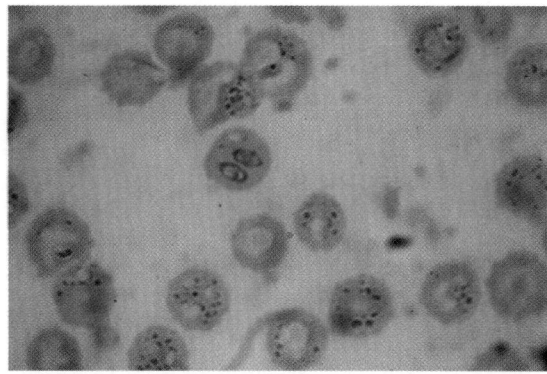

Fig. 33.7 Giemsa-stained blood film from a dog with babesiosis. The red blood cell in the centre contains a pair of *Babesia canis* trophozoites.

red cell membranes which have been antigenically altered by previous exposure to a drug. Administration of trimethoprim–sulphadiazine can induce immune-mediated anaemia as part of a syndrome resembling SLE particularly in Dobermanns (Werner & Bright 1983; Giger *et al.* 1985b).

Isoimmune Haemolytic Disease

Isoimmune haemolytic disease (neonatal isoerythrolysis) occurs when the fetus has a blood type incompatible with that of the mother who has previously been sensitised as a result of an earlier mismatched pregnancy or blood transfusion to produce isoantibodies. The pups become anaemic and icteric when they ingest colostrum within the first 24–72 h of life (Dodds 1977).

Diagnosis of Immune-Mediated Haemolytic Anaemia

Diagnosis of IMHA is based on the following criteria:

- evidence of reduced red cell lifespan,
- evidence of antibodies directed against host's red cells,
- evidence of increased erythropoiesis in response to increased red cell destruction.

Autoagglutination on a Glass Slide
Evidence of autoagglutination of the patient's red cells on a glass slide (Fig. 33.8) precludes the need to perform a direct antiglobulin test (see below). Autoagglutination can be differentiated from clumping of red cells due to rouleaux formation by diluting the blood with 2 or 3 drops of normal saline. True autoagglutination persists whereas rouleaux formation disperses following the addition of saline.

Direct Antiglobulin Test (Coombs' Test)
The direct antiglobulin test remains the cornerstone for the diagnosis of IMHA. It detects antibodies directed against the red cell membrane. The test should be performed at 4°C and 37°C to detect cold (usually IgM) as well as warm (usually IgG) agglutinating antibodies. Positive titres have been reported with a number of infectious, inflammatory, neoplastic and other immune-mediated diseases (Slappendel 1979). Titres less than 1:16 should be interpreted cautiously especially if there is no clinical or laboratory evidence of haemolysis. Some healthy dogs have a low titre of cold agglutinating antibodies (Slappendel 1979). As with most immunological screening tests false negative and false positive results can occur (Klag *et al.* 1993).

Causes of False Negative Results
- Antiserum (usually a polyvalent antiserum against canine IgG, IgM and C3) of inadequate strength.
- Inadequate concentration of antibody or complement on red cell membrane.
- Prozone phenomenon (antiserum contains excess antibody).
- IgM binds to red cells only within a narrow temperature range and may be eluted off cells at higher temperatures.
- Previous corticosteroid therapy.

Causes of False Positive Results
- Inadequate absorption of antiserum with pooled red cells resulting in residual anti-red cell antibody.
- Previous blood transfusion.
- Non-specific absorption of serum proteins on to damaged red cells.

Other Immunological Tests to Detect Red Cell Antibodies
Modifications of the direct antiglobulin test in the form of direct enzyme-linked antiglobulin tests have been developed to enable detection of multiple immunoglobulin classes (IgG, IM and IgA) as well as complement on the surface of red cells (Jones *et al.* 1987; Porter *et al.* 1989; Barker *et al.* 1991).

Bone Marrow Aspiration
Bone marrow aspiration should be considered:

- if there is failure to respond to conventional immunosuppressive therapy;

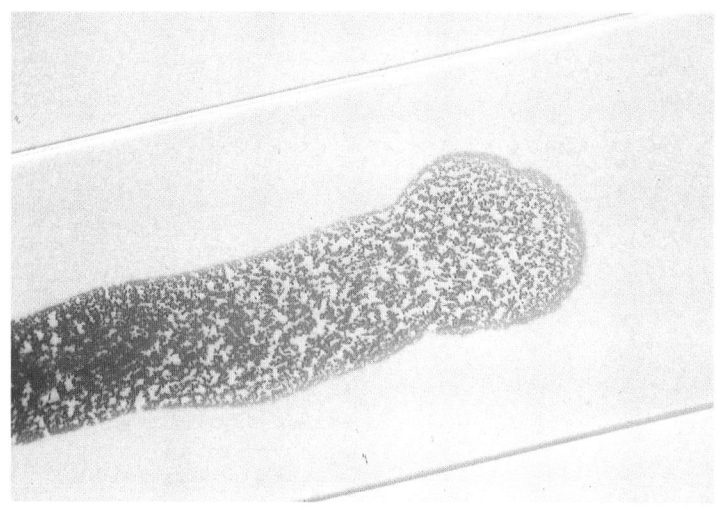

Fig. 33.8 Auto-agglutination of red blood cells on a glass slide. The clumping of erythrocytes persisted after the addition of normal saline.

- if an underlying myeloproliferative or lymphoproliferative disorder is suspected;
- if immune-mediated haemolytic disease is suspected but the anaemia is non-regenerative.

Treatment of Immune-Mediated Haemolytic Anaemia

The treatment of immune-mediated haemolytic anaemia typically involves the use of corticosteroids and other immunosuppressive drugs such as azathioprine and cyclophosphamide. The aim of therapy is to maintain the red cell count and PCV within normal limits using the lowest possible (alternate day) doses of immunosuppressive agents. Some animals require lifelong treatment; in others it may be possible to discontinue all medication.

(1) Initial treatment consists of prednisolone 2–4 mg/kg body weight daily. When a response is noted the dose of prednisolone should be gradually tapered to a low, every other day, maintenance dose over a 3-month period.

(2) The use of cytotoxic drugs such as azathioprine (1–2 mg/kg body weight daily) or cyclophosphamide (50 mg/m² every other day) in combination with prednisolone should be considered in cases showing evidence of autoagglutination or acute intravascular haemolysis or in cases which fail to respond to prednisolone within 5–7 days. The use of these drugs may allow a lower maintenance dose of prednisolone to be used thereby minimising the risk of side effects associated with long-term steroid administration.

(3) Transfusion with whole blood or packed red cells may be necessary if the PCV continues to fall despite appropriate therapy (see Chapter 2).

(4) Danazol (5 mg/kg body weight p.o.) has been used in combination with prednisolone and other immunosuppressive agents to treat refractory cases of IMHA and immune-mediated thrombocytopenia (Holloway *et al.* 1990; Stewart & Feldman 1993b). The onset of action of danazol is slow and an increase in PCV may not be apparent for 1–3 weeks after starting treatment.

(5) A recent study reported the successful treatment with human gamma-globulin of five cases of suspected immune-mediated haemolytic anaemia. In these cases the anaemia was non-regenerative and had failed to respond to conventional immunosuppressive therapy (Scott-Moncrieff *et al.* 1995).

(6) The administration of heparin (100 IU/kg body weight every 6 h) during the acute phase of the disease may minimise the risk of pulmonary thromboembolism and DIC.

(7) Plasmapheresis to remove antibody and immune complexes from plasma has been used occasionally to treat unresponsive cases.

(8) Splenectomy should be regarded as a last resort. It is advocated only for animals that fail to respond to any of the above treatment regimes or in animals that experience frequent relapses.

Fragmentation or Microangiopathic Haemolytic Anaemias

Red cells can be mechanically damaged and distorted as they pass through a meshwork of fibrin in the microvasculature or the abnormal vascular channels of large hepatic or

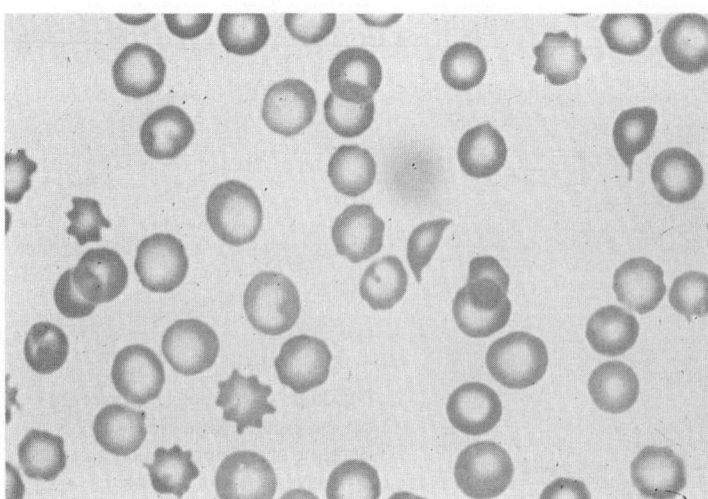

Fig. 33.9 Blood from a dog with splenic haemangiosarcoma. The red cells with irregularly shaped surface projections are acanthocytes. Red cell fragments (schistocytes) are also present. Photo courtesy of Prof. N. T. Gorman.

splenic neoplasms. These fragmented red cells, known as schistocytes (Fig. 33.9), are either destroyed intravascularly or are rendered so abnormal that they become targets for extravascular phagocytosis. Schistocytes are most commonly seen with DIC or splenic haemangiosarcomas.

NON-REGENERATIVE ANAEMIAS

A non-regenerative anaemia is an anaemia of greater than 5 days' duration with an inappropriately low reticulocyte count. They can be classified as either hypoproliferative or maturation defect anaemias.

Hypoproliferative Anaemias

Most non-regenerative anaemias are normocytic, normochromic hypoproliferative anaemias and are insidious in onset. Failure of erythropoiesis may occur as a result of primary bone marrow disease or secondary to some other systemic disease process. Table 33.7 lists the causes of non-regenerative anaemia.

Primary Failure of Erythropoiesis

The main clinical and clinicopathological features of non-regenerative anaemias caused by primary bone marrow disease are as follows:

- Anaemia tends to be slowly progressive with clinical signs becoming apparent only during the later stages of the disease.
- Anaemia is generally severe (PCV < 0.10–0.151/l) and

is often accompanied by a concurrent cytopenia (neutropenia or thrombocytopenia) or in some cases generalised bone marrow suppression results in true pancytopenia. Occasionally the anaemia is caused by selective suppression of red cell precursors (pure red cell aplasia).

- Serum iron concentrations may be increased.
- A bone marrow aspirate and/or trephine biopsy is usually necessary in order to obtain a definitive diagnosis.

Causes of Primary Bone Marrow Failure

Pure Red Cell Aplasia

Pure red cell aplasia (PRCA) is characterised by selective depletion of red cells precursors in the bone marrow. Congenital PRCA (Diamond–Blackfan anaemia) appears to be an extremely rare disorder in dogs (Moore *et al.* 1993). Acquired PRCA is thought to have an immune-mediated pathogenesis on the basis that some cases have positive direct antiglobulin tests and a serum immunoglobulin G inhibitor directed against precursors of erythroid colony forming units can be detected in the serum of some affected dogs (Weiss 1986a). An immune-mediated mechanism is also suspected for dogs with a less severe form of the disease characterised by transient erythroid hypoplasia since affected animals often respond to immunosuppressive drugs, albeit in combination with anabolic steroids and blood transfusion therapy (Weiss *et al.* 1982). Red cell aplasia has been reported as a sequel to canine parvovirus infection.

Bone marrow evaluation is required for a definitive diagnosis. Cytological findings include an increased myeloid : erythroid (M : E) ratio associated with maturation arrest of eythroid precursors at the early to intermediate normoblast stage, increased numbers of plasma cells and in some cases there is evidence of erythrophagocytosis.

Table 33.7 Causes of non-regenerative anaemia.

Primary causes	Secondary causes
- Eythroid hypoplasia	- Chronic inflammatory or neoplastic disease (anaemia of chronic disease)
- Aplastic anaemia	- Chronic renal failure
- Myeloproliferative disease	- Chronic liver disease
- Lymphoproliferative disease	- Endocrine disorders, e.g. hypoadrenocorticism, hypothyroidism
- Myelofibrosis	
- Marrow necrosis	
- Myelodysplasia	

Histological examination of a core biopsy may reveal a variable degree of myelofibrosis or replacement of the haemopoietic spaces with fat.

Aplastic Anaemia

Damage to the bone marrow microenvironment may result in chronic depletion of haemopoietic stem cells. Generalised bone marrow suppression is manifested as a pancytopenia (anaemia, neutropenia and thrombocytopenia). Numerous infectious, chemical and physical agents have been implicated in the pathogenesis (Table 33.8). Sporadic cases of aplastic anaemia have been reported in association with certain drugs (Weiss & Klausner 1990; Fox *et al.* 1993). Toxic doses of oestrogen result initially in a neutrophilic leucocytosis and thrombocytopenia which progresses within 3 weeks to pancytopenia (Farris & Benjamin 1993). The role of an immune-mediated pathogenesis is uncertain.

The cytological appearance of bone marrow varies depending on the time at which it is collected. During the early stages there may be evidence of marrow necrosis. As the disease progresses the marrow becomes progressively more hypocellular and the haemopoietic spaces become replaced by fat or fibrous tissue. Histopathological examination of a core biopsy is usually required to confirm the diagnosis.

Acute drug-induced aplastic anaemia may be reversible if the offending drug is eliminated. The prognosis for chronic aplastic anaemia is generally poor. Severe thrombocytopenic or anaemic animals may show a transient improvement with glucocorticoids. Antibiotic cover (for

Table 33.8 Factors implicated in the pathogenesis of true aplastic anaemia.

- Administration of oestrogenic compounds or hyperoestrogenism resulting from a functional Sertoli cell tumour.
- Drug-induced
  - o Oestrogenic drugs (see above)
  - o Cytotoxic agents such as cyclophosphamide or doxorubicin
  - o Phenylbutazone
  - o Prolonged administration of trimethoprim–sulphadiazine
- Ionising radiation
- Infectious causes
  - o Canine distemper virus
  - o Canine parvovirus
  - o *Ehrlichia canis*
  - o Endotoxin-producing bacteria
- Immune-mediated pathogenesis?

example gentamicin in combination with cephalosporins) should be given especially to dogs that are neutropenic. Immunosuppressive treatment occasionally results in a very transient improvement. Lithium carbonate (11 mg/kg body weight p.o. every 12 h) has been used successfully to treat a few cases of oestrogen-induced aplastic anaemia (Maddux & Shaw 1983; Hall 1992). Serum levels of lithium should be regularly monitored (optimal therapeutic serum lithium concentration in the dog is reported to be 0.5–1.8 mEq/l; Hall 1992). The use of haemopoietic growth factors (e.g. granulocyte–monocyte colony stimulating factor) as bone marrow stimulants has yet to be fully evaluated.

Myelophthisis

Myelophthisis is the term used to describe replacement of normal haemopoietic tissue with neoplastic cells or fibrous tissue (myelofibrosis).

- Lymphoproliferative and myeloproliferative disease (see Chapter 35)
- Myelofibrosis

Myelofibrosis is characterised by fibroblastic proliferation and deposition of reticulin fibres and collagen in the haemopoietic spaces. Myelofibrosis may be classified as primary (idiopathic) or secondary. In humans primary myelofibrosis is associated with myeloid metaplasia of the liver, spleen, and lymph nodes, and proliferation of bone marrow megakaryocytes is often observed. Megakaryocytes may play an important role in the pathogenesis of myelofibrosis since it has been shown that growth factors derived from megakaryocytes and platelets, for example platelet-derived growth factor, stimulate fibroblastic activity and collagen deposition. It has been postulated therefore that some cases of myelofibrosis previously designated as primary are in fact secondary, i.e. myelofibrosis occurs secondary to megakaryocytic hyperplasia or a myeloproliferative disorder involving the megakaryocyte series (megakaryocytic or megakaryoblastic leukaemia).

Primary myelofibrosis appears to be a rare condition in the dog and most cases are probably secondary with the collagen and reticulin fibre deposition occurring as a sequel to prolonged damage to marrow stroma. Myelofibrosis has been reported in association with pure red cell aplasia, aplastic anaemia, marrow necrosis, oestrogen toxicity, exposure to ionising radiation, myeloproliferative disorders, invasion of bone marrow with metastatic tumour and cases of chronic immune-mediated haemolytic anaemia (Thompson & Johnstone 1983; Hoenig 1989; Hoff *et al.* 1991; Scott-Moncrieff *et al.* 1995). In some cases it is associated with osteosclerosis (Dunn *et al.* 1986) and it occurs as a terminal event in Basenjis with red cell pyruvate kinase deficiency.

Splenomegaly and hepatomegaly may be evident on clinical examination. Most cases present with a moderately severe non-regenerative anaemia. White blood cell and platelet numbers initially are often normal or even slightly increased but leucopenia and/or thrombocytopenia may develop as the disease progresses. Examination of a blood film may show marked anisocytosis, tear drop shaped red cells (dacrocytes or ovalocytes) and 'giant' platelets. Repeated 'dry' or hypocellular aspirates are highly suggestive of myelofibrosis and histopathological examination of a core biopsy is required to make a diagnosis. The most common histopathological findings in one study were normal or slightly increased numbers of megakaryocytes, a marked increase in haemosiderin deposition, increased numbers of granulocytic precursors and, in few cases, evidence of erythrophagocytosis (Hoff *et al.* 1991).

The response to treatment depends on the cellularity of the erythroid marrow and not on the degree of fibrosis (Hoff *et al.* 1991). Many cases respond favourably to immunosuppressive therapy and anabolic steroids although repeated blood transfusions may be necessary at the outset to allow the erythroid marrow to become fully active.

Marrow Necrosis

Marrow necrosis in the dog has been reported with oestrogen toxicosis, acute parvoviral enteritis, septicaemia and chronic ehrlichiosis (Weiss *et al.* 1985). The pathogenesis is poorly understood. Necrosis may occur as a result of direct toxic damage. It has also been suggested that damage to the microvasculature of the marrow, for example, endotoxin-induced capillary endothelial damage may lead to thrombosis and ischaemic necrosis.

Haematological abnormalities include non-regenerative anaemia with or without neutropenia or thrombocytopenia; occasionally the animal may be pancytopenic. Bone marrow cytology shows large numbers of degenerate haemopoietic cells and phagocytic macrophages. The cells stain poorly and lack cellular detail. Histologically there is extensive replacement of normal stroma by eosinophilic necrotic debris and haemorrhage. A variable degree of myelofibrosis may be evident (Weiss 1986b).

Myelodysplasia

The term myelodysplasia encompasses a number of non-neoplastic marrow abnormalities which in some cases may precede transition to acute myelogenous leukaemia. Synonyms include preleukaemia or atypical myeloproliferative disease. Myelodysplasia appears to occur much less frequently in the dog than it does in the cat where it is commonly associated with feline leukaemia virus infection. Typical haematological abnormalities include refractory non-regenerative anaemia, neutropenia or thrombocytopenia either singly or in combination, and increased numbers of normoblasts or large granular platelets may appear in the circulation.

Bone marrow cellularity may be normal or increased with alterations in cellular morphology, for example megakaryocytes may be abnormal in nuclear ploidy or cytoplasmic granularity. There may be an increase in the myeloid:erythroid ratio. Maturation arrest of the granulocytic series may result in an apparent excess of myeloblasts and younger myeloid maturation stages or in the case of the erythroid series a disproportionately high percentage of early and intermediate normoblasts.

The clinical signs associated with myelodysplasia are often vague and reflect the haematological and bone marrow abnormalities described above. Inappetence, weight loss, lethargy and intermittent pyrexia are typical signs in dogs that are persistently anaemic and neutropenic; petechial or ecchymotic haemorrhages may be evident in severely thrombocytopenic animals. Treatment of myelodysplasia depends on the severity of the haematological abnormalities and presence or absence of clinical signs. Antibiotic therapy is indicated in cases showing evidence of sepsis; severely anaemic or thrombocytopenic animals may benefit from the administration of prednisolone. Low dose cytosine arabinoside therapy 5–10 mg/m^2 s.c. b.i.d. for 2–3 weeks then every other week) has been advocated to induce differentiation of immature myeloid precursors (Couto 1992). Regular monitoring of blood counts and repeated bone marrow aspiration are essential to ensure that progression of the disease is detected at an early stage.

Secondary Suppression of Erythropoiesis

Anaemia occurs in association with numerous chronic inflammatory, metabolic and neoplastic conditions (see Table 33.7).

Anaemia of Chronic Disease

Anaemia of chronic disease refers to the non-regenerative anaemia associated with numerous chronic infectious, inflammatory, traumatic and neoplastic disease processes. The pathogenesis involves a defect in iron metabolism which results in sequestration of iron stores and a relative unavailability of iron for red cell precursors. Anaemia of chronic disease is normocytic and normochromic and is characterised by low serum iron, normal or increased bone marrow iron stores and decreased red cell survival. *In vitro* inhibitors of colony forming units-erythroid (CFU-E) appear to occur in dogs with infectious diseases (less frequently in dogs with malignancy and renal failure; Weiss 1986c). The role of inflammatory mediators in suppression of erythropoiesis has not been fully investigated. Other mechanisms for anaemia associated with malignancy include haemorrhage, myelophthisis, DIC and haemolysis.

The following clinicopathological features may help to differentiate anaemia of chronic disease from anaemia caused by primary bone marrow disease.

- Anaemia is usually less severe (PCV often between 0.20 and 0.35l/l) and may be accompanied by haematological evidence of acute or chronic inflammation.
- Bone marrow cytology shows a relatively mild degree of erythroid hypoplasia which may be associated with granulocytic hyperplasia and increased numbers of plasma cells and macrophages.
- Serum iron concentration and total iron binding capacity may be normal or decreased despite adequate or increased bone marrow stores of haemosiderin.
- Increased numbers of leptocytes (target cells) may be noted on the blood film.

Renal Disease

The anaemia which is a feature of chronic renal failure (CRF) is typically normocytic and normochromic and is primarily the result of decreased erythropoietin production by the failing kidneys. Other contributory factors include a reduction in red cell lifespan (haemolysis may be associated with uraemic vasculitis) and suppression of the erythroid marrow by uraemic toxins. Gastric ulceration resulting in gastrointestinal haemorrhage and altered platelet function associated with the uraemic state may explain the melaena seen in some dogs with end-stage renal failure. Poikilocytes (acanthocytes or schistocytes; Fig. 33.9) may appear in the circulation. The anaemia of CRF responds well to recombinant erythropoietin therapy (see Chapter 62, page 650). Erthropoietin therapy in humans can cause hypertension and a decrease in serum iron levels. Systemic blood pressure and serum iron concentrations should be determined before erythropoietin therapy commences (Cowgill 1992). Lack of available iron blunts the erythropoietin response therefore iron should be administered concurrently (Giger 1992). Anabolic steroids may have a direct stimulatory effect on committed erythroid stem cells.

Chronic Liver Disease

The anaemia associated with chronic liver disease is multifactorial. Circulating toxins and the anaemia of chronic disease suppress erythropoiesis. Diffuse severe hepatocellular damage may lead to depletion of essential clotting factors and a tendency to bleed, and there may be a microangiopathic haemolytic component especially if hepatic sinusoidal architecture is disrupted for example by a haemangiosarcoma resulting in increased numbers of acanthocytes on a peripheral blood film.

Endocrine Disorders

Decreased oxygen utilisation by peripheral tissues leads to a relatively mild normocytic, normochromic anaemia in some hypothyroid dogs. Most cases of hypoadrenocorticism (Addison's disease) also have a normocytic, normochromic anaemia although this may be masked initially by hypovolaemia. Less frequently an acute Addisonian crisis results in severe gastrointestinal haemorrhage and an intensely regenerative anaemia.

Maturation Defect Anaemias

Anaemias involving abnormalities in nuclear or cytoplasmic maturation are rare. Although the bone marrow is usually hypercellular with increased numbers of red cell precursors, erythropoiesis is ineffective and the red cells are not readily released into the circulation.

Cytoplasmic Maturation Defect Anaemias

- *Iron deficiency*. The anaemia associated with iron deficiency due to chronic blood loss is typically microcytic and hypochromic.
- *Lead poisoning*. Lead interferes with the synthesis of haemoglobin at various points in the haem synthesis pathway. The anaemia is normocytic and normochromic (occasionally microcytic and hypochromic). An inappropriate nucleated red blood cell response may be evident on a peripheral blood film. Basophilic stippling of red cells is a more variable finding and is best demonstrated on a freshly prepared blood film using blood containing no anticoagulant.

Nuclear Maturation Defect Anaemias

Nuclear : cytoplasmic asynchrony of erythroid precursors resulting in the production of large megaloblastic normoblasts in the bone marrow is reflected by the appearance of macrocytic normochromic red cells in the circulation. True megaloblastic or macrocytic anaemias are rare in the dog. Megaloblastosis has been associated with prolonged therapy with anticonvulsive agents (phenytoin, phenobarbital and primidone) and folate antagonists (methotrexate and trimethoprim). Folate-responsive macrocytic anaemia occurs occasionally with small intestinal malabsorption, neoplasia, liver disease and prolonged anorexia.

MANAGEMENT OF ANAEMIA

The management of anaemia is primarily supportive. Specific therapy should be directed at the underlying disease process.

Blood Component Therapy

Blood products used in the treatment of anaemia include:

- fresh whole blood,
- stored blood,
- packed red blood cells,
- stored plasma,
- fresh frozen plasma,
- platelet-rich plasma,
- plasma cryoprecipitate.

The use of a particular blood component is governed by the specific needs of the animal and also to a large extent the facilities available for its collection and preparation. Coagulation factors are preserved for at least 3 months in fresh frozen plasma (plasma frozen within 6 h of collection) stored at −20°C and up to 12 months if frozen at −70°C. The production of platelet-rich plasma or plasma cryoprecipitate is not practical in a practice setting. Platelet-rich plasma should be used within 24 h of collection. Plasma cryoprecipitate is prepared from fresh frozen plasma and may be stored for up to one year. It contains high concentrations of Factor VIII, von Willebrand factor antigen, fibrinogen and fibronectin.

Methods for collection storage and administration of blood products are described in the section on Blood Transfusion in Chapter 2, where also is found a discussion of canine blood groups and complications of blood transfusion.

Indications for Transfusion Therapy in the Treatment of Anaemia

Haemorrhage

Whole blood provides plasma which helps restore oncotic pressure and red cells to correct hypoxaemia. The loss of red cells is generally tolerated better than an acute reduction in plasma volume. Signs of hypovolaemic shock do not become evident until there has been a 30–40% loss of blood volume.

During the first 12 h following an acute haemorrhagic episode the PCV does not provide a reliable indicator of the severity of the anaemia since plasma and red cells are lost in equal proportions and compensatory vasoconstriction and splenic contraction help maintain PCV within normal limits. With acute blood loss therefore signs of hypovolaemic shock (mucosal pallor, prolonged capillary refill time, tachycardia associated with a fast weak femoral pulse, and tachypnoea or dyspnoea) are important factors to consider when determining the need for a blood transfusion.

Acute blood loss associated with a sudden drop in PCV to less than 0.20 l/l probably warrants the transfusion of whole blood especially if there is evidence of continued blood loss.

The recommended dose is 10–20 ml whole blood/kg body weight. In cases of hypovolaemic shock the rate of administration should not exceed 13–22 ml/kg body weight per hour.

If a congenital or acquired disorder of haemostasis is suspected and there is a need to replace clotting factors or platelets, fresh whole blood should be transfused within 8–12 h of collection. Large volumes of fresh whole blood are required to significantly increase platelet numbers in a thrombocytopenic animal (platelet-rich plasma is the blood component of choice). Nevertheless blood transfusion may be effective in temporarily increasing the platelet count sufficiently to stop acute life threatening blood loss. If clotting factors only are required fresh frozen plasma can be given. The transfusion of fresh whole blood is indicated before heparin therapy in the management of DIC. Cases of suspected warfarin toxity should be given vitamin K₁.

Non-Regenerative Anaemias

Most animals with chronic insidious onset anaemias are normovolaemic and there is less of a need for plasma expansion. Transfusion therapy, preferably with *packed red blood cells* resuspended in normal saline to reduce the risk of volume overload, should be considered if signs of hypoxaemia are present. Usually this does not occur until the PCV is less than 0.15–0.10 l/l.

The recommended transfusion rate for a normovolaemic animal is 1–5 ml/kg body weight per hour.

Immune-Mediated Haemolytic Anaemia

Life-threatening circumstances, for example an acute haemolytic crisis, may dictate the transfusion of whole blood despite the fact that in some cases the transfusion may accelerate haemolysis. Where possible a cross match should be performed and donor blood cells that show the least reactivity to the patient's serum should be used.

Iron

Iron supplementation should be given only to animals with confirmed iron deficiency anaemia. Iron is poorly absorbed from the gastrointestinal tract. A single intramuscular injection of iron dextrans (10–20 ml/kg body weight) followed by ferrous sulphate or ferrous gluconate by mouth

(60–300 mg once daily) has been recommended (Squires 1993b).

Immunosuppressive Drugs

Prednisolone (1–2 mg/kg body weight b.i.d.) is indicated for the treatment of immune-mediated haemolytic anaemia or thrombocytopenia, myeloproliferative or lymphoproliferative disease, pure red cell aplasia, aplastic anaemia and some cases of myelodysplasia. Prednisolone may be used in combination with cytotoxic agents such as azathioprine (1–2 mg/kg body weight once daily) or cyclophosphamide (50 mg/m^2 every other day).

Anabolic Steroids

Nandrolone decanoate (1 mg/kg body weight i.m. once weekly for 3 weeks and once every 3 weeks thereafter) and other anabolic steroids are indicated for the treatment of primary erythroid hypoplasia, aplastic anaemia, certain myeloproliferative disorders, cases of myelodysplasia presenting with severe non-regenerative anaemia, and the anaemia associated with chronic renal failure. Prolonged treatment (3–6 months) is often necessary before a response is observed. Danazol (5–10 mg/kg body weight b.i.d. p.o.), a synthetic androgen, has been used in dogs to treat corticosteroid-resistant cases of immune-mediated thrombocytopenia and autoimmune haemolytic anaemia.

REFERENCES

Allard, R.L., Carlos, A.D. & Faltin, E.C. (1989). Canine haematological changes during gestation and lactation. *Companion Animal Practice*, **19**, 3–6.

Andrews, G.A., Smith, J.E., Gray, M. & Chavey, P.S. (1992). An improved canine ferritin assay for canine sera. *Veterinary Clinical Pathology*, **21**, 57–60.

Barker, R.N., Gruffydd-Jones, T.J., Stokes, C.R. & Elson, C.J. (1991). Identification of autoantigens in canine autoimmune haemolytic anaemia. *Journal of Clinical and Experimental Immunology*, **85**, 33–40.

Calvert, C.A. (1982). Valvular bacterial endocarditis in the dog. *Journal of the American Veterinary Medical Association*, **180**, 1080–1084.

Cotter, S.M. (1992). Autoimmune hemolytic anemia in dogs. *Compendium on Continuing Education for the Practicing Veterinarian*, **14**, 53–59.

Couto, C.G. (1992). Leukaemias. In: *Essentials of Small Animal Internal Medicine*, (eds R.W. Nelson & C.G. Couto), pp. 871–878. Mosby Year Book, St. Louis.

Cowgill, L. (1992). Application of recombinant human erythropoietin in dogs and cats. In: *Current Veterinary Therapy XI*, (eds R.W. Kirk & J.D. Bonagura), pp. 484–487. W.B. Saunders, Philadelphia.

Dodds, W.J. (1977). Autoimmune hemolytic disease and other causes of immune-mediated anemia: An overview. *Journal of the American Animal Hospital Association*, **13**, 437–441.

Dunn, J.K., Doige, C.E., Searey, G.P. & Tanke, P. (1986). Myelofibrosis–osteosclerosis syndrome associated with erythroid hypoplasia in a dog. *Journal of Small Animal Practice*, **27**, 799–806.

Dunn, J.K., Jefferies, A.J. & Villiers, E. (1995). Anaemia associated with erythrophagocytosis in the dog: A spectrum of diseases. In: *Proceedings from the 4th ESVIM Congress*, Cambridge. pp. 72–73.

Farris, G.M. & Benjamin, S.A. (1993). Inhibition of myelopoiesis by serum of dogs exposed to estrogen. *American Journal of Veterinary Research*, **54**, 1374–1379.

Feldman, B.F. & Lessard, P. (1992). Hematologic and biochemical analytes in a sporting breed. *Compendium on Continuing Education for the Practicing Veterinarian*, **14**, 1574–1581.

Fox, L.E., Ford, S., Alleman, A.R., Homer, B.C. & Harvey, J.W. (1993). Aplastic anemia associated with prolonged high dose trimethoprim–sulfadiazine administration in two dogs. *Veterinary Clinical Pathology*, **22**, 89–92.

Giger, U. (1992). Erythropoietin and its clinical use. *Compendium on Continuing Education for the Practicing Veterinarian*, **14**, 25–34.

Giger, U., Harvey, J.W., Yamaguchi, R.A., McNulty, P.K., Chiapella, A. & Beutler, E. (1985a). Inherited phosphofructokinase deficiency in dogs with ventilation-induced hemolysis: Increased *in vitro* and *in vivo* alkaline fragility of erythrocytes. *Blood*, **65**, 345–351.

Giger, U., Werner, L.L., Millechamp, N.J. & Gorman, N.T. (1985b). Sulfadiazine-induced allergy in six Doberman pinschers. *Journal of the American Veterinary Medical Association*, **186**, 479–484.

Hall, E.J. (1992). Use of lithium for treatment of estrogen-induced bone marrow hypoplasia in a dog. *Journal of the American Veterinary Medical Association*, **200**, 814–816.

Harvey, J.W., Levin, D.E. & Chen, C.L. (1987). Potential effects of glucocorticoids on serum iron concentration in dogs. *Veterinary Clinical Pathology*, **16**, 46–50.

Hoenig, M. (1989). Six dogs with features compatible with myelonecrosis and myelofibrosis. *Journal of the American Animal Hospital Association*, **25**, 335–339.

Hoff, B., Lumsden, J.H., Valli, V.E.O. & Kruth, S.A. (1991). Myelofibrosis: Review of clinical and pathological features in fourteen dogs. *Canadian Veterinary Journal*, **32**, 357–361.

Holloway, S.A., Meyer, D.J. & Mannella, C. (1990). Prednisolone and danazol for treatment of immune-mediated hemolytic anemia, thrombocytopenia and ineffective erythroid regeneration in a dog. *Journal of the American Veterinary Medical Association*, **197**, 1045–1048.

Jonas, L.D., Thrall, M.A. & Weiser, M.G. (1987). Non-regenerative form of immune-mediated hemolytic anemia in dogs. *Journal of the American Animal Hospital Association*, **23**, 201–204.

Jones, D.E.R., Stokes, C.R., Gruffydd-Jones, T.J. & Bourne, F.J.

(1987). An enzyme-linked antiglobulin test for the detection of erythrocyte-bound antibodies in canine autoimmune haemolytic anaemia. *Veterinary Immunology and Immunopathology*, **16**, 11–21.

Klag, A.R., Giger, U. & Schofer, F.S. (1993). Idiopathic immune-mediated hemolytic anemia in dogs: 42 cases (1986–1990). *Journal of the American Veterinary Medical Association*, **202**, 783–788.

Klein, M.K., Dow, S.W. & Rosychuck, R.A.W. (1989). Pulmonary thromboembolism associated with immune-mediated hemolytic anemia in dogs: Ten cases (1982–1987). *Journal of the American Veterinary Medical Association*, **195**, 246–250.

Moore, A.H., Day, M.J. & Graham, M.W.A. (1993). Congenital pure red cell aplasia (Diamond–Blackfan anaemia) in a dog. *Veterinary Record*, **132**, 414–415.

Maddux, J.M. & Shaw, S.E. (1983). Possible beneficial effect of lithium therapy in a case of estrogen-induced bone marrow hypoplasia in a dog. *Journal of the American Animal Hospital Association*, **19**, 242–245.

Porter, R.E., Weiser, M.G. & Callahan, G.N. (1989). Development of an enzyme-linked immunosorbent assay to detect IgG, IgM and complement (C3) on canine erythrocytes. *American Journal of Veterinary Research*, **50**, 1365–1369.

Scott-Moncrieff, J.C.R., Reagan, W.J., Glickman, L.T., DeNicola, D.B. & Harrington, D. (1995). Treatment of non-regenerative anemia with human alpha-globulin in dogs. *Journal of the American Veterinary Medical Association*, **206**, 1895–1900.

Searcy, G.P., Tasker, J.B. & Miller, D.R. (1979). Animal model of human disease: Pyruvate kinase deficiency. *American Journal of Pathology*, **94**, 689–692.

Slappendel, R.J. (1979). The diagnostic significance of the direct antiglobulin test (DAT) in anaemic dogs. *Veterinary Immunology and Immunopathology*, **1**, 49–59.

Smith, J.E. (1989) Iron metabolism and its diseases. In: *Clinical Biochemistry of Domestic Animals*, (ed. J.J. Kaneko), 4th edn. pp. 256–273. Academic Press, San Diego.

Squires, R. (1993a). Differential diagnosis of anaemia in dogs. *In Practice*, **15**, 29–36.

Squires, R. (1993b). Management of anaemia in dogs. *In Practice*, **15**, 92–94.

Stewart, A.F. & Feldman, B.F. (1993a). Immune-mediated hemolytic anemia: Part I An overview. *Compendium on Continuing Education for the Practicing Veterinarian*, **15**, 372–381.

Stewart, A.F. & Feldman, B.F. (1993b). Immune-mediated hemolytic anemia: Part II Clinical entity, diagnosis and treatment theory. *Compendium on Continuing Education for the Practicing Veterinarian*, **15**, 1479–1491.

Stockham, S.L., Ford, R.B. & Weiss, D.J. (1980). Canine autoimmune hemolytic disease with a delayed erythroid regeneration. *Journal of the American Animal Hospital Association*, **16**, 927–931.

Thompson, J.C. & Johnstone, A.C. (1983). Myelofibrosis in the dog: Three case reports. *Journal of Small Animal Practice*, **24**, 589–601.

Weeks, B.R., Smith, J.E. & Northrop, J.K. (1989) Relationship of serum ferritin and iron concentrations and serum total iron-binding capacity to non-heme iron stores in dogs. *American Journal of Veterinary Research*, **50**, 198–200.

Weiss, D.J. (1986a). Antibody-mediated suppression of erythropoiesis in dogs with red blood cell aplasia. *American Journal of Veterinary Research*, **47**, 2646–2648.

Weiss, D.J. (1986b). Histopathology of canine non-neoplastic bone marrow. *Veterinary Clinical Pathology*, **15**(2), 7–11.

Weiss, D.J. (1986c). Potential role of serum inhibitors of erythropoiesis in the anemia associated with infection, renal disease and malignancy in the dog. *Veterinary Clinical Pathology*, **15**(4), 7–11.

Weiss, D.J. & Klausner, J.S. (1990). Drug-associated aplastic anemia in dogs: Eight cases (1984–1988). *Journal of the American Veterinary Medical Association*, **196**, 472–475.

Weiss, D.J., Stockham, S.L., Willard, M.D. & Schirmer, R.G. (1982). Transient erythroid hypoplasia in the dog. Report of five cases. *Journal of the American Veterinary Medical Association*, **18**, 353–359.

Weiss, D.J., Armstrong, P.J. & Reimann, K. (1985). Bone marrow necrosis in the dog. *Journal of the American Veterinary Medical Association*, **187**, 54–59.

Werner, L.L. & Bright, J.M. (1983). Drug-induced immune hypersensitivity disorders in two dogs treated with trimethoprim–sulfadiazine: Case reports and drug challenge studies. *Journal of the American Animal Hospital Association*, **19**, 783–790.

APPENDIX 1

Normal Red Cell Parameters in the Dog

Parameter	Units	Normal range
Total red blood cells (RBC)	$\times 10^{12}/l$	5.5–8.5
Packed cell volume (PCV)	l/l	0.37–0.55
Haemoglobin (Hb)	g/dl	12–18
Mean cell volume (MCV)	fl	60–77
Mean cell haemoglobin (MCH)	pg	19.5–24.5
Mean cell haemoglobin concentration (MCHC)	g/dl	32–37
Reticulocytes	%	0–15
Nucleated RBCs	number/ 100 WBCs	

Department of Clinical Veterinary Medicine (Central Diagnostic Services), University of Cambridge

Chapter 34

Polycythaemia

J. K. Dunn

Polycythaemia can be defined as an increase in haemoglobin concentration, total red cell count and packed cell volume (PCV).

PATHOPHYSIOLOGY OF POLYCYTHAEMIA

On a pathophysiological basis polycythaemia can be classified as relative or absolute.

Relative polycythaemia is caused by a disturbance in body fluid balance, for example, decreased plasma volume due to severe dehydration.

- PCV and total plasma protein concentration are increased.
- Total red cell mass is normal.

Absolute polycythaemia can be further classified as primary (polycythaemia vera or primary proliferative polycythaemia) or secondary.

- Plasma volume is usually normal or, in some cases of primary polycythaemia, it may be slightly decreased.
- The total red cell mass and PCV are increased but the total plasma protein concentration is normal.

Polycythaemia Vera

- Polycythaemia vera is a chronic myeloproliferative disorder. The total red cell count, haemoglobin concentration and PCV are usually markedly increased (PCV often in the range 0.70–0.80 l/l).
- The neoplastic proliferation of red cells is not dependent on erythropoietin secretion therefore serum erythropoietin levels are usually low or non-detectable.

Secondary Absolute Polycythaemia

- Secondary absolute polycythaemia is associated with certain congenital cardiac disorders resulting in the right to left shunting of blood, chronic pulmonary disease and high altitude acclimatisation. Erythropoietin concentrations are increased in response to chronic hypoxia (low arterial oxygen saturation).
- Secondary absolute polycythaemia may also be associated with an inappropriate erythropoietin response, i.e. it may occur in the absence of tissue hypoxia. This is seen most commonly with renal tumours, for example renal carcinomas and less frequently renal lymphoma (Campbell 1990).

DIAGNOSTIC APPROACH TO POLYCYTHAEMIA

Relative polycythaemia, for example due to severe dehydration, can be confirmed with little difficulty using the criteria given above. The PCV with relative polycythaemia rarely exceeds 0.65 l/l. The primary and secondary forms of absolute polycythaemia are more difficult to differentiate; unlike humans, polycythaemia vera is rarely associated with concurrent leucocytosis, thrombocytosis and splenomegaly. The initial diagnostic plan should therefore be directed towards ruling out possible causes of secondary polycythaemia.

History and Clinical Signs

The history and clinical signs of absolute polycythaemia relate to the increased red cell mass and resultant hyperviscosity. The PCV is often greater than 0.70 l/l.

- Lethargy, weight loss and exercise intolerance.
- Mucous membranes appear intensely congested (Fig. 34.1).
- The retinal vessels appear distended and tortuous (Fig. 34.2).
- Polydipsia and polyuria.
- CNS signs may be present, most frequently hind limb ataxia or collapse.
- Occasionally there is evidence of haemorrhagic diatheses.

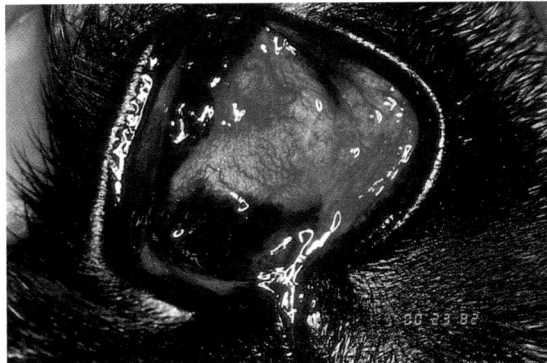

Fig. 34.1   Congested conjunctival mucous membranes of a German Shepherd with polycythaemia secondary to renal lymphoma.

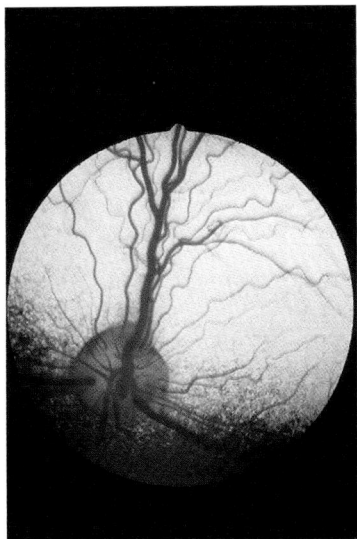

Fig. 34.2   Distended tortuous retinal vessels of dog with primary polycythaemia vera.

Diagnostic Investigations

Plain Radiographs of the Thorax and Abdomen and Intravenous Urography (IVU)

- Plain radiographs of the thorax should be taken to rule out primary cardiac or respiratory disease.
- Radiographs of the abdomen and, if necessary, an IVU should be performed to rule out renal neoplasia as a cause of secondary polycythaemia. Renal angiography is occasionally indicated to detect abnormalities in renal vasculature.

Arterial Blood Oxygen Saturation

Arterial blood oxygen saturation is usually within normal limits (greater than 90%; Pa_{O_2} greater than 60 mmHg) in dogs with polycythaemia vera and cases of secondary absolute polycythaemia associated with an inappropriate release of erythropoietin.

Serum or Urinary Erythropoietin Concentration

The concentration of serum erythropoietin should be measured before phlebotomy.

- Primary polycythaemia is associated with low or unde-tectable erythropoietin concentrations. Erythropoietin levels may be increased in some dogs with poly-cythaemia vera (Cook & Lothrop 1994).
- Erythropoietin levels are usually increased in cases of secondary polycythaemia (although again an area of overlap exists making it difficult in some cases to differ-entiate between the primary and secondary forms of the disease).

Bone Marrow Aspiration and Core Biopsy

Bone marrow aspiration and biopsy is of limited use in confirming a diagnosis of primary polycythaemia.

- The ratio of myeloid cells to erythroid cells may be decreased or normal.
- Erythroid hyperplasia is a consistent finding but the maturation and distribution of erythroid cells is often normal.
- Megakaryocyte numbers may be increased.
- Stores of haemosiderin in cases of primary polycythaemia may be reduced.

MANAGEMENT OF POLYCYTHAEMIA

Relative polycythaemia due to dehydration is treated by the administration of intravenous fluids. The management of polycythaemia vera may require repeated phlebotomy or chemotherapy. Successful management of secondary polycythaemia involves identifying and treating the underlying cause.

Phlebotomy

- Aim to reduce PCV by approximately one-sixth of initial value.
  Replace blood volume and plasma electrolytes with colloidal volume expanders and crystalloid solutions respectively. If facilities are available it is best to separate red cells and return plasma to patient.
- Remove 20 ml/kg body weight every 3–4 weeks thereafter in order to maintain PCV within normal limits or alternatively start on chemotherapy for long-term maintenance (see below).

Chemotherapy

Hydroxyurea is given with an initial loading dose of 30 mg/kg bodyweight p.o. daily for 7–10 days and then 15 mg/kg daily (Peterson & Randolph 1982). Hydroxyurea is a myelosuppressive drug therefore white blood cell and platelet counts should be monitored at 7–14-day intervals until PCV is within normal range and thereafter every 3 months.

REFERENCES

Campbell, K.L. (1990). Diagnosis and management of polycythaemia in dogs. *Compendium on Continuing Education for the Practicing Veterinarian*, **12**, 543–550.

Cook, S.M. & Lothrop, C.D. (1994). Serum erythropoietin concentrations measured by radioimmunoassay in normal, polycythemic and anemic dogs and cats. *Journal of Veterinary Internal Medicine*, **8**, 18–25.

Peterson, M.E. & Randolph, J.F. (1982). Diagnosis of canine primary polycythemia and management with hydroxyurea. *Journal of the American Veterinary Medical Association*, **180**, 415–418.

Lymphoproliferative and Myeloproliferative Disease

J. S. Morris and J. M. Dobson

INTRODUCTION

Haematopoietic neoplasms are the third most common type of tumour diagnosed in the dog, accounting for approximately 8–9% of all canine malignant tumours. They can be divided into neoplastic conditions arising from lymphoid cells, i.e. lymphoproliferative disease (LPD) and both neoplastic and dysplastic conditions arising from myeloid cells, i.e. myeloproliferative disease (MPD). LPD may develop from solid lymphoid organs, e.g. lymphoma, as well as from bone marrow, e.g. lymphoid leukaemias and multiple myeloma. In contrast, all MPD are derived from haematopoietic stem cells in the bone marrow. They include dysplastic or hyperplastic conditions such as myelofibrosis and myelodysplastic syndromes as well as the myeloid leukaemias. Although MPD are derived from red blood cells, platelets, and non-lymphoid white blood cells, only those of the white blood cells will be discussed in this chapter. The term leukaemia is restricted to haematopoietic tumours which are derived from bone marrow and these may be of lymphoid or myeloid origin. For the purposes of this chapter, lymphoid and myeloid leukaemias will be grouped together according to the degree of maturity of the cell type involved, i.e. as either acute or chronic leukaemias.

STRUCTURE AND FUNCTION

Haematopoietic tumours arise either in the bone marrow or solid lymphoid organs. The structure and function of normal bone marrow are discussed in Chapter 32. The lymphoid system consists of lymphocytes, epithelial and stromal cells arranged either in encapsulated organs or as accumulations of diffuse tissue. The system is divided into primary and secondary organs.

Primary organs arise early in fetal life and are the major sites of lymphopoiesis where stem cells proliferate and differentiate to form mature functional lymphocytes. In the fetus, the liver and later the bone marrow are the sources of lymphoid cells and in the adult, the bone marrow continues this function. T cells are further processed by the thymus but there is no other organ in mammals equivalent of the bursa of Fabricius in birds which further processes B cells. The thymus degenerates soon after birth.

Secondary lymphoid organs arise much later in fetal life and persist throughout adult life. They include lymph nodes (Fig. 35.1), spleen (Fig. 35.2) and mucosal associated tissues (Peyer's patches and tonsils). These organs respond to antigenic stimulation and are rich in macrophages and dendritic cells which trap and process antigen and interact with lymphocytes to generate an immune response. Lymphocytes made in the primary organs migrate via the blood to secondary peripheral organs and then return to the blood via the lymphatic system and thoracic duct thus forming a circulating system of lymphocyte traffic.

APPROACH TO THE PATIENT

The general features common to all LPD and MPD will be discussed in this section. Specific details for individual diseases will be considered under separate headings.

History

The majority of cases of multicentric lymphoma (LSA) and chronic lymphocytic leukaemia (CLL) are clinically well and are diagnosed following the discovery of a solid

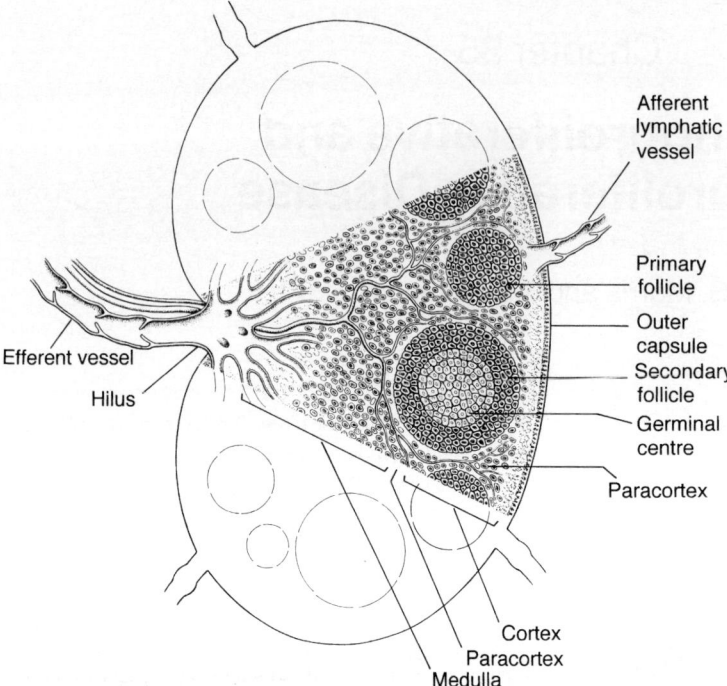

Fig. 35.1 Structure of lymph node (schematic).
Lymph nodes are bean-shaped structures often located at
branches of lymphatic vessels in order to filter antigen from
tissue fluid or lymph, during its passage from the periphery
to the thoracic duct. *Afferent lymphatic vessels* enter the
node at points all over the circumference and *efferent
vessels* leave at the *hilus* where blood vessels also enter
and leave. Below the outer *capsule* there is a *subcapsular
sinus* containing macrophages which trap antigen and
numerous other sinuses pass through the node towards
the hilus. The rest of the node is divided into outer *cortex*,
inner *medulla* and an ill-defined region between the two
called the *paracortex*. The cortex is composed of B cells
arranged either in unstimulated *primary follicles* or if they
have been exposed to antigen, as *secondary follicles* with
germinal centres. The *paracortex* consists of T cells
arranged in poorly defined tertiary follicles. The cells of the

medulla include commited B cells, plasma cells and
reticular cells which are arranged as cellular cords
surrounded by medullary sinuses. Mononuclear
phagocytes in these sinuses screen the efferent lymph
before it joins the efferent lymphatics at the hilus of the
lymph node. Cells of the medulla and cortex turn over very
slowly whereas those of the paracortex are in continuous
flux. Lymphocytes enter the paracortex from the blood by
migrating through post-capillary venules known as high
endothelial venules (HEV) and return to the blood via
efferent lymphatics and the thoracic duct. Some T cells also
enter the lymph node via the afferent lymphatics. In non-
encapsulated lymphoid tissues such as tonsils and Peyer's
patches, lymphocytes leave the blood via HEV in a similar
fashion and then pass via afferent lymphatics to draining
lymph nodes.

mass (lymphoma) or a routine blood screen (CLL). Other
cases of LPD and MPD may present with a history of
vague, non-specific signs such as weight loss, lethargy,
lameness, anorexia, vomiting or diarrhoea.

Examination

A thorough physical examination (Box 35.1) should be
carried out including assessment of overall body condition

to estimate weight loss, body temperature, pulse and respiratory rates followed by examination of each body system
in turn. Particular attention should be paid to those systems
typically involved in LPD/MPD.

Diagnostic Investigation

In most forms of LPD/MPD a series of further
investigations (Box 35.2) will be indicated to confirm

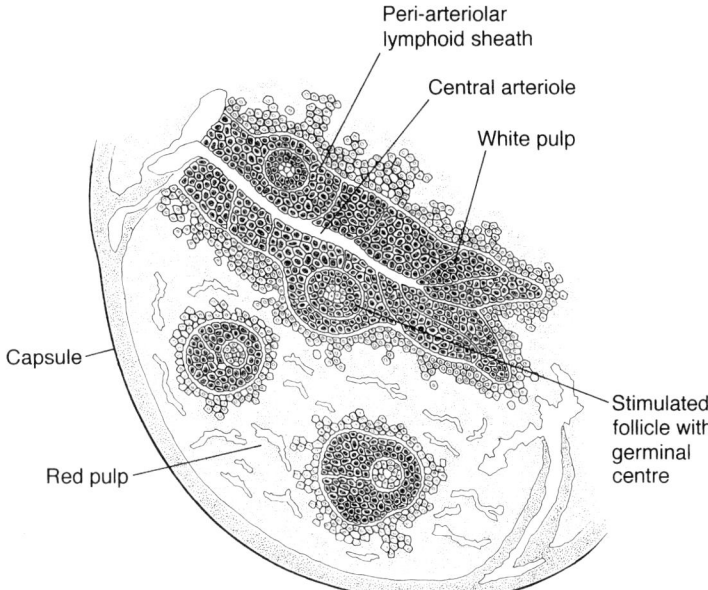

Peri-arteriolar
lymphoid sheath

Central arteriole

White pulp

Capsule

Stimulated
follicle with
germinal
centre

Red pulp

Fig. 35.2 Structure of spleen (schematic).
In the same way that lymph nodes filter antigen from the lymph, the spleen filters the blood. It also provides a system for recirculating small lymphocytes from arteriole to venule through lymphoid tissue without passing through the extensive lymphatic system. The collagenous *capsule* of the spleen contains smooth muscle which penetrates the parenchyma of the organ and together with reticulin fibrils from reticular cells forms a labyrinth of spaces and crevices to support the cells in the organ. There are two main types of tissue: *red pulp* which has many functions including storage of blood, filtration of cells, destruction of effete RBCs, metabolism of iron and removal of intracytoplasmic erythrocyte inclusions and *white pulp* which plays a role in the immune response. Red pulp consists of sinuses lined by phagocytic macrophages, lymphocytes amd plasma cells and white pulp consists of lymphoid tissue arranged around a *central arteriole* to form a *peri-arteriolar lymphoid sheath* (PALS). The T cells form a zone around the central arteriole and the B cells are found beyond this zone either as *primary unstimulated follicles* or as *secondary stimulated follicles* containing *germinal centres.* Many arterioles open directly into stroma or intersinusoidal pulp allowing small lymphocytes to migrate directly to respective lymphoid areas and later rejoin other blood cells passing through the macrophage filter system of the sinusoids to rejoin the blood.

Box 35.1 Physical examination.

Specific systems
- *lymphoid*: examination of all lymph nodes, with comparison of contralateral nodes assessing size, firmness, mobility and painfulness and mechanical obstruction to lymph node drainage, i.e. areas of oedema
- *cardiovascular*: assessment of pulse rate, quality and character, auscultation of heart sounds within chest cavity to detect muffling or caudal displacement and examination of mucous membranes for pallor, petechiae, icterus etc.
- *respiratory*: auscultation of lung sounds to detect loss or caudal displacement, pleural effusion etc.
- *musculoskeletal*: lameness examination and location of bone pain
- *neurological*: if central or peripheral nerve deficits apparent
- *ophthalmic*: examination of iris and ocular chambers for infiltrates, uveitis etc., and retinal examination for signs of hyperviscosity
- *dermatological*: for skin infiltrates or secondary infections
- *gastrointestinal*: for hepatosplenomegaly, abdominal masses, or thickened bowel loops

Box 35.2   Diagnostic investigations.

Haematology

- Blood cell counts (including reticulocytes)
  - Presence of neoplastic cells in blood produces increased cell counts: lymphocytosis, plasmacytosis, granulocytosis or large numbers of immature blast cells.
  - Many of the bone marrow derived neoplasms and stage V lymphoma can suppress normal haematopoiesis leading to non-regenerative cytopenias: anaemia, thrombocytopenia, and leucopenia/neutropenia. A non-regenerative anaemia of chronic disease may also be present.
  - Auto-immune induced cell lysis secondary to LPD or MPD can lead to regenerative cytopenias: anaemia, thrombocytopenia, neutropenia.
  - Regenerative anaemia due to haemorrhage may also be present, particularly if associated with thrombocytopenia.

- Coagulation parameters & fibrin degredation products

  Bleeding disorders may be associated with LPD and MPD for a variety of reasons.
  - Severe thrombocytopenia resulting from myelophthisis may cause spontaneous bleeding.
  - Monoclonal gammopathy with or without hyperviscosity syndrome may give rise to secondary bleeding disorders.
  - Disseminated intra-vascular coagulation resulting from disseminated tumour or immune-mediated haemolytic anaemia may consume platelets and coagulation factors.

Biochemistry

- Liver enzymes

  Liver dysfunction may result from neoplastic infiltration. Elevation of serum alkaline phosphatase (ALP), aspartate aminotransferase (AST), alanine aminotransferase (ALT) or γ-glutamyl transferase (GGT) may indicate liver dysfunction. Confusion may arise if recent corticosteroid therapy has been given since this can also elevate liver enzymes, especially ALP.

- BUN/creatinine

  Renal dysfunction may result from neoplastic infiltration, hypergammaglobulinaemia or hypercalcaemia of malignancy. Renal dysfunction results in elevated blood urea nitrogen (BUN) and creatinine. Dehydration may artificially elevate these parameters.

- Electrolytes

  Hypercalcaemia is common in LPD and some MPD, but it is not pathognomonic and other causes of hypercalcaemia should be investigated.

- Serum protein electrophoresis

  If total protein or globulin is elevated, electrophoresis is indicated in order to differentiate a monoclonal gammopathy associated with LPD from a polyclonal gammopathy associated with inflammation or infection.

- Serum viscosity test) (Appendix 1)

  For high total cell counts, hypergammaglobulinaemia or where clinical signs are suggestive, blood viscosity can be compared with that of water to see if it is increased.

Urinalysis

  Very low S.G. may occur with polydipsia resulting from hypercalcaemia. Elevation of urinary protein (albumin) may indicate severe renal dysfunction and/or glomerulopathy which are possible with prolonged hypercalcaemia or monoclonal gammopathy. Haematuria may be present with bleeding disorders, with cystitis secondary to immunosuppression or if neoplastic infiltration of the kidney disrupts vascular integrity.

Cytology of:

- masses,
- lymph nodes,
- enlarged solid organs (liver, spleen),

  Cytological examination of fine needle aspirates taken from suspicious masses, lymph nodes or bone marrow is indicated to confirm the presence of neoplastic cells of lymphoid or myeloid origin and to assist diagnosis. Patchy infiltration of bone marrow may occur and multiple samples are recommended if initial results

Box 35.2 *Continued*

● bone marrow. (Box 35.3, Figs 35.3–35.6)	are inconclusive. Myelofibrosis or extreme haemodilution of samples in acute leukaemias may prevent diagnostic bone marrow from being obtained by aspiration.
Histopathology/biopsy	Histological examination of a biopsy of a mass, excisional biopsy of a lymph node and needle biopsy of bone marrow may be indicated to make a definitive diagnosis of the disease based on an assessment of tissue architecture as well as cell morphology.
Immunology ● Auto-antibodies	The presence of auto-antibodies demonstrated by a positive Coombs' test, antinuclear antibody (ANA) test or antiplatelet antibody test may indicate auto-immune disease secondary to MPD.
● Immunophenotype	Canine monoclonal antibodies are available to classify lymphocytes by surface antigens. Important prognostic information may be gained from immunophenotype.
Microbiology	The granulocytopenia associated with myelophthisis in LPD and MPD and the reduced immune response associated with neoplastic plasma cells and defective granulocytes can lead to secondary infections of the skin, urinary system etc. Appropriate samples should be submitted for culture and antibiotic sensitivity.
Imaging techniques ● Radiography	*Radiography* of chest and abdomen is necessary for clinical staging of the disease to examine internal lymph nodes, lung infiltrates, organomegaly etc. A skeletal survey is indicated in cases of multiple myeloma to search for bone lesions.
● Ultrasonography	*Ultrasonography* of thymic masses, liver, and spleen will help to confirm hepatosplenomegaly, the presence of focal or diffuse infiltrates and will assist fine needle aspiration or biopsy.
● MRI/ CT	*Specialised imaging techniques* Computed tomography or magnetic resonance imaging may be helpful in assessing thoracic or abdominal organ infiltration and the extent of spinal or cranial masses.
● Scintigraphy	Nuclear scintigraphy using technetium-labelled phosphonate is a sensitive method for detection of bone lesions.

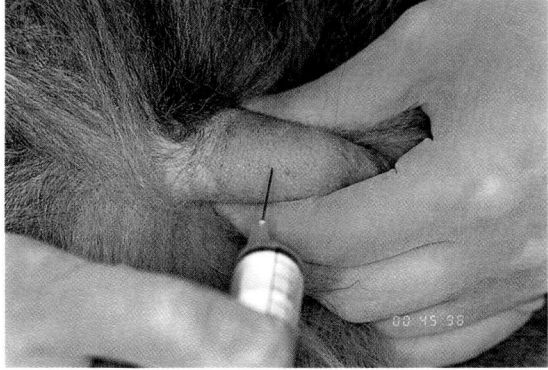
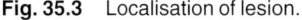

Fig. 35.3   Localisation of lesion.

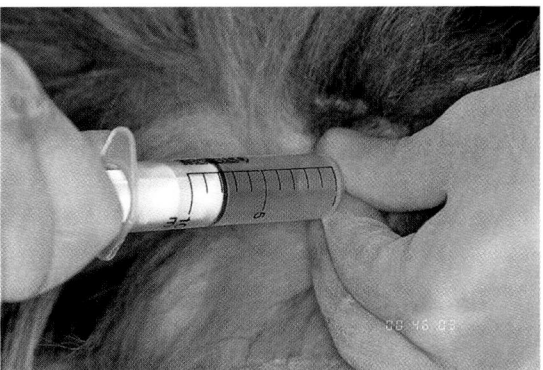

Fig. 35.4   Inserting needle and applying suction.

Box 35.3   Procedures.

FINE NEEDLE ASPIRATE
Indications
Fine needle aspirates are indicated for:

- solitary lymph node enlargement,
- generalised lymphadenopathy,
- cutaneous mass/nodule,
- anterior mediastinal mass/abdominal mass,
- hepatosplenomegaly.

Contraindications
Penetration of an anterior mediastinal or abdominal mass may lead to abdominal or thoracic haemorrhage if there is an underlying coagulopathy or if tumour infiltration is disrupting normal vasculature.

Technique

(1) For superficial masses/lymph nodes
   - Clip the overlying hair to visualise the mass/node more easily.
   - Hold the mass between finger and thumb of one hand and manipulate so that there is minimal overlying tissue (Fig. 35.3).
   - Use a sterile 0.6 mm × 25 mm needle in the other hand, and penetrate the mass, redirecting the needle several times without withdrawing it completely OR with a 10 ml syringe attached to the needle suck back hard several times (Fig. 35.4).
   - Remove the needle and attach a 10 ml syringe full of air OR detach the syringe from the needle and fill it with air before reattaching.
   - Blow out the core of cells within the needle on to a clean, glass slide by expelling the air through the syringe (Fig. 35.5).
   - Place a second glass slide on top of the first at right angles and draw it gently across the first glass slide to smear the tissue sample (Fig. 35.6).
   - The second glass slide carries the smear to be air dried and submitted for cytological staining.
(2) For masses/lymph nodes within body cavities
   - Clipping of the skin and sterile technique should be used.
   - Ultrasonographic guidance will facilitate positioning of the needle within the mass.

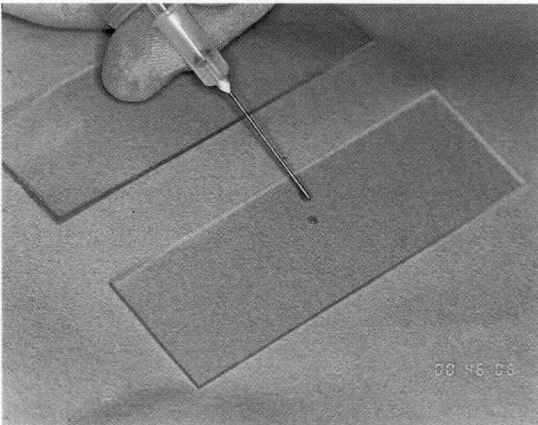

Fig. 35.5   Blowing aspirate on to slide.

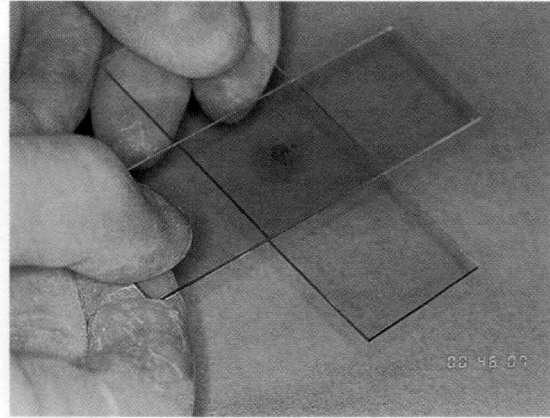

Fig. 35.6   Making smear.

Box 35.4   Differential diagnosis.

Generalised lymph node enlargement	Lymphoma
	Acute/chronic leukaemia
	Multiple myeloma
	Metastatic disease (disseminated MCT)
	Malignant histiocytosis
	Systemic bacterial infection, e.g. *Nocardia, Mycobacteria*
	Systemic parasitic infection, e.g. *Toxoplasmosis*
	Systemic fungal infection, e.g. *Histoplasmosis, Blastomycosis*
	Systemic rickettsial infection, e.g. *Ehrlichiosis*
	Post-vaccination
	Immune-mediated, e.g. Systemic lopus erythematosus
	Mineral-associated lymphadenopathy
Hepato–Splenomegaly	Acute/chronic leukaemia
	Lymphoma
	Multiple myeloma
	Haemangiosarcoma
	Mast cell tumour
	Malignant histiocytosis
	Metastatic neoplasia
	Splenic torsion
Haematological changes (cytopenias etc.)	Acute/chronic leukaemia
	Multiple myeloma
	Lymphoma (stage V)
	Immune-mediated disease
	Haemangiosarcoma
	Sertoli cell tumour/oestrogen toxicity
Hypergammaglobulinaemia (monoclonal)	Multiple myeloma
	Waldenström's macroglobulinaemia (IgM)
	B cell lymphoma
	Chronic lymphocytic leukaemia
	(Chronic infections)
	(Immune-mediated disease)
	(Ehrlichiosis)
Hypercalcaemia	Lymphoma
	Multiple myeloma
	Acute/chronic leukaemia
	Anal sac adenocarcinoma of apocrine glands
	Primary hyperparathyroidism (parathyroid tumour)
	Tumours with primary or metastatic bone invasion, e.g. mammary, prostate, exocrine pancreas
	Other solid tumours, e.g. testicular interstitial tumour, seminoma, thymoma
	Hypoadrenocorticism (Addison's disease)
	Primary renal failure
	Bone lesions, e.g septic osteomyelitis, disuse osteoporosis
	Vitamin D oversupplementation
	Normal finding in young growing animals
	Laboratory error (hyperalbuminaemia / haemoconcentration, lipaemia)

the diagnosis and establish the extent/severity of the disease.

Lymphadenopathy, hepatosplenomegaly, haematological changes, hypercalcaemia and hypergammaglobulinaemia are common findings in LPD/MPD and the differential diagnosis for such conditions includes those listed in Box 35.4.

GENERAL PRINCIPLES OF MANAGEMENT

Supportive Treatment

Fluid Therapy

Many cases of LPD and MPD are dehydrated due to vomiting or anorexia and it is necessary, therefore, to replace the fluid deficit. Cases with hypercalcaemia require urgent fluid therapy for rehydration, promotion of calciuresis and support of renal function (see Box 35.5).

Animals with hypergammaglobulinaemia also may require renal support with fluid therapy (see Box 35.6).

Blood Transfusion

Cases with severe cytopenias may require whole (stored) blood transfusion (or packed red cells) for severe anaemia or fresh blood transfusion if severe thrombocytopenia.

Nutritional Support

Many cancer cases suffer from inability to metabolise foods properly because of altered metabolic pathways in protein, fat and carbohydrate catabolism (Weller 1985; Vail *et al.* 1990; Ogilvie 1993b). It is essential to maintain body weight and improve general condition in order to cope with treatments such as chemotherapy. There is evidence that diets providing energy in the form of fat rather than carbohydrate may be beneficial to cancer patients due to their altered metabolic condition (Ogilvie 1993b). Warming food to just below body temperature or the use of chemical stimulants, e.g. cyproheptadine hydrochloride (Periactin™) may encourage food intake but for severe anorexia, nasogastric tube-feeding provides more satisfactory nutritional support.

Box 35.5 Management of hypercalcaemia.

Hypercalcaemia – aims of management:

- restore circulating volume
  intra-venous fluid therapy with normal (0.9%) saline to replace fluid losses
- promote calciuresis
  intra-venous fluid therapy with normal (0.9%) saline at 2–3 times maintenance (maintenance = 1–2 ml/kg per hour)
  administration of frusemide (Lasix™) at 2 mg/kg two or three times daily. NB: only after circulating volume restored
  administration of prednisolone at 2 mg/kg daily. NB: only after a diagnosis has been obtained since steroid therapy will lyse lymphoid cells and may prevent the correct diagnosis being made
- treat underlying disease
  specific chemotherapy

Once chemotherapy commences, calcium levels should return to normal.
Persistent hypercalcaemia may be treated with

- single intra-venous infusion of mithramycin (plicamycin, Mithracin™) at 25 µg/kg
- biphosphonates, e.g. etidronate sodium (Didronel™) at 15 mg/kg by mouth twice daily.
- (• calcitonin)

Box 35.6   Management.

Hypergammaglobuminaemia
- plasmapheresis to reduce hyperviscosity quickly if very severe
  replace 20 ml blood per kilogram body weight with an appropriate fluid: either centrifuged blood cells from the patient which have been resuspended in crystalloid fluid or cells from a suitable donor
- treat underlying disease
  specific chemotherapy

Specific Treatment

Surgery

Only solitary lymphoid lesions such as lymphoma may be treated adequately by surgery alone. Pathological fractures associated with multiple myeloma may require surgical intervention.

Radiotherapy

Only solitary lymphoid lesions such as thymic or nasal lymphoma may be treated adequately with radiotherapy. Whole body irradiation to include bone marrow is not suitable for dogs because of severe side-effects.

Chemotherapy

This is the established treatment of choice for LPD and MPD. Cytotoxic drugs are administered usually in combinations and numerous protocols which combine drugs of different actions and with varying toxicities have been used to treat LPD and MPD in the dog (see Chapter 5 and later in this chapter). The response to treatment is assessed either as a complete response (CR) (i.e. no clinically detectable disease), a partial response (PR) (i.e. a reduction in detectable disease by at least 50%), no change (NC) or progressive disease (PD). For solid tumours such as lymphoma, this is assessed by palpation, but for other haematopoietic neoplasms, assessment is based on haematological parameters, e.g. reduction in leucocytosis, on biochemical parameters, e.g. presence of monoclonal gammopathy or on the appearance of bone marrow.

Biological Therapy

Biological therapy is a more recent approach to the treatment of cancer and involves the use of biological materials, usually cells or cell products (MacEwen & Helfand 1993). Some of the agents available have a direct cytotoxic effect, e.g. cytokines such as tumour necrosis factor (TNF) while others enhance the natural immune response to tumours, e.g. cytokines such as interleukin 2 (IL-2) or monoclonal antibodies. Other biological agents such as haematopoietic growth factors may be used to reduce the bone marrow toxicity which results from chemotherapy (Ogilvie 1993a). These have the greatest potential for assisting in the treatment of LPD and MPD. Human recombinant granulocyte-colony stimulating factor (G-CSF) and granulocyte monocyte-colony stimulating factor (GM-CSF) are commercially available but their use in the dog leads to antibody production against the foreign protein. Canine recombinant G-CSF and GM-CSF have been tested and shown to be effective in increasing numbers of granulocytes and monocytes (Obradovich *et al.* 1991; Nash *et al.* 1991; Ogilvie *et al.* 1992), but are not yet commercially available.

LYMPHOMA (LYMPHOSARCOMA)

Canine lymphoma may be classified in many different ways, the most common being by anatomical distribution. Of the histological classification schemes which have been applied to canine lymphoma, the World Health Organization scheme (Table 35.1) which was defined for the dog and assesses cell type, is rarely used. Instead, the classification schemes devised for human non-Hodgkin's lymphoma (Tables 35.2–35.4) and which are of great prognostic use in man, have been applied more frequently (Weller *et al.* 1980; Carter *et al.* 1986; Greenlee *et al.* 1990). Many of these assess the growth pattern (follicular or diffuse) within the node as well as cell type (lymphocytic, lymphoblastic etc.). The majority (approximately 85%) of canine lymphomas

Table 35.1   World Health Organization classification of canine lymphoma (Owen 1980).

WHO classification of canine lymphoma
Poorly differentiated
Lymphoblastic
Lymphocytic and prolymphocytic
Histiocytic, histioblastic, histiolymphocytic

are classed as diffuse or minimally follicular. Using the Rappaport scheme (Table 35.2), approximately 70% of canine lymphomas are described as histiocytic (Teske 1993) but little prognostic significance can be attributed to this classification scheme in the dog because of the variable morphological and immunological cell types found. Using the Kiel and National Cancer Institute Working Formulation (WF) schemes (Tables 35.3 and 35.4), the majority of canine lymphomas are found to be of high or intermediate grade malignancy and either large cell (WF) or centroblastic (Kiel). Both schemes are prognostically useful in the dog (Teske *et al.* 1994).

Table 35.2   Rappaport classification of non-Hodgkin's lymphoma (1966).

Rappaport classification of lymphoma
Nodular
Lymphocytic well differentiated
Lymphocytic poorly differentiated
Mixed lymphocytic and histiocytic
Histiocytic
Diffuse
Lymphocytic well differentiated (± plasmacytoid features)
Lymphocytic poorly differentiated
Lymphoblastic
Mixed lymphocytic and histiocytic
Histiocytic
Undifferentiated

Table 35.3   Kiel classification of lymphoma (1974).

Kiel classification of lymphoma
Low grade malignancy
Lymphocytic (CLL, MF, Sezary)
Lymphoplasmacytic, lymphoplasmacytoid
Centrocytic
Centroblastic/centrocytic (follicular/diffuse)
Unclassified
High grade malignancy
Centroblastic
Lymphoblastic (Burkitt's type, convoluted cell type)
Immunoblastic
Unclassified

CLL, Chronic lymphocytic leukaemia; MF, mycosis fungoides.

Table 35.4   National Cancer Institute Working Formulation (1982).

NCI Working Formulation for lymphoma
Low grade malignancy
Small lymphocytic
Follicular predominantly small cleaved
Follicular mixed small cleaved and large cell
Intermediate grade malignancy
Follicular predominantly large cell
Diffuse small cleaved
Diffuse mixed small cleaved and large cell
Diffuse large cell (cleaved/non-cleaved)
High grade malignancy
Immunoblastic
Lymphoblastic (convoluted/non-convoluted)
Small noncleaved (Burkitt's)

The development of canine monoclonal antibodies has enabled the classification of canine lymphomas by immunophenotype. The majority of lymphomas are derived from B cells with estimates of between 10% and 38% derived from T cells. No correlation between immunophenotype and morphological type can be made although T cell lymphomas are often of low or intermediate cytomorphological grade (Teske 1993).

Epidemiology

- *Incidence* Lymphoma is the commonest haematopoietic tumour in the dog accounting for 5–7% of all canine neoplasms and 80–90% of all haematopoietic neoplasms. Incidence is 13–24 cases/100 000 dogs per year.
- *Age* Most cases are middle aged (mean 6–7 years) although young dogs may be affected. 'Histiocytic' lymphoma affects a younger age group (mean 4 years).
- *Sex* Some studies report more males affected, others more females and some report no sex difference.
- *Breed* Breeds reported to be at greater risk include Scottish Terriers, Boxers, Bassett Hounds, Bulldogs, Bernese Mountain Dogs, Airedale Terriers and Saint Bernards.
- *Genetics* A familial incidence has been reported in the Bullmastiff (Onions 1984). Familial clustering has been reported in Rottweilers and Otterhounds (Teske 1993).

Aetiology

Lymphoma is considered to be a multifactorial disease with no clear viral aetiology confirmed in the dog. C-type retroviruses are responsible for the disease in other species, e.g. feline leukaemia virus in the cat.

Pathogenesis

Lymphoma arises from the neoplastic transformation and subsequent proliferation of lymphocytes in solid lymphoid organs. It may originate at one site and progress to others or develop in multiple sites simultaneously. Neoplastic lymphoid cells may circulate in the blood and/or invade bone marrow resulting in myelosuppression. Node enlargement may block lymph drainage and cause regional oedema or compress other structures such as the trachea, oesophagus or intestines resulting in associated clinical signs.

Neoplastic lymphoid cells may secrete factors which act systemically to produce 'paraneoplastic diseases' such as hypercalcaemia and hypergammaglobulinaemia. Hypercalcaemia is present in 10–40% of lymphoma cases and has been associated with mediastinal forms and those thought to be T cell derived (Greenlee *et al.* 1990; Rosenberg *et al.* 1991). Levels of parathyroid hormone-related protein (PTHrP) are slightly elevated in canine lymphoma and may contribute to the hypercalcaemia, but other osteoclast activating factors such as the cytokines interleukin-1, tumour necrosis factor and transforming growth factors may play a greater role (Rosol *et al.* 1992, 1994). Since calcium has important functions in stability and excitability of cellular membranes, hypercalcaemia affects the neuromuscular, gastrointestinal, renal and cardiovascular systems. Hypergammaglobulinaemia is less common than hypercalcaemia. Neoplastic B lymphocytes may secrete immunoglobulins which result in a monoclonal spike detectable in the globulin fraction on serum protein electrophoresis. Clinical signs relate to the hyperviscosity caused by certain types of immunoglobulin, particularly IgM and the resulting poor oxygen perfusion.

Clinical Features

The clinical presentation of lymphoma varies according to the anatomical type. Four anatomical groups are recognised, of which the multicentric form is most common in the dog (Table 35.5).

(1) *Multicentric*: solitary or generalised lymphadenopathy, ± hepatosplenomegaly, ± bone marrow and other organ involvement (see staging system: Table 35.6).

Table 35.5   Anatomical classification of canine lymphoma.

- Multicentric
- Mediastinal (thymic)
- Alimentary
- Cutaneous
- Extranodal (renal, ocular, spinal etc.)

Table 35.6   Clinical staging of canine multicentric lymphoma (Owen 1980).

Stage	Extent of disease
I	Involvement limited to a single lymph node or lymphoid tissue in organ
II	Involvement of many lymph nodes in a regional area (± tonsils)
III	Generalised lymph node involvement
IV	Hepatic and/or splenic involvement (± stage III)
V	Manifestations in the blood and involvement of bone marrow and/or other organ systems (± stage I–IV)

Each stage is subclassified into: (a) without systemic signs, (b) with systemic signs.

- most cases are stage III, IV or V
- lymph nodes massively enlarged, hard, but non-painful (Fig. 35.7)
- majority of cases clinically well
- minority of cases show non-specific signs (weight loss, anorexia, lethargy)
- hypercalcaemia common (20% of cases)

(2) *Mediastinal (thymic)*: anterior mediastinal lymphadenopathy and possible pleural effusion ± bone marrow infiltration (Fig. 35.8).
  - may present with coughing, dyspnoea, regurgitation, Horner's syndrome
  - caudal displacement of heart and lung sounds on auscultation
  - hypercalcaemia common and often associated with T cell immunophenotype

(3) *Alimentary*: solitary, diffuse or multifocal gastrointestinal tract infiltration ± mesenteric lymphadenopathy.
  - abdominal mass or thickened bowel loops may be palpable
  - may present with vomiting, diarrhoea, anorexia, weight loss, dyschezia, tenesmus

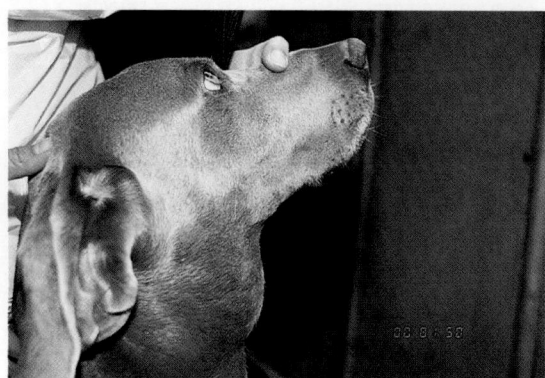

Fig. 35.7   Weimaraner presented with gross generalised lymphadenopathy resulting from lymphoma.

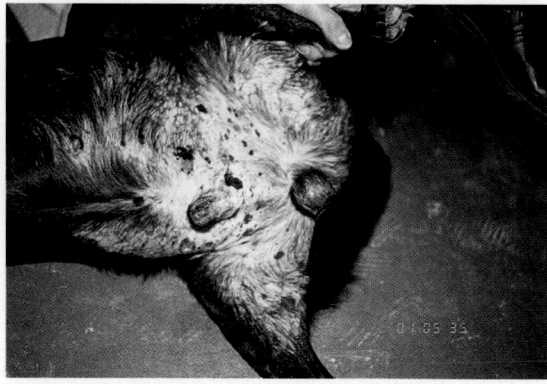

Fig. 35.9   Mycosis fungoides (epitheliotrophic lymphoma). Typical ulcerative skin lesions with patchy alopecia and depigmentation on the ventral abdomen (Black Labrador).

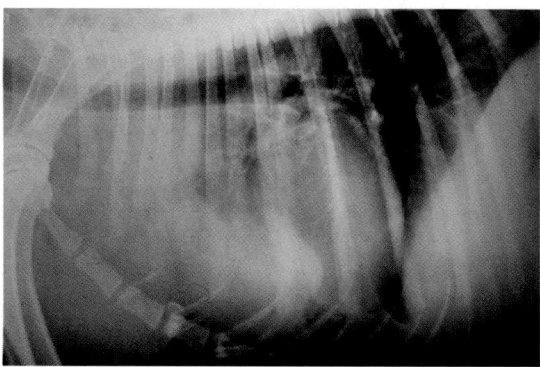

Fig. 35.8   Mediastinal lymphoma. Lateral thoracic radiograph showing the presence of a large anterior mediastinal mass. (Photograph courtesy of Miss Laura Blackwood)

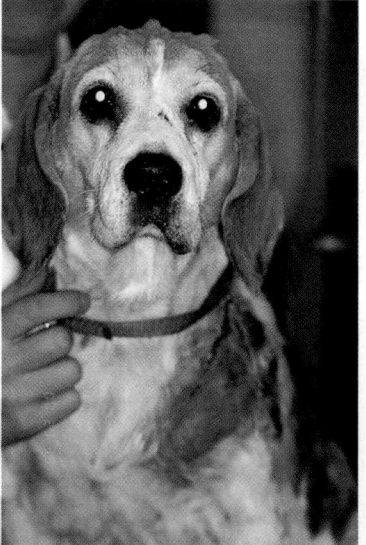

Fig. 35.10   Primary cutaneous lymphoma. Beagle bitch presenting with rapid onset multiple cutaneous lesions, those over the left shoulder region becoming erythematous and ulcerated.

- occasionally get complete obstruction or peritonitis secondary to gastrointestinal rupture

(4) *Cutaneous lymphoma*
- *Primary cutaneous lymphoma*: includes two forms, both of which originate in the skin but may later spread to abdominal viscera, lymph nodes and bone marrow.
  - ○ The *epitheliotropic form*, 'mycosis fungoides' which has a tropism for adnexal structures. This presents with a chronic history of alopecia, depigmentation, desquamation, pruritus, erythema, progressing over months or years to plaque formation characterised by crusting and ulceration and finally to tumour formation (nodules or masses) (Fig. 35.9). Lesions are often around mucocutaneous junctions or in the oral cavity (Kwochka 1986; Walton 1986; Scott *et al.* 1995). Lymphocytes are predominantly CD8+ and CD3+ T cells (Moore *et al.* 1994).
  - ○ *Non-epitheliotropic (dermal) form* which is a more aggressive disease, spreading rapidly

from multiple cutaneous lesions (Fig. 35.10) to involve lymph nodes, abdominal viscera and bone marrow. Lymphocytes are also likely to be T cells.

- *Secondary cutaneous lymphoma*: the dermis is also a site of secondary spread for other forms of lymphoma, e.g. multicentric, especially for those in which the lymphoid cells have morphological features similar to those of histiocytes (histiocytic lymphoma). Immunophenotype may be B or T cell.

(5) *Extranodal lymphoma*:
- Ocular lymphoma: often accompanies the multicentric form. Presents with photophobia, blepharospasm, epiphora, hyphaema, hypopyon, ocular mass, anterior uveitis, chorioretinal involvement, retinal detachment (Fig. 35.11).
- Neural lymphoma: may involve central or peripheral nervous system, be solitary or diffuse and primary or secondary to multicentric form. Variable presenting signs, including paralysis, paresis, lameness, muscle atrophy or central signs (Fig. 35.12).

Paraneoplastic Disease

Hypercalcaemia: Presenting signs include polydipsia, polyuria, anorexia, vomiting, constipation, depression, muscle weakness, cardiac arrhythmias.

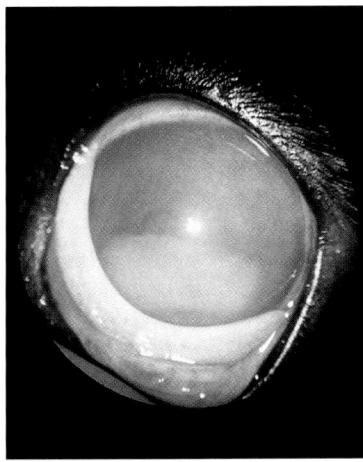

Fig. 35.11 Ocular involvement: lymphoma involving the anterior chamber of the eye. (Photograph courtesy of Dr Simon Peterson-Jones)

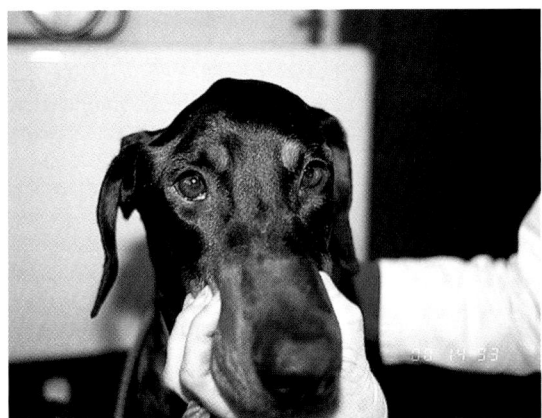

Fig. 35.12 Neurological involvement – young Doberman presented with generalised lymphadenopathy, thrombocytopenia and marked unilateral temporal muscle wastage, the latter thought to be due to lymphomatous infiltration of the fifth cranial nerve.

Monoclonal gammopathy: Presenting signs include bleeding disorders, thromboembolism, ocular lesions (retinal detachment, tortuous blood vessels), neurological signs and infections.

Diagnosis

Diagnosis is made by cytological or histopathological confirmation of the presence of a monomorphic population of neoplastic lymphoid cells in a peripheral lymphoid organ (see Box 35.7).

Management

Management involves general supportive measures if clinically unwell, immediate treatment of paraneoplastic syndromes and then specific treatment of the underlying disease.

Supportive Treatment

Hypercalcaemia: Prolonged hypercalcaemia results in irreversible renal damage and immediate steps should be taken to lower serum calcium levels (Box 35.5).

Hypergammaglobulinaemia: See treatment of multiple myeloma and Box 35.6.

Box 35.7   Diagnostic investigations: (as previously outlined).

Haematology	• Complete blood count to detect anaemia, thrombocytopenia, neutropenia, lymphocytosis and immature lymphoid precursors.
Biochemistry	• liver enzymes to detect liver dysfunction
	• BUN/creatinine to detect renal dysfunction
	• electrolytes to detect hypercalcaemia
	• serum protein electrophoresis to detect monoclonal gammopathy if total protein raised
Cytology	• of mass or lymph nodes to detect neoplastic lymphoid cells and confirm diagnosis, and of bone marrow to stage the disease
Histopathology	• of whole lymph node in preference to excisional biopsy
	• to confirm the diagnosis and staging if cytology inconclusive
	• to classify lymphoma cytomorphologically and by growth pattern.
Immunophenotype	• to assess B or T cell and help with prognosis
Diagnostic imaging	• chest and abdominal radiography to detect lymph node and organ involvement and stage the disease
	• ultrasonography to confirm organ infiltration and to aid biopsy or aspiration

Specific Treatment

Chemotherapy

The most common method of treatment for lymphoma is combination chemotherapy. Without therapy, the mean survival time is only 6–8 weeks. With corticosteroid therapy alone it may be extended to approximately 3 months, but with chemotherapy it is usually 6–9 months. If chemotherapy is intended, corticosteroid therapy should not be started before the chemotherapy, since it induces resistance to the cytotoxic drugs and significantly lowers the response rate and survival time (Dobson & Gorman 1994).

A variety of protocols is available for treating lymphoma but regardless of which is used, approximately 70–80% of cases with multicentric lymphoma achieve remission and remain in remission for a mean of 6–9 months. Survival times, however, may range from one week to several years. It is usually recommended to select a protocol and to keep using the same one, in order to familiarise oneself with the drugs and their toxicities. The 'COAP' and 'COP low dose' protocols (Table 35.7) are often selected for induction because they are inexpensive and of low toxicity, but other protocols based on a 21-day cycle or pulse therapy of a different drug each week are also available (Tables 35.8 and 35.9). Before commencing drug therapy it is essential to establish a base-line of haematological parameters with which to compare future samples in the course of treatment in order to assess the degree of myelosuppression induced by treatment. In most cases of multicentric lymphoma the disease eventually recurrs or relapses, and this is often associated with development of resistance to cytotoxic drugs.

A variety of strategies may be followed for 'rescue' treatment in such cases as summarised in Table 35.10.

The management of *multicentric lymphoma* may be summarised as shown in Box 35.8.

Other anatomic forms of lymphoma are generally managed in a similar manner with the exceptions noted below:

• *Mediastinal*
  ○ as for multicentric
  ○ monitor response of disease to treatment by thoracic radiography
  ○ localised radiotherapy of anterior mediastinum may be an option
  ○ surgical excision at thoracotomy may be indicated if diagnosis cannot be confirmed by fine needle aspirates or needle biopsy.

Box 35.8   Management of multicentric lymphoma.

• Induce remission with chemotherapeutic regime
• Monitor response of disease to treatment by lymph node size
• Monitor for drug side-effects
• Proceed to maintenance treatment once remission is complete or intensify the regime if complete response not achieved
• Resort to rescue regime if relapse occurs (Table 35.10).

Induction

COAP

Cyclophosphamide	50 mg/m^2 p.o. every 48 h or for the first 4 days of each week
Vincristine	0.5 mg/m^2 i.v. every 7 days
Cytarabine	100 mg/m^2 i.v. daily for first 4 days of protocol
Prednisolone	40 mg/m^2 p.o. daily for 7 days then 20 mg/m^2 by mouth every 48 h (with cyclophosphamide)

COP (low dose)

Cyclophosphamide	50 mg/m^2 p.o. every 48 h or for the first 4 days of each week
Vincristine	0.5 mg/m^2 i.v. every 7 days
Prednisolone	40 mg/m^2 p.o. daily for 7 days then 20 mg/m^2 p.o. every 48 h (with cyclophosphamide)

Maintenance

COP

After 8 weeks of induction with COAP / COP, continue COP as alternate week treatment for 4 months, then 1 week in 3 for 6 months, and reduce to 1 week in 4 after 1 year.

MOP

As for COP, but to reduce the risk of haemorrhagic cystitis, substitute melphalan (2–5 mg/m^2 by mouth) for cyclophosphamide after 6 months.

LMP / LP

After 8–10 weeks of induction with COAP or COP, change to different drugs for maintenance, i.e. chlorambucil and prednisolone ± methotrexate

Chlorambucil	20 mg/m^2 p.o. every 14 days
Methotrexate	2.5 mg/m^2 p.o. 2 to 3 times per week
Prednisolone	20 mg/m^2 p.o. every 48 h

Note: doses of cytotoxic agents are calculated for body surface area in m^2 – see Chapter 5 for more detailed explanation.

Table 35.7 Chemotherapy protocols for the treatment of lymphoma (continuous).

- *Alimentary*
  - ○ as for multicentric but risk of bowel perforation if full thickness infiltration of bowel wall
  - ○ surgical excision of affected bowel segment and lymph nodes preferable, followed by chemotherapy
- *Cutaneous*
  - ○ as for multicentric
  - ○ other options reported for mycosis fungoides include retinoids, photodynamic therapy or superficial radiotherapy (DeBoer *et al.* 1990). Topical nitrogen mustard is used in humans but is not recommended for animal use since it is extremely hazardous to the administrator.

Chemo-immunotherapy

A new development in the treatment of lymphoma is chemo-immunotherapy. Using hybridoma technology, a monoclonal antibody called CL/MAb 231 (Synbiotics, California) has been developed in order to prolong remission when used in conjunction with chemotherapy. The monoclonal acts via complement-mediated or antibody-dependent cell cytotoxicity (ADCC) pathways which require an intact host immune system. The chemotherapy regime used, therefore, must avoid immunosuppresion of the patient. Initial trials in the USA by Jeglum (1991) showed a median survival time of 591 days compared with 184 days in controls treated by chemotherapy alone and have led to the monoclonal being commercially available. Further assessment of its activity is ongoing.

Table 35.8 Chemotherapy protocols for the treatment of lymphoma (21 day cycles).

Induction

PACO
Prednisolone	20 mg/m^2 p.o. every 48 h
Actinomycin D	0.75 mg/m^2 i.v. on day 1
Cyclophosphamide	250–300 mg/m^2 p.o. on day 10
Vincristine	0.75 mg/m^2 i.v. on days 8 and 15

COP (high dose)
Cyclophosphamide	250–300 mg/m^2 p.o. every 21 days
Vincristine	0.75 mg/m^2 i.v. every 7 days for 4 weeks, then every 21 days
Prednisolone	1 mg/kg p.o. daily for 4 weeks, then every 48 h

COPA
As for COP, except use:
Doxorubicin	30 mg/m^2 i.v. in place of cyclophosphamide every third cycle, i.e. every ninth week

CHOP
Cyclophosphamide	100–150 mg/m^2 i.v. on day 1
Doxorubicin	30 mg/m^2 i.v. on day 1
Vincristine	0.75 mg/m^2 i.v. on days 8 and 15
Prednisolone	40 mg/m^2 daily for 7 days, then 20 mg/m^2 every 48 h, days 8–21
(Potentiated sulphonamides)	NB: protocol very myelosuppressive, therefore antibiotic cover advised

Maintenance

PAL
After 12 weeks induction with PACO, change to different drugs, i.e. PAL for maintenance:
Prednisolone	20 mg/m^2 by mouth every 48 h
Cytarabine	200 mg/m^2 subcutaneously every 7 days
Chlorambucil	20 mg/m^2 every 14 days

COP/COPA
After 1 year of induction with COP (high dose) or COPA, use the same cycle every 4 weeks for another 6 months

COP/LMP
After 12 weeks of induction with CHOP, change to low dose COP or LMP for maintenance (see Table 35.9)

Prognosis

Using large numbers of animals, and multivariate statistical analysis the following prognostic factors have been defined for multicentric lymphoma:

- *Immunophenotype*: The single most important independent prognostic indicator is a T cell phenotype. This carries a poor prognosis regardless of histological grade (Teske 1993).

- *Clinical stage*: Higher clinical stage carries a worse prognosis and substage (b) leads to shorter disease free interval (DFI) and survival.

- *Histological grade of malignancy*: High grade tumours by Kiel classification have reduced attainment of CR and shorter DFI whereas high grade tumours by the Working Formulation classification have shorter survival time (Teske *et al.* 1994).

- *Sex*: No prognostic value in many studies, but females may have longer DFI and survival (MacEwen *et al.* 1987).

Induction

Week 1 (day 1)	Vincristine	0.5–0.75 mg/m² i.v.
	L-Asparaginase	400 IU/kg i.m.
	±Prednisolone	2.0 mg/kg p.o. daily
Week 2 (day 8)	Cyclophosphamide	200 mg/m² i.v. or p.o.
	±Prednisolone	1.5 mg/kg p.o. daily
Week 3 (day 15)	Vincristine	0.5–0.75 mg/m² i.v.
	±Prednisolone	1.0 mg/kg p.o. daily
Week 4 (day 22)	Doxorubicin	30 mg/m² i.v.
	± Prednisolone	0.5 mg/kg p.o. daily
Week 5 (day 29)	Vincristine	0.5–0.75 mg/m² i.v.
Week 6 (day 36)	Cyclophosphamide	200 mg/m² i.v. or p.o.
Week 7 (day 43)	Vincristine	0.5–0.75 mg/m² i.v.
Week 8 (day 50)	Doxorubicin	30 mg/m² i.v.
	or methotrexate	0.6–0.8 mg/kg i.v.
Week 9 (day 57)	No treatment	

Maintenance

Repeat the 8-week cycle twice with an interval of 2 weeks between each drug administration and then for another two times with an interval of 3 weeks between each drug administration. Chlorambucil (1.4 mg/kg p.o.) may be substituted for cyclophosphamide during maintenance cycles.

Table 35.9 Chemotherapy protocols for treatment of lymphoma (weekly pulse therapy/cyclic combination therapy).

Table 35.10 Rescue chemotherapy for relapsed cases of lymphoma.

If response to initial treatment was good return to original induction protocol until remission achieved and then use maintenance protocol.

COAP	Table 35.7
COP (low or high dose)	Tables 35.7 and 35.8
COPA	Table 35.8
CHOP	Table 35.8
PACO	Table 35.8
Cyclic combination	Table 35.9

If response to initial treatment was slow or for a second relapse, change to new drugs for rescue. Return to maintenance once remission complete.

Single agents
Doxorubicin	30 mg/m² i.v. every 21 days
L-Asparaginase	10 000–20 000 IU/m² i.m. every 14–21 days

ADIC
Doxorubicin &	30 mg/m² i.v. every 21 days
Dacarbazine	1000 mg/m² i.v. infusion (over 6–8 hours) every 21 days
CHOP	Table 35.8
PACO	Table 35.8

MULTIPLE MYELOMA (PLASMA CELL MYELOMA)

Epidemiology

- *Incidence*: Multiple myeloma accounts for 8% of haematopoietic tumours and 4% of all bone tumours but less than 1% of all canine malignant tumours.
- *Age*: Occurs in older dogs (mean 8.3 years, range 2–15 years).
- *Sex*: No sex predisposition.
- *Breed*: No breed predisposition.

Aetiology

No aetiology has been proposed in the dog. Chronic antigen stimulation associated with desensitisation of allergies has been implicated in man and C type retroviruses proposed in other species (MacEwen & Hurvitz 1977; Matus & Leifer 1985).

Pathogenesis

The disease arises from the neoplastic proliferation of plasma cells (B lymphocytes) predominantly in bone marrow, although spill over into blood and infiltration of peripheral lymphoid organs may occur. In classical cases the plasma cells retain their secretory function and produce monoclonal immunoglobulin (sometimes called the M protein). IgA and IgG have equal prevalence in canine multiple myeloma. Proliferation of neoplastic plasma cells may cause:

- skeletal lesions: increased osteoclast activity causes generalised osteoporosis or localised multiple punctate lesions (Fig. 35.13), usually affecting vertebral and long bones;
- occasional spinal compression due to formation of an extra-dural mass;
- hypercalcaemia;
- myelosuppression: normal haematopoiesis depressed resulting in anaemia, thrombocytopenia and leucopenia.

Production of monoclonal immunoglobulin causes:

- Coombs' positive anaemia ± haemolysis due to antibody coating of red cells
- Bleeding disorders due to antibody coating of platelets which leads to poor platelet aggregation and release of PF3, thrombocytopenia, decreased coagulation proteins, abnormal fibrin polymerisation and hyperviscosity syndrome

- Hyperviscosity syndrome, usually associated with the largest immunoglobulin molecule IgM, or with IgA dimers which can polymerise but rarely with IgG. Increased blood viscosity reduces oxygen perfusion due to sludging of blood vessels in the vasculature, interferes with cardiac function due to increased peripheral resistance and inhibits haemostasis.

Other features of myeloma are:

- Renal tubular damage caused by plasma cell infiltration, degradation of immunoglobulin molecules by tubular cells, followed by cast formation in the tubules and exacerbated by hypercalcaemia. Concurrent glomerular amyloidosis rare in dogs although present in humans. Immunoglobulin light chains, known as Bence-Jones proteins are excreted in urine and as glomerular damage proceeds, albumin is also lost. Many dogs are hypoalbuminaemic on presentation. Pyelonephritis is common due to increased susceptibility to infection.
- Increased susceptibility to infection due to depression of normal immunoglobulin levels, impaired phagocytosis and granulocytopenia, and depressed cell mediated immunity.

Clinical Features

- non-specific signs including pyrexia, lethargy, depression
- hepatosplenomegaly ± mild lymphadenopathy
- pallor
- bleeding disorders (one-third of cases) seen as epistaxis, gingival bleeding, bruising, petechiae, echymoses, gastrointestinal bleeding
- hyperviscosity syndrome (20% of cases) seen as bleeding disorders, cerebral dysfunction (ataxia, dementia, coma), ocular changes or sudden blindness (retinal detachment, venous dilation and tortuosity) and congestive heart failure (exercise intolerance, syncope, cyanosis)
- nephrotoxicity and light chain proteinuria (one-third of cases)
- hypercalcaemia (20% of cases)
- skeletal lesions (over 50% of cases) causing lameness, pain, paresis or pathological fracture.

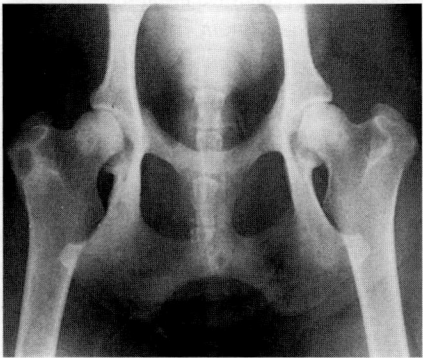

Fig. 35.13   Myeloma: radiograph of the pelvis of a dog with multiple myeloma. Note the multiple 'punched out' lytic skeletal lesions in the proximal femur and the ischium.

Diagnostic Investigations

The diagnostic investigations are listed in Box 35.9.

Box 35.9   Diagnostic investigations for multiple myeloma.

Haematology	• Complete blood count to detect mild to moderate non-regenerative anaemia (70% cases), leucopenia (25% cases), thrombocytopenia (16–30% cases) or peripheral plasmacytosis (10% cases) • coagulation profile to detect bleeding diatheses
Biochemistry	• total protein levels and albumin : globulin ratio to assess immunoglobulin secretion and albumin loss • serum protein electrophoresis to confirm monoclonal gammopathy (Fig. 35.14) • electrolytes to detect hypercalcaemia • BUN/creatinine to assess renal function • urinalysis to assess proteinuria caused by renal damage (albumin seen on dipstick) and Bence-Jones proteins (NB: light chains not detected on dipstick but by heat precipitation test – precipitate forms at 40–60°C, dissolves on boiling and reforms on cooling). Urine electrophoresis
Diagnostic imaging	• *radiography* to screen vertebrae, pelvis and long bones for skeletal lesions
Cytology	• examination of bone marrow aspirates to look for proliferating neoplastic plasma cells and assess the degree of myelosuppression

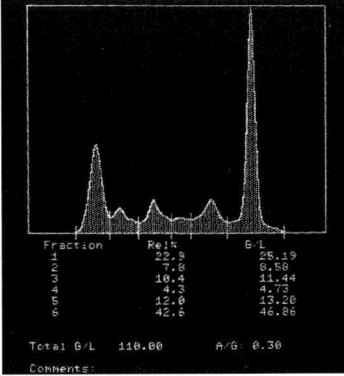

Fig. 35.14   Electrophoretic trace of serum from a dog with a secretory myeloma: showing the characteristic, monoclonal 'spike' in the globulin fraction.

Diagnosis

Three of the following four parameters must be present to confirm the diagnosis of multiple myeloma:

• plasma cells accounting for over 5–10% of bone marrow cells or forming sheets of cells in the bone marrow (essential for definitive diagnosis) (Fig. 35.15);
• osteolytic bone lesions (Fig. 35.13);
• monoclonal immunoglobulin in serum or urine (Fig. 35.14);
• Bence-Jones proteinuria.

Treatment

Supportive Treatment

Supportive therapy may include:

• fluid therapy to reduce hypercalcaemia and support renal function;
• plasmapheresis to reduce hyperviscosity-induced neurological signs, and cardiac changes if very severe (Box 35.6);
• surgical repair of pathological fractures;
• biphosphonate (or mithramycin) therapy to reduce osteoclast activity and prevent further bone lesions – will also reduce hypercalcaemia;
• antibiotic therapy if febrile or evidence of secondary infection.

Specific Treatment

Specific treatment targets the neoplastic plasma cells and usually involves induction with combination chemotherapy based on alkylating agents (melphalan or cyclophosphamide) and corticosteroids (Table 35.11). The response to treatment is assessed by monitoring total protein levels and the presence of a monoclonal spike on serum protein electrophoresis ± examination of bone marrow. Once immunoglobulin concentration is within normal limits, drug doses and frequency are reduced to a maintenance level which keeps the immunoglobulin within these limits.

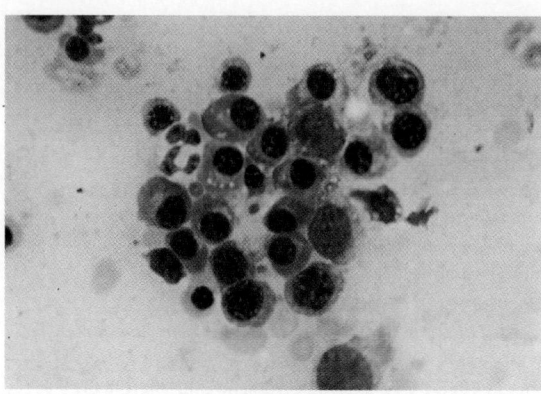

Fig. 35.15 Myeloma – HP photomicrograph (under oil immersion, ×100 objective) cytological preparation of bone marrow from a dog with myeloma, showing clusters of plasma cells.

Radiotherapy may be used to treat localised bone lesions but there is a danger of inducing pathological fracture.

Prognosis

Over 75% of cases respond to treatment with median survival times between 12 –18 months (MacEwen & Hurvitz 1977; Matus & Leifer 1985; Matus *et al.* 1986; Hammer & Couto 1994).

- Immunoglobulin type is not related to prognosis.
- A good initial response to treatment indicates a favourable prognosis.
- Hypercalcaemia, presence of Bence-Jones proteinuria, azotemia or extensive bone lesions reduce survival times.

ACUTE LEUKAEMIAS

The term leukaemia is used to describe any haematopoietic neoplasm derived from bone marrow. These may be of lymphoid or myeloid origin.

Epidemiology

- *Prevalence*: Acute leukaemias account for less than 10% of all haematopoietic neoplasms. The proportion of acute myeloid to acute lymphoid leukaemias is now thought to be 3 : 1 (Couto 1992).
- *Age*: Most cases are young to middle aged (mean 5–6 years for acute lymphoblastic leukaemia (ALL)) but can occur in older animals (range 1–12 years).

Table 35.11 Chemotherapy protocols for the treatment of multiple myeloma.

Induction

Basic protocol

Melphalan	2.0 mg/m² p.o. daily for 7–14 days, then every 48 h
Prednisolone	40 mg/m² p.o. daily for 7–14 days, then 20 mg/m² every 48 h

Additional agent (if response is inadequate)

Vincristine	0.5 mg/m² i.v. every 7 days

Alternative protocols (if response is inadequate)

Cyclophosphamide	50 mg/m² p.o. every 48 h
Prednisolone	40 mg/m² p.o. daily for 7–14 days, then 20 mg/m² every 48 h
±Vincristine	0.5 mg/m² i.v. every 7 days
Chlorambucil	2–5 mg/m² p.o. every 48 h
Prednisolone	40 mg/m² p.o. daily for 7–14 days, then 20 mg/m² every 48 h
±Vincristine	0.5 mg/m² i.v. every 7 days

Maintenance

Use prednisolone in combination with either melphalan, cyclophosphamide or chlorambucil at a dose rate and frequency sufficient to maintain plasma immunoglobulin concentration within normal limits.

- *Sex*: More males than females affected in a 3 : 2 ratio.
- *Breed*: No breed predisposition.

Aetiology

The aetiology of canine acute leukaemias is unknown. Ionising radiation, oncogenic viruses, and benzene exposure proposed for ALL in other species including man (Leifer & Matus 1985). A lentivirus has been isolated from one leukaemic dog (Safran *et al.* 1992).

Pathogenesis

Acute leukaemias arise from the neoplastic transformation and subsequent proliferation of early lymphoid/myeloid precursor cells, leading to the arrest of normal cell lineage differentiation. Depending on the cell type involved, acute myeloid leukaemias can be divided into acute myelogenous without differentiation (AML), acute monocytic/monoblastic (AMoL) or acute myelomonocytic (AMML) leukaemias.

Acute leukaemias are characterised by aggressive biological behaviour and rapid progression. The early blast cells proliferate in the bone marrow at the expense of normal haematopoiesis, spilling over into the blood and infiltrating peripheral organs, e.g. spleen, liver, lymph nodes, bone, nerves. Massive leucocytosis may cause signs of hyperviscosity due to aggregate formation and thrombosis in brain and lungs. Occasionally, neoplastic cells are restricted to the marrow and are not seen in peripheral blood. This is known as an 'aleukaemic leukaemia'.

The effects of cell proliferation include:

- severe myelosuppression, i.e. anaemia, thrombocytopenia and lymphopenia or granulocytopenia;
- increased susceptibility to infection due to reduced humoral and cellular immunity.

Clinical Features

- non-specific signs including weakness, lethargy, anorexia, vomiting and diarrhoea, pyrexia (more common in AML)
- pallor
- mild lymphadenopathy (much less obvious than lymphosarcoma)
- splenomegaly ± hepatomegaly
- bleeding, bruising, joint swelling (haemarthosis)
- disseminated intravascular coagulation (DIC) (more common in AML)
- shifting lameness, bone pain (more common in AML)
- ocular lesions such as retinal and conjunctival haemorrhage, hyphaema, glaucoma, retinal infiltrates (more common in AML)
- neurological signs, neuropathies, paresis (more common in ALL)
- secondary infections, e.g. skin lesions

Diagnostic Investigations

The diagnostic investigations are listed in Box 35.10.

Box 35.10   Diagnostic investigations for acute leukaemias.

Haematology	• Complete blood count to detect cytopenias resulting from myelosuppression, i.e. non-regenerative anaemia, thrombocytopenia, neutropenia (usually more severe in ALL than AML and relatively mild in AMoL); and leucocytosis resulting from atypical neoplastic cells in circulation i.e. lymphoblasts in ALL (often 100–600×10^9/l), myeloblasts in AML (not always present) and monoblasts in AMoL
	• coagulation profile to assess clotting and DIC
Biochemistry	• electrolytes to detect hypercalcaemia
	• liver enzymes to detect liver dysfunction
	• BUN/creatinine to detect renal dysfunction
Cytology	• examination of bone marrow aspirates to look for predominance of blast cells and to assess the level of normal haematopoiesis (Fig. 35.16). Special cytochemical stains essential to differentiate blast cell lineage (Table 35.12).
Diagnostic imaging	• abdominal radiography and ultrasonography to confirm hepatosplenomegaly

	Monocyte marker	Granulocyte markers			
	ANBE	CAE	MPO	LIP	AP
AML	−	+	+	−	+
AMoL	+	−	−	+	−
AMML	±	±	±	±	±
ALL	−(+)	−	−	−	−(+)

Table 35.12 Cytochemical staining reactions for acute leukaemias.

CAE, chloroacetate esterase; ANBE, a-naphthyl butyrate esterase; MPO, myeloperoxidase; LIP, lipase; AP, alkaline phosphatase; AML, acute myeloid leukaemia; AMoL, acute monocytic leukaemia; AMML, acute myelomonocytic leukaemia; ALL, acute lymphoblastic leukaemia.

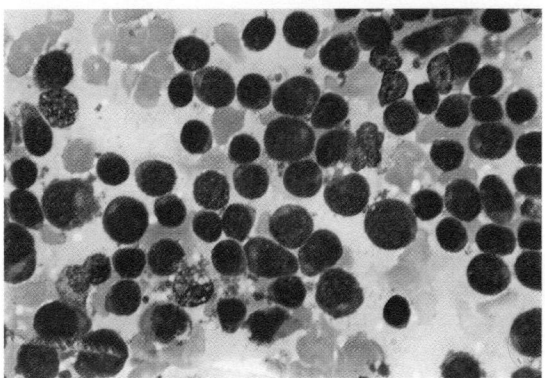

Fig. 35.16 Acute leukaemia – HP photomicrograph (under oil immersion, ×100 objective) – cytological preparation of bone marrow collected from a dog affected by ALL. The marrow is dominated by medium – large lymphoblastic cells.

Diagnosis

The diagnosis of acute leukaemia is based on the predominance (40–50%) of blast cells in the bone marrow, usually accompanied by similar cells in peripheral blood. ALL is differentiated from AML by cytochemical staining (Couto 1985; Facklam & Kociba 1985; Grindem et al. 1985, 1986) and from LSA by much milder lymphadenopathy and much more severe myelosuppression (Leifer & Matus 1985; Morris et al. 1993).

Management

Supportive Treatment

Supportive measures include fluid therapy for dehydration and anorexia, blood transfusion for severe loss of red cells or platelets, and antibiotic therapy for secondary infections.

Specific Treatment

Specific therapy is aimed at destroying the leukaemic cells and allowing normal haematopoiesis to resume. Drugs recommended for ALL are similar to those for lymphoma, i.e. vincristine and prednisolone plus an alkylating agent or another drug whereas those for AML include prednisolone, mercaptopurine or thioguanine in combination with cytosine arabinoside. The latter is used because it may encourage differentiation of the blast cells (Castaigne et al. 1983). Induction protocols for acute leukaemia are given in Table 35.13. These are used until the white blood cell count returns to within the normal range and blast cells are no longer seen in peripheral blood. In theory, drug doses and frequencies can then be reduced to maintenance levels, but in practice, this is rarely achieved. The use of chemotherapy is severely hampered by the degree of myelosuppression which is present with most acute leukaemias and the inability to preserve sufficient levels of normal blood cells during treatment. Intensive medical care, bone marrow transplants and extracorporeal treatment of bone marrow are used in human medicine but are not available, nor are they deemed acceptable for veterinary use. The development of canine recombinant G-CSF and GM-CSF should lead to significant improvements in the treatment of acute leukaemias.

Prognosis

The prognosis is poor for all acute leukaemias due to:

• failure to induce and maintain remission,
• organ failure which enhances the cytotoxic effects of the drugs,
• septicaemia secondary to the disease or treatment.

The prognosis for ALL is slightly better than for AML. Some 20–40% of cases of ALL go into remission, usually

Table 35.13   Chemotherapy protocols for the treatment of acute leukaemia.

Acute lymphoblastic leukaemia

Basic induction protocol
Vincristine	0.5 mg/m^2 i.v. every 7 days
Prednisolone	40 mg/m^2 p.o. daily for 7 days then 20 mg/m^2 every 48 h

Additional agents
Cyclophosphamide	50 mg/m^2 p.o. every 48 h
Cyclophosphamide &	50 mg/m^2 p.o. every 48 h
Cytarabine	100 mg/m^2 s.c. or i.v. daily for 2–4 days (use divided doses if given i.v.)
L-Asparaginase	10 000–20 000 IU/m^2 i.m. every 2–3 weeks

Acute myeloid leukaemia

Basic protocol
Cytarabine	100 mg/m^2 s.c. or i.v. daily for 2–6 days

Additional agents
Prednisolone	40 mg/m^2 p.o. daily for 7 days then 20 mg/m^2 every 48 h
6-Thioguanine	50 mg/m^2 p.o. daily or every 48 h
6-Thioguanine &	50 mg/m^2 p.o. daily or every 48 h
Doxorubicin	10 mg/m^2 i.v. every 7 days
Mercaptopurine	50 mg/m^2 p.o. daily or every 48 h

Alternative protocols
Cytarabine	5–10 mg/m^2 s.c. twice daily for 2–3 weeks, then on alternate weeks
Doxorubicin	30 mg/m^2 i.v. every 3 weeks or 10 mg/m^2 every 7 days

Maintenance

Any of the above combinations of drugs used for induction reduced to a dose and frequency which maintain white blood cell counts within the normal range.

---

with short survival times between 1 and 3 months (Couto 1992) but occasionally for longer (MacEwen *et al.* 1977; Matus *et al.* 1983; Gorman & White 1987). Survival times for AML rarely exceed 3 months (Couto 1985; Grindem *et al.* 1985).

CHRONIC LEUKAEMIAS

Epidemiology

- *Prevalence*: Chronic leukaemias are less common than acute leukaemias. Chronic lymphocytic leukaemia (CLL) is more common than chronic myeloid leukaemia (CML).
- *Age*: Most cases are middle-aged to old (mean 9.4 years for CLL)
- *Sex*: A ratio of male to females of 2:1 is reported for CLL.
- *Breed*: No breed predisposition.

Aetiology

No canine aetiology for chronic leukaemia is reported. Genetic factors but not ionising radiation are implicated for CLL in man and there is an association with auto-immune disease, e.g. systemic lupus ergthematosus, suggesting an immunological aberration (Leifer & Matus 1985, 1986).

Pathogenesis

Chronic leukaemias arise from the neoplastic transformation of late precursor cells in lymphoid and myeloid development leading to proliferation of fairly well differentiated cells. The disease is characterised by slow progression and relatively mild clinical signs. The neoplastic cells proliferate in the bone marrow at the expense of normal haematopoiesis spilling over into the blood and infiltrating peripheral organs, e.g. spleen, liver, lymph nodes. A change from the proliferation of mature cells to blast cells (a blast cell crisis) often occurs as a terminal event with CML but not CLL, months to years after diagnosis.

Effects of cell proliferation include:

- myelosuppression – anaemia, thrombocytopenia and lymphopenia or granulocytopenia but milder than for acute leukaemias;
- secondary infections due to reduced humoral and cellular immunity;
- monoclonal gammopathy associated with 25% of cases of CLL although 10% cases may have reduced immunoglobulin levels.

Clinical Features

In CLL 50% of cases may be asymptomatic and only detected on haematological examination. Remaining cases of CLL and all of CML show mild, progressive disease with vague signs:

- lethargy, anorexia, vomiting, pyrexia, polyuria, polydipsia, weight loss,
- pallor,
- mild lymphadenopathy (more common in CLL),
- splenomegaly ± hepatomegaly,
- skin infiltration,
- hyperviscosity syndrome.

Diagnostic Investigations

The diagnostic investigations are listed in Box 35.11.

Diagnosis

The diagnosis of chronic leukaemia is based on the predominance (40–50%) of relatively mature lymphoid or myeloid cells in the bone marrow, usually accompanied by similar cells in peripheral blood. A marked lymphocytosis ($>20 \times 10^9/l$) is almost pathognomonic for CLL. It is often difficult to distinguish CML from leukaemoid reactions and preleukaemic syndromes because of a lack of specific clinical and laboratory abnormalities characteristic of the disease.

Management

Supportive Treatment

Paraneoplastic complications such as hypercalcaemia and hypergammaglobulinaemia may need to be addressed first.

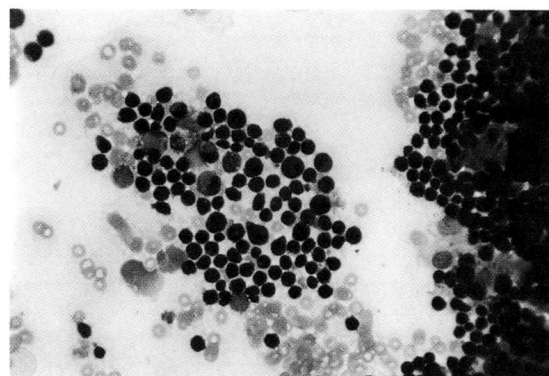

Fig. 35.17   Chronic leukaemia – HP photomicrograph (under oil immersion, ×50 objective) – cytological preparation of bone marrow collected from a dog affected by CLL. The bone marrow is infiltrated by small lymphocytes.

Box 35.11   Diagnostic investigations.

Haematology	• Complete blood count to detect cytopenias, i.e. non-regenerative anaemia and thrombocytopenia resulting from myelosuppression (usually much milder than for acute leukaemias); and leucocytosis resulting from lymphocytosis in CLL (from 5 to over $100 \times 10^9/l$) or granulocytosis in CML with a left shift to myelocytes or occasionally myeloblasts
Biochemistry	• total protein and serum electrophoresis to detect monoclonal gammopathy in CLL
Cytology	• examination of bone marrow aspirates to detect proliferation of mature lymphoid or myeloid cells and to assess the degree of normal haematopoiesis (Fig. 35.17)
Diagnostic imaging	• abdominal radiography and ultrasonography to confirm hepatosplenomegaly

Table 35.14 Chemotherapy protocols for chronic leukaemia.

Chronic lymphocytic leukaemia

Basic induction protocol

Chlorambucil	2–5 mg/m² p.o. daily for 7–14 days then 2 mg/m² every 48 h or 20 mg/m² p.o. as a single dose every 14 days
±Prednisolone	40 mg/m² by mouth daily for 7 days then 20 mg/m² every 48 h

Additional agent

Vincristine	0.5 mg/m² i.v. every 7 days

Alternative protocols

Vincristine	0.5 mg/m² i.v. every 7 days
Cyclophosphamide	50 mg/m² p.o. every 48 hours
Prednisolone	40 mg/m² p.o. daily for 7 days then 20 mg/m² every 48 h
Vincristine	0.5 mg/m² i.v. every 14 days (weeks 2 and 4)
Cyclophosphamide	200–300 mg/m² p.o. or i.v. every 14 days (weeks 1 and 3)
Prednisolone	40 mg/m² p.o. daily for 7 days then 20 mg/m² every 48 h

Chronic myeloid leukaemia

Hydroxyurea	50 mg/kg p.o. daily for 1–2 weeks then every 48 h or 80 mg/kg p.o. every 3 days until remission achieved or 1 g/m² p.o. daily until remission achieved
Busulphan	2–6 mg/m² p.o. daily until remission achieved

Maintenance

Any of the above combinations of drugs used for induction reduced to a dose and frequency which maintain white blood cell counts within the normal range.

Specific Treatment

No treatment may be necessary for asymptomatic cases of CLL although frequent monitoring and haematological screens are advised. Treatment with cytotoxic drugs is usually considered for symptomatic cases of CLL and for CML. The alkylating agent chlorambucil in combination with prednisolone is recommended for treatment of CLL whereas the drug of choice for CML is either hydroxyurea or busulphan (Table 35.14). The aim is to restore the peripheral blood counts to within the normal range and response to treatment is monitored by haematological findings. Once remission is achieved, maintenance therapy is continued at reduced doses and frequencies of the appropriate drugs, in order to keep the white blood cell counts within the normal range.

Prognosis

The prognosis for chronic leukaemias is much more favourable than for acute leukaemias. Mean and median survival times for CLL may exceed 1 year (Leifer & Matus 1985, 1986) but are usually shorter for CML, which has a greater risk of blast cell crisis.

OTHER MYELOID LEUKAEMIAS

Eosinophilic and basophilic leukaemias are rarely reported in the dog. Eosinophilic leukaemias are difficult to distinguish from other hypereosinophilic syndromes and basophilic leukaemias are often confused with mast cell leukaemias. Treatment of both eosinophilic and basophilic leukaemias is with corticosteroids or hydroxyurea.

MYELODYSPLASTIC SYNDROMES (PRELEUKAEMIA)

Certain vague clinical conditions presenting as lethargy, anorexia, depression, and pyrexia are associated with bone marrow which is normocellular or hypercellular but not overtly neoplastic. These conditions are known as myelo-dysplastic syndromes. The bone marrow changes may be reflected by haematological abnormalities such as cytopenias or presence of bizzare cells in the blood and physical findings may include pallor, hepatosplenomegaly, lymphadenopathy, recurrent infections or weight loss. These changes may wax and wane, without ever progressing, but a proportion of cases will develop overt myeloid leukaemia eventually. Treatment of such preleukaemic conditions with chemotherapy is controversial since not all will progress to full leukaemia, but regular monitoring and supportive therapy with fluids and antibiotics is recommended. Differentiating agents (cytosine arabinoside), haematopoietic growth factors or anabolic steroids may also be tried.

REFERENCES

Carter, R.F., Valli, V.E.O. & Lumsden, J.H. (1986). The cytology, histology and prevalence of cell types in canine lymphoma classified according to the National Cancer Institute Working Formnulation. *Canadian Journal of Veterinary Research*, **50**, 154–164.

Castaigne, S., Daniel, M.T., Tilly, H., Herait, P. & Degos, L. (1983) Does treatment with Ara-C in low doses cause differentiation of leukaemic cells? *Blood*, **62**, 85–86.

Couto, C.G. (1985). Clinicopathologic aspects of acute leukemias in the dog. *Journal of the American Veterinary Medical Association*, **186**, 681–685.

Couto, C.G. (1992). Leukemias. In: *Essentials of Small Animal Internal Medicine*, (eds R.W. Nelson & C.G. Couto), pp. 871–878. Mosby Year Book, St. Louis.

De Boer, D.J., Turrel, J.W. & Moore, P.F. (1990). Mycosis fungoides in a dog – demonstration of T cell specificity and response to radiotherapy. *Journal of the American Animal Hospital Association*, **26**, 566–572.

Dobson, J.M. & Gorman, N.T. (1994) Canine multicentric lymphoma 2: Comparison of response to two chemotherapeutic protocols. *Journal of Small Animal Practice*, **35**, 9–15.

Facklam, N.R. & Kociba, G.J. (1985) Cytochemical characterization of leukemic cells from 20 Dogs. *Veterinary Pathology*, **22**, 363–369.

Gorman, N.T. & White, R.A.S. (1987) Clinical management of canine lymphoproliferative diseases. *Veterinary Annual*, **27**, 227–242.

Greenlee, P.G., Filippa, D.A., Quimby, F.W., *et al.* (1990). Lymphomas in dogs. A morphologic, immunologic, and clinical study. *Cancer*, **66**, 480–490.

Grindem, C.B., Stevens, J.B. & Perman, V. (1985). Morphological classification and clinical and pathological characteristics of spontaneous leukemia in 17 dogs. *Journal of the American Animal Hospital Association*, **21**, 219–226.

Grindem, C.B., Stevens, J.B. & Perman, V. (1986). Cytochemical reactions in cells from leukemic dogs. *Veterinary Pathology*, **23**, 103–109.

Hammer, A.S. & Couto, C.G. (1994). Complications of multiple myeloma. *Journal of the American Animal Hospital Association*, **30**, 9–14.

Jeglum, K.A. (1991). Monoclonal antibody treatment of canine lymphoma. *Proceedings of the Eastern States Veterinary Conference*, **5**, 222–223.

Kwochka, K.W. (1986). Cutaneous lymphoma. In: *Contemporary Issues in Small Animal Practice, Vol. 6 Oncology*, (ed. N.T. Gorman), pp. 203–206. Churchill Livingstone, Edinburgh.

Leifer, C.E. & Matus, R.E. (1985). Lymphoid leukaemia in the dog. *Veterinary Clinics of North America: Small Animal Practice*, **15** (4), 723–739.

Leifer, C.E. & Matus, R.E. (1986). Chronic lymphocytic leukaemia in the dog: 22 cases (1974–1984). *Journal of the American Veterinary Medical Association*, **189**, 214–217.

MacEwen, E.G. & Helfand, S.C. (1993). Recent advances in the biologic therapy of cancer. *Compendium on Continuing Education for the Practicing Veterinarian*, **15**, 909–922.

MacEwen, E.G. & Hurvitz, A.I. (1977). Diagnosis and management of monoclonal gammopathies. *Veterinary Clinics of North America*, **7** (1), 119–132.

MacEwen, E.G., Patnaik, A.K. & Wilkins, R.J. (1977). Diagnosis and treatment of canine hematopoietic neoplasms. *Veterinary Clinics of North America*, **7** (1), 105–118.

MacEwen, E.G., Hayes, A.A., Matus, R.E. & Kurzman, I. (1987). Evaluation of some prognostic factors for advanced multicentric lymphosarcoma in the dog: 147 cases (1978–1981) *Journal of the American Veterinary Medical Association*, **190**, 564–568.

Matus, R.E. & Leifer, C.E. (1985). Immunoglobulin-producing tumors. *Veterinary Clinics of North America: Small Animal Practice*, **15** (4), 741–753.

Matus, R.E., Leifer, C.E. & MacEwen, E.G. (1983). Acute lymphoblastic leukaemia in the dog: A review of 30 cases. *Journal of the American Veterinary Medical Association*, **183**, 859–862.

Matus, R.E., Leifer, C.E., MacEwen, E.G. & Hurvitz, A.I. (1986). Prognostic factors for multiple myeloma in the dog. *Journal of the American Veterinary Medical Association*, **188**, 1288–1292.

Moore, P.F., Olivry, T. & Naydan, D. (1994). Canine cutaneous epitheliotropic lymphoma (mycosis fungoides) is a proliferative disorder of CD8+ T cells. *American Journal of Pathology*, **144**, 421–429.

Morris, J.S., Dunn, J.K. & Dobson, J.M. (1993). Canine lymphoid leukaemia and lymphoma with bone marrow involvement: A review of 24 cases. *Journal of Small Animal Practice*, **34**, 72–79.

Nash, R.A., Schnening, F., Appelbaum, F., *et al.* (1991). Molecular cloning and in vivo evaluation of canine granulocyte-macrophage colony factors. *Blood*, **78**, 930–937.

Obradovich, J.E., Ogilvie, G.K., Powers, B.E. & Boone, T. (1991). Evaluation of recombinant canine granulocyte colony-stimulating factor as an inducer of granulopoiesis. *Journal of Veterinary Internal Medicine*, **5**, 75–79.

Ogilvie, G.K. (1993a). Haematopoietic Growth Factors: Tools for a revolution in veterinary oncology and hematology. *Compendium on Continuing Education for the Practicing Veterinarian*, **15**, 851–854.

Ogilvie, G.K. (1993b). Alterations in metabolism and nutritional support for veterinary cancer patients: Recent advances. *Compendium on Continuing Education for the Practicing Veterinarian*, **15**, 925–936.

Ogilvie, G.K., Obradovich, J.E., Cooper, M.F., Walters, L.M., Salman, M.D. & Boone, T.C. (1992). Use of recombinant canine granulocyte colony-stimulating factor to decrease myelosuppression associated with the administration of mitoxantrone in the dog. *Journal of Veterinary Internal Medicine*, **6**, 44–47.

Onions, D.E. (1984). A prospective study of familial canine lymphoma. *Journal of the National Cancer Institute*, **72**, 909.

Owen, L.N. (1980). *TNM Classification of Tumours in Domestic Animals*. WHO, Geneva.

Rosenberg, M.P., Matus, R.E. & Patnaik, A.K. (1991). Prognostic factors in dogs with lymphoma and associated hypercalcaemia. *Journal of Veterinary Internal Medicine*, **5**, 268–271.

Rosol, T.J., Nagode, L.A., Couto, C.G., *et al.* (1992). Parathyroid hormone (PTH)-related protein, PTH, and 1,25-dihydroxyvitamin D in dogs with cancer-associated hypercalcaemia. *Endocrinology*, **131**, 1157–1164.

Rosol, T.J., Chew, D.J., Hammer, A.S., *et al.* (1994). Effect of mithramycin on hypercalcaemia in dogs. *Journal of the American Animal Hospital Association*, **30**, 244–250.

Safran, N., Perk, K. & Eyal, O. (1992). Isolation and preliminary characterisation of a novel retrovirus from a leukaemic dog. *Research in Veterinary Science*, **52**, 250–255.

Scott, D.W., Miller, W.H. & Griffin, C.E. (1995). Neoplastic and non-neoplastic tumors. In: *Muller & Kirk's Small Animal Dermatology*, (eds D.W. Scott, W.H. Miller & C.E. Griffin), 5th edn. pp. 990–1126. W.B. Saunders, Philadelphia.

Teske, E. (1993). *Non-Hodgkin's lymphoma in the dog: Characterization and experimental therapy*. PhD thesis, University of Utrecht.

Teske, E., van Heerde, P., Rutteman, G.R., Kurzman, I.D., Moore, P.F. & MacEwen, E.G. (1994). Prognostic factors for treatment of malignant lymphoma in dogs. *Journal of the American Veterinary Medical Association*, **205**, 1722–1728.

Vail, D.M., Ogilvie, G.K. & Wheeler, S.L. (1990). Metabolic alterations in patients with cancer cachexia. *Compendium on Continuing Education for the Practicing Veterinarian*, **12**, 381–386.

Walton, D.K. (1986). Canine epidermotropic lymphoma. In: *Current Veterinary Therapy IX Small Animal Practice*, (ed. R.W. Kirk), pp. 609–614. W.B. Saunders, Philadelphia.

Weller, R.E. (1985). Cancer-associated hypoglycemia in companion animals. *Compendium on Continuing Education for the Practicing Veterinarian*, **7**, 437–447.

Weller, R.E., Holmberg, C.A., Theilen, G.H. & Madewell, B.R. (1980). Histologic classification as a prognostic criterion for canine lymphosarcoma. *American Journal of Veterinary Research*, **41**, 1310–1314.

White, S.D., Rosychuk, R.A.W., Scott, K.V., *et al.* (1993). Use of isotretinoin and etretinate for the treatment of benign cutaneous neoplasia and cutaneous lymphoma in dogs. *Journal of the American Veterinary Medical Association*, **202**, 387–391.

FURTHER READING

General

Cotter, S.M. (1986). Clinical management of lymphoproliferative, myeloproliferative, and plasma cell neoplasia. In: *Contemporary Issues in Small Animal Practice, Vol. 6, Oncology*, (ed. N.T. Gorman), pp. 169–194. Churchill Livingstone, Edinburgh.

Lymphoma

Carter, R.F., Harris, C.K., Withrow, S.J., Valli, V.E.O. & Susaneck, S.J. (1987). Chemotherapy of canine lymphoma with histopathological correlation: Doxorubicin alone compared to COP as first treatment regimen. *Journal of the American Animal Hospital Association*, **23**, 587–596.

Cotter, S.M. (1983). Treatment of lymphoma and leukemia with cyclophosphamide, vincristine, and prednisolone: 1. Treatment of dogs. *Journal of the American Animal Hospital Association*, **19**, 159–165.

Couto, C.G. (1985). Canine Lymphomas: Something Old, Something New. *Compendium on Continuing Education for the Practicing Veterinarian*, **7**, 291–302.

Couto, C.G., Rutgers, H.C., Sherding, R.G. & Rojko, J. (1989). Gastrointestinal Lymphoma in 20 Dogs. *Journal of Veterinary Internal Medicine*, **3**, 73–78.

Crow, S.E. (1982). Lymphosarcoma (malignant lymphoma) in the dog: diagnosis and treatment. *Compendium on Continuing Education for the Practicing Veterinarian*, **4**, 283–292.

Dobson, J.M. & Gorman, N.T. (1993). Canine multicentric lymphoma 1: Clinico-pathological presentation of the disease. *Journal of Small Animal Practice*, **34**, 594–598.

Hahn, K.A., Richardson, R.C., Teclaw, R.F., *et al.* (1992). Is maintenance chemotherapy appropriate for the management of canine malignant lymphoma? *Journal of Veterinary Internal Medicine*, 6, 3–10.

Leifer, C.E. & Matus, R.E. (1986). Canine lymphoma: clinical considerations. *Seminars in Veterinary Medicine and Surgery (Small Animal)*, 1, 43–50.

MacEwen, E.G., Brown, N.O., Patnaik, A.K., Hayes, A.A. & Passe, S. (1981). Cyclic combination chemotherapy of canine lymphosarcoma. *Journal of the American Veterinary Medical Association*, 178, 1178–1181.

Madewell, B.R. (1975). Chemotherapy for canine lymphosarcoma. *American Journal of Veterinary Research*, 36, 1525–1528.

Price, G.S., Page, R.L., Fischer, B.M., Levine, J.F. & Gerig, T.M. (1991). Efficacy and toxicity of doxorubicin/cyclophosphamide maintenance therapy in dogs with multicentric lymphosarcoma. *Journal of Veterinary Internal Medicine*, 5, 259–262.

Rosenthal, R.C. & MacEwen, E.G. (1990). Treatment of lymphoma in dogs. *Journal of the American Veterinary Medical Association*, 196, 774–781.

Hypercalcaemia

Drazner, F.H. (1981). Hypercalcaemia in the dog and cat. *Journal of the American Veterinary Medical Association*, 178, 1253–1256.

Elliott, J., Dobson, J.M., Dunn, J.K., Herrtage, M.E. & Jackson, K.F. (1991). Hypercalcaemia in the dog: a study of 40 cases. *Journal of Small Animal Practice*, 32, 564–571.

Moreau, R. & Squires, R.A. (1992). Hypercalcaemia. *Compendium on Continuing Education for the Practicing Veterinarian*, 14, 1077–1086.

Weller, R.E. & Hoffman, W.E. (1992). Renal function in dogs with lymphosarcoma and associated hypercalcaemia. *Journal of Small Animal Practice*, 33, 61–66.

Hyperviscosity

Matus, R.E., Leifer, C.E., Gordon, B.R., MacEwen, E.G. & Hurvitz, A.I. (1983). Plasmapheresis and chemotherapy of hyperviscosity syndrome associated with monoclonal gammopathy in the dog. *Journal of the American Veterinary Medical Association*, 183, 215–218.

Biological Therapy

MacEwen, E.G. (1990). Biologic response modifiers: The future of cancer therapy? *Veterinary Clinics of North America: Small Animal Practice*, 20, 1055–1073.

Perren, T. & Selby, P. (1992). Biological therapy. *British Medical Journal*, 304, 1621–1623.

APPENDIX 1 HYPERVISCOSITY MEASUREMENT

Indications

Hyperviscosity measurement is indicated if:

- clinical signs are suggestive,
- serum total protein is elevated,
- red or white blood cell counts are massively elevated.

Technique

Serum is drawn into a capillary tube/volumetric pipette, allowed to flow out under gravity and the rate of flow measured. The procedure is repeated with an equal volume of water. Normal serum viscosity is 1.6 to 1.8 times that of water. Clinical signs of hyperviscosity are present when serum viscosity is five times that of water.

Chapter 36

Bleeding Disorders

A. Mackin

INTRODUCTION

Haemostasis is a complex series of local and systemic homeostatic mechanisms that prevent excessive haemorrhage from damaged blood vessels. Bleeding disorders are characterised by generalised haemorrhage (or predisposition to haemorrhage) associated with a defect in one or more of the components of normal haemostasis.

STRUCTURE AND FUNCTION

Haemostasis is a complicated process involving dynamic interactions between vasculature, platelets and coagulation proteins (Troy 1988; Hackner 1995). Haemostasis is divided into:

- primary haemostasis, the vascular/platelet phase, and
- secondary haemostasis, the subsequent coagulation phase.

The end product of the combination of primary and secondary haemostasis is a solid clot composed of fused platelets enclosed in a tight mesh of fibrin strands.

- Fibrinolysis, the final phase of haemostasis, is the process by which blood clots are dissolved via the dissolution of fibrin.

Primary Haemostasis

Primary haemostasis commences with vasoconstriction triggered by vessel injury, and continues until vessel

integrity is restored and bleeding stops (Feldman 1989). Platelets respond to vessel injury by adhering to exposed vascular subendothelium (adhesion) and other platelets (primary aggregation), changing shape, and releasing substances that promote further vasoconstriction and activate additional platelets (the release reaction). Effective platelet adhesion to vascular subendothelium is facilitated by von Willebrand factor (vWf), a large glycoprotein that circulates in platelets and plasma and links platelet surface membranes to subendothelial proteins such as collagen. Platelet contraction and further aggregation triggered by the substances released by the platelets themselves (secondary aggregation) continue until the original vessel injury is sealed by a relatively fragile platelet plug (Fig. 36.1).

Platelets are small non-nucleated cells composed of membrane-bound cytoplasm (Fig. 36.2) formed via the fragmentation of megakaryocytes. Fragmentation of a single megakaryocyte may produce hundreds of platelets. Following release from the marrow, circulating platelet life span in the normal dog is about one week. Aged and damaged platelets are removed from the circulation by the mononuclear phagocytic system, particularly within the spleen and liver. Thrombopoiesis, the process of platelet production, normally maintains canine platelet numbers at greater than 150×10^9 platelets/l, a count far greater than that needed to prevent spontaneous haemorrhage (about 50×10^9 platelets/l).

Secondary Haemostasis

Primary haemostasis alone will only be temporarily beneficial unless the fragile platelet plug is reinforced by a durable mesh of insoluble fibrin assembled by the coagulation cascade (secondary haemostasis). Secondary haemostasis is dependent on the complex interactions of a number of circulating coagulation proteins within the intrinsic, extrinsic and common pathways of the clotting cascade (Fig. 36.3). Effective secondary haemostasis also requires the presence

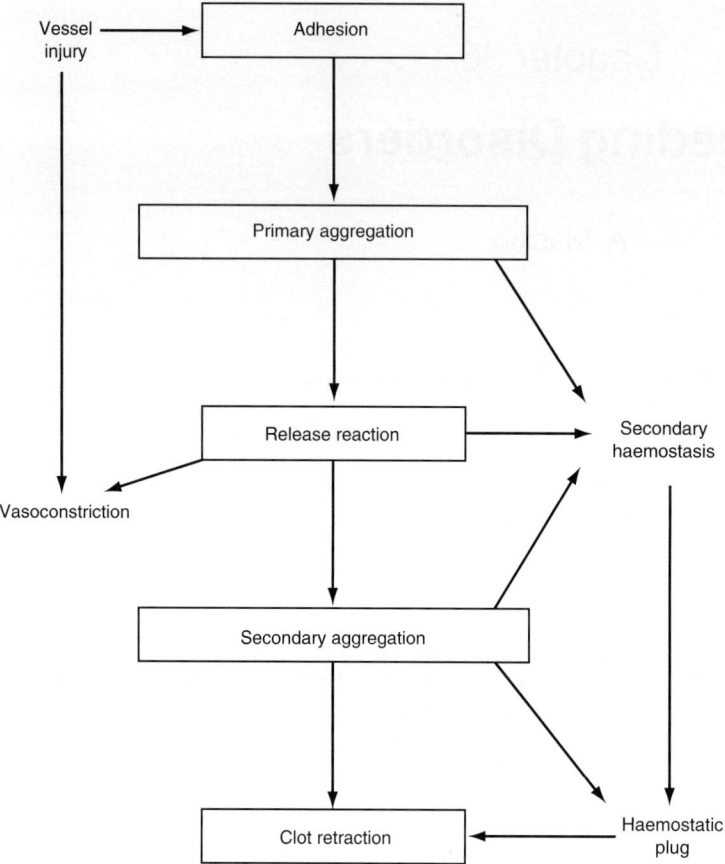

Fig. 36.1 Role of platelets in haemostasis.

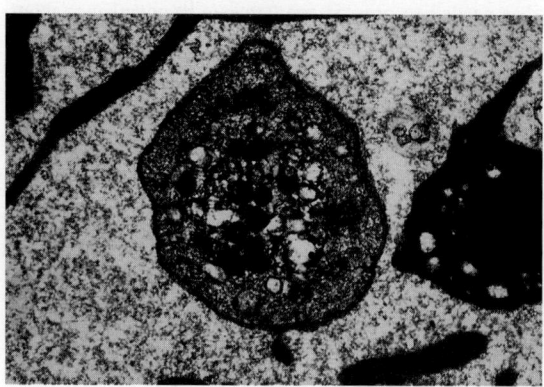

Fig. 36.2 Ultrastructure of a normal canine platelet demonstrated by transmission electron microscopy (photograph courtesy of Malcolm Weir, Ontario Veterinary College).

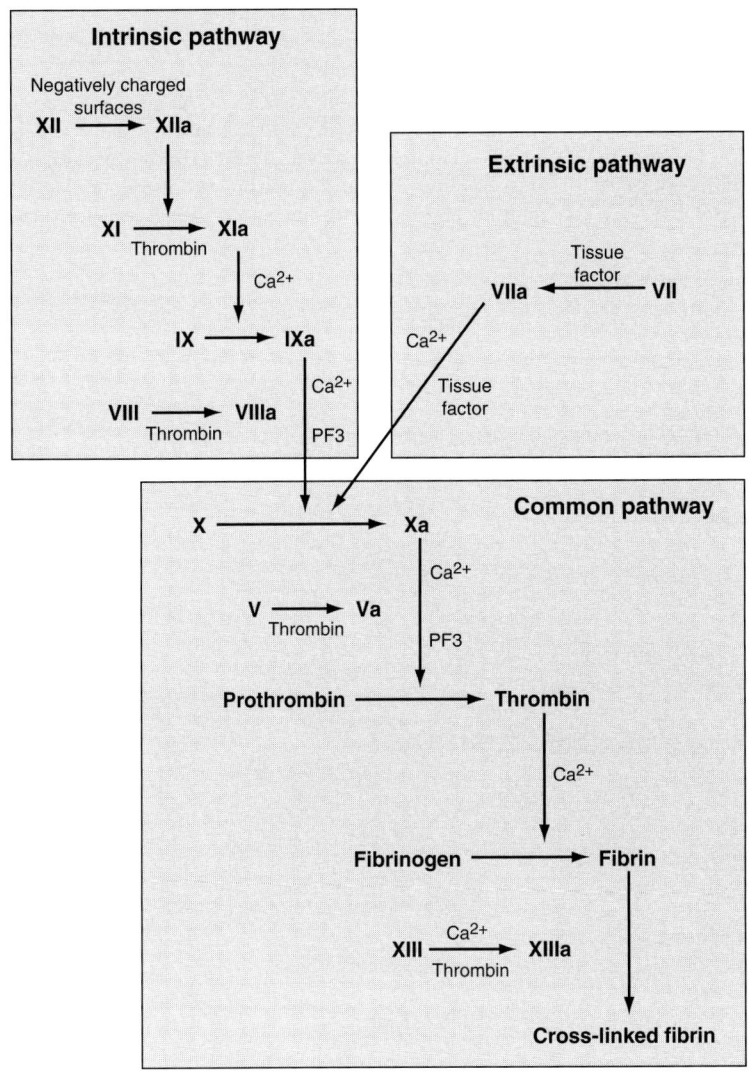

Fig. 36.3 The clotting cascade.

of activated platelets, which provide various substances that bind circulating coagulation proteins and promote the clotting cascade.

The key coagulation proteins (clotting factors) involved in secondary haemostasis are designated by Roman numerals ranging from I to XIII, although factor I is more commonly known as fibrinogen (the precursor of fibrin), factor II as prothrombin (the precursor of thrombin) and factor III as tissue factor. All of the clotting factors are produced by the liver except factor VIII, which is produced by vascular endothelial cells and megakaryocytes.

- The intrinsic pathway contains factors VIII, IX, XI and XII, and is activated when factor XII is exposed to a

negatively charged surface (most likely tissue collagen beneath damaged vessel endothelium).
- The extrinsic pathway contains tissue factor and factor VII, and is activated by the interaction of these two coagulation proteins.
- The common pathway contains fibrinogen, prothrombin, factor V, factor X and factor XIII.

Both the intrinsic and extrinsic clotting pathways activate the common pathway. The central process in the common pathway is the conversion of fibrinogen into fibrin monomers, a process catalysed by thrombin. Fibrin monomers are stabilised by the formation of covalent bonds which cross-link the monomer strands, a process

activated by factor XIII. Contraction of platelets incorpo-
rated within the fibrin meshwork of the blood clot formed
by the combination of primary and secondary haemostasis
(a process called clot retraction) further stablises the
haemostatic plug. Besides the clotting factors, other substances that are essential for efficient secondary haemostasis
include calcium ions and platelet factor 3 (PF3), a phospholipid derived from platelet surface membranes.

Fibrinolysis

The fibrinolytic system consists of plasminogen and a
number of substances (the most well charaterised of which
is tissue plasminogen activator) which convert this inactive
precursor into plasmin. Plasmin breaks down blood clots by
splitting fibrinogen and fibrin into various smaller frag-

Box 36.1 History and examination.

Common features of bleeding disorders

Different bleeding disorders, regardless of whether the major deficiency is affecting primary or secondary
haemostasis (or both), often share many common features:

- Bleeding from multiple unrelated sites:
  Epistaxis
  Haematemesis
  Melaena
  Haematuria
  Anaemia/hypovolaemia (severe defects)
  Neurological signs (intracranial or spinal haemorrhage)

- Excessive bleeding after minor trauma or routine surgery:
  Teething
  Ear cropping
  Tail docking
  Nail clipping
  Neutering

Defective primary haemostasis vs defective secondary haemostasis
Type of haemorrhage can often distinguish defective primary from secondary haemostasis:

Defective primary haemostasis	*Defective secondary haemostasis*
Petechiae/ecchymoses common	Petechiae/ecchymoses extremely rare
Mucous membrane bleeding common	Mucous membrane bleeding rare
Ocular haemorrhage common	Ocular haemorrhage uncommon
Joint haemorrhage uncommon	Joint haemorrhage common
Haematoma formation rare	Haematomas commonly observed
Major body cavity bleeding rare	Body cavity haemorrhage common;
	haemothorax
	haemomediastinum
	haemoperitoneum

Patients with disorders that affect both primary and secondary haemostasis may exhibit a mixture of clinical
features characteristic of both types of haemostatic disorder.

Clinicians must remember that even patients with severe haemostatic defects, although susceptible to life-
threatening haemorrhage, may exhibit no detectable evidence of bleeding at initial presentation.

ments collectively known as fibrin degradation products (FDP).

Summarising haemostasis into three discrete, sequential phases certainly facilitates the clinical and laboratory evaluation of bleeding disorders. However, in reality, haemostasis is a highly complex process composed of non-sequential interactions between platelets, vasculature and a wide variety of proteins with procoagulant or fibrinolytic properties. The major clotting and fibrinolytic pathways are counterbalanced by a complicated array of anticoagulant and antifibrinolytic mechanisms that prevent uncontrolled and fulminant thrombosis or fibrinolysis.

APPROACH TO THE PATIENT

The careful collection of a detailed history and a subsequent meticulous physical examination (Box 36.1) are the cornerstones of the development of a rational diagnostic plan in patients with suspected haemostatic disorders (Johnstone 1988; Hackner 1995).

History

The collection of a detailed history is essential to:

- distinguish a generalised haemostatic defect from local haemorrhage due to a focal disease process,
- differentiate hereditary from acquired conditions,
- discriminate primary from secondary haemostatic disorders.

Careful questioning of the owners of dogs with a chronic generalised haemostatic defect usually reveals a long history of haemorrhage from multiple unrelated sites, although patients with more acute defects may initially present with bleeding from only one site (Fig. 36.4). The veterinarian should be aware that some manifestations of haemostatic disorders may not be recognised by owners as bleeding, particularly petechial and ecchymotic haemorrhages, melaena, and haematemesis (Fig. 36.5). Dogs with severe hereditary haemostatic defects typically develop episodic spontaneous haemorrhage at an early age. Patients with milder defects, however, may not be recognised until significant vessel injury occurs (trauma or surgical procedures such as ear cropping, tail docking or neutering), or a second disease process develops that further compromises haemostasis. Severe hereditary defects are unlikely to be present in a dog that has previously experienced major surgery or trauma without associated excessive bleeding.

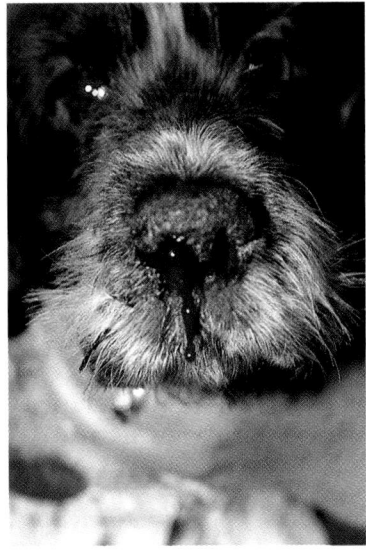

Fig. 36.4 Unilateral epistaxis (the sole site of bleeding) of two days' duration in a dog with a generalised bleeding disorder (immune-mediated thrombocytopenia).

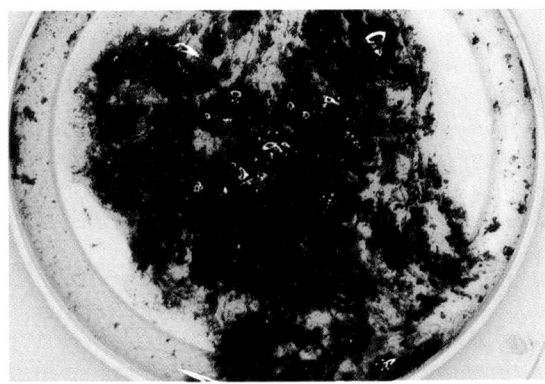

Fig. 36.5 Vomitus from a thrombocytopenic dog with haematemesis (showing the typical 'coffee grounds' appearance of digested blood).

Other important historical details that may be significant in individual cases include information regarding:

- previous or concurrent illnesses,
- potential access to toxins,
- current/recent medications.

Questioning regarding drug history should be carefully directed, since owners may fail to recognise products such as non-steroidal anti-inflammatory drugs (common potential causes of platelet dysfunction) as medications worthy of mention. When available, clinical histories of related dogs should be obtained if a hereditary defect is suspected.

Examination

Dogs with defective *primary haemostasis* typically present with:

- multifocal pinpoint (petechial) haemorrhages affecting the skin and mucous membranes because platelets fail to seal even the tiny traumatic capillary defects associated with normal activity (Fig. 36.6);
- petechiae often merge into small flat bruises (ecchymoses), and occur most commonly at pressure points and on ventral skin surfaces (Fig. 36.7);

- ocular haemorrhage (conjunctival, scleral, iridal and retinal petechiae and, in more severe instances, hyphaema) is common (Fig. 36.8).

Intact secondary haemostasis often prevents major haemorrhage.

Disorders of *secondary haemostasis* typically cause:

- major haemorrhage into joints and body cavities;
- haemothorax, haemoperitoneum or haemarthrosis may respectively cause dyspnoea, abdominomegaly or joint swelling and episodic shifting lameness (Fig. 36.9).

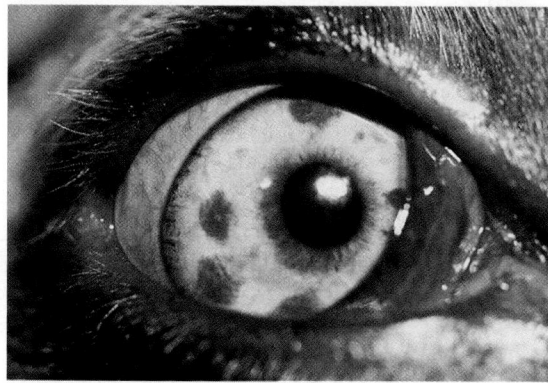

Fig. 36.8   Petechial and ecchymotic haemorrhages on the iris of a thrombocytopenic dog (photograph courtesy of Mark Nasisse, University of Missouri).

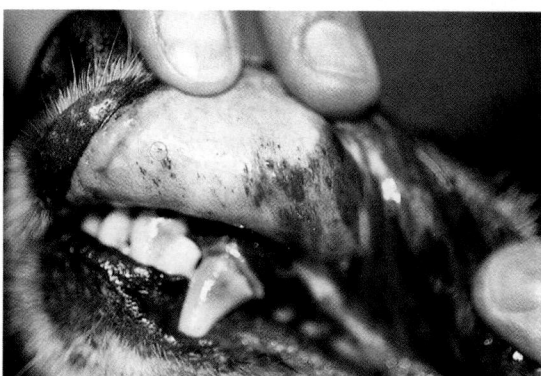

Fig. 36.6   Typical petechial haemorrhages on the mucous membranes of a thrombocytopenic dog.

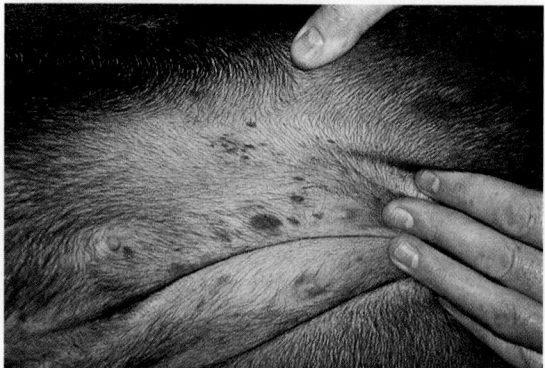

Fig. 36.7   Cutaneous ecchymotic haemorrhage in a dog with thrombocytopenia.

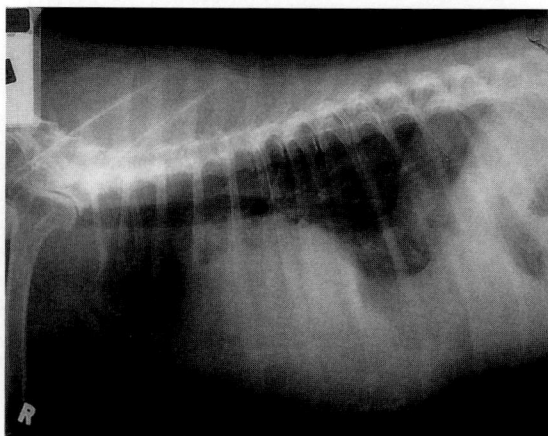

Fig. 36.9   Radiographic appearance of haemothorax in a dog with anticoagulant rodenticide poisoning (photograph courtesy of Helen Whitbread, University of Edinburgh).

Although severe subcutaneous and intramuscular haemorrhages can occur, intact primary hemostasis prevents signs of minor capillary bleeding (petechiae and ecchymoses). Clinicians should be aware that blood that has been present in a body cavity for any appreciable period of time has usually clotted and then become defibrinated via the fibrinolytic system, and is therefore devoid of clotting factors and platelets. The observation that blood obtained by thoracocentesis or abdominocentesis does not clot is therefore not specifically indicative of a bleeding disorder, since blood that is present in a major body cavity for any reason (trauma, for example) typically will not clot on removal.

Patients with abnormalities affecting either *primary or secondary haemostasis* may exhibit signs of external haemorrhage such as epistaxis, haematemesis, melaena and haematuria (Fig. 36.10).

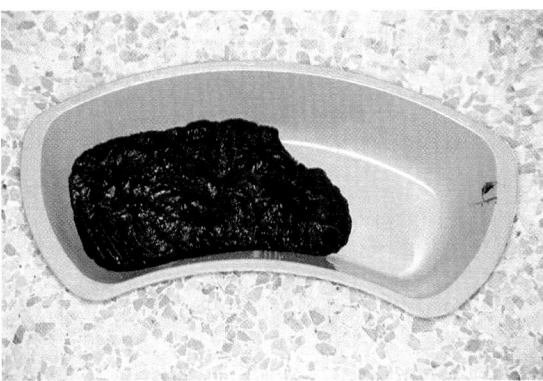

Fig. 36.10 Melaenic faeces produced by a dog with immune-mediated thrombocytopenia.

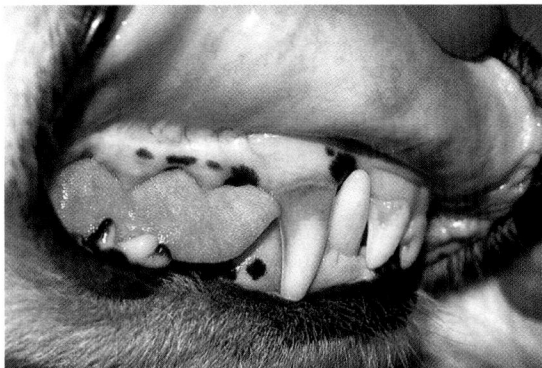

Fig. 36.11 Hypovolaemic shock due to acute blood loss in a dog with haemoperitoneum secondary to disseminated intravascular coagulation associated with haemangiosarcoma.

- Dogs suffering from severe or prolonged blood loss may become obviously hypovolaemic and/or anaemic (Fig. 36.11).
- The presence of relatively small volumes of blood within a sensitive location (for example, the brain, eyes, spinal cord, or pericardial sac) can cause dramatic clinical signs referable to the site of the haemorrhage (Stokol *et al.* 1994).
- Dogs with profound haemostatic defects often appear to be stable or even clinically normal. Such patients, however, are highly susceptible to serious and potentially fatal haemorrhage, and should be regarded as 'ticking time-bombs'.

INVESTIGATION

Disordered haemostasis results from the disruption of any one of the different components previously described. Accurate identification of a specific defect (particularly an uncommon hereditary disorder) may therefore require the performance of a large series of tests, many of which may not be available to the clinician in practice (Johnstone 1988). Common disorders, however, may often be diagnosed with reasonable accuracy using a standard set of simple screening tests, most of which can be performed in practice (see Box 36.2). More specialised haemostatic diagnostic tests require reagents or instrumentation that render them impractical for performance in practice (Johnstone 1988; Parry 1989; Carr & Johnson 1994; Hackner 1995) (see Box 36.3).

The initial investigation of most dogs with suspected bleeding disorders in practice should consist of estimation of platelet numbers, BMBT and ACT, followed by submission of samples to clinical pathology or haemostatic laboratories. More specialised tests that are often of value to practitioners include the activated partial thromboplastin time (APTT or PTT), prothrombin time (PT) and measurement of specific clotting factors, von Willebrand factor (vWf), fibrinogen and fibrin degradation products (FDP).

Box 36.2 In practice screening tests.

Primary haemostasis
  Evaluation of platelet numbers (Box 36.4)
  Buccal mucosal bleeding time (BMBT) (Box 36.5)
Secondary Haemostasis
  Activated clotting time (ACT) (Box 36.6)
  (Whole blood clotting time (WBCT))

Box 36.3 Overview of specialised haemostatic diagnostic techniques.

Important tests that can be requested from the majority of clinical pathology laboratories include:

Activated partial thromboplastin time (APTT or PTT)
(also known as kaolin cephalin clotting time (KCCT) depending upon technique and reagents used)

The APTT evaluates the intrinsic and common clotting pathways. Detection of a prolonged APTT usually indicates a deficit in the clotting factors of the intrinsic (most commonly factors VIII or IX) or common pathways or, less commonly, the presence of a circulating inhibitor of coagulation.

Prothrombin time (PT) or one-stage prothrombin time (OSPT)

The PT evaluates the extrinsic and common pathways of coagulation. Detection of a prolonged PT suggests a deficit in the factors of the extrinsic (most commonly factor VII) or common pathways or, less frequently, the presence of a clotting inhibitor.

von Willebrand factor (vWf)

Von Willebrand factor exists in a range of multimeric forms of varying functional activity. Deficiencies of vWf may be absolute, partial or selective (deficit of functional multimers). Various methods have been developed to evaluate vWf, including quantitative assays (electroimmunoassay or ELISA), qualitative assays (platelet aggregation in response to agonists such as ristocetin and botrocetin) and multimeric analysis (Johnson *et al.* 1988; Kraus & Johnson 1989; Slappendel *et al.* 1992). Most haemostasis laboratories have offered either electroimmunoassay or, more recently, ELISA as routine testing for von Willebrand's disease.

Fibrin degradation products (FDP)

Fibrin degradation products are usually measured using a commercial latex slide agglutination kit developed for human patients, but validated for use in dogs. Blood samples obtained for analysis of FDP must be transferred into a special collection tube, which will usually be provided by the laboratory providing the test. Elevated FDP levels indicate the presence of increased fibrinolytic activity, an abnormality most commonly seen in dogs with disseminated intravascular coagulation (DIC).

Other tests

Other tests that may be indicated but are less widely available, being provided only by specialised haemostatic testing laboratories, include:

- evaluation of thrombin clotting time (TCT or TT),
- fibrinogen levels,
- antithrombin III (AT III) levels,
- specific clotting factors,
- proteins induced by vitamin K absence (PIVKA).

Many clinical pathology laboratories offer as a basic 'haemostatic profile' measurement of platelet numbers (primary haemostasis), and combined measurement of APTT and PT (intrinsic, extrinsic and common pathways of secondary haemostasis). Samples for most specialised haemostatic assays should be collected by clean venipuncture and stored in anticoagulant (most commonly sodium citrate) using the exact proportion of blood to anticoagulant specified by the laboratory. Since clinical pathology laboratories tend to generate normal values using a particular collection, storage and transport protocol, practitioners are strongly advised to contact their particular laboratory for advice before sample collection. Many laboratories recommend paired submission of samples from a healthy control dog, to ensure that sample handling is satisfactory.

Most of the above assays evaluate aspects of the coagulation cascade. Specialised tests of aspects of platelet function, such as adhesion, aggregation and release, are difficult to standardise and often require large numbers of fresh platelets and specialised instrumentation. Such tests are therefore often only used in research situations, and are unlikely to be available to general practitioners.

Box 36.4 Evaluation of platelet numbers.

Platelet numbers may be rapidly and relatively accurately estimated via examination of a stained fresh blood smear, or exactly quantified by use of either a manual counting technique or an automated haematology analyser (Hackner 1995). Blood for evaluation of platelet numbers should be collected into anticoagulant (usually either EDTA or sodium citrate) using a clean venipuncture technique, and preferably processed within a few hours of collection. In some dogs, spontaneous agglutination of platelets can occur following the storage of anticoagulated blood for as little as 1 or 2 hours, and may erroneously lower platelet counts (pseudothrombocytopenia).

Direct smear

Microscopic examination of an air-dried stained blood smear is a quick and reliable method of detecting significant thrombocytopenia.

Normal
In normal dogs, 10–30 platelets will be seen in each oil immersion (1000 power) monolayer field (Figs 36.12 & 36.13).
To obtain an estimated platelet count ($\times 10^9$/l), the number of platelets within 10 consecutive oil immersion fields is counted, divided by 10 (to obtain an average number per field) and then multiplied by 15.

The edges of the blood smear should be scanned (particularly if platelet numbers are estimated to be low) to ensure that thrombocytopenia is not an artefact due to platelet clumping.

Manual count

Exact platelet numbers can be readily determined in practice with a commercial blood dilution system (Unopette, Becton Dickinson) and a standard Nebauer counting chamber (Fig. 36.14), using a technique similar to that used for obtaining manual white cell counts.

Automated haematology analysers

Most clinical pathology laboratories calculate platelet numbers using an automated haematology analyser. Some laboratories will also, if requested, be able to provide further information such as mean platelet volume (MPV) and a histogram displaying the distribution of platelet size (Fig. 36.15). Automated analysers are not infallible, and are prone to reporting erroneous thrombocytopenia when platelet clumping occurs (Fig. 36.16), or when platelet size is unusually large (Fig. 36.17) (see Box 36.9). Evaluation of platelet numbers using an alternative method (direct smear or manual count) should be requested if an unexpectedly low platelet count is obtained using an automated analyser.

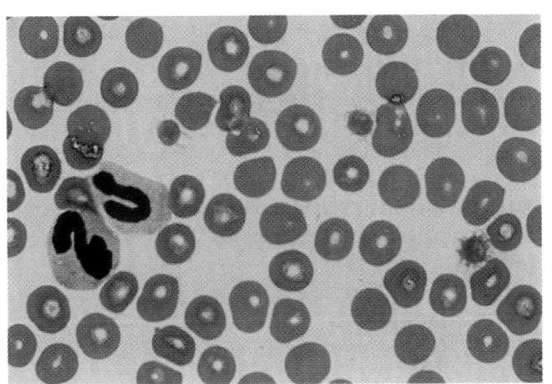

Fig. 36.12 Stained blood smear from a healthy patient demonstrating and adequate number of normal platelets, which are recognised as small (smaller than adjacent red blood cells) anucleate cells that are typically blue or purple in colour (photograph courtesy of Severine Hodson, University of Edinburgh).

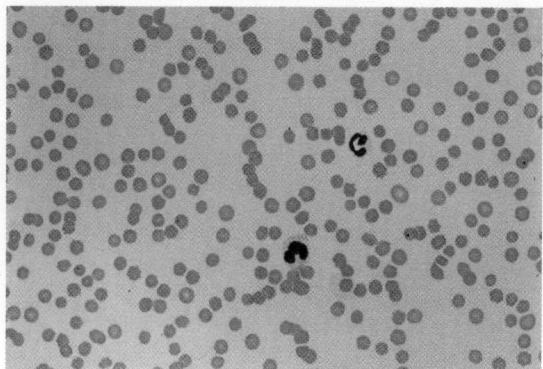

Fig. 36.13   Stained blood smear from a patient with immune-mediated thrombocytopenia, demonstrating the presence of absolutely no platelets on a representative high-power field, a finding consistent with profound thrombocytopenia (photograph courtesy of Severine Hodson, University of Edinburgh).

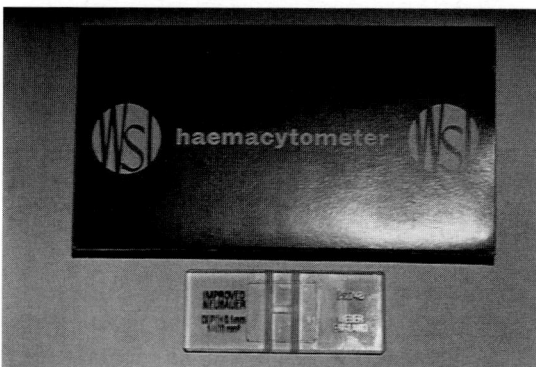

Fig. 36.14   Modified Nebauer haematocytometer, which provides several counting chambers suitable for performing manual platelet counts (photograph courtesy of Severine Hodson, University of Edinburgh).

DIFFERENTIAL DIAGNOSIS

History, physical examination and the results of screening tests can usually separate bleeding disorders into:

- problems that affect primary haemostasis (Box 36.7),
- problems that affect secondary haemostasis (Box 36.8),
- problems that affect both.

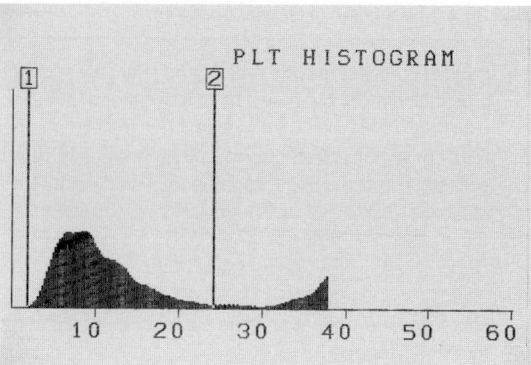

Fig. 36.15   Histogram produced by an automated haematology analyser demonstrating the typical distribution of platelet number and volume in a normal dog. The bottom scale is in femtolitres (fl). In this particular patient, the vast majority of the platelets are between 2 and 20 fl in volume, with a mean platelet volume (MPV) of 9 fl. Setting an upper limit of 25 fl allows for clear distinction between platelets and erythrocytes, since the smallest erythrocytes are not recorded on the histogram until between 30 and 40 fl.

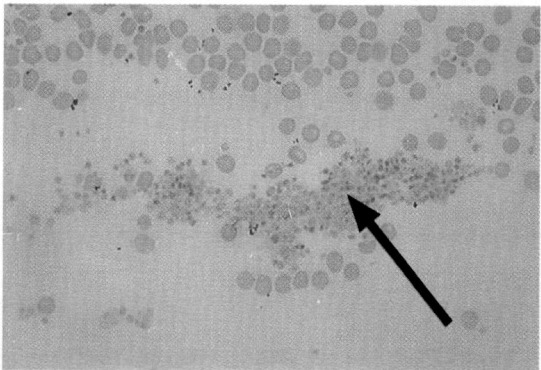

Fig. 36.16   Stained blood smear from a patient with a normal platelet count demonstrating platelet clumping (dark arrow). Few platelets were seen in the central area of the smear. erroneously suggesting the presence of a reduced platelet number, but more thorough evaluation of the smear revealed numerous platelet clumps at the edges of the smear (photograph courtesy of Chris Belford, Cytopath).

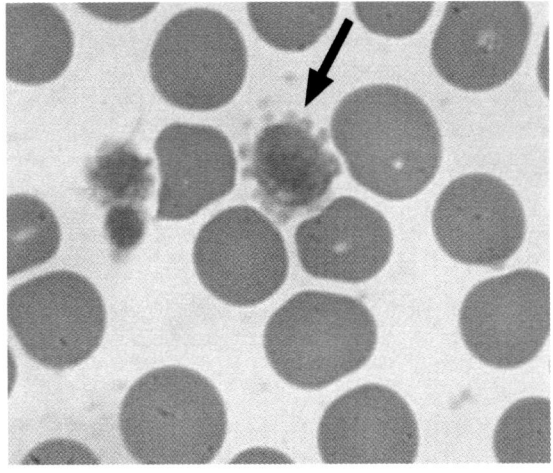

Fig. 36.17   Stained blood smear demonstrating the typical appearance of a megathrombocyte (dark arrow), which is approximately the same size as adjacent red blood cells (photograph courtesy of Severine Hodson, University of Edinburgh).

Box 36.5   Buccal mucosa bleeding time.

The buccal mucosa bleeding time (BMBT) is the time elapsed until cessation of bleeding from a small incision made in the buccal mucosa (Jergens *et al.* 1987; Forsythe & Willis 1989; Kraus & Johnson 1989; Carr & Johnson 1994; Hackner 1995). Since minor vessel injuries may be plugged by platelets alone with minimal need for a functional clotting cascade, a prolonged BMBT usually indicates an abnormality affecting primary haemostasis rather than secondary haemostasis. Since vascular disorders causing defective primary haemostasis are rare in dogs, the BMBT is a simple and relatively specific test of platelet function if platelet numbers are greater than 100×10^9/l. BMBT will progressively prolong as the platelet count drops below this number.

Technique

- The patient is placed in sternal or lateral recumbency (sedation is rarely needed).
- The dog's muzzle is firmly tied shut using a 5 cm wide gauze strip, leaving one top lip folded up under the strip to expose the buccal mucosa.
- A spring-loaded disposable cutting device (Simplate, Organon Teknika) is used to make one or two incisions of a standard length and depth (Fig. 36.18) (a number 12 scalpel blade can be used to make the incisions if the device is not available).
- Excess blood is carefully blotted from below the incision with filter paper, taking care not to touch the incision with the paper (Fig. 36.19).

The BMBT is the time elapsed from the creation of the incision until the complete cessation of bleeding.

Normal
In normal dogs, the BMBT is usually less than 5 min.

Since oozing of blood may persist for many hours in dogs with abnormal primary haemostasis (Fig. 36.20), the BMBT is terminated if bleeding continues for longer than 10 min, and pressure is applied to the incision.

   The BMBT is an insensitive test that may not detect patients with subtle defects in primary haemostasis (for example, dogs with mild von Willebrand's disease). A prolonged BMBT strongly suggests the presence of a clinically significant bleeding disorder.

Toe nail clipping has in the past been used as an alternative means of assessing primary haemostasis. Haemorrhage after nail clipping, however, may be prolonged (up to 8 min in normal dogs), and the procedure is difficult to reproduce in a standard fashion. Furthermore, compared with the BMBT, nail clipping is less specific (it appears to be affected by defects in secondary haemostasis), and is often painful enough to necessitate heavy sedation or light anaesthesia.

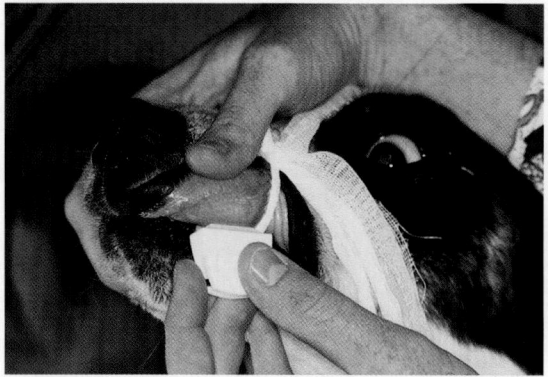

Fig. 36.18 Correct positioning of the gauze strip and disposable cutting device for performing a buccal mucosa bleeding time.

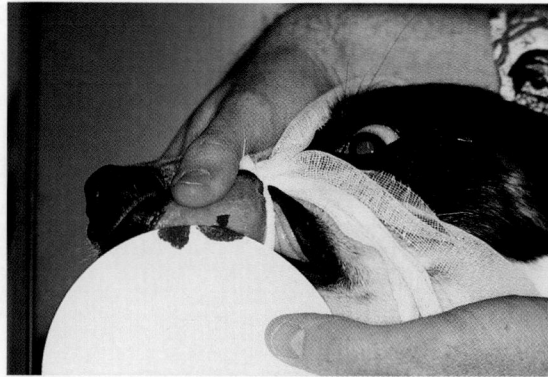

Fig. 36.19 Correct positioning of circular filter paper to enable careful blotting of blood during evaluation of a buccal mucosa bleeding time.

Box 36.6 Activated clotting time.

The activated clotting time (ACT) is the time taken for fresh whole blood to clot within a glass tube containing a contact activator (Parry 1989; Carr & Johnson 1994; Hackner 1995). A prolonged ACT usually indicates an abnormality affecting secondary haemostasis (specifically, the intrinsic and common pathways of the clotting cascade) rather than primary haemostasis. Since traces of platelet factor 3 are essential for activation of the clotting cascade, the ACT may also be prolonged in the presence of severe thrombocytopenia. The ACT is a simple test for abnormalities of the intrinsic and common pathways if platelet numbers are greater than $10 \times 10^9/l$.

Technique

- Using clean venipuncture of a large vessel such as the jugular vein, 2 ml of blood are collected and discarded (leaving the needle in the vein).
- A further 2 ml of blood are then collected and placed in a specialised glass tube containing a small amount of contact activator (ACT Tube, Becton Dickinson).
- The tube is inverted several times to mix the contents, and then left undisturbed for 45 s.
- Thereafter, the tube is gently tilted every 5–10 s until an obvious clot begins to form (Fig. 36.21).

The ACT is the time elapsed from the addition of the blood to the tube until obvious clotting is first noted.

Normal
In normal dogs, the ACT is usually less than 2 min.

The ACT is more reproducible at body temperature (38°C) than at room temperature. ACT testing is therefore performed optimally using a block heater or water bath or, failing that, performed holding the tube within cupped hands.

A prolonged ACT suggests the presence of a severe coagulopathy. The ACT is a relatively insensitive screening test that may miss dogs with mildly defective secondary haemostasis. The ACT does not evaluate the extrinsic pathway, and therefore does not assess all aspects of secondary haemostasis. However, since the most frequent congenital disorders of coagulation (haemophilia A and B) affect the intrinsic pathway, and the commonest acquired defects affect both the intrinsic and extrinsic pathways, the ACT is usually an acceptable screening test of secondary haemostasis as a whole.

The ACT evaluates the same clotting pathways as the activated partial thromboplastin time (APTT). Since the APTT procedure is more sensitive than the ACT test, subtle abnormalities of the intrinsic and/or common pathways may have a prolonged APTT and a normal ACT. APTT testing does not require the presence of platelets and therefore is preferable to the ACT for evaluating secondary haemostasis in dogs with severe thrombocytopenia.

The whole blood clotting time (WBCT) is performed in an identical manner to the ACT except the glass tube does not contain a contact activator. Since glass is a relatively poor activator of clotting, the normal canine WBCT can be as long as 8 min.

Plastic is a very poor activator of clotting, and containers such as plastic syringes should not be used to assess the WBCT.

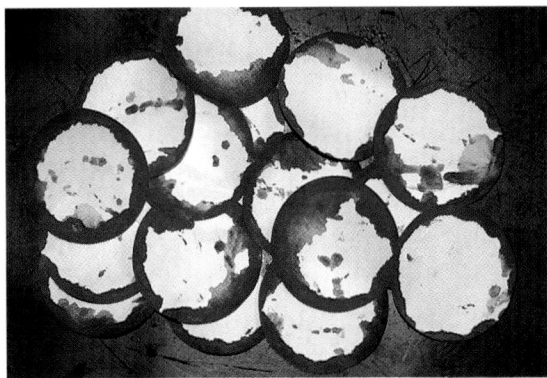

Fig. 36.20 Performance of a buccal mucosal bleeding time in a dog with severe von Willebrand's disease caused a markedly prolonged oozing of blood, with a dramatically increased consumption of filter papers (usually only one or two papers are required).

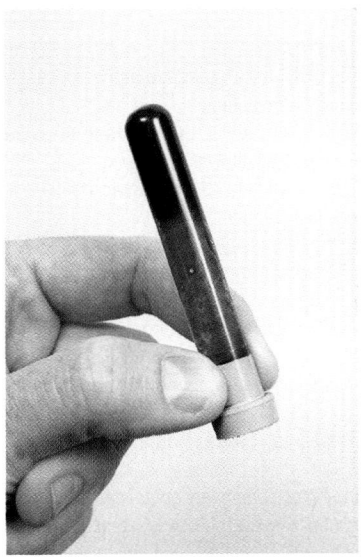

Fig. 36.21 The end point of an activated clotting time test (an obvious whole blood clot).

Box 36.7 Abnormalities affecting primary haemostasis.

Vascular disorders

Vascular disorders rarely cause significant haemostatic defects in the dog.

- Vasculitis
- Ehlers–Danlos syndrome

Thrombocytopenia

Thrombocytopenia is the most common cause by far of clinically significant defects in primary haemostasis in the dog (Davenport & Carakostas 1982; Feldman 1989; Grindem *et al.* 1991 & 1994).

- Decreased platelet production
    Hereditary cyclic haematopoiesis
    Idiopathic aplastic anaemia**
    Myelosuppressive chemotherapy**
    Irradiation
    Ehrlichiosis
    Myelofibrosis and myeloproliferative disorders**
    Pure megakaryocyte hypoplasia (immune-mediated)**
    Drug-induced suppression of bone marrow**:
        oestrogens (exogenous and endogenous)
        phenylbutazone
        phenobarbitone
        antibiotics (sulphonamides, chloramphenicol)
        dapsone

Box 36.7   *Continued*

- Platelet sequestration within vasculature
  - □ Splenic torsion/neoplasia*
  - □ Vascular tumour (haemangioma/haemangiosarcoma)*
- Consumptive coagulopathies
  - □ Disseminated intravascular coagulation (DIC)*
  - □ Haemangiosarcoma*
  - □ Haemolytic uraemic syndrome
- Immune-mediated destruction of platelets
  - □ Immune-mediated thrombocytopenia (IMT)*
  - □ Incompatible transfusion (isoimmune disease)
- Haemorrhage
  - □ Platelet loss due to bleeding only causes mild and transient thrombocytopenia.

A number of *artefacts* may produce an apparently low platelet count

- Platelet clumping or clots in sample 'pseudothrombocytopenia'
- Use of automated cell counters/megathrombocytes (see Box 36.9)

Defective platelet function

Although platelet dysfunction has been associated with numerous drugs and systemic illnesses (Jackson *et al.*
1985; Rackear *et al.* 1986; Catalfamo & Dodds 1988; Helfand 1988; Feldman 1989; Willis *et al.* 1989; Kristensen
et al. 1994), only congenital defects such as von Willebrand's disease commonly cause significant bleeding.

- Congenital defects
  - □ Von Willebrand's disease*
  - □ Hereditary thrombopathias (see Box 36.13)
- Secondary to systemic illnesses
  - □ Uraemia**
  - □ Hepatic diseases**
  - □ Pancreatitis
  - □ Hypothyroidism
  - □ DIC (platelet dysfunction caused by fibrin degradation products)*
  - □ Dysproteinaemia
  - □ Myeloproliferative disorders**
  - □ Ehrlichiosis
- Drug-induced
    Non-steroidal anti-inflammatory drugs (aspirin, phenylbutazone)*
    Antibiotics (penicillins, sulphonamides)
    Heparin
    Phenothiazines
    Dextrans
    Vinca alkaloids (significant platelet dysfunction not proven in the dog)
- Antibody-mediated
    Platelet dysfunction caused by anti-platelet antibodies**

Most of the above disorders of primary haemostasis, although reported or believed to exist, are rarely observed in
clinical situations. Relatively common disorders are denoted with a single asterisk (*) and occasionally (albeit
infrequently) observed disorders are denoted with a double asterisk (**).

Box 36.8   Abnormalities affecting secondary haemostasis.

Clotting factor deficiencies

Clotting factor deficiencies are, by far, the most common causes of defective secondary haemostasis in the dog.

- Decreased production of clotting factors
  - ○ Hereditary coagulopathies:
    haemophilia A (factor VIII deficiency)*
    haemophilia B (factor IX deficiency)**
    other factor deficiencies (see Box 36.15)
  - ○ Deficiency of active vitamin K:
    anticoagulant rodenticide toxicity*
    biliary tract obstruction**
  - ○ Hepatic failure*
- Increased consumption of clotting factors
  - ○ Disseminated intravascular coagulation (DIC)*
  - ○ Haemangiosaroma*
  - ○ Other consumption coagulopathies

Circulating inhibitors of coagulation

Circulating inhibitors of coagulation can cause haemostatic defects despite the presence of normal levels of clotting factors (Stone *et al.* 1994).

- Heparin
- Fibrin degradation products (produced as an end result of DIC)*
- Lupus anticoagulant (antibody against clotting factors)

Relatively common causes of defective secondary haemostasis are denoted with a single asterisk (*) and occasionally (albeit infrequently) observed disorders are denoted with a double asterisk (**).

Box 36.9   Megathrombocytes.

Megathrombocytes ('stress' or 'shift' platelets):

- Very large young platelets
- Functionally superior to mature platelets
- Recognised on microscopic examination of a stained blood smear as platelets with a diameter equal to or greater than that of nearby red blood cells (Fig. 36.17)
- Released from the marrow during periods of increased platelet production
- Often counted by automated haematology analysers as red blood cells rather than platelets, hence platelet numbers may be erroneously reported as decreased by clinical pathology laboratories. Platelet numbers in affected dogs can be more accurately estimated using manual counting techniques.

Increased numbers of megathrombocytes seen in circulation in:

- Dogs with diseases causing an increased rate of platelet destruction, e.g.
  - ○ immune-mediated thrombocytopenia
  - ○ disseminated intravascular coagulation
- Enlarged and bizarre megathrombocytes are sometimes seen in patients with essential thrombocythaemia, a neoplastic disorder of platelets (see Box 36.10).
- Macrothrombocytosis in Cavalier King Charles Spaniels: high numbers of megathrombocytes (sometimes associated with a decreased platelet count) have been reported in apparently healthy Cavalier King Charles Spaniels. The cause and significance is unknown. Affected dogs do not appear to have defective primary haemostasis (Brown *et al.* 1994).

Reduced numbers or absence of megathrombocytes in the presence of thrombocytopenia indicates megakaryocyte failure.

MANAGEMENT OF BLEEDING DISORDERS

Whenever possible collection of samples for diagnostic testing should be performed before instituting therapy because treatments such as transfusion, vitamin K_1 and desmopressin will often affect the results of subsequent haemostatic testing. In order to facilitate potential further specialised testing, it is always advisable to collect and store extra citrated plasma before treatment.

Box 36.10 Thrombocytosis.

Reactive thrombocytosis

Most common cause of thrombocytosis, associated with:

- Acute blood loss
- Iron deficiency anaemia associated with chronic blood loss
- Infectious or inflammatory conditions
- Neoplasia (particularly carcinoma)
- Hyperadrenocorticism
- Splenectomy

Platelet function is usually normal in affected dogs.
Idiopathic mild to moderate elevations in platelet number of no detectable clinical significance are occasionally observed in apparently healthy dogs.

Drug-induced thrombocytosis

Vinca alkaloids (such as vincristine and vinblastine) often induce a transient moderate rise in platelet numbers, without any significant alteration of platelet function (Mackin *et al.* 1995).

Myeloproliferative disorders

- Essential thrombocythaemia
- Polycythaemia vera
- Chronic myelogenous leukaemia
- Other myeloproliferative and myelodysplastic disorders

Essential thrombocythaemia

- A rare myeloproliferative disorder characterised by the uncontrolled neoplastic production of platelets.
- Platelet numbers in affected dogs are often extremely elevated.
- Usually associated with markedly decreased platelet function, affected animals are likely to present with bleeding problems typical of defective primary haemostasis. Treatment of affected dogs has rarely been reported, potential chemotherapeutic agents include hydroxyurea and alkylating agents such as melphalan (Feldman 1989).

Supportive Treatment

- Minimise haemorrhage with strict rest (sedate if necessary), gentle handling, the use of small bore needles and catheters (Fig. 36.22), and avoidance of elective surgery whenever possible.
- Body cavity haemorrhage often does not require drainage. Thoracocentesis or abdominocentesis may exacerbate bleeding, and are usually best avoided. Significant dysponea is an indication for thoracocentesis.

- Consider transfusion (see Box 36.11), especially in emergencies.
- Desmopressin (see Box 36.12) may be useful for the treatment of von Willebrand's disease or haemophilia A.

Specific Treatment

Specific treatments of the more common bleeding disorders are detailed in the following sections on specific diseases.

Box 36.11   Transfusion.

Transfusion of patients with bleeding disorders may be used to:

- address the life-threatening effects of blood loss,
- specifically replace missing platelets and/or clotting factors (Stone & Cotter 1992).

Management of blood loss

Bleeding disorders are often life-threatening because of hypovolaemia, anaemia and hypoproteinaemia. Intravenous correction of these abnormalities can support a patient for a prolonged period even if the underlying bleeding disorder is not rectified. Treatment options include:

- whole blood (fresh or stored),
- packed red blood cells,
- fluids (isotonic crystalloid solutions, hypertonic saline or colloids).

Acute blood loss causing hypovolaemia and shock is best treated with intravenous whole blood or, if blood is not immediately available, rapid infusion of crystalloids, colloids or (especially in a crisis) hypertonic saline. Since dogs with chronic blood loss can maintain an adequate blood volume, fluids are rarely indicated in such patients. Dogs with life-threatening anaemia secondary to chronic haemorrhage are best treated with packed red blood cells or, if packed cells are not available, whole blood. Iron deficiency secondary to prolonged external blood loss may necessitate supplementation with ferrous sulphate (see Chapter 33).

Since blood from body cavities usually does not clot after collection, autotransfusion of blood obtained in a sterile fashion by paracentesis from dogs with haemothorax or haemoperitoneum (given, without anticoagulant, through a standard filtered blood transfusion set) can be used to recycle erythrocytes (but not platelets or clotting factors). Removal of body cavity blood from patients with coagulopathies, however, is associated with a significant risk of precipitating further haemorrhage.

Correction of platelet or clotting factor deficits

(1)   Platelets
      Platelet transfusion may transiently stop bleeding in thrombocytopenic dogs. Blood products that contain viable platelets include:

- fresh whole blood,
- platelet-rich plasma,
- platelet concentrate.

      Transfusion of even large numbers of platelets may only cause a transient, slight (often undetectable) rise in platelet count. Platelet numbers should be measured before and shortly after transfusion. Further transfusions are not indicated if numbers do not remain appreciably elevated for at least 2 hours after the first transfusion. Platelet transfusions may be more effective if thrombocytopenia is due to a failure of platelet production rather than platelet destruction, since the transfused platelets may circulate for up to a week.

(2)   Coagulation proteins
      Transfusion of blood products containing viable clotting factors usually immediately (albeit transiently) improves secondary haemostasis in dogs with factor deficiencies (but may not significantly benefit patients with circulating inhibitors of coagulation). Blood products that may benefit specific conditions include:

- fresh whole blood,
- fresh-frozen plasma,
- frozen plasma,
- cryoprecipitate.

      Fresh whole blood and fresh-frozen plasma (plasma separated from blood immediately after collection, and frozen) provide major clotting factors and von Willebrand factor, while frozen plasma (plasma separated from stored blood) provides minimal amounts of vWf and factors V and VIII, but adequate quantities of other factors, including the vitamin K-dependent clotting factors. Cryoprecipitate, a concentrated plasma product, contains high concentrations of factor VIII and vWf within a relatively small volume of plasma.

Many practices will not have ready access to a blood bank centrifuge or blood products such as packed red cells, plasma, platelet-rich plasma or cryoprecipitate. Transfusion of fresh whole blood (within 12 hours of collection) is therefore often the most practical means of providing blood components. (For further details on the technique and practice of blood transfusion see Chapter 2.)

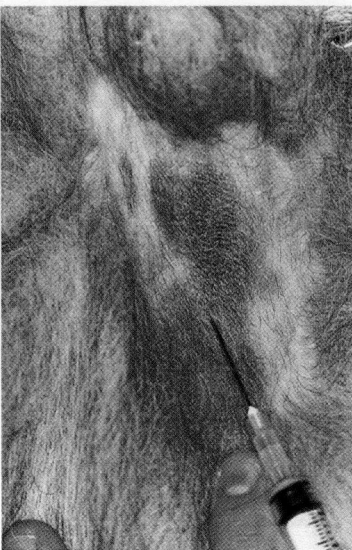

Fig. 36.22   Excessive bruising associated with routine jugular venipuncture in a thrombocytopenic dog.

VON WILLEBRAND'S DISEASE

Aetiopathogenesis

Von Willebrand factor (vWf) is a glycoprotein produced by canine endothelial cells and (to a lesser extent) megakaryocytes that acts as a linking molecule to facilitate binding of platelets to exposed vascular subendothelium (adhesion) and each other (aggregation). Adequate levels of functional vWf are therefore essential for normal primary haemostasis. Von Willebrand's disease (vWD) is a common inherited haemostatic disorder caused by an absolute or partial deficiency of functional vWf (Johnson *et al.* 1988; Kraus & Johnson 1989; Littlewood 1989).

Epidemiology

Von Willebrand's disease has been reported in many different dog breeds world-wide, and in the UK has been

---

Box 36.12   Desmopressin.

- Desmopressin (DDAVP) is a synthetic analogue of antidiuretic hormone (vasopressin), most commonly used to treat diabetes insipidus.
- In human beings, treatment with DDAVP transiently increases blood levels of factor VIII and von Willebrand's factor. DDAVP has therefore been used to complement or replace transfusion during the management of haemophilia A and von Willebrand's disease in people (Johnson *et al.* 1988).
- Dogs with haemophilia A or von Willebrand's disease typically respond poorly to DDAVP (Giger & Dodds 1989; Kraus & Johnson 1989; Mansell & Parry 1991). Any beneficial effect attained is transient (several hours at most), and patients tend to be refractory to repeat treatments.
- DDAVP should not be relied upon as the sole means of improving haemostasis in haemophiliac or von Willebrand's dogs, either in an emergency or before elective surgery.
- DDAVP may occasionally be of some benefit as an adjunctive treatment.
- DDAVP may also be given to healthy donors 30 min before blood collection in order to boost plasma factor VIII and vWf activity within the transfused blood.

Dose

  0.6–2.0 µg/kg intravenously or subcutaneously daily, for up to 4 days.

Human intranasal DDAVP drops (100 µg/ml) can be diluted in sterile saline to produce an administered volume of 1–2 ml.

observed in several breeds including: Dobermann Pinschers, Golden Retrievers and Scottish Terriers (Littlewood 1989).

Disease severity in affected dogs can vary from very mild (causing little or no clinical signs) to very severe (causing, in the most extreme cases, neonatal mortality). Inheritance of vWD is autosomal, and the condition therefore affects dogs of both sexes with equal frequency.

Clinical Features

Dogs with vWD display features consistent with defective primary haemostasis although, for unknown reasons, petechiae are uncommon. Severe vWD causes spontaneous haemorrhage at an early age, whereas milder forms of the disease may not be detected until an episode of vascular injury such as trauma or surgery (often minor or routine procedures such as neutering, tail docking or nail clipping) causes excessive or prolonged haemorrhage. Older dogs with subclinical vWD that are exposed to factors that further impair platelet function (treatment with aspirin, for example) may then develop spontaneous haemorrhage. Dogs with subclinical vWD that then develop concurrent hypothyroidism are also thought to be more susceptible to haemorrhage.

Investigations

- Primary and secondary haemostasis should be evaluated:
  - ○ platelet count,
  - ○ BMBT,
  - ○ ACT, APTT, PT.
- Plasma levels of vWf should be accurately quantified (see Box 36.3).

Diagnosis

Dogs with vWD usually show:

- intact coagulation (normal ACT, PT and APTT),
- adequate platelet numbers,
- abnormal platelet function, i.e. clinical signs consistent with defective primary haemostasis and a prolonged BMBT despite the presence of normal platelet numbers.

Measurement of plasma levels of vWf is usually indicated in such patients, particularly in younger dogs of known breed susceptibility to vWD (such as Dobermanns) with no history or clinical evidence of other causes of platelet dysfunction. Documentation of low levels of vWf confirms the presence of vWD. Other less common hereditary causes of platelet dysfunction (see Box 36.13) should then be considered if vWf levels are normal.

Although dogs with severe vWD will almost invariably have a prolonged BMBT, bleeding times can be normal in patients with mild or subclinical forms of the disease. Since the BMBT is a relatively crude test of primary haemostasis, the documentation of mildly affected dogs or subclinical carriers of vWD requires the measurement of plasma vWf levels.

Box 36.13   Hereditary causes of platelet dysfunction.

Inherited disorders of platelet function (thrombopathias) typically affect one or more of the major aspects of platelet function (adhesion, aggregation, release and clot retraction). Since, apart from vWf assays, specialised testing of platelet function is difficult to obtain in practice, a tentative diagnosis is usually based on finding a prolonged BMBT in a young dog with normal vWf levels and a known breed susceptibility to an hereditary thrombopathia (Davenport & Carakostas 1982; Johnstone 1982; Catalfamo & Dodds 1988; Feldman 1989; Callan *et al.* 1993). Fortunately, apart from vWD, hereditary thrombopathias are uncommonly encountered in practice.

Disorder	Breeds affected	Platelet functions affected
Von Willebrand's disease	Many breeds affected	Adhesion, aggregation
Canine thrombasthenic thrombopathia	Otterhounds	Adhesion, clot retraction
Canine thrombopathia	Basset Hounds	Aggregation, release reaction
Secretion or storage pool disorders	American Cocker Spaniels	Aggregation, release reaction

Box 36.14   Specific management of von Willebrand's disease.

Specific treatment modalities are usually reserved for use either to arrest severe ongoing bleeding or as
prophylaxis before surgery (Johnson *et al.* 1988; Kraus & Johnson 1989).

- Transfusion with fresh or fresh-frozen plasma or, when available, cryoprecipitate (which concentrates vWf) is
  the treatment of choice in the bleeding patient. Transfusion with fresh whole blood, although also providing
  vWf, may sensitise recipient dogs to foreign blood group antigens and thereby increase the risk of a reaction
  associated with subsequent transfusions. Since dogs with vWD are likely to need multiple transfusions, the use
  of whole blood (preferably cross-matched or typed) should if possible be reserved for patients with anaemia or
  hypovolaemia.
- Desmopressin (see Box 36.12).

Management

See page 296 for guidelines on supportive care. Specific
management is outlined in Box 36.14.

Prognosis

Von Willebrand's disease is incurable, and therefore
euthanasia is recommended in severely affected patients
that suffer from multiple life-threatening episodes of
haemorrhage at an early age. Potential causes of disability
and death in severely affected dogs include anaemia and
hypovolameia secondary to blood loss, and haemorrhage
into sensitive locations such as the eyes, brain and spinal
cord. Dogs with milder forms of vWD, however, can have
a normal life expectancy if potential causes of blood loss
(surgery or trauma, for example) are anticipated and
avoided if possible, and if episodes of active haemorrhage
are treated appropriately with transfusion and/or
desmopressin.

Since vWD is inherited, affected dogs should not be
used for breeding.

HAEMOPHILIA A

Aetiopathogenesis

Haemophilia A, the most common hereditary clotting
factor deficiency in the dog, is due to an absolute or partial
deficiency of factor VIII. Factor VIII is a component of the
intrinsic pathway of the clotting cascade, and is produced
by vascular endothelial cells and megakaryocytes (unlike

the other clotting factors, which are produced by the liver).
Adequate levels of factor VIII are essential for normal secondary haemostasis (Fogh 1988; Littlewood 1989).

Epidemiology

Haemophilia A has been reported in most dog breeds, and
in the UK is especially prevalent in German Shepherds
(Littlewood 1989). Haemophilia A is a sex-linked recessive
trait, and therefore is carried by heterozygous females and
clinically affects only males. Disease severity in affected
dogs can vary from mild to severe.

Clinical Features

Haemophiliac dogs display the typical features of defective
secondary haemostasis including subcutaneous and intramuscular haematomas, haemarthroses, haemothorax and
haemoperitoneum. Affected puppies typically have a
chronic history of episodic shifting lameness (sometimes
associated with minor trauma) due to recurrent joint and
muscle haemorrhage. Mild forms of haemophilia A may
not be detected until trauma or routine surgery (particularly castration) causes excessive haemorrhage and
haematoma formation. Occasionally, mildly affected male
dogs have been reported to remain subclinical until they
have sired one or more litters of puppies.

Investigations

- Primary and secondary haemostasis should be
  evaluated:
  o platelet count,
  o BMBT,
  o ACT, APTT, PT.

- When indicated, factor VIII activity should then be specifically quantified (see Box 36.3).

Diagnosis

Haemophiliacs show:

- intact primary haemostasis, i.e. normal platelet numbers and BMBT;
- intact extrinsic pathway of secondary haemostasis, i.e. normal PT;

- an impaired intrinsic pathway, i.e. prolonged APTT and ACT.

Although this particular combination of abnormal test results in a young male dog is highly suggestive of haemophilia A, other less common hereditary coagulopathies such as haemophilia B (see Box 36.15) may cause the same abnormalities (Littlewood 1989). Submission of plasma to a specialised haemostasis laboratory for measurement of specific clotting factors is therefore recommended. Male dogs with haemophilia A typically have extremely low plasma factor VIII activity (often less than 5% of normal).

Box 36.15   Hereditary clotting factor deficiencies.

Hereditary deficiencies of most clotting factors have been reported in dogs (Johnstone 1982; Fogh & Fogh 1988; Feldman *et al.* 1995; Hackner 1995). Fortunately, apart from haemophilia A (factor VIII deficiency) and B (factor IX deficiency), inherited factor deficiencies are either rare or of minimal clinical significance. Some factor deficiencies such as factor XII deficiency may impair haemostatic function tests without actually predisposing affected dogs to bleeding. Clinically significant factor deficiencies cause typical signs of defective secondary haemostasis of varying severity.

Deficient factor (common name of disease)	Breeds affected	Inheritance	Severity of signs
Fibrinogen (Hypofibrinogenaemia)	Saint Bernard	Autosomal recessive and autosomal dominant	Severe
Prothrombin (Hypoprothrombinaemia)	Boxer	Autosomal recessive	Mild to severe
Factor VII (Hypoproconvertinaemia)	Beagle Alaskan Malamute	Autosomal dominant	Mild
Factor VIII (Haemophilia A)	Most dog breeds	Sex-linked recessive	Mild to severe
Factor IX (Haemophilia B)	Many dog breeds	Sex-linked recessive	Mild to severe
Factor X (Stuart-Prower Trait)	Cocker Spaniel	Autosomal dominant (lethal gene)	Neonatal death due to severe bleeding
Factor XI (Plasma thromboplastin antecedent deficiency)	Springer Spaniel Pyrenean Mountain Dog Kerry Blue Terrier	Autosomal recessive	Usually mild, but severe after surgery
Factor XII (Hageman trait)	Miniature Poodle	Autosomal recessive	Subclinical

The abnormalities in haemostatic screening tests (ACT, APTT and PT) caused by the hereditary coagulopathies are highly predictable based upon the location of the deficient factor within the intrinsic, extrinsic or common pathways.

Female carriers of haemophilia typically have approximately 50% of normal plasma factor VIII activity. Since only 10–20% of normal plasma factor VIII activity is necessary to maintain adequate haemostasis, carriers are not susceptible to bleeding and will have normal APTT and ACT results. Quantification of plasma factor VIII activity is therefore necessary to identify female carriers via laboratory methods. Heterozygous carriers can, however, also be identified by genealogical tracing, since affected males can only be produced by carrier females.

Management

See page 296 for guidelines on supportive care. Specific management is outlined in Box 36.16.

Prognosis

Hereditary coagulopathies such as haemophilia A are incurable. Euthanasia should be considered in severely affected dogs suffering from recurrent life-threatening haemorrhage and debilitating and painful haemarthroses. Mild haemophiliacs can have a relatively normal life expectancy if potential causes of haemorrhage are anticipated and avoided, and bleeding episodes are treated with transfusion and/or desmopressin.

Affected males and carrier females should not be used for breeding.

Box 36.16   Specific management of haemophilia A.

Specific therapy is typically only used to stop life-threatening haemorrhage or as prophylaxis before unavoidable surgery.

- Transfusion with fresh or fresh-frozen plasma, cryoprecipitate or human factor VIII products is the recommended treatment for the bleeding patient.
- Fresh whole blood also provides factor VIII, but should ideally be reserved for administration (preferably after cross-matching or typing) to anaemic or hypovolaemic dogs since the use of whole blood also increases the risk of a transfusion reaction associated with future transfusions.
- Desmopressin (see Box 36.12).

ANTICOAGULANT RODENTICIDE POISONING

Aetiopathogenesis

- Anticoagulant rodenticides inhibit an enzyme involved in the process that regenerates active vitamin K (Mount 1988; Rackear 1988; Murphy & Gerken 1989).
- Clotting factors II (prothrombin), VII, IX and X require active vitamin K in order to function effectively.
- The major clotting pathways (intrinsic, extrinsic and common) are typically all affected by anticoagulant toxicity.
- Since all available reserves of active vitamin K must be consumed before haemostasis is affected, bleeding will often not be observed for at least 1 or 2 days after toxin ingestion.

Epidemiology

Anticoagulant rodenticide poisoning is most common in those dogs with access to either bait or rodents that have ingested bait, that is young, active, outdoor dogs (particularly farm dogs).

Various anticoagulants are available as rodenticides, chemically these may be divided into three groups:

(1)   older type hydroxycoumarins (warfarin, coumachlor)
(2)   the indane-diones (pindone, diphacinone), although chemically unrelated to warfarin these compounds have a similar pharmacological action.
(3)   'New generation' anticoagulants (difenacoum, brodifacoum, bromadialone), also hydroxycoumarins but with more potent anticoagulant activity and longer half-life, often with biphasic metabolism (Meehan 1984).

Groups 1 & 2 are sometimes refered to as 'short-acting rodenticides'. It is often stated that multiple exposures to such agents are required before a coagulopathy occurs; however, there is no doubt that toxicity can arise through a single exposure to a rodenticide in this group. Toxic effects (i.e. bleeding) usually become apparent within 1–2 days of ingestion and persist for less than one week.

The 'new generation' compounds are more potent rodenticides and some (e.g. brodifacoum) frequently produce signs of toxicity after a single dose. Whereas others (e.g. bromadialone) rarely cause signs of toxicity except after extremely large or long-term repetitive dosing. In the event of poisoning, the longer half-life of the agent results in haemostatic abnormalities that can persist for 3 weeks or longer.

Clinical Features

Patients with anticoagulant poisoning display features consistent with defective secondary haemostasis, including haemothorax, haemomediastinum and haemoperitoneum (Fig. 36.23). Since haemorrhage is often acute, severe and entirely internal, poisoned dogs can present with unexplained hypovolaemic shock, often accompanied by sudden dyspnoea or abdominomegaly.

Investigations

- Primary and secondary haemostasis should be evaluated without delay:
  - platelet count,
  - BMBT,
  - ACT (WBCT).
- Secondary haemostasis should be evaluated more thoroughly as soon as possible:
  - PT, APTT.
- The location and severity of internal haemorrhage should be determined:
  - abdominal and thoracic radiography,
  - routine haematology.

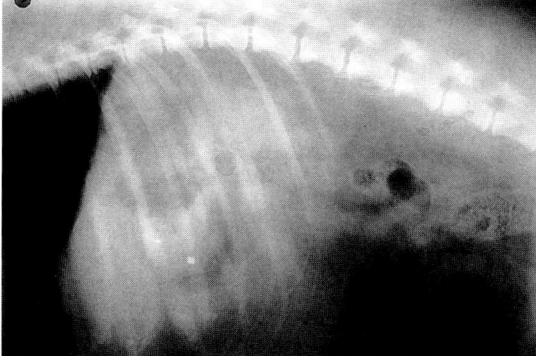

Fig. 36.23 Radiograph demonstrating moderate loss of abdominal detail due to acute haemoperitoneum in a dog with anticoagulant rodenticide poisoning (photograph courtesy of Helen Whitbread, University of Edinburgh).

- Diagnostic thoracocentesis or abdominocentesis is not required (and may be risky) when anticoagulant toxicity is already strongly suspected and can be confirmed by haemostatic testing, and is only indicated when the nature and cause of a body cavity effusion is in doubt.

Diagnosis

A strong presumptive diagnosis of anticoagulant rodenticide toxicity is based on:

- a history of potential access to toxins,
- signs consistent with defective secondary haemostasis and,
- prolongation (often marked) of ACT, PT and APTT (the intrinsic, extrinsic and common pathways are typically all affected in the actively bleeding dog),
- parameters of primary haemostasis (platelet count and BMBT) will usually be normal.

Of the vitamin K-dependent clotting factors, factor VII has the shortest half-life and is therefore the first to be affected by anticoagulant poisoning. Dogs with mild toxicity (particularly those that are not actively bleeding) may therefore have a prolonged PT due to selective impairment of the extrinsic pathway (which contains factor VII) and a normal ACT and APTT. PT is therefore the best test for detecting sub-clinical anticoagulant toxicity and for determining the efficacy of vitamin K_1 therapy.

Anticoagulant rodenticide poisoning leads to an accumulation of non-functional forms of the vitamin K-dependent clotting factors, collectively known as proteins induced by vitamin K absence (PIVKA). Since PIVKA tend to increase markedly with vitamin K antagonism, measurement of PIVKA levels, when available, provides a sensitive screening test for anticoagulant rodenticide toxicity (Mount 1988).

Management

See page 296 for guide-lines on supportive care. Specific management is outlined in Box 36.17.

Prognosis

Anticoagulant poisoning is a highly treatable coagulopathy and, given a correct diagnosis and appropriate treatment, mortalities should be minimal. Veterinarians must ensure that the duration of therapy is adequate (particularly when the exact anticoagulant is unknown), since fatal relapses can occur when treatment is discontinued prematurely.

Box 36.17 Specific management of anticoagulant rodenticide poisoning.

- Vitamin K$_1$ is the specific antidote for anticoagulant toxicity, and must be given until the toxin is cleared from the body. Whenever the specific type of anticoagulant is not identified, vitamin K$_1$ should be given for at least 3 weeks to prevent recurrence of bleeding when treatment is discontinued. Coagulation should be reassessed (via ACT or, preferably, PT) several days after discontinuing therapy.

  Vitamin K$_1$ Dose
  5 mg/kg s.c. is given initially, followed by 2.5–5 mg/kg orally split b.i.d. or t.i.d. for 1 week (short-acting rodenticides) or for at least 3 weeks (long-acting rodenticides)

  Even in emergencies vitamin K$_1$ is best given subcutaneously since intravenous administration can induce anaphylaxis and intramuscular injections may precipitate muscle haemorrhage. An initial dose of vitamin K$_1$ should be given to all dogs with suspected anticoagulant poisoning and a prolonged ACT rather than awaiting the results of further haemostatic tests (PT and APTT). Vitamin K$_3$, although less expensive than vitamin K$_1$, is largely ineffective and should therefore not be used as an antidote to anticoagulant poisoning.

- Since subcutaneous vitamin K$_1$ can taken up to 24 h to correct clotting defects, prompt transfusion with fresh whole blood, fresh-frozen plasma or frozen plasma to immediately replenish vitamin K-dependent clotting factors is indicated if the poisoned dog is suffering from life-threatening haemorrhage.

IMMUNE-MEDIATED THROMBOCYTOPENIA

Immune-mediated thrombocytopenia (IMT), also known as idiopathic thrombocytopenic purpura (ITP), is the most common acquired cause of defective primary haemostasis in the dog (Williams & Maggio-Price 1984; Jackson & Kruth 1985; Mackin 1995a).

Aetiopathogenesis

IMT is characterised by an accelerated rate of destruction of antibody-coated platelets by the organs of the mononuclear phagocytic system, particularly the spleen and (to a lesser extent) liver, leading to a markedly decreased circulating platelet life span. The average platelet life span of a patient with severe IMT is typically less than one day, and can sometimes be as brief as one hour. Thrombocytopenia develops when the rate of platelet destruction overwhelms compensatory platelet production by the bone marrow. Although IMT usually stimulates vigorous thrombopoiesis, in some patients anti-platelet antibodies can cross-react with megakaryocytes and impair platelet production.

Although IMT in the dog is most commonly a typical auto-immune disease, with no recognised precipitating event, antibody-mediated platelet destruction can also occur secondary to a diverse array of underlying disease processes (see Box 36.18).

Epidemiology

IMT most commonly affects middle-aged (average age of onset of 6 years) female dogs. Cocker Spaniels, Poodles and Old English Sheepdogs are particularly predisposed to IMT. However, since secondary IMT can be caused by a diverse range of diseases, the condition can occur in dogs of any sex, breed or age (apart from, arguably, puppies under 6 months of age).

Clinical Features

Severe IMT causes the typical clinical features of defective primary haemostasis, namely petechial and ecchymotic haemorrhages involving the skin and mucous membranes. Since secondary haemostasis is intact and prevents major body cavity haemorrhage, dogs with IMT are often remarkably stable.

Investigations

A presumptive diagnosis of IMT is often based solely on the results of haemostatic screening tests and routine haematology. However, since IMT can occur secondary to a

Many putative associations between various disease processes and IMT in the dog are based on limited clinical evidence or extrapolated directly from experiences in human IMT patients. Processes that are likely to predispose dogs to IMT, based on reasonable experimental, clinical or anecdotal evidence (Helfand 1988; Mackin 1995b), include:

Immune-mediated diseases:	Systemic lupus erythematosus
	Immune-mediated haemolytic anaemia
Infectious diseases:	Ehrlichiosis
Parasitic diseases:	Heartworm
Neoplasia:	Haematopoietic neoplasia
	Solid tumours
Medications:	Sulphonamides
	Cephalosporins
	Penicillins
	Phenylbutazone
	Aspirin
	Gold salts
	Oestrogens
Other:	Modified live-virus vaccination

variety of diseases (some of which can be well hidden), more extensive investigations can usually be justified.

- Primary and secondary haemostasis should be evaluated:
  - platelet count (including a scan for megathrombocytes),
  - PT, APTT.
  Note: ACT is unreliable and BMBT is superfluous in the presence of severe thrombocytopenia.
- Routine haematology should be performed.
- Potential underlying diseases such as immune-mediated disorders, infection, parasites, or neoplasia should be thoroughly pursued. Consider:
  - serum biochemistry,
  - urine analysis,
  - abdominal and thoracic radiography,
  - abdominal ultrasonography,
  - heartworm testing (in endemic areas),
  - rickettsial serology (in endemic areas),
  - immunological testing (Coombs' test, anti-nuclear antibody test).
- Bone marrow should be evaluated via aspiration cytology and/or core biopsy histopathology if haematology reveals concurrent anaemia, leucopenia and thrombocytopenia, or evidence suggestive of marrow disease such as scarce megathrombocytes despite the presence of low platelet numbers (Fig. 36.24). Normal marrow

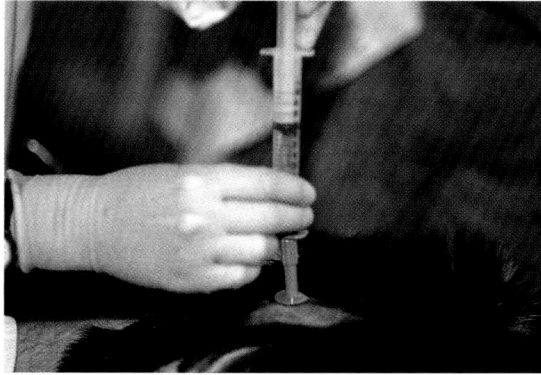

Fig. 36.24 Bone marrow aspiration for cytological analysis in a pancytopenic dog.

aspirates contain about 1 to 3 megakaryocytes per low power (100 power) microscope field (Fig. 36.25).
- Measurement of anti-platelet antibody (see Box 36.19). Anti-platelet antibody assays are not readily available to many veterinarians, and no test as yet has been indisputably proven to be diagnostically accurate.

The diagnosis of IMT in practice remains primarily a presumptive diagnosis based on the balance of clinical

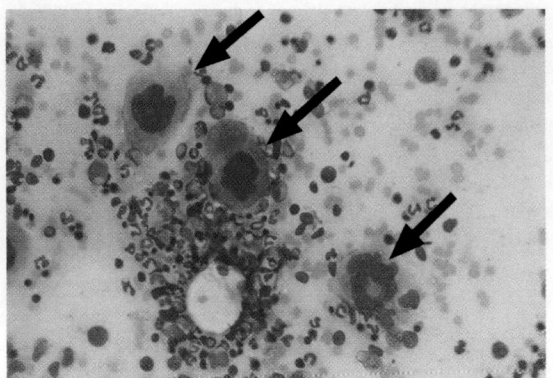

Fig. 36.25 Stained bone marrow smear demonstrating the presence of adequate numbers of large, multi-nucleated megakaryocytes (dark arrows) (photograph courtesy of Chris Belford, Cytopath).

evidence, exclusion of other causes of thrombocytopenia and subsequent response to therapy.

Diagnosis

Since IMT is by far the most common cause of a markedly decreased platelet count in the dog, a strong presumptive diagnosis can be based solely on the detection of severe

thrombocytopenia if history, physical examination and laboratory testing reveal no evidence of other causes of decreased platelet numbers such as DIC or primary bone marrow disorders (see Box 36.7). Treatment should therefore not be withheld in dogs with suspected IMT pending the results of specific anti-platelet antibody testing, particularly as such tests tend to be unreliable. A presumptive diagnosis can usually be confirmed within 1–2 weeks by an appropriate response to immunosuppressive therapy.

Thrombocytopenia in the absence of megathrombocytes (shift platelets) suggests the presence of primary marrow disease, particularly if the patient has concurrent anaemia and leucopenia. Bone marrow analysis in such patients usually reveals diffuse and advanced bone marrow disorders such as neoplasia or fibrosis. The detection of megakaryocyte hypoplasia despite normal numbers of myeloid and erythroid precursors, however, suggests specific antibody-mediated destruction of megakaryocytes, a less common manifestation of IMT in the dog.

Since canine IMT can occur secondary to other diseases, a diagnosis of IMT is not complete without a thorough consideration of potential underlying disorders.

Management

See page 296 for guidelines on supportive care. Specific management is outlined in Box 36.20 and the drugs used are listed in Table 36.1.

Box 36.19 Measurement of anti-platelet antibody.

Absolute confirmation of a diagnosis of IMT requires demonstration of the presence of anti-platelet antibodies (Feldman *et al.* 1988; Mackin 1995b). A number of methods have been developed to evaluate anti-platelet antibody:

- Platelet factor 3 (PF 3) immunoinjury technique.
- Indirect measurement of serum anti-platelet antibody levels via radioactive, enzymatic or fluorescent immunoglobulin labels.
- Direct evaluation of platelet-associated antibody levels using various immunoglobulin labels.
- Detection of megakaryocyte-associated antibodies via the direct immunofluorescent labelling of megakaryocytes on marrow smears.

Measurement of serum anti-platelet antibodies via the PF 3 test and other indirect methods is convenient to practitioners since the techniques can be performed on small volumes of serum which may be frozen for storage and transport. Such techniques, however, have consistently proven to be of very limited diagnostic accuracy. More recently described methods involving direct labelling of platelet-associated antibodies, although diagnostically superior, are unfortunately of very limited availability and not readily transportable.

Bone marrow aspirates can be collected and prepared as air-dried smears to enable convenient transportation and subsequent immunofluorescent labelling. Since anti-megakaryocyte antibodies appear to cross-react with anti-platelet antibodies, immunofluorescent labelling of marrow smears may, if shown to be diagnostically accurate, prove to be the practitioner's diagnostic test of choice for confirming the presence of IMT.

Box 36.20 Specific management of immune-mediated thrombocytopenia.

The initial goal of therapy for canine IMT is to restore platelet numbers to a level sufficient to maintain effective primary hemostasis (greater than approximately 50×10^9 platelets/l). The long-term goal is to restore platelet numbers to normal levels (Mackin 1995b).

- *Standard therapy*
  Oral glucocorticoids (prednisone, prednisolone or dexamethasone, combined with azathioprine in severe cases) are commenced at the time of diagnosis, and continued at immunosuppressive doses until platelet numbers are adequate (usually within 2–4 weeks). Drug doses are then gradually tapered (every 2–4 weeks) if platelet numbers remain adequate. Drug therapy can usually be safely discontinued if complete remission has been maintained for at least 6 months.

- *Emergency care*
  Critical patients may also require treatment with intravenous dexamethasone and/or vincristine. Potential therapeutic options in unresponsive critical cases include splenectomy (ideally just after an emergency platelet transfusion), intravenous high-dose human gamma-globulins or plasmapheresis. Platelet transfusion alone is rarely more than temporarily effective in dogs with severe IMT.

- *Refractory cases*
  Dogs with persistent chronic IMT or unacceptable drug-related side-effects with standard immunosuppressive therapy may respond to danazol, cyclophosphamide or splenectomy (Holloway et al. 1990; Jans et al. 1990). Speculative treatments that may be considered in the extremely refractory patient (which, fortunately, are rarely encountered) include cyclosporin, colchicine and intravenous high-dose human gamma-globulins.

- *Secondary IMT*
  Identification and treatment of underlying primary disorders is the cornerstone of the management of secondary IMT.

Platelet numbers should be monitored every few weeks during the first 2 months of treatment, and then 1–2 weeks after every subsequent reduction in drug dosage. Patients in complete remission (with or without therapy) should have platelet numbers reassessed at least every 3 months.

Prognosis

Although acute IMT is a potentially fatal disorder, with mortality rates of up to 25%, most dogs that survive an initial episode will eventually attain permanent remission without the need for long-term therapy. Appropriate (and, if necessary, aggressive) initial therapy is therefore essential (Williams & Maggio-Price 1984; Jackson & Kruth 1985; Jans *et al.* 1990).

DISSEMINATED INTRAVASCULAR COAGULATION

Disseminated intravascular coagulation (DIC) is a process characterised by accelerated coagulation leading to wide-spread formation of microthrombi (Slappendel 1988). Paradoxically, although DIC is precipitated by accelerated coagulation, the condition is often only recognised when uncontrolled thrombus formation eventually leads to defective haemostasis.

Aetiopathogenesis

- Microthrombus formation can be the end result of a variety of diseases that cause accelerated coagulation.
- Widespread formation of microthrombi can cause depletion of platelets and clotting factors ('consumption coagulopathy') and thereby predispose to haemorrhage.
- Excessive quantities of fibrin degradation products (FDP) may be released as the fibrinolytic system attempts to break down fibrin within microthrombi.
- FDP inhibit both platelet function and various factors

Table 36.1 Drugs commonly used in the treatment of canine IMT.

Agent	Dose rate	Comment
Glucocorticoids		
Prednisolone/Prednisone	initial: 2–4 mg/kg p.o. s.i.d. tapered to maintenance: 0.5–1.0 mg/kg every 48 h.	Prednisone and prednisolone are the most commonly used glucocorticoids although dexamethasone may be more effective in critical or refractory patients
Dexamethasone	0.2 mg/kg i.v. (single dose in critical cases) 0.3 mg/kg p.o. s.i.d. as initial immunosuppressive dose.	
Azathioprine	initial: 2 mg/kg p.o. s.i.d. tapered to maintenance: 0.5–1.0 mg/kg every 48 h.	Immunosuppressive agent of choice for initial treatment of IMT. Used concurrently with glucocorticoids to enable more rapid tapering of glucocorticoid doses
Vincristine	0.02 mg/kg as single i.v. dose	Vincristine can dramatically increase platelet numbers within several days in some dogs
Danazol	initial: 5 mg/kg p.o. b.i.d., slowly tapering to a minimum effective dose	Used concurrently with glucocorticoids
Cyclophosphamide	50 mg/M^2 p.o. daily for the first 4 days of each week or every 48 h. Maximum 6 months	More potent immunosuppressive than azathioprine but the potential for side effects such as myelosuppression, increased susceptibility to infection and haemorrhagic cystitis deters the chronic use of cyclophosphamide
High dose intravenous gamma-globulin	High dose intravenous gamma-globulins have been shown to increase platelet numbers in human patients with critical or refractory IMT. Similar responses have been observed using the human product in dogs without obvious side effects. Cost may be prohibitive	

q 48 h, every other day treatment.
A more detailed consideration of these agents, their mode of action and side effects, is provided in Chapter 5.

within the clotting cascade, and therefore further pre-dispose affected dogs to bleeding.

- In addition to causing blood loss anaemia, DIC may also induce 'microangiopathic haemolytic anaemia', a process by which circulating erythrocytes are mechanically damaged by the fibrin strands within microthrombi, forming fragmented red cells called 'schistocytes' (Fig. 36.26).

Patients with DIC rapidly consume available quantities of a plasma protein called antithrombin III (AT III). Antithrombin III inactivates thrombin and the active forms of clotting factors IX, X, XI and XII, and is the most important natural inhibitor of haemostasis (Green 1988). Deficiencies of AT III therefore further exacerbate the underlying thrombotic tendencies seen in patients with

DIC. Adequate plasma levels of heparin are necessary for efficient functioning of the AT III molecule.

Epidemiology

DIC can complicate any severe systemic disease (Slappendel 1988). Certain diseases strongly predispose affected dogs to DIC (see Box 36.21).

Clinical Features

Since DIC can affect platelet numbers, platelet function and the clotting cascade, the disorder may present with clinical features suggestive of either abnormal primary

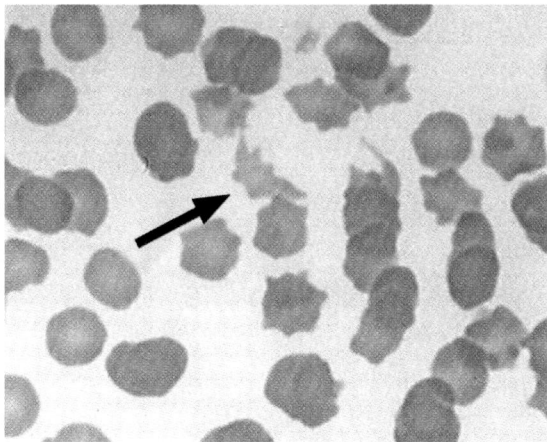

Fig. 36.26   Stained blood smear demonstrating the typical fragmented appearance of a schistocyte (dark arrow), suggesting the presence of microangiopathic haemolysis of red blood cells (photograph courtesy of Guillermo Couto, Ohio State University).

Box 36.21   Diseases commonly associated with DIC in the dog.

Haemangiosarcoma	Septicaemia
Generalised neoplasia	Snake bite
Acute pancreatitis	Shock
Gastric dilation/volvulus	Hypothermia
Immune-mediated haemolytic	
anaemia	Hyperthermia
Liver disease	

haemostasis or abnormal secondary haemostasis, or a highly variable combination of both. Dogs with DIC typically have a serious underlying disorder, and usually present with clinical signs referable to that disorder. Patients with haemangiosarcoma, a common cause of DIC in dogs (Hammer *et al.* 1991; Hargis & Feldman 1991), may however sometimes present solely with unexplained haemorrhage (Fig. 36.27).

Investigations

Extensive screening is usually indicated in dogs with suspected DIC.

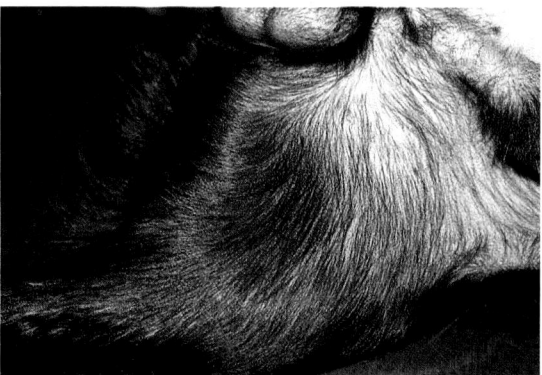

Fig. 36.27   Cutaneous bruising as the sole initial presenting complaint in a dog with disseminated intravascular coagulation associated with haemangiosarcoma.

- Potential underlying diseases (particularly haemangiosarcoma) should be thoroughly pursued. Consider:
  - routine haematology,
  - serum biochemistry,
  - urine analysis,
  - abdominal and thoracic radiography,
  - abdominal and cardiac ultrasonography.
- Primary and secondary haemostasis should be evaluated:
  - platelet count,
  - PT, APTT (and/or ACT),
  - BMBT.
- Other tests of coagulation and fibrinolysis that should be considered if available:
  - fibrinogen,
  - FDP,
  - AT III.

Diagnosis

DIC is one of the few disease processes that can simultaneously affect primary haemostasis, secondary haemostasis and fibrinolysis. DIC should be suspected if:

- haematology reveals evidence of microangiopathic haemolytic anaemia (schistocytes in particular);
- haemostatic screening reveals abnormalities affecting both primary (thrombocytopenia and/or prolonged BMBT) and secondary haemostasis (prolonged PT, APTT and/or ACT);
- the patient has an underlying disease known to be associated with an increased frequency of DIC.

Further haemostatic testing may reveal elevated FDP and decreased fibrinogen and AT III levels.

The haemostatic abnormalities caused by DIC are notoriously variable. Dogs with mild DIC may display only a few of the abnormalities classically associated with the advanced disease. Haemostatic abnormalities most commonly encountered in patients with mild DIC include thrombocytopenia, prolonged APTT, elevated FDP and decreased AT III levels.

Management

See page 296 for guide-lines on supportive care. Specific management is outlined in Box 36.22.

Prognosis

Euphemisms for DIC including 'death is coming' and 'dead in cage' reflect the poor prognosis traditionally associated with this disorder. Early DIC, however, can be a very manageable illness if underlying diseases can be identified and treated. Unfortunately, the prognosis associated with DIC is grave if the primary disease cannot be effectively treated (advanced haemangiosarcoma, for example).

Veterinarians are becoming more aware of the association between DIC and certain diseases, and are therefore more likely to perform haemostatic screening tests in dogs with these diseases. As a result, early DIC may be diagnosed before the onset of overt clinical signs, and therapy consequently has a much greater chance of success. Furthermore, the routine prophylactic use of heparin in dogs with diseases that predispose to DIC may prevent development of the disorder in the first place.

BLEEDING DISORDERS ASSOCIATED WITH LIVER DISEASE

The liver is intimately involved in numerous haemostatic mechanisms, including the production of all of the major clotting factors except factor VIII, important anticoagulants such as antithrombin III and major components of fibrinolysis such as plasminogen, and the degradation of many clotting factors and fibrin degradation products. Liver disease can therefore potentially produce many complex and unpredictable haemostatic derangements (Badylak 1988).

Aetiopathogenesis

Since the liver produces most of the clotting factors, severe hepatic disease can theoretically lead to multiple factor defi-

---

Box 36.22   Specific management of disseminated intravascular coagulation (DIC).

- Identification and treatment (if possible) of underlying disorders is the cornerstone of the management of DIC.

- Heparin, in conjunction with AT III, inhibits a number of factors within the clotting cascade, and may prevent ongoing microthrombus formation in dogs with DIC (Slappendel 1988). The benefits of heparinising dogs that are susceptible to haemorrhage because of a consumption coagulopathy are very controversial, however, as high doses of heparin may actually exacerbate bleeding. Lower doses of heparin are safer, and are probably as effective as high doses at preventing microthrombus formation. Low dose heparin is most effective when used to prevent DIC in dogs suffering from predisposing underlying diseases.

    Heparin dose (low dose regimen)
    75 IU/kg subcutaneously every 8 h

    Heparin, to be effective, requires the presence of adequate amounts of AT III. Heparin may therefore be of little benefit in dogs with depleted AT III levels due to severe DIC unless the AT III is first replaced via transfusion.

- Transfusion with fresh whole blood or with platelet-rich plasma and/or fresh frozen plasma if available (see Box 36.11) to replace depleted platelets, clotting factors and AT III should be considered in dogs with DIC, particularly if the patient is actively bleeding. A single dose of heparin (75 IU/kg) may safely be added to transfused blood or plasma.

ciencies and impairment of the intrinsic, extrinsic and common pathways. In reality, however, significant factor deficiencies are relatively uncommon, and do not correlate well with the severity of hepatic disease. Decreased clotting factor production in patients with hepatobiliary disease may potentially be compounded by a deficiency of vitamin K secondary to poor intestinal absorption of fat and fat-soluble vitamins associated with decreased bile acid secretion, with resultant impairment of vitamin K-dependent factors.

Hepatic disease has also been associated with decreased platelet function (Willis *et al.* 1989) and an increased susceptibility to disseminated intravascular coagulation.

Clinical Features

Since hepatic dysfunction can affect both platelet function and the clotting cascade, dogs with liver disease may potentially present with clinical signs suggestive of either abnormal primary haemostasis or abnormal secondary haemostasis, or a variable combination of both. Spontaneous bleeding in dogs with liver disease is, however, relatively rare. Screening of dogs with liver disease can reveal unexpected subclinical haemostatic disorders that may be of considerable significance if invasive procedures (such as liver biopsies) are performed.

Investigations

Apart from the routine characterisation of the nature and extent of the primary disease process in patients with liver failure, it is also advisable to screen haemostatic function if spontaneous haemorrhage is evident or invasive procedures are contemplated. Primary and secondary haemostasis should therefore be evaluated, and assessment of plasma anticoagulant and fibrinolytic properties should also be considered:

- platelet count,
- PT, APTT (and/or ACT),
- BMBT,
- FDP, fibrinogen, AT III.

Diagnosis

Apart from disseminated intravascular coagulation, liver failure is the only other common disease in the dog that may affect fibrinolysis and primary and secondary haemostasis simultaneously. Liver disease should be considered as an alternative diagnosis to DIC if haemostatic screening reveals abnormalities affecting both primary (prolonged

Box 36.23　Specific management of bleeding disorders associated with liver disease.

- Most patients with liver failure severe enough to cause bleeding disorders will require intensive symptomatic and specific treatment of the many other manifestations of hepatic disease.
- If a haemostatic disorder is detected, transfusion with fresh whole blood or fresh-frozen plasma (see Box 36.11) to temporarily provide clotting factors may be indicated before invasive procedures such as hepatic biopsy.
- Individual patients with a suspected significant component of cholestasis may also benefit from a trial course of vitamin K_1 (by injection rather than orally).

BMBT) and secondary haemostasis (prolonged PT, APTT and/or ACT). Affected patients, however, will usually also be exhibiting obvious clinical signs of advanced hepatic failure.

Management

See page 296 for guide-lines on supportive care. Specific management is outlined in Box 36.23.

Prognosis

Liver disease severe enough to cause haemostatic disorders is usually very advanced and, unless acute and reversible, typically associated with a guarded prognosis, Vitamin K-responsive coagulopathies secondary to cholestasis may potentially be completely reversible following relief of biliary obstruction.

REFERENCES

Badylak, S.F. (1988). Coagulation disorders and liver disease. *Veterinary Clinics of North America. Small Animal Practice*, **18**, 87–93.

Brown, S.J., Simpson, K.W., Baker, S.J., Spagnoletti, M.A. & Elwood, C.M. (1994). Macrothrombocytosis in Cavalier King Charles Spaniels. Proceedings 12th American College of

Veterinary Internal Medicine Forum, San Francisco. p. 1002. ACVIM, Lakewood, Cobrado.

Callan, M.B., Giger, U., Bennett, J.S., Haskins, M.E., Hayden, J.E. & Anderson, J.G. (1993). Platelet storage pool disease in American Cocker Spaniels (Abstract). Proceedings 11th American College of Veterinary Internal Medicine Forum, Washington. p. 940. ACVIM, Blacksburg, Virginia.

Catalfamo, J.L. & Dodds, W.J. (1988). Hereditary and acquired thrombopathias. *Veterinary Clinics of North America. Small Animal Practice*, **18**, 185–193.

Carr, A.P. & Johnson, G.S. (1994). A review of hemostatic abnormalities in dogs and cats. *Journal of the American Animal Hospital Association*, **30**, 475–482.

Davenport, D.J. & Carakostas, M.C. (1982). Platelet disorders in the dog and cat, Part I: Physiology and pathogenesis. *Compendium on Continuing Education for the Practicing Veterinarian*, **4**, 762–772.

Feldman, B.F., Thomason, K.J. & Jain, N.C. (1988). Quantitative platelet disorders. *Veterinary Clinics of North America. Small Animal Practice*, **18**, 35–49.

Feldman, B.F. (1989). Disorders of platelets. In: *Current Veterinary Therapy X*, (ed. R.W. Kirk), pp. 457–464. W.B. Saunders, Philadelphia.

Feldman, D.G., Brooks, M.B. & Dodds, W.J. (1995). Hemophilia B (factor IX deficiency) in a family of German Shepherd dogs. *Journal of the American Veterinary Medical Association*, **206**, 1901–1905.

Fogh, J.M. (1988). A study of hemophilia A in German Shepherd dogs in Denmark. *Veterinary Clinics of North America. Small Animal Practice*, **18**, 245–254.

Fogh, J.M. & Fogh, I.T. (1988). Inherited coagulation disorders. *Veterinary Clinics of North America. Small Animal Practice*, **18**, 231–243.

Forsythe, L.T. & Willis, S.E. (1989). Evaluating oral mucosa bleeding times in healthy dogs using a spring-loaded device. *Canadian Veterinary Journal*, **30**, 344–345.

Giger, U. & Dodds, W.J. (1989). Effect of desmopressin in normal dogs and dogs with von Willebrand's disease. *Veterinary Clinical Pathology*, **18**, 39–42.

Green, R.A. (1988). Pathophysiology of antithrombin III deficiency. *Veterinary Clinics of North America. Small Animal Practice*, **18**, 95–104.

Grindem, C.B., Breitschwerdt, E.B., Corbett, W.T. & Jans, H.E. (1991). Epidemiologic survey of thrombocytopenia in dogs: A report on 987 cases. *Veterinary Clinical Pathology*, **20**, 38–43.

Grindem, C.B., Breitschwerdt, E.B., Corbett, W.T., Page, R.L. & Jans, H.E. (1994). Thrombocytopenia associated with neoplasia in dogs. *Journal of Veterinary Internal Medicine*, **8**, 400–405.

Hackner, S.G. (1995). Approach to the diagnosis of bleeding disorders. *Compendium on Continuing Education for the Practicing Veterinarian*, **17**, 331–350.

Hammer, A.S., Couto, C.G., Swardson, C. & Getzy, D. (1991). Hemostatic abnormalities in dogs with hemangiosarcoma. *Journal of Veterinary Internal Medicine*, **5**, 11–14.

Hargis, A.M. & Feldman, B.F. (1991). Evaluation of hemostatic defects secondary to vascular tumors in dogs: 11 cases (1983–1988). *Journal of the American Veterinary Medical Association*, **198**, 891–894.

Helfand, S.C. (1988). Platelets and neoplasia. *Veterinary Clinics of North America. Small Animal Practice*, **18**, 131–156.

Holloway, S.A., Meyer, D.J. & Mannella, C. (1990). Prednisolone and danazol for treatment of immune-mediated anemia, thrombocytopenia, and ineffective erythroid regeneration in a dog. *Journal of the American Veterinary Medical Association*, **197**, 1045–1048.

Jackson, M.L. & Kruth, S.A. (1985). Immune-mediated hemolytic anemia and thrombocytopenia in the dog: A retrospective study of 55 cases diagnosed from 1969 through 1983 at the Western College of Veterinary Medicine. *Canadian Veterinary Journal*, **26**, 250–255.

Jackson, M.L., Searcy, G.P. & Olexson, D.W. (1985). The effect of oral phenylbutazone on whole blood platelet aggregation in the dog. *Canadian Journal of Comparative Medicine*, **49**, 271–277.

Jans, H.E., Armstrong, P.J. & Sylvester-Price, G. (1990). Therapy of immune mediated thrombocytopenia. *Journal of Veterinary Internal Medicine*, **4**, 4–7.

Jergens, A.E., Turrentine, M.A., Kraus, K.H. & Johnson, G.S. (1987). Buccal mucosa bleeding times of healthy dogs and of dogs in various pathologic states, including thrombocytopenia, uremia, and von Willebrand's disease. *American Journal of Veterinary Research*, **48**, 1337–1342.

Johnson, G.S., Turrentine, M.A. & Kraus, K.H. (1988). Canine von Willebrand's disease. *Veterinary Clinics of North America. Small Animal Practice*, **18**, 195–229.

Johnstone, I.B. (1982). Inherited defects of haemostasis. *Compendium on Continuing Education for the Practicing Veterinarian*, **4**, 483–488.

Johnstone, I.B. (1988). Clinical and laboratory diagnosis of bleeding disorders. *Veterinary Clinics of North America. Small Animal Practice*, **18**, 21–33.

Kraus, K.H. & Johnson, G.S. (1989). Von Willebrand's disease in dogs. In: *Current Veterinary Therapy X*, (ed. R.W. Kirk), pp. 446–451. W.B. Saunders, Philadelphia.

Kristensen, A.T., Weiss, D.J. & Klausner, J.S. (1994). Platelet dysfunction associated with immune-mediated thrombocytopenia in dogs. *Journal of Veterinary Internal Medicine*, **8**, 323–327.

Littlewood, J.D. (1989). Inherited bleeding disorders of dogs and cats. *Journal of Small Animal Practice*, **30**, 140–143.

Mackin, A.J. (1995a). Canine immune-mediated thrombocytopenia – Part I. *Compendium on Continuing Education for the Practicing Veterinarian*, **17**, 353–364.

Mackin, A.J. (1995b). Canine immune-mediated thrombocytopenia – Part II. *Compendium on Continuing Education for the Practicing Veterinarian*, **17**, 515–535.

Mackin, A.J., Allen, D.G. & Johnstone, I.B. (1995). Effects of vincristine and prednisone on platelet numbers and function in clinically normal dogs. *American Journal of Veterinary Research*, **56**, 100–107.

Mansell, P.D. & Parry, B.W. (1991). Changes in factor VIII:coagulant activity and von Willebrand factor antigen concentration after subcutaneous injection of desmopressin in dogs with mild hemophilia A. *Journal of Veterinary Internal Medicine*, **5**, 191–194.

Meehan, A.P. (1984). *Rats and Mice. Their Biology and Control*. The Rentokil Library. Rentokil, East Grinstead, West Sussex.

Mount, M.E. (1988). Diagnosis and therapy of anticoagulant rodenticide intoxications. *Veterinary Clinics of North America. Small Animal Practice*, **18**, 115–130.

Murphy, M.J. & Gerken, D.F. (1989). The anticoagulant rodenticides. In: *Current Veterinary Therapy X*, (ed. R.W. Kirk), pp. 143–146. W.B. Saunders, Philadelphia.

Parry, B.W. (1989). Laboratory evaluation of haemorrhagic coagulopathies in small animal practice. *Veterinary Clinics of North America. Small Animal Practice*, **19**, 729–742.

Rackear, D., Feldman, B., Farver, T. & Lelong, L. (1986). The effect of three different dosages of acetylsalicylic acid on canine platelet aggregation. *Journal of the American Animal Hospital Association*, **24**, 23–26.

Rackear, D.G. (1988). Drugs that alter the hemostatic mechanism. *Veterinary Clinics of North America. Small Animal Practice*, **18**, 67–77.

Slappendel, R.J. (1988). Disseminated intravascular coagulation. *Veterinary Clinics of North America. Small Animal Practice*, **18**, 169–184.

Slappendel, R.J., Frielink, R.A.J., Mol, J.A., Noordzij, A. & Hamer, R. (1992). An enzyme-linked immunosorbent assay (ELISA) for von Willebrand factor antigen (vWf-Ag) in canine plasma. *Veterinary Immunology and Immunopathology*, **33**, 145–154.

Stokol, T., Parry, B.W., Mansell, P.D. & Richardson, J.L. (1994). Hematorrhachis associated with hemophilia A in three German Shepherd dogs. *Journal of the American Animal Hospital Association*, **30**, 239–243.

Stone, M.S. & Cotter, S.M. (1992). Practical guidelines for transfusion therapy. In: *Current Veterinary Therapy XI*, (eds R.W. Kirk & J.D. Bonogura), pp. 475–479. W.B. Saunders, Philadelphia.

Stone, M.S., Johnstone, I.B., Brooks, M., Bollinger, T.K. & Cotter, S.M. (1994). Lupus-type 'anticoagulant' in a dog with hemolysis and thrombosis. *Journal of Veterinary Internal Medicine*, **8**, 57–61.

Troy, G.C. (1988). An overview of hemostasis. *Veterinary Clinics of North America. Small Animal Practice*, **18**, 5–20.

Williams, D.A. & Maggio-Price, L. (1984). Canine idiopathic thrombocytopenia: Clinical observations and long-term follow-up in 54 cases. *Journal of the American Veterinary Medical Association*, **185**, 660–663.

Willis, S.E., Jackson, M.L., Meric, S.M. & Rousseaux, C.G. (1989). Whole blood platelet aggregation in dogs with liver disease. *American Journal of Veterinary Research*, **50**, 1893–1897.

Chapter 37

Fever of Unknown Origin

J. K. Dunn

INTRODUCTION

Fever of unknown origin (FUO) presents one of the most challenging problems in small animal medicine. A logical problem-oriented diagnostic approach is essential in order to obtain a definitive diagnosis.

In practice most fevers are due to transient bacterial or viral infections which resolve spontaneously or in response to appropriate therapy; as such these cannot be regarded as true FUO cases. Many unexplained fevers are due to the early atypical presentations of relatively common diseases. In referral centres a much higher percentage of cases with unresolved febrile episodes are due to immune-mediated disorders or neoplasia. Most diagnoses are made because new clinical or clinicopathological signs develop. This means that in many cases there is a need for repeated physical examinations and laboratory tests and the financial implications of this should be discussed with the owner at an early stage of the diagnostic investigations.

Pathophysiology of Fever

There is a delicate equilibrium between the body's heat production and heat loss mechanisms (Fig. 37.1). Body temperature is determined by the 'set-point' of the thermoregulatory centre situated in the preoptic region of the anterior hypothalamus. Exogenous pyrogens (which include numerous infectious and non-infectious agents) can induce fever via the release of a number of cell-derived mediators (mostly low molecular peptides) known as endogenous pyrogens.

Exogenous pyrogens include Gram-negative and Gram-positive bacteria, bacterial endotoxin, viruses, fungi, parasites, toxins, tumours, bile acids and certain drugs. Endogenous pyrogens are produced by neutrophils, eosinophils, monocytes and fixed mononuclear phagocytes

(e.g. Kupffer cells, splenic and alveolar macrophages). Some tumour cells release endogenous pyrogen without prior stimulation by an exogenous agent.

Endogenous pyrogens increase the thermoregulatory 'set-point'. Several immunological mediators released by endotoxin-activated macrophages can be classified as endogenous pyrogens and, as such, are capable of inducing fever. These mediators include interleukin-1 (IL-1), tumour necrosis factor (TNF), interferons and platelet activating factor (PAF). Both IL-1 and TNF are involved in the generation of the acute phase response and may be directly responsible for many of the systemic effects (anorexia, depression etc.) which are usually associated with fever. Certain chemical mediators, for example prostaglandins (PGE2), cyclic-AMP, 5-hydroxytryptamine and noradrenaline are also thought to play an important role in the generation of the febrile response.

The beneficial effects of fever are often overlooked. Many endogenous pyrogens increase granulocyte function and mobility; both IL-1 and TNF activate T cells and enhance T cell responses during antigen presentation. The decrease in plasma iron that occurs during the acute phase response may inhibit the replication of microbes.

What Constitutes a Fever of Unknown Origin (FUO)?

Fulfilment of certain criteria is necessary to eliminate short-lived fevers associated with infection, postoperative fevers and other non-pyrogenic causes of hyperthermia (see below).

The following criteria, extrapolated from human medicine, can be used to define FUO in small animals.

- Prolonged fever (>3 weeks duration) associated with vague non-specific signs of illness such as lethargy, weight loss and anorexia.

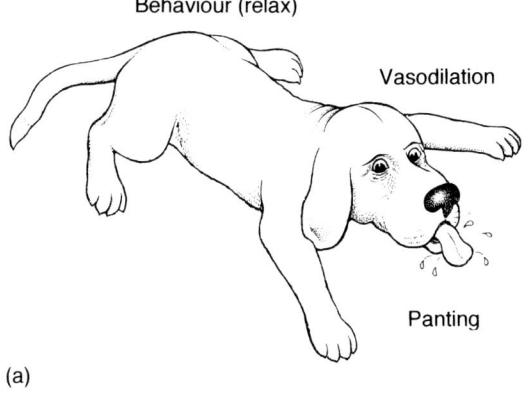

(a)

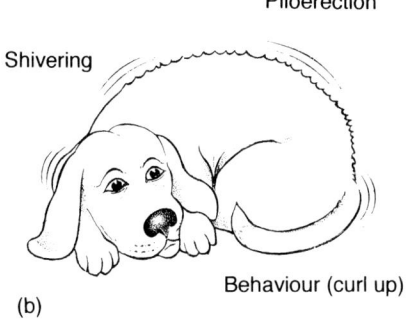

(b)

Fig. 37.1 Behavioural mechanisms for decreasing (A) and increasing (B) body temperature.

- Temperature greater than 1.5°F (0.8°C) above normal on several occasions.
- Diagnosis uncertain after one week of hospitalisation and routine laboratory tests.

Fever can be described as:

- Intermittent, febrile episodes which last one or more days with intervening periods of normal temperature. Fever associated with acute bacterial infections may be characterised by daily temperature 'spikes', sometimes referred to as a 'remittent' fever.
- Persistent (sustained), fever may last for several days with minimal variation between individual measurements.

True fevers must be differentiated from non-pyrogenic causes of hyperthermia such as:

- heat stroke,
- overexertion,

- malignant hyperthermia,
- primary hypothalamic tumours,
- hypermetabolic disorders such as hyperthyroidism and phaeochromocytoma.

In these conditions the thermoregulatory set-point is not increased. Increases in body temperature greater than 41°C are generally not true fevers.

Common Causes of FUO in Dogs and Cats

The list of differential diagnoses for fever, in the absence of more specific localising signs, is extensive. The major causes of FUO can be discussed under four headings (Table 37.1):

- localised or systemic infections;
- immune-mediated disorders;
- neoplasia;
- a miscellaneous group of disorders, many of which are orthopaedic problems associated with pain.

The approximate distribution of FUO cases examined at Cambridge Veterinary School in a recent survey was as shown in Table 37.2.

Infection

- *Bacterial endocarditis* causes intermittent thrombo-embolic bacteraemic episodes. Animals with bacterial endocarditis may present with polyarthritis due to the deposition of immune complexes in the joints. Less frequently, septic polyarthritis develops as a result of direct thromboembolic spread to the joints. A cardiac murmur may be present although in some cases this may develop late in the course of the disease.
- *Bacteraemias* without a primary focus of infection are rare. They may occur in association with lymphoproliferative or myeloproliferative disorders, immunodeficiency syndromes, aplastic anaemia (e.g. oestrogen toxicity, chronic ehrlichiosis) or other causes of bone marrow suppression resulting in persistent neutropenia. A primary (congenital) immunodeficiency syndrome (see below) should be suspected if a young animal presents with a history of recurrent infections.
- *Localised urogenital infections* (stump pyometra, prostatic abscess, pyelonephritis) often present with a history of intermittent or sustained fever. Early cases of pyothorax or inhaled pulmonary (bronchial) foreign bodies may present without obvious respiratory signs.

Table 37.1   Conditions which can present with fever of unknown origin.

Systemic infections	*Localised infections*
Bacterial endocarditis	Bacterial endocarditis
Bacteraemias from an inapparent focus, e.g. secondary to severe neutropenia or other forms of immunodeficiency syndrome	Urogenital infections (e.g. pyelonephritis, chronic prostatitis/prostatic abscess, stump pyometra)
Disseminated toxoplasmosis or *Neospora caninum* infection	Pyothorax and lung infections (e.g. inhaled pulmonary foreign bodies/pulmonary abscess, bronchopneumonia)
Lyme disease (acute)	Occult infections such as hepatic abscess or cholangitis
Leptospirosis	Retrobulbar or tooth root abscesses
Mycobacterial infections	Localised peritonitis
Psittacosis	Discospondylitis
Imported diseases, e.g. ehrlichiosis, leishmaniasis, babesiosis, brucellosis*	Osteomyelitis (especially disseminated haematogenous osteomyelitis in young dogs)
Disseminated mycotic infections (e.g. aspergillosis, histoplasmosis, blastomycosis, cryptococcosis, coccidioidomycosis)	
Immune-mediated disease	*Neoplasia*
Systemic lupus erythematosus (SLE)	Lymphoproliferative or myeloproliferative disease
Immune-mediated polyarthropathy	Large neoplasms (especially hepatic tumours) with necrotic centres
• rheumatoid arthritis (erosive)	
• idiopathic polyarthritis (non-erosive)	
Autoimmune haemolytic anaemia	
Immune-mediated thrombocytopenia	
Steroid-responsive meningitis	
Immunodeficiency syndromes (see Table 37.2)	
Miscellaneous disorders	
Drug reactions: tetracycline, sulphonamides, penicillin, amphotericin B, quinidine	
Metaphyseal osteopathy	
Panosteitis	
Hepatic necrosis	
Pulmonary emboli	
Nodular panniculitis	

* These diseases are not present in the UK but may be occasionally seen in dogs which have passed through quarantine.

- *Discospondylitis.* Bacterial infection of the intervertebral discs results in stiffness and a localised area of pain over the affected disc(s). Larger breeds are more susceptible and the lumbosacral disc space is most frequently involved. Some animals with discospondylitis may present with neurological deficits. *Staphylococcus aureus*, coliforms and, in the United States, *Brucella canis* are the most common organisms isolated from the lesions.
- *Borrelia burgdorferi* infection (Lyme disease). Acute *Borrelia burgdorferi* infection may cause fever especially in young dogs. Polyarthritis resulting in lameness is the most common manifestation of this tick-borne disease.

- *Systemic mycotic diseases* rarely occur in the United Kingdom. Their clinical course tends to be prolonged and fever is often associated with marked weight loss. Many body systems, including skin, joints, bones and eyes, may be affected.

Immune-Mediated Disease

- *Immune mediated polyarthropathies.* Antigen-antibody complexes, deposited in the synovial membrane, activate complement leading to the release of a number of potent inflammatory-inducing agents. Neutrophils and

Table 37.2 Approximate distribution of FUO cases in a Cambridge Veterinary School survey.

Cause of FUO	%
Infection	16
Immune-mediated disease (mostly	
polyarthropathies)	26
Bone marrow disorders	23
myeloproliferative disease	
lymphoproliferative disease	
myelodysplastic conditions	
Solid neoplasms	10
Miscellaneous	8
True FUO	17

(K. J. Dunn, unpublished observations)

macrophages are attracted to sites of immune complex deposition resulting in the release of endogenous pyrogen. Affected animals often have a history of vague shifting lameness. On clinical examination there may be evidence of periarticular soft tissue swelling and pain on manipulation of the joints. A small percentage of dogs may present with fever and cytological evidence of polyarthritis on joint fluid analysis but show little or no evidence of lameness and/or joint pain.

The immune-mediated polyarthropathies may manifest as:
- rheumatoid arthritis (erosive),
- idiopathic (non-septic, non-erosive) polyarthritis,
- polyarthritis/polymyositis syndrome,
- polyarthritis/meningitis syndrome,
- systemic lupus erythematosus,
- polyarteritis nodosa.

Certain breeds, for example Japanese Akitas, appear to be more susceptible to different forms of polyarthritis. Arthritis and amyloidosis of the Chinese Shar-Pei ('Shar-Pei fever' or 'Shar-Pei hock') is characterised by recurrent attacks of fever associated with swelling and inflammation of the hock joints.

Polyarthritis/polymyositis syndrome has been reported most frequently in Spaniel breeds; the incidence of polyarthritis/meningitis syndrome is highest in Weimaraners, German Shorthaired Pointers, Newfoundlands, Boxers and Beagles.
- Immune-mediated haemolytic anaemia or thrombocytopenia (especially if acute). The destruction of red cells results in the release of red cell pyrogens into the circulation and/or activation of splenic and hepatic macrophages.
- Steroid-responsive meningitis. Steroid-responsive meningitis often occurs in association with other

immune-mediated disorders such as arteritis (Beagles) or polyarthritis (Weimaraners) suggesting that this disease also has an immune-mediated pathogenesis. Affected animals are often young and present with fever and acute neck pain. Cerebrospinal fluid analysis typically reveals a marked neutrophilic pleocytosis.
- A syndrome resembling systemic lupus erythematosus has been reported in dogs (particularly Dobermanns) following the administration of potentiated sulphonamides (trimethoprim–sulphadiazine combination). Clinical signs usually regress if the drug is discontinued immediately.

Immunodeficiency Syndromes

Immunodeficiency may be either
- primary (congenital), or
- secondary (acquired).

Primary immunodeficiency should be suspected if a young animal presents with a history of recurrent bacterial infections especially if the infection involves organisms of relatively low virulence and/or becomes refractory to conventional antimicrobial therapy. The infections most frequently involve the skin and urinary and gastrointestinal tracts and affected animals often present with a marked neutrophilia with or without a left shift. Similar infections in littermates or previous litters or evidence of a concurrent immune-mediated disorder may further increase the index of suspicion.

A number of primary immunodeficiency syndromes have been recognised in the dog; many of these occur in certain breeds (Table 37.3). They may affect non-specific immunity (e.g. neutrophil function or mucosal barrier function) or specific components of the immune system (humoral immunity, cellular immunity, complement function, see also Chapter 32).

Acquired immunodeficiency may occur secondary to infection (e.g. generalised demodicosis, certain fungal infections and protracted bacterial infections), drugs (cyclophosphamide, doxorubicin, glucocorticoids, oestrogens), toxins, nutritional factors, stress, endocrine abnormalities (e.g. hyperadrenocorticism or diabetes mellitus) or other systemic diseases.

Neoplasia

- Some tumour cells release endogenous pyrogen without prior stimulation by an exogenous pyrogen.
- Fever may be induced by the interaction of tumour specific or tumour related antigens with sensitised

Table 37.3   Causes of primary and secondary immunodeficiency.

Primary defects in non-specific immunity
- Immotile cilia syndrome resulting in recurrent respiratory infections (Springer Spaniel, Old English Sheepdog, English Setter, West Highland White Terrier, Pointers and other breeds).
- Canine cyclical haemopoiesis (Grey Collies).
- Canine granulocytopathy in Irish Setters (deficiency of leucocyte adhesion proteins).
- Bone marrow dyscrasia in Miniature and Toy Poodles.
- Defective neutrophil bactericidal activity in Dobermanns.
- Complement (C3) deficiency in Brittany Spaniels.
- Pelger–Hüet anomaly (Foxhounds)
- Neutrophil function defect in Collie breeds?

Defects in specific immunity
- Combined immunodeficiency syndrome in Dachshunds and Basset Hounds.
- Thymosin-responsive wasting syndrome in growth hormone deficient Weimaraners.
- Chronic rhinitis and pneumonia in Irish Wolfhounds with low serum IgA levels.
- Immunodeficiency syndrome characterised by low serum IgA and IgG concentrations is Weimaraners.
- Transient hypogammaglobulinaemia (Samoyeds).
- Selective IgA deficiency (Beagles, Chinese Shar-Pei, German Shepherd Dog).
- Selective IgM deficiency (Dobermanns).
- T cell immunodeficiency in Weimaraners.
- Lethal acrodermatitis (Bull Terriers).

Secondary immunodeficiency syndromes
Immunodeficiency may occur secondary to a number of infections (e.g. generalised demodicosis, canine distemper and parvovirus infections, ehrlichiosis, aspergillosis and protracted bacterial infections) and haemopoietic neoplasia. Nutritional problems (e.g. zinc deficiency), drugs (e.g. prolonged glucocorticoid therapy, cytotoxic agents) and endocrinopathies (hyperadrenocorticism and diabetes mellitus) may also predispose to recurrent infection.

lymphocytes. These lymphocytes in turn secrete soluble lymphokines which stimulate the production of endogenous pyrogen by granulocytes and macrophages.
- Fever may be associated with lymphoproliferative or myeloproliferative disease especially if replacement of the bone marrow by neoplastic cells results in persistent neutropenia. Such animals may also be immunosuppressed by virtue of altered cellular or humoral immune function.
- Large (e.g. hepatic) tumours with necrotic centres.

Miscellaneous Diseases

- Painful orthopaedic problems such as metaphyseal osteopathy, panosteitis and nutritional secondary hyperparathyroidism.
- Liver disease, especially active hepatic necrosis, may result in intermittent endotoxaemia and fever.

DIAGNOSTIC APPROACH TO FUO

History and Clinical Examination

The list of differential diagnoses is extensive and *normal* historical and clinical findings can be extremely helpful in ruling out some of the possible causes. The important aspects of the history and clinical examination are summarised in Table 37.4.

The initial presenting signs are generally vague and non-specific; moreover, clinical signs such as shifting lameness associated with the immune-mediated polyarthropathies, often fluctuate in intensity. The type of fever should be established early on during the course of the investigation by recording the animal's temperature twice or three times daily over at least a 72-h period (this can often be done at home by most owners).

Table 37.4   Fever of unknown origin: important points in the history and clinical examination.

History	Clinical examination
Age, sex, breed	Check for:
Vaccination status	Lymphadenopathy
Previous illness or recent operations	Enlargement of liver, spleen or kidneys
Recent trauma or evidence of pain	Petechial/ecchymotic haemorrhages (skin, mucosae, retinae)
Drug administration	Cardiac murmurs (systolic or diastolic)
Previous response to antibiotics	Localised pain (neck, back or abdomen)
Duration and periodicity of clinical signs	Ulcerative/vesicular skin lesions or oral ulcers
Localised or shifting leg lameness	Joint pain, periarticular soft tissue swelling or joint effusion
Geographical location/travel history	Rectal examination (prostatomegaly)
Exposure to infectious agents	Ophthalmoscopy (chorioretinitis, retinal detachment or haemorrhage,
Lifestyle (free roaming)	anterior uveitis)
Exposure to ticks	
Diet	

In the absence of localising signs, it is helpful to perform a series of preliminary screening tests with a view to identifying any septic, inflammatory or neoplastic focus which may be present. An attempt should always be made to rule out infectious causes first.

The indiscriminate use of antibiotics, corticosteroids and non-steroidal anti-inflammatory drugs should be avoided since they may mask clinical signs and interfere with the results of laboratory tests. Although, in general, therapeutic trials should be undertaken only as a last resort, knowledge of a previous response to antibiotics is useful and should prompt more extensive investigation for a septic focus.

Diagnostic Investigations

Preliminary Diagnostic Investigations should include:

- Full haematological examination (including platelet count).
- A complete biochemical screen (to include urea, creatinine, glucose, alanine aminotransferase (ALT), alkaline phosphatase (AP), aspartate aminotransferase (AST), creatinine phosphokinase (CPK), bile salts, sodium, potassium, chloride, calcium and phosphate).
- Total plasma protein and fibrinogen concentrations.
- Routine urine analysis (including microscopic examination of sediment).
- Urine culture and sensitivity.
- Lateral thoracic and abdominal radiographs. Include long bones and joints if there has been a history of a vague shifting leg type of lameness.

- Examination of faeces for parasitic ova, occult blood; submit for bacteriology if history of diarrhoea.

Additional Diagnostic Procedures

The requirement for more specific diagnostic procedures is based on the results of these preliminary screening tests and/or the development of new clinical signs. The major indications for each procedure are summarised in Table 37.5.

Blood Cultures
Blood culture is indicated in most FUO cases. More specific indications include the presence of a systolic or diastolic heart murmur, a history of shifting leg lameness or back, bone or joint pain especially if these signs are accompanied by neutrophilia (with or without a left shift) or neutropenia.

Conditions most frequently associated with bacteraemia in one study (Hirsch *et al.* 1984) were malignant neoplasms and infections of the skeletal, cardiovascular and urogenital systems. The most frequently isolated bacteria are enterobacteriaceae and coagulase positive staphylococci (Hirsch *et al.* 1984; Calvert & Greene 1986). In one study concurrent urinary tract infections were detected in 13% of bacteraemic dogs although it was not determined whether this was cause or effect (Calvert & Greene 1986).

Bacteraemia in dogs with endocarditis is usually continuous and the timing of the blood cultures is probably less important. Bacterial isolation rates between 50% and 80% have been reported (Calvert 1982; Elwood *et al.* 1993). Repeatedly negative results have been reported in confirmed cases of bacterial endocarditis, therefore a negative

Table 37.5 Fever of unknown origin: Indications for diagnostic procedures.

Diagnostic procedure	Indications based on problems identified from the history, clinical examination and initial laboratory and radiographic procedures
Blood culture	Systolic or diastolic cardiac murmur Neutropenia or neutrophilia (± left shift) Shifting leg lameness Back, bone or joint pain
Bone marrow aspiration	Anaemia, thrombocytopenia and/or neutropenia Leucocytosis/suspect leukaemia (e.g. unexplained neutrophilia, lymphocytosis or large numbers of atypical white blood cells in peripheral blood)
Multiple joint aspirates	History of shifting leg lameness with back or joint pain and periarticular swelling Neutrophilia ± hyperfibrinogenaemia
Electrocardiography Echocardiography	Congestive heart failure especially if dysrhythmia (e.g. myocarditis) Cardiac murmur ± dysrhythmia suggestive of bacterial endocarditis
Immunodiagnostic screening tests Rheumatoid factor	As for joint aspirates and blood culture
Antinuclear antibodies	As for joint aspirates and blood culture Ulcerative/vesicular cutaneous or oral lesions Persistent proteinuria
Direct antiglobulin (Coombs') test	Haemolytic anaemia Thrombocytopenia (especially if positive for anti-platelet antibodies)
Anti-platelet antibodies	Thrombocytopenia Coombs' positive anaemia
Serum protein electrophoresis ±immunoelectrophoresis	Abnormal total serum/plasma proteins Hypergammaglobulinaemia Immunodeficiency syndrome suspected
Serology (toxoplasmosis, neosporosis, borreliosis, ehrlichiosis, leishmaniasis, brucellosis, aspergillosis and other systemic mycoses)	Fundic lesions, e.g. chorioretinitis, retinal detachment (toxoplasmosis, FIP, systemic mycoses) Anterior uveitis (toxoplasmosis, systemic mycoses) Discospondylitis (*Brucella canis*) Polyarthropathy (Lyme disease, leishmaniasis) Increased total serum/plasma proteins, especially if increased globulin fraction (FIP, ehrlichiosis, leishmaniasis)
Specialised radiographic techniques Double contrast cystography (with abdominal ultrasound examination)	Prostatomegaly
Barium meal	Persistent melaena
Neutrophil function tests	Unable to establish cause of FUO; indicated especially if an immunodeficiency syndrome is known to exist in the breed.
Radiolabelled leucocyte scan	Unable to establish cause of FUO
Exploratory laparotomy	Abdominal mass Enlarged spleen or liver Unexplained abdominal pain
Tissue biopsy	Abnormal renal or hepatic function tests Ulcerative/vesicular cutaneous or oral lesions (additional immunofluorescent studies may be indicated)
Therapeutic trial	Diagnosis cannot be established after extensive investigation

blood culture does not preclude a diagnosis of bacterial endocarditis. Antibiotics should if possible be discontinued at least 2 days beforehand since they may delay bacterial growth. In order to maximise the chances of obtaining a positive culture two or three blood samples should be collected, preferably at least 1 h apart, over a 24-h period. Each blood sample should be collected from a different vein (jugular or cephalic) using standard aseptic technique. To minimise the risk of contamination a fresh needle should be attached to the syringe before the blood is transferred to an appropriate culture medium (e.g. Bloodgrow™, Medical Wire & Equipment Co, Bath, UK). Each sample should be submitted for aerobic and anaerobic culture. A culture can be considered positive if at least two bottles (each taken at a different time) contain the same bacterial species.

Bone Marrow Aspirates

Bone marrow aspiration is indicated when fever is associated with an unexplained cytopenia (anaemia, neutropenia and/or thrombocytopenia), leucocytosis, (neutrophilia, lymphocytosis or large numbers of atypical white blood cells) or hypergammaglobulinaemia.

Multiple Synovial Fluid Aspirates

Joint aspirates are indicated if there is a history of intermittent or shifting leg lameness, back/joint pain or periarticular soft tissue swelling, especially if such changes are accompanied by neutrophilia and hyperfibrinogenaemia.

Electrocardiography and Echocardiography

Electrocardiography is indicated if there is evidence of congestive heart failure or abnormalities in cardiac rhythm or a pulse deficit are detected on clinical examination. Echocardiography is the most useful diagnostic aid for confirming or ruling out the presence of vegetative thrombi on the heart valves or mural endocardium.

Immunodiagnostic Screening Tests

Results of immunodiagnostic screening tests should always be interpreted in association with clinical signs and results of other laboratory tests since most can produce false negative and false positive results. Consideration should also be given to the titre; the diagnostic significance of the endpoint titre depends on the type of test and the methodology used to perform it. For example with the antinuclear antibody test the titre is dependent on the substrate used. Specific indications for performing rheumatoid factor, antinuclear antibody, direct antiglobulin (Coombs') and anti-platelet antibody tests are summarised in Table 37.5.

Serum Protein Electrophoresis/Immunoelectrophoresis

These tests are indicated when a chronic inflammatory process is suspected or when the total plasma protein concentration is abnormal (usually increased). Polyclonal increases in the globulin fractions are most commonly associated with viral infections, protozoal infections (e.g. ehrlichiosis, leishmaniasis), chronic bacterial infections and immune-mediated disorders. A monoclonal gammaglobulin peak is more consistent with plasma cell myeloma although similar monoclonal peaks are occasionally observed with functional B cell lymphoma (Chapter 35) and chronic ehrlichiosis. Decreased gamma-globulin levels usually occur with a concomitant decrease in the other serum protein fractions and are usually associated with severe debilitating disorders, for example lymphoma.

Serology

Serological tests are currently available for toxoplasmosis, neosporosis, borreliosis (Lyme disease), brucellosis (*B. canis*), aspergillosis and other systemic mycoses. The first of paired serum samples should be collected early in the evaluation of a patient with FUO and stored at −20°C. A second sample can be taken 2–3 weeks later; in most cases a three- to four-fold increase in the titre is significant.

Tests to Assess Neutrophil Function

Some cases of FUO may result from neutrophil dysfunction. Confirmatory diagnosis of neutrophil dysfunction requires *in vitro* evaluation of chemotactic, adhesion and bactericidal properties. Neutrophil function tests must be performed on fresh cells, i.e. within 2 h of collection. A recent study used fluorescent activated cell scanning (FACS) to examine the cell surface expression of leucocyte adhesion molecules (the heterodimer CD18 and CD11) on neutrophils from a group of related dogs, some of which had experienced repeated bouts of pyrexia (Dunn *et al.* 1995). This preliminary investigation suggested that the pyrexic episode in two of these dogs was characterised by a transient decrease in neutrophil adhesion molecule expression (dogs that failed to become pyrexic had normal distribution of these adhesion molecules).

Radionucleotide Studies

Radiolabelled leucocyte scans are used in human medicine as a means of localising various forms of inflammatory disease and infections, for example, inflammatory bowel disease, postoperative sepsis, intra-abdominal and soft tissue sepsis, and acute and chronic osteomyelitis. The essential requirement for their success is that the disease to be localised is associated with a neutrophilic (i.e. purulent or pyogenic) inflammatory response. Their use with regard to the investigation of fever of unknown origin in humans is well established. Preliminary studies in the dog appear to suggest that while technetium[99m]-labelled leucocyte studies may detect areas of hidden infection, other nuclear medicine techniques such as gallium scintigraphy are likely to be more appropriate screening tests (K. J. Dunn, unpublished observations).

REFERENCES

Calvert, C.A. (1982). Valvular bacterial endocarditis in the dog. *Journal of the American Veterinary Medical Association*, **180**, 1080–1084.

Calvert, C.A. & Greene, C.E. (1986). Bacteraemia in dogs: Diagnosis, treatment and prognosis. *Compendium on Continuing Education for the Practicing Veterinarian*, **8**, 179–186.

Dunn, K.J., Bujdoso, R. & Herrtage, M.E. (1995). Decrease in cell-surface expression of CD11 and CD18 by neutrophils isolated from dogs with pyrexia. In: *Proceedings of the 5th Annual Congress of the European Society of Veterinary Internal Medicine*, Cambridge, England, p. 62.

Elwood, C.M., Cobb, M.A. & Stepien, R.L. (1993). Clinical and echocardiographic findings in 10 dogs with vegetative bacterial endocarditis. *Journal of Small Animal Practice*, **34**, 420–427.

Hirsch, D.C., Jang, S.S. & Biberstein, E.L. (1984). Blood culture of the canine patient. *Journal of the American Veterinary Medical Association*, **184**, 175–178.

FURTHER READING

Bennett, D. (1996). Diagnosis of pyrexia of unknown origin. *In Practice*, **17**, 470–481.

Dunn, J.K. & Gorman, N.T.G. (1987). Fever of unknown origin in dogs and cats. *Journal of Small Animal Practice*, **28**, 167–181.

Degen, M.A. & Breitschwerdt, E.B. (1986). Canine and feline immunodeficiency – Part I. *Compendium on Continuing Education for the Practicing Veterinarian*, **8**, 313–323.

Degen, M.A. & Breitschwert, E.B. (1986). Canine and feline immunodeficiency – Part II. *Compendium on Continuing Education for the Practicing Veterinarian*, **8**, 379–386.

Chapter 38

Systemic Lupus Erythematosus

J.K. Dunn

INTRODUCTION

Systemic lupus erythematosus (SLE) is a multisystemic immune-mediated disorder characterised by the presence of circulating antinuclear antibodies (ANA). The disease has been reported in the dog and less frequently in the cat.

In the dog, German Shepherds, Poodles, Shetland Sheepdogs, Collies and Beagles appear to be over-represented (Scott *et al*. 1983). The age of onset is extremely variable ranging from less than one year to greater than ten years. Unlike humans, where there is a definite female predisposition for the disease, male dogs appear to be as susceptible as females (Grindem & Johnson 1983).

PATHOGENESIS

Systemic lupus erythematosus is an immune complex disorder of unknown aetiology. Antinuclear antibodies are produced that bind to components of the nucleus. The interaction of these antinuclear antibodies with their respective antigens results in a Type III hypersensitivity response. Since the nuclear antigens involved are not restricted to a specific cell type SLE is a multisystemic disease. Deposition of immune complexes may occur in glomerular capillaries and basement membrane, in synovial membranes, and in skin at the level of the dermal epidermal junction. Immune complex deposition results in activation of the complement cascade and release of potent inflammatory mediators. Neutrophils are attracted to sites of immune complex deposition resulting in vasculitis and tissue damage. Antibodies may also be directed against cell surface antigens on red blood cells, platelets and leucocytes and occasionally antibodies are produced against clotting factors; a lupus-type anticoagulant which inhibited the activation of thrombin was recently reported in one dog with haemolytic anaemia, thrombocytopenia, membranous glomerulonephritis, polyarthritis and pulmonary thromboembolism (Stone *et al*. 1994). Although the clinical signs were highly suggestive of SLE this dog was ANA negative.

It has been shown that the serological abnormalities associated with spontaneous canine SLE can be transmitted to normal dogs and mice by cell free extracts suggesting the presence of an infectious agent. Indeed there is limited evidence to support a role for C-type viruses in the development of SLE in humans and dogs (Quimby *et al*. 1978). However, it is unlikely that the presence of virus alone is sufficient to provoke clinical disease and that development of the disease requires interaction of the virus with an aberrant immune response in a genetically susceptible host (Scott *et al*. 1983). Dogs with SLE have decreased levels of serum thymic factor (Monier *et al*. 1980), decreased numbers of circulating lymphocytes (Monier 1981) and also lower total haemolytic complement levels (Wolfe & Halliwell 1980). A recent study of 100 cases of canine SLE showed an association with major histocompatability antigen (MHC) Class I dog leukocyte antigen (DLA) 7 and complement genes but not with MHC Class II (Fournel *et al*. 1992).

Certain drugs, for example hydralazine and potentiated sulphonamides (trimethoprim–sulphadiazine), may induce a lupus-like syndrome in dogs. The administration of propylthiouracil to cats is frequently associated with Coombs' positive anaemia, thrombocytopenia and the production of antinuclear antibodies.

CLINICAL SIGNS

The clinical signs of SLE can be conveniently divided into major and minor signs, the major signs representing body systems which are most frequently involved and are therefore more suggestive of SLE (see below). In addition, affected dogs often show non-specific signs such as fever, lethargy, anorexia and weight loss.

Major Signs

- shifting lameness (polyarthritis)
- proteinuria (glomerulonephropathy)
- dermatopathy
- haematological abnormalities (anaemia, thrombocytopenia, leucopenia)

Minor Signs

- polymyositis
- pericarditis/myocarditis
- pleuritis
- generalised lymphadenopathy
- oral ulceration
- CNS signs (behaviour changes, seizures, ataxia)
- gastrointestinal signs (vomiting, diarrhoea)

The clinical signs of SLE vary considerably and reflect the systems involved. They may mimic many other diseases and have a tendency to wax and wane. Fever is common during the acute phase of the disease. Non-septic, non-erosive polyarthritis appears to be the most common manifestation of SLE and is characterised by shifting lameness, joint pain and periarticular soft tissue swelling (Grindem & Johnson 1983). Approximately 50% of dogs have significant proteinuria indicative of glomerular damage (Grindem & Johnson 1983; Scott *et al.* 1983). The skin lesions associated with SLE are extremely variable. The lesions are often erythematous and/or seborrhoeic and most commonly involve the face, ears and limbs. Mucocutaneous ulceration may be evident and the very occasional dog may present with lupus panniculitis, a condition characterised by multiple cutaneous nodules which subsequently ulcerate and develop fistulae (Scott *et al.* 1983). Although previous reports have suggested that immune-mediated (Coombs' positive) haemolytic anaemia is commonly associated with SLE, two of the more recent retrospective surveys have suggested that non-regenerative anaemia may be a more common occurrence (Grindem & Johnson 1983; Scott *et al.* 1983).

DIAGNOSIS

Since the clinical manifestations of SLE are extremely variable opinions vary as to which sets of clinical signs can be used as reliable diagnostic criteria. Several schemes have been proposed. Since neither the major nor minor clinical signs described above are truly specific for SLE a combination of these signs together with supportive serological evidence is helpful in establishing a diagnosis. The following scheme proposed by Gorman & Werner (1986b) offers a degree of flexibility and acknowledges the fact that not every case of SLE has a positive ANA test and that a diagnosis of SLE probably includes numerous overlap syndromes which have some of the clinical signs and/or autoantibodies which are suggestive of the disease.

Definite SLE

- positive ANA test plus two major signs
- positive ANA test plus one major and two minor signs

Probable SLE

- positive ANA test and one major sign
- negative ANA test and two major signs

Antinuclear Antibodies

The ANA test is preferred to the lupus erythematosus (LE) cell test (see below) because it is more sensitive and the results are more consistent on a day-to-day basis. It has been said also that the test is more resistant to corticosteroids (Scott *et al.* 1983). Circulating antinuclear antibodies are most frequently identified using an indirect immunofluorescent antibody test (IFAT). Positive ANA tests have been reported in 75–90% of SLE cases in the dog (Gorman & Werner 1986a). The test is performed using a nuclear substrate (mouse or rat liver/kidney, Vero cell line, HeLa cell line, HEP-2 cell line) and a fluorescein-conjugated species-specific anti-Ig. A polyvalent antiserum should be used since the ANA can be any immunoglobulin class. The cells are examined under fluorescent microscopy for a specific pattern of immunofluorescence. The test serum (1–2 ml usually required) is initially screened at a low dilution, e.g. 1 : 10; if a positive result is obtained serial dilutions should be tested until an end-point titre is established. The result should always be interpreted in conjunction with the clinical signs and results of other laboratory tests. Like most immunological screening tests the ANA test, although sensitive, is not disease specific. A subset of human patients (particularly those with antibodies against cytoplasmic Ro single stranded A antigen and single stranded (ss-) DNA) remain ANA negative throughout the course of their disease and a similar situation may exist in the dog (Kass *et al.* 1985a). A positive ANA titre on its own is not diagnostic of SLE since low ANA titres may be found in normal dogs (usually antibodies against double stranded (ds-)DNA and ss-DNA; Toth & Rebar 1987) and in a variety of infectious, inflammatory and neoplastic disorders. For example positive ANA tests have been reported in dogs with pemphigus erythematosus, pemphigus vulgaris, lymphocytic thyroiditis, idiopathic polymyositis, autoimmune haemolytic anaemia, immune-mediated thrombocytopenia, subacute bacterial endocarditis, dirofilariasis and generalised demodicosis (Scott *et al.* 1983). In cats low ANA titres have been reported with FeLV infection and some cases of lymphocytic cholangiohepatitis (Gorman & Werner 1986b). The significance of an ANA titre depends on the substrate used and the results of the laboratory controls. A titre greater than 1 : 20 is generally regarded as significant if mouse liver is used as the substrate (Gorman & Werner 1986a). It has been suggested that some substrates, e.g. mouse kidney, may not detect certain antinuclear antibodies against soluble nuclear antigens (Toth & Rebar 1987).

In dogs, unlike humans with active SLE, the antinuclear antibodies are not specific for ds-DNA and antibodies may be produced against a wide range of nuclear and cytoplasmic antigens, including DNA histones, denatured or single stranded DNA (ss-DNA), extractable (soluble) nuclear proteins such as Sm and ribonucleoprotein (RNP), phospholipids and RNA (Toth & Rebar 1987; Gorman & Werner 1986b; Costa *et al.* 1984). Anti-DNA histone antibodies are relatively more common in canine SLE. The relationship of a specific type of ANA to a particular presentation has not been determined in dogs. It has been suggested that the titre of ANA, particularly the titre of anti-DNA histone antibodies, may correlate with the severity of the disease (Costa *et al.* 1984). Kass *et al.* (1985b) established a predictive model for SLE in the dog and showed that the risk factors for a positive ANA titre are polyarthritis (with or without lymphadenopathy), anaemia and thrombocytopenia.

Attempts have been made to establish whether different patterns of immunofluorescence within the nucleus or on the nuclear membrane are related to the type of antigen detected or the progression of the disease (Toth & Rebar 1987). These patterns of immunofluorescence are described as (1) homogenous or diffuse, (2) peripheral or rim, (3) speckled or reticulate, (4) nucleolar. Although correlations between staining patterns and different manifestations of SLE have been reported a clear relationship is, as yet, not apparent.

Lupus Erythematosus (LE) Cell Test

The LE cell test is now virtually obsolete for the reasons mentioned above. It detects serum antibodies to DNA-histone complexes (Toth & Rebar 1987). An LE cell is a polymorphonuclear cell which contains a large homogenous inclusion consisting of phagocytosed nuclear mater-

ial that has been opsonised by antinuclear protein antibody. The LE phenomenon does not occur *in vivo* therefore the test involves damaging leucocytes either with glass beads or by mashing them though a wire mesh in order to expose nuclear material to antibodies against nuclear protein. Interpretation of the LE test can be difficult. LE cells should be differentiated from tart cells; these are monocytes or sometimes neutrophils that have phagocytosed a nucleus or a whole cell (usually a lymphocyte). LE cells may also be confused with rosettes consisting of non-phagocytosed LE bodies surrounded by a ring of neutrophils. On their own tart cells or rosettes do not constitute a positive LE cell test.

Approximately 60–80% of dogs with SLE in one survey had positive LE tests at some point during the course of the disease (Grindem & Johnson 1983). The value of the LE test compared with ANA test in monitoring SLE has been questioned since some animals remain consistently LE cell positive or negative despite exacerbations or remissions in their disease (Grindem & Johnson 1983).

Lupus Band Test

Any skin lesions should be biopsied. Histopathological examination (direct immunofluorescence) may show a typical 'lupus band', a zone of immunoglobulin deposition on the basement membrane zone (BMZ), in up to 90% of cases (Scott *et al.* 1983). In one survey IgA was the most commonly detected immunoglobulin in the BMZ followed by IgM. The most commonly detected immunoreactant was C_3; in a few cases this was the only immunoreactant detected (Scott *et al.* 1983).

Other Clinicopathological Findings

The results of routine haematology are generally not specific for SLE; neutrophilia with or without a left shift may be seen in dogs with polyarthritis or skin lesions. Increases in total plasma proteins due to an increased gamma globulin fraction have been reported (Grindem & Johnson 1983). Multiple joint fluid aspirates are helpful in confirming joint involvement. Joint fluid from affected joints is increased in volume and appears turbid. Cytological examination reveals increased numbers of non-degenerate, hypersegmented neutrophils. LE cells are occasionally noted. Routine urine analysis should be confirmed to check for the presence of persistent proteinuria (see above). The significance of persistent proteinuria can be assessed by measurement of the urine protein : creatinine (Up : c) ratio. This ratio is calculated on a spot urine sample and the results correlate well with 24 h urinary protein excretion values. A Up : c ratio greater than 13 is generally regarded as being indicative of glomerular disease. A direct antiglobulin (Coombs') test and direct or indirect fluorescent antibody test to detect anti-erythrocyte and anti-platelet antibodies respectively should be performed in suspected SLE cases which are anaemic and/or thrombocytopenic.

THERAPY

In one study just over 40% of SLE cases were successfully managed with prednisolone alone and long-term remission was achieved on alternate day glucocorticoid therapy. Cases of SLE that present with immune-mediated haemolytic anaemia, immune-mediated thrombocytopenia or glomerulonephritis are more likely to be refractory to prednisolone therapy alone. Combination therapy using prednisolone and azathioprine has proved to be effective in refractory cases or cases in which the maintenance dose of prednisolone produces unacceptable side effects (Scott *et al.* 1983). Induction doses of prednisolone of 2–4 mg/kg body weight should be used reducing to an every other day maintenance dose of 0.5–1 mg/kg body weight. Azathioprine can be given at a dose of 1–2 mg/kg body weight daily reducing to 1 mg/kg body weight every other day (prednisolone can be given on alternate days to the azathioprine). An attempt to stop therapy may be made in dogs that remain disease free for 6 months. The most common causes of death in dogs with SLE are renal failure and infections such as bronchopneumonia and septicaemia.

REFERENCES

Costa, O., Fournel, C., Lotchouang, E., Monier, J.C. & Fontaine, M. (1984). Specificities of antinuclear antibodies detected in dogs with systemic lupus erythematosus. *Veterinary Immunology and Immunopathology*, 7, 369–382.
Fournel, C., Chabanne, L., Caux, C., *et al.* (1992). Canine systemic lupus erythematosus I: A study of 75 cases. *Lupus*, 1, 133–139.

Gorman, N.T. & Werner, L.L. (1986a). Diagnosis of immune-mediated diseases and interpretation of immunologic tests. In: *Current Veterinary Therapy IX*, (ed. R.W. Kirk), pp. 427–435. W.B. Saunders, Philadelphia.
Gorman, N.T. & Werner, L.L. (1986b). Immune-mediated diseases of the dog and cat I: Basic concepts and the systemic immune-mediated diseases. *British Veterinary Journal*, 142, 395–402.
Grindem, C.B. & Johnson, K.H. (1983). Systemic lupus erythematosus: Literature review and report on 42 new canine cases. *Journal of the American Animal Hospital Association*, 19, 498–503.
Kass, P.H., Farver, T.B., Strombeck, D.R. & Ardans, A.A. (1985a). Application of the log-linear and logistic regression models in the prediction of systemic lupus erythematosus in the dog. *American Journal of Veterinary Research*, 11, 2340–2345.
Kass, P.H., Strombeck, D.R., Farver, T.B. & Ardans, A.A. (1985b). Application of the log-linear model in the prediction of the antinuclear antibody test in the dog. *American Journal of Veterinary Research*, 11, 2336–2339.
Monier, J.C. (1981). Le lupus du chien pour mieux comprendre le lupus human. *Pathologie et Biologie*, 29, 261–264.
Monier, J.C., Dardenne, M., Rigal, D., *et al* (1980). Clinical and laboratory features of canine lupus syndromes. *Arthritis and Rheumatism*, 23, 294–301.
Quimby, F.W., Gerbert, R., Datta, S., Andre-Schwartz, J. Tannenberg, W.J. & Lewis, R.M. (1978). Characterisation of a retrovirus that cross-reacts serologically with canine and human systemic lupus erythematosus (SLE). *Clinical Immunology and Immunopathology*, 9, 194–210.
Scott, D.W., Walton, D.K., Manning, T.O., Smith, C.A. & Lewis, R.M. (1983). Canine lupus erythematosus I: Systemic lupus erythematosus. *Journal of the American Animal Hospital Association*, 19, 461–479.
Stone, M.S., Johnstone, I.B., Brooks, M., Bollinger, T.K. & Cotter, S.M. (1994). Lupus-type 'anticoagulant' in a dog with haemolysis and thrombosis. *Journal of Veterinary Internal Medicine*, 8, 57–61.
Toth, L.A. & Rebar, A.H. (1987). Measurement of antinuclear antibodies in the dog: A review. *Veterinary Clinical Pathology*, 16, 76–82.
Wolfe, J.H. & Halliwell, R.E.W. (1980). Total haemolytic complement values in normal and diseased dog populations. *Veterinary Immunology and Immunopathology*, 1, 287–298.

Section 5

Cardiopulmonary Diseases

Edited by Virginia Luis Fuentes

INTRODUCTORY COMMENTS

Diseases of the respiratory system include conditions affecting the nasopharynx, upper and lower airway, lung parenchyma, pleural space and chest wall. As a disease group they constitute an important division of canine medicine, although the exact incidence of respiratory diseases in the dog has not been reported. However, acute tracheobronchitis is probably by far the most common respiratory disease of dogs, with the incidence of more severe conditions, such as chronic bronchitis, bronchopneumonia, and pulmonary neoplasia being relatively low.

Details on diseases affecting the nasopharynx and larynx are included in Chapters 40 and 41. The major features of diseases affecting major airways, bronchi, lung tissue and the pleura and mediastinum are covered in Chapters 42–44.

The pathophysiology of cardiac disease is dealt with in detail in Chapter 45 and covers the principles of the current views on the medical management of cardiac disease. Inherited and acquired cardiac conditions are dealt with in Chapters 46 and 47.

Chapter 39

Clinical Investigation of Respiratory Disease

B. Corcoran

STRUCTURE AND FUNCTION OF THE AIRWAYS AND LUNG

The respiratory system includes the extra-thoracic structures of the nasopharynx, larynx and tracheal, the intrathoracic trachea and communicating airways, lung tissue (interstitium and alveoli) and the associated pulmonary and systemic (bronchial) circulation, the visceral and parietal pleural, and the thoracic cage (ribs and diaphragm). The function of this system is to enable the efficient exchange of gases between atmosphere and the body, and to assist thermoregulation. Clinicians should be familiar with the basic anatomy of the respiratory system and the defence mechanisms that operate to protect against disease. The anatomy of the canine respiratory system is shown in Figs 39.1, 39.2 and 39.3.

The major defence mechanisms in the lower respiratory system include the mucociliary clearance mechanism, which is assisted by coughing, and alveolar macrophages which remove debris in the most distal sites. In the dog the largest number of cough receptors is found in the larynx, in the trachea at the thoracic inlet and carina, and at the major divisions of the airways. The density of receptors diminishes towards the periphery and there are no receptors in the respiratory bronchioles or alveoli.

APPROACH TO THE PATIENT

In addition to the standard clinical procedures used in the investigation of any medical condition there are considerations pertinent to the successful assessment of the respiratory case.

History

The most common clinical presentations are outlined in Table 39.1. Note the severity, frequency, chronicity and rate of development and progression of the presenting sign. If two or more clinical signs are reported, their association, if any, should be determined.

Signalment

The breed and age of the patient are important considerations when investigating the respiratory case.

- Anatomical abnormalities are seen mainly in toy and brachycephalic breeds.
- Chronic bronchitis and chronic pulmonary interstitial disease appear to be more common in terrier breeds.
- Both chronic bronchitis and pulmonary neoplasia are primarily diseases of middle- to old-age dogs.

Environment

The role of environmental factors in respiratory diseases in dogs is undetermined, and the role of environmental pollutants in the aetiopathogenesis of respiratory diseases, such as chronic bronchitis, is unknown.

However, environmental factors that should be considered include the potential for exposure to infective agents (e.g. in boarding kennels), vaccination and worming status, and air quality in the home environment (excessive dust, cigarette smoke etc.).

Physical Examination

The examination of the respiratory system is carried out in conjunction with examination of the cardiovascular system (Chapter 45).

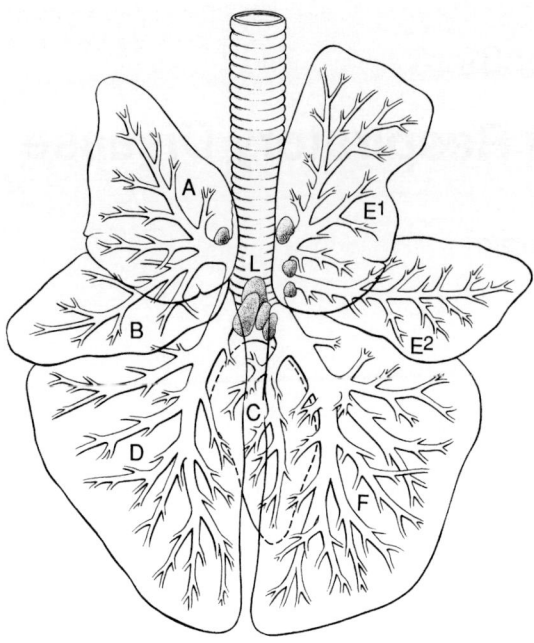

Fig. 39.1 Line drawing demonstrating the gross anatomy of the canine lung. The right lung consists of the cranial (A), middle (B), accessory (C) and caudal (D) lobes. The left lung is divided into the cranial lobe (divided into cranial (E¹) and caudal (E²) divisions) and the caudal (F) lobe. The major lymph node (L) (middle tracheobronchial) is located between the mainstem bronchi.

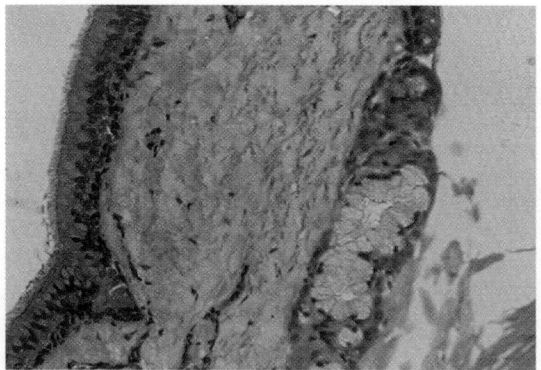

Fig. 39.2 Photomicrograph illustrating the anatomy of the canine trachea. The ciliated columnar epithelium overlies collagen-rich lamina propria containing blood vessels and mucus-secreting glands. Cartilage underlies this layer and is incomplete dorsally. The wings of the cartilage (not shown) are connected by the dorsal membrane, which consists of fibroelastic tissue and the trachealis muscle.

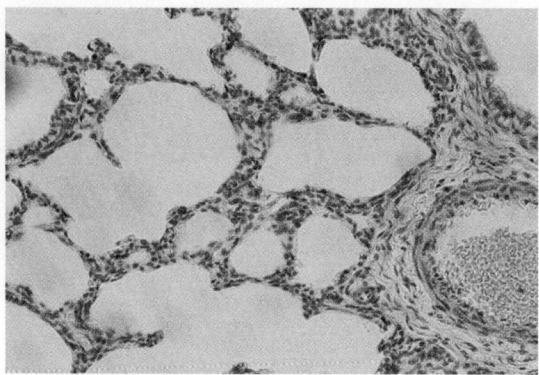

Fig. 39.3 Photomicrograph of dog lung illustrating the normal alveolar structure with associated blood vessel (right lower corner) and part of an intrapulmonary bronchus (right upper corner).

Table 39.1 Clinical signs associated with lower respiratory tract diseases.

Common clinical signs	Minor clinical signs
Cough	Naso-ocular discharges
Dyspnoea and tachypnoea	Vomiting and retching
	Gagging and choking
	Haemoptysis and haematemesis
	Exercise intolerance
	Collapse and syncope
	Cyanosis
	Obesity or cachexia
	Abdominal enlargement

- Pay particular attention to general body condition, noting the presence of obesity or weight loss.
- Assess the colour of the ocular and oral mucosa, and inspect the oropharynx.
- Identify the presence of naso-ocular discharges and assess patency of the external nares.
- Palpate the larynx and extrathoracic trachea.
- Check for lymphadenopathy and other masses close to the extrathoracic airways and at other sites.
- Palpate the abdomen paying particular attention to identification of masses.
- Check body temperature and hydration status and note the overall demeanour of the patient.

Increased respiratory rate (to maintain minute ventilation; tidal volume × frequency)		**Table 39.2** The clinical significance of respiratory distress and difficulty.
Panting	Normal thermoregulatory function
Tachypnoea	Exercise, excitement-associated
	Reduced minute/alveolar ventilation (e.g. alveolar exudates)
	Reduced lung compliance (e.g. lung fibrosis)
	Restriction of lung expansion (e.g. pleural effusion)
Inspiratory difficulty	
Increased noise	Nasal airflow obstruction (*stertor*)
	Upper airway (e.g. larynx) obstruction (*stridor*)
No increased noise	Intrapulmonary airway narrowing (e.g. airway mucus plugging with chronic bronchitis)
Expiratory difficulty	End-expiratory dynamic collapse of larger airway (e.g. compression by extralumenal mass (neoplasm))
Hyperpnoea	Combination of tachypnoea and dyspnoea
Orthopnoea	Adopting a position to ease respiration

Lastly the dog's breathing pattern should be noted, including the *respiratory rate* and the presence of *respiratory effort* or *difficulty* (Table 39.2). The identification of inspiratory and expiratory dyspnoea can be difficult if the dog is also tachypnoeic.

Auscultation

An internationally recognised classification system for respiratory sounds in veterinary species is not yet available, but the author uses the American Thoracic Society/American College of Chest Physicians classification system.

Normal sounds are caused by air flowing through the major airways and the terms *breath* or *bronchovesicular* sounds are used to describe them.

Abnormal sounds (adventitious sounds) include crackles, wheezes and rhonchi.

- *Crackles* are usually inspiratory and are due to re-opening of airways that have closed during expiration (fine or coarse).
- *Wheezes* are high pitched sounds, that can be inspiratory or expiratory, and are due to narrowing of the bronchial lumen.
- *Rhonchi* are low pitched sounds due to high airflow velocity through the larger airways, can be inspiratory or expiratory, and can be normal if exercise or excitement-associated.

- *Stridor* and *stertor* are used to describe rhonchus sounds produced in the larynx and nasal passage respectively.
- It should be noted that a combination of sounds can exist, giving complex harmonics that are not readily identified or classified.

Chest Percussion

Percussion allows identification of variation or changes in chest resonance, and is particularly useful in identifying asymmetric lesions and air–fluid lines. Both sides of the chest must be percussed.

Investigative Techniques

See Tables 39.3 and 39.4.

Figs 39.4 to 39.10 are radiographs showing the main abnormal findings with respiratory diseases. The radiographs are lateral and ventrodorsal views unless otherwise indicated.

Differential Diagnosis Tables

On the basis of the clinical history, physical examination and diagnostic tests the clinician should be able to construct a differential list of possible conditions, and suitable lists

Radiography is a powerful diagnostic tool in respiratory medicine, but depends on good quality images.

Table 39.3 Thoracic radiography.

Radiographic technique (the following are required to get the best diagnostic films):

Equipment	High output (preferably at least 150 mAs) unit
	Good quality films and screens (rare earth)
	Grids (with high output machines only)
Technique	Sedated or anaesthetised
	Properly positioned
	Right lateral and ventrodorsal views (standard)
	Left lateral if indicated
	Standing lateral for pleural effusion
	Inspiratory exposure (standard)
	Expiratory exposure (tracheal collapse)
	Short exposure time (reduces blur)
	High kV, low mAs

Interpretation

Lung patterns (the vessels make up most of the lung density in normal dogs)

Bronchial (Fig. 39.4a, b)	Airway wall calcification (normal ageing process)
	Parallel lines ('tramlines')
	End-on airway wall thickening ('doughnuts')
	Dilated lobar bronchi
Interstitial (Fig. 39.5a, b)	Diffuse non-vascular linear density
Alveolar (Fig. 39.6)	Fluffy coalescing soft tissue densities
	Air bronchograms
Mixed (bronchial, interstitial & alveolar)	Mass lesions
Pleural effusions (Fig. 39.7a, b)	'Scalloping' or 'leafing' of lung lobes
	Interlobar fissures
	Overall increase in fluid density and loss of cardiac silhouette
Mediastinal changes (Fig. 39.8a, b)	Widening or narrowing
	Shift
Thoracic cage integrity (Fig. 39.9a, b)	Fractured ribs
	Ruptured diaphragm
Obesity (Fig. 39.10a, b)	Intrathoracic fat
	Subcutaneous fat

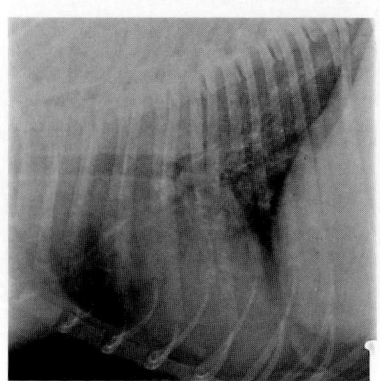
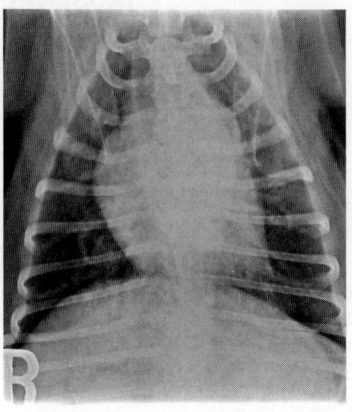

Fig. 39.4a,b A 6-year-old Jack Russell Terrier with dyspnoea and chronic coughing. There is an increase in both interstitial and bronchial markings. The bronchial changes are primarily noted as increased numbers of end-on ring structures ('doughnuts'), and are readily identifiable on both views. This dog had chronic bronchitis which was confirmed on bronchoscopy.

Table 39.4   Bronchoscopy and bronchial sampling.

Bronchoscopy is an invaluable tool in the investigation of respiratory diseases (Venker-van-Haagen 1979), allowing visualisation of the tracheobronchial tree and accurate sampling (Hawkins *et al.* 1990).

Bronchoscopy applications
   Accurate identification of airway changes
   • inflammatory reactions
      ○ mucosal changes
      ○ inflammatory exudates
   • foreign material
   • dynamic movement of airways
   Collection of diagnostic material
   • tracheal and bronchial samples
   • bronchoalveolar lavage
      ○ cytology
      ○ culture and sensitivity testing

Airway sample – interpretation of bronchial and bronchoalveolar lavage fluid samples
   Normal samples (small numbers of cells, Figure 39.11)
   • ciliated epithelium
   • polymorphonuclear leucocytes
   • macrophages
   Abnormal samples (large numbers of cells)
   • goblet cells with undifferentiated epithelial cells
   • non-specific chronic inflammation
   Neutrophils and lymphocytes
   • non-specific inflammatory reaction
   Eosinophils
   • allergic respiratory disease (pulmonary infiltration with eosinophilia)
   • parasitism
   Macrophages
   • lower airway and alveolar inflammation
   Neoplastic cells
   • primary (mainly adenocarcinomas)
   • secondary (mainly carcinomas)
   Increased quantity of mucus
   • non-specific inflammation
   • chronic bronchitis
   Particulate matter
   • inhaled material
   Infectious agents (culture usually required)
   • Gram– and Gram+ bacteria
   • fungal agents
   • microaerophilic agents
   • *Nocardia* spp., *Actinomyces* spp.
   Blood
   • intrapulmonary haemorrhage
   • sampling trauma

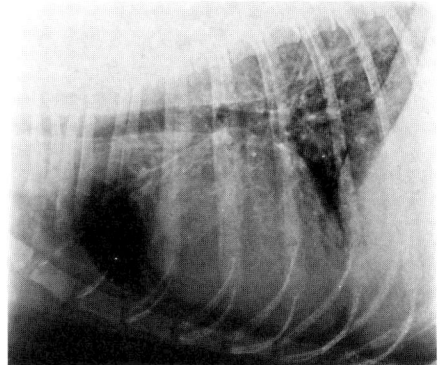

a

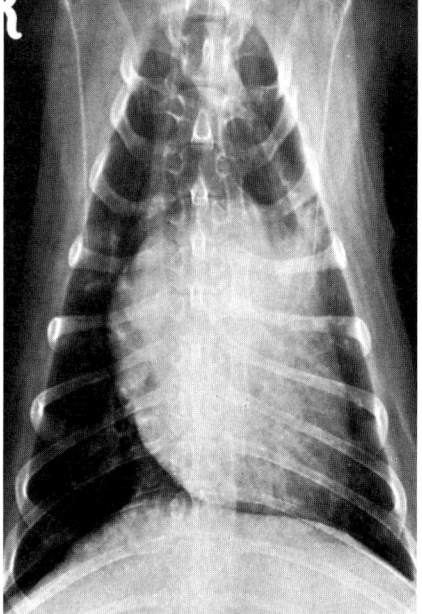

b

Fig. 39.5a,b   A 2-year-old Golden Retriever dog with pulmonary infiltration with eosinophils. There is a moderate to severe diffuse increase in interstitial density, which is more readily appreciated on the lateral view. There is also evidence of increased bronchial markings with peribronchial infiltration. This radiographic pattern is highly suggestive of pulmonary infiltration with eosinophilia (with permission S. Hodgson).

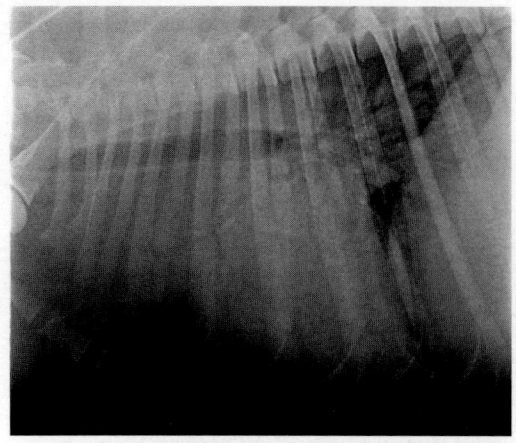

Fig. 39.6 Intrapulmonary haemorrhage in a 2-year-old Labrador (lateral view only). There is marked alveolar pattern in the middle and cranial lung fields with distinctive air bronchograms. This pattern is typical of bronchopneumonia, but in this case blood was found in the airway on bronchoscopy, suggesting haemorrhage as a probable explanation. The dog was subsequently found to have consumed warfarin and responded to therapy.

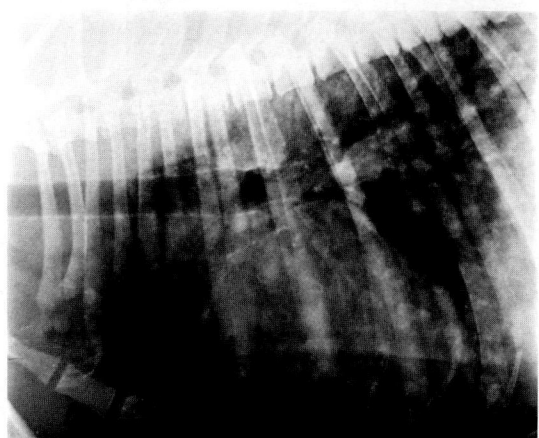

a

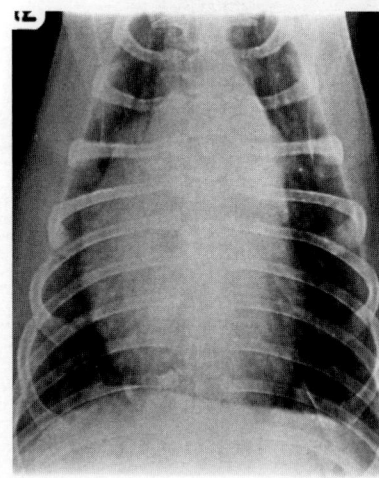

b

Fig. 39.7a,b Metastatic pulmonary haemangiosarcoma in a 10-year-old Labrador. There is a diffuse distribution of small nodular masses throughout the entire lung field. Some of the densities are well delineated, while others have indistinct edges.

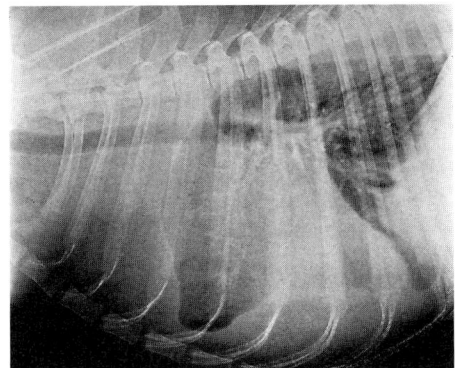

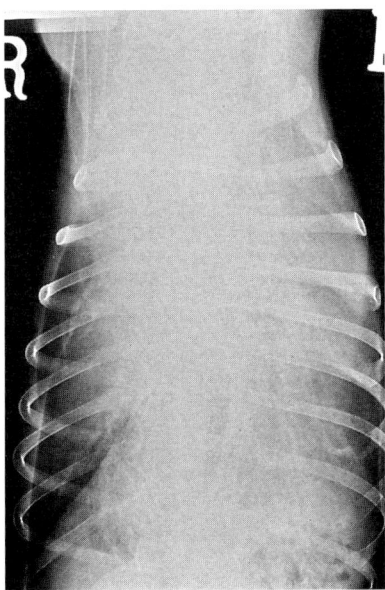

Fig. 39.8a,b Pleural effusion in a Whippet with a right middle lung lobe torsion. All lung lobes are retracted, with the edges showing 'leafing'. Interlobar fissures are readily appreciated on the dorsoventral view, but the cardiac silhouette is obscured.

for the more common clinical presentations in respiratory medicine (cough, tachypnoea and dyspnoea) are given in Tables 39.5 and 39.6.

SPECIFIC DISEASES

Respiratory diseases can be classified according to their anatomical location, pathology and effects on normal physiology (Table 39.7). For example, bronchopneumonia involves the lower airways and lung parenchyma (anatomy), involves a mixed inflammatory cellular reaction (pathology), and restricts lung expansion (physiology).

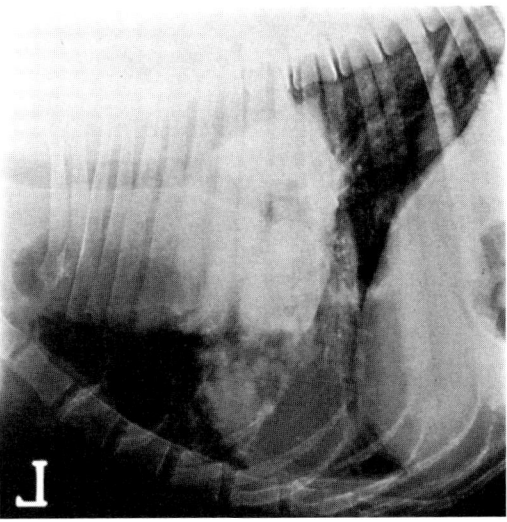

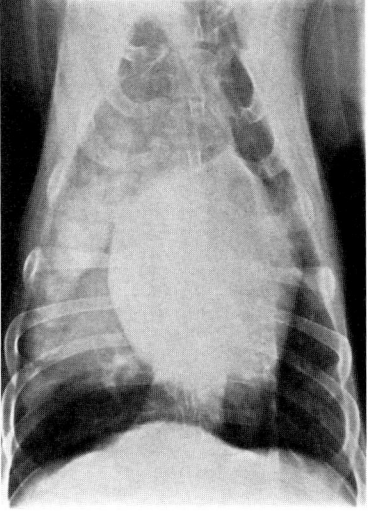

Fig. 39.9a,b Mediastinal shift in an 8-year-old Dobermann with haemoptysis. There is a consolidated mass lesion affecting the right cranial lung field, displacing the trachea towards the midline. There are also numerous nodular masses ventral to this mass visible on the lateral view.

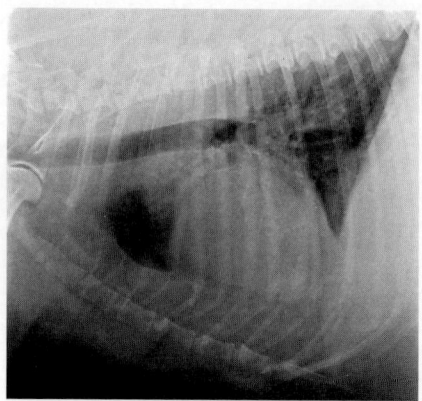

a

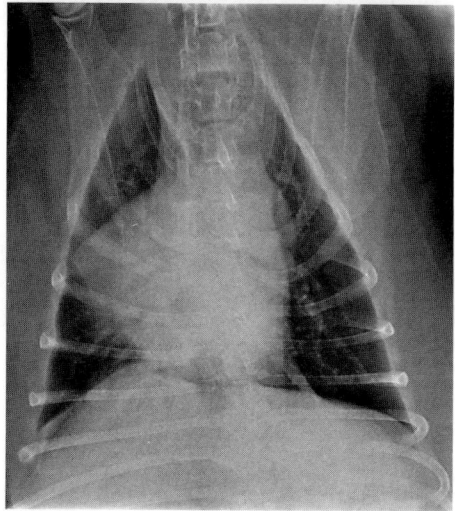

b

Fig. 39.10a,b   A 9-year-old obese cross bred dog with exercise intolerance. There is extensive sternal fat accumulation causing significant cardiac elevation, with widening of the cranial mediastinum. The dog also had extensive subcutaneous fat deposits.

GENERAL THERAPY AND MANAGEMENT OF RESPIRATORY DISORDERS

The therapy and management of specific conditions are covered in the relevant sections, and the broad principles and guide-lines are included here.

Antibacterial Agents

- Antibacterial therapy is used for the treatment of primary respiratory pathogens and control of secondary infections.
- Antibacterial selection should be made on the basis of culture and sensitivity testing, particularly with infectious pleural exudates, but empirical therapy may be initiated before culture results.
- Agents active against Gram-negative organisms and that have good penetrability of lung tissue and airway secretions are preferred. The *tetracyclines*, *potentiated sulphonamides* and *fluoroquinolones* are the first choice, followed by *clavulanate-potentiated penicillins* and the *cephalosporins*.

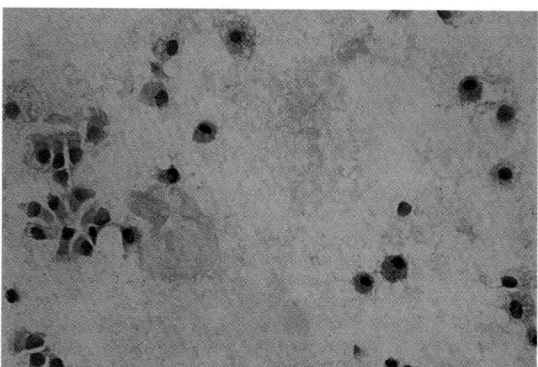

a

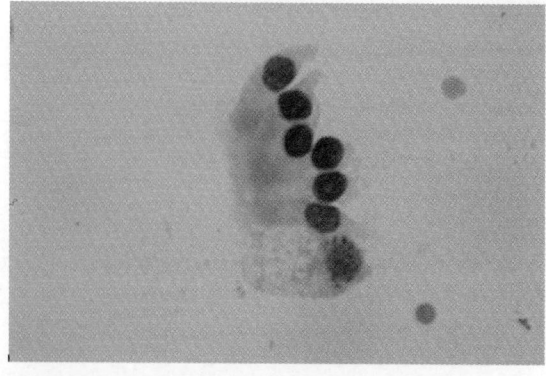

b

Fig. 39.11a,b   Examples of normal airway cytology. (a) Typical normal bronchial sample with small amounts of mucus, groups of ciliated epithelial cells and occasional macrophages and polymorphonuclear leucocytes. (b) High power magnification of a raft of normal epithelial cells with a single goblet cell.

Table 39.5   Differential diagnosis of coughing.

Categories	Examples	Key features	Radiography
Upper airway		Most cause dyspnoea	
Trachea and lower airway	Tracheal collapse	Toy breeds, ± dyspnoea with ↑ respiratory noise, 'goose-honk' cough	Trachea may be narrow or dilated depending on phase of respiration
	Acute tracheobronchitis	History of exposure to other dogs, harsh cough, clinically well, young dogs	Thorax NAD
	Chronic tracheobronchial syndrome	Sequel to kennel cough, persistent cough, minimal abnormalities on investigations	May be mild bronchial markings
	Chronic bronchitis	Terrier breeds, intermittent but progressive, excess mucus on bronchoscopy	Usually bronchial markings, may be interstitial pattern also
	Bronchiectasis	Sequel to chronic bronchitis, recurrent bronchopneumonia	Dilated bronchial lumina often visible
	Bronchial compression		
	Neoplasia	Dyspnoea may be present	Mass may be visible
	Atrial/cardiac enlargement	Murmur often audible	Cardiac enlargement, especially left atrium
	Lymphadenopathy	Other lymph nodes may be enlarged, or signs of pneumonia present	Diffuse soft tissue density around heart base on radiography
	Oslerus osleri (formerly *Filaroides osleri*) infection	Young, kennelled dogs, nodules visible on bronchoscopy	Nodules sometimes visible in trachea
	Airway foreign bodies	Peracute cough, halitosis in chronic stages, visible on bronchoscopy	Diffuse localised soft tissue density changes often in right caudal lobe
Lung parenchymal disease	Pneumonia	Soft cough	Alveolar pattern on radiographs
	Bacterial	Pyrexia, lethargy, anorexia	May be bronchial component also
	Aspiration	May be history of regurgitation	Alveolar pattern dependent lung lobes
	Pulmonary infiltration with eosinophilia/ parasites	Eosinophils in bronchial wash	Interstitial/bronchial pattern
	Chronic pulmonary interstitial disease	Terrier breeds, inspiratory crackles, variable dypsnoea, progressive	Diffuse interstitial pattern
	Pulmonary neoplasia	Middle aged older dogs, progressive	Mass lesions may be visible
	Primary	± Expiratory dyspnoea, ± haemoptysis	Solitary mass lesion ± consolidation ± hypertrophic pulmonary oesteopathy
	Secondary	± Coughing; may be asymptomatic	Metastases visible on radiography
	Intrapulmonary haemorrhage	Blood in airways, ± bleeding elsewhere	Alveolar pattern on radiographs

NAD, no abnormalities detected.

Table 39.6 Differential diagnosis of dyspnoea.

Categories	Examples	Key features	Radiography
Upper airway		↑ Noise, ↑ inspiratory effort	
	Brachycephalic syndrome	Characteristic breed, stertor, stridor, ± cyanosis on exertion	Often long hypertrophied soft palate
	Laryngeal paralysis	Labradors, Setters; stridor, gradual onset and progression, dysphonia	NAD
	Upper airway neoplasia	Rare: stridor. Mass may be visible on inspection	Soft tissue mass may be visible
	Foreign bodies	Severe inspiratory dyspnoea ± cyanosis; foreign body may be visible	Foreign body may be visible
Trachea and lower airway	Tracheal collapse	Toy breeds, coughing with ↑ respiratory noise, 'goose-honk' cough	Trachea may be narrow or dilated depending on phase of respiration
	Hypoplastic trachea	Brachycephalic breeds, young dogs	Trachea < diameter of 3–4th rib
	Tracheal stenosis	Rare: history of trauma.	Focal narrowing of trachea
	Chronic bronchitis	Terrier breeds, coughing, mucus hypersecretion	Increased bronchial markings
	Bronchial neoplasia/ foreign bodies	Coughing, visible on bronchoscopy	Tracheal foreign bodies visible
Lung parenchymal disease		Tachypnoea, no ↑ respiratory noise	
	Pulmonary oedema	May cough frothy oedema fluid if severe	Interstitial/alveolar pattern
	Cardiogenic	Cardiac signs on physical examination	Left atrial enlargement often with distended pulmonary veins
	Non-cardiogenic	Sudden onset, concurrent systemic disease/trauma (electrocution)	Normal cardiac silhouette, marked alveolar pattern
	Severe pneumonia	Cough, pyrexia, lethargy, anorexia	Alveolar pattern ± increased bronchial markings
	Chronic pulmonary interstitial disease	Terrier breeds (West Highland White), inspiratory crackles, ± coughing, progressive	Diffuse interstitial markings
	Pulmonary neoplasia	Coughing, expiratory dyspnoea	Solitary mass lesions or consolidation
	Intra-pulmonary haemorrhage	Signs of trauma or bleeding elsewhere	Patchy alveolar pattern
	Pulmonary thromboembolism	Peracute dyspnoea, concurrent primary systemic disease	Variable changes from alveolar pattern to NAD
	Smoke inhalation	History of exposure, external burns	Mixed pattern
	Near-drowning	History	Alveolar pattern

Table 39.6 *Continued.*

Categories	Examples	Key features	Radiography
Pleural/mediastinal disease		'Barrel-shaped' chest if severe	
	Pleural effusion	Ventral dullness on percussion	'Leafing' of lung lobes, interlobar markings
	Pneumothorax	Hyper-resonance dorsally on percussion	Retraction of lung lobes, increased lucency of periphery with absence of vascular markings
	Ruptured diaphragm	History of trauma ± muffled heart, empty abdomen	Loss of diaphragmatic integrity, ± abdominal organs in thorax, ± pleural effusion
	Mediastinal masses	± Regurgitation, ± Horner's syndrome, incompressible cranial chest	Widened cranial mediastinum, displacement of trachea, ± pleural fluid
Neurological abnormalities	Polyneuropathies	Generalised muscle wasting, exercise intolerance/weakness, ± laryngeal/pharyngeal dysfunction	Thorax may be NAD, megaoesophagus may be present
	CNS disease: reduced consciousness	Hypoventilation	Thorax NAD
$\downarrow O_2$ carrying capacity	Anaemia	Pale mucous membranes	Thorax NAD
	Right-to-left shunts	Cyanosis	Thorax NAD
	Carboxyhaemoglobinaemia	Cherry-red mucous membranes	Thorax NAD unless smoke inhalation
Metabolic	Metabolic acidosis	Concurrent disease, e.g. ketoacidosis	Thorax NAD
	Fear, pain	Behavioural signs	Thorax NAD

NAD, no abnormalities detected.

Classification	Examples
Anatomical classification	
Upper airway	Tracheal collapse
Lower airway	Chronic bronchitis
Lung parenchyma	Pneumonia
Pleural space	Pleural effusions
Pathological classification	
Acute inflammation	Acute tracheobronchitis
Chronic inflammation	Chronic pulmonary interstitial disease
Neoplasia	Primary pulmonary neoplasia
Infective Processes	Bacterial pneumonia
Physiological classification	
Obstructive respiratory disease	Tracheal collapse
Restrictive pulmonary disease	Pulmonary oedema
Restrictive chest bellows disease	Obesity
Pulmonary vascular disease	Thromboembolism

Table 39.7 Classification systems for respiratory diseases (with examples).

- Antibacterial agents used for pyothorax must have anaerobic activity and *clindamycin* is currently the most widely used agent for this purpose. This is also active against *Actinomyces* and *Nocardia* spp.
- Acute bacterial bronchopneumonia should be treated vigorously and pyothorax may have to be treated for several months

Anti-inflammatory Agents

It is well recognised that anti-inflammatory agents have an important role to play in the immediate treatment and the long-term management of respiratory diseases.

- *Glucocorticosteroids* are widely used in the treatment of pulmonary infiltration with eosinophilia (Corcoran *et al.* 1991), chronic bronchitis and chronic pulmonary interstitial disease.
- *Non-steroidal anti-inflammatory* agents have been used to assist in controlling the acute inflammatory component of bronchopulmonary diseases (e.g. flunixin meglumine).

Bronchodilators

Bronchodilators seem to be beneficial when used in combination with glucocorticosteroids, in the control of chronic bronchitis and chronic pulmonary interstitial disease. Their efficacy in the treatment of acute tracheobronchial and bronchopulmonary diseases is questionable.

- The methylxanthine agents aminophylline, theophylline and etamiphylline campsylate are widely used.
- β_2-adrenoreceptor agonists (terbutaline, clenbuterol) are less widely used.

Anti-tussives

Suppression of coughing is acceptable if it is non-productive or causing exhaustion and distress. The use of anti-tussives is contraindicated in chronic bronchitis and bronchopneumonia.

Commonly used anti-tussives include *butorphanol*, *codeine* and *dextromethorphan*.

Mucolytics and Expectorants

Expectorant agents are of doubtful efficacy.

Mucolytics such as bromhexine can be beneficial in the management of chronic bronchitis. However, assisting movement and removal of secretions can be best achieved with physiotherapy (Hawkins *et al.* 1989).

FURTHER READING

Corcoran, B.M., Thoday, K.L., Henfrey, J.I., Simpson, J.W., Burnie, A.G. & Mooney, C.T. (1991). Pulmonary infiltration with eosinophils in 14 dogs. *Journal of Small Animal Practice*, 32, 494–502.

Hawkins, E.C., Ettinger, S.J. & Suter, P.F. (1989). Disease of the lower respiratory tract (lung) and pulmonary oedema. In: *Textbook of Veterinary Internal Medicine*, (ed. S.J. Ettinger), pp. 816–866. W.B. Saunders, Philadelphia.

Hawkins, E.C., Denicola, D.B. & Kuehn, N.F. (1990). Bronchoalveolar lavage in the evaluation of pulmonary disease in the dog and cat. *Journal of Veterinary Internal Medicine*, 4, 267–274.

Venker-van-Haagen, A.J. (1979). Bronchoscopy of the normal and abnormal canine. *Journal of the American Animal Hospital Association*, 15, 397–410.

Chapter 40

Nasal Discharge in the Dog

M. Sullivan

INTRODUCTION

The diagnosis of disease always presents a challenge to the clinician because of the diversity of signs that may be presented by any particular disease, so that the *classical* list of signs, historical or clinical, is rarely present in its entirety. One simple method to overcome the avalanche of information that a case may present is to try and categorise diseases and place them into mental boxes.

Diseases of the upper respiratory tract can be broadly grouped into those that produce nasal discharge, which are dealt with in this chapter, and those that lead to respiratory obstruction or embarrassment, which are dealt with in subsequent chapters.

ANATOMICAL CONSIDERATIONS

The entrances to the nasal cavity are the external nares. The nostrils are composed of flexible cartilage supporting a rich epithelial covering. In the normal dog the nares are comma-shaped and once inside the large alar fold causes air entering to veer medially to the beginning of the common meatus. The nasal cavity is divided into two chambers by the nasal septum. The septum is composed of a sheet of cartilage supported ventrally by the vomer bone. Although the vomer bone produces the bulk of the radio-opacity that is the nasal septum on radiographs, the cartilaginous part is a significant contributor and can be clearly seen if there is deviation of the cartilage. Rostrally, the bulk of the nasal cavity is filled with ventral concha or turbinates. A small extension of the ethmoidal concha lies dorsally. The root of the ventral concha is located at approximately the level of the carnassial tooth. It is only with difficulty and with a very

fine endoscope that one is able to get past this root to reach the ethmoturbinate area that lies beyond in the normal animal. On radiographs the border between the ventral concha and the ethmoturbinates is evident as a coarse area with a poorer turbinate pattern, which can be mistaken for a destructive lesion. The turbinates are fine scrolls of bone supporting a mucous membrane that is extremely rich in blood vessels and mucous glands (Fig. 40.1). The dog has a highly developed sense of smell and the olfactory neuroepithelium is located deep in the ethmoturbinates. The sinuses of the dog are few in number. The sphenoidal sinus is not relevant and the maxillary sinus is merely a lateral diverticulum of the nasal cavity and not a true sinus. The frontal sinuses start above the ethmoidal concha and extend caudally over the cribiform plate and then the cranial vault. The frontal sinus has rostral and caudal compartments that drain through narrow ostia into the ethmoidal concha.

Nasal breathing is normal in the quiescent animal. Mouth breathing becomes necessary:

- when temperature and humidity rise,
- during strenuous physical activity,
- in brachycephalic breeds,
- in some disease processes.

Obstruction to air flow in a disease process may occur because there has been significant disruption of the normal anatomy, or where there is a physical mass.

Thus in the normal resting dog the incoming air is split and channelled by the turbinates and therefore fed over the large surface area of mucus-secreting ciliated epithelium that covers the turbinate bones. Passing over the turbinates the air is warmed to body temperature and humidified – thus the need for a profuse blood supply and abundant mucous glands. During the process of warming and humidification the air is filtered of most particulate matter. This particulate material is trapped by the mucus carpet and carried by the ciliated epithelium from the nasal cavity.

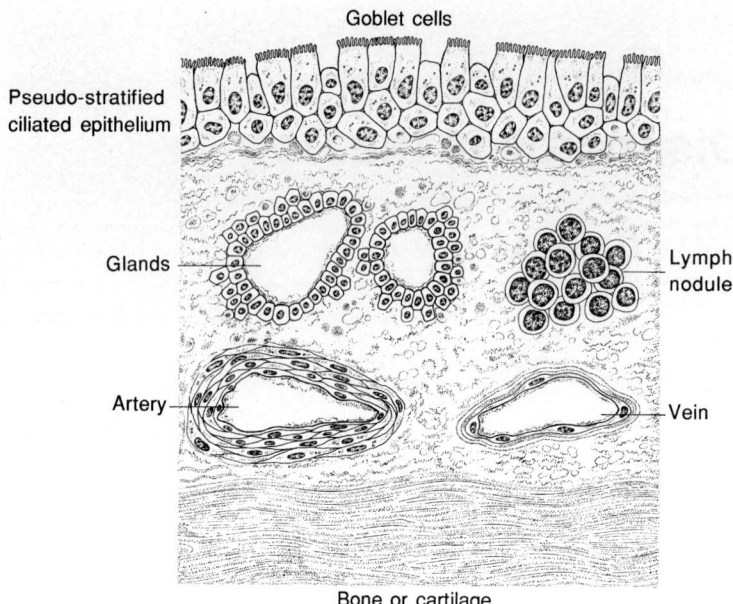

Fig. 40.1 Diagram of the elements of a turbinate.

Table 40.1 Differential diagnosis of chronic nasal discharge.

Common	Less common	Rare
Neoplasia	Cleft or hypoplastic palate	Idiopathic destructive rhinitis
Chronic hyperplastic rhinitis	Foreign body	Oronasal fistula
Aspergillosis	Rhinarial ulceration	Bleeding disorders
		Macroglobulinaemia
		Nasal polyp

ACUTE VERSUS CHRONIC NASAL DISCHARGE

Acute

- Acute nasal discharge is usually a sign of systemic or non-nasal disease with the exception of acute allergic rhinitis.

Chronic

- An animal may be considered as having a chronic nasal discharge if it has been present for more than 7–10 days. It is at this stage that further investigation should

be undertaken if the history and clinical examination suggest that it is warranted.

- Chronic nasal discharge in some animals secondary to disease of other organs such as megaoesophagus or severe systemic illness such as distemper. These will not be pursued further as they will be distinguished by the competent clinician on history and clinical examination.

When presented with a dog suffering from chronic nasal discharge there are a bewildering array of diseases that may be the cause. It is useful to have a list of differential diagnoses, which are weighted on the basis of their relative frequency of occurrence. With these in mind one can be more confident that a disease is not being overlooked at each stage of the diagnostic process (Table 40.1).

Susceptibility

Dolicocephalic and mesaticephalic breeds are susceptible to chronic nasal disease where, in contrast, brachycephalic breeds are largely spared intranasal disease, which may be due, in part, to a more mouth-breathing nature. The age of the dog is useful in trying to weight the possible diagnoses when starting to consider the cause of the discharge. Knowledge of the age range of the three most frequently encountered diseases; nasal neoplasia, aspergillosis and chronic hyperplastic rhinitis is helpful.

The majority of nasal tumours occur in older dogs, while aspergillosis and chronic hyperplastic rhinitis are found in younger dogs, but as can be seen there is considerable overlap (Fig. 40.2). It is mandatory to integrate the history, clinical examination and information gained from ancillary aids to enable an accurate diagnosis to be confirmed.

INVESTIGATION OF NASAL DISEASE

History

The features that owners first notice and lead them to seek veterinary attention are sneezing, snorting, possibly gagging or the appearance of a nasal discharge. The speed of onset, the type of discharge, the side or sides affected and the type of terrain over which the dog is exercised are all important and should be discovered at this stage. Questioning the owner to ascertain the presence or absence of:

- sneezing,
- coughing,
- gagging,
- facial pain,
- mouth breathing,

provides very useful data.

Table 40.2 Character of nasal discharge.

Type	Suggests
Serous	Lack of significant inflammation
Mucopurulent	Inflammatory or necrotic process
Mucohaemorrhagic	Erosion of blood vessels
Epistaxis	Significant vascular damage

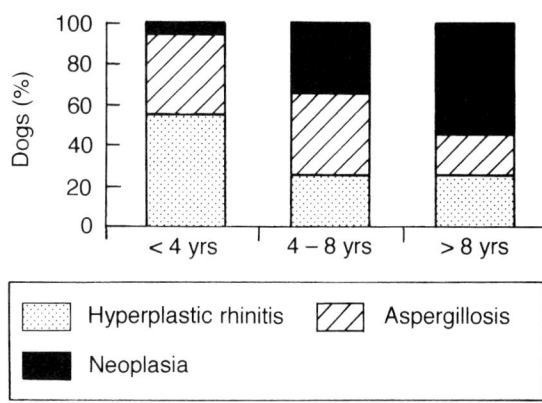

Fig. 40.2 Cumulative bar chart of age distribution of three commonest nasal diseases.

The type and pattern of discharge is equally important (Table 40.2). In addition, changes in these signs over a period of time are important. For example a change from a unilateral discharge to a bilateral discharge, indicates in many cases that the continuity of the nasal septum has been lost. In most diseases the discharge starts as a serous discharge that is accompanied by pronounced sneezing, but, the discharge becomes more purulent as the disease proceeds with the sneezing tending to abate. The discharge in the early stages may not be apparent as many dogs lick their noses so frequently that discharge is not present for long enough to be observed by the owner or the discharge drains caudally to the nasopharynx and is swallowed.

Clinical Examination

The nature of the discharge and side(s) involved should be assessed when it is present. However, in many dogs the intermittent nature of the discharge means that it is frequently absent at the time of examination. A full clinical examination of the head region is necessary to avoid missing significant features.

Nasal Portion

Look for:

- Ulceration and depigmentation of the rhinarium,
- Ocular discharge,
- Alteration in the nasal contour (particularly at the medial canthus of the eye),
- Softness of overlying nasal or maxillary bones indicates erosion.

- The presence of facial pain can be detected by moving a hand quickly towards the animal's face and/or by tapping the nasal cavity and frontal sinuses on each side. A dog with facial pain will shy away or cringe.

Loss of nasal airway patency will define obstruction and may demonstrate an undisclosed bilateral lesion. This can be assessed simply by using a thread, long hair or wisp of cotton wool suspended in front of each nostril. The force with which the thread is sucked towards and blown from each nostril during inspiration and expiration is noted.

Oral Portion

Look for:

- convexity of the hard palate,
- defects in the palate,
- condition of the teeth, in particular the upper canines.

Convexity of the hard palate indicates that a tumour has eroded the palatine bone and is pushing the mucoperiosteum of the hard palate orally. Defects in the hard palate permit food material to move from the oral into the nasal cavity and foreign material will stimulate a purulent rhinitis. Periapical abscess of the canine can erode the medial alveolar wall and allow drainage into the nasal cavity.

This is as far as the clinical examination can be taken without recourse to ancillary aids. However, at this stage a tentative diagnosis should have been reached. A resumé of the typical features of the diseases listed above will help in deciding what the specific diagnosis is or at least narrow the range of possibilities.

NASAL NEOPLASIA

Key features: reduced airflow and alteration in shape of bony case.

Tumours are the most common cause of the chronic nasal discharge in the dog. Many different cell types have been identified, but the clinical behaviour of all these tumours is similar. Tumours generally arise in the ethmoturbinate region and spread rostrally. They are locally invasive but rarely metastasise until quite late in the disease process. Initially, the discharge will be unilateral but can become bilateral as the tumour erodes through the septum (Fig. 40.3). Owners may complain that the dog excessively

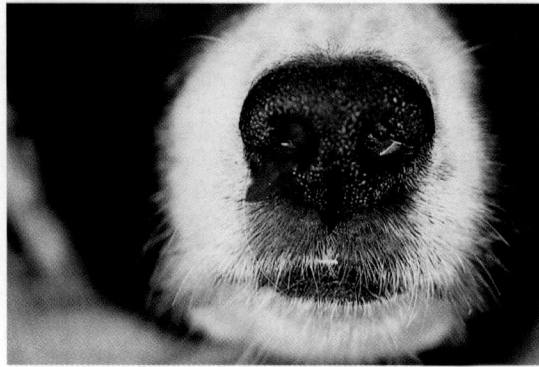

Fig. 40.3   The bilateral haemorrhagic discharge that one might see in a dog with a nasal tumour. The discharge is more prominent on the right with staining of the muzzle of the left.

mouth-breathes, snorts when eating and has difficulty sleeping due to occlusion of the nasal passages or caudal choanae. Reduction in airflow is often, though not always, present. The tumour can erode through the bony case and appear as a soft painless swelling at the medial canthus of the eye, or produce convexity of the mucoperiosteum of the hard palate. Some tumours arise in the frontal sinuses rather than the nasal cavity. These tumours are characterised by the destruction of overlying sinus bone, in addition to nasal discharge. Where a tumour is suspected as arising primarily from the frontal sinus, rostrocaudal (RCd) frontal sinus and lateral views of the calvarium and sinuses are the most valuable in confirming the diagnosis and extent of the lesion.

NASAL ASPERGILLOSIS
(SEE ALSO CHAPTER 14 PAGE 140)

Key feature: rhinarial depigmentation/ulceration and facial pain.

This mycotic infection is seen more frequently in dogs classified as suburban, with no demonstrable access to heavy concentrations of fungal spores. However, in the urban environment grass cuttings at the bottom of the garden carry a heavy concentration of spores and spores can be recovered from the nasal cavity of most dogs. What triggers active infection in the nasal cavity of dogs is unclear. Trauma and immune-incompetence have been implicated in some dogs, but the immune status of most cases has not

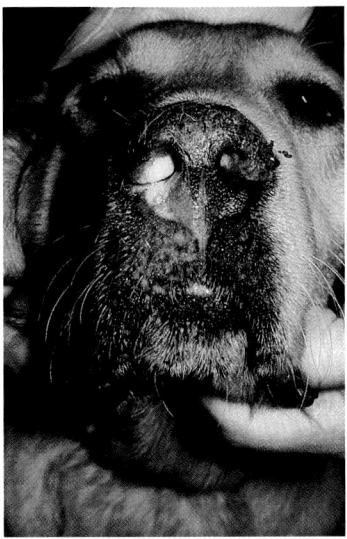

Fig. 40.4 Profound rhinarial ulceration and depigmentation that is characteristically seen in dogs with aspergillosis.

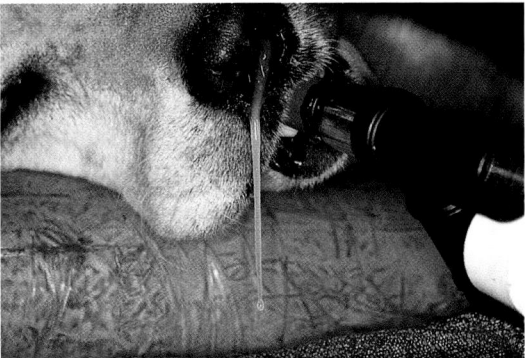

Fig. 40.5 Purulent stringy disharge from dog with chronic hyperplastic rhinitis.

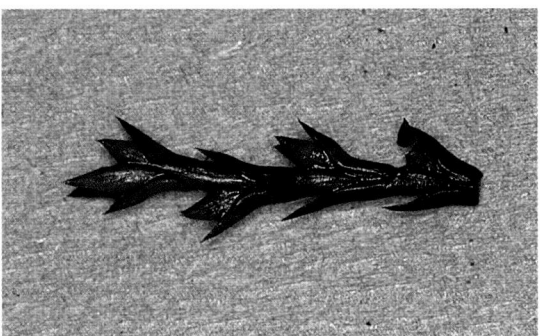

Fig. 40.6 Caudal choanal foreign body (seed head) removed from a Lhaso Apso with nasal discharge and upper airway obstruction.

been adequately investigated. Certain breeds seem to be predisposed such as the Golden Retriever, Labrador, Border Collie and German Shepherd Dog. Other breeds are seen sporadically.

Dogs are usually presented with a history of unilateral nasal discharge or a sudden bout of epistaxis. The owner often reports an ocular discharge, some dullness and loss of appetite. Pain is frequently present when the affected side is touched or when the dog is seen chewing food. Rhinarial depigmentation/ulceration is a characteristic feature (Fig. 40.4). Airflow is normal.

CHRONIC HYPERPLASTIC RHINITIS

Key feature: mucopurulent discharge worst early morning.

Although this condition can affect many breeds Whippets and Dachshunds are more susceptible for as yet unexplained reasons. Dogs are presented with a nasal discharge that is more often bilateral than unilateral. However, if unilateral the side may vary and where bilateral the side predominantly affected also varies. The discharge never contains blood and airflow is normal (Fig. 40.5). The underlying pathology is hypersecretion of abnormal mucus from hypertrophied mucosa.

FOREIGN BODY

Key features: (a) seasonal, nasal frenzy; (b) gagging.

There are two types of foreign body, those that enter rostrally and those retrograde from behind the soft palate. Dogs that work in rough cover are at risk of running on to a twig or plant stem. They may also inhale grass awns. These animals present with acute onset nasal frenzy and violent sneezing often accompanied by epistaxis. These features subside and a mucopurulent discharge supervenes as a secondary bacterial rhinitis develops when the problem is untreated.

Dogs, if eating grass or plant heads, can forcibly reflux these into the naso-pharynx and nasal cavity through the caudal choanae (Fig. 40.6). They may presumably do this if the material irritates the larynx in passing. They are more likely to have a history of severe snorting, gagging or retching.

RHINARIAL ULCERATION

Key features: lack of other signs associated with aspergillosis.

A number of young dogs have been seen with a chronic nasal discharge, which is frequently unilateral, rhinarial ulceration and depigmentation accompanied by a swollen alar fold. Ancillary aids return normal results and biopsies are often inconclusive. The early stages of squamous cell carcinoma and mast cell tumours of the nostrils would have to be considered as potential differential diagnoses. However, these both produce a more extensive lesion extending on to the philtrum and over the nasal sill. The ulceration is excavating and the adjacent tissue is indurated.

IDIOPATHIC DESTRUCTIVE RHINITIS

Key features: similar to aspergillosis, but no facial pain.

A few dogs have been seen with signs clinically (no rhinarial lesions) and radiologically largely indistinguishable from dogs with aspergillosis. Serological study of blood returns negative results for antibodies to *Aspergillus* and *Penicillium* species. No fungal plaques are detected endoscopically, or recovered by mycological investigation. It is possible that these are dogs that have sustained damage to the turbinate scrolls that stimulates a severe turbinate necrosis.

ORONASAL FISTULAE

Key features: communication between oral and nasal cavity.

These dogs will have a cleft palate or dental problem (usually periodontal disease) seen on clinical examination. The various forms of cleft palate cause a bilateral mucopurulent discharge, in contrast to dental disease where the discharge is unilateral. The tooth most often responsible is the canine, rarely the incisors and the carnassial tooth may be the cause.

RARE CAUSES OF EPISTAXIS

Key features: epistaxis alone.

Some systemic diseases can cause epistaxis that is the main clinical presentation. Coagulopathies such as auto-immune thrombocytopenia, von Willebrand's disease, haemophilia and macroglobulinaemias with cryoglobulins are examples (Fig. 40.7). These conditions should only be considered if general clinical examination fails to reveal co-existing clinical signs and there are no other features attributable to primary intranasal disease. Dogs suspected of any of these conditions require a thorough haematological and biochemical evaluation.

ANCILLARY INVESTIGATIONS
Radiography

Radiography is the main ancillary aid in the investigation of intranasal disease because it can deliver positive informa-

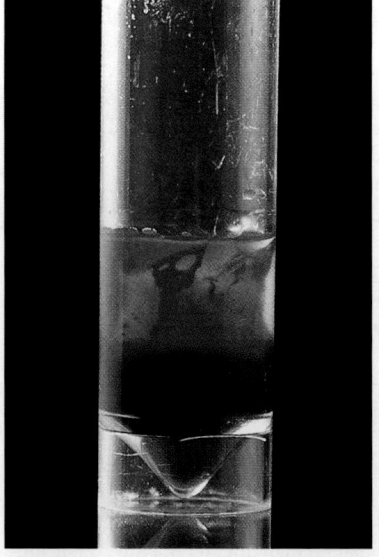

Fig. 40.7 Blood sample from a dog suffering from macroglobulinaemia with cryoglobulins, which has been allowed to stand and cool. It shows a white clot of precipitated immunoglobulins in the centre of the serum above the red cells.

tion on more of the diseases than any other method of further investigation (Table 40.3). Quality radiographs with good definition and accurate positioning are essential since positional artefacts are easily created.

The dorsoventral intra-oral view is the most informative as this allows comparison of both sides of the nasal cavity. This view is best achieved with non-screen film, which gives very good definition because of the fine grain. A typical exposure would be 70–75 kV and 30 mAs. Alternatively, screen film and a high definition screen supported by rigid cardboard can be placed in a black plastic envelope, a smaller exposure is needed. It should be noted

Table 40.3 Radiographic views.

Views	Use
Dorsoventral intra-oral	General
Ventro20°-dorsal intra-oral	General when non-screen film or equivalent is unavailable
Rostrocaudal frontal sinuses	Aspergillosis
Lateral	Neoplasia
Dorsoventral skull	Cribiform area

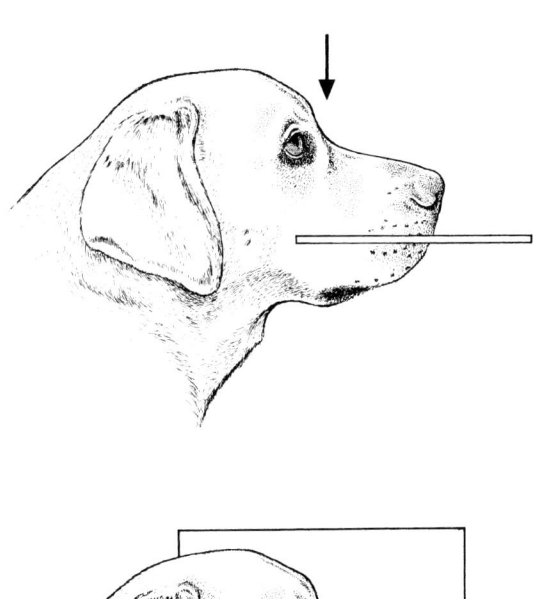

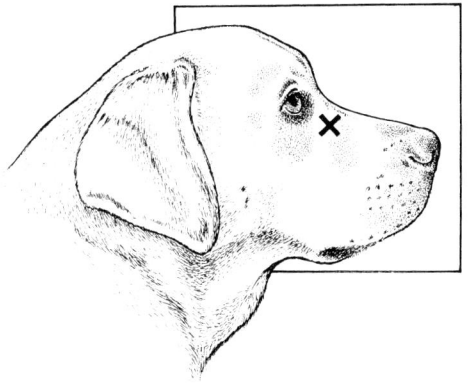

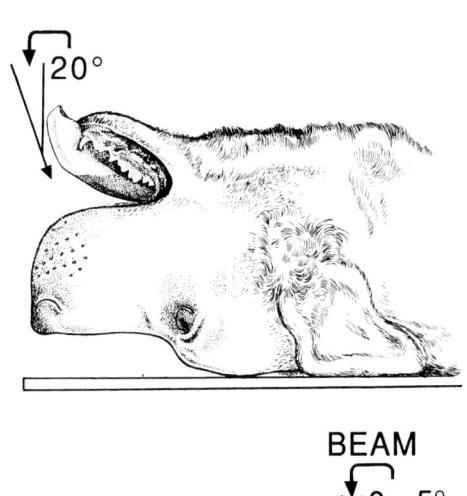

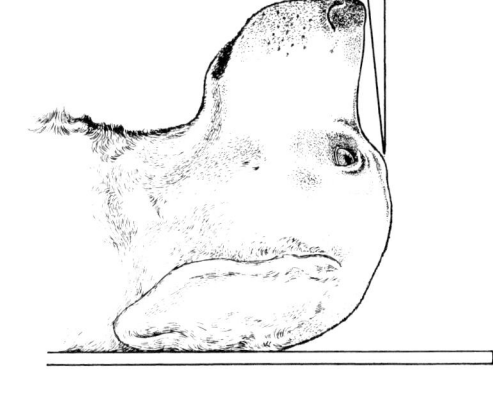

Fig. 40.8 Diagram to show the views that are commonly used to obtain radiographic images of the nasal cavity of the dog. The dorsoventral intra-oral view is the most useful as it allows comparison of both sides. A poorer alternative is the ventro20°-dorsal intra-oral. The rostrocaudal view of the frontal sinuses is very useful to identify involvement of the frontal sinuses in the management of aspergillosis. The lateral view has limited value due to superimposition but does identify destruction of the bony case. (Redrawn with permission of *In Practice*.)

that this will shorten the life-span of the intensifying screen as it will not be protected from the rigours of use by being enclosed in a cassette. Cassettes are too bulky to reach far enough into the mouth to assess the caudal parts of the nasal cavity and so the Ventro 20°-dorsal–intra-oral view allows a cassette to be utilised. The beam is angled to project the open mandible on to the calvarium as it would otherwise intrude on the image of the nasal turbinates. The other views are optional and are really of value when directed at a specific area/condition that has been defined by the intra-oral views (Fig. 40.8). The lateral view is restricted to evaluating the cribiform plate and the bony case as the two sides are superimposed. The dorsoventral skull view causes superimposition of the mandibles on to a

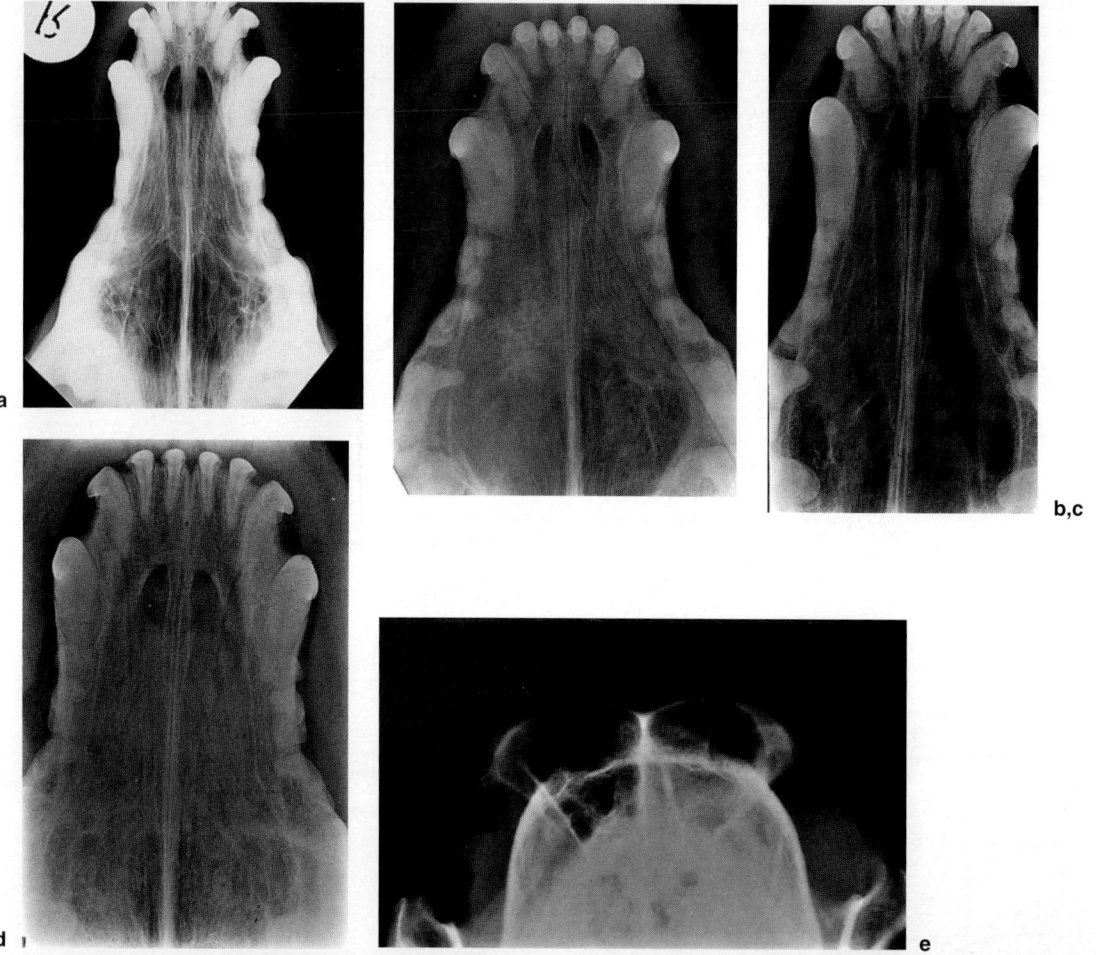

Fig. 40.9 (a) Dorsoventral intra-oral view of a normal nasal cavity. Note the fine turbinate pattern rostrally and caudally, with a coarser pattern at the level of the carnassial teeth. (b) Dorsoventral intra-oral view of a nasal tumour. There is substantial destruction of the turbinates centred at the level of the carnassial tooth on the left. The turbinates have been replaced by a homogenous soft tissue opacity, which unusually has a mineralised element embedded rostrally. (c) Dorsoventral intra-oral view of a nasal aspergillosis. There is turbinate destruction on the left rostrally causing an increase in radiolucency. Caudally there is also some increased radiolucency but the pattern here is of a mixed opacity. (d) Dorsoventral intra-oral view of chronic hyperplastic rhinitis. The turbinate pattern is still present but has been masked by a fluffy increase in opacity. (e) Rostrocaudal view of frontal sinuses of a dog with aspergillosis. The left sinus is partially opacified by fungus ventrally and the sky-lined bone is thickened and mottled.

large part of the nasal cavity, but is effective for the cribiform area. The RCd skull to skyline view of the frontal sinuses is most useful where aspergillosis has been diagnosed as it demonstrates involvement of the frontal sinuses and the need to treat that area as well as the nasal cavity. It is not an easy view to obtain and repeat.

The radiographic features of the normal nasal cavity and the various diseases are shown in Figs. 40.9a–e (Gibbs *et al.* 1979; Sullivan *et al.* 1986, 1987).

Other imaging systems such as computed tomography and magnetic resonance imaging have been used to evaluate chronic nasal disease in the dog but their availability is very limited at the moment (Koblik & Berry 1990; Codner *et al.* 1993).

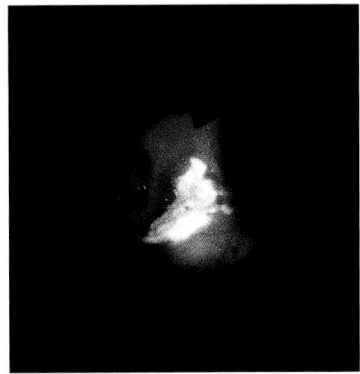

Fig. 40.10 Rostal endoscopic view of a fungal plaque sited on a truncated turbinate.

Rhinoscopy

Every animal anaesthetised for further investigation of nasal discharge should be examined endoscopically (Sullivan 1991). The nasal passages can be examined from two directions. Rostral rhinoscopy is quick and allows identification of foreign bodies and fungal plaques, with removal of the former and sampling of the latter for mycological investigation (Fig. 40.10). The fungus has a variable appearance with plaques sitting on the turbinates being white or a dirty yellow/green. It can be distinguished from mucus by its very dry non-reflective appearance. Occasionally a nasal tumour can be seen projecting into the common meatus. However, in many conditions discharge will hinder examination, or the lack of observable change fails to contribute to the clinical diagnosis.

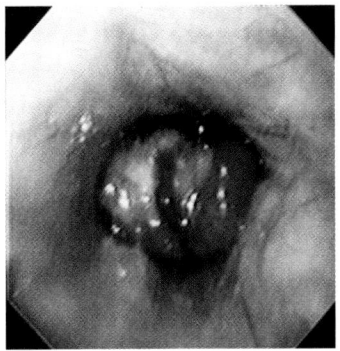

Fig. 40.11 Caudal rhinoscopic view of a large tumour extending from the nasal cavity through and obstructing the caudal choanae into the nasaopharynx.

> Note: arthroscopes can be used in examinations as they are thin, but their sharp ends tend to damage the sensitive mucosa and cause haemorrhage that clouds the nasal passages. Paediatric bronchoscopes (3.5 mm diameter) are excellent where there has been some turbinate destruction and can reach the ethmoturbinates, but are very expensive. A cheap and comparatively effective instrument is an otoscope with a long speculum.

extending into the nasopharynx as large friable and ulcerated masses (Fig. 40.11).

Serology

A 5–10 ml clotted blood sample, preferably spun to retrieve the serum allows competent laboratories to test for antibodies to particular fungi, specifically *Aspergillus fumigatus*. Currently the fastest and most sensitive test is counter-immunoelectrophoresis. The laboratory should test the sample against at least three, preferably six, different antigens and must maintain a quality control on the antigens used (Lane & Warnock 1977; Richardson *et al.* 1982). In this way false negatives should be avoided. This test is disease specific as a positive result confirms aspergillosis, a

The speculum must be directed medially to lever the alar fold laterally allowing the speculum to pass into the common meatus. Caudal rhinoscopy is best achieved with the use of a flexible fibre-optic endoscope that can be hooked around the soft palate and pulled rostrally to view the caudal choanae. Foreign bodies can be identified and retrieved. Nasal tumours that have extended in this direction can also be seen occluding the caudal choanae or negative generally rules it out, but fails to provide information about any other potential diagnosis. Serial sampling to evaluate treatment of aspergillosis is unrewarding as the titre takes many months to fall and bears no relationship to the success or otherwise of treatment.

Histopathology and Cytology

Examination of tissue samples is often the sole way to distinguish neoplasia from chronic hyperplastic rhinitis. The best samples are those obtained by rhinotomy, but this involves significant surgical intervention that is not warranted in chronic hyperplastic rhinitis. Good samples can be obtained through an otoscope or with an arthroscopic biopsy forceps (Fig. 40.12). Another simple technique is to use a large male urinary catheter or intravenous drip tubing attached to a 50-ml syringe to obtain a suction biopsy of intra-nasal material.

Haematology and Biochemistry

Haematological and biochemical profiles are only of value in specific diseases where the common causes of intra-nasal disease have been ruled out. Haematology will define the bleeding disorder causing the epistaxis. In dogs with macroglobulinaemias and cryoglobulins an assay of blood spun down at as near body temperature as possible will show profound rise in serum globulin levels caused by the overproduction of immunoglobulins. If the sample is allowed to cool precipitation of cryoglobulins can be seen as plugs or flocculations (Fig. 40.7).

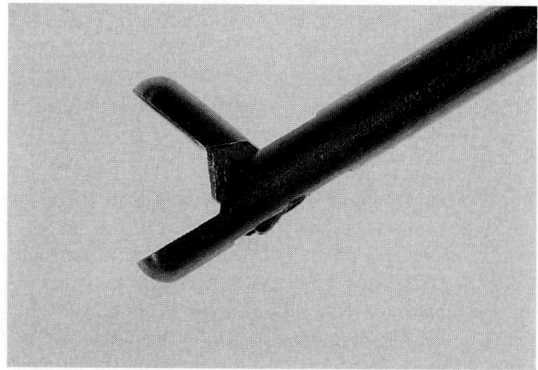

Fig. 40.12   Arthoscopic biopsy forceps are an excellent method of obtaining samples of nasal tissue.

Microbiology

Bacteriology from nasal swabs is of doubtful value as any bacteria recovered are usually normal commensals or opportunistic invaders. However, culture of nasal swabs is worthwhile where a secondary bacterial infection needs to be tackled. For fungal isolation direct endoscopic biopsy is recommended, as nasal washings or blind swabbing frequently return false negatives.

TREATMENT

Nasal Neoplasia

Neoplasia is rarely detected at an early stage suggesting that there are no clinical signs or that they are so subtle as to go unobserved. Rhinotomy and radical surgery does not alter the life-expectancy of the animal, and even as a palliative procedure it is unrewarding, staying the clinical signs for only a couple of months. Some recent studies have indicated that radical surgery combined with radiotherapy can increase the life expectancy in some animals. The restriction on this method of treatment is that the radiation is delivered as fractionated doses and thus requires a facility to which the owner is prepared to travel (Adams *et al.* 1987).

Chronic Hyperplastic Rhinitis

Some response can be gained from administering a broad-spectrum antibiotic in combination with oral bromhexine hydrochloride (Bisolvon™). Owners should be encouraged to let the dog out of the house first thing in the morning when the discharge will be at its worst, as it will have gathered overnight in the nasal chambers. Surgery should be avoided, as there is a significant residual nasal discharge after turbinectomy. The prognosis is guarded as the owners dislike the discharge. It is a most benign condition yet troublesome to treat. This is the intranasal disease that needs a significant amount of work to understand the condition more fully and to improve the management.

Nasal Aspergillosis

Prognosis is good following aggressive therapy with the current treatment of choice enilconazole (Imaverol™) instilled into the nasal cavity via drains implanted in the frontal sinuses (Fig. 40.13a, b). This avoids turbinectomy and prolonged oral courses of antimycotic agents (Sharp *et al.* 1993). Animals should be re-evaluated one month after

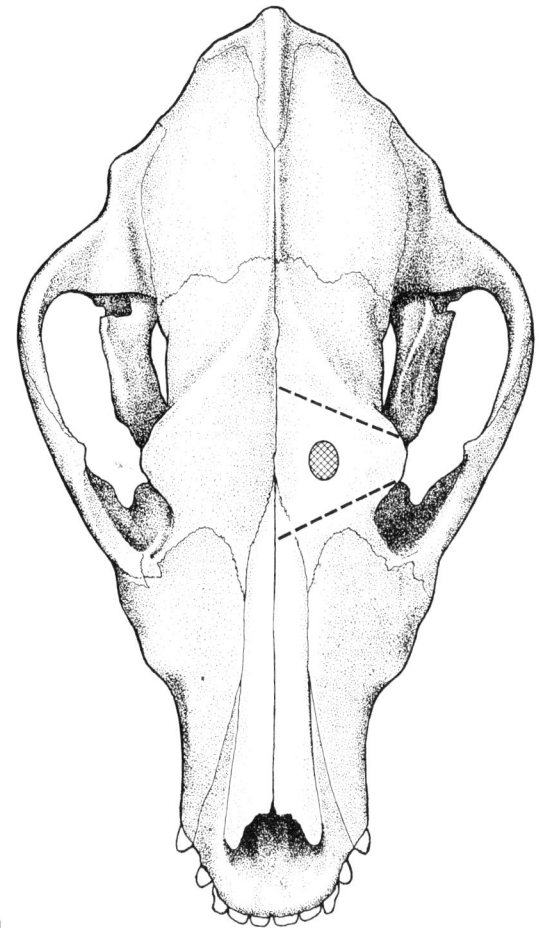

a

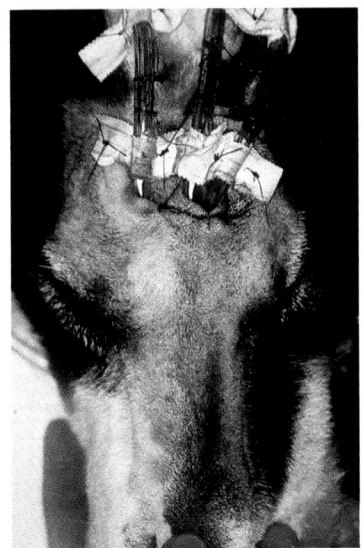

b

Fig. 40.13 (a) The landmarks, supra-orbital ridge, external frontal crest and midline suture line, represent a triangle the centre of which is the point of entry for drainage tubes. (b) Three drains have been placed in the nasal cavities on both sides and into the left frontal sinus.

treatment. Recurrence of discharge should initiate general anaesthesia and endoscopy. If fungal plaques are visible the treatment can be repeated and if necessary supplemented with oral ketoconazole at 5 mg/kg for 6 weeks (Sharp & Sullivan 1989a). Where ketoconazole is to be used pre-treatment evaluation of hepatic and renal function is advised as this drug is hepatotoxic (Sharp & Sullivan 1989b). If no plaques are evident the cause of the discharge may be a superimposed bacterial infection and a broad-spectrum antibiotic (2 weeks) should clear the problem.

Rhinarial Ulceration

As the biopsy results are often inconclusive, the old standby of broad-spectrum antibiotic and corticosteroid, started at an immunosuppresive dose then reduced over 4 weeks, does seem to manage this condition satisfactorily.

Idiopathic Destructive Rhinitis

Since no cause is established for the destruction, treatment of the secondary bacterial rhinitis causes an improvement in the level of discharge.

ORO-NASAL FISTULAE

These should be corrected by closing the defect in the cleft palate with the sandwich technique. If dental disease is responsible the diseased tooth needs to be removed and the underlying defect reconstructed.

REFERENCES

Adams, W.M., Withrow, S.J., Walshaw, R., *et al.* (1987). Radiotherapy of malignant nasal tumours in 67 dogs. *Journal of the American Veterinary Medical Association*, **191**, 311.

Codner, E.C., Lurus, A.G., Miller, J.B., Gavin, P.R., Gallina, A. & Barnee, D.D. (1993). Comparison of computer tomography with radiography as a noninvasive diagnostic technique for chronic nasal disease in dogs. *Journal of the American Veterinary Medical Association*, **202**, 1106.

Gibbs, C., Lane, J.G. & Denny, H.R. (1979). Radiological features of intra-nasal lesions in the dog: a review of 100 cases. *Journal of Small Animal Practice*, **20**, 515.

Koblik, P.D. & Berry, C.R. (1990). Dorsal plane computed tomographic imaging of the ethmoid region to evaluate chronic nasal disease in the dog. *Veterinary Radiology*, **31**, 92.

Lane, J.G. & Warnock, D.W. (1977). The diagnosis of *Aspergillus fumigatus* infection of the nasal chambers of the dog with partic-ular reference to the value of the double diffusion test. *Journal of Small Animal Practice*, **18**, 169.

Richardson, M., Warnock, D.W., Bovey, S.E. & Lane, J.G. (1982). Rapid serological diagnosis of *Aspergillus fumigatus* infection of the frontal sinuses and nasal chambers of the dog. *Research in Veterinary Science*, **33**, 167.

Sharp, N.J.H. & Sullivan, M. (1989a). Treatment of canine aspergillosis with systemic ketoconazole and topical enilcona-zole. *Veterinary Record*, **118**, 560.

Sharp, N.J.H. & Sullivan, M. (1989b). Ketoconazole therapy for nasal aspergillosis: a reduced dose regime. *Journal of the American Veterinary Medical Association*, **194**, 782.

Sharp, N.J.H., Sullivan, M., Harvey, C.E. & Webb, T. (1993). Treatment of canine nasal aspergillosis with enilconazole. *Journal of Veterinary Internal Medicine*, **7**, 40.

Sullivan, M. (1991). Rhinoscopy. In: *A Colour Atlas of Small Animal Endoscopy*, (eds M.J. Brearley, J.E. Cooper & M. Sullivan), pp. 19–30. Wolf Publications, London.

Sullivan, M., Lee, R., Jakovljevic, S. & Sharp, N.J.H. (1986). The radiological features of aspergillosis of the nasal cavity and frontal sinuses in the dog. *Journal of Small Animal Practice*, **27**, 167.

Sullivan, M., Lee, R. & Skae, K. (1987). The radiological features of canine nasal neoplasia: a review of 60 cases. *Journal of Small Animal Practice*, **28**, 575–586.

Chapter 41

Obstructive Upper Airway Disease

M. Sullivan

INTRODUCTION

Trauma to the airway has the potential to cause obstruction to airflow in the dog. These animals present acutely because of the sudden onset. The nares may be damaged, fractures to the bones of the nasal case and also the turbinates are more common. The subsequent haemorrhage, swelling and possible displacement are responsible for the airway obstruction. However, the obstruction is usually temporary and normal first aid measures provide adequate relief, such that more invasive or long-term management is not needed. Due to its position in the neck the larynx is well protected and trauma to it is uncommon. However, punctures to the area from dog bites or stick penetrations do occur. Excessive use of the check chain has the potential to fracture the hyoid apparatus or crush the laryngeal cartilages, but this type of injury is extremely rare, and the apparent defects produced by incomplete mineralisation of the hyoid apparatus seen in older dogs should not be mistaken for a fracture. With soft feeding, fractured hyoid bones are best left to heal themselves. Depending on the injury tracheotomy and or steroid therapy may be needed to re-establish an airway and suppress oedema. Where there has been an open wound antibiotic cover should be instituted.

Iatrogenic injury to the laryngeal membranes can be caused by attempting to intubate while the glottic reflex is still present, or forcibly intubating with a tube that is too large. The result is a cough that arises due to the oedema and mucous membrane erosion. In severe cases, also seen as a consequence of acute laryngitis, this may progress to fibrosis of the laryngeal tissues and stenosis, which is not amenable to partial laryngectomy.

UPPER AIRWAY OBSTRUCTION SYNDROME

For the sake of classification it is possible to broadly define animals presenting primarily with obstruction to airflow as suffering from upper respiratory obstruction syndrome (UROS). Some authors use the phrase brachycephalic obstruction syndrome (BOS). Others name it canine asphyxia, a broader term to include laryngeal paralysis that is seen in larger non-brachycephalic dogs.

Initially discussion of upper airway obstruction will be confined to the brachycephalic obstruction syndrome as laryngeal paralysis presents in a different and discrete manner. This syndrome consists of a group of conditions affecting primarily the brachycephalic breeds, it is both congenital and hereditary. The breeds most commonly affected are English Bulldogs, Pugs, Pekingese, Yorkshire Terriers, Boston Terriers and the Boxer. A variety of abnormalities contribute to this syndrome, though not all are present in every case (Table 41.1).

The clinical signs vary and depend on the number and severity of the conditions that are contributing to the syndrome in a particular animal. Fortunately, in many a single abnormality predominates. The clinical signs may include:

- noisy respiration characterised as snuffling,
- noisy respiration, coughing and gagging,
- respiratory distress,
- respiratory distress and collapse with or without cyanosis.

These conditions may cause chronic hypoxia and consequent pulmonary hypertension, leading to cor pulmonale.

Table 41.1   Conditions contributing to upper respiratory obstruction syndrome.

Primary	Secondary
Stenotic nares	
Soft palate elongation	Soft palate hypertrophy
Tracheal stenosis/ hypoplasia	Laryngeal saccule eversion
Tracheal collapse	Laryngeal collapse
	Displacement of the glosso-epiglottic mucosa
	Tonsillitis

Anaesthesia

From the anaesthetic point of view, these dogs are frequently hypoxic and are somewhat acidotic due to the respiratory embarrassment. Some have cardiac abnormalities, but auscultation is made difficult due to the referred upper airway noises. Many of these conditions are a consequence of the creation of brachycephalic breeds, but the conditions are exacerbated by the fact that the pharynx has become smaller and flattened in a craniocaudal direction.

   As a consequence any surgery on the upper respiratory tract should be done as early in the day as possible to allow maximum monitoring following surgery. Equipment and facilities for temporary tracheotomy and care thereof are a prerequisite for undertaking surgery in these cases. All animals should be given peri-operative injections of corticosteroid and a further injection at the end of surgery.

SPECIFIC CONDITIONS

Stenotic Nares

Only rarely are stenotic nares caused by severe trauma, it is as a rule a congenital defect. The dorsal parietal cartilage and its epithelial covering collapse medially and obstruct the airflow at the external nares. The normal comma shaped appearance of the lumen is lost and replaced by an L-shaped slit. The nares are collapsed and on inspiration the degree of occlusion worsens. They can sometimes be seen to vibrate. On occasion slight serous nasal discharge is seen as a bead on the nasal sill. Although this can occur alone, as it does in the Boxer, it is generally present with other conditions of the syndrome that contribute to the obstruction. As an example of ubiquity many Pekingese have stenotic nares. The diagnosis is made by inspection.

Treatment

Stenotic nares should be treated as early as possible to prevent the exacerbating effect that the secondary conditions have on the animal's respiratory obstruction. There are at least three techniques described for correcting stenotic nares, but the author's preferred technique is to remove a vertical wedge of epithelium and cartilage from the ventral aspect of the wing of the nostril. The wedge is best removed with a no.11 scalpel blade. The profuse haemorrhage is controlled by appositional sutures of 1.5 metric (410) polyglactin 910. An immediate improvement should be evident (Fig. 41.1).

Soft Palate Elongation with Hypertrophy

Soft palate elongation is not seen exclusively in the brachycephalic breeds. It is frequently seen in Labradors and Spaniels. Although the owner is often aware of the dog

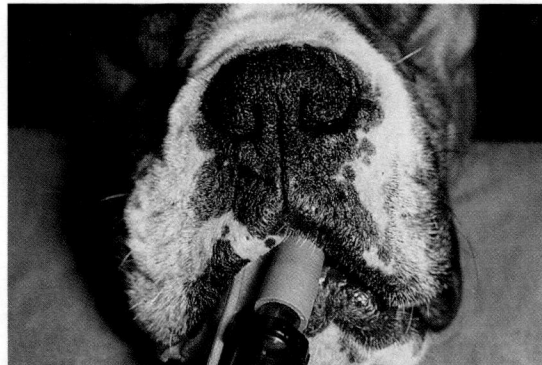

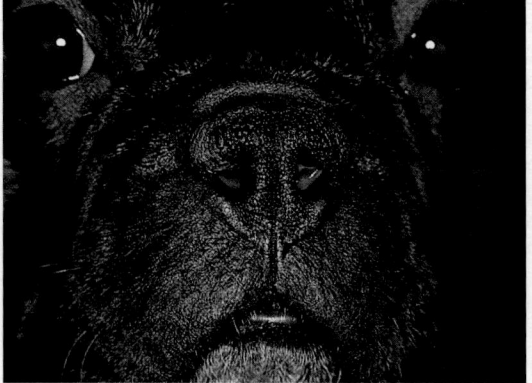

Fig. 41.1   (a) Young Boxer with stenotic nares. (b) Staffordshire Bull Terrier 1 month after wedge resection of epithelium and cartilage.

occasionally 'choking up' during exercise it seldom worries owners and attention is rarely sought for soft palate elongation in these breeds. However, it is important to recognise its presence in animals with laryngeal paralysis as it will compromise the laryngeal airway and affect the results of surgery, such that it should be corrected if present in animals undergoing corrective surgery for laryngeal paralysis.

The excessively long palate is sucked into the larynx by the negative pressure of inspiration. This is exacerbated by and exacerbates the increased negative inspiratory pressure that results from the other abnormalities, which make up the syndrome. The repeated trauma of plugging the larynx leads to hypertrophy of the mucosa and palatine muscles. On inspection the normal soft palate lies just on top of the epiglottis. Resection is indicated if it is hypertrophied and elongated.

Treatment

It is possible to remove too much soft palate and leave the animal unable to adequately protect the nasopharynx during deglutition so that nasal regurgitation of food material arises. This will cause a chronic rhinitis. However, in the brachycephalic breeds with elongated soft palate it is unlikely that too much will be removed. The landmark for estimating the amount of tissue to be removed is the caudal pole of the tonsil. There are several techniques described (Table 41.2).

Although the technique that involves suturing the palate after resection is the most time-consuming, it is the safest technique as it avoids the potential hazard of aspiration of blood and the significant postoperative swelling that electrocautery causes. Temporary tracheotomy is an optional measure, but in most brachycephalics it is not necessary. The pharynx should be packed with dampened swabs to prevent inhalation of blood. The soft palate is drawn forward and the excess tissue removed with scissors, care should be taken to ensure that equal amounts of oral and nasal mucosa are removed as it is easy to resect oral

mucosa and leave a long tail of nasal mucosa. Coughing, gagging and vomiting are common in the postoperative period.

Dorsal Displacement of the Glosso-epiglottic Mucosa

The small, somewhat compressed pharynx of the brachycephalic breeds contributes to the syndrome and the excess negative pressure can also cause collapse of the pharyngeal airway and displacement of the glosso-epiglottic mucosa. The mucosa underneath the epiglottis in affected dogs can be drawn forwards, upwards and over the epiglottis to demonstrate filling of the laryngeal aditus (Fig. 41.2). This should be sectioned with scissors to prevent the tissue continuing to dynamically occlude the airway. Care should be taken not to damage the epiglottal cartilage. There have been no long-term studies to assess the efficacy of this procedure or whether the mucosa with time will elongate and

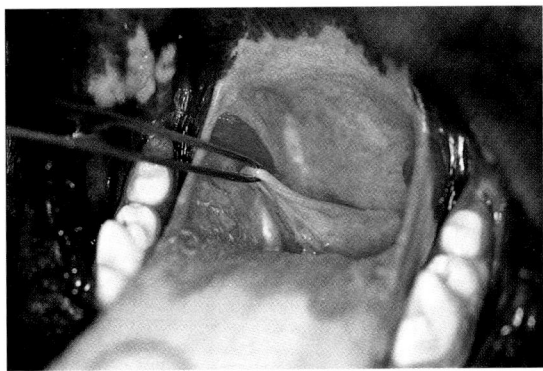

Fig. 41.2 Under anaesthesia the excessive glosso-epiglottic mucosa has been drawn up to demonstrate how it can envelop the epiglottis and compromise the glottic opening.

Table 41.2 Treatment of soft palate elongation with hypertrophy.

Technique	Negative aspect
Resect and oversew with an interrupted or continuous polyglactin 910 sutures	Time-consuming
Clamping the soft palate with curved artery forceps and resecting along the crush line	Risk of haemorrhage
Electrocautery to section the mucosa and muscle, and thus prevent haemorrhage	Significant oedema induced

dorsally displace again. It is important not to overlook this mucosal displacement, but equally it is important to check that there is not also a laryngeal collapse (Bedford 1983).

Tonsillitis

Since the airway obstruction forces these animals to mouth-breathe and the distorting anatomy of the pharynx alters the normal conformation, many of these dogs have normal tonsils that are large with respect to the small pharynx or have a degree of secondary tonsillitis. Tonsillectomy is of definite value in these animals as part of the correction process.

Everted Laryngeal Saccules

Another effect of the excess negative pressure drawing mucosal tissue into the glottides is that the laryngeal saccules evert and plug the ventral portion of the glottides, perhaps by 50–60%. As well as being seen in brachy-cephalic dogs it is also occurs in Miniature Poodles. The diagnosis cannot be made on clinical signs alone but requires general anaesthesia and laryngoscopy, and full evaluation for other associated conditions.

Laryngoscopy

In the normal animal the entrance to the laryngeal saccules is seen as a dark slit between the vocal cords and the ventricular folds (Fig. 41.3). In general both saccules evert to the same extent. The vocal cords (if still visible) will be thickened and oedematous, otherwise they are obscured by two translucent oedematous globes that are the everted saccules. The airway is reduced to a small diamond dorsally between the corniculate cartilages. The obstruction is exacerbated by the accumulated secretions that are often present cranial to the saccules.

Treatment

These can be removed per os or by laryngotomy. However, whichever technique is used the animal really needs to have a bypass tracheotomy as the endotracheal tube significantly obstructs the surgical site. Removal per os can be achieved with the use of fine Metzenbaum scissors, with care taken not to section the vocal cords. Haemorrhage is minimal because the everted saccules are relatively avascular.

Laryngeal Collapse

Key features: snorting, choking, respiratory noise, collapse.

Laryngeal collapse is an under-diagnosed condition and is more often responsible for the snuffling and respiratory noise seen in Cavalier King Charles Spaniels than for example elongated soft palate. On endoscopy, the cuneiform and corniculate tubercles of the arytenoid are seen to be inverted or scrolled inwards to severely narrow the laryngeal lumen (Fig. 41.4). This medial displacement is accompanied by scrolling of the epiglottis in severe cases. This condition is progressive, yet surgery to the larynx to

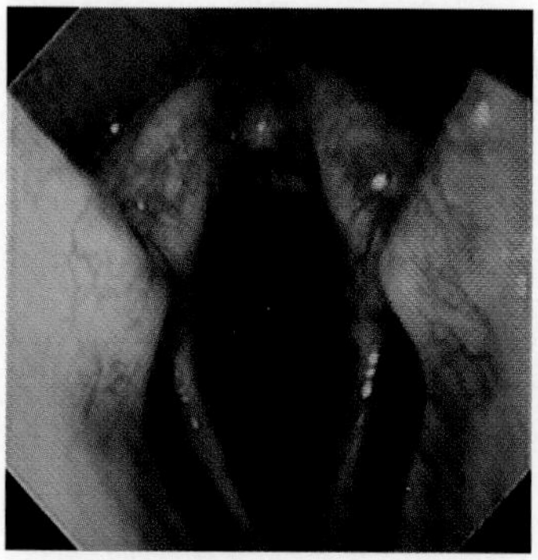

Fig. 41.3 Endoscopic view of a normal larynx. The corniculate process of the arytenoid can be seen diverging dorsally and the large wings of the cuneiform processes in the foreground. The glottis is a large diamond shape bordered ventrolaterally by the vocal cords.

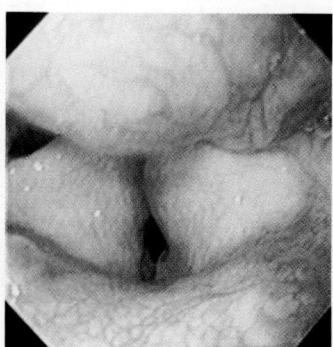

Fig. 41.4 The glottis is reduced to a small diamond. The cuneiform cartilages have collapsed to midline and are starting to overlap one another (stage 2 moving to stage 3). The corniculate cartilages are obscured by an elongated soft palate.

correct the collapse has given poor results with a significant mortality associated with surgery. Current opinion is that other aspects of the BOS should be addressed and corrected before surgery for laryngeal collapse is contemplated. This is on the basis that often surgery elsewhere will sufficiently alleviate the respiratory distress to render surgery for collapse avoidable.

Treatment

As a staged procedure, correct other conditions causing the BOS that may be present. Only if this fails should further surgery be contemplated. Partial laryngectomy with removal of the arytenoid processes can be done but conspicuous postoperative monitoring and care are required, and postoperative fibrosis and webbing are serious complications. The alternative is to bypass the larynx and carry out a permanent tracheostomy. However, one should be aware that some of these dogs will have a co-existing tracheal collapse that will preclude permanent tracheostomy as an option, and the tracheostomy wound must be managed assiduously for 10–14 days after surgery to prevent occlusion with the profoundly increased bronchial secretions that are stimulated by the removal of the modifying influence of the nasal chambers.

Laryngeal Disease

The larynx is innervated by two nerves: the cranial laryngeal nerve, which exits the vagus at the nodose ganglion and supplies the cricothyroideus muscle. The caudal laryngeal nerve – the terminal portion of the recurrent laryngeal nerve – innervates the remaining muscles. In a number of large breed old dogs such as the Irish Setter, Labrador and Afghan an acquired neurogenic atrophy occurs. In the Bouvier and Siberian Husky a congenital and hereditary paralysis has been identified. Though the Bouvier is a rare breed in the UK a disproportionate number of cases have been seen from this breed.

Examination

The larynx is prominent in all but the most obese dogs and is normally movable from side to side. On manipulation, the larynx is bilaterally symmetrical and is not markedly sensitive, a cough can be induced by firm digital pressure on the larynx. Detailed examination of the larynx is only possible under general anaesthesia. Laryngoscopy can only be adequately carried out using a laryngoscope. Where paralysis is suspected light anaesthesia is required with the animal in sternal not lateral recumbency. The larynx can then be inspected at induction or during recovery.

Laryngeal Paralysis

Key features: inspiratory stridor, exercise intolerance, cough, change in bark.

Laryngeal paralysis is more common than is generally recognised and some cases are incorrectly diagnosed as lower respiratory disease in aged animals. Although most cases in the adult are due to an acquired idiopathic neurogenic atrophy of the laryngeal muscles, cases have been seen resulting from surgery to the ventral cervical region, polyneuropathy, and due to tumours or space-occupying lesions in the neck or cranial mediastinum, e.g. thyroid tumours or thymomas.

Clinical Signs

As the animal is unable to abduct the arytenoids, the history and signs are related to this failure:

- exercise intolerance,
- respiratory difficulty when excited (which can cause collapse),
- cyanosis (generally exacerbated by a hot environment),
- a moist cough is frequently present,
- a loss or change in the dog's bark.

The animal will have a hoarse or harsh inspiratory noise, which is most dramatic when the proximal trachea or larynx is auscultated in preference to the thorax. In a few cases a laryngeal fremitus will be palpable.

Diagnosis

Although the breed, history and clinical signs are often adequate confirmation can be made by laryngoscopy. The examination must be done under light anaesthesia with the dog in sternal recumbency. Endoscopy will show a laryngitis, the corniculate tubercles being most obviously affected, the vocal cords are inflamed and oedematous. On inspiration there will be failure of abduction, in severely affected cases there may be complete collapse, and the vocal cords will be pulled into mid-line. It is usually bilateral in nature. An elongated soft palate should also be looked for. The paradoxical abduction seen on expiration should not be mistaken for inspiratory abduction.

Treatment

Treatment is outlined in Table 41.3.

In a recent cadaver surgery study (Lussier *et al.* 1996) the authors found that the cricoarytenoid lateralisation

Table 41.3   Treatment of laryngeal paralysis.

Technique	Comment
Conservative management with weight loss	Is often very successful in fat Labradors where there is no respiratory difficulty
Laryngectomy, removing part or all of the arytenoids	There are almost always complications to this technique. Persistent inhalation tracheitis and a chronic cough leading to bronchopneumonia. Laryngeal webbing occurs though rarely a significant problem – resection is indicated
Laryngoplasty	Suture replaces the dorsal cricoarytenoid muscle. Technique similar to that in the horse and most anatomically correct
Arytenoid lateralisation	Most popular surgical treatment currently

(laryngoplasty) provided a greater increase in glottic opening than did thyroarytenoid lateralisation (see below). However, work demonstrating the transfer of this effect to the clinical case has not been published.

Arytenoid Lateralisation (White 1989)

Through a left or right lateral approach ventral to the jugular vein, the thyroid lamina is identified and will serve as a landmark throughout the approach. The thyropharyngeus muscle is identified and sectioned level with the top of the thyroid lamina. This exposes the fascia that must be punctured to access the various articulations, which must be destroyed. A suture placed in the craniodorsal aspect of the thyroid cartilage acts as a most useful retractor for the rest of the procedure. Directing curved scissors caudally the cricothyroid articulation is cut and further retraction of the thyroid lamina will allow the muscular process of the arytenoid to be identified, as a small triangular projection of cartilage lying on the cricoid cartilage. If the muscular process is lifted the cricoarytenoid articulation can be easily sectioned by introducing scissors underneath and into the joint (Fig . 41.5). The most difficult part of the procedure is to section the interarytenoid sesamoid. One publication suggests that it is not necessary to section this sesamoid cartilage. The sesamoid is palpable as a thin piece of cartilage between the two muscular processes through overlying soft tissue. Great care must be taken when sectioning to avoid penetrating the mucosa of the laryngopharynx. Once done the muscular process is freed and can be pulled caudally, thus abducting the larynx on that side. There are several suture patterns described and each represents the personal choice of the surgeon, but may be dictated by the degree of calcification of the muscular process:

- single bite in the muscular process,
- mattress suture in muscular process,
- either of above re-inforced with a laryngoplasty (cricoid to muscular process suture).

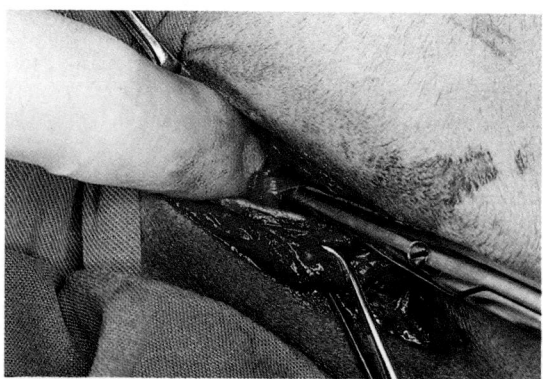

Fig. 41.5   Arytenoid lateralisation. The thyropharyngeus muscle has been sectioned highlighting the edge of the thyroid cartilage. The cricothyroid articulation has been broken down. For the sake of the illustration the atrophied dorsal cricoarytenoid muscle has not been sectioned and is seen overlying the scissors that have been pushed between the muscular process, highlighted by the finger, and the cricoid to split the cricoarytenoid articulation.

Monofilament nylon, polypropylene or polyester (3 m) can all be used as the suture material; more important is a fine trocar pointed swaged-on needle.

Mattress Pattern

Using 3 m non-absorbable synthetic material, the suture is passed through the most caudodorsal part of the thyroid cartilage above the notch and the free end isolated with a haemostat. The needle is then passed through the muscular process towards the articular surface of the cricoid and back up through the muscular process. The suture is completed by passing the suture material through the thyroid cartilage 5 mm cranial to the first bite. Tying the suture is crucial because the throws are being placed against the solid surface of the thyroid. It is essential when laying the first throw to apply gentle upward traction on the ends of the suture material to ensure that the throw does not snare against the thyroid cartilage. The suture is tightened to take up the slack and the process repeated several times. This should be done carefully to ensure that the suture material does not break or pull through the muscular process.

The thyropharyngeus muscle and overlying subcutaneous tissue is closed to remove dead space and the skin closed in a routine manner.

In most cases it is only necessary to carry out the procedure on one side; where there is doubt about the improvement in the lumen the contralateral side should be lateralised.

Reasons for Failure

- The muscular process has disintegrated – caused by aggressive tension being placed on the cartilage or too many bites being attempted.
- The suture has pulled through the cartilage (avoid using cutting needles as the triangular points can create a cleavage line in the cartilage).

The risk of the suture pulling out is exacerbated by a dog that, in the postoperative period, spends its time howling and barking, so good postoperative analgesia is important.

Postoperative Management

The dog should be given water and a gruel-like diet for 5–7 days, avoiding milk and dry food, to prevent inhalation pneumonia in a situation where the laryngeal protective mechanism may be impaired. Exercise should be minimal for 21 days followed by a further 21 days restricted lead exercise. This is to encourage rapid fibrosis of the cartilages and reduce dependence on the suture.

Laryngeal Neoplasia

Malignant tumours of the larynx are very rare in the dog and benign laryngeal polyps are more frequently encountered, although they also are rare. The dog presents with progressive respiratory embarrassment. On endoscopy a red tonsil-like mass can be seen occluding the laryngeal lumen. This can be grasped and removed with long handled scissors and forceps to cause an immediate improvement in the airways. However, the origin of the polyp needs to be searched for and extirpated to prevent recurrence. This can be done per os or preferentially through a ventral laryngotomy. The prognosis is good.

REFERENCES

Bedford, P.G.C. (1983). Displacement of the glosso-epiglottic mucosa in canine asphyxia disease. *Journal of Small Animal Practice*, **24**, 199.

Lussier, B., Flanders, J.A. & Erb, H.N. (1996). The effect of unilateral arytenoid lateralisation on rima glottidis area in canine cadaver larynges. *Veterinary Surgery*, **25**, 121.

White, R.A.S. (1989). Unilateral arytenoid lateralisation: An assessment of technique and long term results in 62 dogs with laryngeal paralysis. *Journal of Small Animal Practice*, **20**, 169.

Chapter 42

Tracheobronchial Diseases

B. Corcoran and M. Sullivan

Diseases of the trachea and bronchi can be divided broadly into anatomical problems or inflammatory conditions although one can lead to the other.

TRACHEAL HYPOPLASIA

Tracheal hypoplasia is seen mainly in English Bulldogs and can contribute to the obstruction caused by other elements of the brachycephalic obstructive described fully in Chapter 41 page 353. However, it may not cause sufficiently abnormal signs for the owner to seek veterinary attention and may only be noticed incidentally on radiographs of the thorax. There is no satisfactory treatment (Bedford 1982).

Radiographic Appearance

On lateral views of the thorax that include the thoracic inlet and caudal neck the trachea is seen to have a very narrow lumen. Compared with the normal dog where the tracheal lumen may be two to three times the diameter of the proximal third of the third to fourth ribs, it is less than the diameter of the rib in these animals. This narrowing is subjectively aggravated by a large neck, broad cranial thorax and the profusion of skin folds that these dogs have (Fig. 42.1).

TRACHEAL COLLAPSE

The key features of tracheal collapse are:

- honking noise,
- respiratory distress,
- flattened tracheal lumen.

Tracheal collapse is seen in many small breed dogs. The underlying cause is a failure of mineralisation of the cartilage that makes up the tracheal rings. As a consequence the rings lose the normal C shape and start to flatten, this has the effect of stretching the dorsal tracheal membrane. As the membrane stretches, it may become 'sucked' into the lumen of the trachea, narrowing the airway during respiration. As the animal ages and other problems with the cardiorespiratory systems supervene, the membrane becomes wider and the impingement on the lumen becomes greater. So although the changes to the cartilaginous rings can be detected in young dogs, most only show clinical signs once they have reached 7 years of age. Characteristically these dogs (and most are Yorkshire Terriers) honk like a goose and it not unusual for this noise to have been present for years without the tracheal collapse actually causing respiratory embarrassment. The best way to confirm the diagnosis is by tracheobronchoscopy (Fig. 42.3). The mucous membrane can be thickened in places and a wide membrane is evident between the edges of the flattened tracheal rings. The change is most severe at the thoracic inlet, but it is also worthwhile inspecting the main bronchi for involvement. The diagnosis can be confirmed by radiography. The tracheal collapse can be imaged dynamically with fluoroscopy. As fluoroscopy is rarely available, plain radiographs can be used and will show pronounced narrowing of the trachea centred on the thoracic inlet but extending up the cervical trachea. If this is not present a profound widening to the thoracic trachea caused by ballooning of the dorsal membrane is more often visible on plain radiographs.

Treatment

Management of tracheal collapse is contentious with there being two schools of thought. Most of the dogs with this problem can and should be managed conservatively (White & Williams 1994).

Conservative management includes:

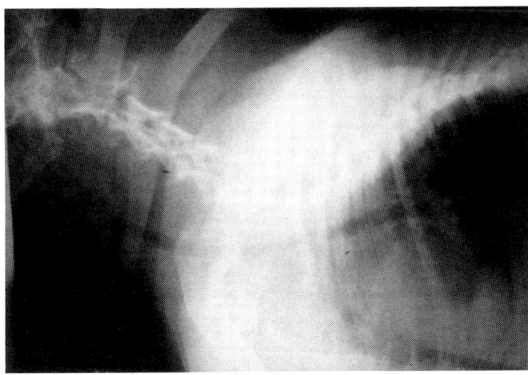

Fig. 42.1   Lateral radiograph of neck and cranial thorax of a dog with tracheal hypoplasia. The trachea is narrower than normal and this narrowing is accentuated by the broad cranial thorax and excessive skin folds at the thoracic inlet.

- weight loss,
- avoidance of excitement and excessively hot environments,
- support for co-existing cardiorespiratory problems such as chronic bronchitis and compensated heart failure,
- avoidance of smoky atmospheres.

Only if such tactics fail should surgical correction be considered (Table 42.1).

The fact that there are a diverse number of surgical techniques described for the correction of tracheal collapse stands testament to the failure, in many cases, of surgery to improve the animal's condition in the long term.

All the techniques in Table 42.1 have been used but it is essential to appreciate that both the cervical and thoracic portions of the trachea must be supported. However, the

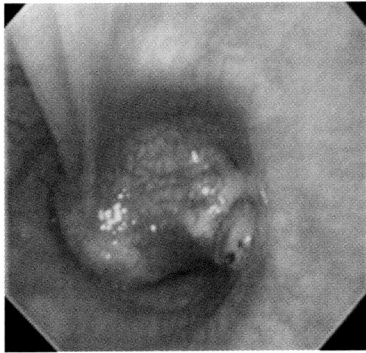

Fig. 42.2   Endoscopic view of a large osteochondroma that has grown into the lumen from a dorsolateral aspect and is compromising the airway. This was successfully removed. Tracheal neoplasia is very rare and can cause significant obstruction of the airflow.

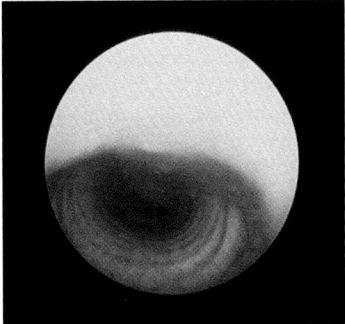

Fig. 42.3   Endoscopic view demonstrating marked collapse of the trachea. The dorsal membrane is widened and impinging on the lumen. The cartilages are flattened producing a D shape rather than a C shape.

Table 42.1   Surgical correction for tracheal collapse.

Technique	Comment
Dorsal plication	Pleats the stretched ligament, but does not address the underlying tracheal ring problem, so that over time the membrane stretches again
Intraluminal support	Causes erosion and ulceration of the mucous membrane
Ring support & dorsal plication	Plication prevents the membrane collapsing intra-luminally and by suturing incomplete plastic rings along the trachea the cartilaginous rings are supported
Extraluminal spiral prosthesis	Lack of published cases to support this procedure

area worst affected, at the thoracic inlet, is also the most difficult to approach. Unfortunately the animals in most need of surgery are those where the cartilage has become so affected that the cartilage is almost flat rather than being C-shaped. For these animals the prognosis is poor.

ACUTE TRACHEOBRONCHITIS (KENNEL COUGH) AND ACUTE BRONCHITIS
(SEE CHAPTER 12)

Acute tracheobronchitis is the most common cause of coughing in dogs, and is an enzootic condition in most countries (Hawkins *et al.* 1989). Transmission is by direct contact as aerosolised infective respiratory secretions, and via fomites and animal handlers and is increased where dogs congregate, such as in boarding kennels, dog rescue pounds, shows and training classes and veterinary surgery waiting rooms and kennel areas.

The aetiological agents implicated in kennel cough were discussed in Chapter 12. In brief, acute tracheobronchitis is an infectious and contagious disease, but a proportion of cases may be due to non-infectious causes.

- *Bordetella bronchiseptica.*
- Parainfluenza III virus, canine distemper virus, canine adenovirus II and canine herpes virus.
- Simultaneous infection with several agents is a possibility.
- Secondary bacterial and mycoplasma organisms can be implicated.
- The importance of environmental pollutants and allergens is unknown.

The key clinical features are:

- paroxysmal harsh nonproductive coughing;
- mild pyrexia, lethargy and inappetance, and naso-ocular discharge may be noted;
- clinical signs persist for up to 3 weeks;
- complications include purulent nasal discharge, bronchopneumonia, and gastrointestinal and neurological signs (suspect canine distemper).

The accurate diagnosis of *acute bronchitis* in the dog is problematic, in that acute inflammation of the bronchi could be a manifestation of a more readily identified disorder. For example, as part of acute tracheobronchitis, an active inflammatory component of chronic bronchitis, or in association with tracheal collapse, foreign body reactions, bronchopneumonia etc. Acute bronchitis probably does occur on its own in dogs, but in the majority of instances it presents as part of a more complex disease process. In uncomplicated cases it is probably indistinguishable from kennel cough.

The typical clinical presentation and history of contact support the diagnosis, and investigative procedures are rarely used to aid the diagnosis of kennel cough. In general the following points apply:

- The condition is self-limiting and antibacterial therapy is not necessarily required, although the tetracycline and potentiated sulphonamides are often effective.
- Anti-tussives, avoidance of dusty environments and restriction of exercise will alleviate excessive coughing.
- Keep affected dogs separate from susceptible animals.

Control and prevention of infection in dog kennels and pounds is difficult, and the expense involved may preclude control programmes. In the case of pet dogs some precautions can be taken but are not always effective.

- Vaccination against *Bordetella bronchiseptica* (intra-nasal) before anticipated challenge (e.g. boarding) will reduce the chances of infection.
- Vaccination against PI III, canine distemper and CAV II is now routine.
- Avoidance of enzootic areas is advised.

The prognosis for uncomplicated kennel cough is excellent, unless canine distemper virus is involved. In a small proportion of cases the tracheobronchitis will not resolve fully and as a result residual coughing may persist and present as a chronic management problem (see 'Chronic tracheobronchial syndrome' below).

CHRONIC TRACHEOBRONCHIAL SYNDROME

Chronic tracheobronchial syndrome is a sporadically occurring condition (Corcoran *et al.* 1992). The aetio-pathogenesis of this condition is not understood, but is usually a sequel to acute trachebronchitis (Hawkins *et al.* 1989).

The clinical signs usually appear several weeks after apparent resolution of acute tracheobronchitis.

- Paroxysms of harsh, non-productive cough are often associated with excitement and lead-pulling.

Table 42.2 Clinical investigations in chronic tracheobronchial syndrome.

Radiography	Usually demonstrates a mild to moderate increase in bronchial markings is noted in most cases
Bronchoscopy	Findings are normal in the majority of dogs
Bronchial cytology	Findings are normal in the majority of dogs

- No other clinical abnormalities are present in uncomplicated cases.
- In some cases persistence of the syndrome may precede development of chronic bronchitis.

The typical clinical presentation is usually diagnostic (Table 42.2) and is supported by the exclusion of all other possible causes. There is no recommended specific therapy and spontaneous resolution over a period of months may occur. The use of anti-tussives, a harness rather than a dog collar, and avoidance of dusty environments may help to ameliorate the clinical signs.

The prognosis for such cases is generally good but some dogs can continue to cough for several years. In others spontaneous resolution can occur, while in a small minority chronic bronchitis may develop (Corcoran *et al.* 1992).

CHRONIC BRONCHITIS

Chronic bronchitis is a mucus hypersecretory disorder affecting the trachea and bronchi (Wheeldon *et al.* 1974; Hawkins *et al.* 1989). The excessive mucus production is a reaction to airway inflammation and a cause of further bronchopulmonary problems, and is associated with increased epithelial goblet cell numbers and mucous gland hyperplasia.

Chronic bronchitis is primarily a condition of middle-aged to old dogs, and the incidence appears highest in small to medium sized dogs and in terrier breeds. The exact cause of chronic bronchitis in the dog is not known. The mucus hypersecretion, however, is inappropriate and causes further airway damage. The common aetiologies include:

- possible sequel to acute tracheobronchitis, acute bronchitis and chronic tracheobronchial syndrome (Brownlie 1990; Corcoran *et al.* 1992);
- recurrent or persistent airway damage by infections, airway irritants and inhaled allergens;

- complication of primary ciliary dyskinesia and acute and chronic bronchopneumonia;
- complication of anatomical airway abnormalities including brachycephalic airway syndrome, tracheal collapse and hypoplastic trachea.

If there is prolonged insult to the airways, the inflammatory reaction persists with irreparable damage to the airway mucosal surface (Wheeldon *et al.* 1974).

- squamous cell hyperplasia
- loss of ciliated epithelium
- deposition of fibrous tissue
- increased goblet cell numbers
- mucus glands hyperplasia
- smooth muscle hypertrophy

Excessive quantities of viscid mucus coats the mucosa and entraps debris, compromising airway hygiene, plugs smaller airways, and leaves the dog prone to recurrent bouts of bacterial bronchitis and bronchopneumonia. This causes irreversible damage to the lung with alveolar fibrosis and eventually results in respiratory failure.

Chronic bronchitis is an insidious and progressive disease with a wide range of clinical signs and degrees of severity, and can be complicated by secondary bacterial bronchopneumonia (Hawkins *et al.* 1989; Ford 1990). The signs include:

- coughing for at least 2 of the previous 12 months;
- quiescent periods punctuated by episodes of acute bronchopneumonia with pyrexia, inappetance and lethargy;
- tachypnoea, dyspnoea and exercise intolerance, depending on disease severity;
- general debility and cachexia develops over a prolonged period of time.

The clinical investigations in such cases are highlighted in Table 42.3.

Bronchoscopic demonstration of mucus hypersecretion is highly supportive of a diagnosis of chronic bronchitis, but confirmation is only possible on histopathology.

- Treatment of the underlying cause, if identified, should be attempted.
- Antibacterial therapy should be used to deal with acute bacterial bronchitis and bronchopneumonia episodes (with oxygen therapy and in-hospital nursing care).
- Combined bronchodilator and glucocorticosteroid therapy can be effective in controlling uncomplicated chronic bronchitis.
- Mucolytics, chest physiotherapy (four 10-min sessions of simple chest coupage sessions a day) and airway humidification can be beneficial.

Table 42.3　Clinical investigations in chronic bronchitis.

Chest auscultation	A wide range of respiratory sounds can be detected, including low pitched rhonchi, wheezes and crackles
Haematology	Polycythaemia in response to chronic hypoxaemia may be present
Radiography	Prominent bronchial pattern with discrete parallel bronchial markings, tortuous and twisted bronchi, and bronchial dilatation (bronchiectasis). Secondary lung (interstitial and alveolar changes) and cardiac (right-sided changes) may also be noted
Bronchoscopy (Fig. 42.4)	Marked airway changes with excessive quantities of airway mucus and roughened and nodular mucosal surface. Mucosal blanching may also be seen with indistinct mucosal vessels. Bronchoscopy is required for a definitive diagnosis to be made
Bronchial cytology	Excessive quantities of mucus, with a variable and mixed cellular component

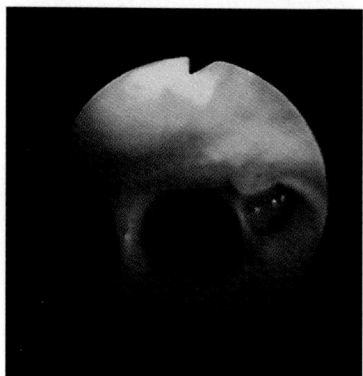

Fig. 42.4　Chronic bronchitis. Bronchoscopic image showing mucosal blanching and nodular changes on the mucosal surface.

● Anti-tussives are contra-indicated.
● Expectorant agents are of doubtful value.

The long-term prognosis is poor, as the condition is progressive and can result in terminal respiratory failure. In the short- to medium-term prognosis is good if there is a satisfactory response to therapy. Accurate diagnosis and appropriate therapy is the key to success.

BRONCHIECTASIS

This is a pathological dilatation of bronchi, with consequent entrapment of purulent material in the affected airway (Hawkins *et al.* 1989). It is often a sequel to chronic bronchitis, and will have similar clinical features. The dilated airway can be appreciated on radiography and confirmed by bronchoscopy. The presence of significant dilatation is a very poor prognostic sign.

CILIARY DYSKINESIA (IMMOTILE CILIA SYNDROME)

Primary ciliary dyskinesia is a rare inherited (autosomal recessive) condition characterised by abnormal development of ciliary ultrastructure (Hawkins *et al.* 1989; Vaden *et al.* 1991). A combination of situs inversus (complete transposition of the viscera), bronchiectasis (chronic bronchitis) and sinusitis (Kartagener's syndrome) can also be present. The consequences of ciliary dyskinesia are rhinitis, sinusitis, tracheobronchitis, chronic bronchitis and bronchiectasis. Thus the clinical signs can be complex and difficult to manage (Vaden *et al.* 1991).

AIRWAY PARASITES (PARASITIC TRACHEOBRONCHITIS)
(SEE CHAPTER 13)

Parasitic tracheobronchitis is caused by *Oslerus osleri* (formerly known as *Filaroides osleri*). The incidence appears to be low, but the prevalence of infection is not known. It is primarily a disease of kennelled dogs, such as Greyhounds and Foxhounds, but does occur in pet dogs (Brownlie 1990). Infection is by ingestion of larvae; the adult worms form nodules at the carina which cause a reac-

Table 42.4 Investigations in parasitic tracheobronchitis.

Haematology	Circulating eosinophilia may be present
Radiography	Reactive nodules might be seen at the carina
Bronchoscopy	Grey-brown to whitish reactive nodules visible at carina, with associated mucosal inflammatory reaction
Bronchial cytology (Fig. 42.5)	Adult worms, larvae and embryonated eggs, with a mixed inflammatory or eosinophil-rich reaction

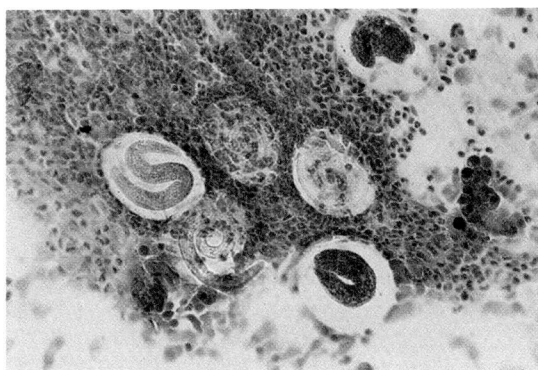

Fig. 42.5 *Oslerus osleri* infection. Haematoxalin and eosin stain of material collected by tracheal sampling from a dog with a chronic cough. There are several embryonated eggs and emerging *Oslerus osleri* larvae with attendant polymorphonuclear leucocyte inflammatory reaction.

tive tracheitis and bronchitis. Transmission is mainly from dam to offspring (sputum/saliva), with horizontal transmission by faecal contamination. Patent infection should develop within the first 2 years of life, and parasitic tracheobronchitis is rarely seen in dogs over 5 years of age.

The key clinical presentation includes:

- paroxysmal episodes of a harsh cough (similar to acute tracheobronchitis);
- dyspnoea if nodules are large;
- transient response to antibacterial or glucocorticosteroid therapy may occur, complicating diagnosis.

The clinical investigation is shown in Table 42.4.

The identification of adult, free larval or embryonated eggs in tracheobronchial samples is the most clear diagnosis as faecal samples can give false negative results. The management is centred around appropriate anthelmintic treatment and a complete cure should be achieved.

- Benzimidazole anthelmintics are effective (e.g. fenbendazole).
- Treat dam, siblings and close contacts.

AIRWAY FOREIGN BODIES

For respiratory disease caused by inhalation of food, fluid, gastric contents and liquid medications, see 'Pneumonia' page 368. This section deals with inhalation of discrete objects. The majority of incidents occur during exercise and inquisitive playing with small objects.

- Typical inhaled objects include grass seed heads (cereal heads), small twigs/sticks, small stones and other solid inanimate objects (Hawkins *et al.* 1989; Brownlie 1990).
- The majority pass the carina and lodge in the mainstem or lobar bronchi (Dobbie *et al.* 1986).
- Larger objects may get caught at the rima glottis or rostral to the carina, causing severe inspiratory airflow obstruction (Dobbie *et al.* 1986).

An inflammatory reaction develops in response to the presence of the foreign body:

- Marked mucopurulent reaction occurs in the vicinity of the foreign body.
- Chronic localised bronchial changes and localised bronchopneumonia can develop.
- Pleurisy and pyothorax can develop if it migrates.

The clinical features can be varied but include:

- acute onset of coughing, (sometimes with haemoptysis) that can be continuous, harsh and very distressing to the dog;
- the coughing becomes chronic and paroxysmal over subsequent days;
- pronounced halitosis will develop over the following weeks to months;
- signs of acute bronchopneumonia or pleural effusion in complicated cases.

The key diagnostic features are:

- typical history of acute onset coughing in typical circumstances (e.g. dog running through a wheat field),
- halitosis with chronic coughing,
- confirmed by bronchosocopy.

Table 42.5   Investigations of suspect tracheal or bronchial foreign body.

Radiography (Fig. 42.6a,b)	Radiodense objects are identified. Radiolucent foreign bodies (e.g. grass seed heads) will not be seen. A localised bronchial or interstitial reaction may develop close to the foreign body and an alveolar pattern if localised bronchopneumonia develops
Bronchoscopy (Fig. 42.7)	Allows identification, localisation and retrieval
Bronchial cytology	Mixed inflammatory cell population will be present

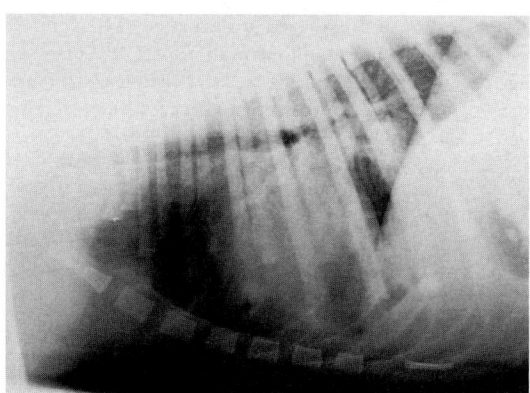

a

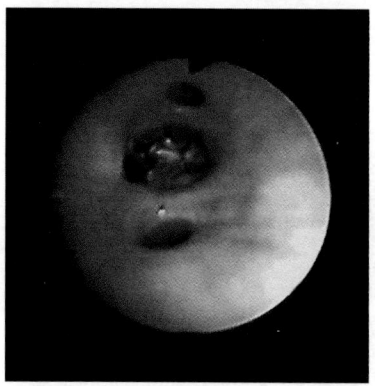

Fig. 42.7   Airway foreign body. Bronchoscopic image of a wheat head foreign body located in the right caudal lobe bronchus of a Springer Spaniel.

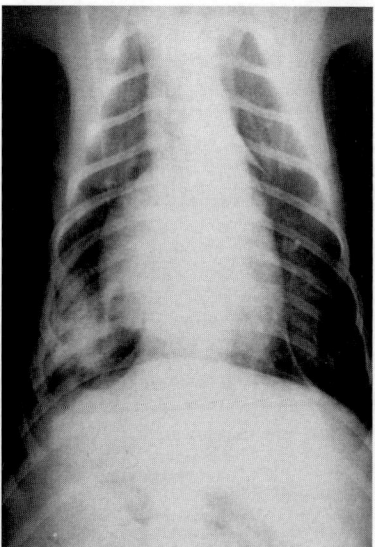

b

Fig. 42.6a,b   Foreign body bronchopneumonia in a 5-month- old Labrador. There is a discrete area of increased radiodensity in the right caudal lobe. This was associated with an inhaled grass seed head in the right caudal lobe bronchus.

It is essential to remove the foreign body.

- Retrieval by bronchoscopy is the preferred method.
- Failure to retrieve by bronchoscopy will necessitate thoracotomy and possibly lung lobectomy.
- Immediate intervention is required if there is significant airflow obstruction.
- Antibacterial and glucocorticosteroid therapy is used to counteract secondary infections and the inflammatory response.

The prognosis is good provided there has been no extension from the bronchial tree into the pleural space. Pleural contamination is a grave complication and has a guarded to grave prognosis. Fortunately this is uncommon and retrieval using bronchoscopy is usually successful at the first attempt. If thoracotomy and lobectomy are required, the patient recovery rate is very good.

REFERENCES

Bedford, P.G.C. (1982). Tracheal hypoplasia in the English bulldog. *Veterinary Record*, **110**, 58–59.

Brownlie, S.E. (1990). A retrospective study in 109 cases of diagnosis of canine lower respiratory disease. *Journal of Small Animal Practice*, **31**, 371–376.

Corcoran, B.M., Luis Fuentes, V. & Clarke, C.J. (1992). Chronic tracheobronchial syndrome in eight dogs. *The Veterinary Record*, **130**, 485–487.

Dobbie, G., Darke, P.G.G. & Head, K.W. (1986). Intrabronchial foreign bodies in dogs. *Journal of Small Animal Practice*, **27**, 227–238.

Ford, R.B. (1990). Chronic lung disease in old dogs and cats. *The Veterinary Record*, **126**, 399–402.

Hawkins, E.C., Ettinger, S.J. & Suter, P.F. (1989). Disease of the lower respiratory tract (lung) and pulmonary oedema. In: *Textbook of Veterinary Internal Medicine*, (ed. S.J. Ettinger), pp. 816–866. W.B. Saunders, Philadelphia.

Vaden, S.L., Breitschwerdt, E.B., Henrikson, C.K., Metcalf, C.K., Cohn, L. & Craig, W.A. (1991). Primary ciliary dyskinesia in Bichon Frise litter mates. *Journal of the American Animal Hospital Association*, **27**, 633–640.

Wheeldon, E.B., Pirie, H.M., Fisher, E.W. & Lee, R. (1974). Chronic bronchitis in the dog. *The Veterinary Record*, **94**, 466–471.

White, R.A.S. & Williams, J.M. (1994). Tracheal collapse in the dog – is there really a role for surgery? A survey of 100 cases. *Journal of Small Animal Practice*, **35**, 191–196.

Chapter 43

Lung Parenchymal Diseases

B. Corcoran

PNEUMONIA

Inflammatory diseases of the lung parenchyma including the interstitium, alveolar spaces and the smaller bronchi, bronchioles and respiratory bronchioles are grouped together as pneumonia (Thayer & Robinson 1983). Further classification of pneumonias can be based on:

- aetiology (e.g. aspiration),
- anatomy (e.g. lobar, bronchopneumonia),
- inflammatory cell type (e.g. eosinophilic).

Pneumonitis is synonymous with interstitial pneumonia, where there is little or no extension of the disease into the alveoli or lower airways.

Pneumonia is a complex inflammatory cellular reaction (Coogan & Carpenter 1989) with production of material that is removed either by rostral movement up the tracheobronchial tree where it is expectorated by coughing, or phagocytosed by alveolar macrophages in the lung periphery. If the system is overwhelmed, macrophages become sequestrated in the alveolar walls, resulting in fibroblast proliferation and loss of functional alveoli.

The aetiologies of pneumonia are outlined in Tables 43.1 and 43.2.

The clinical features can show marked variability in the clinical presentation, depending on the severity of the pathology and its extent, and the duration of clinical signs and the speed of their development (Thayer & Robinson 1983; Hawkins *et al.* 1989; Brownlie 1990).

- coughing which is usually soft and ineffectual;
- airway material can appear as a nasal discharge;
- varying degrees of tachypnoea, dyspnoea and exercise intolerance;
- pyrexia, lethargy and inappetance or anorexia with acute bronchopneumonia;

- debility and cachexia can occur with chronic pneumonia;
- cyanosis only occurs in very severe acute pneumonia, or if chronic recurrent pneumonia has destroyed large areas of functional lung;
- a history of dysphagia, regurgitation or vomiting (inhalation pneumonia) (Tams 1985; Hawkins *et al.* 1989).

Diagnosis and Management

Diagnosis is made on the basis of the clinical, radiographic and bronchoscopic features (Thayer & Robinson 1983). The approach to management depends on (1) the primary problem and (2) the severity of clinical signs. With a localised lobar bronchopneumonia there is little danger to the patient, while acute bronchopneumonia with diffuse pathology is potentially fatal.

- Deal with the primary problem.
- Intensive antibacterial therapy (preferably based on culture and sensitivity testing) is used and continued for 3 weeks after resolution.
- *Tetracyclines, potentiated sulphonamides, fluoroquinolones, clavulanate-potentiated amoxycillin* and the *cephalosporins* are usually effective.
- Bronchodilator therapy is of questionable value.
- Anti-tussives are contraindicated.
- Mucolysis using nebulised solutions and steam vapour can be useful, but simple chest physiotherapy is often as effective. The use of mucolytic agents can give variable results.
- Flunixin meglumine may be beneficial in peracute bronchopneumonia.
- Glucocorticoids are the drugs of choice in treating eosinophilic pneumonia.
- Hospitalisation, supplemental oxygen and good nursing care, are required for acute bronchopneumonia cases.

Table 43.1 Infectious agents implicated in pneumonia.

Primary viral
  Canine distemper virus
  Canine adenovirus II
  Parainfluenza III
Primary bacterial
  Bordetella bronchiseptica
  β-haemolytic streptococci.
Secondary bacterial
  Pasteurella
  Klebsiella
  Proteus
  Escherichia coli
  Actinomyces and *Nocardia* spp.
Mycoplasma spp.
Fungi (histoplasmosis and blastomycosis in enzootic
  areas).

Table 43.2 Non-infectious causes of bronchopneumonia (result in significant secondary bacterial infection).

Inhaled foreign material
  Pharyngeal, laryngeal, oesophageal disorders
  Iatrogenic (administration of medications)
  Discrete foreign bodies
Inhaled allergens (pulmonary infiltration with eosinophilia (PIE))
Parasitic diseases
  Migrating ascarid larvae
  Oslerus osleri
  Crenosoma vulpis
Systemic illnesses (pneumonitis)
  Toxaemia
  Uraemic pneumonitis
  Septicaemia
Other respiratory diseases (predisposing to bronchopneumonia)
  Primary ciliary dyskinesia
  Chronic bronchitis
  Chronic pulmonary interstitial disease

The prognosis for most forms of pneumonia is good if the underlying cause can be corrected, intervention is rapid with vigorous therapy, and therapy is continued for a sufficient period of time.

SMOKE INHALATION

It should be presumed that any dog rescued from a house fire has been affected (Tams 1985). The products of combustion are toxic causing severe bronchitis and bronchopneumonia. In addition to the toxic effect severe thermal injury can occur. Laryngospasm and bronchospasm cause severe dyspnoea, choking and coughing. Airway wall oedema and epithelial necrosis predispose to further respiratory embarrassment and respiratory infections.

Carbon monoxide toxicity (>10% in inspired air) is a common feature and characterised by:

- cherry-red mucosa;
- tachypnoea and dyspnoea, after mild exertion, can occur with low CO concentrations;

Table 43.3 Investigation in cases of pnuemonia.

Haematology	Leucocytosis with a neutrophilia and left shift in acute bacterial bronchopneumonia
Radiography (Figs 43.1 and 43.2)	Radiographic changes tend to lag behind the clinical development and progression of the disease. Alveolar patterns with air bronchograms (bronchopneumonia). Interstitial pattern (PIE, aspiration pneumonia (dependent lung areas)). Mixed bronchial, interstitial and alveolar patterns.
Bronchoscopy (Fig. 43.3)	Mucopurulent material is present in the airways, without evidence of chronic airway mucosal changes
Bronchial cytology	Variable number of leucocytes and macrophages. Large numbers of eosinophils support a diagnosis of eosinophilic pneumonia (PIE). Pathogenic organisms should be isolated from the airway sample.

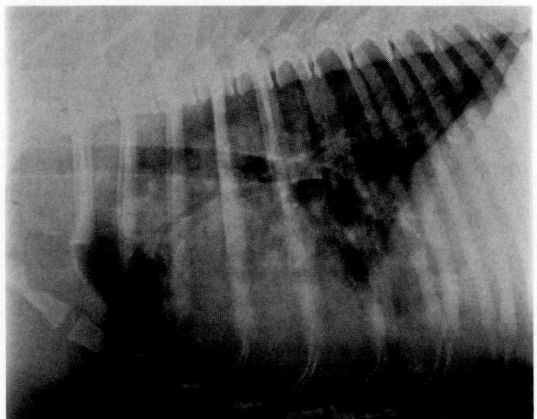

a

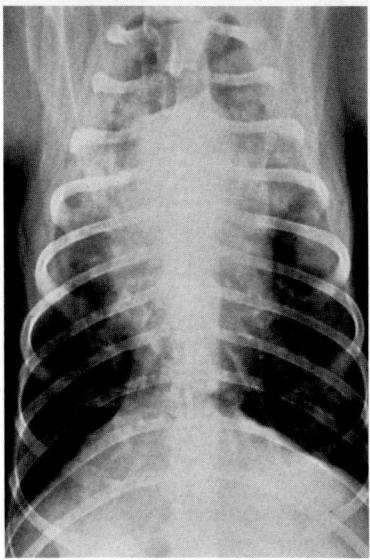

b

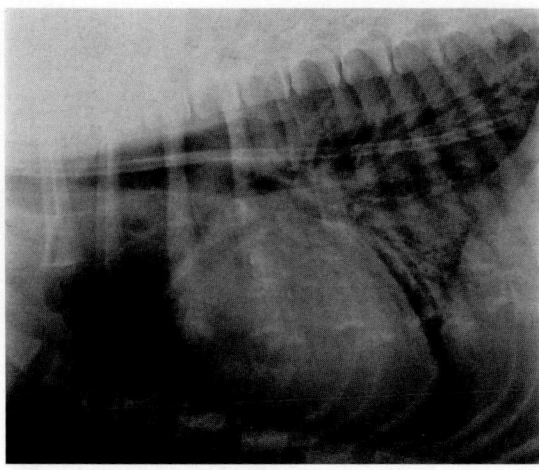

a

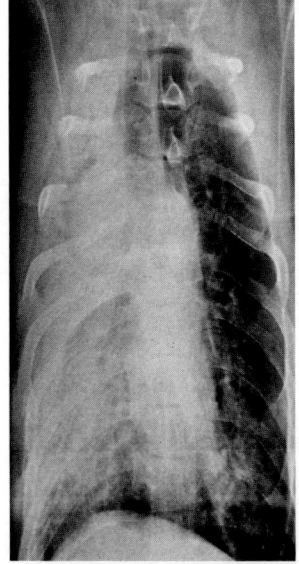

b

Fig. 43.1a,b Bronchopneumonia in a 3-year-old Border Collie. There is a generalised alveolar pattern in the cranial and middle lung lobes with distinct air bronchograms visible on the lateral view. These are radiographic changes typically associated with bacterial bronchopneumonia. This dog recovered completely after antibacterial therapy. The distribution of the changes is also typical of aspiration pneumonia (with permission A. French).

Fig. 43.2a,b Bronchopneumonia in a 7-month-old Irish Wolfhound. There is extensive lung consolidation on the right side of the chest with distinctive air bronchograms. This dog had recurrent bacterial pneumonia and required intermittent antibiotic therapy.

- vomiting, confusional states, ataxia, convulsions and coma occur at higher concentration.

Note: The major concern in the first 24 h is CO toxicity. Pathological changes are important after 24 h.

Radiography, bronchoscopy and bronchial sampling are used to investigate airway and lung inflammation, but are rarely of use in the first 24 h. Blood gas analysis is key as it confirms:

- carboxyhaemoglobinaemia,
- arterial hypoxaemia and hypercapnia.

Note: The half-life COHb is 4 h when breathing room air and 30 min when breathing 100% oxygen.

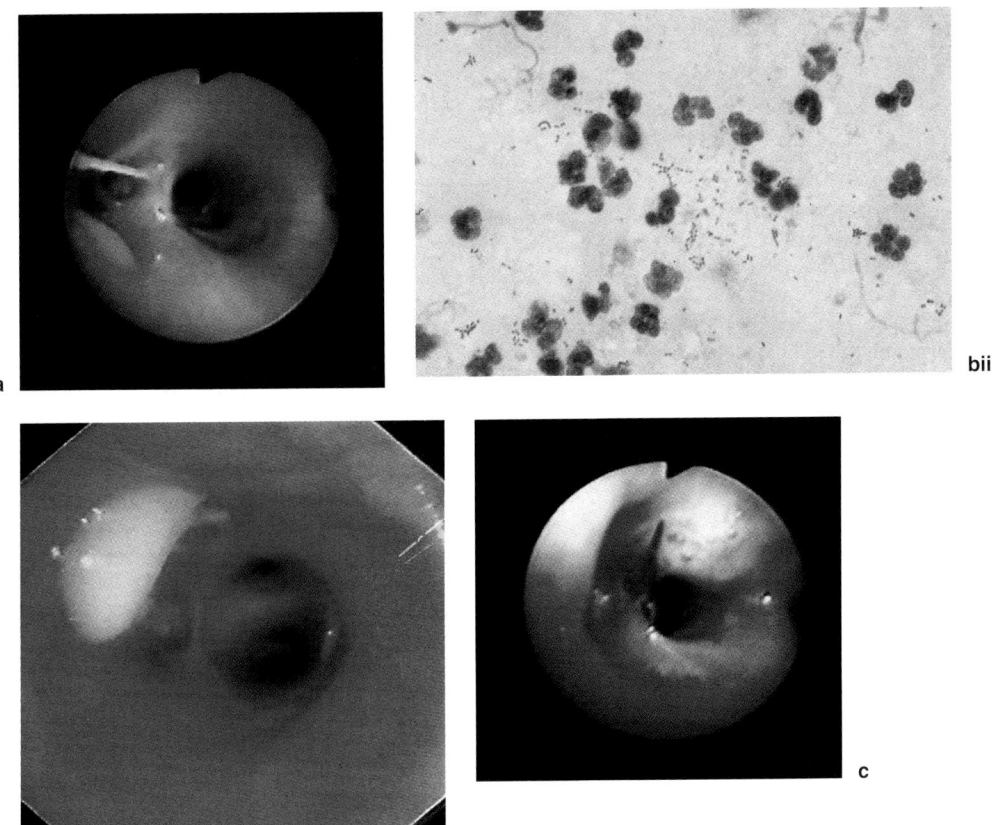

a

bii

bi

c

Fig. 43.3 Bronchopneumonia bronchoscopic images. (a) Mucopurulent material can be seen exiting a bronchus. The airway mucosa appears normal and the material was found to be eosinophil-rich. (b) Mucopurulent material in a dog with lobar pneumonia (i). The material is exiting the right middle lobe bronchus, and contains polymorphonuclear leucocytes and coccal bacteria (ii). (c) Foreign body reaction in the right mainstem bronchus. The associated radiographic changes are shown in Fig. 42.6.

Diagnosis and Management

A dog is assumed to have smoke inhalation injury if it has been rescued from a house fire, has evidence of burn injuries or has cherry red mucous membranes (CO toxicity). It is essential to reverse the carboxyhaemoglobinaemia and hypoxia and manage airway and lung inflammation.

- 100% oxygen is used to speed up the removal of COHb and reverse hypoxaemia.
- Intravenous fluids are used to maintain cardiac output.
- Antibacterial agents are given for secondary bacterial infections.
- Bronchodilators may be beneficial in countering reflex bronchoconstriction.
- Glucocorticoids might actually increase morbidity and mortality.
- Intermittent or continuous positive pressure ventilation is applied, particularly if there is severe laryngeal damage.

The prognosis for smoke inhalation injury varies, but there is poor survival if bronchopneumonia develops or body surface burns have occurred (Hawkins *et al.* 1989).

PULMONARY INFILTRATION WITH EOSINOPHILIA

Pulmonary infiltration with eosinophilia (PIE) is a group of diseases in which the eosinophil is the predominant cell type found in bronchial washes (Corcoran *et al*. 1991). The forms in which PIE presents are difficult to distinguish from acute tracheobronchitis, chronic tracheobronchial syndrome, chronic bronchitis and pneumonia. However, there are clinical features specific to the PIE diseases. The precise aetiology remians unresolved but includes:

- a hypersensitivity reaction to inhaled allergens or migrating ascarid parasites;
- airway eosinophilia is also noted with respiratory and cardiac parasitic infections.

The clinical features of pulmonary eosinophilic infiltrate are comparable to acute tracheobronchitis, chronic tracheobronchial syndrome, chronic bronchitis and pneumonia:

- coughing is seen in the majority of cases;
- tachypnoea and dyspnoea, and exercise intolerance, with severe lung inflammation;
- concurrent cutaneous signs typical of canine atopic dermatitis in a minority of cases;
- cases are usually otherwise clinically normal.

Treatment with glucocorticoids is usually effective, and an appropriate response supports the diagnosis.

- Intravenous methyl prednisolone succinate is used in severe acute cases.

- Oral prednisolone, reducing to the lowest possible dose that controls symptoms, is used on an alternate day therapy regime.
- Some individuals may require continuous therapy.

The prognosis with PIE is excellent although continuous therapy may be required in some dogs. Pulmonary eosinophilic granulomatosis (often associated with *Dirofilaria immitis* in enzootic areas) may show a transient improvement, but becomes refractory to therapy.

NON-CARDIOGENIC PULMONARY OEDEMA

Cardiac diseases are the most common cause of pulmonary oedema and the reader is referred to Chapters 45–47 for more detailed discussion. However, non-cardiogenic causes of pulmonary oedema occur, but the incidence is not well documented (Kerr 1989).

The majority of cases of non-cardiogenic pulmonary oedema are due to altered vascular permeability, and not elevated pulmonary venous capillary pressures (Hawkins *et al*. 1989). The aetiologies include:

- pulmonary vascular damage (toxins, such as paraquat, organophosphates, ANTU (alpha-naphthylurea), and multi-systemic inflammatory diseases, toxaemia and septicaemia (shock-lung syndrome));
- electrocution and neurogenic oedema secondary to cranial trauma and convulsions;
- hypoproteinaemia (reduced plasma oncotic pressures);
- acute upper airway obstruction (increased negative pleural pressures).

Haematology	A mild to marked circulating eosinophilia may be present (1.5 to 50.0 × 10⁹ cell/1) in some cases (Hawkins *et al*. 1989; Corcoran *et al*. 1991). The presence of a circulating basophilia is probably more significant
Radiography	A diffuse increase in interstitial and bronchial markings is often found with PIE (Hawkins *et al*. 1989), although other changes (such as alveolar patterns) may also be noted (Corcoran *et al*. 1991)
Bronchial cytology	The predominance of eosinophils in samples is diagnostic, providing parasitism is excluded
Transthoracic needle biopsy	Can yield diagnostically useful material in PIE (Teske *et al*. 1991)

Table 43.4 Investigations in pulmonary eosinophilic disease.

The clinical signs are similar to cardiogenic pulmonary oedema:

- respiratory impairment;
- coughing and expectoration of pink-tinged frothy fluid, varying degrees of exercise intolerance, tachypnoea, dyspnoea and cyanosis;
- crackles can be heard on auscultation;
- evidence of the underlying cause (see above).

The biochemical changes are attributable to systemic illness and radiographic examination of the lungs shows diffuse alveolar or interstitial pattern, without evidence of pulmonary vascular engorgement or left atrial enlargement.

Non-cardiogenic pulmonary oedema will resolve spontaneously if the underlying cause is corrected and the patient can be adequately supported in the meanwhile by:

- oxygen supplementation, cage rest and good nursing care advisable;
- frusemide, venodilators and anti-inflammatory agents are ineffective;
- fluid therapy to reverse dehydration and excessive fluid loss and plasma or synthetic colloids to improve oncotic pressure;
- surgical correction of upper airway obstruction.

The prognosis depends on the underlying cause, and if this cannot be controlled, the outcome is grave.

CHRONIC PULMONARY INTERSTITIAL DISEASE (FIBROSIS)

Chronic pulmonary interstitial disease is a poorly understood condition characterised by chronic coughing, dyspnoea and exercise intolerance. Increased interstitial changes are seen on chest radiographs, caused by interstitial fibrosis. It is a commonly recognised chronic disease of terrier breeds, and in particular the West Highland White Terrier,

and may be similar to *idiopathic pulmonary fibrosis* in man (Coogan & Carpenter 1989).

The condition is seen mainly in terrier breeds, particularly the West Highland White and Cairn Terrier, but can also occur in other small to medium sized dogs. The aetiology is not known, but the radiographic changes of an increased interstitial pattern may be secondary to underlying chronic respiratory disease:

- secondary to chronic bronchitis and bronchopneumonia;
- idiopathic (possibly immune-mediated) in terrier breeds;
- toxins, such as paraquat and other unidentified environmental pollutants (Darke *et al.* 1977; O'Sullivan 1989);
- a normal ageing change in the lungs of older dogs;
- chronic low-grade respiratory viral infections;
- endocrinopathies such as hyperadrenocorticalism, and obesity, may complicate the clinical picture, and result in apparent increased interstitial density (Crawford *et al.* 1986).

Fibroblast proliferation occurs in the alveolar walls, with replacement of the alveolar architecture by fibrous tissue (Coogan & Carpenter 1989). The resultant loss of functional alveolar tissue explains the clinical features of this condition.

There is marked variability in the severity of clinical signs.

- Onset is gradual and progressive deterioration occurs over a period of months to years.
- Coughing is usually present.
- Tachypnoea, dyspnoea and exercise intolerance are found in most cases.
- Cyanosis occurs in the terminal stages.
- Marked crackles are audible on chest auscultation.

Diagnosis and Management

Diagnosis of chronic pulmonary interstitial disease is difficult and tends to be made on the basis of exclusion of all other possible conditions:

Table 43.5   Investigations in cases of chronic pulmonary fibrosis.

Radiography (Fig. 43.4)	Generalised and diffuse increase in interstitial density, correlating with the degree of respiratory impairment
Bronchoscopy	Dynamic end-expiratory collapse of lobar bronchi may be seen
Bronchial cytology	Non-specific inflammatory reaction

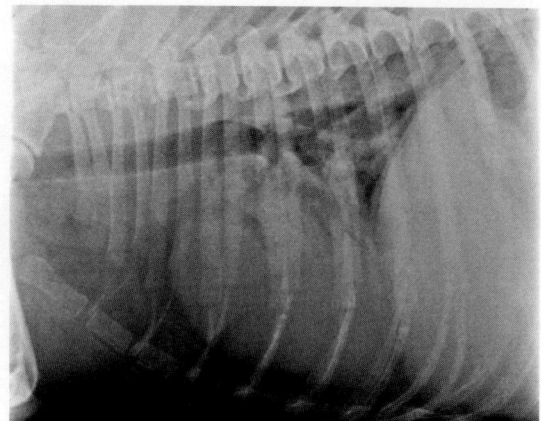

a

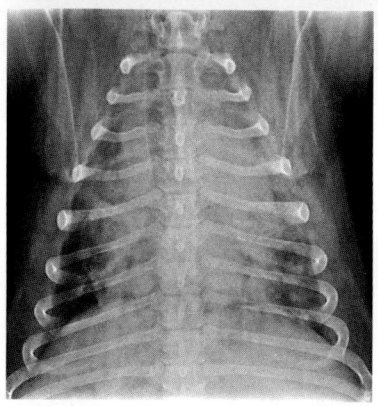

b

Fig. 43.4a,b Chronic pulmonary interstitial disease (fibrosis) in an 11-year-old West Highland White Terrier. There is an overall increase in radiodensity in the entire lung field, partially obscuring the cardiac silhouette. The pattern is mixed with diffuse interstitial and some alveolar changes.

- susceptible breeds with marked crackles on chest auscultation;
- radiographic evidence of increased interstitial pattern;
- dynamic collapse of airways visible on bronchoscopy.

The condition is irreversible and progressive. Reliance on long-term glucocorticoid therapy is standard practice in both humans and dogs.

- Alternate day glucocorticoid therapy is used, although there can be marked variability in the individual response.
- Some dogs seem to benefit from additional bronchodilator therapy.
- Antibacterial therapy may be required if there are complications of bronchitis or bronchopneumonia.

The prognosis is guarded as the lung changes are permanent and the disease appears to be progressive.

PULMONARY NEOPLASIA

The incidence of (detected) pulmonary neoplasia is low (Mehlhaff & Mooney 1985), but in the author's experience, it appears to be highest in large breeds. The majority of primary neoplasms are of epithelial origin (adenocarcinomas), while the lung is the major metastatic site for malignant neoplasms elsewhere in the body (Miles 1988; Hawkins *et al*. 1989).

Neoplastic tissue results in destruction and loss of functional lung tissue. Most neoplasms cause coughing by compression of adjacent bronchi, and minimal inflammatory reaction occurs in the airways themselves. Vessel erosion by the mass will, however, cause bleeding into the airway and lung. Paraneoplastic changes, such as debility and cachexia and hypertrophic pulmonary osteoarthropathy occur.

The appearance and severity of clinical signs depends on the stage of the disease (Mehlhaff & Mooney 1985).

- Dogs are usually over 5 years of age.
- Coughing is a common finding with primary neoplasms (Miles 1988), with expectoration of blood in some cases, but is not consistently found with metastatic disease.
- Tachypnoea, dyspnoea and exercise intolerance suggest advanced disease and are poor prognostic signs.
- Expiratory dyspnoea can be a particularly useful finding, suggesting a mass is compressing a large airway.
- Debility, cachexia and inappetance are paraneoplastic signs suggestive of advanced disease.
- Hypertrophic pulmonary osteoarthropathy (Marie's disease) with limb pain is seen in a minority of cases.
- Rarely the lung primary tumour metastasises to other organs in the body with associated clinical signs.

Diagnosis and Management

Pulmonary neoplasia should be suspected in middle-aged to old dogs presenting with chronic cough and progressive deterioration. The diagnosis is confirmed by collecting neoplastic material from bronchial washes or biopsy samples (Mehlhaff & Mooney 1985; Miles 1988).

Pulmonary neoplasia is usually diagnosed in an advanced stage and lung lobectomy can be attempted if the mass is localised to single lobes, and may give survival of 12–18 months in exceptional cases (Miles 1988). The scope

Table 43.6 Investigations in cases of pulmonary neoplasia

Biochemistry	Paraneoplastic changes, such as hypercalcaemia, may be present
Radiography (Fig. 43.5)	It is important to take both a right and left lateral radiograph. Well delineated consolidated masses, lung lobe consolidation and hilar and sternal lymphadenopathy are often found. However, diffuse interstitial and alveolar changes with air bronchograms can also be seen
Bronchoscopy (Fig. 43.6)	Blood-tinged mucus and dynamic collapse of major airways on expiration is often seen. A tumour may distort the shape of adjacent airway walls
Bronchial cytology	Neoplastic cells can be found in a significant number of cases
Thoracocentesis	Transthoracic needle sampling of a mass will allow diagnosis, but is not successful in all instances (Teske *et al.* 1991).

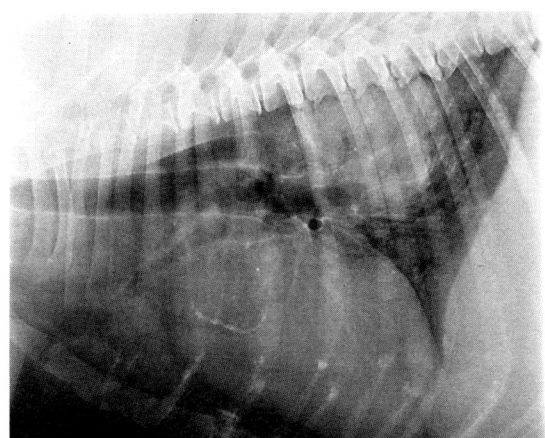

a

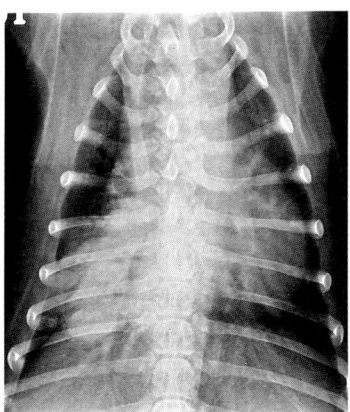

b

Fig. 43.5a,b Primary pulmonary neoplasia in an 11-year-old Golden Retriever. There is a well-defined large mass in the right caudal lobe and several smaller masses in the cranial lung fields.

for chemotherapy is limited, although glucocorticoids can alleviate clinical signs for several weeks to months (Miles 1988). Therapy for metastatic pulmonary neoplasia is not currently feasible.

The prognosis for well defined lobar neoplasia can be fair if adequate surgery can be performed. This form is eventual terminal but lacks the aggressive nature of the human equivalent. Metastatic spread is presumed to have occurred by the time a diagnosis is made. Amelioration of the symptoms can be achieved for weeks to months, but if metastatic disease is present at the time of diagnosis the survival time is usually short.

PULMONARY THROMBOEMBOLISM

The incidence of pulmonary thromboembolism is not known and it is rarely diagnosed. It is characterised by acute onset tachypnoea/dyspnoea and is predisposed to by the following conditions (Hawkins *et al.* 1989):

- trauma and surgery,
- sepsis and disseminated intravascular coagulation,
- haemolytic anaemia,
- hyperadrenocorticalism and hypothyroidism,
- glomerulonephropathy,
- heart worm infection,
- hypoalbuminaemia.

Radiography findings can include no discernible change (despite profound respiratory signs), hyperlucent areas in the lung that have lost their vascular markings and consolidated areas with air bronchograms, similar to pneumonia or neoplasia. Blunted pulmonary arteries may be visible.

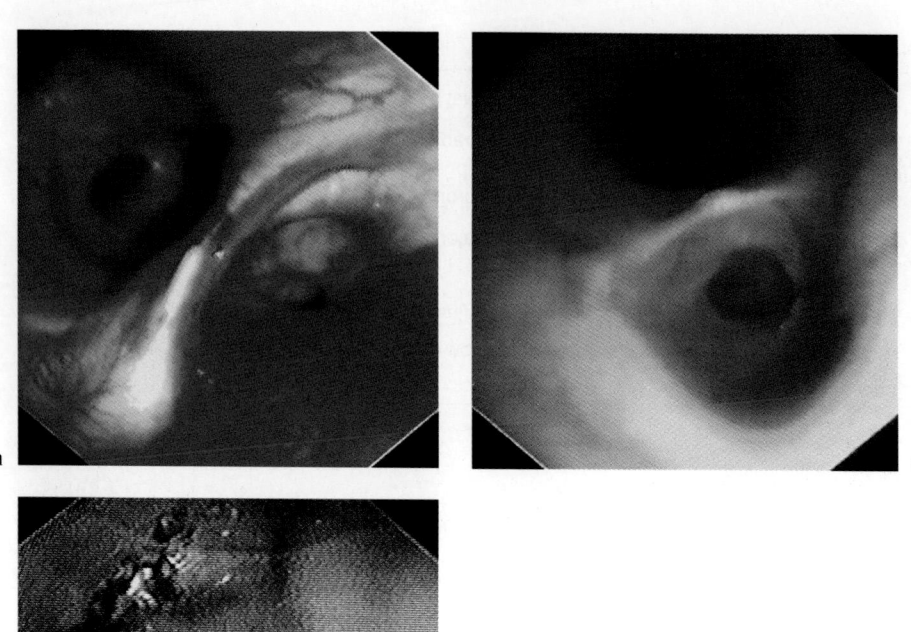

Fig. 43.6 Pulmonary neoplasia bronchoscopic images.
(a) Bronchoscopic image from a 10-year-old Dobermann with a right-middle lung lobe mass. A large pool of blood-tinged material can be seen in the airway on the right of the image, but the airway mucosa is normal. (b) This dog had a neoplasm confined to the accessory lobe. There is distortion of the airway wall such that it is significantly occluding the bronchial lumen. (c) This bronchoscopic image appears relatively normal, but on closer inspection significant narrowing of the lumen of the lower airway can be appreciated. The radiographs for this dog are shown in Fig. 43.5.

Diagnosis and Management

The clinical features centre around an acute respiratory embarrassment usually associated with a concurrent disease process as listed above. The common feature of these conditions is a failure in the homeostasis of the haemostatic mechanisms due to consumption (DIC, heart worm), loss (glomerulonephropathy) or failure to function (hypothyroidism). The prognosis in these cases is very guarded and the management involves managing the crisis while the underlying disease is being controlled. Managing the crisis alone is in itself insufficient.

- Improve oxygen tension as far as possible with oxygen supplementation.
- High dose glucocorticoid therapy is used to control lung tissue damage.

- Heparinisation and warfarin therapy are used if a hypercoagulopathy disorder is suspected.
- Surgical removal of the thrombus is not feasible.
- Antibacterial cover is given to protect against secondary bacterial infections.

PULMONARY CAVITARY LESIONS

Cavitary lesions in the lung are rare, usually found incidentally at post-mortem and only occasionally cause clinical problems. The main types of cavitary lesions are cysts, bullae, sub-pleural blebs, abscesses, pneumatocoeles, parasitic cysts and cystic bronchiectasis (see 'Bronchiectasis' and 'Chronic bronchitis' in Chapter 42).

EMPHYSEMA

Similarly to the cavitary lesions, emphysema is found mainly as an incidental finding on post-mortem and rarely causes clinical signs. Rare instances of lobar and bullous congenital forms have been reported. If clinically significant emphysema occurs the major clinical findings are end-expiratory dyspnoea and pronounced inspiratory crackles.

THORACIC TRAUMA AND PULMONARY CONTUSION

These conditions are grouped together as thoracic trauma is often the underlying cause, although there are non-traumatic causes which should be considered. More likely than not, a trauma patient will present with two or more of these problems. Damage to other body organs should also be suspected in trauma cases.

The majority of thoracic trauma cases are the result of road-traffic accidents. Flail chest segments are more obvious in young dogs where the costochondral junctions are not calcified. Diagnosis is usually achieved with thoracic radiography.

Chest wall injuries are invariably a result of direct trauma:

- *fractured ribs* and *flail segments* with paradoxical chest wall motion during inspiration;
- *penetrating wounds* resulting in *pneumothorax*;
- results in respiratory distress due to pain and compromised lung expansion (pneumothorax);
- control of pain is often the only effective means of treatment of such injuries, but restrictive bandaging of the rib cage is not advised.

INTRA-PULMONARY HAEMORRHAGE

Intra-pulmonary haemorrhage can be caused by *trauma*, *ingestion of coumarin-based rodenticides* and *coagulopathies*.

- Clinical presentation depends on the severity of haemorrhage into the lung.

- Coughing, with possible expectoration of blood tinged mucus might be present.
- Tachypnoea, dyspnoea and exercise intolerance appears if there is severe haemorrhage.
- Other evidence of trauma and bleeding elsewhere in the body may be apparent (see Chapter 36).
- On radiography there can be increased interstitial and alveolar densities, with air bronchograms, indistinguishable from most types of pneumonia.
- Haematology profiles may be normal unless there has been severe blood loss. Coagulation profiles should be performed.
- Blood tinged material might be visible on bronchoscopy.
- Therapy includes whole blood transfusion, plasma volume expanders or plasma to treat clotting disorders, vitamin K_1 analogues for warfarin poisoning, and cage rest with oxygen therapy.

REFERENCES

Brownlie, S.E. (1990). A retrospective study of diagnosis of canine lower respiratory disease. *Journal of Small Animal Practice*, **31**, 371–376.

Coogan, D.C. & Carpenter, J.L. (1989). Diffuse alveolar injury in two dogs. *Journal of the Veterinary Medical Association*, **194**, 527–530.

Corcoran, B.M., Thoday, K.L., Henfrey, J.I., Simpson, J.W., Burnie, A.G. & Mooney, C.T. (1991). Pulmonary infiltration with eosinophils in 14 dogs. *Journal of Small Animal Practice*, **32**, 494–502.

Crawford, M.A., Robertson, S. & Miller, R. (1986). Pulmonary complications of Cushing's syndrome: metastatic mineralization in a dog with high-dose chronic corticosteroid therapy. *Journal of the American Animal Hospital Association*, **23**, 85–87.

Darke, P.G.G., Gibbs, C., Kelly, D.F., Morgan, D.G., Pearson, H. & Weaver, B.M.Q. (1977). Acute respiratory distress in the dog associated with paraquat poisoning. *The Veterinary Record*, **100**, 275–277.

Hawkins, E.C., Ettinger, S.J. & Suter, P.F. (1989). Disease of the lower respiratory tract (lung) and pulmonary oedema. In: *Textbook of Veterinary Internal Medicine*, (ed. S.J. Ettinger), pp. 816–866. W.B. Saunders, Philadelphia.

Kerr, L.Y. (1989). Pulmonary edema secondary to upper airway obstruction in the dog: a review of nine cases. *Journal of the American Animal Hospital Association*, **25**, 207–211.

Mehlhaff, C.J. & Mooney, S. (1985). Primary pulmonary neoplasia in the dog and cat. *Veterinary Clinics of North America: Small Animal Practice*, **15**, 1061–1068.

Miles, K.G. (1988). A review of primary lung tumours in the dog and cat. *Veterinary Radiology*, **29**, 122–128.

O'Sullivan, S.P. (1989). Paraquat poisoning in the dog. *Journal of Small Animal Practice*, **30**, 361–364.

Schaer, M., Gamble, D. & Spencer, C. (1981). Spontaneous pneumothorax associated with bacterial pneumonia in the dog-two case reports. *Journal of the American Animal Hospital Association*, **17**, 783–788.

Tams, T.R. (1985). Aspiration pneumonia and complications of inhalation of smoke and toxic gases. *Veterinary Clinics of North America*, **15**, 971–989.

Teske, E., Stokhof, A.A., Van Den Ingh, T.S.G.A.M., Wolvekamp, W.Th.C., Slappendel, R.J. & deVries, H.W. (1991). Transthoracic needle aspiration biopsy of lung in dogs with pulmonic diseases. *Journal of the American Animal Hospital Association*, **27**, 289–294.

Thayer, G.W. & Robinson, S.K. (1983). Bacterial bronchopneumonia in the dog: a review of 42 cases. *Journal of the American Animal Hospital Association*, **20**, 731–735.

Chapter 44

Pleural and Mediastinal Diseases

B. Corcoran

The major condition affecting the pleural space is pleural effusion (Suter & Zinkl 1982; Noone 1985; Forrester *et al.* 1988), and in general primary pleural diseases are relatively rare.

Additional information on the aetiopathogenesis of diseases that cause pleural effusion is available in the chapters covering cardiac, hepatic and gastrointestinal diseases.

PLEURITIS

Primary inflammation of the visceral and parietal pleurae is rare and pleuritis (*dry pleuritis, fibrinous pleuritis, pleural thickening, pleural adhesions*) in the dog is usually associated with lung parenchymal disease (pleuropneumonia) or is a consequence of a pleural effusion. This usually results in pleural scarring, with well defined pleural lines or scalloping of the lung lobe borders being visible on thoracic radiographs (Suter & Zinkl 1982).

PLEURAL EFFUSIONS

The incidence of the different pleural effusions is not known, but they constitute an important category of diseases causing respiratory impairment (Noone 1985; Forrester 1990). There are several different types of effusion (Noone 1985) and the features of each effusion are outlined in Table 44.1. Pneumothorax and haemorrhage into the pleural space will also cause respiratory symptoms similar to pleural effusion (see 'Thoracic trauma' in Chapter 43). Five types of effusion are recognised as shown in Table 44.1 and the distinguishing features are indicated in Table 44.2.

It should be noted that different effusion types can be caused by the same disease processes. As an example, neoplastic diseases can cause transudates, exudates and chylous effusions.

Clinical Features

The clinical features all relate to two components. First, a decreased pleural space and the impact that has on the functional lung volume. Second, the pleural fluid has a dramatic effect upon cardiac function due to compression of major vascular intrathoracic structures and intrapleural vascular beds. The end result is:

- Restriction of lung expansion resulting in varying degrees of tachypnoea, dyspnoea and exercise intolerance (Forrester *et al.* 1988).
- With severe effusions, cyanosis, either at rest or after mild exertion, may develop.
- Debility and cachexia develops with long-standing pleural effusion due to increased work of breathing and chronic loss of proteins lipids.
- Pyrexia may be present with pyothorax.
- Muffling of respiratory and cardiac sounds occurs, and alteration in chest percussion.
- Abdominal distension with ascites is present, or the abdomen may feel empty with diaphragmatic hernia.

Diagnosis and Management

Radiography will allow identification of an effusion. Identification of the underlying cause can be difficult. For specific types of effusion, therapy is usually directed at the underlying cause (Noone 1985), but for dogs presenting with severe respiratory distress a standard approach to therapy applies irrespective of the effusion type.

Management of Pleural Effusion Causing Severe Respiratory Distress

- On initial presentation avoid unnecessary excitement and provide supplemental oxygen if tolerated (e.g.

Table 44.1   Types of Pleural Effusion.

True transudate	Translucent, colourless, serous effusion, mainly caused by hypoalbuminaemia and congestive heart failure
Modified transudate	True transudates become modified (increased cell numbers and protein content) the longer they are in the pleural space. In addition to cardiac disease and hypoalbuminaemia, obstruction of lymphatic drainage secondary to inflammatory reactions, neoplasia and herniation of abdominal contents can cause this type of effusion
Exudate	These arise either because of infections (pyothorax) or as a cellular reaction to destructive inflammatory disease such as neoplasia
Chyle	This is a milky-white, lymphocyte and lipid-rich effusion that leaks from lymphatics (thoracic duct). Chylothorax can result from trauma, neoplasia, infectious and right heart failure, although idiopathic and congenital forms are also recognised
Pseudochylous effusion	This is differentiated from true chyle by having fewer lymphocytes, and not staining with Sudan III or clearing with ether. However, there is increasing opinion that use of the term pseudochyle should be discontinued, and the term *chylous* used to describe all types of milky-white effusions

Table 44.2   Differentiation of effusion types.

Effusion type	Specific gravity	Protein content (g/l)	Cell count (µl)	Triglyceride levels (mg/ml)	C:T ratio	Lipid content	Colour and opacity
Transudate	<1.018	<25	<500	<1.0	>2.0	Low	Pale yellow, clear
Modified transudate	>1.018	>25	>200	<1.0	>2.0	Low	Yellow/pink, translucent
Exudate	High	>30	>2000	<1.0	>2.0	Moderate	Yellow, opaque
Chyle	High	>25	>400	≥1.0	<1.0	Very high	White/pink, opaque

C:T ratio, cholesterol:triglyceride ratio

face-mask). Over-zealous investigation of a dog with severe respiratory distress can be fatal.

- Only perform thoracic radiography if it is safe to do so. The objective of radiography at this stage is to confirm the presence of effusion and not to obtain a diagnosis.
- Perform thoracocentesis and withdraw sufficient fluid to allow a noticeable improvement in respiratory function. Retain some fluid for analysis, cytology and culture.
- Pleural catheter placement will allow intermittent or continuous drainage and pleural lavage (Turner & Breznock 1988).
- Continue draining until only small quantities of a serous effusion can be collected.
- Only when the patient is stabilised should further radiographs, right and left lateral, be taken to identify if there is any clear aetiology present within the thorax, such as a neoplastic disease.

Table 44.3 Investigations in cases of pleural effusion.

Thoracocentesis	For effusion identification and culture of infective organisms (aerobic and anaerobic)
Biochemistry	To identify hypoalbuminaemia
Radiography (Fig. 44.1a & b)	Should be carried out with caution. Typical findings include a homogenous ground-glass appearance, pleural fluid lines, lung lobe border delineation, lung lobe retraction

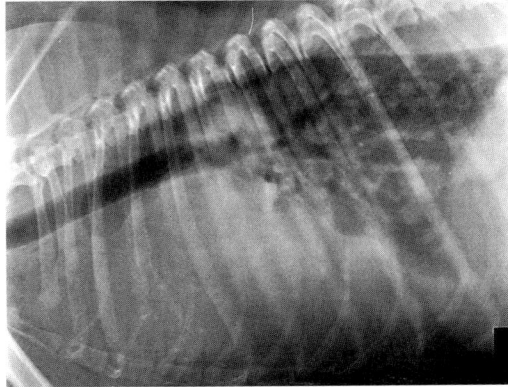

a

b

Fig. 44. 1a,b Thoracic radiographs of a 10-year-old Labrador with a pleural effusion. Initial radiographs showed a marked pleural effusion which made it difficult to determine the underlying aetiology. These films were taken after significant quantities of fluid had been removed by thoracocentesis. There is still a large amount of fluid in the chest, but now there are distinct nodular masses visible throughout the aerated regions of lung field. In addition, there is destruction and deviation of the ventral portion of the fourth rib, which is the site of the primary tumour. (Reproduced with permission of V. Luis Fuentes.)

Prognosis

The outcome of a pleural effusion and its management depends on the underlying cause. In general, pleural effusions can be difficult to treat and manage. Control of the accumulation of pleural fluid rather than achieving an overall cure, is usually the aim of therapy. Undoubtedly, progressive diseases such as neoplasia and cardiac conditions causing right-sided heart failure will eventually prove difficult to control. By contrast, infectious processes can be cured provided appropriate drainage and flushing is instigated. In a proportion of patients chylothorax can be controlled.

Ruptured Diaphragm

Ruptured diaphragm is usually the result of trauma:

- respiratory signs might not appear for weeks to months after the incident;
- all trauma cases should have the integrity of the diaphragm checked, even if there are no signs of respiratory distress;
- the rupture should be surgically repaired.

Lung Lobe Torsion

Lung lobe torsion can be associated with trauma, but often the underlying cause is not identified. It may be secondary to other problems such as pleural effusion.

- This is a rare condition, but is seen more commonly in deep-chested dogs, with the right middle and caudal part of the left cranial lobes most likely to be affected.

- Pleural effusion is usually present and is often restricted to the area of the affected lobe.
- The presence of air bronchograms suggest the torsion is recent.
- Clinical signs of respiratory distress and coughing can occur.
- Lung lobectomy is required.

Table 44.4   Management of specific types of pleural effusion.

Type	Condition	Treatment
True transudate and modified transudate		An underlying cause, such as hypoproteinaemia or congestive heart failure, is often identified, and should be treated accordingly (see relevant chapters for detailed discussion).
Exudate	Pyothorax	Use intermittent or continuous chest drainage (the latter gives a higher survival rate long term), particularly important in *Nocardia* spp. Antibacterial therapy (up to 3 months after drain removal) should be instituted on the basis of culture and sensitivity testing. The penicillins and clindamycin are very effective in dealing with anaerobic infections such as *Nocardia* spp. Chest lavage with warmed normal saline is beneficial
	Neoplasia	Therapy is usually limited to palliative thoracocentesis and pleural drainage to alleviate respiratory symptoms. Euthanasia should be considered if frequent pleural drainage is required. Chemotherapy is restricted to the treatment of lymphoma. Pleurodesis may be a last resort option in those dogs where dyspnoea alone, due to pleural effusion, is the sole clinical complaint (Birchard & Gallagher 1988). Treatment of underlying infections and neoplastic diseases should be attempted if feasible
Chylothorax		Chylothorax cases are usually managed by a combination of dietary control of fat intake and surgical ligation of the thoracic duct. In very few cases the underlying cause can be identified and treated – feed a low fat diet, with medium chain triglyceride fats to reduce the development of chylothorax. Thoracic duct ligation may be successful in up to 50% of cases and pleurodesis is only successful if combined with thoracic duct ligation. Benzopyrone agents may be of potential benefit, but their efficacy is still being assessed

Pneumothorax

Pneumothorax can arise from chest wall penetration (trauma, iatrogenic puncture [Teske *et al.* 1991]), rupture of *cysts*, *bullae*, *blebs*, alveoli and intrapulmonary bronchi, or be spontaneous (Schaer *et al.* 1981). *Tension pneumothorax* will develop if the air cannot escape from the pleural space via the route of entry. Diagnosis is confirmed by radiography.

- Mild to moderate pneumothorax might not cause appreciable respiratory distress, and can resolve spontaneously.
- Severe pneumothorax, and in particular tension pneumothorax, cause tachypnoea and dyspnoea due to pronounced lung compression.
- Thoracocentesis is required if the dog is symptomatic or there is persistent reappearance of air in the pleural space.
- Surgical correction of an identifiable cause of recurrent pneumothorax should be considered.

MEDIASTINAL DISEASE

The clinical presentation of most mediastinal abnormalities can be attributed to their effects on structures present within the mediastinum (Suter & Zinkl 1982):

- extension to involve the thoracic vertebra and spinal cord causing pain and hindlimb paresis;
- interference with the trachea, mainstem bronchi and oesophagus causing coughing, dyspnoea, dysphagia and regurgitation;
- compression of major vessels causing head, neck and fore-limb oedema (cranial vena cava), ascites and hind limb oedema (caudal vena cava) or chylothorax (thoracic duct);
- damage to sympathetic ganglia, the vago-sympathetic trunk and recurrent laryngeal nerves causing Horner's syndrome and laryngeal dysfunction.

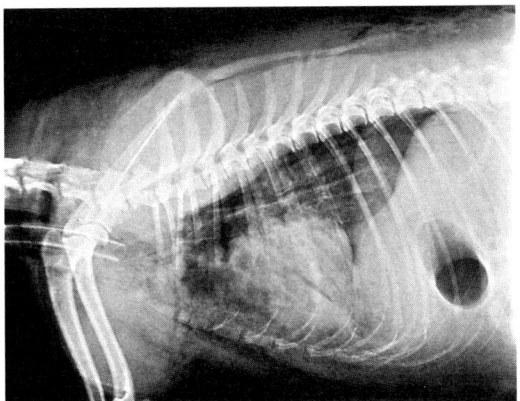

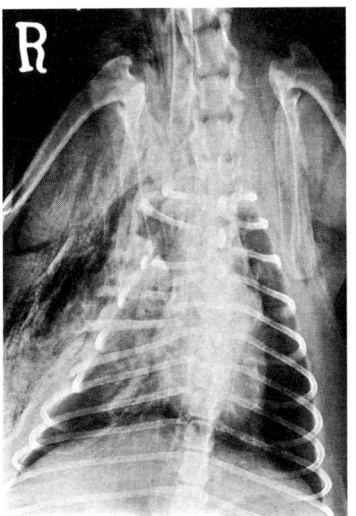

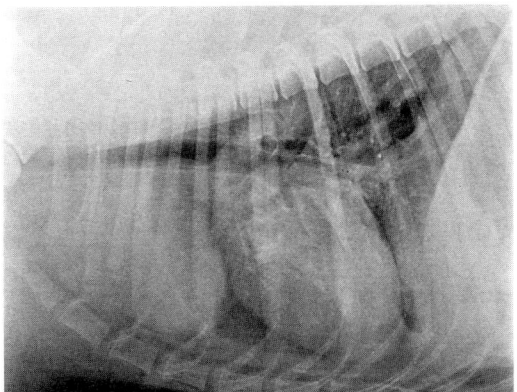

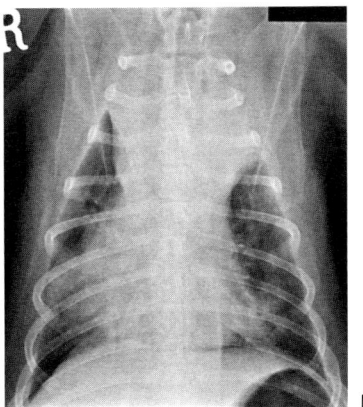

Fig. 44. 3a,b A 12-year-old Border Collie dog with cranial mediastinal widening and megoesophagus. There is a well defined mass in the cranial mediastinum resulting in widening, with dorsal displacement of the trachea.

Fig. 44. 2a,b Pneumomediastinum secondary to trauma. Both borders of the oesophagus can be seen, as well as both tracheal walls. There is a flail chest, with fracture of ribs 2 to 6 on the right hand side. The lung lobe beneath the flail segment is partially collapsed, and there is extensive subcutaneous emphysema with minimal pneumothorax.

pleural adhesions, atelectasis, unilateral pleural effusions and pneumothorax, diaphragmatic hernia and uneven lung lobe inflation (Suter & Zinkl 1982).

Pneumomediastinum

The presence of free gas within the mediastinum enables visualisation of the outer walls of the trachea, the oesophagus, cranial vena cava and azygous vein.

The causes of pneumomediastinum include:

- idiopathic pneumomediastinum;
- tracheal or oesophageal rupture;
- iatrogenic puncture of the trachea or bronchi during airway samplingl;
- deep neck wounds, with air migrating along the neck muscle fascial planes.

The presence of inflammatory disease in the mediastinum itself, in addition to the signs caused by damage to adjacent structures, might also result in pain, discomfort and pyrexia.

Mediastinal Shift

Mediastinal shift is a displacement of the mediastinum, either to the right or left, and is often associated with

In uncomplicated cases, pneumomediastinum is not harmful and is usually self-limiting (7–10 days to resolve). However, marked increases in mediastinal pressure can compromise venous return to the heart, and in the event of mediastinal rupture a life-threatening pneumothorax may occur (see Fig. 44.2).

Mediastinal Widening

Mediastinal widening (Fig. 44.3) can be due to:

- obesity or an enlarged thymus (normal young dogs);
- neoplasia, including lymphoma, heart base tumours, lipomas, thymoma, thyroidal (ectopic) tumours and metastases from other tumour sites (Suter & Zinkl 1982);
- abscesses, granulomas and other infectious/inflammatory disorders (mediastinitis);
- oesophageal dilation, impaction and foreign bodies;
- oedema (in association with pleural effusion) and haemorrhage.

Mediastinal Narrowing

Chronic mediastinitis can result in scar healing and narrowing of the mediastinal space. This might be appreciated on thoracic radiographs. If this narrowing impairs tracheal or oesophageal function or compresses the major vessels, clinical signs associated with such effects can be appreciated.

REFERENCES

Birchard, S.J. & Gallacher, L. (1988). Use of pleurodesis in treating selected pleural disease. *Compendium on Continuing Education for the Practicing Veterinarian*, **10**, 826–832.

Forrester, S.D. (1990). Pleural effusion in the dog and cat. *Veterinary Annual*, **30**, 283–297.

Forrester, S.D., Troy, G.C. & Fossum, T.W. (1988). Pleural effusions: pathophysiology and diagnostic considerations. *Compendium on Continuing Education for the Practicing Veterinarian*, **10**, 121–136.

Noone, K.E. (1985). Pleural effusion and disease of the pleura. *Veterinary Clinics of North America*, **15**, 1069–1084.

Suter, P.F. & Zinkl, J.G. (1982). Mediastinal, pleural, and extrapleural thoracic diseases. In: *Veterinary Internal Medicine*, (ed. S.J. Ettinger), pp. 841–883. W.B. Saunders, Philadelphia.

Turner, W.D. & Breznock, E.M. (1988). Continuous suction drainage for management of canine pyothorax. A retrospective study. *Journal of the American Animal Hospital Association*, **24**, 485–494.

Chapter 45

Cardiac Disease

V. Luis Fuentes

INTRODUCTION

Cardiac disease is relatively common in dogs, with acquired cardiac disease comprising the majority of such cases (Buchanan 1992). In contrast congenital heart disease is much less common (Buchanan 1992), although a number of systemic diseases may also give rise to cardiac abnormalities. It is important to distinguish *cardiac disease* from *cardiac failure*. The latter only occurs when cardiac function is sufficiently compromised to result in clinical signs; compensatory mechanisms ensure that many dogs remain asymptomatic despite the presence of cardiac disease. The clinician must recognise when intervention is appropriate.

Structure and Function

The Myocardium

The myocardium is composed of bundles of myofibrils consisting of actin and myosin filaments. The filaments are linked by cross-bridges which can be broken and reformed to allow the myofibrils to change length. Breaking and reforming of the cross-bridges requires ATP and calcium ions, so that an influx of calcium into the myocardial cell induces contraction of the myocyte (Levick 1995).

The Conduction System

Calcium ions move into the myocytes during depolarisation, which leads to opening of the calcium channels. There is therefore a slight delay between electrical depolarisation and mechanical contraction.

- Depolarisation usually begins in the *sinoatrial (SA) node* (see Fig. 45.1), which is situated in the right atrium. Parasympathetic stimulation slows down the rate of discharge of these pacemaker cells, and sympathetic stimulation speeds up the rate.
- Depolarisation spreads from the SA node to the rest of the atrial myocardium, and reaches the *atrioventricular (AV) node*. Conduction is particularly slow through the AV node, to allow time for atrial contraction to fill the ventricles before ventricular contraction occurs.
- Conduction of the impulse from the AV node to the ventricles occurs through the specialised conduction fibres of the *bundle of His*. The bundle of His passes through the electrically insulated *annulus fibrosus* which separates the atria from the ventricles.
- The bundle of His divides into *left and right bundle branches*, which supply the left and right ventricles respectively.
- The bundle branches divide into smaller and smaller fibres called *Purkinje fibres*, which extend into the myocardium.

The SA node is the dominant pacemaker, but all of the specialised conduction tissue has innate automaticity, i.e. will spontaneously discharge. The SA node has the highest rate of discharge, and the Purkinje fibres have the slowest rate of discharge (Levick 1995).

Cardiac Output (Box 45.1)

The heart is the powerhouse of the circulatory system, and together with the autonomic, renal, and endocrine components of circulatory control, it must ensure adequate distribution of oxygenated blood to the organs of the body under a wide range of loading conditions. The complex homeostatic interactions of different parts of the circulatory system allow the body to compensate for a diseased heart up to a certain degree. This also means that it may be possible for the clinician to approach a clinical problem from a number of different therapeutic angles.

Box 45.1   Determinants of cardiac output.

Cardiac output is determined by *heart rate* and *stroke volume.*

Stroke volume is determined by *myocardial contractility*, *preload*, and *afterload.*

- *Contractility* is defined as the intrinsic ability of the myocardial fibres to contract.
- *Preload* is defined as the forces distending the ventricles at the end of diastole ('end-diastolic wall stress'). According to Starling's law of the heart, an increase in preload results in increased contractile force (Braunwald *et al.* 1992).
- *Afterload* is defined as the *forces opposing ejection from the ventricles during systole* ('*systolic wall stress'*)

Systolic wall stress is affected by:

- systemic arterial pressure,
- ventricular diameter,
- ventricular wall thickness,
- aortic wall stiffness.

Increases in heart rate, contractility, and afterload usually result in increased myocardial oxygen consumption; i.e. they result in increased cardiac work. Factors affecting cardiac performance are summarised in Table 45.1.

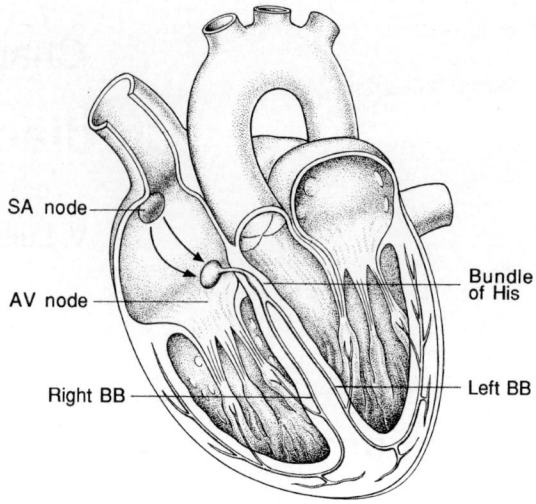

Fig. 45.1   The conduction system.

Backward failure may also be termed *congestive failure*. Forward and backward failure are actually intimately related, as most of the mechanisms that result in fluid retention are activated by a decrease in cardiac output. The neuroendocrine mechanisms involved are listed in the Table 45.2.

Box 45.2   Types of cardiac failure.

Forward failure is another term sometimes used for the situation where there is inadequate blood supply to the tissues.

Signs of forward failure

- weakness
- syncope
- peripheral vasoconstriction (pallor, cold extremities)

Backward failure may also be termed congestive failure and will usually occur when filling pressures (or atrial pressures) are raised.

Signs of backward failure

- dyspnoea (pulmonary oedema, pleural effusion)
- coughing (left atrial enlargement)
- ascites

This means that the walls of a *dilated ventricle* experience *more* systolic wall stress than a normal-sized heart at the same systemic arterial pressures, whereas a ventricle with hypertrophied walls experiences *less* systolic wall stress.

Heart Failure

Heart disease becomes *heart failure* when the heart is unable to supply blood to the tissues at an adequate rate, or when it can only achieve this at raised filling pressures. Filling pressures will be raised with increased ventricular end-diastolic pressures or increased atrial pressures. There are two types of heart failure: forward failure and backward failure (see Box 45.2).

Factors resulting in ↑ contractility	Factors resulting in ↓ contractility
β₁ adrenergic stimulation	Negative inotropes
Positive inotropes	Dilated cardiomyopathy
	Secondary to volume overload:
	advanced endocardiosis
	mitral dysplasia
	patent ductus arteriosus
Factors resulting in ↑ preload	**Factors resulting in ↓ preload**
Na⁺, H₂O retention	Hypovolaemia
Venoconstriction	Pericardial effusion
↑ Venous return:	Tachycardias
left-to-right shunts	Diuretics, venodilators
mitral regurgitation	
aortic regurgitation	
Bradycardias	
Factors resulting in ↑ afterload	**Factors resulting in ↓ afterload**
Any dilated ventricle with	LV hypertrophy
normal/thin walls	Arteriodilators
Aortic and pulmonic stenosis	Mitral regurgitation
Systemic or pulmonary hypertension	

Table 45.1 Factors affecting cardiac performance.

Table 45.2 Neuroendocrine effects in heart failure.

	Pathway	Mediator	Effects
Sympathetic nervous system	α-adrenoceptor stimulation		• Peripheral vasoconstriction diverts blood flow from skin, gut, muscle, kidney
	β-adrenoceptor stimulation		• ↑ Heart rate
			• ↑ Contractility
Kidneys	Changes in renal perfusion		• Retention of sodium and water
			• Secretion of renin
Endocrine	Activation of renin–angiotensin–aldosterone axis	Angiotensin II	• Vasoconstriction (↑ afterload)
			• Sympathetic activation
			• Increased thirst
			• Aldosterone release
			• Vasopressin release
		Aldosterone	• Sodium and water retention (↑ preload)
			• Potassium loss
		Vasopressin	• Antidiuresis
	Raised atrial pressures	Atrial Natriuretic Peptide	• ↑ Renal excretion of sodium
			• Slight arteriolar dilation

The signs of congestive failure are different according to whether the left or right heart is predominantly affected.

Left Heart Failure

The *key sign* of left heart failure is *pulmonary oedema*.

The causes of left heart failure are listed in Table 45.3.

An increase in left-sided filling pressures may result in raised left atrial pressure. This increased pressure is transmitted to the pulmonary veins and pulmonary capillaries, where the increased hydrostatic pressure leads to exudation of fluid into the pulmonary interstitium, or *interstitial pulmonary oedema*. This excess fluid in the interstitial tissue is drained by an increase in lymphatic drainage.

If the left atrial pressure remains high, and the lymphatics are unable to cope with the increased fluid transport, then fluid passes from the interstitial tissue to the alveolar spaces, causing *alveolar pulmonary oedema*.

Right Heart Failure

The *key signs* of right heart failure are *ascites* and *pleural effusion*.

The causes of right heart failure are listed in Table 45.4.

An increase in right atrial pressure leads to similar problems to left-sided failure, but the pressure rises in the systemic veins instead. This can be seen as distension of the jugular veins, but distension of the portal and hepatic veins leads to exudation of fluid into the abdomen, and hepatomegaly. Although *ascites* is the most common sign of right-sided failure, *pleural effusion* may also sometimes occur.

Acute Heart Failure

Acute heart failure results in a rapid reduction in cardiac output, without time for many of the neuroendocrine mechanisms to become activated. Systemic blood pressure therefore falls, leading to profound weakness. Examples would include a sudden sustained ventricular tachycardia, or even a ruptured chordae tendinaea (which would also involve a sudden rise in filling pressures).

Chronic Heart Failure

In chronic heart failure, many mechanisms contribute to the maintenance of normal systemic arterial pressure, which is the main homeostatic priority. This is primarily achieved by:

- stimulation of the sympathetic nervous system;
- preload augmentation (by activation of the renin-angiotensin system and retention of sodium and water).

The various neuroendocrine effects of heart failure are summarised in Table 45.2.

Causes of Heart Failure

Cardiac failure may be the end-result of a number of different pathological mechanisms. This is relevant when deciding on therapy, as treatment will be most effective when directed at the weakest link in the chain of cardiac performance. Examples of functional categories of disease resulting in cardiac failure are listed in Table 45.5.

Classification of Severity of Heart Failure

It is helpful to be able to categorise the severity of heart failure. The main human classification (New York Heart Association classification) is often used in small animals, but is based on exercise tolerance and can be difficult to apply. A newer alternative is the International Small Animal Cardiac Health Classification (International Small

---

Table 45.3   Causes of left heart failure.

Mitral endocardiosis
Dilated cardiomyopathy
Patent ductus arteriosus
Mitral dysplasia
Ventricular septal defect
Dysrhythmias
Aortic stenosis with myocardial failure
Bacterial endocarditis

Table 45.4   Causes of right heart failure.

Tricuspid endocardiosis
Dilated cardiomyopathy
Pericardial disease
Pulmonic stenosis
Tricuspid dysplasia
Dysrhythmias
Secondary to left heart failure

Table 45.5 Causes of heart failure.

Category	Primary disturbance	Examples
Myocardial failure	↓ Contractility	• Dilated cardiomyopathy • End-stage endocardiosis
Volume overload	↑ End-diastolic volume	• Mitral regurgitation • Left-to-right shunts
Pressure overload	↑ End-systolic pressure	• Aortic/pulmonic stenosis • Systemic hypertension
Diastolic dysfunction	Inadequate ventricular filling	• Pericardial effusion
Dysrhythmias	↓ Output through inadequate filling or inadequate heart rate	• Tachycardias • Bradycardias

Class I	*Asymptomatic* Signs of heart disease on examination (e.g. murmur) No clinical signs	IA Minimal/no cardiac enlargement IB Some cardiac enlargement present
Class II	*Mild-moderate heart failure*	Signs of cardiac failure: exercise intolerance, coughing, dyspnoea, ascites
Class III	*Advanced heart failure* Severe dyspnoea/ marked ascites/ hypoperfusion at rest	IIIA Home care is possible IIIB Hospitalisation is mandatory: life-threatening pulmonary oedema/ pleural effusion

Table 45.6 The International Small Animal Cardiac Health Council (ISACHC) system of heart failure classification.

Animal Cardiac Health Council 1995), summarised in Table 45.6.

HISTORY AND PHYSICAL EXAMINATION OF THE PATIENT WITH CARDIAC DISEASE

The importance of a physical examination in cases of heart disease cannot be over-emphasised (Gompf 1988). Although echocardiography is required in the majority of cases for definitive diagnosis, it should only serve to confirm a suspected diagnosis if a careful physical examination is combined with logical interpretation of radiographs and ECGs. Congenital heart disease is more difficult to diagnose without more sophisticated tests such as Doppler echocardiography. These are dealt with in subsequent sections in this chapter.

History

A good history should help to establish whether or not there is a cardiac problem. The common presenting signs with heart disease are coughing, dyspnoea, exercise intolerance and syncope.

Coughing

Coughing is often caused by left atrial enlargement, and may be one of the first signs noted in chronic mitral insufficiency or dilated cardiomyopathy. Care must be taken to distinguish coughing from left atrial enlargement from coughing caused by chronic airway disease in small dogs with murmurs (see Table 39.5).

Dyspnoea

Dyspnoea is generally associated with congestive heart failure. It may be caused by pulmonary oedema, or pleural effusion. It may also be present with right-to-left shunts and with pericardial effusions (see Table 39.6).

Table 45.7   Differential diagnosis of syncope.

Categories	Examples	Key features
Cardiac causes		Occur on exertion
Outflow tract obstruction	Aortic stenosis	Loud left base murmur
	Pulmonic stenosis	Loud left base murmur
	Hypertrophic obstructive cardiomyopathy	Prominent apex beat, diagnosis on ultrasound
	Atrial tumour / ball thrombi	Diagnosis on ultrasound
Cardiac tamponade	Pericardial effusions	Quiet/muffled heart sounds, large cardiac silhouette on radiographs
Dysrhythmias	Supraventricular tachycardias	Rapid regular heart rate, normal QRS complexes on ECG
	Ventricular tachycardias	Audible dysrhythmias, wide bizarre complexes on ECG
	Bradycardias (e.g. 3rd degree AV block)	May occur on rising from resting position, slow heart rate
Right-to-left shunts	Tetralogy of Fallot, septal defects with pulmonary hypertension	Cyanosis, polycythaemia, under-circulated lung field on radiography
Acquired valvular disease	Endocardiosis	Small breed, pansystolic murmur left apex
	Bacterial endocarditis	Variable: often malaise, pyrexia ± many other clinical signs
Myocardial disease	Dilated cardiomyopathy	Large breed, ± soft pansystolic murmurs, ± gallop sounds ± dysrhythmias
Vascular causes	Vasovagal	Excitement/exercise-induced, NAD on all investigations (boxers?)
Metabolic	Hypoglycaemia	Low blood glucose
	Hypovolaemia	Underperfused lung fields on radiography
Respiratory	Upper respiratory tract obstruction	Cyanosis, induced by exertion / excitement, respiratory noise
	Pulmonary hypertension	Rare: usually right ventricular enlargement, tortuous pulmonary vessels
	Pulmonary thromboembolism	Sudden onset dyspnoea, variable radiographic changes
Haematological	Anaemia	↓PCV
	Polycythaemia	↑PCV
Iatrogenic	Drug-induced hypotension	History of drug administration

Exercise Intolerance

Exercise intolerance may be an early sign of decompensation with heart disease, but may be attributed to other factors by the owner. Exercise intolerance is more likely to be noticed in working dogs.

Syncope

Syncope has many causes (see Table 45.7), but clues to a cardiac origin include:

- syncope on exertion (including getting up after lying down),
- rapid recovery (back to normal in minutes),

- lack of salivation,
- no pre-ictal signs (although may appear unsteady shortly before – 'presyncope').

Other Cardiac Presenting Signs

- Anorexia
- Weight loss
- Lethargy

Physical Examination

Physical examination is probably the most important part of the investigation of any dog with heart disease.

General Condition

Dogs with advanced congestive heart failure may be in poor body condition, with muscle wastage. Note should obviously be made of any non-cardiac abnormalities that might indicate other systemic disease, as cardiac dysfunction can be secondary to a number of non-cardiac conditions.

Mucous Membranes

- *Pallor*. Peripheral vasoconstriction caused by poor cardiac output may lead to pale mucous membranes. Conversely, severe anaemia can *result* in murmurs, or even cardiac enlargement.
- *Cyanosis*. Generally cyanosis indicates severe respiratory compromise. In cardiac disease this usually indicates severe pulmonary oedema or pleural effusion. Congenital right-to-left shunts may also cause cyanosis, usually with concurrent polycythaemia so that the mucous membranes are dark purplish-maroon.
- *Capillary refill time*. Blanching of the mucous membranes may persist for longer than 2 s following digital pressure if there is marked peripheral vasoconstriction due to poor cardiac output.

Pulse

Pulse quality varies according to stroke volume as shown in Table 45.8.

The pulse rate can be taken to measure heart rate, although a discrepancy will exist with some dysrhythmias (pulse deficit).

Respiratory Rate

The respiratory rate is a useful indicator of congestive heart failure; usually the respiratory rate will rise with pulmonary oedema or pleural effusion.

normal = 15–30 breaths/min

Table 45.8 Pulse quality.

Pulse characteristic	Associated conditions
Weak	Poor stroke volume
Bounding	High output states
Rapid rise and fall	Patent ductus arteriosis
Brief	Aortic stenosis

Jugular Veins

The jugular veins may become distended with right-sided cardiac failure, as the raised right atrial pressures are transmitted to the jugular veins. Jugular pulsation may be seen as high as the angle of the jaw with right-sided failure.

Hepatojugular Reflux

Pressure on the liver and cranial abdomen will increase venous return to the right atrium, and may induce jugular distension if the pressure is already critically raised in the right atrium. A positive hepato-jugular reflux test therefore indicates raised right atrial pressures.

Abdomen

Right-sided failure may cause hepatomegaly, or cause ascites.

Precordium

Palpation of the precordium is an underestimated part of the physical examination. Information can be obtained about:

- heart rate,
- heart rhythm,
- cardiac size,
- strength of the apical impulse,
- thrills associated with loud murmurs,
- large pleural effusions ('barrel-shaped chest').

Percussion

Percussion of the chest may be effected by tapping the chest wall directly, or using the middle finger as a plexime-

Table 45.9 Valve location.

Valve	Dog
Mitral	Left 5th intercostal space, at costochondral junction
Aortic	Left 4th intercostal space, just above costochondral junction
Pulmonic	Left 2nd–4th intercostal space, just above sternum
Tricuspid	Right 3rd–5th intercostal space, just above costochondral junction

ter. The resulting sound will be dull when overlying fluid or soft tissue, or resonant when overlying air or air-filled lung. It is particularly useful when pleural effusions are suspected.

Auscultation

Auscultation is a vital part of the examination of the cardiac patient. When auscultating the heart, attention must be paid to each of the valve areas (Table 45.9).

Heart Sounds
Normally two heart sounds are heard.

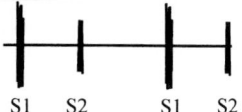

S1   1st sound – 'lub'

- associated with closure of the mitral/tricuspid valves
- heard loudest over the apex

S2   2nd sound – 'dup'

- associated with closure of the aortic/pulmonic valves
- heard loudest over the heart base

Heart Rate. Normal rate = 65–150/min (or higher in puppies and nervous/very excited dogs). In dogs with congestive heart failure, the rate tends to be increased and the rhythm becomes regular, with loss of sinus arrhythmia.

Audibility of Heart. It should be noted that to some extent, the audibility of the heart will depend on thoracic conformation (Table 45.10).

Abnormal Sounds – Murmurs
Cardiac murmurs indicate turbulent blood flow, which is generally the result of high velocity blood flow within the

Table 45.10   Audibility of the heart.

Increased audibility	Decreased audibility
Cardiac enlargement	Pericardial effusion
Hyperdynamic heart	Pleural effusion
	Thoracic mass
	Diaphragmatic hernia
	Severe myocardial failure

heart. The characteristics of a murmur can be used to identify the probable cause of the turbulent flow.

Intensity. Murmur intensity is graded from 1 to 6, with 6/6 being the loudest and 1/6 being the quietest. Grades 5/6 and 6/6 are associated with precordial thrills. Very loud murmurs are usually clinically significant, although not all quiet murmurs are insignificant.

Character. The character or quality of the murmur sound will vary according to the cause. Descriptions are often taken from their appearance on a phonocardiogram.

Plateau–shaped murmur ('soft', 'blowing')

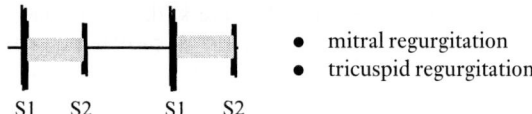

- mitral regurgitation
- tricuspid regurgitation

Crescendo–decrescendo ('harsh')

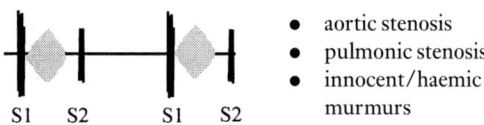

- aortic stenosis
- pulmonic stenosis
- innocent/haemic murmurs

Point of Maximum Intensity. The point of maximum intensity often indicates the site of intracardiac turbulent flow, e.g. murmurs of mitral regurgitation are usually heard best over the mitral valve, at the left apex.

Radiation. Many loud murmurs radiate widely, so that the murmur can be heard over other parts of the thorax. However, murmurs associated with some conditions may radiate in specific directions; e.g. aortic stenosis murmurs often radiate to the right hemithorax and the thoracic inlet.

Timing. The majority of murmurs in dogs are systolic.

Pansystolic/holosystolic

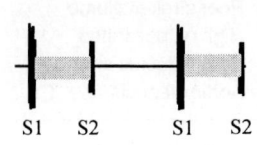

- mitral regurgitation
- tricuspid regurgitation
- ventricular septal defects
- severe aortic/ pulmonic stenosis

Midsystolic

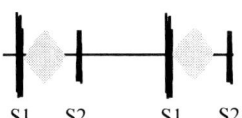

- aortic stenosis
- pulmonic stenosis
- innocent/haemic murmurs

Diastolic

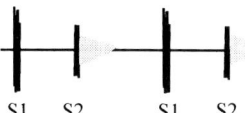

- rare in dogs
- aortic regurgitation (bacterial endocarditis)

Continuous

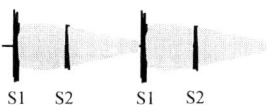

- patent ductus arteriosus
- (severe aortic stenosis with aortic regurgitation)

Abnormal Sounds – Gallops

It is not normal to hear more than two heart sounds in dogs.

S3 – Third heart sound

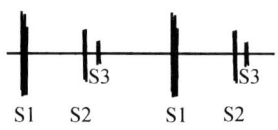

- associated with increased early ventricular filling
- elevated left atrial pressure

S4 – Fourth heart sound

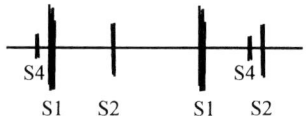

- associated with atrial filling
- stiff/dilated ventricle

Lung Sounds

Respiratory sounds are generally normal in cardiac disease unless there is *severe pulmonary oedema*, or *pleural effusion*.

Severe Pulmonary Oedema. End-inspiratory crackles may be auscultated when alveolar oedema is present, and in this setting indicate serious respiratory compromise. However, end-inspiratory crackles may also be caused by airway disease, which may often be present in small dogs.

Pleural Effusion. Breath sounds may be reduced ventral to the fluid line, although they may be easily audible dorsal to this.

ANCILLARY DIAGNOSTIC AIDS

Once a history and physical examination are obtained, a reasonable differential diagnosis can usually be obtained. However, further investigations are nearly always necessary to confirm a diagnosis. The most commonly-used diagnostic aids for evaluating cardiac disease in dogs are radiography, electrocardiography, and echocardiography.

Cardiac Radiology

Radiology is still an essential part of the diagnostic procedure for dogs with cardiac disease (Suter 1984). It can be used to provide information about:

- cardiac shape/chamber enlargement,
- cardiac size,
- congestive cardiac failure and the pulmonary circulation,
- intercurrent disease.

Radiographic Technique

Warning: Although many dogs with cardiac disease are well-compensated, dogs with congestive heart failure *must be handled with care*. Restraint for radiography is stressful for dogs with minimal cardiac reserves, and it is all too easy to lose a patient during radiography. Restraint should always be minimal, and positioning should be carried out quietly and patiently. Chemical restraint is usually necessary, but minimal doses should be used where possible. Radiography of dogs with severe heart failure should either be delayed until the animal's condition is more stable, or obtained without sedation if the dog will lie quietly for views to be obtained. Manual restraint is not acceptable.

To obtain good quality radiographs, the exposure time must be short.

- low mAs (milliamp seconds)
- high kVP (kilovoltage peak)
- use grid (in large chests) only if short exposure time can be maintained
- accurate positioning
- dorsoventral and right lateral views preferred

Radiographic Interpretation

Cardiac Size

As there is enormous variation in normal chest conformation, it is difficult to be categoric about changes in cardiac size. One technique which appears to be more flexible than others is the vertebral heart scoring system (Buchanan 1992). The apico-basilar length of the heart (labelled L in Fig. 45.2) is measured in vertebral bodies starting from the cranial edge of the fourth thoracic vertebra. The width of the heart (labelled W in Fig. 45.2) is measured in the same way, and the sum of both measurements gives the vertebral body score.

Normal hearts should not measure more than 8–10 vertebral bodies.

Cardiac Shape

It is often easier to recognise changes in shape which indicate chamber enlargement (see Figs 45.3–45.7). Recognition of left atrial enlargement is an essential key to the diagnosis of left-sided heart failure. Radiology is much more sensitive than electrocardiography in the identification of chamber enlargement, and can still be useful even when echocardiography is available.

Changes in the Great Vessels

The major vessels should be assessed for changes in size (see Figs 45.8–45.10), as clues may be present which can assist in the recognition of congenital conditions or right heart failure.

Recognition of Heart Failure

Radiography is an invaluable tool for the assessment of cardiac failure, and can only be beaten by invasive measurement of right atrial and pulmonary capillary wedge pressures. Recognition of congestive failure centres on assessment of pulmonary vessels, the lung parenchyma, and the pleural space (see Figs 45.11–45.15).

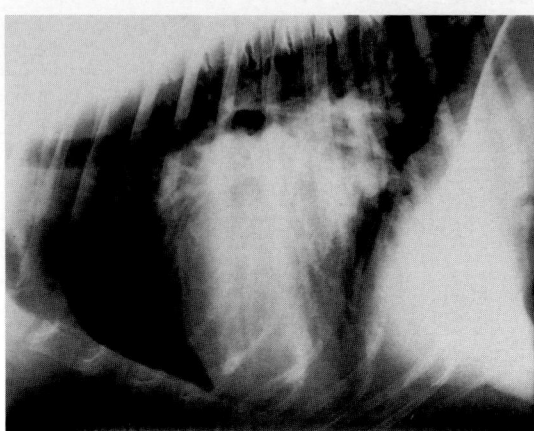

a

b

Fig. 45.3   Left atrial enlargement. A grossly enlarged left atrium in a Dobermann with dilated cardiomyopathy. Typical features of left atrial enlargement on *lateral* view:
- an acute angle between the caudal cardiac border and the terminal trachea,
- splitting of the mainstem bronchi with compression.

Typical features on the *dorsoventral*:
- widening of the angle of the mainstem bronchi with a rounded soft tissue density between them (open arrow),
- a bulge at the 2–3 o'clock position from the left auricular appendage (white arrow).

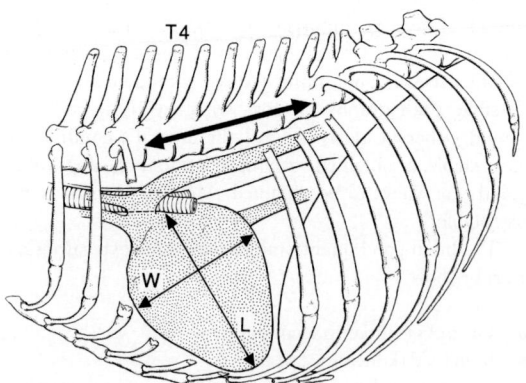

Fig. 45.2   Measurement of the heart in relation to vertebral bodies.

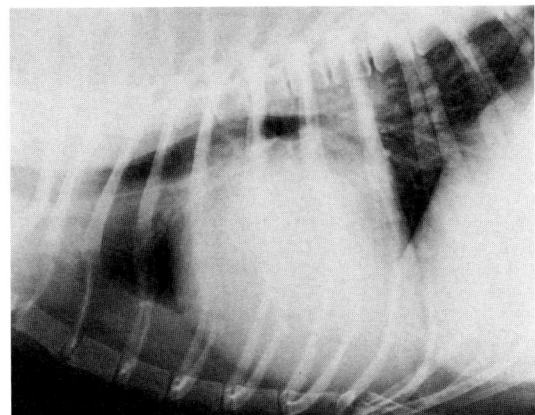

a

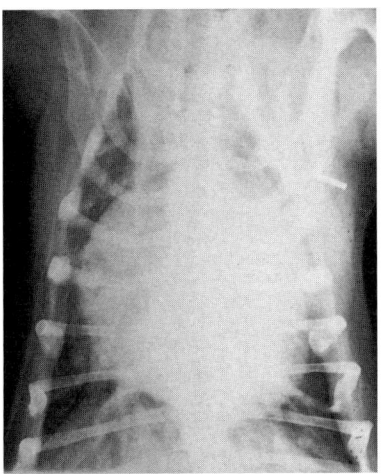

b

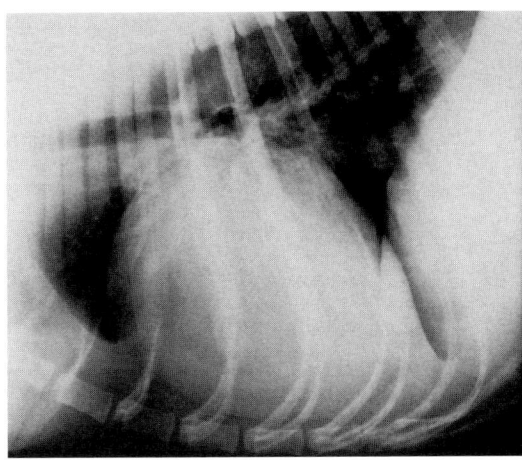

a

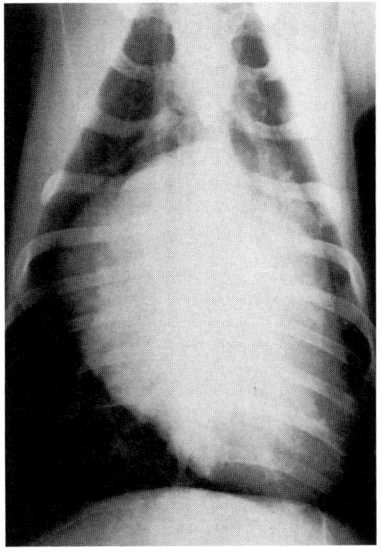

b

Fig. 45.4   Left ventricular enlargement. Left-sided enlargement in a 10-year-old Dachshund with endocardiosis.
Typical features of left ventricular enlargement on *lateral* include:
- increase in apico-basilar height,
- straightening of caudal border.

Typical features of left ventricular enlargement on *dorsoventral* include:
- rounding of the cardiac outline from 3 to 6 o'clock,
- increase in apico-basilar length.

Fig. 45.5   Right atrial enlargement. Marked right atrial enlargement in Labrador Retriever with tricuspid dysplasia.
Typical features of right atrial enlargement on lateral include:
- elevation of the trachea cranial to the carina,
- increased width.

Typical features of right atrial enlargement on dorsoventral include:
- rounding of the cardiac outline from 9 to 12 o'clock.

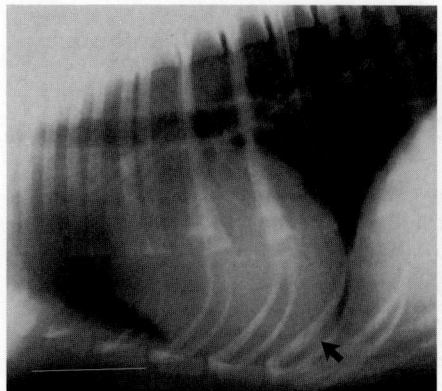

a

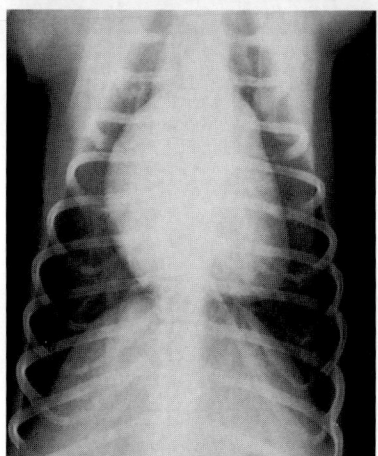

b

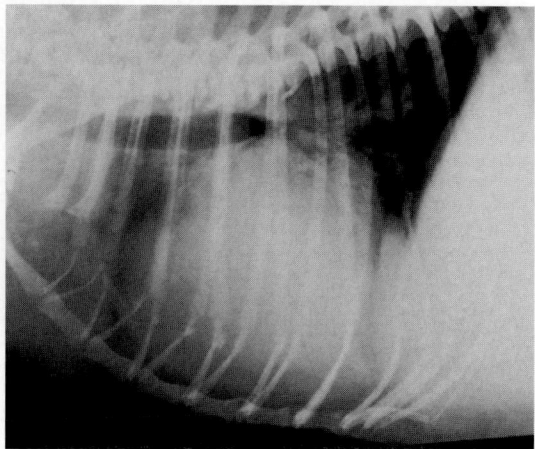

a

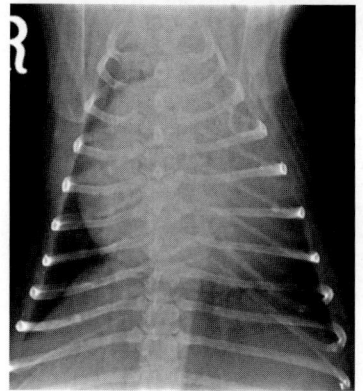

b

Fig. 45.6   Right ventricular enlargement. Right ventricular enlargement in a 5-month-old Jack Russell Terrier with a right-to-left shunting ventricular septal defect.
Typical features of right ventricular enlargement on lateral include:

- increase in sternal contact,
- increase in cardiac width,
- in addition, 'apex-tipping' may be seen when right ventricular hypertrophy is present (arrow).

Typical features of right ventricular enlargement on dorsoventral include:

- rounding of the cardiac outline from 6 to 9 o'clock,
- rounding of the cardiac apex or shift to the left.

Fig. 45.7   Biventricular enlargement. Both sides of the heart are enlarged (in particular, the right side) in this Cavalier King Charles spaniel with endocardiosis affecting both atrioventricular valves.

Electrocardiography

The Electrocardiogram (ECG)

The cardiac cycle is usually referenced to the electrocardiogram, which is a graphical display of the potential difference across the body measured at the skin surface during the cardiac cycle (see Fig. 45.16). The positive electrode records a deflection above the baseline when the wave of depolarisation travels towards it, and a negative deflection when the baseline travels away from it.

Electrocardiography is essential for the diagnosis of dysrhythmias (Tilley 1992), and can provide additional information regarding chamber enlargement as well as some forms of electrolyte imbalance. It can also be used to provide a permanent record of heart rate and rhythm.

Technique

See Table 45.11.

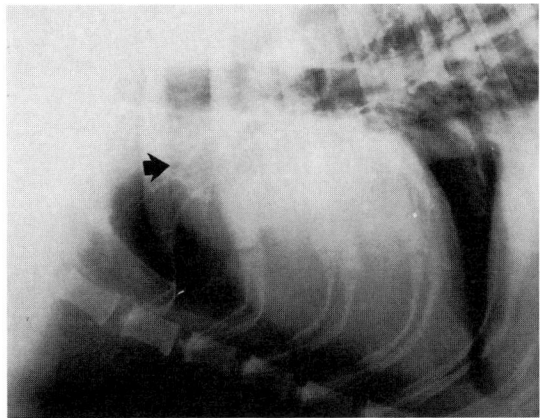

a

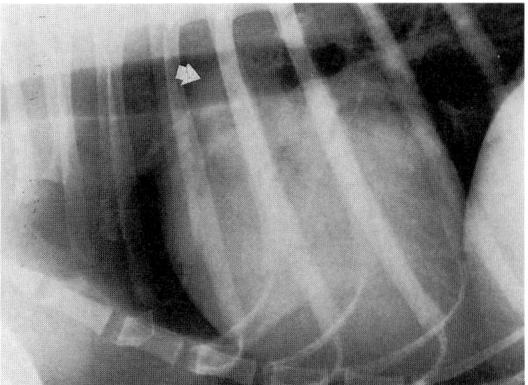

a

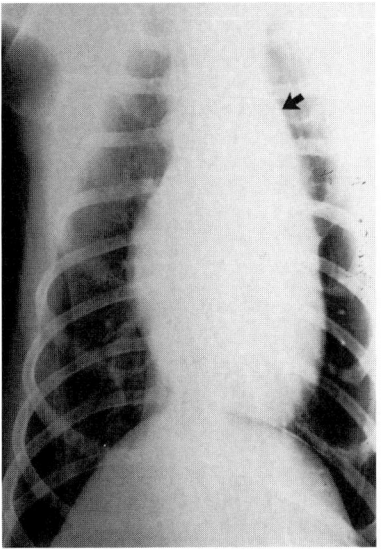

b

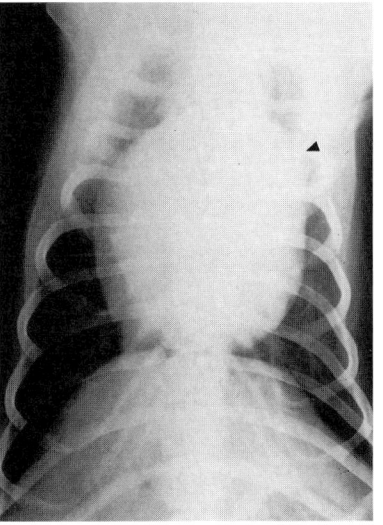

b

Fig. 45.8 Aortic bulge. A widening of the aortic root on the lateral (arrow) and a prominent bulge at the 12–1 o'clock position on the dorsoventral (arrow) may be seen with this Golden Retriever with subaortic stenosis and a post-stenotic dilatation.

Fig. 45.9 Pulmonary artery bulge. These films from a dog with pulmonic stenosis show a visible soft tissue density 'cap' overlying the trachea on the lateral view (arrow) and a bulge at the 1–2 o'clock area on the dorsoventral (arrow). (With permission from J. Dukes-McEwan.)

ECG Interpretation

It is often best to work from first principles when attempting to interpret ECGs (Fig. 45.17). If one understands what the P–QRS deflections represent, it is often possible to unravel dysrhythmias which appear unfathomable on initial inspection. By applying a set of seven basic questions (Box 45.3) it is possible to distinguish sinus rhythms from ectopic rhythms, supraventricular rhythms from ventricular rhythms/abnormal conduction.

After assessing the ECG by answering the questions in Box 45.3, it should be possible to identify the rhythm or rhythms. The waveforms should be measured in detail, selecting sinus complexes from a lead II recording. Normal waveform measurements are given in Table 45.12. Examples of common dysrhythmias are shown in Table 45.13.

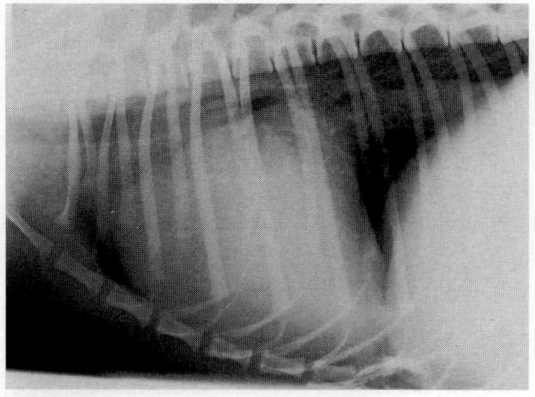

a

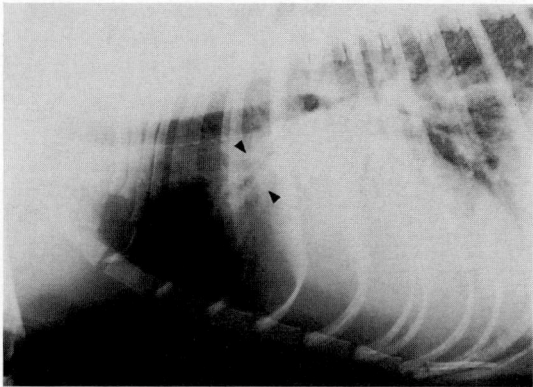

a

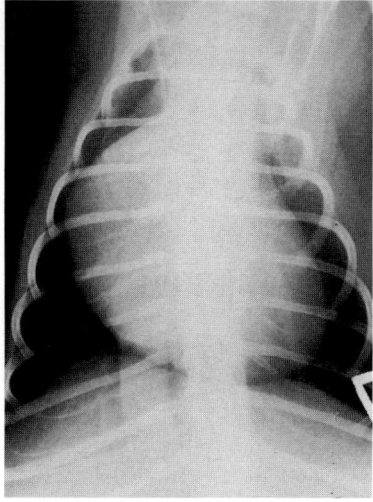

b

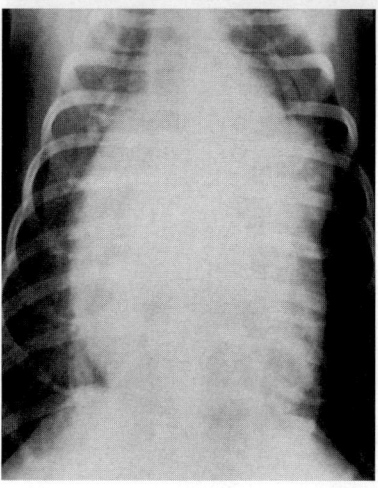

b

Fig. 45.10   Distended caudal vena cava. Gross widening of the caudal vena cava is visible on both these views of a Cavalier King Charles Spaniel with tricuspid dysplasia and right heart failure.

Fig. 45.11   Distended pulmonary arteries and veins (pulmonary overcirculation). Both the pulmonary veins and pulmonary arteries are distended in this Springer Spaniel with a patent ductus arteriosus. This is typical of pulmonary over-circulation secondary to a left-to-right shunt. The cranial lobe vessels are best seen in the lateral view (arrows) and the caudal lobe vessels are best seen in the dorsoventral view.

Table 45.11   Recording an ECG

- Place dog in right lateral recumbency on insulated surface
- Attach electrodes to loose skin on limbs with plenty of gel
    red (RA) right forelimb
    yellow (LA) left forelimb
    green (LF) left hindlimb
    black (RF) right hindlimb
- Record calibration mark
- Record a few complexes of each lead at 50 mm/s
- Record a longer rhythm strip of lead II at 25 mm/s
- LABEL with patient details/date!

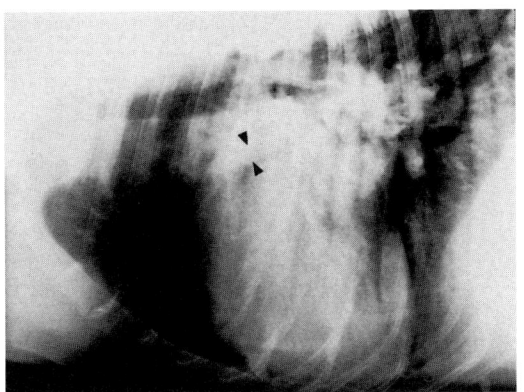

a

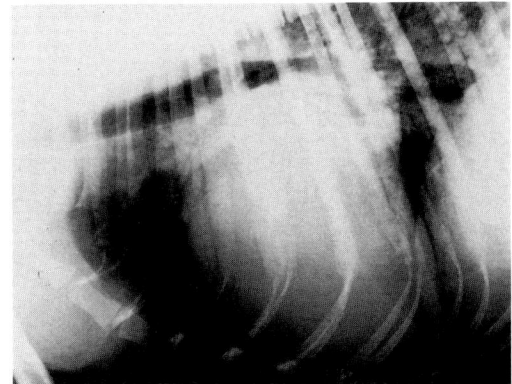

a

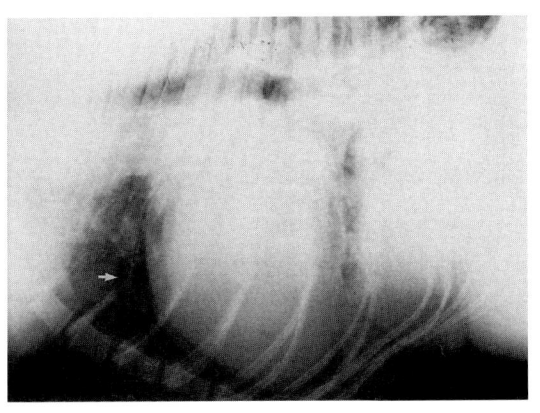

b

Fig. 45.12 Distended pulmonary veins. The pulmonary veins are much wider than the pulmonary arteries in this Dobermann with dilated cardiomyopathy (pulmonary veins = open arrows, pulmonary arteries = closed arrows). This is typical of left heart failure, with increased left atrial pressures transmitted to the pulmonary veins.

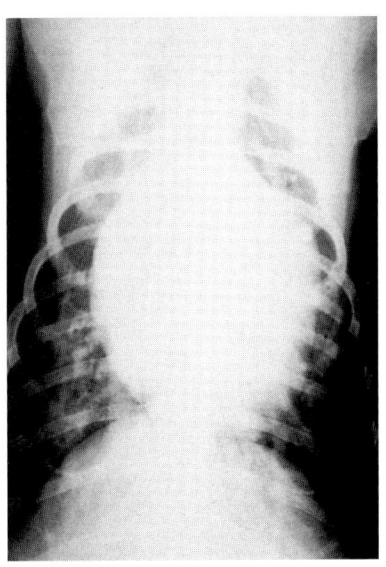

b

Fig. 45.13 Hilar interstitial oedema. This 2-year-old Labrador with mitral dysplasia has a hazy interstitial pattern around the hilus, obscuring the borders of the left atrium and the clarity of the vessels in this region. The cranial and ventral areas appear normal. This distribution of pulmonary oedema is often seen with chronic left-sided failure.

Fig. 45.14 Alveolar oedema. The cardiac silhouette is itself somewhat obscured in this Dobermann with dilated cardiomyopathy, with fluffy opacities affecting most of the lungfields, including the cranial lobes and the periphery. Air bronchograms can be seen in the ventral cranial lobe on the lateral view (arrow).

Table 45.12 Lead II measurements.

Rate	70–160/min (adults)	
	60–140/min (giant breeds)	
	70–180/min (toy breeds)	
	Up to 220/min (puppies)	
P duration	<0.04 s	2 boxes wide
P amplitude	<0.4 mV	4 boxes tall
PR interval	0.06–0.13 s	3 to 6½ boxes
R amplitude	3.0 mV in large breeds	30 boxes
	2.5 mV in small breeds	25 boxes
QRS	0.06 s in large breeds	3 boxes
duration	0.05 s in small breeds	2½ boxes
QT interval	0.15–0.25 s (depending on heart rate)	7½ to 12½ boxes
T amplitude	0.05–1.0 mV (or <¼ R wave height)	½ to 10 boxes
ST segment	<0.2 mV depression	<2 boxes depression
	<0.15 mV elevation	<1½ boxes elevation
MEA	+40° to +100°	

All measured at 50 m/s and 1 cm = 1 mV, i.e. one box = 0.02 s wide × 0.1 mV tall.

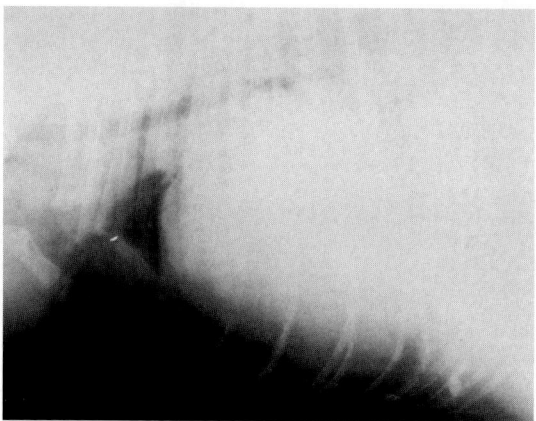

a

Fig. 45.15 Pleural effusion. The outline of the heart is obscured, and there is 'leafing' or 'scalloping' of the lung lobes, where they are retracted from the chest walls. Interlobar fissures can be seen (arrow).

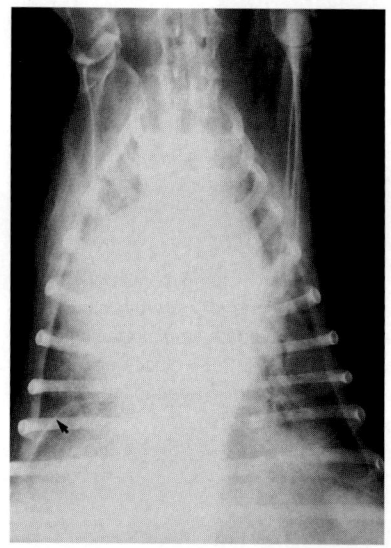

b

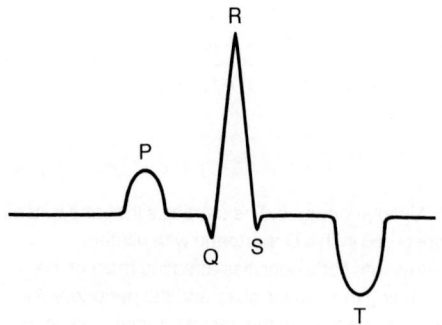

P wave – represents atrial depolarisation

P–Q – conduction through the AV node

QRS complex – ventricular depolarisation

ST segment – period between ventricular depolarisation and repolarisation

T wave – repolarisation of the ventricles

Fig. 45.16 Basic electrocardiogram.

Box 45.3 Basic questions for ECG interpretation.

- Question 1 – Are there P waves visible?

P waves indicate atrial depolarisation.

Absence of P waves suggests either
- no normal atrial depolarisation, e.g. *atrial fibrillation, atrial standstill*, or
- the P waves are hidden within the QRS complexes, e.g. *ventricular tachycardial junctional tachycardia*
- Question 2 – Is there a P wave for every QRS complex, and a QRS complex for every P wave?

P waves without associated QRS complexes indicate atrial depolarisation which has not been conducted through the atrioventricular node to the ventricles, i.e. *atrioventricular block*.

QRS complexes without P waves are either ectopic complexes (premature or escape), atrial fibrillation or sinoventricular complexes (atrial standstill).

- Question 3 – What is the relationship between the P waves and QRS complexes?

Normal PQ interval which remains constant = sinus rhythm

Long PQ interval = first degree atrioventricular (AV) block

PQ interval is long and varies = vagal influence on SA node – Wenckebach phenomenon

No consistent relationship of any sort = third degree (complete) atrioventricular block

- Question 4 – Are the QRS complexes narrow (normal) or wide (bizarre-looking)?

Narrow complexes indicate rapid conduction through the ventricular myocardium, which can only occur when conduction spreads via the bundle branches and Purkinje system.

Narrow complexes therefore indicate complexes of supraventricular origin.

Wide complexes suggest that the ventricles have taken more time than normal to become depolarised. This means that spread of conduction has not taken place via the bundle branches and Purkinje system, but instead by passive cell-to-cell conduction, which is much slower.

Wide complexes indicate
- *ventricular ectopic complexes* (premature or escapes)
- *bundle branch block*

- Question 5 – Is the rhythm regular or irregular?

Some rhythms are usually very regular, e.g. *supraventricular tachycardias, sustained ventricular tachycardia.*

Some rhythms are always irregular, e.g. *sinus arrhythmia, atrial fibrillation, sinus rhythm interrupted by ectopics.*

- Question 6 – Do all the complexes look the same?

If there is more than one form of QRS complex, one should attempt to identify to classify the complexes as:

Sinus in origin	normal, narrow QRS complexes consistently associated with P waves and a normal PQ interval
Supraventricular	normal, narrow complexes
Ventricular	wide, and bizarre

- Question 7 – What is the heart rate?

Slow heart rates (<65/min)	sinus arrhythmia
	sinus bradycardia
	2nd/3rd degree AV block
	atrial standstill
	sinus arrest
Fast heart rates (>160/min)	sinus tachycardia
	atrial fibrillation
	supraventricular tachycardias
	some ventricular tachycardias

Rhythm	Key features	Treatment
Normal rhythms		
Sinus rhythm Fig. 45.18	• Regular • 60–160/min • Normal P waves • Normal QRS complexes	None required
Sinus arrhythmia Fig. 45.19	• Heart rate varies with respiration • 60–140 beats/min • Normal P waves (height may vary) • Normal QRS complexes	None required
Sinus tachycardia Fig. 45.20 Seen with increased sympathetic tone, fear, fever, etc.	• Regular fast rhythm • >160 beats/min • Normal P waves • Normal QRS complexes	None – treat underlying cause
Sinus bradycardia Fig. 45.21 Often seen with cranial injury/disease, hypothyroidism	• Regular slow rhythm • <70 beats/min • Normal P waves • Normal QRS complexes	None – treat underlying cause
Pathological bradycardias		
Sinus arrest Fig. 45.22	• Normal P waves & QRS complexes but periods >2 × normal RR intervals with no complexes at all • Pauses may be interrupted by escapes (= narrow or bizarre complexes without P waves)	• Treat hyperkalaemia • Atropine • Propantheline • Terbutaline • Pacemaker
Atrial standstill Fig. 45.23 Associated with hyperkalaemia, muscular dystrophies	• No P waves • Slow rate • QRS complexes may be normal and narrow, or wide (hyperkalaemia)	• Atropine • Propantheline • Terbutaline • Pacemaker
'Brady-tachy' syndrome Sometimes called 'sick sinus syndrome' Fig. 45.24a	• Periods of sinus arrest interspersed with supraventricular tachycardias	• Pacemaker if symptomatic, may require subsequent therapy for tachycardias
Atrioventricular block		
1st degree Fig. 45.24b Increased vagal tone	• PQ interval >0.13 s • Normal P-QRS complexes	None

Table 45.13 Common canine rhythms.

Table 45.13   *Continued.*

Rhythm	Key features	Treatment

2nd degree
Fig. 45.25
Increased vagal
  tone/AV node
  disease
	• Some P waves
	  unassociated with QRS
	  complexes
	• PQ interval may vary
	  (Mobitz type I)
	• Normal (type A) or wide
	  (type B) QRS complexes
		• Often none with
		  type A / Mobitz
		  type I
		• Pacemaker if
		  symptomatic
		  (usually type B)

3rd degree
Fig. 45.26
AV node disease
  (neoplasia,
  cardiomyopathy,
  idiopathic)
	• P waves not associated
	  with QRS complexes
	• QRS complexes may be
	  wide and bizarre
		• Pacemaker
		
		• Terbutaline

Supraventricular tachycardias		

Supraventricular
  premature
  complexes
Fig. 45.27
Atrial stretch/disease
	• Ectopic complexes
	  closely following sinus
	  complexes
	• Normal configuration
	  ectopic QRS complexes
	• P wave of ectopic
	  abnormal (if visible)
		Treat underlying
		  cause

Supraventricular
  tachycardia
Fig. 45.28
Atrial stretch/disease,
  idiopathic
	• Rapid, regular rate
	  (often >300/min)
	• Normal QRS complexes
	• P waves hidden or
	  abnormal
		• Beta-blocking
		  drugs
		• Calcium
		  channel
		  blockers
		• Digoxin

Atrial fibrillation Fig. 45.29 Atrial stretch	• Rapid rate • Irregular • No P waves	Digoxin
Ventricular tachycardias		

Ventricular premature
  complexes
Fig. 45.30
Ventricular disease,
  metabolic disease
	• Wide and bizarre
	  premature ectopic QRS
	  complexes
		• Treat underlying
		  disease

Ventricular tachycardia
Fig. 45.31
Ventricular disease,
  metabolic disease
	• Wide and bizarre
	  complexes
	• No consistent
	  associated P waves
	• Rate >120/min
		• Lignocaine if
		  sustained
		• Treat underlying
		  disease
		• Procainamide,
		  mexiletine, beta
		  blockers if
		  symptomatic

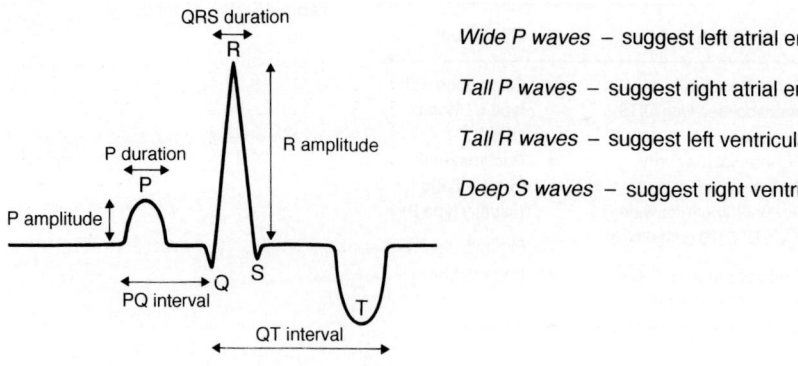

Fig. 45.17   Normal electrocardiogram pattern.
Note: all ECGs are recorded at 50 mm/s, 1 cm = 1 mV, unless otherwise stated.

Wide P waves – suggest left atrial enlargement

Tall P waves – suggest right atrial enlargement

Tall R waves – suggest left ventricular enlargement

Deep S waves – suggest right ventricular enlargement

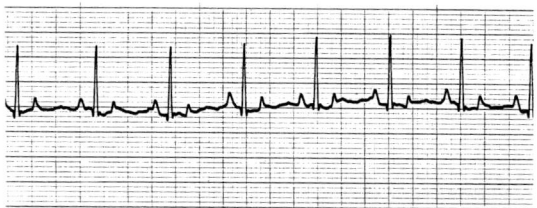

Fig. 45.18   Sinus rhythm.

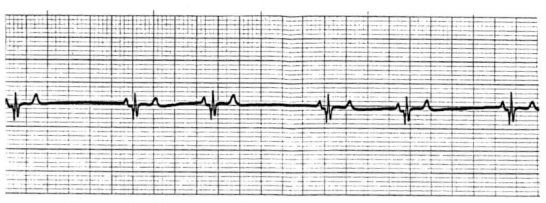

Fig. 45.21   Sinus bradycardia (25 mm/s).

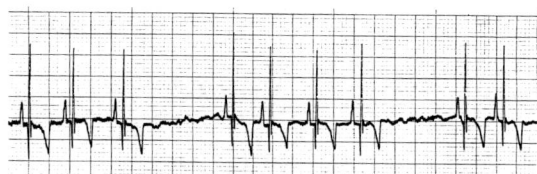

Fig. 45.19   Sinus arrhythmia (25 mm/s).

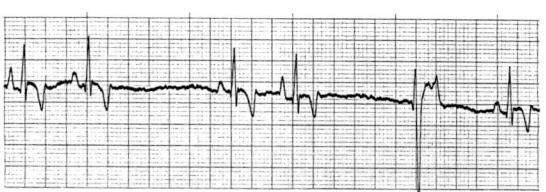

Fig. 45.22   Sinus arrest (25 mm/s).

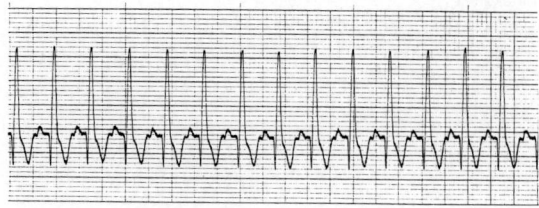

Fig. 45.20   Sinus tachycardia.

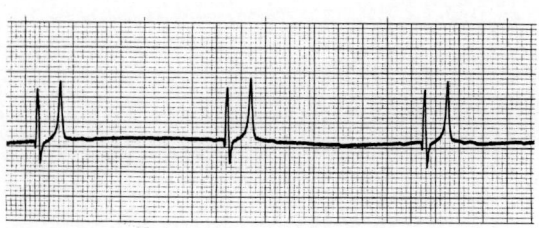

Fig. 45.23   Atrial standstill (25 mm/s).

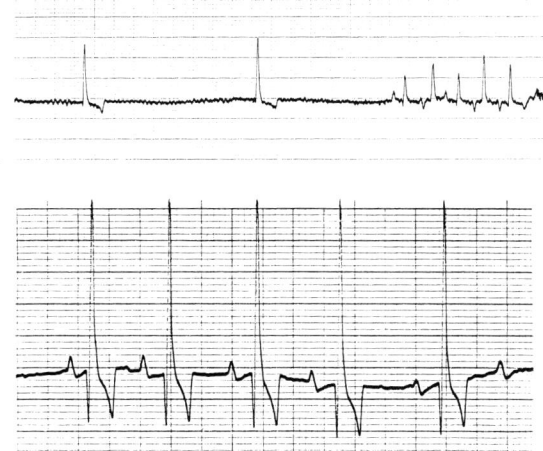

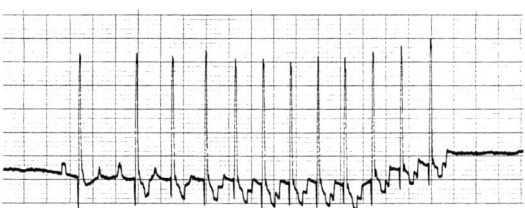

Fig. 45.28 Supraventricular tachycardia (25 mm/s).

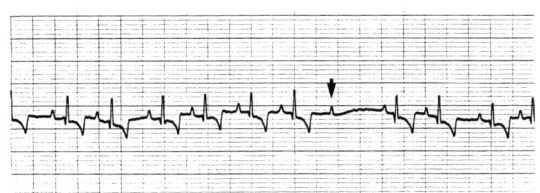

Fig. 45.24 **a** 'Brady-tachy' syndrome (25 mm/s). **b** First degree atrioventricular block.

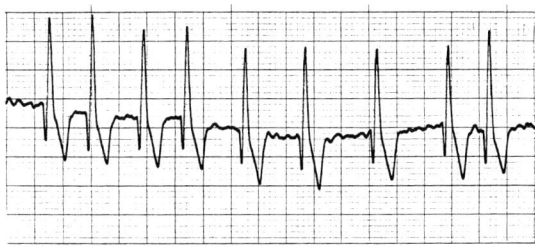

Fig. 45.29 Atrial fibrillation.

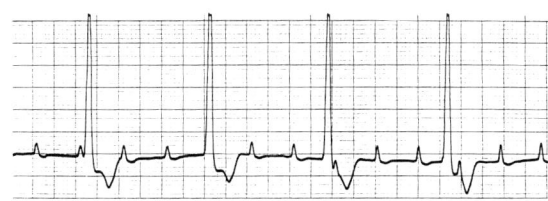

Fig. 45.25 Second degree atrioventricular block (25 mm/s).

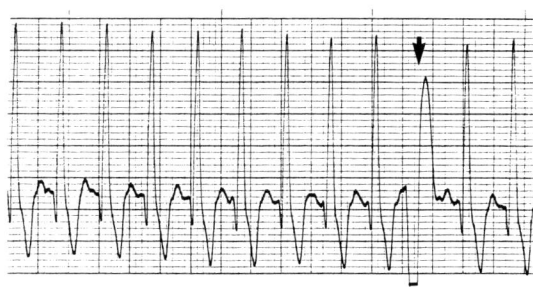

Fig. 45.30 Ventricular premature complexes.

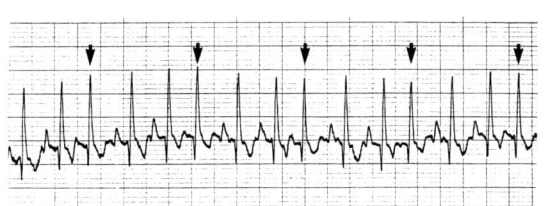

Fig. 45.26 Third degree atrioventricular block (25 mm/s).

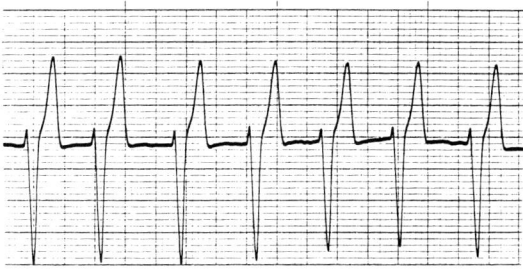

Fig. 45.27 Supraventricular premature complexes.

Fig. 45.31 Ventricular tachycardia.

Echocardiography

Echocardiography has revolutionised veterinary cardiology. It is now possible to diagnose complex congenital anomalies completely non-invasively using Doppler echocardiography, and even basic two-dimensional echocardiograpy machines will allow definitive diagnosis of myocardial failure or pericardial effusions (Moise 1988).

Echocardiography is particularly useful for delineating soft tissue–fluid interfaces, and as images can be produced in real-time, it is a modality ideally suited to the study of the heart. Echocardiography can be used to image lesions, to measure cardiac dimensions, and to assess cardiac function.

Types of Echocardiography

In all forms, the transducer acts as both an emitter of ultrasound waves, and a receiver.

Two-dimensional echocardiography (2D echo) is usually carried out with a sector probe, which produces a fan-shaped beam and a fan-shaped image on the monitor. The image moves in real-time. This is the most accessible form of echocardiography, but it still requires a tomographic understanding of cardiac anatomy.

M-mode echocardiography uses a single ('ice-pick') beam of ultrasound, and produces a graphical display of the points of the heart crossed by the beam against time. This is the most accurate modality for timed cardiac events.

Doppler-echocardiography uses the Doppler principle to give information about the velocity and direction of blood flow within the heart. This allows the non-invasive assessment of pressure gradients between cardiac chambers and across valves. *Colour-flow Doppler* is an added sophistication which overlays information about the direction and nature of blood flow on top of the black-and-white 2D image using colour.

Transducers

The tremendous size variation between breeds means that one transducer is unlikely to produce optimal images in all dogs. For small puppies 7.5 MHz transducers are ideal, whereas 3.5 MHz may be more suitable for large broad-chested dogs. A 5 MHz probe is a compromise.

Technique

- Clip the coat over the apex beat on both sides of the chest.
- Try to scan without sedating the dog (but sedation may be used in difficult patients).
- Ideally the dog should be placed in lateral recumbency, with the probe placed underneath the chest (via a cut-out portion of the table).
- Use liberal amounts of coupling gel.
- Employ a consistent routine, and attempt to obtain all images in every dog to encourage familiarity with standard views (see Table 45.14).

Table 45.14   Standard echocardiographic views.

Right parasternal long-axis views
   Fig. 45.32. 4-chamber view
   Fig. 45.33 Left ventricular outflow view
Right parasternal short-axis views
   Fig. 45.34 Level of papillary muscle
   Fig. 45.35 Level of chordae tendineae
   Fig. 45.36 Mitral valve level
   FIg. 45.37 Aortic valve level
Left caudal parasternal views
   Fig. 45.38 Long-axis 2-chamber view
   Fig. 45.39 Long-axis left ventricular outflow view
   Fig. 45.40 4-chamber (inflow) view
   Fig. 45.41 5-chamber (LV outflow) view
Left cranial parasternal views
   Fig. 45.42 Long-axis view 1
   Fig. 45.43 Long-axis view 2
   Fig. 45.44 Long-axis view 3

LV, left ventricle; LA, left atrium; RA, right atrium; RV, right ventricle; Ao, aorta; PA, pulmonary artery; MV, mitral valve; TV, tricuspid valve; R, right coronary cusp; L, left coronary cusp; NC, non-coronary cusp.

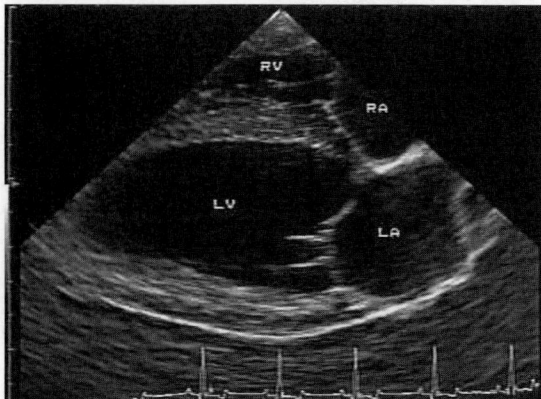

Fig. 45.32   Four-chamber view.

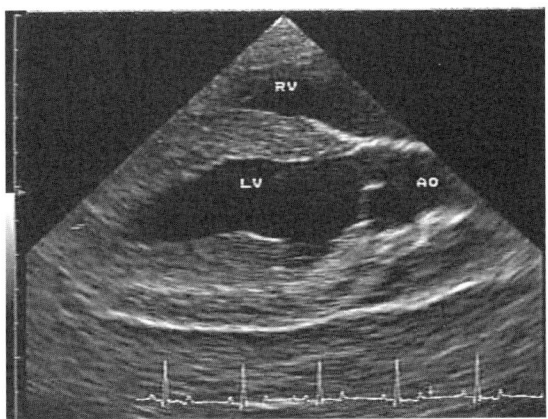

Fig. 45.33 Left ventricular outflow view.

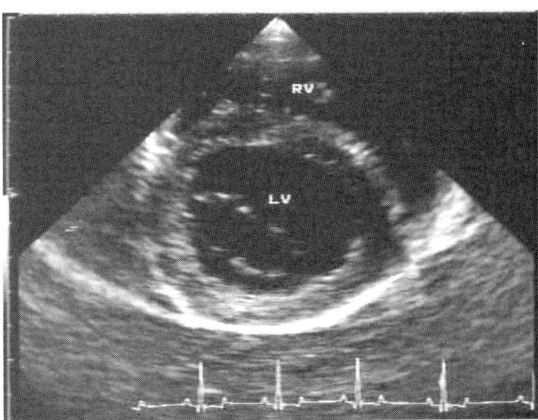

Fig. 45.36 Mitral valve level.

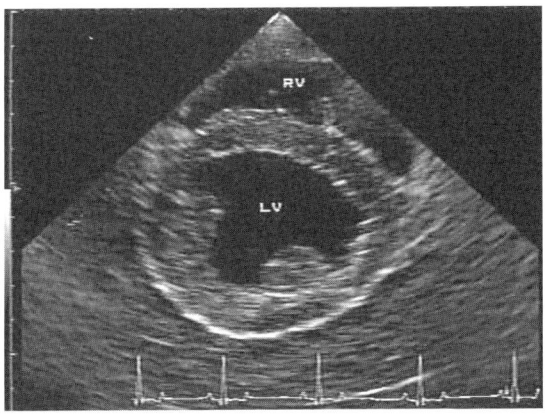

Fig. 45.34 Level of papillary muscles.

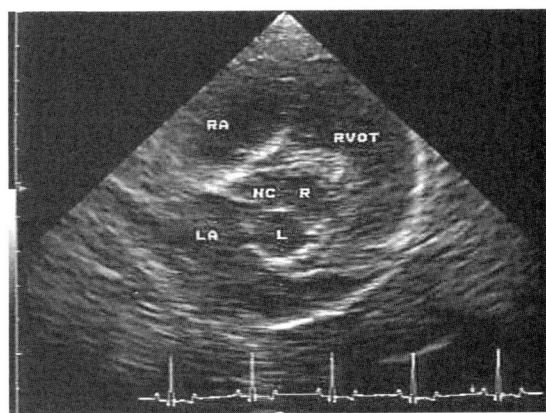

Fig. 45.37 Aortic valve level.

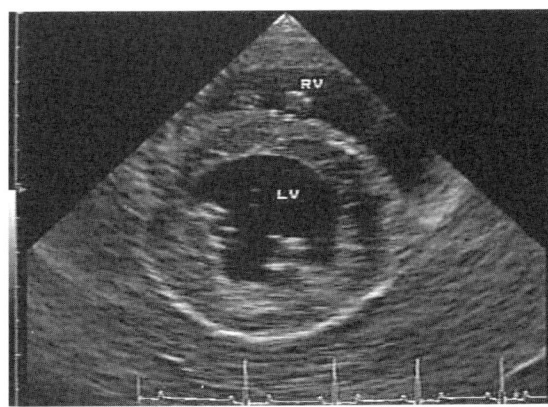

Fig. 45.35 Level of chordae tendineae.

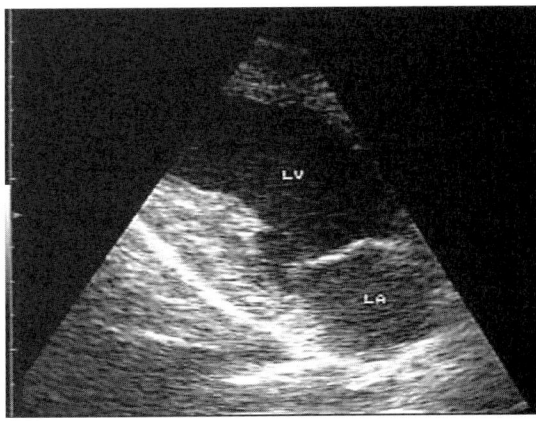

Fig. 45.38 Long-axis two-chamber view.

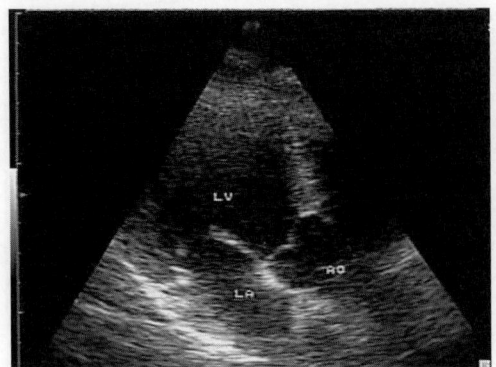

Fig. 45.39   Long-axis left ventricular outflow view.

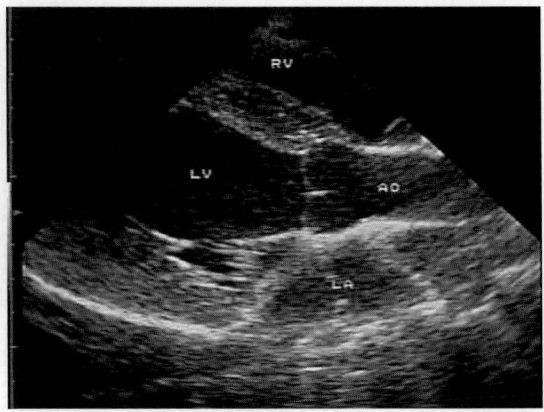

Fig. 45.42   Long-axis view 1.

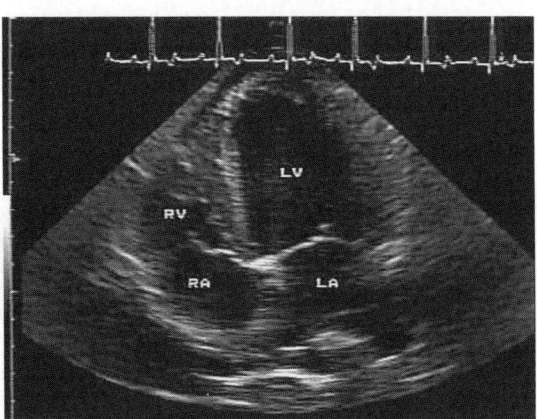

Fig. 45.40   Four-chamber (inflow) view.

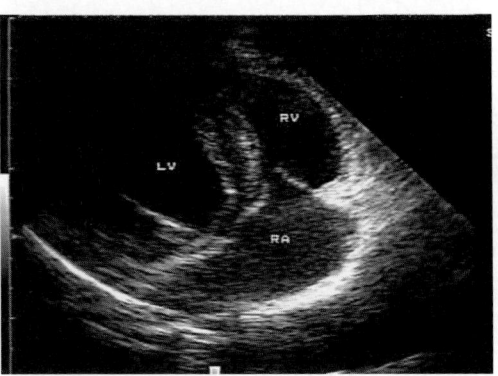

Fig. 45.43   Long-axis view 2.

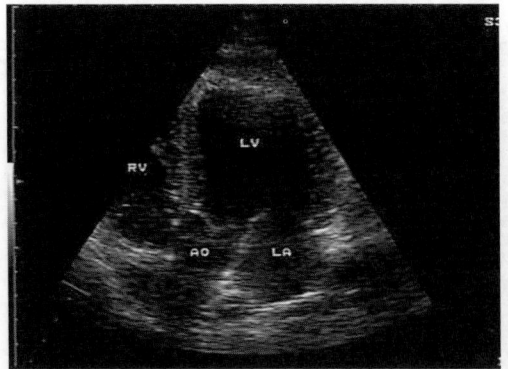

Fig. 45.41   Five-chamber (LV outflow) view.

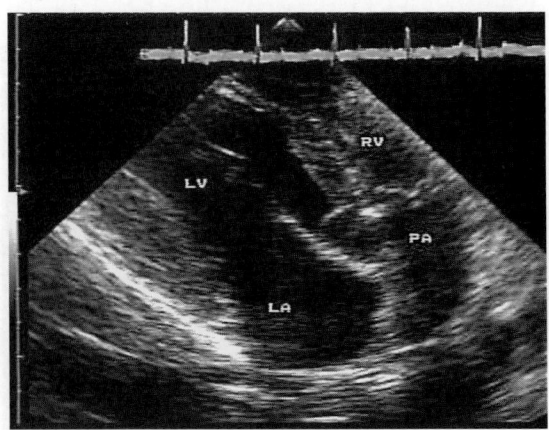

Fig. 45.44   Long-axis view 3.

Echocardiographic Interpretation

Interpretation of morphological abnormalities is usually based on assessment of two-dimensional images. A summary of two-dimensional echocardiographic interpretion is described in Table 45.15. Accurate measurement of wall thickness and chamber diameter should be made from M–mode images (see Table 45.16). Normal values have been published according to bodyweight (Bonagura *et al.* 1985) and on a breed basis for Toy Poodles, Pembroke Corgis, Afghan Hounds and Golden Retrievers (Morison *et al.* 1992), and Cocker Spaniels (Gooding *et al.* 1986).

Doppler Echocardiography

Doppler echocardiography can be used to obtain a definitive diagnosis in the majority of cases with cardiac disease

Table 45.15 Interpretation of two-dimensional echocardiographic images.

Site	Abnormality	Causes
Left atrium	Dilation	Mitral endocardiosis
		Dilated cardiomyopathy
		Patent ductus arteriosus
		Ventricular septal defect
		Mitral dysplasia
Mitral valve	Leaflet thickening	Endocardiosis
		Mitral dysplasia
		Endocarditis
Left ventricle	Dilation	Mitral endocardiosis
		Dilated cardiomyopathy
		Patent ductus arteriosus
		Ventricular septal defect
		Mitral dysplasia
Left ventricle	Hypertrophy	Aortic stenosis
		Systemic hypertension
		(Hypertrophic cardiomyopathy)
Left ventricular outflow tract	Outflow tract lesions	Subaortic stenosis
Aortic valves	Leaflet thickening	Aortic stenosis
		Endocarditis
Right atrium	Dilation	Tricuspid endocardiosis
		Dilated cardiomyopathy
		Pulmonic stenosis with tricuspid regurgitation
		Tricuspid dysplasia
		Atrial septal defect
Tricuspid valve	Leaflet thickening	Endocardiosis
		Tricuspid dysplasia
Right ventricle	Dilation	Tricuspid endocardiosis
		Dilated cardiomyopathy
		Pulmonic stenosis with tricuspid regurgitation
		Tricuspid dysplasia
		Ventricular septal defect
Right ventricle	Hypertrophy	Pulmonic stenosis
		Pulmonary hypertension
Right ventricular outflow tract	Outflow tract lesions	Subvalvular pulmonic stenosis
Pulmonic valve	Leaflet abnormalities	Pulmonic stenosis

Chordae tendineae level Fig. 45.45	LV diameter at end-systole (LVDs) LV diameter at end-diastole (LVDd) LV free wall thickness at end-systole (LVFWs) LV free wall thickness at end-diastole (LVFWd) Interventricular septal thickness at end-systole (IVSs) Interventricular septal thickness at end-diastole (IVSd)	**Table 45.16** M-mode measurements.
Mitral valve level Fig. 45.46	E-point to septal separation (EPSS)	
Aortic valve level Fig. 45.47	Aortic diameter in diastole (Ao) Left atrial diameter in systole (LA)	

Derived M-mode indices

Fractional shortening (FS%) $\dfrac{\text{LVDd} - \text{LVDs}}{\text{LVDd}} \times 100$

% Free wall thickening $\dfrac{\text{LVFWs} - \text{LVFWd}}{\text{LVFWs}} \times 100$

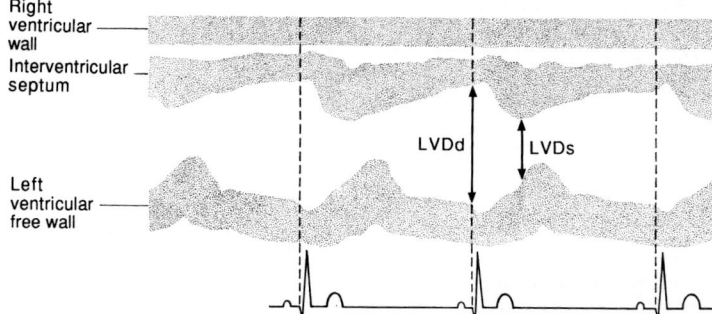

Fig. 45.45   Chordae tendineae level.

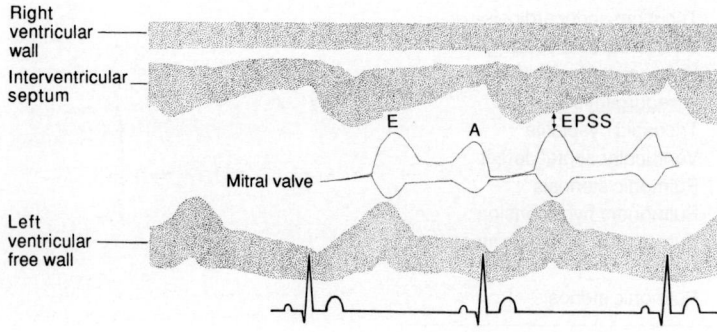

Fig. 45.46   Mitral valve level.

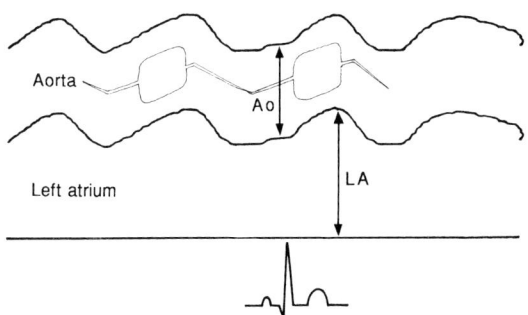

Fig. 45.47 Aortic valve level.

(particularly if colour flow mapping is available). Whereas invasive techniques such as cardiac catheterisation, intra-cardiac pressure measurement and selective angiography were previously necessary for accurately defining lesions, the same ends can now be achieved by echo-Doppler in even unsedated dogs (Darke 1992). Doppler echocardiography is based on the Doppler principle, so that the frequency of the reflected ultrasound wave is increased or decreased according to whether the target (red blood cells) are moving towards or away from the transducer. The velocity of the target red blood cells can also be calculated from the change in frequency, although the alignment of the ultrasound beam is critical for accurate calculations.

Main Applications

Detection of High Velocity Flow:

- aortic stenosis
- pulmonic stenosis
- mitral regurgitation
- tricuspid regurgitation
- ventricular septal defects

The measured blood flow velocity can be used to determine the pressure gradient between two chambers or vessels, which is of particular interest in aortic stenosis, pulmonic stenosis, septal defects and pulmonary hypertension.

Detection of Abnormal Blood Flow Direction:

- mitral regurgitation
- tricuspid regurgitation
- aortic regurgitation
- septal defects
- patent ductus arteriosus

Assessment of Systolic and Diastolic Function:

- systolic time intervals
- mitral filling patterns (diastolic function)

MANAGEMENT OF CONGESTIVE HEART FAILURE

The most effective way to treat congestive cardiac failure is to treat the underlying cause. This can be achieved surgically with patent ductus arteriosus, but is difficult in most veterinary situations. Logical therapy requires a definitive diagnosis, but in the initial stages treatment can be initiated before a diagnosis is reached if congestive heart failure is recognised. Pericardial effusion is an important separate case, where the condition should be recognised and the effusion drained as soon as possible.

Management of Acute Cardiac Failure

- Minimise stress.
- Ensure adequate oxygenation.
- Reduce preload.
- Obtain definitive diagnosis.
- Give specific treatment.

Management of Chronic Cardiac Failure

- Obtain definitive diagnosis.
- Control pulmonary oedema/ascites with diuretics.
- Reduce activation of renin–angiotensin system.
- Give specific treatment (e.g. surgery, positive inotropes, reduce afterload).
- Keep exercise within realistic limits.

The commonly used cardiac drugs are listed in Tables 45.17–45.20 and their application is covered in specific cardiac therapy in Chapters 46 and 47.

Other Management Strategies

Exercise Restriction

Rest is vital in the early stages of acute heart failure, to reduce oxygen consumption and improve renal perfusion.

Table 45.17   Drugs that reduce preload.

Drug type	Examples	Actions
Diuretics	Frusemide	Loop diuretic, i.e. potent Can lead to hypokalaemia, and hyponatraemia Give minimum dose that will relieve clinical signs Can stimulate renin–angiotensin system
	Spironolactone	Weak diuretic Potassium-sparing Aldosterone antagonist Slow onset of action Insufficient as a sole diuretic, but may be effective in conjunction with other diuretics and angiotensin converting enzyme inhibitors in refractory cases
Venodilators	Nitroglycerine (glyceryl nitrate)	Useful in acute cardiogenic pulmonary oedema 2% ointment absorbed through skin Avoid contact with hands Also available as transdermal glyceryl trinitrate patches (0.1 mg/h for small dogs, 0.2 mg/h for larger dogs)
Angiotensin converting enzyme (ACE) inhibitors	Enalapril	Effects include vasodilation of arteries and veins Inhibits aldosterone release, thereby reducing sodium and water retention Dilation of renal efferent arterioles, reducing glomerular filtration pressures Inhibits release of arginine vasopressin Reduces effects of sympathetic stimulation by inhibiting release of noradrenaline from sympathetic nerve terminals Enalapril has proven efficacy in mitral insufficiency and dilated cardiomyopathy in dogs (The COVE Study Group 1995)
	Benazepril	As for enalapril, with similar beneficial effects but 50% biliary excretion

Table 45.18   Drugs that reduce afterload.

Drug type	Examples	Actions
Arteriolar dilators	Hydralazine	May be particularly beneficial in mitral insufficiency May cause symptomatic hypotension May cause reflex tachycardia
ACE inhibitors		See Table 45.17

Table 45.19   Drugs that increase contractility.

Drug type	Examples	Action
Positive inotropes Cardiac glycosides	Digoxin	Do not give loading dose – start on maintenance dose Steady-state levels achieved within 5 days Therapeutic levels (obtained 6–8 h after last tablet) = 0.8–2.4 ng/ml Always stop digoxin if gastrointestinal signs or development of dysrhythmias Decrease dose proportionately for obese dogs, fluid retention and renal failure,
	Digitoxin	Metabolised by liver (safer for animals with renal failure) Available preparations inconvenient for large dogs
Sympathomimetic amines	Dobutamine	Only available as intravenous infusion Main indication severe myocardial failure Start at low doses Some beneficial effects persist after cessation of infusion

Drug	Trade name	Dose p.o.
Frusemide	Lasix*	2–4 mg/kg s.i.d.–t.i.d.
Spironolactone	Aldactone	2–4 mg/kg per day
Glyceryl trinitrate (nitroglycerine)	Percutol	5–40 mm ($1/_4$–$11/_2$ inch) length of ointment t.i.d. on the skin
Hydralazine	Apresoline	0.5–2.0 mg/kg b.i.d.
Enalapril	Cardiovet*	0.5 mg/kg s.i.d.–b.i.d.
Benazepril	Fortekor*	0.25 mg/kg s.i.d.–b.i.d.
Digoxin	Lanoxin	0.01 mg/kg b.i.d.
		0.22 mg/m^2 b.i.d.
Digitoxin		0.03–0.06 mg/kg b.i.d.–t.i.d.
Dobutamine	Dobutrex	5–20 µg/kg per min i.v.
Diltiazem	Tildiem	0.5–1.0 mg/kg t.i.d.
Propranolol	Inderal	0.2–1.0 mg/kg t.i.d.
Atenolol	Tenormin	0.25–1.0 mg/kg s.i.d.–b.i.d.
Atropine		0.01–0.04 mg/kg s.c., i.m., i.v.
Propantheline	Pro-Banthine	3.75–7.5 mg b.i.d.–t.i.d.
Lignocaine		2 mg/kg i.v. bolus repeated up to 3 times
		25–80 µg/kg per min infusion
Procainamide	Pronestyl	5–15 mg/kg q.i.d.
		10–20 mg/kg i.m.
Mexiletine	Mexitil	5–8 mg/kg b.i.d.–t.i.d.

Table 45.20 Drug dosages.

* Licensed for use in dogs.

In the long-term management of heart failure, strict rest serves no purpose. However, it is important to avoid extremes of exercise, as excessive exertion results in reduced renal blood flow and increased sodium and water retention.

Dietary Sodium Restriction

Low salt diets have been advocated for many years for dogs with congestive heart failure, although there have been no studies examining their efficacy. Recent studies suggest that low sodium diets may actually stimulate the renin–angiotensin system, which could be interpreted as a potentially undesirable effect. The place of low sodium diets in the management of canine congestive heart is at present under scrutiny.

Management of Specific Cardiac Conditions

This is covered under the specific diseases in Chapters 46 and 47.

REFERENCES

Bonagura, J.D., O'Grady, M.R. & Herring, D.S. (1985). Echocardiography. Principles of interpretation. *Veterinary Clinics of North America*, **15**, 1177–1194.

Braunwald, E., Sonnenblick, E.H. & Ross, J. (1992). Mechanisms of cardiac contraction and relaxation. In: *Heart Disease*, (ed. E. Braunwald), pp. 351–392. W.B. Saunders, Philadelphia.

Buchanan, J.W. (1992). Causes and prevalence of cardiovascular disease. In: *Current Veterinary Therapy XI*, (eds R.W. Kirk & J.D. Bonagura), pp. 647–654. W.B. Saunders, Philadelphia.

The COVE Study Group (1995). Controlled clinical evaluation of enalapril in dogs with heart failure: results of the Cooperative Veterinary Enalapril Study Group. *Journal of Veterinary Medicine*, **9**, 243–252.

Darke, P.G.G. (1992). Doppler echocardiography. *Journal of Small Animal Practice*, **33**, 104–112.

Gompf, R. (1988). The clinical approach to heart disease: history and physical examination. In: *Canine and Feline Cardiology*, (ed. P.R. Fox), pp. 29–42. Churchill Livingstone, New York.

Gooding, J.P., Robinson, W.F. & Mews, G.C. (1986). Echo-cardiographic assessment of left ventricular dimensions in clinically normal English Cocker spaniels. *American Journal of Veterinary Research*, **47**, 293–300.

International Small Animal Cardiac Health Council (1995). Recommendations for the diagnosis and the treatment of heart failure in small animals (Appendix 1). In: *Manual of Canine and Feline Cardiology*, (eds M.S. Miller & L.P. Tilley), 2nd edn. pp. 469–502. W.B. Saunders, Philadelphia.

Levick, J.R. (1995). *An Introduction to Cardiovascular Physiology*, 2nd edn. Butterworth-Heinemann, Oxford.

Moise, N.S. (1988). Echocardiography. In. *Canine and Feline Cardiology*, (ed. P.R. Fox), pp. 113–156. Churchill Livingstone, New York.

Morison, S.A., Moise, N.S., Scarlett, J., Mohammed, H. & Yeager, A.E. (1992). Effect of breed and body weight on echocardiographic values in four breeds of differing somatotype. *Journal of Veterinary Internal Medicine*, **6**, 220–224.

Suter, P.F. (1984). *Thoracic radiography. A Text Atlas of Thoracic Diseases of the Dog and Cat.* Peter F. Suter, Wettswil, Switzerland.

Tilley, L.P. (1992). *Essentials of Canine and Feline Electrocardiography*, 3rd edn. Lea & Febiger, Philadelphia.

Chapter 46

Congenital Heart Disease

M. Cobb

The purpose of this chapter is to review the various forms of congenital heart disease in the dog. For each condition an overview of the pathophysiology is given. The descriptions of the clinical features, investigation, management and prognosis are given in tables and clear lists. Congenital heart disease is rare, occurring in 0.46–0.85% of dogs surveyed (Buchanan 1992). It is usually identified when a heart murmur is discovered on clinical examination in a young dog. If the lesion is severe the patient may be stunted. Occasionally the patient presents with evidence of forward or backward cardiac failure. Diagnosis and assessment of the severity of a particular lesion and therefore the prognosis, usually requires ancillary diagnostic tests such as Doppler echocardiography, cardiac catheterisation, pressure measurement, angiography and blood gas analysis. Multiple defects may co-exist in an individual. Individual lesions vary in their severity.

PATENT DUCTUS ARTERIOSUS

Patent ductus arteriosus (PDA) is one of the most common congenital cardiac defects. The predisposed breeds include Pomeranian, Shetland Sheepdog, English Springer Spaniel, Maltese Terrier, Poodles, Yorkshire Terrier, Border Collies and Collie Crosses, German Shepherd Dog, and Cavalier King Charles Spaniel. PDA is one of the few cardiac conditions seen more frequently in females than in males. An autosomal dominant mode of inheritance has been proposed (Patterson 1968).

Pathogenesis and Pathophysiology

The ductus arteriosus fails to close after birth, so that blood flows through the persistent connection from the descend-ing aorta into the main pulmonary artery *throughout* the cardiac cycle. Overcirculation of the pulmonary vasculature results, leading to volume overloading of the left heart. Mitral insufficiency and myocardial failure may develop secondary to this chronic volume overload. The end result in most cases is left-sided congestive heart failure, often before the animal reaches maturity. Very rarely, flow through a PDA is reversed, either because of failure of the pulmonary circulation to develop correctly or as a result of chronic pulmonary overcirculation resulting in the development of pulmonary hypertension (Eisenmenger's physiology). Reversal of flow results in flow of de-oxygenated blood to the caudal half of the body, consequently 'differential cyanosis' (cyanosis of the mucous membranes of the caudal half of the body only) may be seen.

Clinical Features

Affected animals may be presented with dyspnoea, coughing or exercise intolerance from left-sided heart failure (pulmonary oedema), or a murmur may be detected as an incidental finding. The findings on clinical examination include:

- characteristic 'machinery' murmur, continuous throughout the cardiac cycle over the left heart base (NB the diastolic component may be very localised);
- ± murmur of secondary mitral insufficiency;
- hyperkinetic ('water hammer') femoral pulse;
- murmur may be low grade and systolic only with a 'reverse' PDA.

Investigations are outlined in Table 46.1.

Management

The mainstay for treatment is surgical correction of the defect.

Table 46.1 Investigations into suspected cases of patent ductus arteriosus.

Radiography	Possible changes include: • left heart enlargement • dilation of the pulmonary artery / aorta / left atrial appendage on the dorsoventral view • evidence of pulmonary overcirculation
Electrocardiography	There are no specific changes, but common findings include: • evidence of left atrial and/or left ventricular enlargement (wide P waves, tall R waves) • dysrhythmias (especially atrial fibrillation)
Echocardiography	2D echocardiography may demonstrate left atrial and ventricular dilation, and eccentric hypertrophy due to volume overload. Dilation of the main pulmonary artery may be evident, but it is often difficult to image the ductus itself. Doppler echocardiography (and contrast echocardiography and/or selective angiography) may be necessary to diagnose PDA definitively (especially if shunting right to left) and rule out co-existing defects.

- Surgical ligation is curative and described in detail in Eyster 1993.
- Dogs with left-sided congestive heart failure are managed medically before surgery as described in Chapters 45 and 47.
- Surgery is contraindicated in right to left shunting PDAs as this may lead to right-sided failure due to the fibrosis in the pulmonary vasculature.

Prognosis

The prognosis is good if the defect is corrected early before secondary change has occurred, but poor once left-sided congestive failure develops. Surgery should be carried out as soon as a murmur is detected.

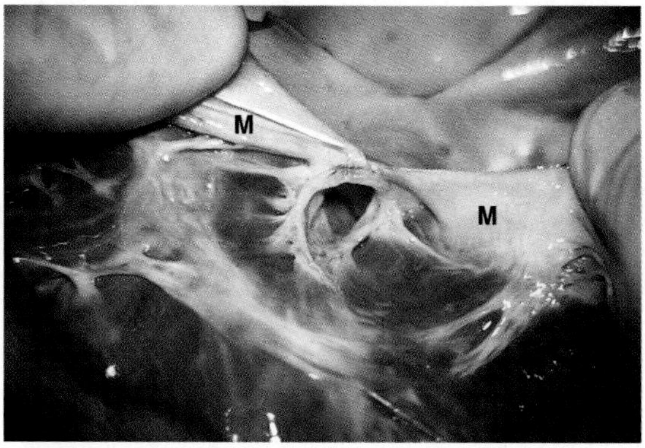

Fig. 46.1 Post-mortem specimen showing the left ventricular outflow tract of a dog with subvalvular aortic stenosis opened to show the fibrous subvalvular stenotic lesion below the aortic valve. (M: anterior mitral valve leaflet sectioned to show the lesion.)

AORTIC STENOSIS

Aortic stenosis (AS) is one of the most common congenital cardiac defects in the UK. Predisposed breeds include Boxers, Golden Retreivers, Rottweilers, German Shepherd Dogs and Newfoundlands. An autosomal dominant mode of inheritance has been proposed in the Newfoundland breed (Pyle *et al.* 1976).

Pathogenesis and Pathophysiology

Aortic stenosis is usually the result of a fibrous band or ring which develops below the valve (subaortic stenosis, Fig. 46.1) but can be the result of malformation of the valve itself, or, rarely, supravalvular lesions. Lesion severity, and therefore the resulting clinical syndrome, is very variable (Sisson 1992). The haemodynamic effect and the murmur associated with the lesion can increase with age until maturity. The lesion increases resistance to left ventricular ejection, resulting in concentric myocardial hypertrophy, which develops in proportion to the severity of the stenosis. If severe, this results in compromised myocardial perfusion, and ischaemia and ventricular dysrhythmias develop. Consequently, syncope and sudden death can occur with severe aortic stenosis. Secondary mitral insufficiency may occur, but congestive left heart failure is rare. Dogs with mild AS are usually asymptomatic.

Clinical Features

Dogs with severe AS may present with syncope on exertion, or can be asymptomatic. Occasionally sudden death may be the only sign. Findings on clinical examination include:

- harsh systolic heart murmur loudest over the left heart;
- the murmur may radiate to the thoracic inlet, the neck (over the carotid arteries) and along the spine;
- hypokinetic ('flat') femoral pulse in severe cases;
- dysrhythmias are common in severe AS.

Investigations are outlined in Table 46.2.

Management

Management and prognosis are determined by severity (Kienle *et al.* 1994). Mild cases do not require any treatment. Options for severe cases include:

- β adrenergic blocking drugs to reduce wall stress and improve myocardial oxygenation in patients with severe left ventricular concentric hypertrophy;
- anti-arrythmic drugs for dogs with ventricular dysrhythmias;
- balloon dilation (DeLellis *et al.* 1993) and surgical correction utilising cardiopulmonary bypass (Orton 1994).

The success with balloon dilation and surgery is still relatively unproven.

Prognosis

Mild lesions are associated with normal quality and duration of life, severe lesions associated with a high pressure gradient across the valve are associated with shorter life span, and a risk of sudden death.

PULMONIC STENOSIS

Predisposed breeds include Boxer, English Bulldog, Mastiff, Samoyed, Cocker Spaniel and Miniature Schnauzer.

Pathogenesis and Pathophysiology

Valvular, subvalvular and supravalvular lesions have all been described. The stenosis increases impedence to right ventricular ejection and results in concentric myocardial hypertrophy. In patients with severe stenosis, myocardial hypertrophy can result in dynamic obstruction, worsening the outflow obstruction. Secondary tricuspid regurgitation may develop as a result of right ventricular hypertrophy and atrioventricular valve distortion. Right-sided congestive failure may ultimately develop, and right atrial enlargement may lead to dysrhythmias.

Clinical Features

Affected dogs may present with right-sided heart failure (ascites), syncope on exertion, or may be asymptomatic. Findings on physical examination include:

- systolic heart murmur over the left heart near the sternum;
- murmur may be audible over the right heart base and may radiate widely (particularly dorsally) if loud;
- pulse quality is usually good.

Investigations are outlined in Table 46.3.

Table 46.2   Investigations in suspected cases of aortic stenosis.

Radiography	Plain radiography is rarely helpful, as the heart frequently appears normal. In severe cases there may be a post-stenotic dilation in the region of the ascending aorta
Electrocardiography	There may be electrocardiographic changes consistent with left atrial and/or left ventricular enlargement (wide P waves and tall R waves). ST segment changes as a result of ischaemia and dysrhythmias may be found, but are often only seen on an ECG recorded post-exercise
Echocardiography	If severe, AS may be diagnosed with 2D echocardiography. Findings include: • abnormal aortic valve cusps and/or subvalvular fibrous lesions, • concentric left ventricular hypertrophy. Doppler echocardiography or selective angiography may be necessary to diagnose AS definitively. Doppler echocardiography can also be used to assess the severity of the stenosis, as well as to rule out complicating co-existing lesions

Table 46.3   Investigations in suspected cases of pulmonic stenosis.

Radiography	Right heart enlargement Post-stenotic dilation in the main pulmonary artery Normal or hypovascular lung fields
Electrocardiography	There is often electrocardiographic evidence of right ventricular enlargement (deep S waves in leads I, II and III see Fig. 46.2)
Echocardiography	Changes on 2D echocardiography may be pronounced. The secondary effects of the right ventricular pressure overload may be more obvious than the stenosis itself. Typical features include: ● concentric right ventricular hypertrophy and flattening of the interventricular septum, ● abnormal valve cusps or subvalvular lesions. Doppler echocardiography or selective angiography may be necessary to diagnose definitively, assess severity and rule out-co-existing lesions (particularly septal defects)

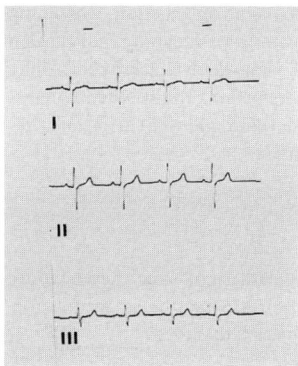

Fig. 46.2   ECG leads I, II and III recorded from a dog with right ventricular concentric hypertrophy secondary to severe pulmonic stenosis showing prominent S waves in all three leads.

Management

As with AS, the management and prognosis are determined by severity. Dogs with mild PS may not require any treatment. In patients with more severe stenosis, some form of correction may be indicated. There are two main types of correction:

● balloon valvuloplasty (Brownlie *et al.* 1991; Martin *et al.* 1992);
● surgical correction (Eyster 1993).

A number of methods of surgical correction have been described, and are particularly indicated in severe cases complicated by infundibular muscle hypertrophy. The potential risks of surgery are greater than with balloon valvuloplasty.

Prognosis

Mild lesions are associated with normal quality and duration of life. Severe lesions with a high pressure gradient across the outflow tract are associated with a poorer prognosis, with eventual development of right-sided heart failure or sudden death.

VENTRICULAR SEPTAL DEFECT

Pathogenesis and Pathophysiology

Ventricular septal defects (VSDs) are usually high in the membranous interventricular septum. Blood shunts left-to-right during systole resulting in pulmonary overcirculation, volume overloading of the left heart and sometimes secondary mitral insufficiency. Small ('restrictive') defects offer high resistance to flow. A high pressure gradient is maintained between the ventricles and a loud murmur results. Larger ('non-restrictive') defects are associated with a greater degree of left-to-right shunting, leading to equilibration of ventricular pressures and relatively low intensity murmurs. Increased blood flow through the pulmonic valve may result in turbulence and a murmur due to 'relative' pulmonic stenosis. Some defects 'close' spontaneously. In some cases there is an associated aortic insufficiency. Large left-to-right shunts may result in left-sided congestive failure. With some VSDs, there is persistence of elevated pulmonary artery pressures from the fetal state (or theoretically, chronic pulmonary overcirculation could also result in increased pulmonary vascular resistance). This reduces the degree of left-to-right flow, and in some cases the direction of flow may even reverse, resulting in cyanosis (Eisenmenger's physiology). Cyanosis may also be seen in patients with co-existing pulmonic stenosis. Dogs with significant right-to-left shunts are usually polycythaemic.

Clinical Features

Dogs with a VSD may present with left-sided heart failure (pulmonary oedema), they may be asymptomatic, or (rarely) they may be cyanotic and exercise intolerant.

Auscultatory findings include:

- a systolic murmur heard loudest on the right side, near the sternum, and radiating to the left;
- a murmur of relative pulmonic stenosis may be audible over the left heart base;
- a diastolic murmur may be audible over the heart base in cases with an associated aortic insufficiency.

Investigations are outlined in Table 46.4.

Cardiac catheterisation, blood gas analysis and selective angiography may be necessary to diagnose definitively, especially if shunting right to left, and rule out co-existing lesions.

Management

Restrictive ventricular septal defects rarely require any therapy. Corrective surgery has been attempted, but requires cardiopulmonary bypass. Pulmonary artery banding has been suggested as a palliative procedure to reduce the amount of left-to-right shunting. The obstruction to right ventricular outflow increases the right ventricular pressure and therefore reduces the pressure gradient between the two ventricles. Patients with significant right-to-left shunting may require periodic phlebotomy if the associated polycythaemia becomes excessive.

Prognosis

The prognosis is good for restrictive defects which exist as the only lesion; life-expectancy and quality may be normal. The prognosis is much poorer if there is significant left-to-right shunting through a large, non-restrictive defect, or if Eisenmenger's physiology develops.

ATRIAL SEPTAL DEFECT

Atrial septal defects (ASD) rarely exist as an isolated defect in the dog, and usually occur in association with other defects.

Pathogenesis and Pathophysiology

ASDs may be found in one of a number of sites as a result of abnormal development of the interatrial septum. As isolated defects they are often not haemodynamically signifi-

Table 46.4 Investigations in cases of ventricular septal defects.

Radiography	Generalised cardiac enlargement Signs of pulmonary overcirculation Signs of right ventricular hypertrophy and pulmonary undercirculation if shunting right-to-left
Electrocardiography	There may be electrocardiographic evidence of left atrial and/or left ventricular enlargement (wide P waves and tall R waves) with large left-to-right shunts. Right ventricular enlargement patterns (deep S waves in leads I, II and III) may be seen in patients with pulmonary hypertension Intraventricular conduction defects are sometimes evident
Echocardiography	Secondary changes may be evident on 2D echocardiography, such as left atrial and ventricular dilation. Right ventricular hypertrophy may be seen in patients with pulmonary hypertension. It may be possible to image the defect itself, although small defects may not be evident in all views. Doppler echocardiography (colour flow mapping in particular) will demonstrate turbulent flow associated with the defect. A high velocity of flow through the defect suggests a restrictive defect and a better prognosis. Measurement of the velocity of any tricuspid regurgitant jet may be helpful in assessing the likelihood of Eisenmenger's physiology. Diastolic aortic regurgitation may be evident in cases with an associated aortic insufficiency. Contrast echocardiography is a useful method for identifying right-to-left shunts, and negative contrast may sometimes identify a left-to-right shunt

Table 46.5   Investigations in suspected cases of atrio-septal defects.

Radiography	Plain radiography may show right heart enlargement
Electrocardiography	With large isolated ASDs there may be electrocardiographic evidence of right ventricular enlargement
Echocardiography	The secondary changes may be more obvious on 2D echocardiography than the defect itself. Right atrial and ventricular dilation and eccentric right ventricular hypertrophy may be seen from a number of views, but the defect itself may only be imaged from a right parasternal long axis view. Contrast echocardiography is a useful method for identifying right-to-left shunting, negative contrast may sometimes identify a left-to-right shunt. Doppler echocardiography, cardiac catheterisation, blood gas analysis and selective angiography may be necessary to diagnose definitively and rule out co-existing lesions

cant, although large defects may result in significant left-to-right shunting, right atrial enlargement and a volume overload of the right heart.

Clinical Features

An isolated ASD is usually detected as an incidental finding. A low intensity murmur is sometimes heard on auscultation, which may be a murmur of 'relative' pulmonic stenosis as a result of increased blood flow through the pulmonic valve.

Investigations are outlined in Table 46.5.

TETRALOGY OF FALLOT

Tetralogy of Fallot is rare in the dog. The defect has been reported in Golden Retrievers, Keeshund, Wire Haired Fox Terriers, Labrador Retrievers, Siberian Husky, and Toy Poodles (Ringwald & Bonagura 1988). In the Keeshund it is inherited as an autosomally-dominant trait with variable penetrance.

Pathogenesis and Pathophysiology

Tetralogy of Fallot consists of:

- a ventricular septal defect,
- pulmonic stenosis (often pulmonary artery hypoplasia),
- secondary right ventricular hypertrophy,
- dextropositioned aorta.

The main effect is for deoxygenated blood to be shunted from the right ventricle into the aorta and systemic circulation. Cyanosis and polycythaemia may be marked.

Clinical Features

Most dogs with cyanotic heart disease present with exercise intolerance or tachypnoea. Occasionally an affected dog will be asymptomatic, and appear to cope with the defect. Alternative presentations include signs referable to the polycythaemia (hyperviscosity syndrome).

The main physical findings are:

- cyanosis of all visible mucous membranes, particularly with exercise;
- variable systolic heart murmur, which may be low intensity (or even absent).

Investigations are outlined in Table 46.6.

Management

Corrective surgery has been attempted, using cardiopulmonary bypass. Palliative transposition of a major artery (usually the subclavian) to the pulmonary artery will divert blood from the aorta to the pulmonary circulation (Eyster 1993). Patients with significant polycythaemia may require periodic phlebotomy to prevent problems associated with hyperviscosity.

Prognosis

The prognosis is generally guarded, but will depend on the degree of right-to-left shunting. Some animals will tolerate the defect into middle age.

Table 46.6 Investigations in suspected cases of tetrology of Fallot.

Radiography	The key features of plain radiographs include: • right heart enlargement (particularly 'apex-tipping', where the apex is lifted off the sternum on the lateral view by the hypertrophied right ventricle), • signs of pulmonary undercirculation
Electrocardiography	The ECG features may be similar to those found with PS, and referable to right ventricular enlargement (deep S waves in leads I, II and III)
Echocardiography	2D echocardiography can be very useful in the diagnosis of tetralogy of Fallot. The key features of the defect can often be identified: • right ventricular hypertrophy, • ventricular septal defect, • the dextropositioned aorta may be seen over the VSD. The hypoplastic pulmonary artery and pulmonic stenosis may be difficult to identify. Contrast echocardiography is useful for identifying right to left shunting. Doppler echocardiography, cardiac catheterisation, blood gas analysis and selective angiography may be necessary to diagnose definitively. Arterial blood gas analysis will confirm hypoxaemia, and polycythaemia may be evident on routine haematology

ATRIOVENTRICULAR VALVE DYSPLASIA

Mitral dysplasia has been reported in Bull Terriers (Lehmkuhl *et al.* 1994), German Shepherd Dogs, and Great Danes (Dear 1971) In some young dogs the lesion appears to 'resolve'.

Tricuspid dysplasia has been reported in various breeds (Liu & Tilley 1976) including Labrador Retrievers (Buchanan 1992). Ebstein's anomaly is a particular form of tricuspid dysplasia in which the attachment of the valve is ventrally-displaced within the ventricle.

Pathophysiology

The affected atrioventricular valve may have abnormal chordae tendineae or papillary muscles, and is usually incompetent. The atrioventricular regurgitation results in atrial enlargement and ventricular dilation (eccentric hypertrophy). Congestive heart failure may develop with time, which may be worsened by progressive secondary myocardial failure. Mitral dysplasia will lead to left-sided failure (pulmonary oedema) and tricuspid dysplasia leads to right-sided failure.

Some cases of mitral dysplasia may be further complicated by a degree of mitral stenosis, which results in even greater left atrial enlargement. Atrioventricular valve dysplasias may be present with other defects.

Clinical Features

Affected animals often develop congstive heart failure, and will be presented for signs of exercise intolerance, dyspnoea or coughing. Occasionally a murmur will be detected as an incidental finding.

Auscultatory findings include:

• a systolic heart murmur loudest over the affected valve;
• dysrhythmias – especially atrial fibrillation.

Investigations are outlined in Table 46.7.

Management

Management is as for mitral and tricuspid regurgitation due to endocardiosis; therapy is primarily aimed at relieving the congestive signs.

Prognosis

The prognosis depends on the severity of the valvular incompetence, and whether there is any exacerbating valvular stenosis. Many animals will develop signs of congestive failure by early adulthood.

Table 46.7   Investigations in suspected cases of atrioventricular valve dysplasias.

Radiography	The radiographic signs of mitral dysplasia may be indistinguishable from those of dilated cardiomyopathy or endocardiosis (i.e. left atrial and left ventricular enlargement). Dogs with tricuspid dysplasia may have very prominent right atrial enlargement
Electrocardiography	The electrocardiographic changes may reflect enlargement of the left or right side, depending on the valve affected. With tricuspid dysplasia, the waveform changes are not usually as marked as with conditions associated with right ventricular concentric hypertrophy (e.g. PS). Dysrhythmias such as atrial fibrillation are common
Echocardiography	2D echocardiography usually demonstrates atrial and ventricular dilation, with eccentric ventricular hypertrophy. The abnormalities of the affected valve may be quite obvious, or fairly subtle. Hyperkinesis of the ventricle early in the disease may progress to hypokinesis if myocardial failure develops.
	Doppler echocardiography or selective angiography may be necessary to diagnose definitively and assess severity and rule out complicating co-existing lesions

Table 46.8   Investigations in suspected cases of congenital peritoneo-pericardial hemias defects.

Radiography	Abnormalities on thoracic radiographs include overlap of the caudal border of an enlarged, well-defined cardiac silhouette and the diaphragm. Occasionally gas-filled loops of bowel are seen within the pericardial sac as shown in Fig. 46.3 (identification can be established by the oral administration of barium)
Echocardiography	Definitive diagnosis is often readily achieved with ultrasonography

VASCULAR RING ANOMALIES

Abnormal development of the aortic arch can result in the formation of a vascular ring, which causes occlusion of the oesophagus over the heart base. The most common vascular ring anomaly is persistence of the right aortic arch.

Affected animals typically present with regurgitation of solid food from the time of weaning. Diagnosis is by thoracic radiography or fluoroscopy following a barium swallow, which will identify oesophageal dilation cranial to the obstruction.

Treatment is by surgical section if possible. In some cases of persistence of the right aortic arch, the ductus arteriosus remains patent. Oesophageal function may not return to normal after surgery and in these cases regurgitation persists.

CONGENITAL PERITONEO-PERICARDIAL HERNIA

Epidemiology

Congenital peritoneo-pericardial diaphragnatic hernias (PPDH) are rarely found in the dog. Most cases are diagnosed as puppies, but a significant number are diagnosed in dogs older than one year old.

Clinical Features

Clinical signs are typically gastrointestinal or respiratory; signs suggestive of cardiovascular disease are rare. On examination the heart sounds may be muffled, and intestinal sounds may be heard in the thorax. Concurrent defects, such as sternal malformations or abdominal hernias frequently co-exist.

Investigations are outlined in Table 46.8.

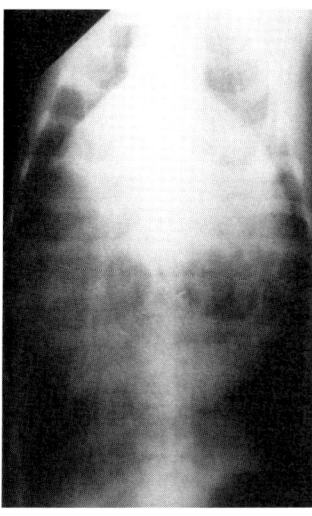

Fig. 46.3 Dorsoventral radiograph of the thorax of a dog with a congenital peritoneo-pericardial hernia. Gas-filled loops of bowel are evident within the enlarged, well defined cardiac silhouette.

Management

Treatment, where necessary, is by surgical correction via a laparotomy.

REFERENCES

Brownlie, S.E., Cobb, M.A., Chambers, J., Jackson, G. & Thomas, S. (1991). Percutaneous balloon valvuloplasty in four dogs with pulmonic stenosis. *Journal of Small Animal Practice*, **32**, 165–169.

Buchanan, J.W. (1992). Causes and prevalence of cardiovascular disease. In: *Current Veterinary Therapy XI*, (eds R.W. Kirk & J.D. Bonagura), pp. 647–655. W.B. Saunders, Philadelphia.

Dear, M.G. (1971) Mitral incompetence in dogs of 0–5 years of age. *Journal of Small Animal Practice*, **12**, 1–10.

Delellis, L.A., Thomas, W.P. & Pion, P.D. (1993). Balloon dilation of congenital subaortic stenosis in the dog. *Journal of Veterinary Internal Medicine*, **7**, 153–161.

Eyster, G.E. (1993). Basic cardiac surgical procedures. In: *Textbook of Small Animal Surgery*, (ed. D. Slatter), 2nd edn. pp. 893–918. W.B. Saunders, Philadelphia.

Kienle, R.D., Thomas, W.P. & Pion, P.D. (1994). The natural clinical history of canine congenital subaortic stenosis. *Journal of Veterinary Internal Medicine*, **8**, 423–431.

Lehmkuhl, L.B., Ware, W.A. & Bonagura, J.D. (1994). Mitral stenosis in 15 dogs. *Journal of Veterinary Internal Medicine*, **8**, 2–17.

Liu, S.-K. & Tilley, L.P. (1976). Dysplasia of the tricuspid valve in the dog and cat. *Journal of the American Veterinary Medical Association*, **169**, 623–630.

Martin, M.W.S., Godman, M., Luis, Fuentes, V., Clutton, R.E., Haigh, A. & Darke, P.G.G. (1992). Assessment of balloon valvuloplasty in six dogs. *Journal of Small Animal Practice*, **33**, 443–446.

Orton, C.E. (1994). Current techniques in cardiac surgery. In: *Proceedings of the Twelfth Annual Forum of the American College of Veterinary Internal Medicine*. San Francisco, USA.

Patterson, D.F. (1968) Epidemiologic and genetic studies of congenital heart disease in the dog. *Circulation Research*, **23**, 171–202.

Pyle, R.L., Patterson, D.F. & Chacko, S. (1976). The genetics and pathology of discrete subaortic stenosis in the Newfoundland dog. *American Heart Journal*, **92**, 324–334.

Ringwald, R.J. & Bonagura, J.D. (1988). Tetralogy of Fallot in the dog. Clinical findings in 13 cases. *Journal of the American Animal Hospital Association*, **24**, 33–43.

Sisson, D. (1992). Fixed and dynamic subvalvular aortic stenosis in dogs. In: *Current Veterinary Therapy XI*, (eds R.W. Kirk & J.D. Bonagura), pp. 760–766. W.B. Saunders, Philadelphia.

Chapter 47

Acquired Heart Disease

M. Cobb

The purpose of this chapter is to detail the major acquired cardiac diseases found in the dog. Acquired cardiac disease is an important entity and around 11% of all dogs have reliable evidence of heart disease (Buchanan 1992). The basic prinicples and therapeutic agents have been covered in Chapter 45 and the reader is referred to that chapter for specific information on drug actions and doses.

CHRONIC ACQUIRED DEGENERATIVE VALVE DISEASE (ENDOCARDIOSIS)

Endocardiosis is the most common acquired cardiac abnormality in the dog. The aetiology is unknown, although particular breed predispositions suggest a hereditary component. The frequency of endocardiosis increases with advancing age. Evidence of disease may be present for years before clinical signs develop. Overt heart failure is more common in middle-aged and older dogs. Endocardiosis is seen most often in smaller breeds of dog, especially the Cavalier King Charles Spaniel, Poodle, Chihuahua, Cocker Spaniel, Whippets and Yorkshire Terrier (Thrusfield *et al.* 1985; Beardow & Buchanan 1993). Occasionally larger breeds are affected, such as Setters.

Gross Pathology (Whitney 1974)

The lesions develop over many years and are most frequently seen on the left atrioventricular valve, often in association with less severe lesions of the right atrioventricular valve. Grey-white nodules or plaque-like thickening of the valve cusps due to deposition of excess extracellular matrix (glycosaminoglycans) in the upper layer of the valve leaflets, results in the valve cusps becoming shorter and

thicker (Fig. 47.1). The chordae tendinae are often thickened near their attachment to the valve (Fig. 47.2). Physical irritation of the atrial endocardium by the regurgitant blood flow results in 'jet lesions' developing at the site of impact. Hyalinisation of the intramural myocardial vessels occurs, resulting in myocardial ischaemia, necrosis and fibrosis (microscopic intramural infarction) in some patients.

History

Not all affected dogs develop heart failure. A murmur may be present for many years without signs of failure. Lesions are frequent incidental post-mortem findings in older dogs. In patients that do develop cardiac failure, typical presenting complaints include:

- exercise intolerance,
- coughing,
- dyspnoea,
- syncope/collapse,
- weight loss (usually with advanced disease),
- ascites,
- nocturnal restlessness.

Clinical Features

Patients usually present with signs of left-sided (sometimes with right) congestive heart failure.

Findings on physical examination include:

- a systolic murmur over the left cardiac apex which typically increases in intensity, duration and radiation as the disease progresses;
- a precordial thrill may be palpable in severe cases;
- a murmur is also frequently heard over the right hemithorax, a result of radiation of the mitral murmur

or of concomitant tricuspid regurgitation;
- dysrhythmias, especially in more advanced cases;
- gallop sounds;
- prominent apex beat;
- normal pulse in the early stages of the disease, or hypo-kinetic in cases which develop myocardial failure.

Diagnosis and Management

A tentative diagnosis is often based on the identification of a systolic murmur audible over the left cardiac apex, typically in small- and medium-sized dogs.

Investigations are outlined in Table 47.1.

Management

The management of these patients is dependent upon the level of valvular damage and the success or failure of the compensatory mechanisms to overcome the haemodynamic changes. It is worth considering the management of these patients in four groups: (1) patients with murmur but no signs of cardiac failure; then, once backward or congestive heart failure develops, patients with: (2) mild failure; (3) progressing failure; (4) severe failure. Once there has been progression from no signs of cardiac failure to the early stages of congestive heart failure, therapy requires individual assessment of each patient with respect to severity and adjustment of therapeutic regime according to response. The recommendations in Box 47.1 are guidelines for treatment.

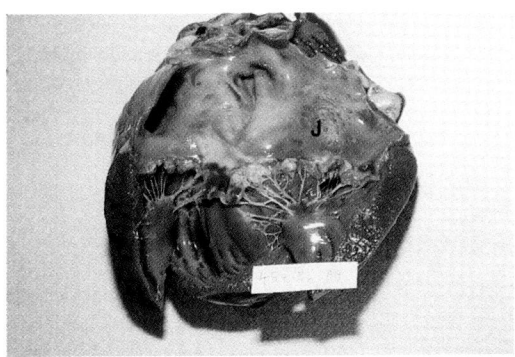

Fig. 47.1 Heart from a small breed dog showing typical post-mortem lesions of endocardiosis. Thickening and shortening of the valve cusps is evident and the regurgitant blood flow has resulted in a jet lesion developing on the atrial wall (J).

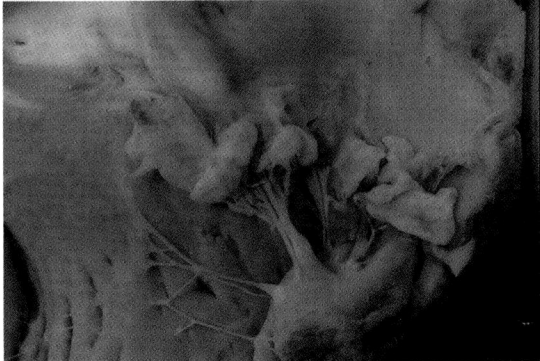

Fig. 47.2 Close-up of an atrioventricular valve affected with severe endocardiosis. There is gross distortion of the valve cusps, the chordae tendinae are thickened near their attachment to the valve and the physical irritation of the atrial endocardium by the regurgitant blood flow has resulted in the development of a jet lesion.

Table 47.1 Investigations in cases of endocardiosis.

Radiography	Thoracic radiography will typically demonstrate progressive left-sided (or global) cardiomegaly and, as the disease progresses, signs of left heart failure. A definitive diagnosis of mitral insufficiency can be made by left-sided cardiac catheterisation and angiography or Doppler echocardiography
Electrocardiography	ECGs may show evidence of (usually left) atrial and/or ventricular enlargement, with wide P waves and tall R waves. Dysrhythmias are common in more advanced cases, including atrial fibrillation and atrial premature complexes
Echocardiography	Echocardiography will identify more advanced valvular endocardiosis lesions (see Fig. 47.3), along with progressive atrial and ventricular enlargement and eccentric ventricular hypertrophy as the disease progresses. Initially, myocardial function remains good and the left ventricle appears to be hyperkinetic as a result of the large total stroke volume. In time, however, myocardial failure may develop

Box 47.1   Guide-lines for management of endocardiosis.

Management of patients with murmur but *no signs of cardiac failure*:

- Make a definitive diagnosis.
- Assess severity of disease/complications.
- Reassess regularly.
- Control weight in obese individuals.

Management of patients with murmur and *mild cardiac failure*:

- Dietary sodium excesses should be avoided.
- Exercise control.
- Low dose of diuretic is introduced to control oedema, dose titrated to effect; this may be reduced or discontinued once signs of failure are controlled.
- ACE inhibitors are usually introduced with diuretic.
- Reassess regularly for progression/complication.

Management of patients with murmur with *progressive cardiac failure*:

- Stricter exercise control.
- Diuretic dose increased as necessary.
- May require combination of diuretics.
- Regular checks of renal function and electrolyte levels.
- ACE inhibitors are maintained, dose may be increased if necessary.
- Digoxin as antidysrhythmic or if myocardial failure is evident.
- Antidysrhythmic therapy if indicated.

Management of patients with a murmur and in *severe heart failure*:

- Correct any precipitating/complicating factor.
- Cage rest.
- Intravenous frusemide.
- May require combination of diuretics.
- Vasodilators (e.g. topical nitroglycerine, hydralazine, ACE inhibitor or intravenous sodium nitroprusside).
- Digoxin as antidysrhythmic or if myocardial failure is evident.
- Oxygen administration.
- Sedation (opiate) may help in some cases.
- Intravenous dobutamine may improve output in cases with myocardial failure.
- Dysrhythmias may require specific management.
- Monitor renal function and electrolyte levels.
- Drain life-threatening effusions.

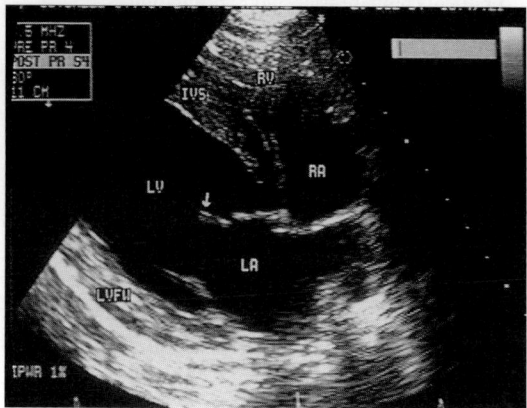

Fig. 47.3   Long axis echocardiographic view of the left ventricle (LV) and the left atrium (LA) from a right paracostal transducer location showing a thickened, echodense anterior mitral valve leaflet (marked with an arrow) in a patient with endocardiosis. (IVS, interventricular septum; LVFW, left ventricular free wall; RV, right ventricle; RA, right atrium.)

Prognosis

Patients with compensated mitral insufficiency may be free of clinical signs for years. Once cardiac failure develops the outlook is poor. Careful management can extend the comfortable life of some patients with mild or moderate failure for years, but sudden death or acute decompensation may develop at any time.

CANINE DILATED CARDIOMYOPATHY

Epidemiology and Aetiology

The aetiology of dilated cardiomyopathy (DCM) is unknown. DCM probably represents a common end-stage myocardial failure resulting from a wide variety of insults. The pronounced breed predispositions in dogs suggest a hereditary component. DCM is characterised by impaired ventricular function and dilation of one (typically the left) or both ventricles. Isolated right-sided DCM is rare.

Evidence suggests that insidious systolic failure progresses gradually over a period of years with mild ventricular dysfunction and frequently cardiac dysrhythmias evident for months, even years before cardiac failure develops (Brownlie 1991; Calvert 1992). Patients may develop acute, severe forward failure with signs of reduced tissue perfusion and hypotension.

Prevalence

Myocardial disease is recognised with increasing frequency, 1.1% of all dogs examined were found to have DCM in a 1988 survey (Fioretti & Delli Carri 1988) compared with 0.45% in 1965 (Detweiler & Patterson 1965). This increase is due in part to improved ability to diagnose myocardial disease, but also seems to reflect a genuine increase in the prevalence of the disease. DCM is primarily a disease of young and middle-aged dogs, although a wide range of age groups may be affected. Giant and large breed dogs are predominantly affected, with some medium-sized breeds. Small breeds and cross-breds are relatively spared. Breed differences in presentation and progression suggest that different causes and/or genetic factors play a role (Gooding *et al.* 1982; Hazlett *et al.* 1983).

Gross Pathology and Histopathology

The heart exhibits a variable degree of dilation, usually of all four chambers, although the disease process may affect the left side predominantly (Fig. 47.4). The ventricular walls appear thin, pale and soft but eccentric hypertrophy is

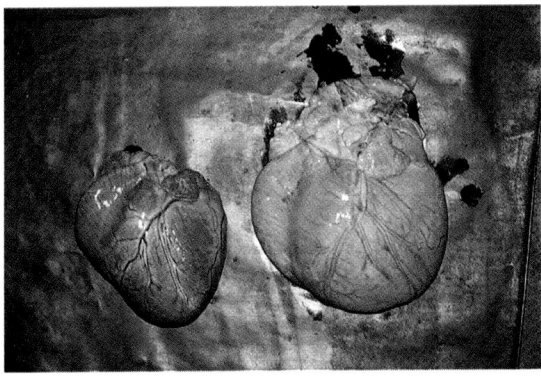

Fig. 47.4 Hearts removed at post mortem from two dogs of the same breed and similar age. The specimen on the right is from a dog affected with dilated cardiomyopathy and shows the generalised cardiomegaly typically seen in patients affected with this condition, the specimen on the left from a dog free of signs of cardiac disease before death.

invariably present. There may be coexistent valvular endocardiosis, especially in the smaller breeds. Scattered pale foci representing areas of necrosis or fibrosis may be evident grossly.

Histopathological findings are variable and nonspecific, and include areas of myocyte hypertrophy and degeneration, varying degrees of myocardial necrosis as well as areas of interstitial oedema and fibrosis. Much of the myocardium, however, may appear normal.

History

Patients with 'occult' disease, free of signs of cardiac failure may be identified on routine clinical, ECG or echocardiographic examination/screening.

When heart failure develops the onset of clinical signs is frequently acute and presenting signs typically include:

- dyspnoea,
- cough,
- syncope/collapse, anorexia and weight loss,
- reduced exercise tolerance, lethargy, weakness,
- ascites if concomitant right-heart failure,
- sudden death.

Clinical Features

There are breed differences in the presentation and progression of the disease:

- Dobermanns typically present with acute-onset left-sided failure, ventricular tachydysrhythmias, a short clinical course, and a high incidence of sudden death (Calvert *et al.* 1982).
- Boxer DCM principally affects the left heart, ventricular tachydysrhythmias are common and are often the only early sign (Harpster 1983).
- Cocker and Springer Spaniels usually present with congestive heart failure but prognosis is often good if carefully managed (Staaden 1981).
- Giant breeds, especially Irish Wolfhound, St Bernard, Great Dane, Newfoundland, often present with a subclinical dysrhythmia, usually atrial fibrillation, that is well tolerated for months or years before congestive cardiac failure develops.

Presentation with signs of left-sided (and sometimes right-sided) congestive heart failure is common, as are dysrhythmias (both ventricular and supraventricular).

Other physical findings include:

- gallop sounds,
- apex beat may be weak or strong,
- normal or hypokinetic pulse as a result of the poor stroke volume,
- systolic murmurs due to secondary valvular incompetence in the region of the atrioventricular valves.

Investigations and Diagnosis

A tentative diagnosis is usually made based on the patient details, the history and the results of the physical examination.

Investigations are outlined in Table 47.2.

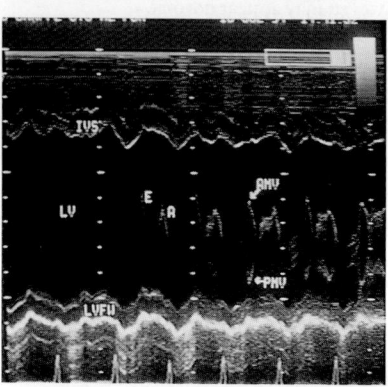 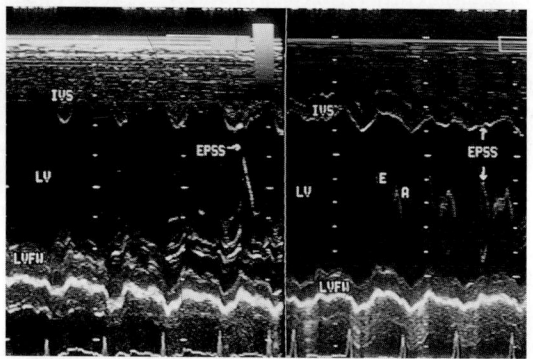

a   b

Fig. 47.5a,b   (a) M-mode echocardiogram at the level of the left ventricular lumen and the mitral valve from an Old English Sheepdog with dilated cardiomyopathy. Cardiac chamber dimensions are above the upper limits of normal and the E-point to septal separation is increased. (IVS, interventricular septum; LVFW, left ventricular free wall; LV, left ventricular lumen; E, mitral valve E-point; A, mitral valve A point; AMV, anterior leaflet of the mitral valve; PMV, posterior leaflet of the mitral valve; the scale on the left is in centimetres.) (b) M-mode echocardiogram at the level of the left ventricular lumen and the mitral valve from a normal dog (left) and a dog of the same breed and approximate age with dilated cardiomyopathy (right). The figure on the right shows some of the echocardiographic changes typically associated with the disease, the cardiac chamber dimensions and E-point to septal separation (EPSS) are all increased. (IVS, interventricular septum; LVFW, left ventricular free wall; LV, left ventricular lumen; E, mitral valve E-point; A, mitral valve A point; the scale on the left is in centimetres.)

Table 47.2   Investigations into suspected cases of dilated cardiomyopathy.

Electrocardiography	There may be electrocardiographic evidence of atrial and/or ventricular enlargement or conduction abnormalities. Dysrhythmias are common, especially atrial fibrillation in larger breeds and ventricular dysrhythmias in the Dobermann and the Boxer. Long-term dysrhythmia-monitoring or ambulatory electrocardiography (Holter monitoring) may help to identify paroxysmal dysrhythmias not detected on routine electrocardiography, and may be indicated in patients exhibiting syncope and to identify 'occult' disease in breeds in which the primary disease is commonly complicated by life-threating dysrhythmias (e.g. the Dobermann and Boxer).
Radiography	Thoracic radiographs will demonstrate progressive left-sided (or global) cardiomegaly and signs of heart failure as the disease progresses. In some cases of acute-onset left heart failure, especially in deep-chested breeds, cardiomegaly may be difficult to appreciate.
Echocardiography	M-mode echocardiography permits accurate assessment of chamber size and myocardial function. Cardiac chamber dimensions are usually above the upper limits of normal, end-systolic diameter is increased as a result of reduced myocardial contractility, there is a secondary increase in end-diastolic diameter and eccentric myocardial hypertrophy. E point to septal separation (EPSS) is often increased and left ventricular shortening fraction is depressed (Fig. 47.5a,b).

Management

Each patient requires individual assessment of the severity of the disease and adjustment of the therapeutic regime according to response. Patients can be divided into four groups: (1) those with 'occult' disease; (2) those with congestive heart failure; (3) as cardiac failure progresses; (4) severe failure. Guide-lines for treatment are given in Box 47.2.

Box 47.2 Guide-lines for management of dilated cardiomyopathy.

Management of patients with a DCM with *'occult' disease*:

- Definitive diagnosis is made.
- Assess severity of disease.
- ECG diagnosis of any dysrhythmia.
- Regular reassessment.
- If a deficiency is truly documented (e.g. carnitine or taurine) patient may benefit from supplementation although this is tenuous.

Management of patients with a DCM in *congestive heart failure*:

- Exercise control.
- Dietary sodium excesses should be avoided.
- Supplement if deficiency is identified.
- Diuretic is introduced to control oedema, dose titrated to effect, may be reduced or discontinued once signs of congestive failure are controlled.
- ACE inhibitors are usually introduced with the diuretic.
- Digoxin.
- Specific antidysrhythmic therapy may be required, e.g. digoxin (often with an additional negative chronotrope) to control the ventricular rate in atrial fibrillation.
- Monitor renal function and electrolyte levels.

Management of patients with a DCM *as cardiac failure progresses*:

- Stricter exercise control.
- Maintain ACE inhibitor/dietary/supplements/digoxin.
- Dose of ACE inhibitor may need to be increased.
- Higher doses of diuretic may be needed.
- May require combination of diuretics.

Box 47.2 *Continued*

Management of patients with a DCM and in *severe heart failure*:

- Correct any precipitating/complicating factor.
- Cage rest.
- Intravenous frusemide.
- May require combination of diuretics.
- Vasodilators (e.g. topical nitroglycerine, hydralazine, ACE inhibitor or intravenous sodium nitroprusside).
- Digoxin.
- Oxygen administration.
- Sedation (opiate) may help in some cases.
- Intravenous dobutamine may improve output.
- Dysrhythmias may require specific management.
- Monitor renal function and electrolyte levels.
- Drain life-threatening effusions.

Prognosis

The prognosis appears to vary with the breed and severity at presentation. Patients identified as a result of the discovery of a dysrhythmia (especially giant breed dogs) may remain free of clinical signs and compensated for years. Once cardiac failure develops, however, the outlook is poor. Most patients die or are euthanased within 6–12 months of the development of overt cardiac failure, although with careful management some patients will survive for years. The prognosis in the Dobermann seems particularly poor, with most patients living only 3–6 months after the development of cardiac failure. In all cases sudden death or acute decompensation are possible (see Monnet *et al.* 1995).

SPECIFIC HEART MUSCLE DISEASES

A number of specific heart muscle diseases, which may manifest as DCM, have been described. In these cases the cause of the myocardial disorder is known or the myocardial damage is the result of an identifiable primary systemic or metabolic disorder. Diagnosis of a specific myocardial disorder may require endomyocardial biopsy.

In addition, compromised cardiovascular function can occur as a result of the use of drugs or anaesthetics and may be a feature of a number of systemic conditions. These include obesity, anaemia, pregnancy, hypoxia, chronic respiratory tract disease, toxaemia (for example due to pyometra, gastric dilatation/volvulus, renal failure etc.), other major organ failures, CNS disease, endocrinopathies, hypertension and acid–base or electrolyte imbalances, particularly potassium and calcium imbalance. These conditions can be associated with rhythm abnormalities and/or compromised myocardial function (Atkins 1991). While these conditions often may not affect the cardiovascular system directly, in the presence of significant primary cardiac disease, they may increase the workload of the heart sufficiently to precipitate decompensation.

BACTERIAL ENDOCARDITIS

Bacterial endocarditis (BE) is a condition characterised by bacterial infection of the heart valves or mural endocardium following transient or persistent bacteraemia. The disease can affect any age, breed or sex. The prevalence seems to increase with advancing age. It is said to be more common in medium and large breed male dogs. Preexisting valve damage is not a pre-requisite for infection, and dogs with endocardiosis do not seem to be at increased risk.

There are two syndromes that are generally recognised:

- a quickly progressive, acute, ulcerative septic condition with rapid tissue destruction and necrosis;
- a subacute or chronic form characterised by the development of a friable vegetation with evidence locally of necrosis associated with an attempt at repair.

History

Unfortunately, the history rarely suggests a previous or current bacterial infection, or an opportunity for bacteria to gain access to the circulation. The history is usually vague and non-specific. The signs are multi-systemic and include anorexia, malaise, lethargy, shaking or trembling, weight loss, lameness (may be variable – shifting), syncope, abdominal pain and CNS signs.

Clinical Features

The clinical signs are referable to:

- sepsis and bacteraemia,
- thromboembolic disease and metastatic infection,

- valve lesions and the development of heart failure,
- secondary immune-mediated disease.

Presenting signs are usually non-specific, often variable, and chronic or intermittent, signs of cardiovascular disease are rare (Elwood *et al.* 1993).

Typical findings on physical examination include:

- poor physical condition,
- weakness,
- persistent or recurrent pyrexia,
- joint swelling or pain, spinal pain,
- petechiation or haemorrhage,
- abdominal pain,
- signs of CNS disease,
- dysrhythmia,
- new cardiac murmurs.

A heart murmur developing in an individual in which none had been previously detected, particularly a diastolic murmur of aortic regurgitation, is suggestive of BE, especially if accompanied by other signs consistent with the disease. The characteristics of such murmurs (timing, character, grade etc.) may vary between examinations and they must be differentiated from physiological murmurs associated with any concurrent pyrexia or anaemia. Signs of overt congestive heart failure are rare; however, secondary thromboembolic and/or immune-mediated disease is common.

Investigations and Diagnosis

Investigations are outlined in Table 47.3.

Definitive Diagnosis

The history, physical examination and the results of laboratory investigations may alert the clinician to the possibility of BE, particularly if a high index of suspicion is maintained.

Blood culture may document the presence of bacteraemia and identify the organism(s) involved and their sensitivity to anti-bacterials. Ideally at least three or four samples are taken, at least one hour apart, if possible from different sites. Skin preparation at the venepuncture site is as for surgery and samples should be incubated aerobically and anaerobically; growth of the same organism from two or more samples is very suggestive of bacteraemia. Any site suspected of being the primary source of a bacteraemia, e.g. the urinary tract, should also be cultured.

Echocardiography, especially 2D, may demonstrate vegetations, the secondary effects of valvular damage and other

Table 47.3 Investigations in suspected cases of bacterial endocarditis.

Haematology	The haematological findings are variable, although abnormalities are frequently present. Evidence of acute or chronic inflammatory disease may be present. Anaemia of chronic disease or a secondary auto-immune haemolytic anaemia may develop. Thrombocytopenia may be evident with DIC or secondary immune-mediated thrombocytopenia
Clinical biochemistry	Chronic inflammation may result in an elevation of serum globulin. Albumin levels may be low if there is significant haemorrhage, renal or gastrointestinal protein loss or reduced hepatic protein synthesis. There may be biochemical evidence of dysfunction in organs affected by embolisation or metastatic infection, e.g. kidneys/liver
Urinalysis	Urinary tract infections may be primary or secondary, renal infarction is common, there may be pyuria, haematuria, evidence of cells and casts in the sediment, significant proteinuria may accompany secondary glomerulonephropathy.
Joint fluid/CSF analysis	This may be indicated where there is an index of suspicion of infective arthritis or bacterial menigitis
Tests for immune-mediated disease	This may be indicated where there is an index of suspicion of secondary immune disease
Electrocardiography	Abnormalities of rate and rhythm are common; waveform changes are less so. There is no specific rhythm associated with bacterial endocarditis
Radiography	Radiography affected joints is often indicated and is some cases spinal radiographs. Chest radiographs may be necessary to document cardiomegaly, overt or impending congestive cardiac failure

cardiac complications. Aortic valve lesions are more reliably identified, as differentiating mitral valve lesions from lesions due to endocardiosis can be difficult.

In some cases, definitive diagnosis is only obtained at post-mortem examination.

Management

Management of BE is expensive, and often unrewarding to investigate and treat. It is important for the clinician to make the correct judgement and often treat based upon limited substantive data. Waiting for all data to be collated is, in general, too late.

(1) Treat any active infection.
  - Long courses of high doses of bactericidal antibiotics are indicated.
  - Begin once blood sampling for culture is completed if index of suspicion is high.
  - A useful antibacterial combination for use while culture results are pending and in culture-negative individuals is ampicillin, combined with an aminoglycoside (monitor renal function) or a quinolone such as enrofloxacin.
  - Treat intravenously if possible for the first 7 days.
  - Change anti-bacterial if indicated by blood culture results.
  - Follow up with a 6 week course of non-aminoglycoside oral antibiotics.
  - Check efficacy with follow-up blood cultures.
(2) Identify and deal with any potential sources of infection (abscesses, osteomyelitis, pyometra etc.).
(3) Consider and treat as necessary any cardiac complications, e.g. dysrhythmias, overt congestive cardiac failure.
(4) Consider and treat as necessary any extra-cardiac complications.
(5) Frequent reassessment for signs of improvement or the development of further complications.

Prognosis

Even if the primary infection is controlled, permanent valve damage is to be expected. The prognosis seems to be especially poor if the disease is associated with large vegetations, overt congestive cardiac failure, evidence of DIC or severe tachydysrhythmias.

Prophylactic antibiotic treatment is indicated if signifi-cant bacteraemia is likely, especially in the patient with pre-existing valvular disease.

PERICARDIAL DISEASE

Epidemiology and Aetiology

Pericardial disease is rare in small animals (Lombard 1983). Most pericardial disease is manifested as an accumulation of fluid within the pericardial sac, known as pericardial effusion. The effusion is categorised on the basis of the type of fluid present. The two most frequent causes of peri-cardial effusion in the dog are intrapericardial neoplasia and idiopathic pericardial haemorrhage (Berg & Wingfield 1984), both of these conditions result in a sanguinous effu-sion. Exudative (purulent) pericarditis has been described rarely in the dog. Transudates or modified transudates are found in right-sided heart failure, hypoproteinaemia, peri-toneopericardial hernias, etc.

Pathophysiology

The haemodynamic effect of a pericardial effusion is determined principally by the rate and volume of fluid accumulation and the elasticity of the pericardium. The pericardium will expand to accommodate slowly develop-ing fluid accumulations. As a result pressure within the pericardium does not increase significantly until later in the disease process. When the intrapericardial pressure reaches a critical level, the right atrium (and sometimes the right ventricle) collapses in diastole, right ventricular filling is compromised, therefore cardiac output falls (pericardial tamponade) and compensatory mechanisms are activated. Signs of right heart failure predominate because the thinner-walled chambers are affected earlier by a rise in intrapericardial pressure.

Clinical Features

History

Typical presenting complaints:

- reduced exercise tolerance, lethargy or weakness,
- syncope,
- ascites,
- dyspnoea/tachypnoea.

Clinical Signs

Patients typically present with signs of congestive right heart failure. Specific features include:

- muffling of the heart sounds,
- weak, hypokinetic pulses,
- pale mucous membranes,
- signs of right heart failure,
- apex beat difficult to palpate.

Investigations and Diagnosis

Investigations are outlined in Table 47.4.

Table 47.4 Investigations into cases of pericardial effusion.

Pericardiocentesis	Pericardiocentesis provides fluid for analysis and the relief of tamponade, although cytological examination of pericardial fluid is an unreliable method for distinguishing neoplastic from non-neoplastic pericardial disorders (Sisson *et al.* 1984)
Radiography	Global enlargement of a well defined cardiac silhouette may be evident, although the radiographic findings in many cases of acquired pericardial disease are not 'typical'
Electrocardiography	The QRS complexes may be of diminished voltage (an unreliable predictor of pericardial effusion). Electrical alternans may be present where complexes alternate in size. This is caused by swinging of the heart within the effusion. S-T segment elevation is another electrocardiographic feature often associated with pericardial effusion. Other cases of pericardial effusions will show none of these changes
Echocardiography	Echocardiography may be required to differentiate pericardial effusion (and identify any primary intrapericardial mass lesions) from cardiomegaly due to primary cardiac disease, especially dilated cardiomyopathy (Fig. 47.6)

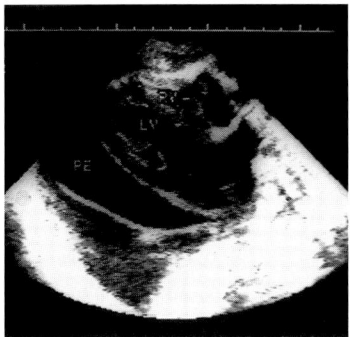

Fig. 47.6 Ultrasound image of the heart from a right paracostal transducer location showing an echo-free space round the heart typical of a pericardial effusion (PE). (LV, left ventricle; RV, right ventricle.)

Management

Pericardiocentesis will relieve any tamponade and drainage of the effusion usually results in prompt resolution of the clinical signs over the next few days. Diuretic therapy should be used with caution in cases exhibiting signs of congestive heart failure since their use may result in further reduction in ventricular filling. Thoracotomy and subtotal pericardectomy are indicated in patients with evidence of intrapericardial neoplasia, and is often an effective procedure for recurrent idiopathic haemorrhagic effusions. The use of corticosteroids to try and prevent recurrence of idiopathic pericardial haemorrhage after the effusion has been drained has been advocated.

Prognosis

Generally the prognosis is poor if an intrapericardial tumour is the cause of the effusion, although surgical resection and pericardectomy has been described and may improve the short-term outlook in some patients. Idiopathic pericardial haemorrhage generally recurs despite repeated drainage, and thoracotomy with subtotal pericardectomy is often effective in preventing recurrence of effusions.

VASCULAR DISEASE

Thrombosis of arteries and veins is described as a result of vascular damage associated with a number of primary conditions. Aortic thromboembolism occurs less frequently in the dog than it does in the cat

Pulmonary thromboembolism does occur, typically secondary to systemic diseases such as hyperadrenocorticism, auto-immune haemolytic anaemia, nephrotic syndrome etc. Patients typically present with acute-onset dyspnoea, cough, haemoptysis and cyanosis, thoracic radiographic findings are variable, but often show little to account for the respiratory distress.

ARTERIOVENOUS FISTULAE

Extracardiac arteriovenous shunts are rare. They may be congenital, but are more commonly acquired, usually secondary to trauma, surgery or neoplasia. Shunting of blood directly from artery to vein results in audible turbulence and sometimes a thrill. The affected area may be warm and swollen, other changes seen depend on the organ affected. Continuous shunting results in volume overloading which can progress to high output heart failure.

HEARTWORM

Dirofilaria Immitis (see also Chapter 28)

Heartworm disease resulting from infestation with *Dirofilaria immitis* occurs in parts of the USA, Europe, Australia and Japan. It does not occur in the UK except in imported dogs. The adult worms live in the pulmonary arteries and right ventricle, and release microfilariae into the bloodstream. Mosquitoes are an essential part of the life cycle, and they ingest the microfilariae which develop into an infective stage within the mosquito. Mosquitoes re-infect the next host with infective larvae, which migrate through the tissues to the right ventricle. This stage usually takes around 6 months.

A number of clinical syndromes may be seen in patients, including pulmonary hypertension and right heart failure. Presenting signs include coughing, exercise intolerance and weight loss.

Diagnosis of *Dirofilaria* is by immunological detection with an ELISA test or detection of circulating microfilariae in stained blood smears.

Treatment of dirofilariasis is difficult and can be hazardous, thiacetarsamide sodium is the drug typically recommended for removal of adult worms. This should be followed by microfilaricidal therapy (e.g. dithiazanine iodide, ivermectin, levamisole). Preventative measures can be taken to prevent tissue-stage larvae reaching the heart; effective drugs include diethyl-carbamazine and ivermectin.

ANGIOSTROGYLUS VASORUM

Angiostrogylus vasorum is an intravascular parasite that is found in the UK, particularly in the south-west of England and in dogs imported from Eire.

The adult worms live in the pulmonary arteries and the presenting clinical features can be very variable although evidence of haemorrhage or peripheral oedema are fairly common. *Angiostrongylus* is diagnosed by detecting larvae in the faeces. Levamisole and fenbendazole have been suggested as effective treatments for *Angiostrongylus*.

HYPERTENSION

Systemic hypertension may be primary or, much more commonly in small animal practice, secondary to underlying diseases particularly renal disease (Dukes 1992). Hypertension is typically only recognised after the acute development of ocular signs, such as intra-ocular haemorrhage.

REFERENCES

Atkins, C.E. (1991). The role of non-cardiac disease in the development and precipitation of heart failure. *Veterinary Clinics of North America*, **21**, 1035–1080.

Beardow, A.W. & Buchanan, J.W. (1993). Chronic mitral valve disease in Cavalier King Charles Spaniels: 95 cases (1987–1991). *Journal of the American Veterinary Medical Association*, **203**, 1023–1029.

Berg, J.R. & Wingfield, W. (1984). Pericardial effusion in the dog: a review of 42 cases. *Journal of The American Veterinary Medical Association*, **20**, 721–730.

Brownlie, S.E. (1991). An electrocardiographic survey of cardiac rhythm in Irish Wolfhounds. *Veterinary Record*, **129**, 470–471.

Buchanan, J.W. (1992). Causes and prevalence of cardiovascular disease. In: *Current Veterinary Therapy XI*, (eds R.W. Kirk & J.D. Bonagura), pp. 647–655. W.B. Saunders, Philadelphia.

Calvert, C.A. (1992). Update: Canine dilated cardiomyopathy. In: *Current Veterinary Therapy XI*, (eds R.W. Kirk & J.D. Bonagura), pp. 773–779. W.B. Saunders, Philadelphia.

Calvert, C.A., Chapman, W.L. & Toal, R.L. (1982). Congestive cardiomyopathy in Doberman Pinscher dogs. *Journal of the American Veterinary Medical Association*, **181**, 598–602.

Detweiler, D.K. & Patterson, D.F. (1965). Prevalence and types of cardiac disease in dogs. *Annals of the New York Academy of Science*, **127**, 481–516.

Dukes, J. (1992). Hypertension: A review of the mechanisms, manifestations and management. ical and echocardiographic findings in 10 dogs with vegetative bacterial endocarditis. *Journal of Small Animal Practice*, **33**, 119–129.

Elwood, C.M., Cobb, M.A. & Stepien, R.L. (1993). Clinical and echocardiographic findings in 10 dogs with vegetative bacterial endocarditis. *Journal of Small Animal Practice*, **34**, 420–427.

Fioretti, M. & Delli Carri, E. (1988). Epidemiological survey of dilatative cardiomyopathy in dogs. *Veterinaria*, **2**, 81.

Gooding, J.P., Robinson, W.F., Wyburn, R.S. & Cullen, L.K. (1982). A cardiomyopathy in the English Cocker Spaniel: a clinico-pathological investigation. *Journal of Small Animal Practice*, **23**, 133–149.

Harpster, N.K. (1983). Boxer cardiomyopathy. In: *Current Veterinary Therapy VIII*, (ed. R.W. Kirk), pp. 329–337. W.B. Saunders Company, Philadelphia.

Hazlett, M.J., Maxie, M.G., Allen, D.G. & Wilcock, B.P. (1983). A retrospective study of heart disease in Doberman Pinscher dogs. *Canadian Veterinary Journal*, **24**, 205–210.

Lombard, C.W. (1983). Pericardial disease. *Veterinary Clinics of North America*, **13**, 337–353.

Monnet, E., Orton, C., Salman, M. & Boon, J. (1995). Idiopathic dilated cardiomyopathy in dogs: Survival and prognostic indicators. *Journal of Veterinary Internal Medicine*, **9**, 12–17.

Sisson, D., Thomas, W.P., Ruehl, W.W. & Zinkl, J.G. (1984). Diagnostic value of pericardial fluid analysis in the dog. *Journal of the American Veterinary Medical Association*, **184**, 51–55.

Staaden, R.S. (1981). Cardiomyopathy of English Cocker Spaniel. *Journal of the American Veterinary Medical Association*, **178**, 1289–1292.

Thrusfield, M.V., Aitken, C.G.G. & Darke, P.G.G. (1985). Observations on breed and sex in relation to canine heart valve incompetence. *Journal of Small Animal Practice*, **26**, 709–717.

Whitney, J.C. (1974). Observations on the effect of age on the severity of heart valve lesions in the dog. *Journal of Small Animal Practice*, **15**, 511–522.

Section 6

Gastroenterology

Edited by Kenny W. Simpson

Chapter 48

Oropharyngeal and Oesophageal Diseases

R. J. Washabau

INTRODUCTION

The structures of the oral cavity and oesophagus are involved in the prehension, chewing, lubrication and swallowing of food. Dysphagia (difficulty in swallowing) and hypersalivation are the most important clinical signs associated with diseases of the oral cavity. Regurgitation is the most important clinical sign associated with diseases of the oesophagus; dysphagia and odynophagia (pain on swallowing) are less frequently reported clinical signs with oesophageal disease. Other clinical signs will depend upon the site, pathogenesis, and severity of the lesion (Table 48.1).

STRUCTURE AND FUNCTION

Oral Cavity

Swallowing is a complex process involving many different structures. The *oral* stage of swallowing begins with the prehension of food with teeth and tongue, and the formation of the bolus at the base of the tongue. In the *pharyngeal* stage, pharyngeal contractions propel the bolus from the base of the tongue to the opening of the cricopharyngeal sphincter. The cricopharyngeus muscle relaxes during the *cricopharyngeal* stage, and the bolus passes into the cranial oesophageal body. The cricopharyngeus muscle subsequently contracts, pharyngeal muscles relax, and the oropharyngeal phase is repeated (Watrous & Suter 1979). Salivation, which is essential in the lubrication of ingested food, is a less complicated process than swallowing. Saliva is secreted from the parotid, mandibular, sublingual and zygomatic salivary glands in anticipation, or during ingestion, of food.

Oesophagus

The oesophagus is involved in the transport of ingested liquids and solids from the oropharynx to the stomach. In the dog, the anatomic structures that permit this function are the striated muscle of the cricopharyngeal sphincter and oesophageal body, and the smooth muscle of the gastro-oesophageal sphincter. Striated muscle is innervated by somatic branches (glossopharyngeal, pharyngeal and recurrent laryngeal) of the vagus nerve arising from the brainstem nucleus ambiguus. The smooth muscle of the gastro-oesophageal sphincter is innervated by autonomic branches (oesophageal) of the vagus nerve arising from the dorsal motor nucleus of the vagus. During fasting, the elevated pressures of the cricopharyngeal sphincter and gastro-oesophageal sphincter prevent movement of food and chyme into the oesophageal body from the oral cavity and stomach, respectively. When a dog swallows, the cricopharyngeal sphincter relaxes to permit the movement of liquids and solids into the proximal oesophageal body. Swallowing also initiates a wave of peristaltic contractions (primary peristalsis) in the oesophagus that sweeps food into the distal oesophageal body. Primary peristaltic contractions are reinforced by a secondary wave of contraction (secondary peristalsis) mediated physiologically by intraluminal distension. The gastro-oesophageal sphincter relaxes in advance of the propagated pressure wave to permit food to empty into the stomach. Once the bolus of food has passed into the stomach, the gastro-oesophageal sphincter resumes its high resting pressure.

An important species difference between the dog and cat is in the musculature of the oesophageal body. The full length of the canine oesophageal body is composed of striated muscle, whereas the distal one-third to one-half of the feline oesophageal body is composed of smooth muscle. The practical importance of this species difference is that smooth muscle prokinetic agents (e.g. cisapride) will stimulate lower oesophageal peristalsis in cats but not in dogs (Washabau & Hall 1995).

Table 48.1   Localisation of clinical signs – oral cavity vs. oesophageal vs. gastric disease.

Clinical sign	Oral cavity	Oesophagus	Stomach
Dysphagia	Always present	Sometimes present	Absent (with oesophagitis or obstruction)
Regurgitation	Absent	Present	Absent
Vomiting	Absent	Absent	Present
Hypersalivation	Usually present	May be present	May be present
Gagging	Often present	Usually absent	Absent
Ability to drink	Abnormal	Normal	Normal
Ability to form a solid bolus	Abnormal	Normal	Normal
Dropping of food from the mouth	Present	Absent	Absent
Time of food ejection	Immediate	Delayed, minutes to hours	Delayed, minutes to hours
Character of food ejected	Undigested	Undigested	Partially digested, bile-stained, acidic pH
Odynophagia	Occasionally seen	Frequent, particularly with oesophagitis	Absent
Number of swallowing attempts	Multiple	Single to multiple	Usually single
Associated signs	Nasal discharge	Dyspnoea, cough	Abdominal pain, retching
Reluctance to eat	May be present	May be present	May be present
Muscle atrophy	May be present	May be present	Usually absent
Ptosis/lip droop/enophthalmos	May be present	May be present	Usually absent

APPROACH TO THE PATIENT

History

Diseases of the oral cavity and oesophagus may affect dogs of any age, sex or breed. However, known breed predispositions may help formulate a differential diagnosis (Table 48.2).

History is very important in differentiating clinical signs associated with disease of the oral cavity, oesophagus, and stomach, and in planning diagnostic tests. Dysphagia and hypersalivation are the most important clinical signs in oral cavity disorders. Dysphagia (difficulty in swallowing) is frequently seen with oral cavity disease because of pain, obstructive lesions, or neuromuscular disturbances. Hypersalivation is observed with diseases of the oral cavity because of inability to swallow saliva, or because of inflammation-induced stimulation of salivation. Depending upon the pathogenesis of the disease, the pet owner may also describe difficulty or pain in chewing food, trismus (difficulty in opening the mouth), gagging, difficulty in drinking water or forming a solid bolus, excessive mandibular or head motion, persistent forceful ineffective swallowing efforts, dropping of food from the mouth, coughing, failure to thrive, or reluctance to eat. Regurgitation, a common sign of oesophageal disease, is less frequently observed with diseases of the oral cavity (Table 48.1).

Regurgitation is the primary sign of oesophageal disease. The presence and severity of other clinical signs is dependent upon the pathogenesis of oesophageal disease (Table 48.1). For example, dogs affected with vascular ring anomaly may have severe regurgitation with normal to excessive appetite. Dogs affected with oesophagitis, on the other hand, may have complete anorexia, dysphagia, odynophagia (painful swallowing) and hypersalivation, with little evidence of regurgitation. Regurgitation should be differentiated from vomiting associated with gastric or intestinal disease. Regurgitation is characterised by the passive retrograde evacuation of undigested food from the oesophagus. Vomiting, on the other hand, is characterised by co-ordinated contractions of the abdominal, diaphragmatic, and gastrointestinal musculature culminating in the active evacuation of digested or partially digested food from the stomach or intestine (Table 48.1). The investigation and diagnosis of vomiting disorders is outlined in Chapter 49.

Examination

Physical examination should include general systemic examination, oral cavity and neck examination, chest aus-

Table 48. 2   Known breed predispositions for diseases of the oral cavity or oesophagus.

Condition	Breed
Oral neoplasia	Golden Retriever, Weimeraner, Boxer, Cocker Spaniel
Oropharyngeal dysphagia	Bouvier des Flandres
Oral eosinophilic granuloma	Siberian Husky
Hiatal hernia	Chinese Shar-Pei, Chow, Bulldog
Persistent right aortic arch	German Shepherd
Anamolous coronary artery like PRAA	Bulldog
Congenital mega-oesophagus	Miniature Schnauzer, Fox Terrier, Irish Setter, Great Dane, German Shepherd, Labrador Retriever, Chinese Shar-Pei and Newfoundland
Myasthenia gravis-associated megaesophagus	German Shepherd, Golden Retriever, Smooth Fox Terrier, Jack Russell Terrier, Springer Spaniel
Gastro-oesophageal intussusception	German Shepherd
Oesophageal fistula	Cairn Terrier
Craniomandibular osteopathy	West Highland White Terrier

PRAA, persistent right aortic arch.

cultation, and abdominal palpation. Significant findings that may be present are outlined in Table 48.3. As with history, physical examination findings are dependent upon the site, pathogenesis, and severity of the lesion.

Many abnormalities of the oral cavity (e.g. neoplasia, inflammation, trauma, foreign body) are fairly obvious. Dogs with neuromuscular disorders, on the other hand, may have very few morphological abnormalities. Focal or generalised muscle atrophy and diminished or absent gag reflex may be the only abnormal findings in the latter group of animals.

Dogs affected with mild oesophageal disease may have minimal abnormalities. However, severe regurgitation may result in cachexia, aspiration pneumonia and fever. It is important to palpate the cervical oesophagus during the physical examination. An occasional foreign body or oesophageal dilation may be detected during examination. While there may be few definitive findings, the physical examination is none the less important from the standpoint of excluding other gastrointestinal or systemic disease.

Investigation

General Investigation

Initial laboratory testing should include haematology, biochemistry and urinalysis. This database will be useful in excluding systemic and metabolic disease, and will provide information about the animal's hydration status.

Table 48. 3   Physical examination – diseases of the oral cavity and oesophagus.

General examination
  Hydration status
  Body condition – cachexia, obesity
  Fever
  Lymphadenopathy
  Muscle atrophy – diffuse or focal (m. temporalis)
  Cranial nerve abnormalities (V, VII, IX, X, XII) – ptosis, lip droop, enophthalmos

Oral cavity examination
  Mucous membranes – colour, ulceration, capillary refill time
  Neoplasia
  Inflammation or infection
  Trauma – physical injury, chemical burns, foreign body
  Dental or periodontal disease
  Diminished or absent gag reflex
  Trismus or pain evinced during opening of the mouth

Neck examination
  Cervical oesophageal foreign body
  Cervical oesophageal dilation

Chest auscultation
  Pulmonary wheezes or crackles

Abdominal palpation
  Absence of gastrointestinal contents (stomach, liver) – gastro-oesophageal intussusception

Haematology

- Haemoconcentration with dehydration.
- Normocytic, normochromic non-regenerative anaemia with hypothyroidism.
- Leukocytosis, neutrophilia, ± left shift with aspiration pneumonia or severe oesophagitis.
- Basophilic stippling of erythrocytes and nucleated erythrocytes with lead poisoning.

Biochemistry

- Urea, sodium, phosphorus, and albumin elevated with dehydration.
- Na^+/K^+ ratio abnormal with hypoadrenocorticism (occasional cause of mega-oesophagus). (See also Chapter 59 page 611)

- Hypoalbuminaemia and hypoglobulinaemia with severe malnutrition.
- Hypercholesterolaemia with hypothyroidism.
- Creatine phosphokinase activity increased with polymyositis.

Investigation of Oropharyngeal Disease

An approach to the diagnosis of dysphagia and hypersalivation is depicted in Fig. 48.1. Diagnosis of morphological abnormalities is usually straightforward and, except for tissue biopsy or culture, does not usually require any additional diagnostic testing. Survey radiography should be performed to assess for severity of local traumatic injury, trismus, suspected temperomandibular joint disease, or distant metastasis. The diagnosis of neuromuscular disease

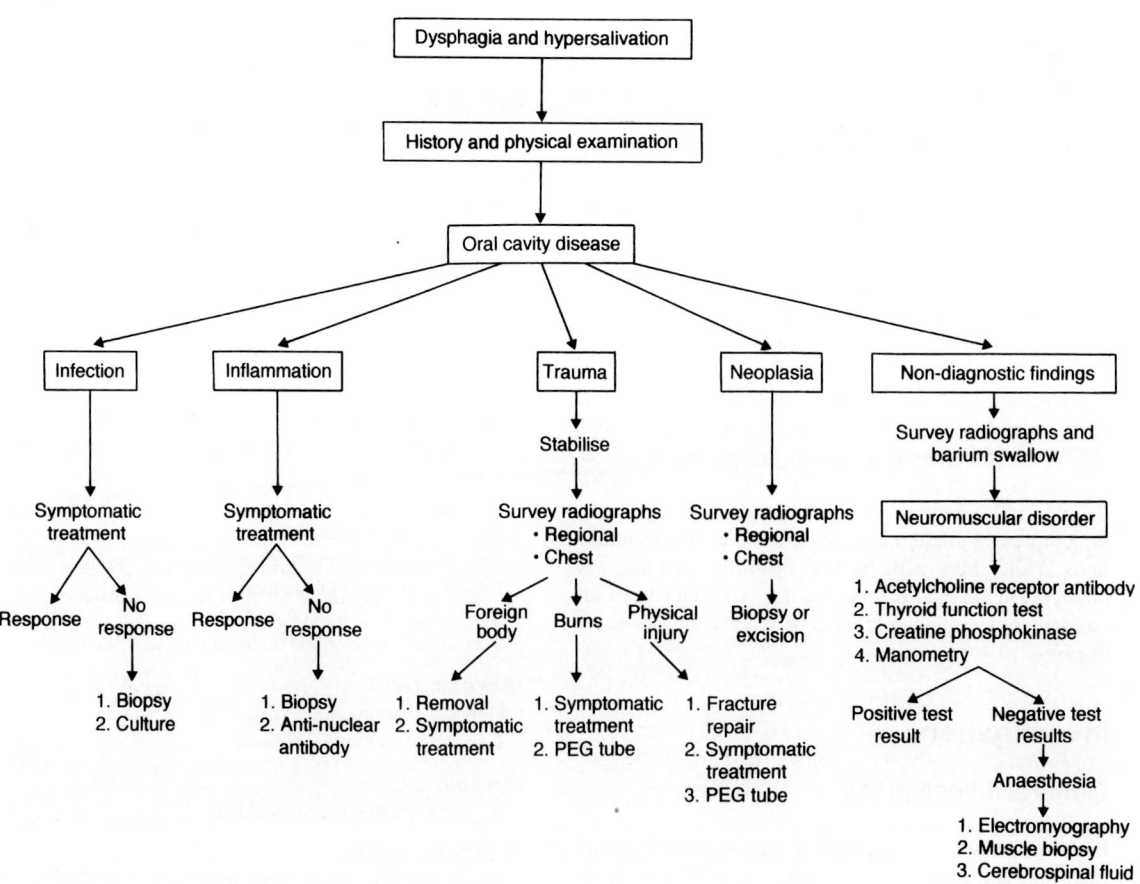

Fig. 48.1 Diagnostic approach to dysphagia and hypersalivation. (PEG, percutaneous endoscopic gastrostomy)

is more difficult and will require additional diagnostic testing.

Diagnostic Imaging

- Dynamic contrast studies (barium swallow videofluoroscopy) should be used instead of static radiographs whenever possible.
- The oral cavity and oesophageal phases of swallowing should be carefully studied in animals with dysphagia.
- Contrast studies are often useful in differentiating oral, pharyngeal and cricopharyngeal stage swallowing disorders (Table 48.4; Suter & Watrous 1980).

Serology

- Nicotinic acetylcholine receptor antibody.
- Some cases of acquired myasthenia gravis may have dysphagia as the only clinical sign (Shelton *et al.* 1990).
- Serum antibody titre >0.6 nmol/l is considered diagnostic of the disease.

Endocrine Function Testing

- Thyroid function test, e.g. thyroid-stimulating hormone (TSH), TSH stimulation T_4, T_4, auto-antibody.
- There may be an association between hypothyroidism, peripheral neuropathy and oropharyngeal dysphagia.

Table 48.4 Radiographic findings in swallowing disorders involving the oral cavity.

Oral stage dysphagia
  Weak tongue-thrust action
  Retention of contrast medium in oropharynx
  Loss of contrast medium from the mouth

Pharyngeal stage dysphagia
  Incomplete pharyngeal contraction
  Slow induction and slow progression of the peristaltic-like contraction from the rostral to the caudal pharynx
  Laryngotracheal aspiration

Cricopharyngeal stage dysphagia
  Failure of relaxation of the cricopharyngeus (achalasia)
  Inappropriate relaxation of the cricopharyngeus following pharyngeal contraction (inco-ordination)

Cricopharyngeal Manometry

- Useful in documenting cricopharyngeal achalasia (Rosin 1986; Lang *et al.* 1991).
- Available only in university teaching hospitals or major referral centres.
- Requires a co-operative animal for this study to be performed.

Electrophysiology and Muscle Biopsy

- Repetitive nerve stimulation may show decrement in the amplitude of the muscle action potential with myasthenia gravis.
- Fibrillation and positive sharp waves may be observed in the oropharyngeal musculature of animals with primary muscle disease, neurological disease or neuromuscular junction disease.
- Findings may be useful in distinguishing neuromuscular disease of the oral cavity from cricopharyngeal or oesophageal disease.
- Requires general anaesthesia.
- Muscle biopsy may be useful in diagnosing myositis or other degenerative muscle disorders.

Cerebrospinal Fluid Analysis, Brainstem Magnetic Resonance Imaging

- Should be performed in animals with suspected brainstem disease.
- Requires general anaesthesia.

Investigation of Oesophageal Disease

An approach to the diagnosis of regurgitation and odynophagia is depicted in Fig. 48.2. Survey radiography, contrast radiography, and oesophageal endoscopy are the diagnostic methods of choice for disorders of the oesophagus.

Survey Radiography

- Survey radiographs may be diagnostic for several disorders, including gastro-oesophageal intussusception, oesophageal foreign body, neoplasia, mega-oesophagus and hiatal hernia.
- Survey radiographs may also identify complications of oesophageal disease, including aspiration pneumonia, pleural effusion, mediastinitis and pneumothorax.

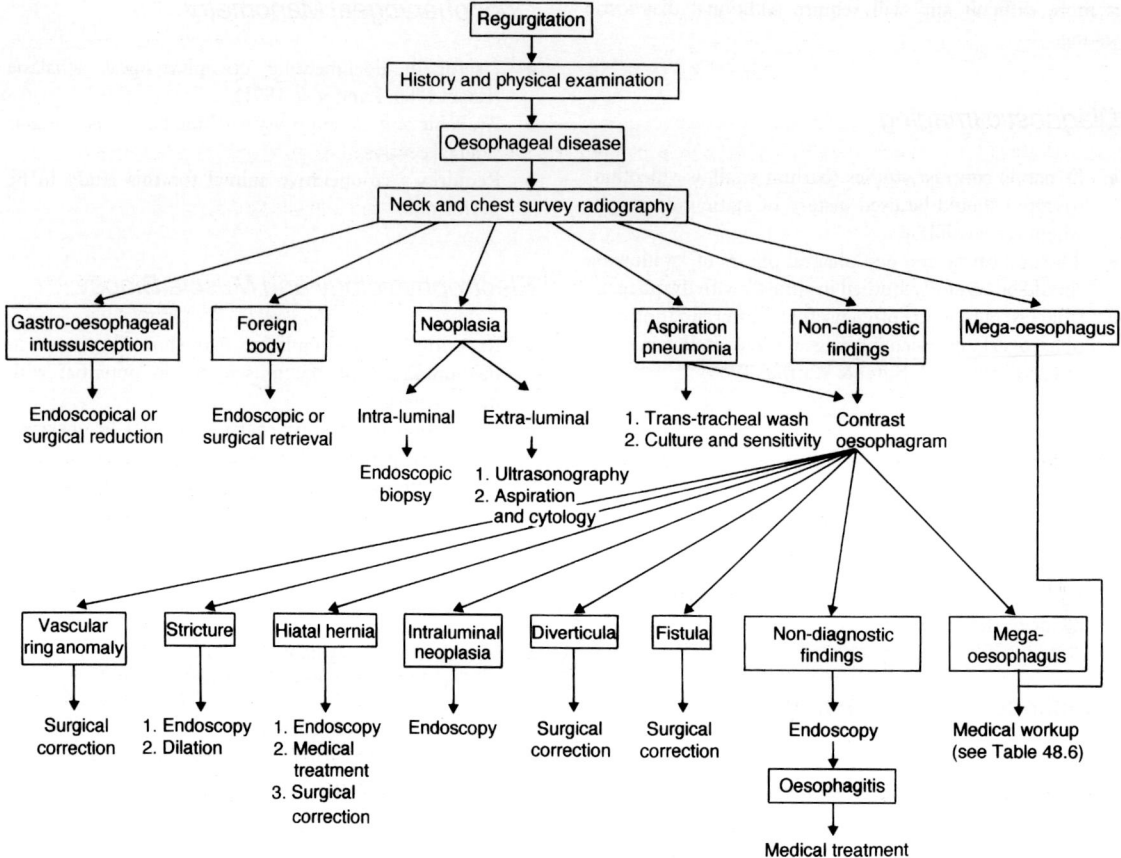

Fig. 48.2 Diagnostic approach to regurgitation.

- If survey radiographs are non-diagnostic, contrast radiography or endoscopy should be performed.

Contrast Radiography

- Barium swallow should be performed with video-fluoroscopy instead of static radiographs whenever possible.
- Contrast agents include barium paste (80–100% weight/volume), barium suspension (30% weight/volume), barium-coated meals, or iodinated contrast agents.
- Iodinated contrast agents should not be used in cases of suspected oesophageal fistula since they are hyperosmolar and chemically irritating to the lung.
- Barium should be not used in cases of suspected oesophageal perforation to avoid barium pleuritis; iodi-

nated contrast agents should be used if oesophageal perforation is suspected.
- Contrast radiography is more sensitive than survey radiography in detecting radioluscent foreign body, oesophagobronchial fistula, oesophagitis, diverticula and stricture.
- Contrast radiography also provides some information about oesophageal motility.
- The survey and contrast radiographic findings associated with oesophageal disease are outlined in Table 48.5.

Endoscopy

- Endoscopy is an increasingly important diagnostic and therapeutic tool in the management of oesophageal disease.

Table 48.5 Radiographic and endoscopic findings in swallowing disorders involving the oesophagus.

Oesophageal disorder	Radiographic findings	Endoscopic findings
Oesophageal foreign body	Radio-opaque foreign bodies are usually detected on survey radiography. Contrast radiography may be required to document radioluscent foreign bodies	Many radio-opaque and radioluscent foreign bodies are readily identified and treated with endoscopy
Oesophageal fistula	Lobar pneumonia is a common finding. The oesophagus may appear normal on survey radiographs unless a foreign body has become lodged near the fistula. Contrast radiography usually demonstrates the abnormal communication between oesophagus and bronchus, lung, or trachea	Large fistulae are usually visible, but small fistulae may not be readily apparent. Fistulae appear as round lesions on the oesophageal mucosa with raised hyperaemic margins
Vascular ring anomaly	In severely affected cases, proximal oesophageal dilation may be apparent on survey radiographs. The oesophageal stricture at the base of the heart is usually only apparent with contrast radiography	Narrowing is observed near the base of the heart; pulsations of the major arteries can be observed in the region of oesophageal narrowing
Oesophageal neoplasia	Peri-oesophageal neoplasia arising from the lung, thyroid, heart base or other structures may be readily apparent on survey radiographs. Contrast radiography and endoscopy are often required to document intraluminal neoplasia	Peri-oesophageal neoplasia are not visible with endoscopy, but oesophageal narrowing may be apparent due to extraluminal compression. Intraluminal neoplasia may appear focal, pedunculated and polypoid, or they may appear diffuse with mucosal haemorrhage and ulceration
Oesophagitis	Mild to moderate oesophageal dilation may be apparent on survey or contrast radiographs in some cases. Minimal change or no abnormalities may be observed in other cases. The latter cases be further investigated by endoscopy	Erythaema, ulceration, constriction, bleeding evidence of reflux
Oesophageal diverticulum	Focal or segmental sacculations are observed on survey or contrast radiographs	Sacculations of the oesophageal wall may be evident with endoscopy, but it may be necessary to aspirate food and fluid from the sacculated segment to visualise the defect
Mega-oesophagus	Variable degrees of oesophageal dilation will be observed on survey radiographs. Contrast radiographs will confirm the oesophageal dilation as well as provide some limited information about oesophageal motility. Endoscopy is usually not needed to make the diagnosis	Variable degrees of oesophageal dilation will be apparent at endoscopy. Oesophagitis or oesophageal obstruction may be observed in some cases
Hiatal hernia	Survey radiographs are usually diagnostic (e.g. caudodorsal gas-filled opacity in the thoracic cavity) in congenital forms of the disease. Several contrast studies may be required to document the same findings in animals with acquired hiatal herniae	Findings consistent with the diagnosis include cranial displacement of the gastro-oesophageal sphincter, a large oesophageal hiatus, and oesophagitis

Table 48.5 *Continued*

Oesophageal disorder	Radiographic findings	Endoscopic findings
Gastro-oesophageal reflux	Survey radiographs are usually non-remarkable. The contrast radiographic findings of irregular mucosal surface and oesophageal dilation are consistent with oesophagitis secondary to gastro-oesophgeal reflux. Gastro-oesophageal reflux of barium may or may not be abnormal. Endoscopy should be performed for definitive diagnosis mass	Endoscopic findings will be similar to those of oesophagitis
Gastro-oesophageal intussusception	Proximal oesophageal dilation, consolidation or mass effect between the cardiac silhouette and diaphragm and gastric rugal folds within the intrathoracic oesophagus are findings consistent with the diagnosis of gastro-oesophageal intussusception	An intra-oesophageal mass completely obstructing the lumen of oesophagus is evident. Gastric rugal folds may be visible

- Usually performed after contrast radiography, endoscopy is now often performed instead of contrast radiography except for mega-oesophagus.
- Endoscopy is particularly useful in diagnosing oesophageal stricture, oesophagitis, intraluminal mass, foreign body and diverticula.
- Endoscopy may also be used therapeutically to remove foreign bodies, dilate oesophageal strictures, or to place gastrostomy feeding tubes.
- Technique requires general anaesthesia.
- The endoscopic findings associated with oesophageal disease are outlined in Table 48.5.

Ultrasonography

- Ultrasonography does not have a traditional role in the diagnosis of primary oesophageal disease.
- However, it has proved useful in the diagnosis of peri-oesophageal (e.g. neoplasia) or other mediastinal disease.

Oesophageal Manometry

- Manometry may be useful in diagnosing cricopharyngeal achalasia and gastro–oesophageal sphincter incompetence.
- The technique is currently limited to university teaching hospitals.

ORAL CAVITY: DIFFERENTIAL DIAGNOSIS AND SPECIFIC DISEASES

The differential diagnosis for dysphagia and hyper-salivation is depicted in Table 48.6 and the management of oral cavity disease is outlined in Box 48.1 and Box 48.2. The clinical features of specific diseases are outlined below.

Neuromuscular Dysphagia

The aetiology is unknown in most cases, but some have been associated with brainstem disease, peripheral (cranial nerves V, VII, IX, X, XII) neuropathy, myasthenia gravis, myositis or hypothyroidism (Suter & Watrous 1980; Peeters 1995). Rabies is an occasional cause of neuro-muscular dysphagia in the United States and Western Europe. Neuromuscular dysphagias other than cricopharyngeal achalasia are treated medically; treatment is mostly supportive with a gastrostomy tube feeding on a temporary or permanent basis. Cricopharyngeal achalasia is best treated by cricopharyngeal myotomy. The prognosis for neuromuscular dysphagia is guarded to poor. Only those disorders associated with myasthenia gravis, polymyositis, or hypothyroidism show some clinical improvement with treatment.

Box 48.1 Management of oral cavity disease.

Supportive treatment

Fluids

- Assess dehydration and electrolyte status
- Calculate fluid deficit and maintenance requirements
- Balanced electrolytes solutions most useful; potassium supplementation may be necessary if animal is anorectic

Dietary manipulation

- A short fast (24–48 h) may be beneficial in animals with inflammation, infection, or trauma
- Liquid diets are handled better in animals with neuromuscular dysphagia

Nutritional support

- Gastrostomy feeding tubes may be placed surgically, or by endoscopic guidance (Fig. 48.3; Bright & Burrows 1988; Armstrong & Hardie 1990)
- Gastrostomy feeding may be maintained for several weeks or months

Specific treatment

Neuromuscular disease

- Gastrostomy tube feeding if necessary
- Cricopharyngeal myotomy for cricopharyngeal achalasia
- Thyroid replacement therapy for documented cases of hypothyroidism
- Acetylcholinesterase inhibitors for documented cases of acquired myasthenia gravis
- Corticosteroids for documented cases of polymyositis or myasthenia gravis

Oropharyngeal neoplasia

- Surgical excision likely to yield best outcome
- Radiation therapy for acanthomataous epulis and squamous cell carcinoma

Oropharyngeal eosinophilic granuloma

- Oral (prednisone), intralesional (triamcinolone), or subcutaneous (methylprednisolone) corticosteroids
- Surgical resection for corticosteroid non-responsive lesions

Box 48.1 *Continued.*

Oropharyngeal trauma

- Removal of foreign bodies
- Anatomic defects resulting from physical injury should be surgically corrected
- Thermal, electrical, or chemical injury may require surgical debridement
- Tissue necrosis should be managed with dilute chlorhexidine solution and broad-spectrum antibiotics

Oropharyngeal inflammation

- Broad-spectrum antibiotics for documented cases of bacterial infection
- Antifungal agents for documented cases of fungal infection
- Corticosteroids for inflammation or immunological disease (systemic lupus erythematosus, bullous pemphigoid)

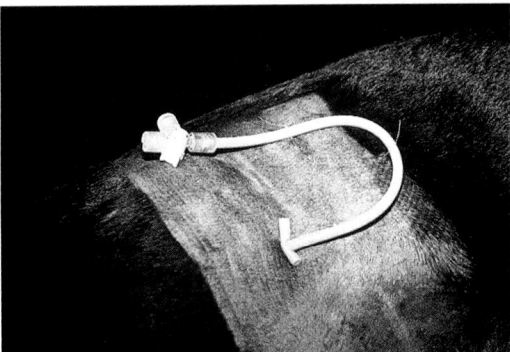

Fig. 48.3 Percutaneous endoscopic gastrostomy tube. (Photo courtesy of Dr Kenneth W. Simpson, Cornell University, Ithaca, NY, USA.)

Oropharyngeal Neoplasia

The oropharynx is a common site for the development of neoplasia with the most common tumours being melanoma, squamous cell carcinoma, periodontal epulis and fibrosarcoma (Withrow & MacEwen 1989a). Definitive diagnosis by tissue biopsy and histopathological examination of primary tumour and regional lymph nodes. In general squamous cell carcinoma, associated with either the

Box 48.2 Oral cavity and oesophageal disease: therapeutics.

Broad-spectrum antibiotics (see page 53 for antibiotic dosages)

- Aminoglycosides (gentamicin, amikacin), ampicillin, cephalosporins (cefoxitin, cephalexin, cephalothin), clindamycin, enrofloxacin, metronidazole, trimethoprim–sulfa

Oesophageal diffusion barriers

- Sucralfate 0.5–1.0 g p.o. t.i.d. – should be given as oral suspension, much less effective when given as intact tablet

Gastric acid secretory inhibitors

- Cimetidine 5–10 mg/kg p.o. or i.v. t.i.d.–q.i.d.
- Ranitidine 1.0-2.0 mg/kg p.o. or i.v. b.i.d.–t.i.d.
- Famotidine 0.1–0.2 mg/kg p.o. or i.v. b.i.d.
- Nizatidine 1.0–3.0 mg/kg s.c. or i.m. or i.v. t.i.d.
- Omeprazole 0.7 mg/kg p.o. s.i.d.

Smooth muscle prokinetic agents

- Cisapride 0.1–0.5 mg/kg p.o. b.i.d.–t.i.d.
- Metoclopramide 0.2–0.4 mg/kg p.o. t.i.d.–q.i.d.

Corticosteroids

- Prednisone 0.5–1.0 mg/kg s.c. or i.m. b.i.d. for oesophageal strictures
- Prednisone 1.0–2.0 mg/kg p.o. b.i.d. for systemic lupus erythematosus, bullous pemphigoid or oral eosinophilic granuloma

Thyroid replacement therapy

- Levothyroxine 0.22 µg/kg p.o. b.i.d.

Acetylcholinesterase Inhibitors

- Pyridostigmine 1.0–3.0 mg/kg p.o. b.i.d.–t.i.d.

Oral irrigants

- 0.1% chlorhexidine, 15–30 ml oral lavage b.i.d.–t.i.d. for oropharyngeal necrosis or mucositis

mandible or maxilla can be treated either by various forms of mandibulectomy or maxillectomy, some carry a good prognosis and cures can be achieved. Squamous cell carcinoma of the tonsil is considered unresponsive to all forms of treatment. Fibrosarcomas can be resected and have significant disease free periods but tend to recur at the site, albeit after 12 months (White & Gorman 1989). Melanomas can be managed palliatively by radical or local surgery but carry a poor prognosis of under 6 months. Radiation therapy is also of use in the management of the principal tumour types although nothing seems to affect tonsillar carcinomas in the dog (Theilen & Madewell 1987).

Oropharyngeal Eosinophilic Granuloma

This primarily affects young dogs and may be heritable in the Siberian Husky and is usually seen on the lateral

Table 48.6 Differential diagnosis of dysphagia and hypersalivation.

Congenital
   Cleft palate
   Facial malformation

Infection
   Many primary bacterial infections, Gram positive and
      negative
   Candida albicans
   Periodontal disease

Inflammation
   Idiopathic
   Systemic lupus erythematosus
   Bullous pemphigoid

Neoplasia
   Melanoma
   Squamous cell carcinoma
   Periodontal epulis
   Fibrosarcoma
   Eosinophilic granuloma

Trauma
   Physical injury
   Chemical, thermal, and electrical burns
   Foreign bodies

Neuromuscular
   Cricopharyngeal achalasia
   Myasthenia gravis
   Hypothyroidism
   Myositis
   Idiopathic peripheral neuropathy
   Brainstem disease

Musculoskeletal
   Temperomandibular joint disease
   Craniomandibular osteopathy

and ventral aspects of the tongue. Lesions may appear indistinguishable from malignant neoplasia. Peripheral eosinophilia may be recognised in haematology, but diagnosis should always be based on biopsy and histopathological examination. Spontaneous remissions may occur, but corticosteroid therapy is generally required for control or cure in most cases. Corticosteroid non-responsive lesions may be successfully treated with surgical excision. Treatment with corticosteroids or surgical excision is generally curative in the dog.

Oropharyngeal Trauma

Trauma may result from direct physical injury (animal fights or blunt head trauma), burns (electrical, thermal, or chemical) and foreign bodies. The inciting causes may differ, but the pathogenesis (tissue destruction) is similar. A tranquiliser or short-acting anaesthetic agent may be necessary to examine the oral cavity. Physical abnormalities consistent with trauma are usually straightforward. The most difficult problem is that of tracking foreign bodies, particularly wooden sticks, that penetrate the oral mucosa and can migrate to a number of sites around the head. Sites include the retropharyngeal area, the lateral pharynx and beneath the eye, where abscesses form and then subsequently track to the skin and discharge persistently. The management of these cases is by surgical exploration and removal of the foreign body and is reviewed in detail by White & Lane 1988.

Tissue necrosis from some electrical, thermal or chemical burns may not become evident for 3–5 days after the injury. Pulmonary oedema may be a complication of electrical burns in the oral cavity; chest radiographs should be obtained in such cases. Prognosis ranges from poor to excellent depending upon the severity of the injury.

Oropharyngeal Inflammation

Primary stomatitis/pharyngitis has several important aetiologies, including infectious (e.g. *Candida albicans*), immunological (systemic lupus erythematosus, bullous pemphigoid, pemphigus vulgaris) and chemical causes but may occur secondarily with gingivitis and glossitis, or as a consequence of uraemia. Oral examination may require use of a short-acting intravenous anaesthetic agent and definitive diagnosis may require tissue culture and/or biopsy in many instances. Once a diagnosis has been made antimicrobial, antifungal, and immunosuppressive therapy should be instituted when appropriate.

OESOPHAGUS: DIFFERENTIAL DIAGNOSIS AND SPECIFIC DISEASES

The differential diagnosis for regurgitation is depicted in Table 48.7 and the management of oesophageal disease is outlined in Box 48.3 and Therapeutics Box 48.2. The clinical features of specific diseases are outlined below.

Oesophageal Foreign Bodies (Fig. 48.4)

Most common foreign bodies found in dogs are bones or bone fragments. The severity of damage is dependent upon foreign body size, angularity or sharp points, and the duration of obstruction (Houlton *et al.* 1985). Oesophageal foreign bodies should be removed promptly; prolonged retention increases the likelihood of oesophageal mucosal damage, ulceration and perforation. A rigid endoscope is most useful in retrieving large foreign bodies, e.g. bones. The flexible fibre-optic endoscopes are more useful with small foreign bodies, e.g. fish hooks (Michels *et al.* 1995). Surgery is only indicated if endoscopy fails, or to treat oesophageal perforation. Complications of foreign bodies

Table 48.7   Differential diagnosis of regurgitation.

Oesophageal foreign bodies

Oesophageal fistulae

Oesophageal inflammation
    Oesophagitis
    Gastro-oesophageal reflux

Oesophageal neoplasia
    Fibrosarcoma
    Osteosarcoma
    Leiomyosarcoma
    Metastatic tumours – thyroid, pulmonary and gastric
      carcinomata

Mechanical obstruction of the oesophagus
    Vascular ring anomaly – persistent right aortic arch most
      common
    Stricture – fibrosing or malignant
    Gastro-oesophageal intussusception
    Hiatal hernia
    Compression from peri-oesophageal neoplasia

Functional obstruction of the oesophagus
    Idiopathic mega-oesophagus
    Non-idiopathic congenital or acquired megaoesophagus
    Oesophageal diverticula

Box 48.3 Management of oesophageal disease.

Supportive treatment

Fluids

- Assess dehydration and electrolyte status
- Calculate fluid deficit and maintenance requirements
- Balanced electrolytes solutions most useful; potassium supplementation may be necessary if animal is anorectic

Dietary manipulation

- A short fast (24–48 h) may be beneficial in animals with oesophagitis or oesophageal foreign body
- Low fat diets are beneficial in animals with gastro-oesophageal reflux
- Liquid diets are handled better in animals with oesophageal stricture
- Dietary consistency should be formulated to produce the fewest clinical signs in animals affected with mega-oesophagus. Some animals handle liquids quite well, while others do better with solids

Nutritional support

- Gastrostomy feeding tubes may be placed surgically, or by endoscopic guidance (Bright & Burrows 1988; Armstrong & Hardie 1990)
- Gastrostomy feeding may be maintained for weeks or months

Specific treatment

Foreign bodies

- Endoscopic removal (rigid endoscope for large foreign bodies, flexible fibre-optic endoscope for smaller foreign bodies)
- Surgery if endoscopic failure, or if oesophageal perforation
- 24–48 h fast following removal (longer if severe mucosal ulceration or necrosis)
- Percutaneous gastrostomy tube feeding if necessary
- Oral sucralfate suspensions and broad-spectrum antibiotics after foreign body removal

Fistulae

- Surgical excision of the fistula, closure of oesophageal defect
- Resection of affected lung lobe
- Broad-spectrum antibiotics

Vascular ring anomalies

- Ligation of anomalous blood vessel (left intercostal approach for persistent right aortic arch; right intercostal thoracotomy for persistent right ductus arteriosus, aberrant right subclavian artery, and double aortic arch), reduction of peri-oesophageal fibrosis
- Dilation of stricture site if necessary
- Postoperative forced elevated feedings; percutaneous gastrostomy tube feeding if necessary

Neoplasia

- Resection of benign tumours (e.g. leiomyoma)
- Chemotherapy or radiation therapy for malignant tumours. Surgical resection is complicated by inadequate surgical exposure, lengthy resection, tension on the anastomosis, and poor healing properties of the oesophagus

Oesophagitis

- Withhold oral food intake for 2–3 days; percutaneous gastrostomy tube feeding if necessary
- Oral sucralfate suspensions
- Gastric acid secretory inhibitors (e.g. cimetidine, ranitidine, omeprazole)
- Broad-spectrum antibiotics

Stricture

- Liquid feedings if tolerable; withhold oral food intake if not tolerable
- Percutaneous gastrostomy tube feedings if necessary
- Balloon dilation or bougienage – may require multiple dilations
- Surgical resection usually not successful
- Oral sucralfate suspensions
- Gastric acid secretory inhibitors
- Corticosteroids (prednisone) to prevent fibrosis and re-stricture

Diverticula

- Liquid to semi-liquid feedings
- Surgical excision and reconstruction of the oesophageal wall

Box 48.3 *Continued.*

Idiopathic mega-oesophagus

- Dietary management – high-calorie, small frequent feedings, of liquid or solid consistency from an elevated or upright position
- Treat aspiration pneumonia with broad-spectrum antibiotics

Gastro-oesophageal reflux

- Dietary management – low fat diets, avoid late night feedings
- Oral sucralfate suspensions
- Gastric acid secretory inhibitors
- Smooth muscle prokinetic agents (e.g. cisapride, metoclopramide)

Congenital hiatal hernia

- Surgical repair – diaphragmatic crural apposition, oesophagopexy, gastropexy (Prymak *et al.* 1989)

Acquired hiatal hernia

- Oral sucralfate suspensions
- Gastric acid secretory inhibitors
- Smooth muscle prokinetic agents

Gastro-oesophageal intussusception

- Brief period of stabilisation
- Emergency surgery – reduction of the intussusception, gastropexy

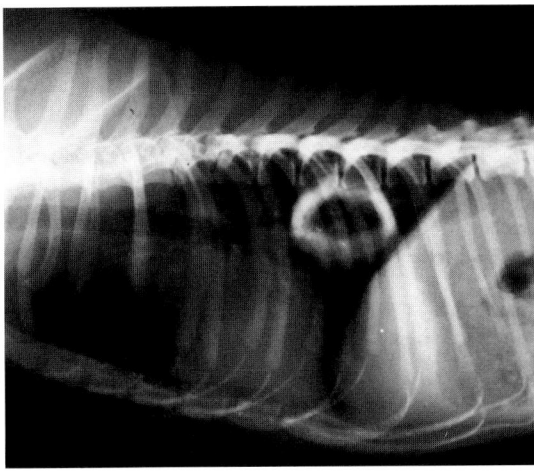

Fig. 48.4 Bone foreign body in the distal oesophageal body of a 7-year-old mixed breed dog.

include fistulation, mediastinitis, diverticula or stricture formation.

Oesophageal Fistula

Most fistulae involve the lungs or airway structures. Congenital fistulae have been reported in the Cairn Terrier (Twedt 1994). Acquired oesophageal fistulae typically result from foreign body ingestion, oesophageal perforation, and extension of inflammation into adjacent tissues with bones and awned grass seeds being most commonly incriminated. The clinical signs are more related to bronchopneumonia and pulmonary abscess with the right caudal, right intermediate and left caudal lung lobes most often involved. The definitive diagnosis of oesophageal fistulae requires contrast radiography or endoscopy. Fortunately surgical excision and repair provide the most successful outcomes.

Vascular Ring Anomalies (Fig. 48.5a & b)

These are congenital malformations of the major arteries of the heart that, because of altered anatomic relationships, entrap the oesophagus and trachea. The reported anomalies include persistent right aortic arch, persistent right or left subclavian arteries, persistent right dorsal aorta, double aortic arch, left aortic arch and right ligamentum arteriosum and aberrant intercostal arteries (Patterson 1968). The most common anomaly is the persistent right aortic arch, puppies develop regurgitation and failure to thrive shortly after weaning. The diagnosis is based on barium contrast radiographic finding of oesophageal body dilation cranial to the base of the heart. Surgery is essential with persistent right aortic arch best managed using a left intercostal approach whereas a peristent right ductus arteriosus, aberrant right subclavian artery, and double aortic arch are best approached by right intercostal thoracotomy. Prognosis is generally favourable if the condition is recognised early. However, the clinical signs may persist after surgery in long-standing undiagnosed cases and some cases may require placement of percutaneous gastrostomy tubes to maintain nutritional support.

Oesophageal Neoplasia (Fig. 48.6a & b)

Tumours of the oesophagus are uncommon and may be of primary oesophageal, peri-oesophageal or metastatic origin. The most common primary oesophageal tumours are osteosarcoma and fibrosarcoma, particularly in areas of *Spirocerca lupi* endemicity (Ridgway & Suter 1979). It is

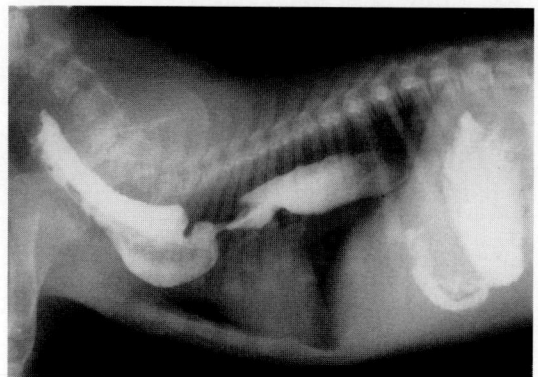

a

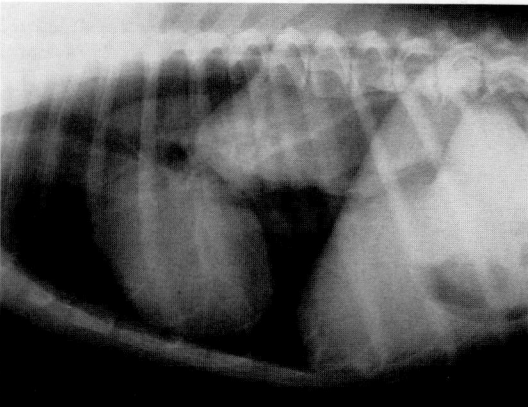

a

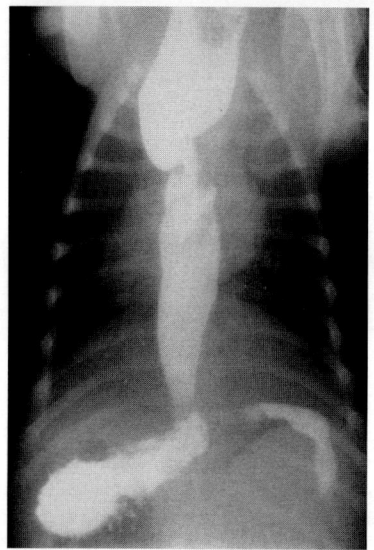

b

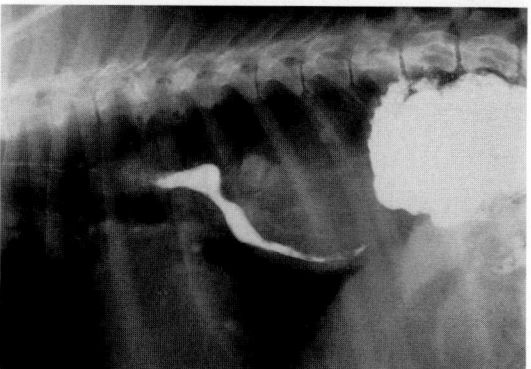

b

Fig. 48.6a & b   Peri-oesophageal tumour (sarcoma) in a 10-year-old mixed breed dog.

Fig. 48.5a & b   Persistent right aortic arch in a 5-month-old Great Dane puppy.

recognised that metastatic lesions are the most common oesophageal tumours in dogs. The primary tumours include thyroid, pulmonary, and gastric carcinoma, which are usually malignant and bear a poor prognosis. Chemotherapy, radiation therapy, or surgical resection may be attempted with malignant tumours, but the prognosis is poor (Withrow & MacEwen 1989b). In contrast benign tumours, e.g. leiomyoma, have a more favourable prognosis following surgical resection.

Oesophagitis

This may result from chemical injury from swallowed substances, oesophageal foreign bodies, or gastro-oesophageal

reflux during anaesthesia. On survey thoracic radiographs the oesophagus often appears normal. Contrast radiographic findings include irregular mucosal surface, segmental narrowing, oesophageal dilation, and/or diffuse oesophageal hypomotility. The most reliable means of diagnosing oesophagitis are endoscopy and biopsy. The best outcomes are obtained with medical treatment (e.g. sucralfate) and the prognosis for mild oesophagitis is generally favourable; ulcerative oesophagitis warrants a more guarded prognosis. The most important complication is oesophageal stricture.

Oesophageal Stricture

The important causes of oesophageal stricture are chemical injury from swallowed substances, oesophageal foreign bodies, oesophageal surgery, and intraluminal or extralumi-

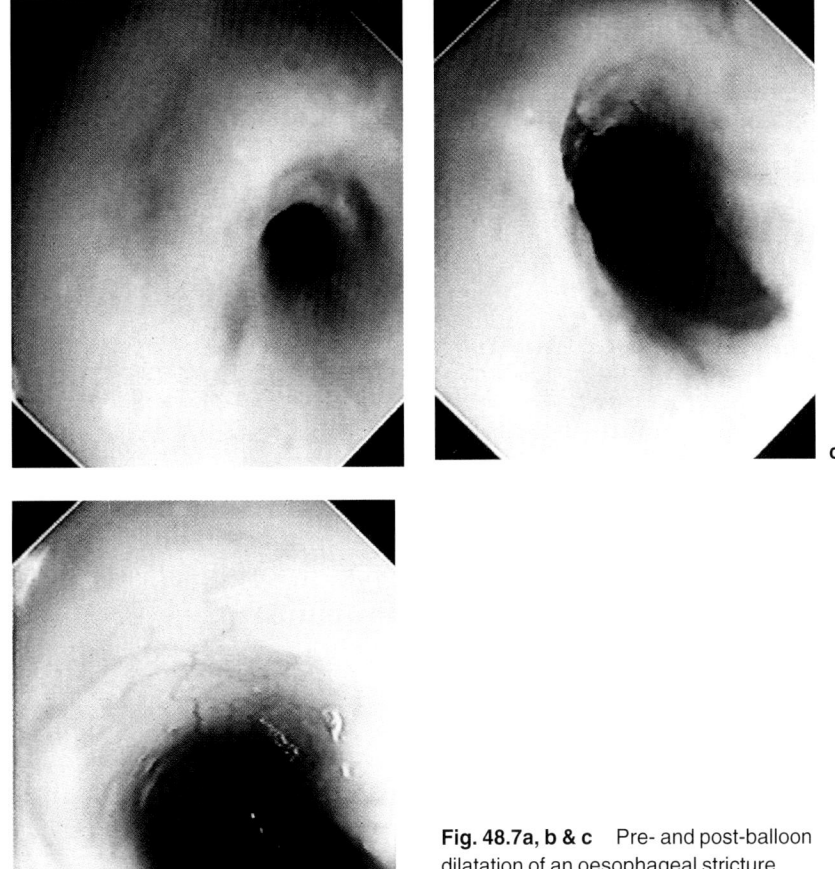

Fig. 48.7a, b & c Pre- and post-balloon dilatation of an oesophageal stricture. (Photographs courtesy of Dr Kenneth W. Simpson, Cornell University, Ithaca, NY, USA.)

nal mass lesions (neoplasia or abscesses). Anaesthesia, poor patient preparation and poor patient positioning during anaesthesia place some animals at risk for gastro-oesophageal reflux, oesophagitis and subsequent stricture formation (Pearson *et al.* 1978; Harai *et al.* 1995). Segmental or diffuse narrowing observed with barium contrast radiography is usually diagnostic of the disorder. Endoscopy should be performed to confirm the site and severity of stricture, and to exclude the possibility of intraluminal malignancy. Balloon dilation of the stricture is the preferred method of treatment (Fig. 48.7; Burk *et al.* 1987; Harai *et al.* 1995). The prognosis for recovery is guarded; recurrences are common.

Oesophageal Diverticula

These are circumscribed sacculations in the wall of the oesophagus and can be congenital or acquired.

- Congenital diverticula result from herniation of the mucosa through a defect in the oesophageal muscularis.
- Acquired diverticula result from inflammatory diseases involving the oesophagus or other mediastinal structures; adhesions to adjacent tissue distort the oesophageal lumen and create sacculations.

Contrast radiography will demonstrate a focal dilated segment of oesophageal lumen but endoscopy will confirm the diagnosis. Diverticula are best treated by surgical excision and reconstruction of the oesophageal wall.

Mega-oesophagus (Fig. 48.8)

- Congenital idiopathic mega-oesophagus is a generalised dilation and hypomotility of the oesophagus causing regurgitation and failure to thrive in puppies shortly after weaning; a defect in the vagal afferent innervation is involved in the pathogenesis (Tan & Diamant 1987; Holland *et al.* 1994).
- Acquired secondary mega-oesophagus may develop in association with a number of other conditions (see Table 48.8); localised versus generalised myasthenia

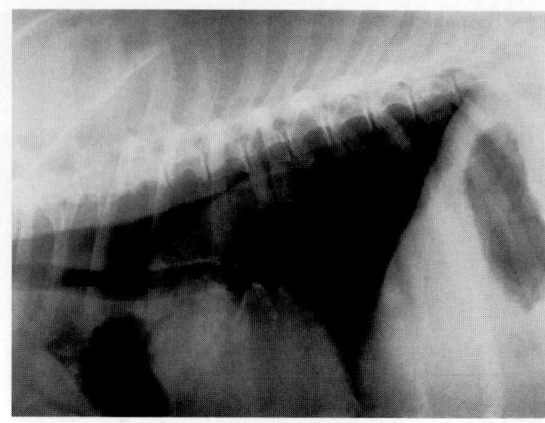

Fig. 48.8   Idiopathic acquired mega-oesophagus in a 9-year-old German Shepherd Dog.

Table 48.8   Medical investigation of acquired mega-oesophagus.

Cause	Evaluation
Congenital mega-oesophagus	
Myasthenia gravis	Edrophonium response ± electrophysiology
Neuropathy	Oesophageal manometry ± electrophysiology
Hiatal hernia	Survey and contrast chest radiography
Glycogen or lipid storage disease	Muscle or liver biopsy, serum enzyme activities
Acquired idiopathic mega-oesophagus	
Neuropathy	Oesophageal manometry ± electrophysiology
Acquired secondary mega-oesophagus	
Myasthenia gravis	Nicotinic acetylcholine receptor antibody, edrophonium response, ± electrophysiology, oesophageal motility, decreased gag and blink reflexes. Generalised weakness.
Polymyositis/polymyopathy	Serum creatine phosphokinase, muscle biopsy ± electrophysiology
Hypothyroidism	Thyroid function test (e.g. T_4, TSH stimulation)
Systemic lupus erythematosus	Anti-nuclear antibody
Hypoadrenocorticism	ACTH stimulation
Hiatal hernia	Contrast radiography and oesophageal endoscopy
Gastric dilation/volvulus	Survey and contrast radiography
Lead toxicity	Haematology, blood lead concentrations
Organophosphate toxicity	Blood organophosphate concentrations, serum cholinesterase activity
Oesophagitis	Oesophageal endoscopy
Dermatomyositis	Skin and muscle biopsy
Distemper	Distemper serology, cerebrospinal fluid analysis
Thymoma	Chest radiography, thymic aspirate and/or resection

T_4, thyroxine; TSH, thyroid-stimulating hormone; ACTH, adrenocorticotrophic hormone.

gravis may account for as many as 25% of these cases. There may also be facial nerve paralysis (ptosis), loss of gag reflex, loss of bark in some dogs or muscle atrophy with myasthenis gravis.

Acquired idiopathic mega-oesophagus accounts for most of the adult-onset disease; the pathogenesis may involve a defect in the afferent neural response to oesophageal distension (Washabau 1992). Malnutrition and aspiration pneumonia are common complications. Diagnosis is straightforward and can usually be made on survey or contrast radiographs. The prognosis for the congenital form is fair to good; prognosis for the acquired idiopathic form is fair to poor. Unfortunately, cisapride, a smooth muscle prokinetic agent, has little effect on the striated muscle of the canine oesophageal body.

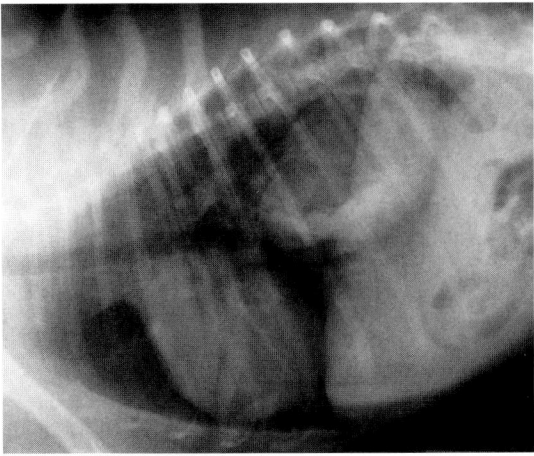

a

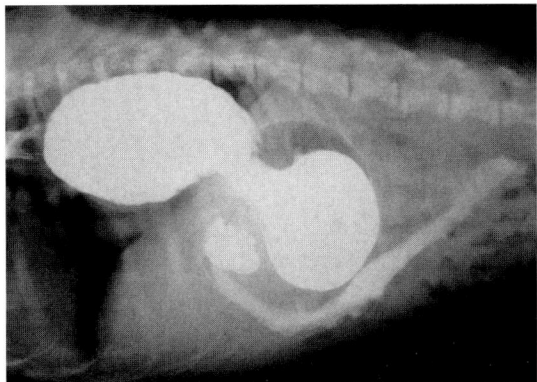

b

Fig. 48.9a & b   Congenital hiatal hernia in a 3-month-old Chinese Shar-Pei puppy.

Gastro-oesophageal Reflux

Chronic vomiting, disorders of gastric emptying, hiatal hernia, and anaesthesia-induced decreases in gastro-oesophageal sphincter pressure are the major causes. The frequency of reflux and composition of the refluxed material determines the severity of the oesophagitis (Cassidy *et al.* 1992; Evander *et al.* 1987). Diagnosis may be based on little more than clinical suspicion since survey and contrast radiographs may be non-remarkable. Endoscopy is the current best means of documenting mucosal inflammation. Medical therapy includes dietary manipulation, oesophageal diffusion barriers, gastric acid secretory inhibitors and drugs to improve the tone of the gastro-oesophageal sphincter.

Hiatal Hernia (Fig. 48.9a & b)

Congenital hiatal herniae have been reported in the Chinese Shar-Pei and Chow breeds. The affected animals develop clinical signs shortly after weaning (Callan *et al.* 1993). Survey radiographs may be sufficient to diagnose the congenital form. Congenital hiatal hernia generally requires surgical correction (Prymak *et al.* 1989). The acquired form of hiatal hernia may occur in any breed of dog and frequently results from increased intra-abdominal pressure with chronic vomiting disorders. Contrast radiographs are usually required to make the diagnosis. Acquired hiatal herniae are generally responsive to medical treatment (oesophageal diffusion barriers, gastric acid secretory inhibitors).

Gastro-oesophageal Intussusception (Fig. 48.10a & b)

Gastro-oesophageal intussusception is a rare condition of young dogs characterised by invagination of the stomach into the oesophagus (Leib & Blass 1984). Many affected animals have pre-existing idiopathic mega-oesophagus. Survey radiographs are usually sufficient to make the diagnosis. Gastro-oesophageal intussusception is a true gastrointestinal emergency; animals quickly deteriorate without emergency treatment. The recommended treatment is a brief period of stabilisation followed by endoscopical or surgical reduction. The prognosis is poor unless the disorder is quickly recognised and treated.

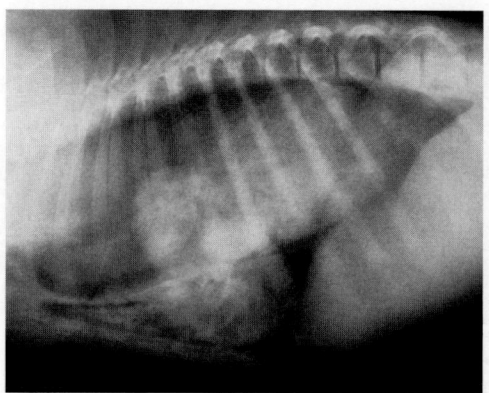

a

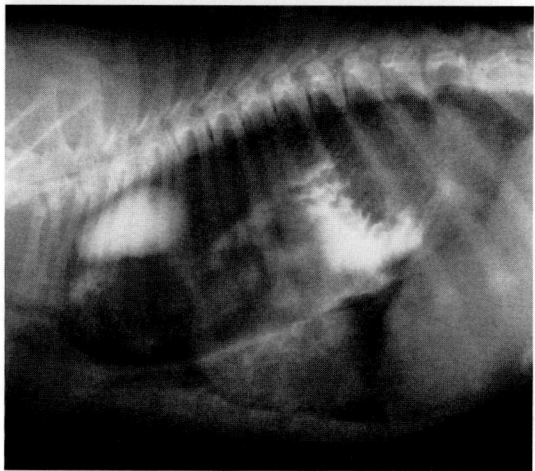

b

Fig. 48.10a & b   Gastro-oesophageal intussusception in a 12-month-old mixed breed dog.

REFERENCES

Armstrong, P.J. & Hardie, E.M. (1990). Percutaneous endoscopic tube gastrostomy: a retrospective study of 54 clinical cases in dogs and cats. *Journal of Veterinary Internal Medicine*, **4**, 202.

Bright, R.M. & Burrows, C.F. (1988). Percutaneous endoscopic tube gastrostomy in dogs. *American Journal of Veterinary Research*, **49**, 629.

Burk, R.L., Zawie, D., *et al.* (1987). Balloon catheter dilation of intramural esophageal strictures in the dog and cat. *Seminars in Veterinary Medicine and Surgery*, **2**, 241.

Callan, M.B., Washabau, R.J., Saunders, H.M., Kerr, L., Prymak, C. & Holt, D. (1993). Congenital esophageal hiatal hernia in the Chinese Shar-pei dog. *Journal of Veterinary Internal Medicine*, **7**, 210–215.

Cassidy, T.K., Geisinger, K.R., Kraus, B.B. & Castell, D.O. (1992). Continuous versus intermittent acid exposure in the production of oesophagitis in a feline model. *Digestive Diseases and Sciences*, **37**, 1206–1211.

Evander, A., Little, A.G., Riddle, R.H., Walther, B. & Skinner, D.B. (1987). Composition of the refluxed material determines the degree of reflux esophagitis in the dog. *Gastroenterology*, **93**, 280–286.

Harai, B.H., Johnson, S.E. & Sherding, R.G. (1995). Endoscopically guided balloon dilatation of benign esophageal stricture in 6 cats and 7 dogs. *Journal of Veterinary Internal Medicine*, **9**, 332–335.

Holland, C.T., Satchell, P.M. & Farrow, B.R.H. (1994). Vagal afferent dysfunction in naturally occurring canine esophageal motility disorder. *Digestive Diseases and Sciences*, **39**, 2090–2098.

Houlton, J.E.F., Herrtage, M.E., Taylor, P.M. & Watkins, S.B. (1985). Thoracic oesophageal foreign body in the dog: a review of ninety cases. *Journal of Small Animal Practice*, **26**, 521–536.

Lang, I.M., Dantas, R.O., Cook, I.J. & Dodds, W.J. (1991). Videoradiographic, manometric, and electromyographic analysis of canine upper esophageal sphincter. *American Journal of Physiology*, **260**, G911–G919.

Leib, M.S. and Blass, C.E. (1984). Gastroesophageal intussusception in the dog. *Journal of the American Animal Hospital Association*, **20**, 783.

Michels, G.M., Jones, B.D., *et al.* (1995). Endoscopic and surgical retrieval of fishhooks from the stomach and esophagus in dogs and cats: 75 cases (1977–1993). *Journal of the American Veterinary Medical Association*, **207**, 1194.

Patterson, D.F. (1968). Epidemiologic and genetic studies of congenital heart disease in the dog. *Circulation Research*, **23**, 171.

Pearson, H., Darke, P.G., Gibbs, C., Kelly, D.F. & Orr, C.M. (1978). Reflux oesophagitis and stricture formation after anesthesia. *Journal of Small Animal Practice*, **19**, 507–519.

Peeters, M.E. (1995). *A clinical study of dysphagia in the dog with emphasis on dysphagia in bouviers.* Doctoral Thesis, Universiteit Utrecht.

Prymak, C., Saunders, H.M. & Washabau, R.J., *et al.* (1989). Hiatal hernia repair by restoration and stabilization of normal anatomy. *Veterinary Surgery*, **18**, 386–391.

Ridgway, R.L. & Suter, P.F. (1979). Clinical and radiographic signs in primary and metastatic esophageal neoplasms of the dog. *Journal of the American Veterinary Medical Association*, **174**, 700.

Rosin, E.R. (1986). Quantitation of the pharyngoesophageal sphincter in the dog. *American Journal of Veterinary Research*, **47**, 660.

Shelton, G.D., Willard, M.D., Cardinetgh, B. & Lindstrom, J. (1990). Acquired myasthenia gravis: selective involvement of esophageal, pharyngeal, and facial muscles. *Journal of Veterinary Internal Medicine*, **4**, 281–284.

Suter, P.F. & Watrous, B. (1980). Oropharyngeal dysphagias in the dog: a cinefluorographic analysis of experimentally induced and spontaneously occurring swallowing disorders. *Veterinary Radiology*, **21**, 24.

Tan, B.J.K. & Diamant, N. (1987). Assessment of the neural defect in a dog with idiopathic megaesophagus. *Digestive Diseases and Sciences*, **32**, 76.

Theilen, G.H. & Madewell, B.R. (1987). Tumors of the digestive tract. In: *Veterinary Cancer Medicine*, (eds G.H. Theilen & B.R. Madewell), 2nd edn. pp. 499–534. Lea & Febiger, Philadelphia.

Twedt, D.C. (1994). Diseases of the esophagus. In: *Textbook of Veterinary Internal Medicine*, (eds S.J. Ettinger & E.C. Feldman), 4th edn. pp. 1124–1142. W.B. Saunders Company, Philadelphia.

Washabau, R.J. (1992). Canine megaesophagus: pathogenesis and therapy. *Proceedings of the American College of Veterinary Internal Medicine*, **10**, 671.

Washabau, R.J. & Hall, J.A. (1995). Clinical pharmacology of cisapride. *Journal of the American Veterinary Medical Association*, **207**, 1285.

Watrous, B. & Suter, P.F. (1979). Normal swallowing in the dog: a cineradiographic study. *Veterinary Radiology*, **20**, 99.

White, R.A.S. & Gorman, N.T. (1989). Surgical treatment of acanthomatous epulis in twenty five dogs. *Veterinary Surgery*, **18**, 12–14.

White, R.A.S. & Lane, J.G. (1988). Pharyngeal stick penetration injuries in the dog. *Journal of Small Animal Practice*, **29**, 13–35.

Withrow, S.J. & MacEwen, E.G. (1989a). Tumors of the oral cavity. In: *Clinical Veterinary Oncology*, pp. 177–189.

Withrow, S.J. & MacEwen, E.G. (1989b). Esophageal cancer. In: *Clinical Veterinary Oncology*, pp. 190–192.

Chapter 49

Diseases of the Stomach

R. C. DeNovo, Jr and C. C. Jenkins

FUNCTIONAL ANATOMY

Macroscopic Anatomy

The stomach is a pouch-shaped organ that extends from the lower oesophageal sphincter proximally to the pylorus distally (Miller *et al.* 1964). The stomach lies mostly in a transverse position, more to the left of midline, and when empty is located within the rib cage. It is divided into several functionally distinct parts:

- The cardia is the gastric inlet which blends with the muscles of the oesophagus; it allows entry of ingesta into the stomach but prevents excessive gastro-oesophageal reflux.
- The fundus is a dome-shaped portion of the stomach located left and dorsal to the cardia which dilates to accommodate volumes of ingesta without increasing intragastric pressure.
- The body is the large middle portion of the stomach extending from the cardia and fundus to the antrum. The body stores ingesta and secretes hydrochloric acid, pepsin and other digestive enzymes.
- The funnel-shaped antrum is the distal third of the stomach which extends from the incisura angularis on the lesser curvature to the proximal limit of the pylorus; it grinds food into smaller particles.
- The pylorus is the most distal and narrowly tubular part of the stomach; its thick muscular wall forms the pyloric sphincter which limits the size of food particles that pass into the duodenum and prevents duodenogastric reflux.
- The pyloric canal is the short lumen passing through the sphincter which connects to the duodenum.

The stomach has a blood supply from the coeliac, hepatic and splenic arteries with the venous return to the hepatic portal vein via the gastrosplenic and gastroduode-nal veins. The lymphatic drainage is via the hepatic and mesenteric lymph nodes to the cisterna chyli and thoracic duct. There are two innervation pathways extrinsic and intrinsic. The extrinsic autonomic innervation consists of sympathetic afferents and efferents from the coeliac plexus, and parasympathetic vagal efferents. The intrinsic innervation consists of a myenteric plexus which innervates muscular layers, and a submucosal plexus which controls mucosal secretion.

GASTRIC MOTILITY

The oesophageal myenteric nerve plexus is continuous with that of the stomach and the gastric myenteric plexus is continuous with that of the pylorus and small intestine, features which facilitate co-ordinated oesophagogastric and gastroduodenal contractions (Russell & Bass 1985; Hall *et al.* 1988; Smout & Akkermans 1992).

Movements of the stomach facilitate storage, mixing, grinding and transport of food: stretch receptors in the gastric fundus and body are activated when food arrives, causing gastric relaxation which facilitates reservoir function without causing increased intragastric pressure. There are several peristaltic contractions per minute, which travel from the body to the antrum to mix and grind food and transport liquid and small food particles to the pylorus. The pylorus remains slightly opened most of the time to allow easy passage of liquid chyme. As a peristaltic wave approaches the pylorus, several millilitres of chyme pass into the duodenum; the pylorus then closes and larger particles are propelled back into the gastric body. High concentration of carbohydrate, protein or fat in the duodenum stimulates pyloric closure to prevent small intestinal overload.

Antral–duodenal co-ordination is central to normal gastric emptying:

- Liquids begin to empty from the stomach immediately, depending on osmotic and caloric content.
- Solids require 1–3 h to empty.
- Disordered movements of the stomach, pylorus and duodenum cause symptoms such as anorexia, nausea, bloating and pain.

GASTRIC MUCOSAL DEFENCE

Several physical and chemical components, collectively referred to as the gastric mucosal barrier, protect the stomach from cell-damaging effects of gastric acid, pepsin, bile acids and digestive enzymes, i.e. prevent autodigestion. A number of gastric conditions arise when this barrier is compromised and a clear understanding of the barrier is clearly important (Lacy & Ito 1984; Silen & Ito 1985; Konturek & Pawlik 1986; Flemstrom 1987; Silen 1987; Wallace & Bell 1992; Lichtenberger 1993) (Table 49.1).

PATHOPHYSIOLOGY OF VOMITING

The Vomiting Reflex

Vomiting is a centrally mediated neurological reflex that requires co-ordinated actions of the gastrointestinal, musculoskeletal and nervous systems (Washabau 1995). The vomiting centre, located within the medulla oblongata, controls vomiting and is activated by humoral or neural stimulation of receptors sensitive to chemicals, inflammation and changes in osmolality. There are four different pathways which stimulate vomiting:

(1) The chemoreceptor trigger zone (CRTZ), located in the area postrema of the fourth ventricle, is sensitive to humoral emetogenic substances such as uraemic and bacterial toxins, cardiac glycosides, general anaesthetics, dopaminergic agonists, antineoplastic drugs and apomorphine.
(2) Impulses from the vestibular semicircular canals to the CRTZ and vomiting centre are responsible for vomiting from vestibulitis and motion sickness.

Table 49.1   Gastric mucosal barrier.

Mucus–bicarbonate layer	A thick layer of mucus is secreted by surface epithelial cells; soluble mucus acts as a lubricant to prevent mechanical damage; soluble gel glycoprotein adheres to the mucosa to impede back-diffusion of acid and pepsin from the lumen into the epithelium. Bicarbonate is trapped in this mucous gel to maintain surface mucosal pH above 6, even when the pH of the lumen is as low as 1.5. This layer provides a diffusion barrier to protons (H^+ ions) and protects the surface epithelium from luminal acid
Epithelial cells and restitution	Gastric epithelial cells are characterised by low permeability to water and ions, tight intercellular junctions, and continual and rapid cell renewal, features that promote resistance to high acid concentration. Superficial injury to the gastric mucosa repairs within a few hours by epithelial restitution, a process whereby intact cells at the edge of the damaged area migrate over the defect
Mucosal blood flow	A dense network of capillaries supplies oxygen and nutrients to maintain mucus and bicarbonate secretion and to support the rapid cellular renewal. A high rate of mucosal blood flow removes toxic substances such as acid that have breached the mucosal barrier
Prostaglandins	Type E prostaglandins increase mucus and bicarbonate secretion, regulate mucosal blood flow, stimulate epithelial cell growth, and inhibit acid secretion; the collective effect is to enhance rapid epithelial restitution and prevent progression of damage deeper into the mucosa

(3) Abdominal visceral receptors send impulses via vagal and sympathetic nerves to the vomiting centre. Visceral receptors are sensitive to distension of the gastrointestinal tract and biliary ducts, inflammation or irritation of the viscera, peritoneum and pharynx, and hypertonicity of gastric and small intestinal content.

(4) Input from the cerebral cortex causes vomiting associated with anxiety, pain or behavioural influences.

Antiemetic therapies are designed to diminish either the humoral or neural pathways of the vomiting. (Table 49.2).

Metabolic Consequence of Vomiting
(Johnson 1992; Twedt & Magne 1989)

Vomiting for short duration does not cause significant fluid, electrolyte or acid–base losses, whereas profuse and protracted vomiting can lead to significant imbalances:

(1) Dehydration is the most common problem caused by vomiting.
(2) Hypokalaemia from loss of potassium in the vomitus and urine, coupled with lack of dietary intake is the most common, and potentially life-threatening, electrolyte abnormality.

Table 49.2   Antiemetic drugs and dosages.

Drug	Primary site of action	Dosage	Side-effects
Prochlorperazine (Compazine)	CRTZ Vomiting centre	0.5 mg/kg every 8 h s.c., i.m.	Hypotension Sedation
Chlorpromazine (Thorazine)	CRTZ Vomiting centre	0.25–0.4 mg/kg every 8 h s.c.	Hypotension Sedation
Phenylethylpirazine (Torecan)	CRTZ Vomiting centre		Hypotension Sedation
Yohimbine (Yobine)	CRTZ Vomiting centre	0.25–0.5 mg/kg every 12 h s.c., i.m.	Hypotension Sedation
Diphenhydramine (Benedryl)	CRTZ	2–4 mg/kg every 8 h p.o., i.m.	Sedation
Dimenhydrinate (Dramamine)	CRTZ	4–8 mg/kg every 8 h p.o.	Sedation
Haloperidol (Haldol)	CRTZ	0.02 mg/kg every 12 h	Sedation
Metoclopramide (Reglan)	CRTZ Gastrointestinal smooth muscle (facilitates gastric emptying)	0.25–0.4 mg/kg every 6 h p.o., s.c., i.m. 1–2 mg/kg per day as continuous i.v. infusion	Extrapyramidal signs
Domperidone (Motilium)	Gastrointestinal smooth muscle cells (facilitates gastric emptying)	0.1–0.3 mg/kg every 12 h i.m., i.v.	None reported
Cisapride (Propulsid)	Gastrointestinal smooth muscle Myenteric neurons (facilitates gastric emptying)	0.1–0.5 mg/kg every 8 h p.o.	None reported
Scopolamine (Hyoscine)	Vestibular system CRTZ	0.03 mg/kg every 6 h s.c., i.m.	Ileus Xerostomia Sedation
Ondansetron (Zofran)	CRTZ Blocks vagal afferent neurons	0.5–1.0 mg/kg every 12–24 h or 30 min before chemotherapy p.o.	Sedation Head shaking

CRTZ, chemoreceptor trigger zone.

(3) Hypochloraemia can occur from loss of chloride-rich gastric secretions; concurrent hypokalaemia causes reduction of distal nephron chloride reabsorption which exacerbates hypochloraemia.

(4) Plasma bicarbonate concentration and blood pH may be increased, normal or decreased depending on the cause of the vomiting, the acidity of the vomitus and presence of dehydration, lactic acidosis or renal insufficiency.

Many vomiting dogs have normal acid–base status due to simultaneous loss of gastric HCl and bicarbonate-rich duodenal juice. Some will have metabolic acidosis caused by dehydration, prerenal azotemia and lactic acidosis from decreased tissue perfusion. Metabolic alkalosis usually occurs secondary to pyloric outflow obstruction, but can develop secondary to profuse, frequent vomiting in the absence of obstruction; hypochloraemia contributes to the alkalosis. Causes of vomiting associated with alkalosis are listed in Table 49.3.

Table 49.3 Causes of vomiting associated with increased plasma bicarbonate (TCO_2).

Gastric outflow obstruction
   Gastric foreign body
   Pyloric hypertrophy syndrome
   Gastric neoplasm
   Gastric dilatation-volvulus
Gastric hypomotility
Gastrinoma (rare)
Acute pancreatitis
Duodenal obstruction
   Foreign body
   Neoplasia
Biliary obstruction

Table 49.4 Causes of vomiting associated with hyperkalaemia.

Hypoadrenocorticism
Renal failure
   Oliguric
   Anuric
Pseudo-hypoadrenocorticism
Trichuriasis
Salmonellosis

Increased urinary H$^+$ secretion, known as paradoxical aciduria, can occur if hypochloraemic metabolic alkalosis develops. Renal reabsorption of sodium is normally accompanied by chloride. If hypochloraemia exists, sodium is reabsorbed in exchange for H$^+$ and K$^+$ which are secreted. For each H$^+$ secreted, bicarbonate is reabsorbed. The net effect is to reabsorb sodium (and water) to maintain intravascular volume at the expense of acid–base balance. Causes of vomiting associated with hyperkalaemia are listed in Table 49.4.

INVESTIGATION OF GASTRIC DISEASE

History

Vomiting, haematemesis, melaena, anorexia, abdominal pain and/or abdominal distension are predominant signs of gastric disease; diarrhoea and weight loss occur less frequently. The characteristics of vomiting that are helpful in localisation and diagnosis of disease are listed in Tables 49.5 and 49.6.

Vomiting is the hallmark of gastric disease, however many non-gastric diseases cause vomiting. Owners often confuse vomiting with regurgitation, dysphagia and occasionally with coughing (Table 49.7).

(1) Vomiting is associated with nausea, retching and forceful abdominal contractions; subtle signs of nausea are anorexia, salivation and repeated swallowing.

(2) Vomitus varies from partially digested food to clear or bile-stained fluid that usually has an acid pH.

(3) Regurgitation is a passive retrograde movement of ingesta, usually before it reaches the stomach, that localises disease to the oesophagus. It occurs suddenly and without retching and appears to look like undigested food.

(4) Dysphagia is characterised by difficulty swallowing and indicates a disorder of the oral cavity, pharynx or oesophagus (page 437).

Vomiting is a major diagnostic challenge because of the wide variety of intestinal and metabolic disorders that cause this symptom (Tables 49.8 and 49.9). Although vomiting does not always indicate a serious disorder, it is frequently the first sign of parvovirus, haemorrhagic gastroenteritis, pancreatitis, intestinal obstruction, Addison's disease, renal failure, toxicities, and many other life-threatening diseases. Because not all animals with gastric disease vomit, a detailed history and thorough physical examina-

Table 49.5   Important characteristics of vomiting.

Characteristic	Significance
Soon after eating	Dietary indiscretion
	Overeating
	Food intolerance
	Acute gastritis
	Oesophageal or hiatal disorder
Hours after eating	Gastric motility disorder
	Gastric outflow obstruction (partial or complete)
	Intestinal disease
Chronic intermittent	Chronic gastritis
	Motility disorder
	Inflammatory bowel disease
	Metabolic disease
Undigested food	Gastric motility disorder
	Gastric outflow obstruction
	Oesophageal or hiatal disorder
Bile in vomitus	Enterogastric reflux syndrome
	Pancreatitis
	Inflammatory bowel disease
	Intestinal foreign body
	Metabolic disease
Blood in vomitus	Erosion or ulceration
	Coagulopathy
	Neoplasia
Faecal or fetid odour	Intestinal obstruction
	Intestinal stasis with bacterial overgrowth
	Ischaemic intestinal injury

Table 49.6   Important questions to ask in the history of the vomiting patient.

Duration	Recent and acute
	Chronic and intermittent
	Static or progressive
Associated signs	Appetite change
	Diarrhoea
	Abdominal pain
	Weight change
Past pertinent history	Vaccinations
	Worming
	Pancreatitis
	Garbage ingestion
Dietary history	Type
	Recent changes
Recent drug history	Non-steroidal anti-inflammatory drugs
	Cardiac drugs
	Antibiotics
Environment	Free roaming
	Scavenging
	Travel history
Systems review	Activity and attitude
	Polyuria/polydipsia
	Coughing, sneezing
	Regurgitation, dysphagia
	Diarrhoea
	Reproductive status

Vomiting characteristics – see Table 49.5.

Table 49.7   Features of dysphagia, regurgitation and vomiting.

Symptom	Characteristics	Significance
Dysphagia	Difficult swallowing Repeated swallowing Drooling	Localise disease to oral cavity or less commonly pharynx or oesophagus
Regurgitation	Passive expulsion of non-digested food and fluid. Occurs soon after meal. No prodromal nausea or retching	Localises disease to oesophagus
Vomiting	Forceful expulsion of ingesta and/or fluid. Preceded by salivation, retching, abdominal contractions. No consistent temporal relation to eating	Localises disease to stomach or proximal intestine or caused by metabolic disease

Usually self-limiting	Potentially life-threatening
Acute gastritis	Gastric-duodenal foreign body
Dietary indiscretion	Gastric-duodenal ulcer
Abrupt dietary change	Intussusception
Ingested foreign material	Canine parvovirus enteritis
Drugs (antibiotics, NSAIDs)	Canine distemper virus enteritis
Ingested chemicals	Infectious canine hepatitis
	Leptospirosis
Ascaris infection (puppies)	Haemorrhagic gastroenteritis
	Acute gastric dilatation-volvulus
Giardia	Acute pancreatitis
	Acute renal failure
Motion sickness	Acute hepatic failure
	Hypoadrenocorticism
	Pyometra
	Peritonitis
	Sepsis
	Salmon poisoning – *Neorickettsia*
	helminthoeca
	Splenic torsion

Table 49.8 Causes of acute vomiting in the dog.

Table 49.9 Causes of chronic vomiting in the dog.

Metabolic disease
  Renal disease
  Pancreatitis
  Hepatic disease
  Biliary disease
  Hypoadrenocorticism
  Diabetic ketoacidosis
  Hypercalcaemia
  Hypokalaemia
  Mastocytosis

Gastric disease
  Partial obstruction
    foreign body
    mucosal hypertrophy
  Chronic non-specific gastritis
    superficial, hypertrophic,
    atrophic
  Helicobacter-associated gastritis
  Mycotic gastritis
    phycomycosis
    histoplasmosis
  Parasites
    Physaloptera spp.
  Gastric neoplasia
    lymphosarcoma
    adenocarcinoma
  Benign gastric polyps
  Gastric hypomotility
  Enterogastric reflux
  Gastric dilatation

Oesophageal disease
  Hiatal hernia
  Gastro-oesophageal reflux
  Distal-oesophagitis

Small intestinal disease
  Parasites
    Giardia
    nematodes
  Inflammatory bowel disease
  Obstruction
    foreign body
    neoplasia
  Diffuse neoplasia
  Fungal disease
  Ileus

Large intestinal disease
  Chronic colitis
  Obstipation

Neurological disease
  Vestibular disease
  Autonomic epilepsy
  Neoplasia

Table 49.10 Predisposing causes of gastrointestinal ulcer disease in dogs.

Non-steroidal anti-inflammatory drugs (NSAIDS)
  Aspirin
  Phenylbutazone
  Indomethacin
  Ketoprofen
  Meclofenamic acid
  Piroxicam
  Naproxen
  Ibuprofen
  Indoprofen
  Flunixin meglumine

Corticosteroids

Metabolic diseases
  Liver failure
  Hypoadrenocorticism
  Neurologic disease
  Renal failure
  Acute pancreatitis

Inflammatory bowel disease

Altered gastric blood flow/stress-related factors
  Hypotension
  Shock
  Sepsis
  Surgery
  Spinal cord disease
  Gastric dilatation-volvulus

Conditions of increased HCl secretion
  Gastrin-secreting tumour
  Mast cell tumour
  Pyloric outflow obstruction

Toxic/traumatic agents
  Bile salts
  Pancreatic enzymes
  Lead
  Foreign bodies
  Alcohol
  Corrosive compounds

Gastric neoplasia
  Leiomyoma
  Adenocarcinoma
  Lymphosarcoma

tion with emphasis on body systems is essential to determine a diagnostic and therapeutic plan.

Haematemesis and *melaena* are important signs of gastric disease that usually indicate gastric bleeding caused by erosion or ulceration (Table 49.10).

- Digested blood in the vomitus, often described as resembling coffee grounds or dirt, is typical of gastric bleeding.
- Fresh blood is more likely to be of oral or oesophageal origin.
- Black or tarry stool, referred to as melaena, can be caused by bleeding anywhere in the upper gastro-intestinal tract and usually indicates significant haemorrhage. Gastric bleeding is the most common cause of melaena.
- Coagulopathy must be ruled-out as a cause for haematemesis or melaena.

Abdominal distension is a less common, yet important, sign of gastric disease. Abdominal distension accompanied by unproductive retching in a large breed dog should alert the clinician to the likelihood of gastric dilatation/volvulus. In this instance, distension is primarily caused by air in the stomach. Postprandial abdominal distension occurs due to gastric retention disorders.

Physical Examination

The physical examination findings of animals with primary gastric disease are usually non-specific. Cranial abdominal pain, distension or mass, or the presence of melaena on digital rectal examination are most consistent with gastric disease. It is most important to assess the overall condition and hydration status of the patient and to rule out non-gastric causes of vomiting. Abdominal palpation can be helpful in some cases.

Laboratory Evaluation

Initial diagnostic testing is aimed at distinguishing primary gastrointestinal causes from metabolic causes. Metabolic causes are usually eliminated by a complete blood count, serum biochemical profile, and urinalysis.

Complete Blood Count

Complete blood counts (CBCs) are usually normal with primary gastric diseases; however a CBC can provide clues to the cause of vomiting.

- Chronic gastric bleeding causes a non-regenerative anaemia, often with characteristics of iron-deficiency (microcytosis, thrombocytopenia, hypochromasia).
- Acute gastric haemorrhage can cause either a regenerative or non-regenerative anaemia, depending on severity and duration of bleeding.

- Parvovirus causes neutropenia, whereas other enteric viruses cause no characteristic change in the haematological picture and values.
- Acute pancreatitis, bacterial gastroenteritis, and inflammatory bowel disease often cause a neutrophilic leukocytosis.
- Eosinophilia can occur from eosinophilic gastroenteritis, adrenocortical insufficiency and infrequently from gastric nematodes.

Serum Biochemistry

Serum biochemistries provide useful information in the vomiting patient both from diagnostic and therapeutic perspectives. Normal biochemical tests eliminate metabolic causes of vomiting. Electrolyte and acid–base disorders are common if vomiting has been severe or chronic; however they do not reliably indicate the cause of the problem.

- Hypokalaemic, hypochloraemic metabolic alkalosis suggests substantial loss of gastric content, most indicative of gastric outflow obstruction. Acute pancreatitis or renal failure can also cause such changes from loss of large quantities of gastric juice.
- Hyperkalaemia in the vomiting patient is most indicative of hypoadrenocorticism, oliguric or anuric renal failure; occasionally severe intestinal disease caused by trichuriasis or by salmonellosis mimics hypoadrenocorticism (Table 49.4).
- Vomiting caused by gastric disease does not always cause electrolyte or acid–base imbalance; absence of such abnormalities has no diagnostic significance.

The plasma total CO_2 (TCO_2) should be included in the assessment of any vomiting patient as an accurate indicator of plasma bicarbonate concentration.

Urinalysis

Urinalysis is used to rule out non-gastrointestinal causes of vomiting such as renal failure or diabetic ketoacidosis. Urine pH may also be a diagnostic clue (see Metabolic consequences of vomiting, above). The presence of an acid urine in the hypochloraemic, alkalotic patient (paradoxic aciduria) indicates substantial loss of gastric content, as would occur with a pyloric outflow obstruction.

Diagnostic Imaging

Plain and contrast radiographs are valuable when evaluating the stomach (Leib *et al*. 1985; Arnbjerg 1992).

Survey radiographs identify foreign bodies, gastric distension with fluid or gas, and displacement or malposition of the stomach. Gastric distension with air is common in the excited, dyspnoeic or struggling patient due to aerophagia; this is also seen secondary to gastric dilatation/volvulus syndrome.

- Simple aerophagia can cause a large but normally positioned and non-tympanic stomach and no clinical signs.
- Gastric dilatation/volvulus causes a tense and malpositioned stomach; dorsal displacement of the pylorus creates a shelf-like partition of tissue across the gastric shadow.

A fluid-distended stomach can be caused by gastric outflow obstruction, but is also seen soon after drinking large volumes of fluid. Gastric wall thickness, gastric ulcers and gastric masses are difficult to identify with plain radiographs unless outlined by intraluminal air. Pneumoperitoneum indicates rupture of a hollow viscus such as a penetrating gastric or intestinal ulcer, abdominal infection with gas-forming bacteria, or less commonly from perforation of the vagina or uterus.

Contrast radiographs of the stomach and duodenum are indicated when laboratory data and survey radiographs have not revealed the cause of persistent vomiting. Contrast radiographs help to identify gastric or proximal duodenal foreign bodies, gastric wall masses or infiltrative disease, mucosal ulceration, delayed gastric emptying or gastroparesis. Negative contrast gastrography can be performed by filling the stomach with air which may help to identify foreign bodies, gastric wall masses or deep ulcers. Positive contrast gastrography using premixed barium sulphate is more reliable (Box 49.1).

Nuclear scintigraphy, used to evaluate gastric emptying of liquids versus solids, is limited in availability to referral institutions.

Ultrasonography has limited use in evaluating the stomach wall for masses or infiltrative lesions (Pennick *et al*. 1990). Air in the lumen interferes with evaluation of the gastric wall; this can be eliminated by filling the stomach with water via gastric tube.

Endoscopy

Gastroduodenoscopy is one of the most useful methods of diagnosis of gastric disease because it allows direct inspection and gives the ability to biopsy of the surface of the stomach and duodenum (see Figs 49.1–49.10).

- Small lesions not detected by radiographs are easily seen with an endoscope and foreign bodies can be removed.

Box 49.1 Contrast gastrography with barium sulphate.

- Barium should be given by stomach tube to the fasted patient; recommended doses are 8–12 ml/kg for small dogs and cats and 5–7 ml/kg in large dogs.
- Ventrodorsal, right lateral and left lateral radiographs should be taken within 5 min of giving the barium and repeated in 20–30 min.
- Liquid barium should be observed in the duodenum within 5–20 min and the stomach should be nearly empty within 3 h.
- If barium does not enter the duodenum within 30 min, or if the stomach remains barium-filled with no evidence of peristalsis, gastroparesis or gastric outflow obstruction should be suspected.
- The presence of a narrowed stream of barium at the pylorus, referred to as a 'beak sign' is suggestive of pyloric obstruction from hypertrophy, neoplasia or inflammatory disease.
- Atropine, aminopentamide, ketamine and xylazine will decrease gastric motility, giving the false impression of gastric outlet obstruction.
- If a tranquiliser is needed, acetylpromazine is recommended.
- Gastric emptying of solids can be evaluated by mixing barium with food and observing emptying with a fluoroscope.

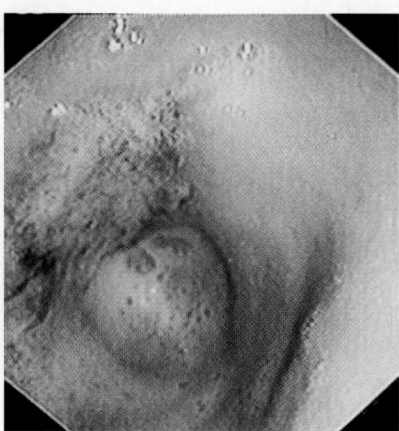

Fig. 49.2 Endoscopic appearance of an antral ulcer as a result of asprin administration. (Courtesy of K. W. Simpson.)

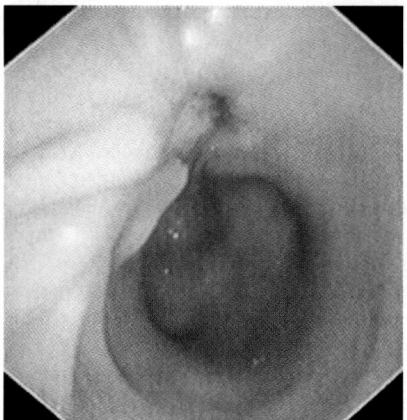

Fig. 49.3 Endoscopic appearance of hypertrophic pylorogastropathy associated with hypergastrinaemia. (Courtesy of K. W. Simpson.)

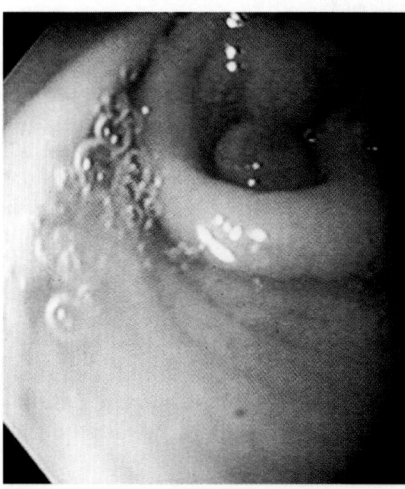

Fig. 49.1 Endoscopic appearance of a pyloric polyp. (Courtesy of K. W. Simpson.)

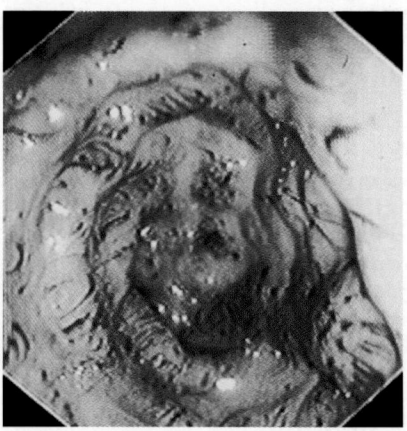

Fig. 49.4 Case in Fig. 49.3 following treatment with sucralphate and ranitidine. (Courtesy of K. W. Simpson.)

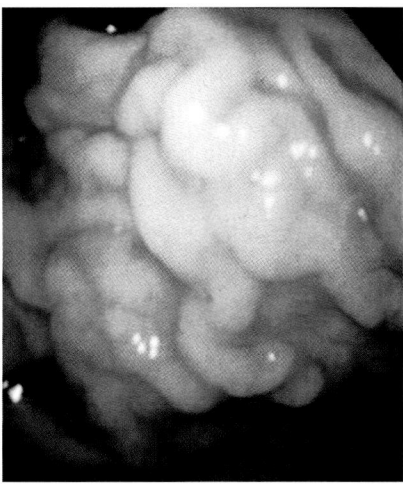

Fig. 49.5   Endoscopic appearance of a gastric lymphosarcoma. (Courtesy of K. W. Simpson.)

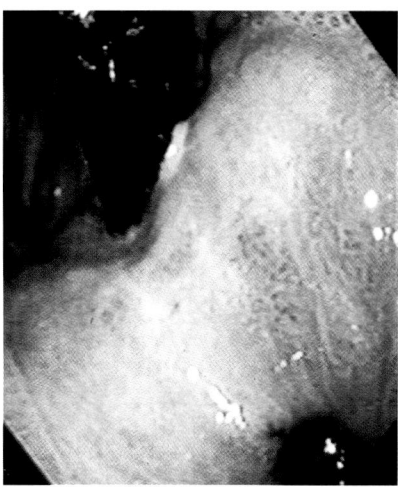

Fig. 49.7   Endoscopic appearance of a gastric carcinoma. (Courtesy of K. W. Simpson.)

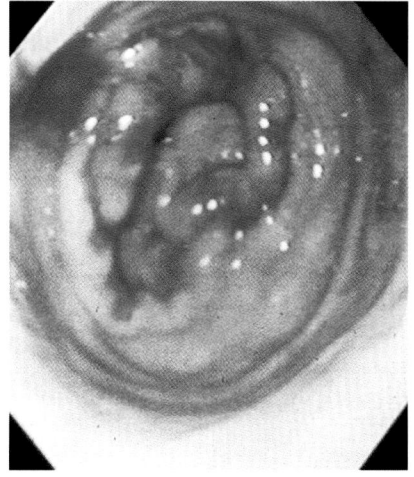

Fig. 49.6   Endoscopic appearance of a gastric lymphosarcoma. (Courtesy of K. W. Simpson.)

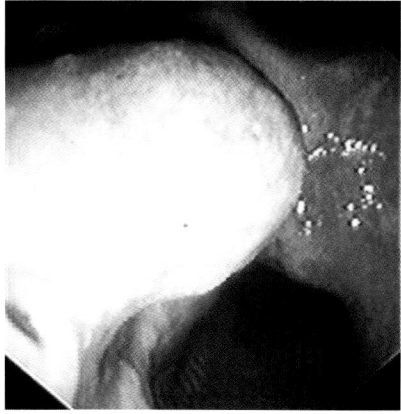

Fig. 49.8   Endoscopic appearance of a gastric tubular carcinoma. (Courtesy of K. W. Simpson.)

- Histolopathological lesions can be present in what appears as a normal appearing stomach or duodenum; multiple biopsies should always be obtained from the stomach and duodenum, even if the gross appearance is normal.
- If endoscopy is not available, exploratory surgery must be done to facilitate inspection and to obtain biopsies.

ACUTE GASTRITIS AND GASTRODUODENAL ULCER DISEASE

Acute gastritis occurs commonly in dogs and cats and is caused by numerous factors that result in gastric mucosal damage and inflammation (Stanton & Bright 1989). Dietary indiscretion, food intolerance or allergy, ingestion of foreign material, chemical and plant irritants, viral and

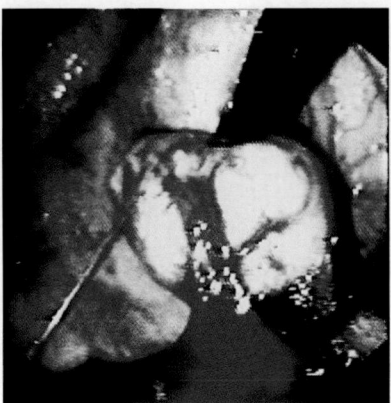

Fig. 49.9　Endoscopic appearance of a bleeding gastric leiomyoma. (Courtesy of K. W. Simpson.)

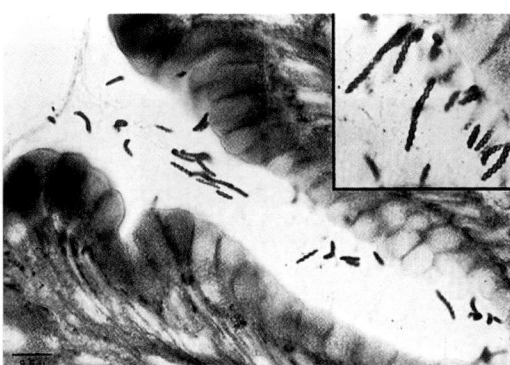

Fig. 49.10　Photomicrograph of *Helicobacter* sp. (Courtesy of K. W. Simpson.)

Table 49.11　Causes of acute gastritis in dogs.

Dietary
　Spoiled foods
　　Bacterial toxins
　　Mycotoxins
　Food sensitivity
　Foreign body

Infectious
　Viral
　　Parvovirus
　　Distemper
　　Infectious hepatitis
　　Coronavirus
　Bacterial
　　Helicobacter sp.*
　Parasitic
　　Physaloptera sp.*

Drugs
　NSAIDs*
　Corticosteroids*
　Antibiotics
　　Cephalosporins
　　Doxycycline
　　Tetracycline

Chemicals/toxins
　Cleaning products
　Ethylene glycol
　Herbicides
　Fertilisers
　Petroleum distillates
　Organophosphates
　Heavy metals
　Plant toxins

* Can cause chronic gastritis and has yet to be confirmed as a major cause of acute gastritis.

parasitic infections and drugs are common causes of acute gastritis (Table 49.11). Repeated exposure to dietary antigens, drugs, chemicals, toxins or infectious agents may initiate allergic or immune-mediated response, causing chronic gastritis. In many instances, acute gastritis is self-limiting and the aetiology is not determined. Diagnostic features of acute non-specific gastritis are listed in Table 49.12.

Gastric and duodenal ulcer disease (GDUD) is a common complication of many diseases and drug therapies (Table 49.10). Symptoms can be acute or chronic. The treatment of dogs with non-steroidal anti-inflammatory drugs (NSAIDs) is the most common cause of gastric mucosal injury and ulceration in dogs; NSAIDs cause direct damage to the mucosa and inhibit synthesis of gastroprotective prostaglandins. All the commonly used NSAIDs, including aspirin, ibuprofen and indomethacin have the potential to cause gastric and duodenal ulcer disease (Graham 1990). High doses of corticosteroids have been associated with gastric and duodenal ulcers in dogs (Sorjonen *et al.* 1983). In most instances, corticosteroids alone do not cause ulceration; rather corticosteroids enhance the damaging effects of NSAIDs, bile acids and other factors of mucosal damage.

Chronic liver diseases and cirrhosis are commonly associated with GDUD. The diminished gastric mucus production, decreased epithelial cell renewal, reduced gastric blood flow secondary to portal hypertension, and bile acid stimulation of gastrin have been identified as causative factors (Twedt 1985). Acute and chronic renal failure cause gastric mucosal damage (Cheville 1979). Uraemic toxins cause direct injury to gastric epithelial cells and mucosal vessels and decreased renal metabolism of gastrin causes excess acid secretion. Adrenocortical insufficiency infrequently causes gastric ulceration; mucosal damage is likely caused by hypotension and loss of vascular tone (DiBartola et al. 1985).

Shock, sepsis, hypovolaemia, spinal trauma, and surgery, are common but often unrecognised causes of GDUD (Gottlieb 1986). Gastric mucosal ischaemia caused by reduced mucosal blood flow impairs epithelial cell renewal. Secretion of vasoactive catecholamines and corticosteroids coupled with administration of exogenous corticosteroids further potentiate ulcer formation. All critically ill patients, especially those with severe trauma, major surgery, organ failure or sepsis should be considered likely candidates for development of ulcers.

Mast cell tumours, pancreatic gastrin-secreting and pancreatic polypeptide-secreting tumours can cause GDUD in dogs, presumably by induction of gastric acid hypersecretion (Carrig & Seawright 1968; Jones et al. 1976; Drazner 1981; Zerbe et al. 1989).

The diagnostic features of gastric ulceration are listed in Table 49.13.

MEDICAL MANAGEMENT OF ACUTE GASTRITIS, GASTRIC EROSION AND GASTROINTESTINAL ULCERS

Management of gastritis, erosions and ulceration requires treatment and elimination of underlying causes and supportive therapy to enhance mucosal defences (Box 49.2). In general the key features are:

- Fluid therapy is given to prevent dehydration and maintain mucosal perfusion.
- If vomiting is persistent, oral intake of food and water should be stopped for several days.
- Debilitated patients and those in poor nutritional condition may need parenteral or enteral nutrition.
- Blood transfusion is required in anaemic patients with evidence of active gastrointestinal bleeding.
- Surgical treatment is indicated when uncontrolled haemorrhage, gastric obstruction or perforation occurs.

Drugs used for non-specific medical management of gastritis and GDUD include potent histamine H_2-receptor

Table 49.12 Diagnostic features of acute non-specific gastritis.

History	Acute onset of vomiting, exacerbated by eating or drinking; diarrhoea may be present
Physical examination	Usually normal; may be dehydrated or febrile
Laboratory	May reveal systemic cause, electrolyte or acid–base imbalance
Recovery	Rapid response to symptomatic treatment; often spontaneous recovery
Biopsy	Erosion and/or ulceration with variable neutrophilic infiltrate. Biopsy is seldom necessary for the diagnosis of acute gastritis

Table 49.13 Diagnostic features of gastric ulceration.

History	Intermittent vomiting, variable haematemesis, melaena, acute onset of weakness or collapse; recent NSAID and/or corticosteroid therapy
Physical examination	Usually normal; may have signs of anaemia, abdominal pain, melaena
Laboratory	Anaemia is common, ranging from regenerative to non-regenerative microcytic-hypochromic anaemia. Biochemistries may reveal systemic disease such as renal failure, liver disease, hypoadrenocorticism
Radiographs	Survey radiographs are usually normal but allow evaluation of renal and hepatobiliary systems. Peritonitis is indicative of perforation. Contrast studies might confirm deep ulceration
Endoscopy	Appearance of benign ulcers varies from punctate superficial erosive lesions to deep ulcer crater with smooth margins. Malignant ulcers have thickened and irregular margins, often associated with mass lesions. Biopsy of ulcer margin needed to differentiate benign from neoplastic lesions.

Box 49.2 Symptomatic management for acute gastritis of unknown cause.

Dietary	Nil per os for 24–48 h Feed small portions of low-fat, single source protein, highly digestible diet starting 6–12 h after vomiting has resolved.
Fluids	Deficits, maintenance and ongoing losses must be provided via parenteral route: If dehydration is <5%, give subcutaneously If dehydration is >5%, or if vomiting is persistent, give intravenously 0.9% normal saline if electrolyte and acid–base status are unknown; lactated Ringer's solution is a good alternative.
Electrolytes	Potassium supplementation is usually not necessary unless vomiting is frequent and persists for >24 h. If serum potassium is not known, 20 mEq KCl added to 1 litre of 0.9% saline can be used for replacement and maintenance fluid therapy. If serum potassium is known, supplement as:

Serum potassium (mEq/l)	Potassium added/litre (mEq KCl)
<2.0	80
2.0–2.5	60
2.5–3.0	40
3.0–3.5	30

	– Do not exceed 0.5 mEq potassium/kg per hour intravenously.
Anti-emetics	Phenothiazines for 24–72 h if vomiting is severe or persistent; to avoid hypotension, do not use until dehydration is corrected. Metoclopramide may be more effective if gastric stasis or ileus is suspected, as in parvovirus gastroenteritis, to restore upper gastrointestinal motility. Do not use if gastrointestinal obstruction is suspected.

Box 49.2 *Continued.*

Antisecretory drugs	H_2-receptor blocker for 7–10 days if haematemesis or melaena is present. Omeprazole if severe erosive/ulcerative gastritis or oesophagitis is suspected, or if response to histamine H_2-receptor therapy has been unsatisfactory.
Cytoprotective drugs	Sucralfate if vomiting is not persistent Misoprostol is indicated in patients with suspected NSAID-induced gastritis

antagonists, a proton-pump inhibitor, cytoprotective agents, and prostaglandin analogues. These drugs, specifically intended for treatment of ulcer disease, can be used to treat a broad variety of disorders including oesophagitis, gastritis and gastrointestinal bleeding as well as GDUD (Table 49.14).

Histamine H_2-Receptor Antagonists

(Stanton & Bright 1989; Feldman & Burton 1990; Freston 1990)

The histamine H_2-receptor antagonists bind to H_2-receptors on acid-producing parietal cells to inhibit acid-stimulating effects of histamine and to render the cell less responsive to stimulation by acetylcholine and gastrin. Cimetidine, ranitidine, nizatidine and famotidine have been used to treat gastritis and gastric ulcer disease in dogs. All are efficacious and differ primarily in potency and frequency of dosing. The incidence of side-effects from H_2-receptor antagonists is low. Cimetidine can cause vomiting and diarrhoea, whereas lethargy, confusion and seizures have infrequently been observed with all of the H_2-receptor antagonists. Cimetidine and ranitidine interfere with hepatic metabolism of theophylline, phenytoin and warfarin and should not be used concurrently with these drugs.

Proton Pump Inhibitors (Wallmark et al. 1985; Jenkins et al. 1991; Jenkins & DeNovo 1991)

The final step in hydrochloric acid secretion from the parietal cells is mediated by the enzyme hydrogen-potassium

Table 49.14 Drugs used in the treatment of gastritis and gastrointestinal ulcer disease.

Generic name	Mechanism	Proprietary name	Suggested dosage	How supplied for dogs	Strength	Side effects
Histamine H$_2$-receptor antagonists	Decrease acid secretion					
Cimetidine		Tagamet™	5–10 mg/kg every 6 h p.o., i.v., i.m.	Tablet	200 mg 300 mg 400 mg 800 mg	Inhibition of hepatic microsomal enzymes may cause drug interactions; mental depression
				Liquid Injection	60 mg/ml 150 mg/ml	
Ranitidine		Zantac™	2 mg/kg every 8–12 6 h p.o., i.v., i.m., s.c.	Tablet	150 mg 300 mg	Similar to cimetidine, but to lesser extent
				Liquid Injection	15 mg/ml 25 mg/ml	
Nizatidine		Axid™	5 mg/kg once daily p.o.	Capsule	150 mg 300 mg	None reported
Famotidine		Pepcid™	0.5 mg/kg once daily p.o., i.v.	Tablet	20 mg 40 mg	Similar to ranitidine
				Liquid Injection	8 mg/ml 10 mg/ml	
Proton pump Inhibitor	Blocks acid secretion					
Omeprazole		Prilosec™	20 mg once daily PO (>20 kg) 10 mg once daily p.o. (5–20 kg) 5 mg once daily p.o. (<5 kg) must be repackaged	Capsule	20 mg (>20 kg)	Prolonged use can cause reversible gastric mucosal hypertrophy. No clinically significant side-effects reported with short-term (2–4 weeks) use
Mucosal protectant	Forms protective barrier, inactivates pepsin, adsorbs bile acids, stimulates prostaglandins	Carafate™	1 g/30 kg every 6–8 h p.o.	Tablet	1 g	Constipation
Prostaglandin analogue	Cytoprotective: stimulates mucus-bicarbonate secretion, enhances mucosal blood flow, decreases acid secretion					
Misoprostol		Cytotec™	2–5 µg/kg every 8 h p.o.	Tablet	200 mg 100 mg	Diarrhoea, abdominal cramping, vomiting, abortion
Prokinetic drug	Enhances gastric emptying, anti-emetic – blocks CRTZ					
Metoclopramide		Reglan™	0.25–0.5 mg/kg every 8 h p.o., s.c.	Tablet	5 mg 10 mg	Hyperactivity, restlessness, constipation
				Liquid Injection	1 mg/ml 1–2 mg/kg every 24 h as slow i.v. infusion	5 mg/ml

CRTZ, chemoreceptor trigger zone.

adenosine-triphosphatase (H+K+-ATPase) located in the secretory membrane of gastric parietal cells. This is referred to as the parietal cell proton pump. Substituted benzimidazoles such as omeprazole specifically block the parietal cell proton pump to inhibit gastric acid secretion. As the proton-pump inhibitors block the final step of hydrogen ion secretion, hydrochloric acid secretion stimulated by histamine, acetylcholine and gastrin is blocked. These drugs are more effective than the H_2-receptor blockers in acid inhibition.

Omeprazole is the most effective drug for the treatment of oesophagitis, erosive gastritis and gastric ulcer disease that have not responded to therapy with histamine H_2-receptor antagonists and sucralfate.

Sucralfate (Tarnawski *et al.* 1987)

Sucralfate is a sulphated disaccharide complex with aluminum hydroxide that accelerates gastric mucosal healing by several mechanisms:

- adherence to mucosal erosions and ulcers provides a barrier to acid penetration;
- inactivation of pepsin and adsorption of gastric-damaging bile acids refluxed from the duodenum;
- stimulation of endogenous prostaglandin synthesis with subsequent increased secretion of mucus and bicarbonate;
- binding to and concentration of epidermal growth factor in the ulcer where it stimulates cellular proliferation.

Sucralfate is effective in acidic or near neutral pH and can therefore be used concurrently with anti-secretory drugs such as histamine H_2-receptor antagonists. Other orally administered drugs can be absorbed by sucralfate and should not be given orally within 2 h of treatment with sucralfate. Sucralfate is recommended for the treatment of oesophagitis, gastritis and gastric ulcer of any cause in dogs and cats; safety is well established, with constipation being the only reported side-effect.

Synthetic Prostaglandins (Graham *et al.* 1988; Murtaugh *et al.* 1992; Johnson *et al.* 1995)

Synthetic prostaglandin analogues such as misoprostol have been developed to prevent and heal gastroduodenal injury caused by NSAIDs. These drugs impart protection to gastric mucosa by stimulating gastric mucus secretion, increasing bicarbonate secretion, increasing gastric mucosal blood flow, inhibiting gastric acid secretion and by inhibiting release of histamine from gastric mucosal mast cells. NSAIDs are used frequently in dogs, especially to control chronic inflammation and pain from degenerative joint disease, as a result, misoprostol is a valuable drug to help prevent GDUD in patients requiring long-term NSAID therapy. Clinical studies of human and canine arthritic patients have shown misoprostol to be effective in preventing NSAID-induced gastric haemorrhage, erosion or ulceration. Diarrhoea and vomiting are potential side-effects and misoprostol will cause abortions and should not be used in pregnant patients. No adverse hematological or biochemical effects have been reported with the use of misoprostol in dogs.

Prokinetic and Antiemetic Drugs (Albibi & McCallum 1983)

Metoclopramide is an effective anti-emetic with both central nervous system and peripheral effects on the gastrointestinal system. The central antidopaminergic action blocks stimulation of the chemoreceptor trigger zone. Peripherally, metoclopramide enhances upper gastrointestinal motility, resulting in decreased gastroesophageal reflux, accelerated gastric emptying, and decreased duodenogastric reflux. It is contraindicated if gastric outlet obstruction or gastrointestinal perforation is suspected. Some patients appear to be sensitive to the effects of this drug and will actually have increased vomiting caused by gastrointestinal spasm. Behavioural changes have been found in some patients ranging from lethargy to hyperactivity and agitated behaviour; these effects occur most frequently at high dosages but can occur in some patients at low dosages. Metoclopramide is excreted by the kidneys and therefore should not be used by patients with renal insufficiency.

Summary

In general, histamine H_2-receptor antagonists and/or sucralfate are effective first-choice drugs in treating gastritis, erosions and ulcers. Omeprazole should be considered for those patients not responding to therapy and in those patients with hypersecretory disorders. Misoprostol should be considered for patients that require NSAID therapy, and possibly for the critically ill patient. The duration of treatment varies depending on the underlying cause. In most veterinary patients, treatment with anti-ulcer medications for 2–3 weeks is adequate providing predisposing factors have been eliminated. Relapse is uncommon.

CHRONIC VOMITING

Chronic vomiting is characterised by intermittent episodes of vomiting, sometimes with acute exacerbations, that has not responded to symptomatic treatment. Associated clinical signs are non-specific and include inappetence, anorexia and weight loss; abdominal pain, pica and melaena are less commonly observed and diarrhoea is uncommon. Differential diagnosis of chronic vomiting is listed in Table 49.9.

Table 49.15   Aetiological classification of chronic gastritis in dogs.

Dietary	Food intolerance
Drug-induced	NSAIDs
Infectious	Spiral bacteria
	Phycomycosis
	Histoplasmosis
	Physaloptera
Ulcerative	See Table 49.10
foreign body	

Chronic Gastritis

Chronic gastritis is an important cause of chronic vomiting in the dog (Twedt & Magne 1986). The prevalence of chronic gastritis is unknown; however the increased use of endoscopy has led to a significant increase in the diagnosis of chronic gastritis. Suspected causes of chronic gastritis include food allergy, chronic NSAID therapy, fungal or parasitic infection, and infection with gastric spiral bacteria (*Helicobacter* sp., Fig. 49.10) (Table 49.15). In many cases however, a cause is never identified. In this circumstance, chronic gastritis is characterised by histological appearance which may point to an aetiological diagnosis as listed in Table 49.16. Although histological classification is non-specific, it can assist the clinician in making therapeutic and prognostic decisions.

Chronic gastritis, regardless of cause, is characterised by *clinical signs* including (Table 49.17):

- Intermittent episodes of vomiting of gastric juice, bile-stained mucoid fluid or ingesta occur, sometimes with acute exacerbation of persistent vomiting.
- Blood is present if erosive-ulcerative disease is present (see Table 49.10).
- Inappetence, weight loss, abdominal pain, melaena and pale mucous membranes and poor haircoat may be present.

Predominant histologic type*	Possible causes to consider

Eosinophilic	Immune response to:
	    dietary antigens
	    migrating parasites
	    foreign material
	Idiopathic eosinophilic gastroenteritis
	Mast cell tumour

Granulomatous	Chronic infections:
	    histoplasmosis
	    phycomycosis
	    mycobacteria
	    parasitic
	Immune response to foreign material
	Response to gastric neoplasia
	Chronic NSAID therapy

Lymphocytic/plasmacytic	*Helicobacter* (lymphoid nodules common) Immune response to dietary antigens Idiopathic lymphocytic-plasmacytic gastroenteritis Lymphosarcoma

Table 49.16   Histological classification of chronic gastritis in dogs.

* Many gastric diseases cause mixed inflammatory cell reaction.

Table 49.17 Diagnostic features of chronic gastritis

History	Persistent intermittent vomiting
	Inappetence
	Variable weight loss
Physical examination	Usually normal
	Poor haircoat
	Pale mucous menbranes
Laboratory	Systemic disease ruled out as cause of vomiting
Radiographs	Survey radiographs usually normal
	Contrast studies may reveal gastric mass, foreign body, or gastric retention
Biopsy	Variable inflammatory cell infiltration (lymphocytes, plasma cells, eosinophils, macrophages); see Table 49.16
	Spiral organisms (*Helicobacter* sp.)

- Diarrhoea is uncommon in uncomplicated gastritis but is frequently observed in patients with concomitant inflammatory bowel disease.

Diagnosis

Diagnosis of chronic gastritis is based on laboratory tests to exclude chronic vomiting secondary to metabolic disease, radiography, and endoscopic or surgical biopsy. Laboratory abnormalities that might occur with chronic gastritis include:

- Regenerative to non-regenerative microcytic hypochromic anaemia from chronic GI blood loss; thrombocytosis is also characteristic of iron deficiency anaemia.
- Leukocytosis and absolute eosinophilia occur in most cases of eosinophilic gastritis.
- Panhypoproteinemia occurs infrequently.

Survey radiographs help to identify gastric foreign bodies but seldom identify primary gastric lesions. Contrast radiographs may show:

- Thickened gastric wall or prominent mucosal folds.
- Mucosal ulceration.
- Single or multiple nodules or mass lesion.
- Delayed gastric emptying.

Features of chronic gastric diseases are outlined below.

Chronic Non-Specific Gastritis (Lymphocytic-Plasmacytic)

(Guilford & Strombeck 1996b)

This commonly diagnosed type of gastritis is characterised by an infiltrate of gastric mucosa predominantly with lymphocytes and plasma cells; erosions and ulcerations may occur. Three general types are observed:

(1) Diffuse superficial gastritis characterised by mucosal infiltrate with lymphocytes and plasma cells, often involving full thickness of the mucosa, with variable fibrosis.
(2) Atrophic gastritis characterised by severe inflammatory infiltrate with reduced mucosal parenchyma, loss of gastric glands and shallow gastric pits; fibrosis is prominent in some.
(3) Hypertrophic gastritis characterised by diffuse or focal mucosal hypertrophy or hyperplasia with variable inflammatory infiltrate and fibrosis. Focal proliferation of antral mucosa is its most common form (see CHPG – chronic hypertrophic pylorogastropathy).

The aetiology is unknown but it is generally agreed that a defect in gastric mucosal barrier from any cause might allow absorption of lumen contents into mucosa, with stimulation of immune-mediated response. In many cases the severe infiltration of mucosa with lymphocytes can be difficult to distinguish from lymphosarcoma. Clinical, laboratory and radiographic findings are non-specific; diagnosis is based on biopsy. The treatment includes symptomatic management (Box 49.3) coupled with immunosuppressive therapy (Box 49.4). Focal antral hypertrophy may require surgery to improve gastric outflow.

Eosinophilic Gastritis

This is characterised by a mucosal infiltration predominantly with eosinophils; diffuse granulomatous lesions or discrete granulomas with ulceration and necrosis can occur (Hayden & Fleischman 1977). The aetiopathogenesis is unknown but hypersensitivity to dietary antigens may be a cause in some; an immune response to migrating parasites or microbial antigens are other suggested but unproven causes. Many cases of eosinophilic gastritis have a peripheral eosinophilia but this is by no means all cases. The differential diagnosis for a vomiting dog with an eosinophilia includes:

- gastrointestinal parasitism,
- eosinophilic gastroenteritis,
- hypoadrenocorticism,

Box 49.3   Symptomatic management of chronic gastritis of unknown cause.

Dietary	Nil per os for 24–48 h Feed limited antigen/ hypoallergenic (novel protein) diet for at least 4–6 weeks. Depending on response, continue or change to another diet with a different protein source.
Antisecretory drugs	Histamine H$_2$-receptor blocker or omeprazole for 2–4 weeks, especially if haematemesis or melaena is observed.
Locally acting protectants	Sucralfate is well-tolerated long term and enhances healing of gastric mucosa; it should be used whenever haematemesis or melaena is observed.
Prokinetic drugs	Metoclopramide or cisapride may be helpful to decrease chronic vomiting and can be used indefinitely.
Antibiotics	May be helpful, particularly if *Helicobacter*-associated gastritis is suspected.
Corticosteroids	Generally not used unless histological diagnosis has confirmed lymphocytic- plasmacytic or oeosinophilic gastritis; or if no response to controlled diets, protectants and antibiotics has occurred.

Box 49.4   Immunosuppressive therapy for lymphocytic-plasmacytic gastritis and eosinophilic gastritis.

Corticosteroids	Prednisone (1–2 mg/kg every 12 h) for 1–2 weeks. Decrease dose by 50% every 2–3 weeks during next 2–3 months to lowest alternate- day dose required to maintain remission. Steroids can be discontinued in many patients that are then managed long term with dietary control.
Azathioprine	Used if response to steroids is inadequate, and as adjunct to steroids in severe lymphocytic-plasmacytic disease: 1 mg/kg once daily for 2 weeks, followed by alternate-day therapy. For long-term maintenance, alternate the azathioprine treatment with the steroid treatment on alternate-day schedule. Monitor CBC for neutropenia or thrombocytopenia every 2 weeks for first 2 months of therapy and monthly thereafter. Decrease dose or discontinue drug if bone marrow suppression occurs.

Also refer to Chapter 5, page 73, cytotoxic and immunosuppressive drugs.

- mastocytosis,
- incidental parasitism, e.g. heartworm disease, fleas.

Dietary change to a hypoallergenic, limited antigen diet or oligoantigenic diet (novel protein such as fish, venison, rabbit, cottage cheese) may help control the disease, but is seldom effective alone. Most respond well to corticosteroids; azathioprine is occasionally needed (Box 49.4); granulomatous masses require surgical resection. The prognosis is good.

Parasitic Gastritis

Physaloptera species are infrequently diagnosed as a cause of chronic vomiting in dog, perhaps because ova are difficult to find consistently using routine faecal flotation. The diagnosis is made by routine faecal flotation or direct examination via endoscopy. The adults are easily identified as 1–4-cm long nematodes in the fundus or antrum; smaller larvae are easily overlooked; small bleeding erosions are caused. The treatment is a single dose of pyrantel pamoate

(5 mg/kg); because of difficulty diagnosing this disease consideration should be given to empiric therapy before in-depth work-up.

Ollulanus tricuspis is a gastric nematode of cats occasionally identified in dogs; clinical significance uncertain. It is diagnosed by a microscopic examination of vomitus for adult parasites. Therapy is uncertain but fenbendazole (10 mg/kg every 12 h for 2 days) is effective in cats.

Bacterial Gastritis

The spiral bacteria of the genus *Helicobacter* infect the stomachs of many mammalian hosts, most notably humans, dogs, cats, ferrets, primates, cheetahs and laboratory rodents (Marshall & Warren 1984; Fox *et al.* 1990; Radin *et al.* 1990; Fox *et al.* 1991; Lee *et al.* 1992; Eaton *et al.* 1993; Otto *et al.* 1994; Skirrow 1994). *Helicobacter pylori* infection has been determined to be the primary cause of chronic gastritis and gastric and duodenal ulcers disease in humans; recent studies have confirmed a relationship between *H. pylori* infection and development of gastric adenocarcinoma and gastric lymphoma in humans (Parsonnet *et al.* 1994).

Gastric spiral bacteria are commonly found in the stomachs of dogs, however the clinical significance is not as well-defined as in humans. *Helicobacter heilmannii*, *H. felis* and *H. bizzozenonii* are the most common spiral bacteria found in dogs, having been identified in clinically normal dogs as well as in dogs with clinical and histologic gastritis. In the authors' hospital, approximately 50% of dogs that have had gastroscopy for upper gastrointestinal symptoms have *Helicobacter* infection. As some infected dogs appear to develop gastritis whereas others do not, the full pathogenic and clinical significance of infection is not clear.

- Anecdotal reports of resolution of clinical disease following antimicrobial therapy exist, however information is limited by lack of controlled study.
- Many patients in the authors' practice with clinical signs of gastritis have had biopsy-confirmed *Helicobacter*-associated gastritis, with no other aetiology for the gastritis being identified. Symptoms and histological disease have resolved following combination antibiotic antacid therapy.
- *H. felis* has been used to cause follicular lymphocytic-plasmacytic gastritis in laboratory-raised dogs (Lee *et al.* 1992).
- Many infected dogs have some degree of histological gastritis that varies in severity from vacuolisation of surface epithelium to necrosis of gastric glands; most have mucosal inflammation with lymphocytic-plasmacytic and neutrophilic infiltrates; macroscopic and microscopic follicular lymphoid nodules occur in more severely affected dogs. *Helicobacter* produces large amounts of urease which converts urea to ammonia, thereby producing an alkaline microenvironment around the organism to ensure survival in the acidic stomach. Ammonia, mucolytic and cytotoxic substances secreted by the organism are damaging to gastric epithelial cells. Diagnosis is best made by histological examination of gastric mucosal biopsies:

- Silver stains (Warthin–Starry method) facilitate identification of spiral organisms located deep in the gastric glands.
- Wet mounts of mucosal scrapings can be examined by dark field microscopy for motile helical organisms.
- Gastric biopsies can be placed in a urea broth containing a pH-indicator to detect presence of urease. A positive reaction is indicated by a colour change to deep pink caused by the production of ammonia from by urease-producing organisms. Commercial urease test media with a pH indicator are available as screening tests (Campylobacter-like organisms (CLO) test).
- *Helicobacter* spp. are extremely difficult to culture.
- Definitive identification of species is done by polymerase chain reaction (PCR) amplification.

Treatment of *Helicobacter*-associated gastric disease in humans requires combination of antibiotic and antisecretory drugs given for 10–14 days (Bayerdorffer *et al.* 1992; Neri *et al.* 1992; Anon. 1994). Triple-therapy protocols using various combinations of metronidazole and bismuth with either tetracycline, amoxycillin or the acid-stable macrolide azithromycin, given for 10–14 days, are considered to be the most effective to eradicate the organism. Dual therapy with amoxycillin–omeprazole or with azithromycin–omeprazole for 10–14 days has been reported to be equally effective. The authors recommend that dogs with biopsy-confirmed *Helicobacter*-associated gastritis should be treated with combination antibiotic–antisecretory drugs for at least 14 days. Suggested protocols are:

- Initial therapy: amoxicillin 22 mg/kg every 8 h (or azithromycin) plus omeprazole 0.7 mg/kg QD
- If incomplete response or relapse occurs: add metronidazole 10 mg/kg every 8 h to the above therapy for an additional 7 days.

H. heilmannii and *H. felis* may have zoonotic potential; these organisms have been isolated from humans with chronic gastritis, most of whom have had close contact with dogs or cats. Additionally, *H. pylori* has been isolated from the stomach of cats, where it causes a low-grade antral gastritis (Handt *et al.* 1994; Fox & Lee 1993).

DELAYED GASTRIC EMPTYING AND GASTRIC MOTILITY DISORDERS

Abnormal retention of food in the stomach is caused by gastric-outlet obstruction, disorders of gastric motility, or a combination of both. Lesions of the pylorus that cause partial obstruction include mural thickening from mucosal hyperplasia and/or muscular hypertrophy, neoplasia, eosinophilic granuloma, or infiltrative mycoses. Foreign bodies in the pylorus cause partial to complete gastric-outlet obstruction. Less frequently, lesions external to the pylorus such as pancreatic inflammation or abscess will compress the pylorus and cause delayed gastric emptying. Gastric motility disorders can occur secondary to a variety of metabolic diseases, inflammatory disease of the peritoneum or gastrointestinal tract, electrolyte imbalances, neurological disease, or drug therapy. Primary gastric motility disorders occur but are infrequently diagnosed in dogs. Specific causes of delayed gastric emptying from gastric-outflow obstruction and from gastric motility disorders are listed in Table 49.18.

Clinical Signs

Clinical signs of gastric-outlet obstruction and gastric motility disorders are similar, characterised by vomiting of large amounts of partially digested food and fluid, usually greater than 8–10 h after eating. Abrupt vomiting of poorly digested food without retching sometimes occurs and is incorrectly interpreted to be regurgitation rather than vomiting. Onset of signs is gradual, with intermittent vomiting observed initially, but changing to predictable postprandial vomiting, especially if gastric-outflow obstruction is present. Gastric foreign bodies are the exception, usually causing acute and persistent vomiting. Postprandial abdominal distension and discomfort relieved by vomiting may be reported by the owner.

Most dogs are normal between episodes of vomiting, with no consistent physical or laboratory abnormalities occurring unless metabolic complications occur. Moderate weight loss, abdominal distension and dehydration may be detected on physical examination. Some will become anorectic and lose weight if an inflammatory or neoplastic disease is present. Haematemesis and melaena are typical of

Table 49.18 Causes of delayed gastric emptying.

Gastric outlfow obstruction
  Chronic hypertrophic pyloric gastropathy
  Chronic hypertrophic gastritis
  Gastric ulcer
  Gastric neoplasia
  Gastric foreign body
  Gastric antral polyps
  Granulomatous gastritis/granuloma
  Fungal
  Eosinophilic
  Idiopathic
  External compression
  Pancreatic abscess, tumour
  Abdominal mass

Gastric motility disorders

Subacute
  Gastroenteritis
  Pancreatitis
  Peritonitis
  Abdominal pain
  Trauma
  Stress
  Hypercalcaemia
  Hypocalcaemia
  Hypokalaemia
  Drugs: anticholinergics,
  narcotics,
  β-adrenergic agonists

Chronic
  Dysautonomia
  Gastric dilatation-volvulus
  Gastric ulcer
  Chronic gastritis
  Gastric neoplasia
  Gastric arrhythmias
  Idiopathic
  Hypothyroidism
  Diabetes mellitus
  Hypoadrenocorticism
  Uraemia
  Liver failure
  Inflammatory bowel disease
  Constipation

Table 49.19   Diagnostic features of delayed gastric emptying.

History	Vomiting of food at times greater than 8 h after eating; food is often partially digested; large volumes of liquified food or fluid vomited without usual prodromal signs of vomiting; postprandial abdominal distension and discomfort
Physical examination	Usually normal or non-specific findings such as dehydration or abdominal discomfort; abdominal distension or tympany may be present
Laboratory	Usually normal; gastric outflow obstruction may cause hypochloraemic metabolic alkalosis.
Radiography	Fluid-distended stomach on survey radiographs; contrast studies confirm abnormal gastric emptying
Endoscopy or coeliotomy	Confirms gastric outflow obstruction, the absence of which implies presence of a gastric motility disorder

gastric-outlet obstruction from gastric adenocarcinoma, or less frequently from gastric ulcer.

Diagnosis

Diagnosis of delayed gastric emptying is made on the basis of history, physical examination, and exclusion of metabolic diseases that cause chronic vomiting. Radiographs and assessment of gastric emptying studies are helpful to determine if delayed gastric emptying is present and to identify the cause (Table 49.19).

Laboratory Evaluation

Laboratory changes caused by delayed gastric emptying are mild and non-specific. Because concurrent metabolic diseases can cause gastric motility disorders, complete haematologic, biochemical and urinary tests are necessary for accurate diagnosis. Anaemia, often with iron deficiency, may occur with leiomyoma and gastric adenocarcinoma. Electrolyte and acid–base imbalances are uncommon unless complete or near-complete pyloric obstruction is present: Hypochloraemic alkalosis, sometimes with paradoxical aciduria, occurs with complete or near-complete pyloric obstruction. Hypokalaemia can result from chronic vomiting or can be a cause of gastric hypomotility. Mild acidosis may occur from dehydration.

Diagnostic Imaging

There are a number of methods to evaluate gastric emptying. The most commonly used is radiography. Survey abdominal radiographs can be normal or reveal an enlarged stomach, depending on the cause, duration and severity of delayed emptying. In general:

- Obstructive lesions cause a distended, fluid-filled stomach, in contrast to gaseous distension that typically occurs with gastric volvulus.
- Primary gastric motility disorders are usually normal on survey abdominal radiographs.

Contrast radiographs, using barium sulphate liquid, are used to outline the lumen of the stomach and to subjectively evaluate gastric emptying (Miyabayshi & Morgan 1984; Burns & Fox 1986). Mixing barium with food will more accurately estimate gastric emptying of food. Although neither type of study is quantitative and both vary markedly in normal animals, useful information can be determined. Fluoroscopic examination helps to identify sequential changes in the shape of the stomach and pylorus and movement of contrast through the pylorus.

- Liquid barium normally enters the duodenum within 15 min of administration; gastric emptying should be complete within about 1–4 h. Emptying of a barium meal may not be complete in some dogs until 15 h after feeding, although most normal dogs empty a meal in about 8 h.
- Retention of most of the liquid barium after 4 h, presence of liquid barium in the stomach longer than 12 h, or retention of a large amount of a barium meal longer than 8–10 h is abnormal and indicates delayed gastric emptying.
- Initial delay of gastric emptying may be of no significance because fear, anxiety and physical restraint can cause transient delay in gastric emptying.
- Anticholinergic drugs cause gastric atony that can delay gastric emptying for several hours.
- Restrictive mural diseases of the pylorus such as muscular hypertrophy, neoplasia or granulomatous disease produce annular narrowing; barium may only fill the narrow entrance to the pylorus, resulting in a thin

stream of barium often referred to as having a 'beak-like' appearance; this is a common finding with antral hypertrophic gastropathy.

- Polyp-like filling defects are caused by benign mucosal hypertrophy, inflammatory granuloma, neoplasia or foreign body.
- Primary gastric motility disorders are characterised by delayed gastric emptying in the absence of morphologic lesions.

Barium-impregnated polyspheres (BIPS, Arnolds, Shrewsbury, UK) are radiopaque markers used as a convenient alternative to barium studies for evaluation of gastric emptying (Guilford & Strombeck 1996b; Burns & Fox 1986). BIPS are given with a canned-food meal, approximately 25% of the daily caloric intake, and abdominal radiographs taken at 4–6 h intervals over the next 12–24 h. The percentage of BIPS that have left the stomach is compared with a standard curve for normal gastric emptying that is provided by the manufacturer.

Scintigraphic studies using radioactive tracers mixed with food are the method of choice for measuring gastric emptying; this technique is limited to facilities with nuclear medicine facilities (Van den Brom & Happe 1986). Electrogastrograms are useful to detect abnormal gastric motility patterns such as tachygastria and bradygastria. This technique is not widely available.

Other Diagnostic Procedures

Once delayed gastric emptying is confirmed, additional diagnostic procedures such as ultrasound, endoscopy or coeliotomy are necessary to determine if an obstructive lesion is present. In the absence of a gastric-outlet obstruction, gastric motility disorders are likely causes of the delayed emptying.

- Ultrasonography is useful to detect foreign bodies, mural thickening and masses not detected by radiographs.
- Endoscopy and mucosal biopsies are useful if chronic inflammatory gastric or intestinal disease, neoplasia or foreign body are suspected causes of delayed gastric emptying.
- Surgical examination and biopsy should be considered if the cause of delayed emptying is less certain. Full-thickness gastric biopsy allows examination of muscle and nerve plexuses not included in endoscopic pinch biopsy. Surgery provides opportunity for resection of masses and for procedures to relieve gastric-outlet obstruction.

Features of specific diseases causing delayed gastric emptying are covered in the following sections.

Hypertrophypertrophic Gastropathy or Antral Pyloric Hypertrophy Syndrome or Hypertrophy Pyloric Gastropathy (Table 49.20) (Matthieson & Walter 1986; Sikes *et al*. 1986; Walter & Matthiesen 1993)

This occurs most frequently in brachycephalic breeds, most notably Boxers, Boston Terriers, Lhasa Apso, Maltese, Pekingese and Shih Tzu dogs and young to

Table 49.20 Clinical characteristics of chronic antral pyloric hypertrophy syndrome.

History	Chronic vomiting, especially in small breed and brachycephalic breed dogs
	Postprandial abdominal distension and discomfort, often relieved by vomiting
	Normal to increased appetite
Physical examination	Usually normal
	Weight loss occurs infrequently
Laboratory	Usually normal
Radiography	Fluid-filled distended stomach
	Contrast study reveals gastric-outlet obstruction; narrowed pyloric lumen has typical 'beak-like' appearance
Endoscopy	Thickened pyloric mucosal folds, sometimes with punctate erosions
	Protuberant pylorus that is difficult to intubate with the endoscope
Coeliotomy	Pylorus feels stiff and thickened
	Gastrotomy reveals thickened mucosal and/or muscular layers

middle-age adult male dogs are most frequently affected. The clinical and radiographic signs are of delayed gastric emptying with intermittent gastric dilation; projectile vomiting occurs in many; physical examination and laboratory findings are usually normal. Contrast radiographs show abrupt narrowing of the pyloric canal with a narrow stream of barium passing through; fluoroscopy may reveal hypermotility. The pyloric mucosa appears thickened and redundant, or may appear as a protuberant mass, often with multifocal erosions although the pylorus may appear normal in some. Mucosa are histologically normal to thickened with oedema and hyperplasia; muscularis may be hypertrophied.

Treatment (Box 49.5)

Surgical treatment is necessary. In most instances, pyloroplasty with submucosal resection to remove thickened mucosal folds is required to re-establish gastric outflow; Y-U antral flap pyloroplasty is most effective and preserves normal pyloric function. The prognosis is good following pyloroplasty; some may require treatment with metoclopramide or cisapride to enhance gastric emptying; small frequent meals are necessary in some.

Gastric Tumours and Antral Polyps
(Murray *et al*. 1972; Patniak *et al*. 1977; Couto 1993)

Gastric tumours can obstruct pyloric outflow causing insidious and progressive anorexia, vomiting, haematemesis, melaena and weight loss. Carcinomas and leiomyomas are the most common gastric neoplasms in dogs, followed by lymphosarcoma and leiomyosarcoma, fibroma, squamous cell carcinoma and plasmacytoma. Benign polyps are often asymptomatic but can cause delayed gastric emptying. Diagnosis is based on radiographic, endoscopic and surgical findings. Contrast radiographs may reveal a thickened and ulcerated gastric wall. Endoscopic findings vary from normal to discoloured and thickened mucosa to single large ulcers with thick, raised margins. Biopsy is needed for definitive diagnosis.

Solitary gastric carcinomas are best treated by surgical resection; diffuse or extensive lesions are not usually resectable. Metastasis of carcinomas to lymph nodes, liver or lungs has often occurred by the time of diagnosis and adjunctive chemotherapy has not been successful. Lymphosarcoma can be treated with chemotherapy but the prognosis is guarded. Benign tumours, adenomatous polyps and hyperplastic polyps can be resected, which resolves the outflow obstruction, thus the prognosis is good.

Box 49.5 Management of delayed gastric emptying.

Nutritional management	Frequent feeding of small meals
	Low fat diets
	Limited fibre diets
	Blenderised diets
Prokinetic drugs*	Metoclopramide
	Dopamine antagonist at chemoreceptor trigger zone (central anti-emetic) and at gastrointestinal receptors (stimulates gastrointestinal motility)
	Potential for CNS side-effects
	0.25–0.4 mg/kg every 8 h p.o., s.c., i.m.
	Cisapride
	Stimulates enteric cholinergic transmission†
	No adverse effects
	0.25–0.50 mg/kg every 8 h p.o.
	Erythromycin
	Stimulates gastrointestinal smooth muscle motilin receptors
	Stimulates gastrointestinal cholinergic receptors‡
	0.5–1 mg/kg every 8 h p.o.
Surgical management	Various pyloroplasty and pyloromyotomy procedures indicated for pyloric outflow obstruction.

* Contraindicated in gastric outlet obstruction.
† May be more effective than metoclopramide to enhance gastric emptying of solids.
‡ Higher dosages stimulate vomiting.

Pylorospasm

This is a syndrome of delayed gastric emptying in which no morphological or metabolic cause is found. Contrast radiography may reveal normal antral contractions with episodic abnormal pyloric sphincter contraction; probably caused by lack of antral, pyloric and duodenal co-ordination. It is infrequently diagnosed and must be differentiated from antral pyloric hypertrophy syndrome. Medical management with metoclopramide, cisapride or erythromycin may improve function, but efficacy in dogs is not documented.

Abnormal Gastric Contractions (Gastric Dysrhythmias) (Hall *et al.* 1990; Kim *et al.* 1986)

A delayed gastric emptying can be caused by abnormally slow gastric contraction (bradygastria), rapid rhythm (tachygastria), or irregular rhythm (dysrhythmia); which is thought to be caused by abnormal gastric pacemaker activity or by an ectopic pacemaker. Bradygastria causes infrequent gastric contraction, whereas tachygastria and arrhythmia cause reversed propagation of motor activity which prevents normal emptying. Gastric arrhythmias have been observed to occur normally in healthy dogs during fasting; feeding abolishes the dysrhythmia. Symptomatic dogs have abdominal discomfort, vomiting and gastric stasis. Diagnosis requires measurement of gastric electrical activity, generally limited to referral institutions. The treatment is limited to the use of promotility drugs and dietary changes to enhance gastric emptying.

Delayed Gastric Emptying Caused by Other Diseases

Many disorders can cause acute or chronic gastric motility disorders (Table 49.18). Treatment depends on diagnosis and treatment of the primary cause.

GASTRIC DILATATION-VOLVULUS SYNDROME

Acute gastric dilatation-volvulus (GDV) occurs most frequently in large-breed dogs such as Great Danes, German Shepherds, Irish Setters, Saint Bernards, and Doberman Pinchers. GDV occurs occasionally in smaller-breed dogs such as Bassets, Bulldogs, Miniature Poodles, Dachshunds, and Pekingese, and rarely in cats. Age range is wide, from 2 months to 15 years, with a mean of about 6 years. No sex predilection is apparent.

Causes of GDV

No single cause of GDV has been identified, however multiple risk factors appear to be important in the development of this condition (Van Kruiningen *et al.* 1987; Van Sluys 1987). The key factors are listed below:

- Conformation – deep-chested breeds of dogs are definitely predisposed to GDV, possibly by increased potential of volvulus.
- Laxity of hepatoduodenal and hepatogastric ligaments may cause rotational instability.
- Large volume intake of food and water causes gastric distension and delayed gastric emptying. Chronic overdistension can potentially cause impaired gastric emptying. Exercise by dogs with a distended stomach, particularly deep-chested dogs, may cause the stomach to be displaced and result in volvulus.
- Dietary composition, particularly feeding dry-food diets, has been suggested as a contributing factor to GDV, however a direct relationship has not been established. The incidence of GDV at one hospital has been reported to decline when dry food was dampened before feeding; presumably this prevents swelling of dry food with water in the stomach.
- Increased intake or production of gastric gas may contribute to GDV in some instances. Aerophagia occurring from rapid eating, hyperventilation, and oesophageal motility abnormalities have been associated with recurrent GDV.
- Impaired eructation has been suggested as a predisposing cause of GDV, possibly resulting from an anatomically or functionally abnormal gastro-oesophageal junction (GEJ), which normally prevents gastro-oesophageal reflux. In deep-chested dogs, the oblique angle of the GEJ may be exaggerated, especially if the stomach is distended following a large meal, preventing normal eructation.
- Delayed gastric emptying may predispose to GDV in some instances.

Pathophysiology of Gastric Dilatation-Volvulus (Wingfield *et al.* 1976; Orton & Muir 1983; Horne *et al.* 1985)

Gastric dilatation and volvulus trap ingesta, fluid and gas in the stomach that quickly leads to an extreme increase of intragastric pressure. A cascade of life-threatening effects occurs that, if not corrected rapidly and aggressively, will cause death of the patient. Increased intragastric pressure impedes gastric blood flow leading to gastric wall oedema, vasoconstriction and thrombosis. Subsequently, gastric ulceration, necrosis and perforation will occur rapidly. The splenic malposition leads to splenic congestion, thrombosis, and eventually necrosis. Venous return from viscera is decreased and the tidal volume of the lung reduced resulting in impaired respiration, acidosis, decreased cardiac output, vascular collapse and shock. This is further exacerbated by ischaemia of the splanchnic viscera which releases endotoxins further contributing to hepatic, renal, pancreatic and cardiac damage. The end result is that shock, sepsis and disseminated intravascular coagulation (DIC) occur.

Treatment by gastric deflation and derotation and by the rapid administration of fluids, although very necessary, can have further detrimental effects. Reperfusion injury, coupled with release of endotoxins and cardiodepressant factors, haemodilution and metabolic acidosis can further contribute to metabolic and cardiovascular dysfunction.

Metabolic Consequences of Gastric Dilatation-Volvulus

Several different acid–base and electrolyte imbalances may be seen with gastric dilatation volvulus syndrome (Muir 1982):

- Imbalances may be absent initially but develop subsequent to gastric intubation, fluid therapy and anesthesia; frequent monitoring of these parameters is necessary until the patient is stabilised.
- Metabolic acidosis commonly occurs from decreased circulating blood volume, arterial hypoxaemia and lactic acidosis.
- Metabolic alkalosis, caused by sequestration and loss of gastric H^+, Cl^- and K^+, occurs less frequently.
- Hyperventilation may cause respiratory alkalosis.

- Hypoventilation from gastric distension can interfere with diaphragm function and cause respiratory acidosis.
- Electrolyte abnormalities occur infrequently, hypokalaemia being the most common.

Diagnosis

GDV is diagnosed on the basis of clinical findings and is confirmed by gastric decompression and radiographic findings consistent with dilatation and/or volvulus. Laboratory tests are helpful to assess status of the patient (Table 49.21). The characteristic clinical signs are acute onset of depression in association with retching, but without vomiting. Some dogs are reluctant to stand, whereas others are in lateral recumbency. Abdominal distension and tympany are obvious. There is a rapid, weak pulse, prolonged capillary refill time, and pale mucous membranes are indicative of cardiovascular failure; arrhythmias may be present. Radiographs, taken *only* following initiation of fluid therapy and decompression, will determine if volvulus is present; right lateral recumbent position is the view of choice.

- The stomach usually has residual dilation with gas and fluid.
- A dorsal soft-tissue fold that appears to compartmentalise the stomach and/or a gas-filled pylorus located dorsal to the fundus of the stomach are key indicators of the presence of volvulus.

Table 49.21 Clinical features of gastric dilitation-volvulus.

History	Acute onset of non-productive retching without vomiting
	Acute onset of abdominal distension
Physical examination	Severe depression to collapse and shock
	Reluctant to stand or walk
	Severe abdominal tympany
	Cardiavascular failure characterised by rapid weak pulse or arrhythmia: pale mucous membranes prolonged capillary refill time
	Rapid and shallow respirations
Laboratory	Haemoconcentration
	Metabolic acidosis and hypochloraemia most common; may see metabolic alkalosis, respiratory acidosis, respiratory alkalosis, hypochloraemia and hypernatraemia
	Variable increases in BUN, creatinine and ALT
Radiographs	Right lateral recumbent position, large gas and fluid-filled stomach. Soft tissue fold compartmentalises the stomach. Gas-filled pylorus located dorsal to fundus. Oesophagus dilated with air or fluid

BUN, blood urea nitrogen; ALT, alanine aminotransferase.

- Abdominal fluid is suggestive of peritonitis or haemorrhage.
- Free abdominal gas indicates perforation.
- Mega-oesophagus is a common finding.

Treatment

The successful treatment begins with rapid intravenous fluid therapy and gastric decompression, followed by surgical repositioning of the stomach and gastropexy. Concurrent therapy for electrolyte imbalances, arrhythmias, DIC and gastrointestinal hypomotility are necessary.

Intravenous Fluid Therapy

Intravenous fluid therapy should be started immediately. Lactated Ringer's solution should be given at a rate of 45 ml/kg within the first 15 min to re-establish adequate cardiac output; an additional 45 ml/kg is then given over the next 30–45 min; depending on response, this may need to be repeated during the second hour. Pulse quality, capillary refill, central venous pressure and urinary output should be used as a guide for continued fluid needs; PCV and serum total protein should be monitored to avoid haemodilution (total protein should not decrease <3.5 g/dl).

After gastric decompression, the fluid rate can usually be decreased to 10–20 ml/kg per hour for the next 2 h and then to 5 ml/kg per hour, depending on patient stability. If the plasma protein decreases to <3.5 g/dl, colloidal fluids such as plasma or combination dextran-70/hypertonic saline (Allan *et al.* 1991) can be used.

- Plasma dose = 20 ml/kg given over 1–2 h
- Dextran-70/hypertonic saline (prepared by adding 33 g of powdered NaCl to 500 ml of 6% dextran-70 and autoclaving) is a good alternative to plasma and should also be considered for initial shock therapy instead of lactated Ringer's solution.
  Dose = 4–6 ml/kg given at a rate of 1 ml/kg per minute; followed by maintenance lactated Ringer's solution.

Gastric Decompression

Gastric decompression must be accomplished immediately, occurring as soon as intravenous fluid therapy has begun. Decompression is achieved by either passage of a stomach tube or by gastric trocharisation.

Trocharisation is easier and better tolerated by the patient than gastric intubation; rarely does it cause peritonitis. A 16 G, 5 cm needle or 14–16 G over-the-needle catheter is used; trocharising the stomach on the left side at the site of maximal distension is best. Partial decompression using trocharisation often facilitates passage of a large-bore oral–gastric tube for more complete decompression and gastric lavage. Once a gastric tube is passed, gastric contents should be removed. If possible, the tube should be left in place while radiographs are taken.

If the stomach tube is difficult to pass, attempt to pass the tube while holding the animal in an upright or sitting position. Gently shaking the patient while in the upright position may help. Forcing the tube can cause oesophageal or gastric perforation. An inability to pass the tube does not necessarily mean that volvulus is present, neither does the ability to pass the tube mean volvulus is not present.

Gastric decompression can also be achieved by gastrostomy (Pass & Johnston 1973), usually performed under sedation and local anaesthesia. This is a temporary procedure that fixes the stomach caudal to the right costal arch, but does not return the stomach to normal position. It is indicated for stabilisation if a gastric tube cannot be placed or if the patient needs several days of stabilisation before surgical repositioning and gastropexy.

Surgical Correction

As soon as the clinical condition has been stabilised by gastric decompression and correction of haemodynamic, fluid and electrolyte abnormalities, surgery should be done to re-position and stabilise the stomach. The optimal time for surgery is variable, depending on patient condition and response to initial therapy. In general, surgery should not be delayed beyond the initial period of time required for stabilisation:

- If gastric content is noted to contain digested blood suggestive of gastric ulceration and/or necrosis, if there is radiographic evidence of perforation or peritonitis, if decompression cannot be achieved, or if decompression is difficult to maintain, surgery should not be delayed for more than 1–2 h.
- If the patient responds well to initial therapy and decompression is sustained, surgery can be delayed for 12–24 hours if necessary. In this circumstance, decompression must be maintained, either by nasogastric or pharyngostomy tubes, gastrostomy, or by repeated orogastric intubation.

Infrequently, spontaneous reposition of the stomach occurs after decompression. In this circumstance, surgery can be delayed or may not be necessary. Surgical treatment has three main goals: correct gastric malposition, assess and treat gastric and spenic injury, and prevent recurrence of malposition. The reader is refered to general surgery texts for description of techniques.

Medical Management

Antibiotics should be given to dogs with GDV because shock, mucosal damage and portal hypertension predispose to sepsis. Antibiotics should be effective against Gram-positive, Gram-negative and anaerobic organisms. A combination of ampicillin (20 mg/kg i.v.) and enrofloxacin (2.5–5 mg i.m.), or of ampicillin and an aminoglycoside (gentamicin 2.2 mg/kg slowly i.v. every 8 h or amikacin 5 mg/kg s.c. every 8 h) are good choices. Administration of aminoglycosides must be delayed until after initial fluid therapy has been given to avoid nephrotoxicity. Second generation cepahlosporins or trimethoprim–sulfa antibiotics can be used in less severely affected dogs.

Corticosteroids may be beneficial in the initial management of shock to improve capillary blood flow, to decrease capillary permeabilbity, to reduce intestinal absorption of endotoxin, and to inhibit tissue damaging phospholipases. Short-term, high dose therapy is recommended such as prednisolone sodium succinate (30 mg/kg i.v.) or dexamethasone sodium phosphate (10–15 mg/kg) i.v.

Histamine H_2-receptor blockers can be given to help diminish gastric ulceration; this therapy can be started during initial therapy and continued for 7–10 days. If gastric mucosal damage has been severe, omeprazole should be used as soon as oral medication can be tolerated because of its increased gastric antisecretory activity.

Management of Complications

Cardiac arrhythmias, disseminated intravascular coagualtion (DIC), and gastrointestinal motility disorders are common complications occurring during the acute and convalescent phases of disease.

Cardiac arrhythmias can occur at the time of presentation, but may not develop until as long as 72 h after onset of GDV; as such, frequent ECG monitoring is required from presentation until the dog is discharged from the hospital. Ventricular premature contractions (VPCs), paroxysmal ventricular contractions and ventricular tachycardia are common. Correction of acid–base, electrolyte (especially potassium) and fluid balance is the first step in control of arrhythmias.

Anti-arrhythmic therapy is indicated if ventricular tachycardia with a heart rate of 150 beats per minute or greater is present, or if multifocal VPCs are present (see also page 385). Recommended therapy for ventricular arrhythmias are:

Lidocaine   2–4 mg/kg slow i.v. bolus followed by infusion of 50–100 µg/kg per minute is used for initial control and can be continued for several days.

Procainamide   used as a supplement to lidocaine if arrhythmia is refractory or as longer-term maintenance therapy. 12–20 mg/kg i.m. every 6 h followed by same dose given p.o.

Supraventricular arrhythmias occur infrequently and can be treated with quinidine sulfate 6 mg/kg i.m. every 6 h or 15 mg/kg every 6 h p.o. DIC is a frequent complication of GDV and is detected initially by thrombocytopenia and prolonged coagulation times. As this progresses DIC is detected by bruising, bleeding, decreasing platelet counts, or progressively prolonged coagulation times despite fluid therapy. Treatment of DIC has been covered elsewhere (page 307) but the authors' recommendation is that these cases should treated with:

- plasma (10–20 ml/kg) in combination with heparin (100 units/kg every 8 h s.c.) until platelets begin to increase and other coagulation parameters stabilise;
- heparin should then be decreased slowly by giving doses every 12 h for 24 h and then every 24 h for the next day to avoid rebound hypercoagulation.

Gastric atony, delayed gastric emptying and ileus frequently occur following GDV; in most instances these are transient. If intermittent vomiting persists, therapy with promotility drugs (metoclopramide or cisapride) are helpful to re-establish more normal gastric emptying. Treatment with antisecretory drugs and sulcralfate may also be beneficial.

Overall the prognosis for GDV is guarded, especially if gastric damage is severe and requires gastrectomy. Mortality is reported to be from 23% to 60%. Poor prognostic signs at presentation include a pulse rate >180 beats per minute, arrhythmia, cyanotic mucous membranes, prolonged capillary refill time and severe coagulopathy.

REFERENCES AND FURTHER READING

Albibi, R. & McCallum, R.W. (1983). Metoclopramide: Pharmacology and clinical application. *Annals of Internal Medicine*, **98**, 86–95.

Allan, D.A., Schertel, E.R., Muir, W.W. & Valentine, A.K. (1991). Hypertonic saline/dextran resuscitation of dogs with experimentally induced gastric dilatation-volvulus shock. *American Journal of Veterinary Research*, **52**, 92–96.

Anonymous (1994). Antibacterial therapy of *Helicobacter pylori*-associated peptic ulcer disease: A new strategy [editorial]. *Journal of Clinical Gastroenterology*, **19**(1), 6–10.

Arnbjerg, J. (1992). Gastric emptying time in the dog and cat. *Journal of the American Animal Hospital Association*, **28**(1), 77.

Bayerdorffer, E., Mannes, G.A., Sommer, A., *et al.* (1992). High dose omeprazole treatment combined with amoxicillin eradicates *H. pylori*. *Gastroenterology* **102**, A38.

Burns, J. Fox, S.M. (1986). The use of a barium meal to evaluate total gastric emptying time in the dog. *Veterinary Radiology*, **27**, 169–172.

Carrig, C.B. & Seawright, A.A. (1968). Mastocytosis with gastrointestinal ulceration in a dog. *Australian Veterinary Journal*, **44**, 503–506.

Cheville, N.F. (1979). Uremic gastropathy in the dog. *Veterinary Pathology*, **16**, 292–309.

Couto, C.G. (1993). Gastrointestinal neoplasia in dogs and cats. In: *Current Veterinary Therapy XI*, (ed. R.W. Kirk), pp. 595–601. W.B. Saunders, Philadelphia.

DiBartola, S.P., Johnson, S.E., Davenport, D.J., *et al.* (1985). Clinicopathologic findings resembling hypoadrenocorticism in dogs with primary gastrointestinal disease. *Journal of the American Veterinary Medical Association*, **187**, 60–63.

Drazner, F.H. (1981). Canine gastrinoma: A condition analogous to the Zollinger–Ellison syndrome in man. *California Veterinary*, **11**, 6–11.

Eaton, K.A., Radin, M.J., Kramer, L., *et al.* (1993). Epizootic gastritis associated with gastric spiral bacilli in cheetahs (*Acinonyx jubatus*). *Veterinary Pathology*, **30**, 55–63.

Feldman, M. & Burton, M.E. (1990). Histamine$_2$-receptor antagonists. Standard therapy for acid-peptic diseases. *New England Journal of Medicine*, **323**, 1672, 1749.

Flemstrom, G. (1987). Gastric and duodenal mucosal bicarbonate secretion. In: *Physiology of the Gastrointestinal Tract*, (ed. L.R. Johnson), pp. 1011–1029. Raven Press, New York.

Fox, J.G. & Lee, A. (1993). Gastric *Helicobacter* infection in animals: Natural and experimental infections. In: *Helicobacter Pylori: Biology and Clinical Practice*, (eds S. Goodwin & B.W. Worsley), pp. 407–430. CRC Press, Boca Raton, Florida.

Fox, J.G., Correa, P., Taylor, N.S., Lee, A., Otto, G., Murphy, J.C., *et al.* (1990). *Helicobacter mustelae*-associated gastritis in ferrets. An animal model of *Helicobacter pylori* gastritis in humans. *Gastroenterology*, **99**, 352–361.

Fox, J.G., Lee, A., Otto, G., Taylor, N.G. & Murphy, J.C. (1991). *Helicobacter felis* gastritis in gnotobiotic rats: An animal model of *Helicobacter pylori* gastritis. *Infection and Immunity*, **59**, 785–791.

Freston, J.W. (1990). Overview of medical therapy of peptic ulcer disease. *Gastroenterology Clinics of North America*, **19**, 121–139.

Gottlieb, J.E. (1986). Gastrointestinal complications in critically ill patients: The internist's overview. *American Journal of Gastroenterology*, **81**, 227–238.

Graham, D.Y. (1990). The relationship between nonsteroidal anti-inflammatory drug use and peptic ulcer disease. *Gastroenterology Clinics of North America*, **19**, 171.

Graham, D.Y., Agrawal, N.M. & Roth, S.H. (1988). Prevention of NSAID induced gastric ulcer with misoprostol: Multicentre, double-blind, placebo-controlled trial. *Lancet*, **ii**, 1277–1280.

Guilford, W.G. & Strombeck, D.R. (1996a). Gastric structure and function. In: *Strombeck's Small Animal Gastroenterology*, (eds G.W. Guilford, *et al.*), 3rd edn, pp. 239–255. W.B. Saunders, Philadelphia.

Guilford, G.W. & Strombeck, D.R. (1996b). Chronic gastric diseases. In: *Strombeck's Small Animal Gastroenterology*, (eds G.W. Guilford, *et al.*), 3rd edn, pp. 276–283. W.B. Saunders, Philadelphia.

Hall, J.A., Burrows, C.F. & Twedt, D.C. (1988). Gastric motility in dogs. Part I. Normal gastric function. *Compendium on Continuing Education for the Practicing Veterinarian*, **10**(11), 1282.

Hall, J.A., Twedt, D.C. & Burrows, C.F. (1990). Gastric motility in dogs. II. Disorders of gastric motility. *Compendium on Continuing Education for the Practicing Veterinarian*, **12**, 247–261.

Handt, L.K., Fox, J.G. & Dewhirst, F.D. (1994). *Helicobacter pylori* isolated from the domestic cat: Public health implications. *Infection and Immunity*, **62**, 2367–2374.

Hayden, D.W. & Fleischman, R.W. (1977). Scirrhous eosinophilic gastritis in dogs with gastric arteritis. *Veterinary Pathology*, **14**, 441–448.

Horne, W.A., Gilmore, D.R., Dietze, A.E., Freden, G.O. & Short, C.E. (1985). Effects of gastric distension-volvulus on coronary blood flow and myocardial oxygen consumption in the dog. *American Journal of Veterinary Research*, **46**, 98–104.

Jenkins, C.C. & DeNovo, R.C. (1991). Omeprazole: A potent antiulcer drug. *Compendium on Continuing Education for the Practicing Veterinarian*, **13**, 1579–1582.

Jenkins, C., DeNovo, R.C., Patton, C.S., Bright, R.M. & Ruhrback, B.W. (1991). Comparison of the effects of cimetidine and omeprazole on mechanically created ulceration and on aspirin-induced gastritis in dogs. *American Journal of Veterinary Research*, **52**, 658–661.

Johnson, S.E. (1992). Fluid therapy for gastrointestinal, pancreatic and hepatic disease. In: *Fluid Therapy in Small Animal Practice*, (ed. S.P. DiBartola), pp. 507–528. W.B. Saunders, Philadelphia.

Johnson, S.A., Leib, M.S., Forrester, S.D., *et al.* (1995). The effect of misoprostol on aspirin-induced gastroduodenal lesions in dogs. *Journal of Veterinary Internal Medicine*, **9**(1), 32–38.

Jones, B.R., Nicholls, M.R. & Badman, R. (1976). Peptic ulceration in dog associated with an islet cell carcinoma of the pancreas and an elevated plasma gastrin level. *Journal of Small Animal Practice*, **17**, 593–598.

Kim, C.H., Azpiroz, F. & Malagelada, J.R. (1986). Characteristics of spontaneous and drug-induced gastric dysrhythmias in a chronic canine model. *Gastroenterology*, **90**, 421–427.

Konturek, S.J. & Pawlik, W. (1986). Physiology and pharmacology of prostaglandins. *Digestive Diseases and Sciences*, **31**, 6S–19S.

Lacy, E.R. & Ito, S. (1984). Rapid epithelial restitution of the rat gastric mucosa after ethanol injury. *Laboratory Investigation*, **51**, 573–583.

Lee, A., Krakowka, S., Fox, J.G., *et al.* (1992). Role of *Helicobacter felis* in chronic canine gastritis. *Veterinary Pathology*, **29**, 487–494.

Leib, M.S., *et al.* (1985). Gastric emptying of liquids in the dog: Serial test meal and modified emptying-time techniques. *American Journal of Veterinary Research*, **46**(9), 1876.

Lichtenberger, L.M. (1993). Mechanisms of gastric mucosal protection. *Proceedings 11th ACVIM Forum*, 74–79.

Marshall, B.J. & Warren, J.R. (1984). Unidentified curved bacilli in the stomach of patients with gastritis and peptic ulceration. *Lancet*, **i**, 1311–1315.

Matthieson, D.T. & Walter, M.C. (1986). Surgical treatment of chronic hypertrophic pyloric gastropathy in 45 dogs. *Journal of the American Animal Hospital Association*, **22**, 241–247.

Miller, M.E., Christenson, G.C. & Evans, H.E. (1964). The digestive system and abdomen. In: *Anatomy of the Dog*, pp. 681–685. W.B. Saunders, Philadelphia.

Miyabayshi, T. & Morgan, J.P. (1984). Gastric emptying in the normal dog. *Veterinary Radiology*, **25**, 187–191.

Muir, W.W. (1982). Acid-base and electrolyte disturbances in dogs with gastric dilatation-volvulus. *Journal of the American Veterinary Medical Association*, **181**, 229–231.

Murray, M., Robinson, P.B., McKeating, F.J., *et al.* (1972). Primary gastric neoplasia in the dog. A clinicopathologic study. *Veterinary Record*, **91**, 474–479.

Murtaugh, R.J., Matz, M.E., Labato, M.A., *et al.* (1992). The use of misoprostol for prevention of gastroduodenal haemorrhage and ulceration associated with aspirin therapy. *Journal of Veterinary Internal Medicine*, **6**(2), 129.

Neri, M., Susi, D., Bovani, I., Pindo, R. & Cullorollo, F. (1992). Omeprazole, bismuth and clarythromycin: A new approach to the treatment of *H. pylori* related gastritis. *Gastroenterology*, **102**, A134.

Orton, E.C. & Muir, W.W. (1983). Hemodynamics in experimental gastric dilatation-volvulus in dogs. *American Journal of Veterinary Research*, **44**, 1512–1515.

Otto, G., Hazell, S.H., Fox, J.G., *et al.* (1994). Animal and public health implications of gastric colonization of cats by *Helicobacter*-like organisms. *Journal of Clinical Microbiology*, **32**, 1043–1049.

Parsonnet, J., Hansen, M.D., Rodriguez, L., *et al.* (1994). *Helicobacter pylori* infection and gastric lymphoma. *New England Journal of Medicine*, **330**, 1267–1271.

Pass, M.A. & Johnston, D.R. (1973). Treatment of gastric dilation torsion in the dog. Gastric decompression by gastrotomy under local analgesia. *Journal of Small Animal Practice*, **14**, 1131–1142.

Patniak, A.K., Hurvity, A.I. & Johnson, G.V. (1977). Canine gastrointestinal neoplasms. *Veterinary Pathology*, **14**, 547–555.

Pennick, D.G., Nyland, T.G., Kerr, L.Y. & Fisher, P.E. (1990). Ultrasonographic evaluation of gastrointestinal diseases in small animals. *Veterinary Radiology*, **31**(30), 134–141.

Radin, M.J., Eaton, K.A., Krakowka, S., *et al.* (1990). *Helicobacter pylori* gastric infection in gnotobiotic beagle dogs. *Infection and Immunity*, **58**, 2606–2612.

Robert, A. (1979). Cytoprotection by prostaglandins. *Gastroenterology*, **77**, 761.

Russell, J. & Bass, P. (1985). Canine gastric emptying of fiber meals: Influence of meal viscosity and antroduodenal motility. *American Journal of Physiology*, **249**, G622.

Sikes, R.I., Birchard, S., Patniak, A. & Bradley, R. (1986). Chronic hypertrophic pyloric gastropathy: A review of 16 cases. *Journal of the American Animal Hospital Association*, **22**, 99–104.

Silen, W. (1987). Gastric mucosal defense and repair. In: *Physiology of the Gastrointestinal Tract*, (ed. L.R. Johnson), pp. 1055–1069. Raven Press, New York.

Silen, W. & Ito, S. (1985). Mechanisms for rapid re-epithelialization of the gastric mucosal surface. *Annual Review of Physiology*, **47**, 217–229.

Skirrow, M.B. (1994). Diseases due to *Campylobacter*, *Helicobacter* and related bacteria. *Journal of Comparative Pathology*, **111**, 113–149.

Smout, A.J. & Akkermans, L.M. (1992). *Normal and Disturbed Motility of the Gastrointestinal Tract*, pp. 11–39. Wrightson Biomedical Publishing, Peterfield, UK.

Sorjonen, D.C., Dillon, A.R., Powers, R.D. & Span, J.S. (1983). Effects of dexamethasone and surgical hypotension on the stomach of dogs: Clinical, endoscopic, and pathologic evaluations. *American Journal of Veterinary Research*, **44**, 1233–1238.

Stanton, M.E. & Bright, R.M. (1989). Gastroduodenal ulceration in dogs. *Journal of Veterinary Internal Medicine*, **3**, 238–244.

Tarnawski, A., Hollander, D. & Gergely, H. (1987). The mechanism of protective, therapeutic and prophylactic actions of sucralfate. *Scandinavian Journal of Gastroenterology*, **22** (Suppl. 140), 7–13.

Twedt, D.C. (1985). Cirrhosis: A consequence of chronic liver disease. *Veterinary Clinics of North America*, **15**, 151.

Twedt, D.C. & Magne, M.L. (1986). Chronic gastritis. In: *Current Veterinary Therapy IX*, (ed. R.W. Kirk), pp. 852–855. W.B. Saunders, Philadelphia.

Twedt, D.C. & Magne, M.L. (1989). Diseases of the stomach. In: *Textbook of Veterinary Internal Medicine*, (ed. S.J. Ettinger), 3rd edn, pp. 1289–1322. W.B. Saunders, Philadelphia.

Van den Brom, W.E. & Happe, R.P. (1986). Gastric emptying of a radionuclide-labeled test meal in healthy dogs: A new mathematical analysis and reference values. *American Journal of Veterinary Research*, **47**, 2170–2174.

Van Kruiningen, H.J., Wajan, L.D., Stake, P.E., *et al.* (1987). The influence of diet and feeding frequency on gastric function in the dog. *Journal of the American Animal Hospital Association*, **23**, 145–152.

Van Sluys, F.J. (1987). *Gastric dilatation volvulus in the dog*. Thesis, Department of Small Animal Medicine and Surgery, University of Utrecht.

Van Sluys, F.J. & Wolvenkamp, W.T.C. (1993). Abnormal esophageal motility in dogs with recurrent gastric dilatation-volvulus [abstract]. *Proceedings of the European College of Veterinary Surgeons*, p. 250.

Wallace, J.L. & Bell, C.J. (1992). Gastroduodenal mucosal defense. *Current Opinion in Gastroenterology*, **8**, 911–917.

Wallmark, B., Lorentzon, P. & Lorsson, H. (1985). The mechanism of action of omeprazole – A survey of its inhibitory actions *in vitro*. *Scandinavian Journal of Gastroenterology*, **20** (Suppl. 108), 37–51.

Walter, M.C. & Matthiesen, D.T. (1993). Acquired antral pyloric hypertrophy in the dog. *Veterinary Clinics of North America*, **23**, 547–554.

Washabau, R.J. & Elie, M.S. (1995). Antiemetic therapy. In: *Kirk's Current Veterinary Therapy XII*, (eds J.D. Bonagura, *et al.*), pp. 679–684. W.B. Saunders, Philadelphia.

Wingfield, W.E., Betts, C.W. & Rawlings, C.A. (1976). Pathophysiology associated with gastric dilatation-volvulus in the dog. *Journal of the American Animal Hospital Association*, **12**, 136–142.

Zerbe, C.A., Boosinger, T.R., Grabau, J.H., Pletcher, J.M. & O'Dorisio, T.M. (1989). Pancreatic polypeptide and insulin-secreting tumor in a dog with duodenal ulcers and hypertrophic gastritis. *Journal of Veterinary Internal Medicine*, **3**, 178–182.

Chapter 50

Small Intestinal Disease

E. J. Hall

INTRODUCTION

The small intestine has paradoxical roles as both a barrier and an absorptive surface. It normally performs and co-ordinates secretion, digestion, absorption, motility, and tolerance and immunity in order to digest and absorb nutrients and egest faecal waste in an acceptable form. Although not invariably present, diarrhoea is considered the cardinal sign of malfunction of this complex system. However, diarrhoea may also be a manifestation of disease elsewhere in the gastrointestinal tract or even in other organ systems (Table 50.1). Similarly, vomiting is a sign not only of gastric disease, but also disease of the small intestine as well as other organ systems.

Diarrhoea, an increase in frequency, fluidity or volume of faeces, is often divided for convenience into acute and chronic as their differential diagnosis and treatment often vary. Some causes of chronic diarrhoea result in malabsorption of nutrients with consequent weight loss or failure to thrive. Melaena may also be a sign of small intestine disease, while severe small intestine diseases termed protein-losing enteropathies (PLE) may result in ascites and/or peripheral oedema.

FUNCTIONAL ANATOMY

Macroscopic Anatomy (Fig. 50.1)

The small intestine is a tubular structure beginning at the pylorus on the right side of the cranial abdomen and ending at the ileo-colic valve some 1.5–4.5 m later (depending on the size of the dog). It is divided anatomically into three segments duodenum, jejunum and ileum:

(1) Duodenum
   - turns caudally from pylorus, in contact with right flank and right limb of pancreas,
   - caudal flexure at pelvic brim,
   - ascending limb ends at level of L6 close to root of mesentery near left kidney,
   - turns ventromedially into jejunum.
(2) Jejunum
   - forms majority of small intestine,
   - loosely suspended in mid-abdomen in mesentery, forming mobile loops.
(3) Ileum
   - approximately last 30 cm of small intestine, but not clearly demarcated from jejunum,
   - ends at ileo-colic valve in close association with caeco-colic junction.

The small intestine has a blood supply from coeliac and cranial mesenteric arteries and a venous drainage to liver via hepatic portal vein. The lymphatic drainage is via mesenteric nodes to cisterna chyli and thoracic duct. Innervation is from vagal and sympathetic innervation which co-ordinate with intrinsic neuropeptides and enteric hormones to regulate small intestine motility and function.

Microscopic Anatomy (Fig. 50.1)

The general layered structure of the intestinal wall is constant throughout its length. The mucosa is adapted to provide a digestive and absorptive surface as well as a physical and immunological barrier and these are documented below.

(1) Digestive adaptations
   - mucosal folds and cylindrical villi about 1 mm long to increase surface area,

Table 50.1   Causes of diarrhoea.

Gastrointestinal disease	Primary small intestinal disease (see Table 50.13)
	Dietary-induced (see Table 50.11)
	Gastric disease
	achlorhydria*
	dumping syndromes*
	Pancreatic disease
	exocrine pancreatic insufficiency
	pancreatitis
	Liver disease
	liver failure
	intrahepatic and extrahepatic
	bilary duct obstruction
	Large intestinal disease
Polysystemic infectious diseases	Distemper
	Parvovirus
	Leptospira
	Infectious canine hepatitis
	Histoplasma
Non-gastrointestinal disease	Endocrine disease
	hypoadrenocorticism
	hyperthyroidism*
	APUDomas* (gastrinoma/ Zollinger–Ellison syndrome, VIPomas, functional carcinoids)
	Renal disease
	uraemia
	nephrotic syndrome (in association with PLE in Soft Coated Wheaten Terriers)
Miscellaneous	Toxaemias
	pyometra
	peritonitis
	Congestive heart failure
	Various toxins and drugs

* Rare conditions or not even reported in dogs.
PLE, protein-losing enteropathies.

- specialised enterocytes, arising from crypts, on surface of villi, enterocyte surface folded into microvilli (brush border),
- digestive hydrolases and carrier proteins carried on microvillar membrane.
(2) Barrier adaptations
   - secretory immunoglobulin A (IgA),
   - mucus secretion by goblet cells,
   - continual renewal of enterocytes from crypts,

Fig. 50.1   Functional anatomy of the small intestine.
(a) Anatomical arrangement of the small intestine. The duodenum arises from the pylorus of the stomach and is in close association with the pancreas, both being supplied by the cranial pancreatico-duodenal artery from the coeliac artery. Digestive enzymes are secreted into the duodenal lumen via one or two pancreatic ducts. After the caudal duodenal flexure, the duodenum merges into the jejunum which is approximately 2–5 m in length, depending on the breed. Loops of jejunum are suspended in a mesentery through which pass the caudal pancreatico-duodenal and the jejunal arterial branches of the cranial mesenteric artery as well as the jejunal veins leading to the hepatic portal vein. The terminal part of the small intestine is the ileum, and is distinguished by the anti-mesenteric path of the ileo-caeco-colic artery. The ileum enters the large intestine at the ileo-colic valve. (Redrawn from Miller *et al.* 1964, Figs 4.54 p. 353 and 4.59 p. 361.)
(b) The small intestine is basically a tube with a serosal surface covered by visceral peritoneum, and an inner absorptive and digestive surface, the mucosa. (Redrawn from Simpson & Else 1991, Fig. 5.2 p. 103.)
(c) Beneath the outer serosa, longitudinal and circular muscle layers produce peristaltic and segmental contractions for propelling and mixing the luminal contents. The submucosa is rich in blood and lymphatic vessels. The mucosa comprises the thin muscularis mucosa, the lamina propria and the columnar epithelium, and is thrown into folds and covered by finger-like villi to increase the digestive and absorptive surface area. (Redrawn from Freeman & Bracegirdle 1966, Fig. 39 p. 69.)
(d) Enterocytes are shed from the villus tip, but are continually replaced by division of crypt cells, and are the site of nutrient digestion and absorption. Goblet cells secrete protective mucus. Water-soluble nutrients pass into the rich capillary network of the lamina propria, and fat is passed as chylomicrons into the lacteals. Immunocytes in the lamina propria are involved in maintaining tolerance to luminal antigens. (Redrawn from Simpson & Else 1991, Fig. 5.3 p. 104.)
(e) The luminal membrane of the enterocyte is thrown into processess called microvilli which increase the luminal surface area, and are known as the brush border. Tight junctions between enterocytes maintain epithelial integrity. Absorbed nutrients are passed from the enterocyte into the intercellular space for distribution to the body. (Redrawn from Batt 1984, Fig. 1 p. 93.)
(f) A schematic representation of a microvillus showing digestive hydrolases anchored in the phospholipid cell membrane and buli protruding into the intestinal lumen. Carrier proteins within the membrane are believed to act as 'pores', shuttling nutrients across the membrane by conformational changes in their structure often induced by sodium influx at the expense of energy utilisation through a Na/K ATPase on the basolateral membrane.

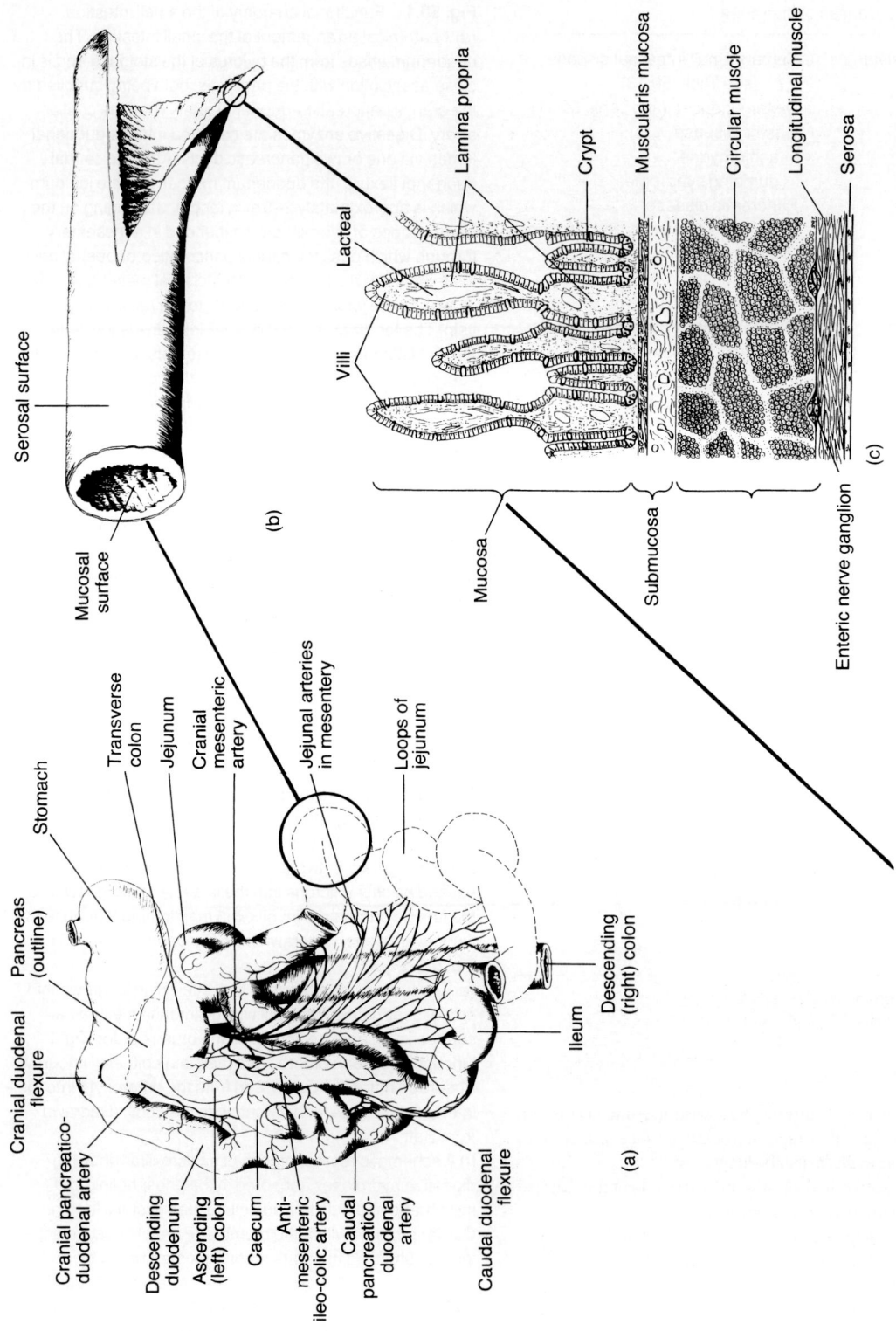

Serosal surface

Mucosal surface

(b)

Lamina propria

Crypt

Muscularis mucosa

Circular muscle

Longitudinal muscle

Serosa

Lacteal

Villi

Mucosa

Submucosa

Enteric nerve ganglion

(c)

Stomach

Transverse colon

Jejunum

Cranial mesenteric artery

Jejunal arteries in mesentery

Loops of jejunum

Pancreas (outline)

Cranial duodenal flexure

Cranial pancreatico-duodenal artery

Descending duodenum

Ascending (left) colon

Caecum

Anti-mesenteric ileo-colic artery

Caudal pancreatico-duodenal artery

Caudal duodenal flexure

Ileum

Descending (right) colon

(a)

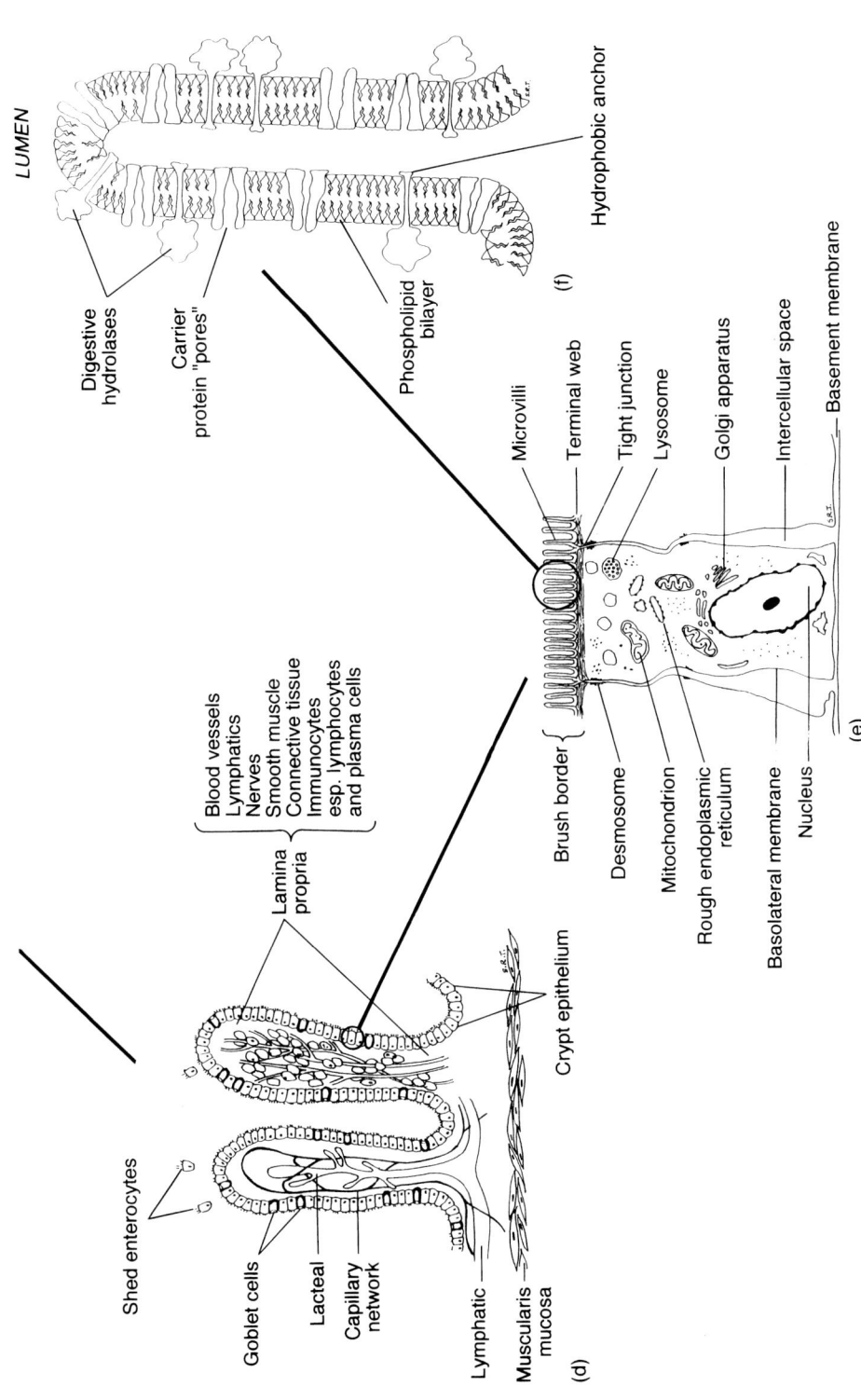

Fig. 50.1a–f *Continued*

- inter-enterocyte tight junctions,
- gut-associated lymphoid tissue – sample luminal antigens at Peyer's patches and mount local IgA response and systemic T cell mediated tolerance.

Digestion

Mixing of luminal contents occurs between areas of segmental contraction (Fig. 50.2), while peristaltic waves propel ingesta. Small intestine transit time is normally about 30–120 min. Between meals, migrating motor complexes send periodic waves of peristalsis along the intestinal tract to sweep all residual ingesta and many bacteria to the colon.

Maldigestion can arise in a number of situations. This may reflect hepatic or pancreatic disease because digestion of chyme begins within the small intestine lumen with solubilisation of fat by bile salts and hydrolysis of macromolecules by pancreatic peptidases, amylase, lipase and nucleases; the small intestine provides optimum temperature and pH, and mechanical agitation. However, small intestine disease also causes maldigestion as well as malassimilation because both completion of digestion and absorption is performed by the mucosa (Fig. 50.1). The digestion of maltose, sucrose-isomaltose, lactose, and di- and tri-peptides occurs on microvillar membrane. There is active absorption via carrier-mediated uptake of glucose, galactose, amino acids, dipeptides, nucleic acids, bile acids, and perhaps minerals (iron, copper, zinc) and facilitated (carrier-mediated) diffusion of fructose and folate. There is passive diffusion of monoglycerides, free fatty acids, most vitamins and receptor-mediated endocytosis of cobalamin. Enterocytes utilise mostly glutamine for energy, transferring luminal glucose and amino acids to portal circulation. Protein-rich chylomicrons are assembled in enterocytes and transported by lymphatics (lacteals), but C8–C10 fats (medium chain triglycerides (MCTs)) pass to the portal blood. There is a constant entero-hepatic recycling of bile salts which is important in the overall digestion of fat.

There is great functional reserve capacity, and adaptation following gut resection occurs. However, structure and functions normally vary along the small intestine:

(1) Duodenum
- receives chyme from stomach and pancreatic secretions,
- water and electrolyte secretion by crypts,
- primary site of maximum intraluminal digestion.
(2) Jejunum
- main site of digestion and absorption,
- longest villi,
- water uptake driven by monosaccharide absorption.

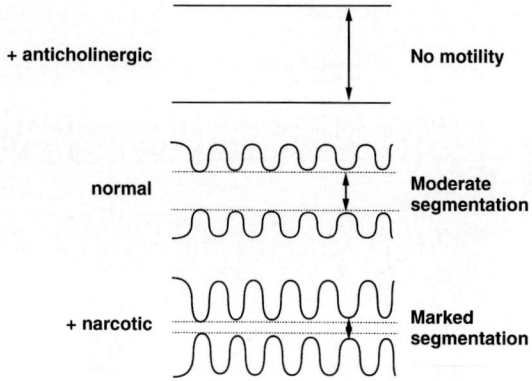

Fig. 50.2   Patterns of segmental contraction in the intestine.

(3) Ileum
- decreased height of villi and more prominent lymphoid tissue,
- site of cobalamin and bile acid absorption,
- water uptake driven by sodium absorption.

PATHOGENESIS OF DIARRHOEA

The pathogenesis of diarrhoea may be considered as separate pathophysiological mechanisms, i.e. osmotic secretory permeability and motility (Table 50.2), although most cases are complex (Fig. 50.3). Each day over 2.5 l of fluid enters the small intestine of a 20-kg dog from the diet and gastrointestinal secretions (Strombeck & Guilford 1991). The normal jejunum reabsorbs approximately 50% of this fluid and the ileum 75% of the remainder. Increased secretion or malabsorption in small intestine disease can easily overwhelm the small colonic absorptive reserve and produce diarrhoea, even assuming the colon is not diseased as well. The fluid fluxes can be so great that dehydration, electrolyte losses (especially potassium) and acid–base disturbances may become life-threatening.

INVESTIGATION OF SMALL INTESTINE DISEASE

Many small intestine diseases are self-limiting and do not need a precise diagnosis, but any case has the potential to be life-threatening or to be communicable to other pets or

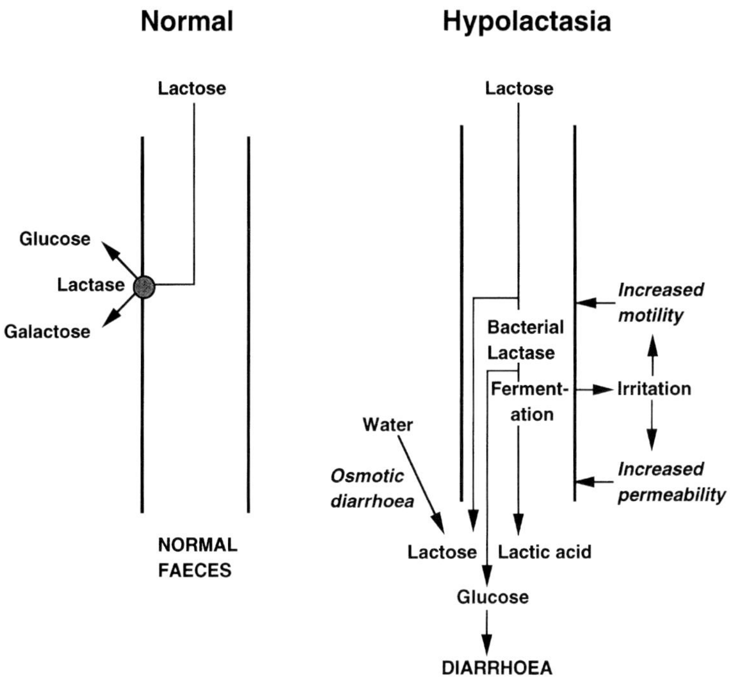

Normal

Hypolactasia

Fig. 50.3 Diagram to illustrate the interaction of the major pathophysiological mechanisms in hypolactasia.

Table 50.2 Pathogenesis of diarrhoea.

Osmotic	Probably most common mechanism in dog, undigested and/or unabsorbed solutes drag water into small intestine, e.g. • dietary overload • malabsorption – exocrine pancreatic insufficiency, small intestine mucosal disease
Secretory	Hypersecretion usually in response to microbial toxins, less common mechanism in dogs than man, e.g. • bacterial enterotoxins and endotoxins • *Giardia* • bacterial deconjugation of bile salts and hydroxylation of fatty acids • hormonal
Abnormal permeability	To fluid and electrolytes • invasive bacteria • mucosal inflammation • portal hypertension, e.g. liver disease, congestive heart failure etc. To plasma proteins • mucosal ulceration by infectious agents • lymphangiectasia • obstruction by inflammation or neoplasia
Abnormal motility	Transit rate decreased • partial obstruction / stagnant loop • ileus Transit rate increased • absence of segmentation, i.e. hypomotility • spasm and hypermotility a rare primary cause, e.g. hyperthyroidism

Breed	Condition
Basenji	Lymphocytic–plasmacytic enteritis (syn. Immunoproliferative enteropathy)
Beagle	Idiopathic SIBO (usually asymptomatic)
German Shepherd Dog*	Idiopathic (antibiotic-responsive) SIBO Inflammatory bowel disease
Giant Schnauzer	Defective cobalamin absorption
Irish Setter	Gluten-sensitive enteropathy
Lundehund	Lymphangiectasia
Retrievers	Dietary allergy†
Rottweiler	Susceptibility to parvovirus
Shar-Pei	Lymphocytic–plasmacytic enteritis
Toy breeds	Haemorrhagic gastroenteritis
Yorkshire Terriers	Lymphangiectasia

Table 50.3 Known or suspected breed predispositions for small intestine disease.

* Exocrine pancreatic insufficiency is common and should be ruled out.
† Suspected.
SIBO, small intestinal bacterial overgrowth.

man. A logical diagnostic approach, founded on history and physical examination, is required to rule out potential problems without performing unnecessary tests. Known breed predispositions may help formulate a differential diagnosis (Table 50.3), but either a 'trawling expedition' or following hunches can be wasteful and expensive. Attention must always be given to the hydration status of the patient.

History and Physical Examination

Questions concerning general health are always relevant but, in the context of small intestine disease, certain pertinent information should be obtained (Table 50.4). Diarrhoea is a primary sign of small intestine disease; secondary signs are listed in Table 50.5.

It can be useful to classify diarrhoea as small intestine in origin based on clinical signs and faecal characteristics (Table 50.6). Signs of large intestinal diarrhoea are discussed in Chapter 51. Failure to pass faeces may indicate complete small intestine obstruction, although vomiting is most likely to be the presenting complaint. While vitally important, complete obstructions are surgical conditions that will not be discussed. Segmental adynamic ileus or pseudo-obstruction, mimics complete obstruction, but may respond to prokinetic agents (metoclopramide, 0.2–0.4 mg/kg p.o. t.i.d.–q.i.d.; cisapride, 0.1–0.5 p.o. b.i.d.–t.i.d.). Intestinal sclerosis has been identified as one cause of this very rare condition (Strombeck & Guilford 1991). However, generalised adynamic ileus or failure of

Table 50.4 Important historical information in small intestine disease.

Background
  Complete dietary intake
  Possibility of access to non-food substances
  Scavenging
  Coprophagy
  Vaccination and worming history

Signs
  Nature of diarrhoea (see Tables 50.5 & 50.6)
  Vomiting
  Appetite
  Abdominal pain
  Borborygmi & flatulence
  Polydipsia
  Skin disease (pruritus, otitis, pedal dermatitis)

Characteristics of signs
  Duration
  Severity
  Progression
  Frequency, periodicity
  Response to treatment

Systems review
  Hydration status
  Organ systems (cardiovascular, locomotor, neurological, reproductive, respiratory, urinary)

Table 50.5   Signs associated with small intestine disease.

Diarrhoea (see Table 50.6)

Abdominal discomfort / pain	Inappetence or polyphagia
Abdominal distension	Melaena
Borborygmi	Polydipsia
Dehydration	Vomiting
Flatulence	Weight loss
Halitosis	Coprophagy and/or scavenging
Oedema	Protein-losing enteropathy

Table 50.6   Characteristics of small intestine diarrhoea.

Faeces
   Volume – markedly increased
   Consistency – poorly formed to watery
   Mucus – rarely present
   Melaena – may be present
   Fresh blood – absent except in acute haemorrhagic
      diarrhoea
   Steatorrhoea – present with malabsorption
   Undigested food – may be present
   Colour – colour variations occur

Defecation
   Urgency – absent except in acute or very severe disease
   Tenesmus – absent unless secondary colitis
   Frequency – two to three times normal for the patient
   Dyschezia – absent
   Haematochezia – absent unless acute haemorrhagic
      diarrhoea

Table 50.7   Abnormalities that may be noted during physical examination that may be relevant in primary small intestine disease.

General examination
   Dehydration
   Lethargy
   Fat/thin/muscle wasting
   Lymphadenopathy
   Mucous membranes – colour, CRT, ulceration etc.
   Linear foreign body around base of tongue
   Oedema

Abdominal palpation
   Abdominal pain/discomfort
   Ascites
   Borborygmi
   Fluid/gas-filled bowel loops
   Thickened bowel loops
   Intussusception
   Masses

Rectal examination
   Faecal colour, consistency
   Melaena

Skin
   Pruritic rash
   Scurf and seborrhoea

CRT, capillary refill time.

peristalsis more commonly reflects hypokalaemia, tox-aemia, peritonitis or postoperative complications. Physical examination should include oral inspection, careful palpa-tion of the abdomen and rectal examination in all cases of intestinal disease. Significant findings that may be present are listed in Table 50.7.

Laboratory Testing

The extent of any laboratory testing in gastrointestinal disease is a balance between the acuteness and severity of the illness and economic considerations. There are various levels of investigation including a minimum database, functional tests of the small intestine, diagnostic imaging and intestinal biopsy. A logical approach is essential to arrive at the correct diagnosis but a minimum database will rule out the majority of systemic causes of diarrhoea, and also suggest possible primary gastrointestinal causes.

Ideal Minimum Database

- Haematology
  - Haemoconcentration if dehydrated or haemor-rhagic gastroenteritis (HGE).
  - Mild anaemia of chronic disease sometimes seen in malabsorption.
  - Microcytic iron-deficiency anaemia if chronic blood loss; microcytosis is also seen in congenital porto-systemic shunt.
  - Mild neutrophilia ± left shift ± monocytosis sometimes seen in inflammatory bowel disease (IBD).
  - Eosinophilia may reflect parasitism, hypoadreno-corticism or sometimes eosinophilic enteritis.
  - Lymphopenia characteristic of lymphangiectasia.
  - Neutropenia frequently seen in parvovirus infec-tion and sometimes in salmonellosis.
- Biochemistry
  - Urea, creatinine and electrolytes for hydration status.

○ Urea: creatinine ratio sometimes raised by small intestine bleeding.

○ Na:K ratio abnormal in primary hypoadrenocorticism and, rarely, in secretory diarrhoea (whipworms, salmonellosis).

○ Calcium not usually increased in small intestine lymphoma.

○ Pan-hypoproteinaemia (decreased albumin and globulin) characteristic of PLE.

○ Mild elevations in alanine amino transferase (ALT) and alkaline phosphatase (ALP) secondary to disturbed intestinal integrity and possible absorption of hepatotoxins.

○ Cholesterol and triglycerides may be low if prolonged inappetence, PLE or malabsorption.

○ Glucose not altered by primary small intestine malabsorption.

- Urinalysis
  ○ No significant changes except increased specific gravity if dehydrated.
- Faecal examination
  ○ Bacterial culture.
  ○ Only helpful when known pathogens, such as *Salmonella* and *Campylobacter*, are found. Pathogenic coliforms are only beginning to be characterised in dogs (Sancak *et al.* 1995).
  ○ Faecal flora does not reflect small intestine flora and cannot diagnose small intestinal bacterial overgrowth (SIBO).
- Faecal virology
  ○ By direct electron microscopy or immunological tests to confirm viral enteritis, but usually too late to be of clinical relevance to individual patient.
- Parasitology
  ○ Ideally three faecal samples should be examined.
  ○ Fresh direct smear for parasites including *Giardia* trophozoites and *Strongyloides*.
  ○ Sugar or salt flotation or formol–ether sedimentation for endoparasitic ova.
  ○ Zinc sulphate flotation for *Giardia* oocysts.
- Faecal content
  ○ Faecal proteolytic activity (gelatin digestion) superseded by trypsin-like immunoreactivity (TLI) test for exocrine pancreatic insufficiency.
  ○ Presence of fat droplets, starch granules or muscle fibres may indicate malabsorption but too non-specific to be valuable.
  ○ 72-h faecal fat analysis quantitates steatorrhoea, but is very unpleasant to perform.
  ○ Occult blood tests detect gastrointestinal bleeding if dog will eat a blood-free meal for 3 days to prevent false positives.
- Rectal cytology

○ May reveal inflammatory disease, but more relevant to large intestinal disease.

Functional Tests

- Absorption tests
  ○ Glucose absorption test – unreliable
- Tolerance tests
  ○ Starch tolerance test – unreliable
  ○ Lactose tolerance test – unreliable
  ○ D-xylose tolerance test
  ○ D-xylose is a pentose sugar probably absorbed by facilitated diffusion on the fructose carrier. Reputedly not metabolised after absorption and completely excreted in urine, in fact almost 50% is metabolised (Hall & Batt 1996). Apparent xylose malabsorption may also be caused by intra-luminal bacterial degradation. The test is often normal despite significant mucosal disease (Burrows *et al.* 1995).
  ○ Fat tolerance test – observation of lipaemia or measurement of serum triglyceride peak after administration of 3 ml/kg corn oil.
- Serum-trypsin like immuno-reactivity concentration
  ○ To rule out exocrine pancreatic insufficiency (Williams 1987).
- Serum folate and cobalamin concentrations
  ○ May permit detection of SIBO and proximal and distal small intestine disease (Batt & Morgan 1982).
  ○ The principle is that folate absorption occurs in proximal intestine and is reduced by proximal damage. Cobalamin is absorbed by ileum and is reduced by distal damage; bacteria in small intestinal bacterial overgrowth synthesise excess folate but bind cobalamin. For interpretation see Table 50.8.
- Intestinal permeability
  ○ Unmediated, passive permeability as an index of mucosal integrity measuring ^{51}Cr-EDTA absorption or differential absorption of different sized probe sugars (e.g. cellobiose/mannitol, lactulose/rhamnose) to detect intestinal damage, and monitor to treatment (Hall & Batt 1990, 1991; Quigg *et al.* 1993; Rutgers *et al.* 1995)
- Differential sugar absorption
  ○ Ratio of D-xylose/3-*O*-methyl glucose absorption may be a marker of carbohydrate absorptive capacity. Can be combined with lactulose/rhamose test (Sørensen *et al.* 1994; Rutgers *et al.* 1995)
- Faecal protein loss to diagnose PLE
  ○ ^{51}Cr-labelled albumin excretion. Distasteful and potentially hazardous test. Faecal excretion of

Table 50.8 Interpretation of serum folate and cobalamin in dogs with chronic diarrhoea and without exocrine pancreatic insufficiency (normal trypsin-like immunity).

Use	Folate concentration	Cobalamin concentration	Interpretation
Potentially helpful results	Increased	Decreased	SIBO
	Increased	Normal or increased	Possible SIBO Vitamin supplementation
	Normal	Decreased	Possible SIBO Possible distal small intestine disease Cobalamin absorption defect
	Decreased	Normal (or increased)	Possible proximal small intestine disease: perhaps dietary sensitivity
	Decreased	Decreased	Diffuse small intestine disease Possible SIBO and mucosal damage Malnutrition
Unhelpful results	Normal	Normal	Does *not* rule out small intestine disease or SIBO
	Normal/increased	Increased	Vitamin supplementation or unknown significance

SIBO, small intestinal bacterial overgrowth.
N.B. Serum folate and cobalamin may be affected by age, diet, exocrine pancreatic insufficiency, neoplasia, systemic diseases, and drugs such as sulphonamides.

serum α_1 protease inhibitor. This plasma protein is resistant to bacterial degradation after loss into the small intestine (not validated in dogs)
- Breath hydrogen
  - Exhaled H_2 is derived from intestinal bacterial fermentation, and normally arises in the colon. Increased or more rapid production of H_2 after a test meal or administration of a test sugar (e.g. xylose, lactulose, glucose) may indicate carbohydrate malabsorption or rapid small intestine transit (Washabau *et al.* 1986). SIBO may be indicated by an early or double peak of H_2 excretion, although interpretation remains controversial.

Imaging

- Plain radiographs
  - Always taken before any contrast study, as masses, foreign bodies or gravel signs (indicating partial obstruction) may be obscured.
  - Look for displacement, bunching, distension or thickening of small intestine.
  - Loss of detail may reflect significant weight loss, peritonitis or ascites.
- Contrast radiography
  - Contrast studies in malabsorption cases usually unrewarding unless severe mucosal disease.

  - If necessary, sedation with acetylpromazine will not significantly affect small intestine motility.
  - Give micropulverised barium sulphate suspension (10 ml/kg), preferably by stomach tube, and take ventrodorsal and right lateral views at intervals [5, 15–30, 60 min, then 2, 3, 6, (24) h], stopping only when all the intestine is adequately visualised.
  - Use iodinated contrast agents if small intestine perforation is suspected, but they are hypertonic and may cause dehydration, and give poorer mucosal detail and abnormally rapid transit.
  - Contrast should be unnecessary to detect complete intestinal obstruction, and may miss partial obstructions.
  - Barium-impregnated poly spheres (BIPS, Arnolds) to evaluate gastric emptying and small intestine transit times and to detect partial obstructions have recently been developed (Guilford 1994a).
- Ultrasonography
  - May demonstrate diffuse or focal thickening of the small intestine wall and the presence of masses.

Intestinal Biopsy

Biopsy is rarely indicated in acute diarrhoea, but may provide a definitive diagnosis in chronic cases, although

Table 50.9 Chronic small intestine diseases where intestinal biopsies may appear normal.

Small intestinal bacterial overgrowth
Dietary indiscretion
Food intolerance
Type 1 hypersensitivity to food (if dog starved before
   biopsy)
Toxigenic and secretory diarrhoeas
Motility disorders
Brush border enzyme deficiency (e.g. hypolactasia)
Patchy mucosal disease not sampled
Intestinal sclerosis if biopsies not full thickness
Undiagnosed exocrine pancreatic insufficiency, or colonic
   or systemic disease

N.B. detection of abnormalities depends on size and quality of biopsy, quality of processing, and expertise of pathologist.

common histopathological descriptions such as lymphocytic enteritis give no clue as to the underlying aetiology (Batt & Hall 1989). Furthermore, in approximately half of patients with chronic small intestine disease, intestinal biopsies will be histologically normal (Loth *et al.* 1990; Van der Gaag & Happé 1990). Conditions where biopsies may be relatively normal are listed in Table 50.9.

Biopsy specimens may be obtained without surgery by endoscopy or peroral suction biopsy using a single (Crosby capsule) or multiple shot (Quinton) instrument (Batt 1979; Hall 1994a). An exploratory laparotomy is an acceptable alternative diagnostic procedure provided biopsies are always taken even when the gut appears grossly normal. The relative merits of the three methods are listed in Table 50.10.

Empirical Treatment

An empirical dietary trial may be worth while when practical or financial constraints preclude a definitive diagnosis in chronic diarrhoea, or where attempts at a diagnosis have failed. However, empirical use of drugs can never be wholeheartedly recommended as signs may be masked and definitive treatment delayed, and the unjustified use of immunosuppressive drugs is potentially dangerous.

ACUTE DIARRHOEA

By definition, acute diarrhoea is sudden in onset. It is often associated with acute vomiting and may be part of a generalised gastro-entero-colitis. Non-fatal, self-limiting acute diarrhoea is common and often resolves before a definitive diagnosis can be made (e.g. dietary indiscretion). Acute diarrhoea can also be secondary to extraintestinal and systemic disease (e.g. distemper, liver disease), and occasionally is a severe, potentially, life-threatening problem (e.g. hypoadrenocorticism, parvovirus, haemorrhagic gastroenteritis, intussusception). Therefore, on presentation a number of decisions must be made:

Table 50.10 Relative merits of three methods of intestinal biopsy.

Method	Advantages	Disadvantages
Endoscopy	Minimally invasive Visualise and biopsy focal lesions Multiple biopsies Minimal adverse reactions Can start steroids early	Requires general anaesthetic Only duodenum (distal ileum) accessible Small, superficial (and crushed) biopsies Expensive equipment Technically demanding
Suction	Minimally invasive Sedation only Reach proximal jejunum Larger biopsies Multiple biopsies (Quinton) Can start steroids early	Requires fluoroscopy Blind biopsy Suction artefacts Single biopsies (Crosby capsule) Biopsies only reach muscularis Equipment no longer manufactured
Laparotomy	Biopsy multiple sites Large full thickness biopsies Inspect other organs Potential for corrective surgery	Requires general anaesthetic Surgical risk Convalescence Delay before starting steroids

- Is intensive emergency treatment needed (fluid–electrolyte, acid–base balance)?
- Is the patient systemically unwell?
- Is there an underlying non-enteric cause of diarrhoea?
- Is an infectious cause likely?
- Is hospitalisation needed?
- Is surgery indicated?
- Is non-specific/symptomatic anti-diarrhoeal treatment sufficient?

An approach to diagnosis is depicted in Fig. 50.4 and the differential diagnosis for acute diarrhoea is shown in Table 50.11. Specific treatments are available for some of these causes of acute diarrhoea (e.g. antibacterials, antiprotozoals, surgery etc.). Most cases, however, respond to symptomatic treatment as detailed in Box 50.1.

CHRONIC DIARRHOEA

Chronic diarrhoea may start either as an acute episode that fails to respond to treatment, or more insidiously.

Diarrhoea may be constant, or intermittent; SIBO and IBD sometimes show waxing and waning. If significant malabsorption exists, weight loss and failure to thrive may occur, although other differential diagnoses must be considered (Table 50.12). Rarely, significant malabsorption occurs without overt diarrhoea. Malabsorption often results in increased appetite, often associated with coprophagy and other forms of pica. However, severe inflammatory bowel disease and neoplasia are usually characterised by decreased appetite. The differential diagnosis for chronic diarrhoea is listed in Table 50.13. Severe small intestine disease may result in PLE (see page 507).

The techniques for investigation of chronic diarrhoea are described earlier, and an approach is depicted in Fig. 50.5.

Features of specific diseases are noted below.

Parasitism

- Helminths (treatment – see Tables 50.14 and 50.15)
- Nematodes
  - Roundworms (*Toxocara canis*, *T. cati*, *Toxascaris leonina*, *Strongyloides stercoralis*) generally problem of young dogs causing ill thrift, pot belly, vomiting and diarrhoea.

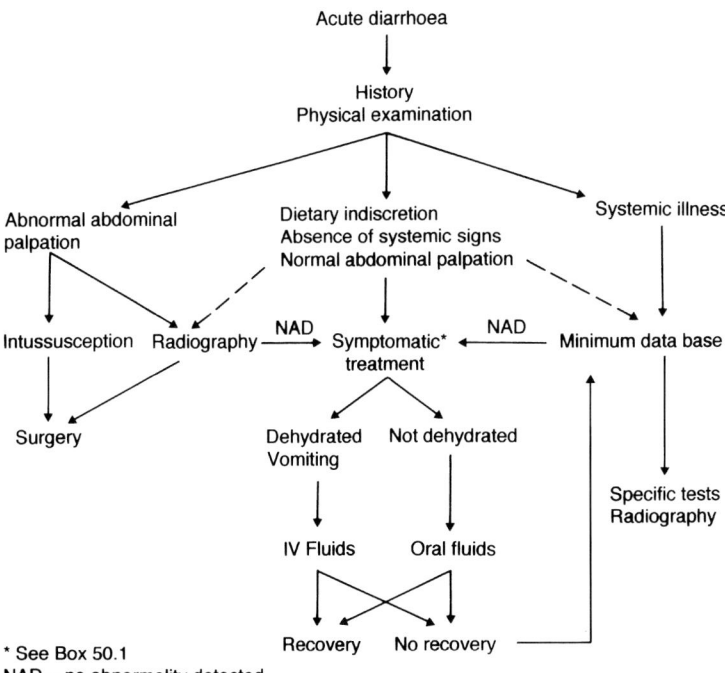

Fig. 50.4 Approach to a case of acute diarrhoea. History and physical examination will usually indicate whether a dog has a systemic illness, and any abnormal findings on abdominal palpation can be confirmed by radiography if necessary before exploratory laparotomy. Most other cases are treated symptomatically, unless radiographs and a minimum database are desired as a precaution. Correction of fluid and electrolyte status is initially the most important consideration. However, if symptomatic therapy fails, a re-evaluation of the patient and more specific tests are indicated.

Box 50.1 Symptomatic management of acute diarrhoea.

Fluid and electrolytes
- Assess dehydration and electrolyte status.
- Calculate fluid deficit and maintenance requirement, including continuing gastrointestinal losses.
- i.v. Hartmann's solution (lactated Ringer's) most useful, but extra K^+ probably required.

Serum potassium (mmol/l)	Amount to be added to 250 ml 0.9% NaCl (not > 0.5 mmol/kg/per hour) (mmol)
<2	20
2–2.5	15
2.5–3	10
3–3.5	7

- Oral rehydration fluids if animal is drinking and not vomiting.

Prevent access to toxins and withdraw any drugs

Dietary manipulation
- Withhold food for 12–36 h depending on severity and age of patient.
- 'Feeding through diarrhoea' is beneficial in human infants, but has little advantage for dogs because of frequent concurrent vomiting and increased faecal volume.
- Gradually introduce a bland easily digestible food in small frequent meals (see Box 50.3).

Oral protectants and absorbents
- Efficacy unproven; cannot physically coat whole mucosal surface, but probably bind toxins and excess water.
- Bismuth has antibacterial and anti-secretory effects.
- Often in combination products with antibiotics:
  - ☐ kaolin (Kaopectate), kaolin–pectin (Kaogel) 1–2 ml/kg q.i.d.
  - ☐ bismuth compounds:
    - tripotassium dicitratobismuthate (De-Nol) 10–30 ml q.i.d.
    - bismuth subsalicylate (Pepto-Bismol) 2 ml per 10 kg q.i.d.
    - combination products, e.g.
      - BCK = bismuth subnitrate/calcium phosphate/charcoal/kaolin
      - Carsub = bismuth subnitrate/charcoal/kaolin
      - Forgastrin = bismuth subnitrate/charcoal
  - ☐ activated charcoal 0.3–5.0 g t.i.d.
  - ☐ magnesium trisilicate 10–30 ml t.i.d.

Motility modifiers (see Fig. 50.2)
- Should never be used for >3 days without re-evaluating patient.
- Opiates act by decreasing peristalsis but increased segmentation delaying transit, and by decreasing secretion.
  - ☐ diphenoxylate (Lomotil) 0.05–0.1 mg/kg t.i.d.-q.i.d. p.o.
  - ☐ loperamide (Imodium) 2 mg/25 kg t.i.d. p.o.
  - ☐ kaolin–morphine may be a useful combination product for mild cases
- Anticholinergics/antispasmodics less effective as they decrease resistance to flow.
  - ☐ atropine 0.02–0.04 mg/kg s.c. t.i.d.
  - ☐ hyoscine/dipyrone (Buscopan) 1–2.5 ml i.v., i.m.
  - ☐ propantheline romide (Pro-Banthine) 0.25 mg/kg p.o. every 8–12 h

Antibiotics – see Box 50.2
- Not routinely in diarrhoea. Appropriate if:
  - ☐ acute haemorrhagic diarrhoea
  - ☐ culture of known pathogen
  - ☐ evidence of sepsis
  - ☐ profound neutropenia ($<3 \times 10^9/l$)
- Present in combination products.
  - ☐ Kaobiotic = neomycin/kaolin

Probiotics
- live yoghurt or *Lactobacillus* preparations may aid recolonisation of small intestine.
- unproven efficacy

All Proprietary drug names are trademarks.

Table 50.11   Differential diagnosis of acute diarrhoea.

Type	Cause	Frequency	Comments
Dietary	Sudden change Incorrect diet Scavenging Gluttony	Probably common	
	Inadequate fibre	Hospitalisation problem	Hospitalised dogs fed low-fibre 'intestinal diets' may develop diarrhoea through proliferation of toxin-producing *Clostridia* (Burrows *et al.* 1995)
	Food allergy or intolerance	Uncommon?	Frequently suspected but rarely proven (see page 502)
	Brush border enzyme deficiency	Not yet proven	
Viral	Canine parvovirus	Common	Major cause of haemorrhagic gastroenteritis. Preferentially targets rapidly dividing cells, i.e. crypts and granulocytes; potentially fatal through dehydration/shock and leukopenia
	Canine distemper virus	Common if unvaccinated	
	Infectious canine hepatitis	Uncommon	
	Coronavirus	Probably common	Generally only cause mild diarrhoea – important in kennel situations
	Rotavirus	Unknown	Generally only cause mild diarrhoea – important in kennel situations
Bacterial	*Salmonella*	Uncommon	Can be isolated from asymptomatic dogs, but always a zoonotic risk. Isolation significant if dog has systemic illness or is immunosuppressed; antibiotic treatment may lead to carrier state (Box 50.3)
	Campylobacter	Frequent isolate	Frequent isolate from asymptomatic dogs. May not be a primary pathogen in isolation; erythromycin is antibiotic of choice
	Yersinia	Rare in UK	
	Bacillus piliformis (Tyzzer's disease)	Rare	
	Escherichia coli	Unknown significance	Normal isolate but presence of pathogenic species in dogs uncertain. Enterotoxigenic, enteroadherent, enteropathogenic, enteroaggregative and entero-invasive strains found in other species also likely in dogs (Sancak *et al.* 1995).
Protozoa	*Giardia*	Probably quite common	May cause acute enterocolitis. Can persist as cause of chronic diarrhoea; metronidazole-resistant isolates reported
	Coccidia	Problem in puppies	
Metabolic	Hypoadrenocorticism	Seen in younger dogs	
Toxicities	Numerous toxins	Probably common	
Others	Haemorrhagic gastroenteritis	Quite common in certain breeds	Thought to be a clostridial enterotoxaemia. Characterised by vascular collapse and marked increase in PCV (often >0.70); responds to shock doses of crystalloid fluids ± albumin, and antibiotics; tendency to recur
	Intussusception	Quite common in young dogs	Life-threatening condition that must be ruled out in any dog with haemorrhagic diarrhoea

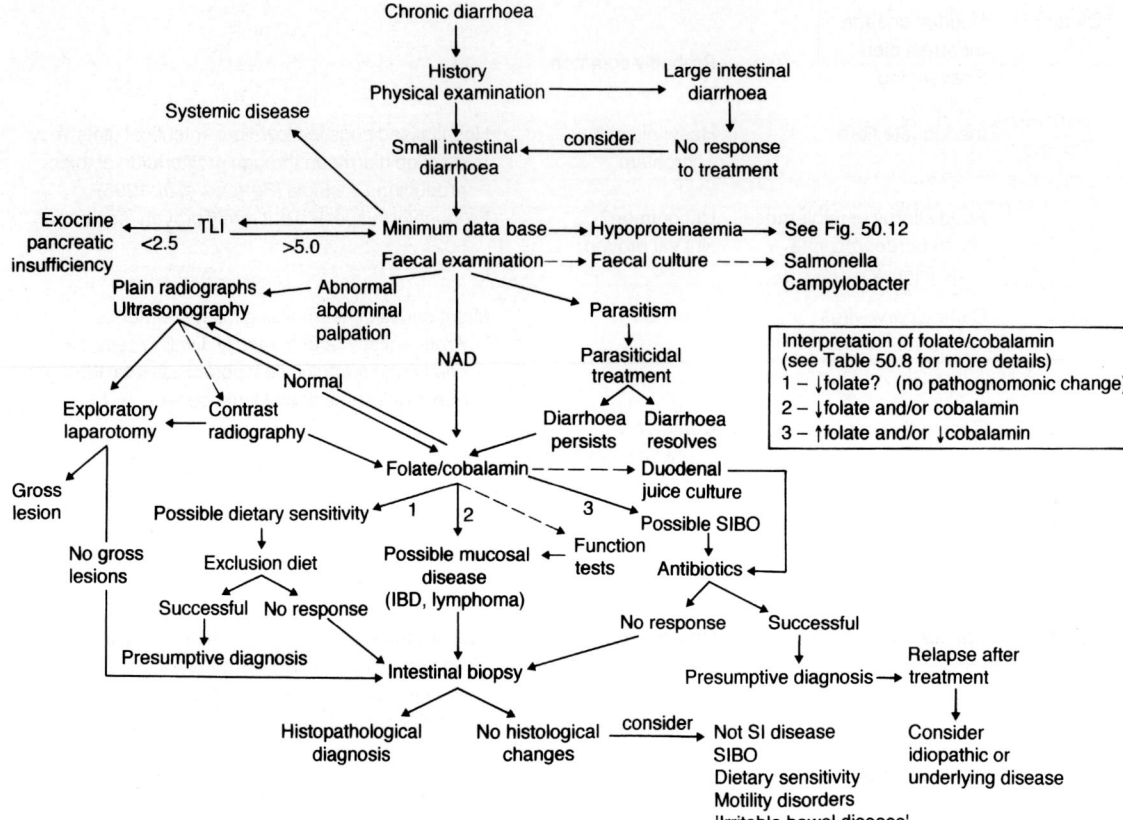

Fig. 50.5 Approach to a case of chronic diarrhoea.
History and physical examination will usually identify a
small intestinal problem, but failure of specific therapy for
an apparent large intestinal problem should also make the
clinician consider small intestine disease. A minimum
database may provide evidence of systemic disease
(leading the investigation away from the small intestine) or
a protein-losing enteropathy (see Fig. 50.12). Faecal
examination and culture will identify gastrointestinal
parasites and pathogenic bacteria, but they may not
necessarily be the only cause of the problem. If abdominal
palpation is abnormal, plain radiographs and ultrasound
are indicated. Contrast radiography is rarely helpful,
especially in cases of diffuse mucosal disease, and

exploratory laparotomy with mandatory biopsy is usually
preferred. Trypsin-like immunoreactivity (TLI) should
probably be measured in all cases where there are no
abnormalities on abdominal palpation, as the signs of
exocrine pancreatic insufficiency (EPI) are not always
typical and serum folate/cobalamin concentrations are
altered. Serum folate and cobalamin concentrations may
give clues as to the most likely diagnosis, although
intestinal biopsy will provide more definitive evidence.
However, in a number of cases there will be no histological
diagnosis and, if folate/cobalamin concentrations are
suggestive and the nature of the case permits, empirical
trials of antibiotics and exclusion diets at this stage are an
acceptable pragmatic approach.

o *Trichuris vulpis* whipworms generally cause enterocolitis (see Chapter 51, page 512).
o *Uncinaria stenocephala* is hookworm in UK.
   Interdigital lesions may be noted.
o *Ancylostoma caninum* hookworms are significant

cause of small intestine disease, anaemia and even
death in USA and tropics.
o Controversial association of visceral larva migrans
   with eosinophilic enteritis (Hayden & Van
   Kruiningen 1973).

Table 50.12 Differential diagnosis of weight loss/failure to thrive.

Young dog

   Inadequate/inappropriate diet*

   Parasitism*

   Small intestinal bacterial overgrowth (SIBO)*

   Exocrine pancreatic insufficiency

   Dietary sensitivity

   Undiagnosed intussusception

   Congenital cardiovascular anomaly including vascular
     ring

   Congenital portosystemic shunt

   Juvenile liver fibrosis

   Juvenile renal disease

   Endocrinopathy (hypoadrenocorticism, diabetes
     mellitus, dwarfism)

Adult dog

   Inflammatory bowel disease ± secondary SIBO*

   Dietary sensitivity ± secondary SIBO*

   Giardia

   Exocrine pancreatic insufficiency

   Hypoadrenocorticism (<6 years)

   Chronic hepatitis

   Renal disease

   Neoplasia

* Most common small intestine diseases diagnosed.

- Cestodes
  - Tapeworms rarely cause small intestine disease.
  - Zoonotic potential of *Dipylidium caninum* and *Echinococcus granulosus*.
  - Involvement of flea cycle for *Dipylidium*.
- Protozoa
  - *Giardia lamblia* probably under-diagnosed as cause of chronic diarrhoea (Fig. 50.6).
  - May be associated with immunosuppression and SIBO.
  - Intermittent excretion of trophozoites and oocysts make diagnosis difficult.
  - Empirical treatment with metronidazole may suggest diagnosis, but resistant strains exist.
- Coccidia
  - Treatment – see Table 40.15.
  - *Isospora* treated with sulphonamides.
  - Cryptosporidia are small coccidia-like organisms.
  - Questionable efficacy of paromomycin, but usually self-limiting; potential zoonotic risk.
- Toxoplasma
  - See Chapter 26.

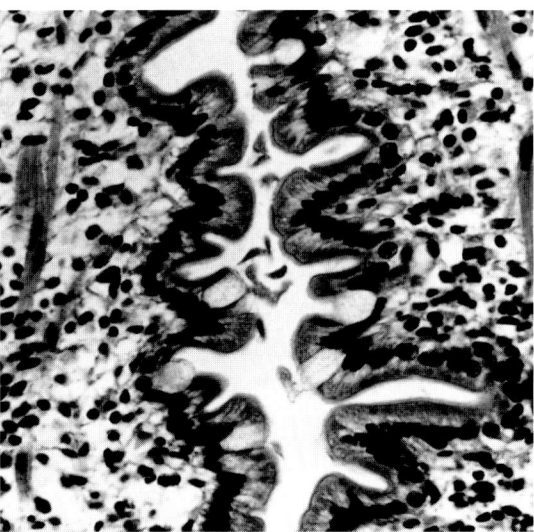

Fig. 50.6 Photomicrograph demonstrating numerous *Giardia* trophozoites (crescent-shaped in section) on the surface of two adjacent villi. (Haematoxylin and eosin.)

Small Intestinal Bacterial Overgrowth

Small intestinal bacterial overgrowth (SIBO) has been defined as $>10^4$ anaerobic bacterial or $>10^5$ total bacterial colony-forming units per millilitre of duodenal juice during fasting, and in some dogs is associated with clinical signs that are antibiotic responsive (Batt *et al.* 1983b, 1988). However, equally high numbers of bacteria may be found in dogs with no clinical signs (Batt *et al.* 1992; Willard *et al.* 1994; Simpson 1996), although the differences in methodology and patient IgA status may explain reported contradictory findings. It is crucial to consider SIBO as a sign rather than a specific disease, except perhaps in young dogs (especially German Shepherd Dogs) where a primary cause cannot be found and response to antibiotics is good. The presence of SIBO (antibiotic-responsive diarrhoea that relapses when antibiotics finish) appearing in an adult should prompt search for underlying cause; may be secondary to IBD, dietary sensitivity, partial obstruction (tumour, intussusception, foreign body) or EPI (Williams *et al.* 1987). Idiopathic, antibiotic-responsive, SIBO may be related to decreased secretory IgA in small intestine, or abnormal motility (Batt *et al.* 1991) and is associated with minimal histological changes (Batt *et al.* 1983b, 1988) or occasional inflammatory infiltrate (Rutgers *et al.* 1988).

SIBO causes chronic diarrhoea, polyphagia, coprophagy and stunting and weight loss and definitive diagnosis is made by culture of $>10^5$ aerobes or 10^4 anaerobes per mil-

Table 50.13 Differential diagnosis of chronic diarrhoea of primary small intestine origin.

Parasitism	Giardia*
	Ascarids and hookworms
Small intestinal bacterial overgrowth	Idiopathic*
	Secondary (exocrine pancreatic insufficiency, inflammatory bowel disease, dietary sensitivity, partial obstruction)
Dietary sensitivity	Food allergy
	Food intolerance
Inflammatory bowel disease	Lymphocytic – plasmacytic enteritis*
	Eosinophilic enteritis
	Granulomatous enteritis
Lymphangiectasia	
Neoplasia	Lymphosarcoma
	Adenocarcinoma
Fungal, algae and rickettsial gastroenteritis†	Candidiasis (secondary to antibacterials)
	Histoplasmosis
	Aspergillosis
	Mucormycosis
	Prototothecosis
	Salmon poisoning (*Neorickettsia helminthoeca*)

* Most common diagnoses.
† Rarely or never reported in UK.

litre duodenal juice; mixed flora containing coliforms is usually found. Examination of breath hydrogen is likely to be abnormal. The use of folate and cobalamin may aid diagnosis (Table 50.8) although its value is disputed (Simpson 1996). The sensitivity and specificity in dogs with chronic diarrhoea has been reported (Rutgers *et al.* 1996):

	Sensitivity (%)	Specificity (%)
↑folate	51	79
↓cobalamin	24	87
↑ folate & ↓ cobalamin	5	100

Once a diagnosis is made, treatment with a broad-spectrum antibiotic is started and may control signs but relapse is common. The initial choice is oxytetracycline 10 mg/kg p.o. t.i.d. for 4–6 weeks but metronidazole, tylosin and amoxycillin are suggested alternatives (Box 50.2). Diet should be modified to a low-fat, easily digested diet and in some mild cases this alone may control signs (Box 50.3). The great variability that is seen means that continued low-dose antibiotics may be necessary for control in some cases. Long-standing, untreated SIBO may result in severe villus atrophy resembling tropical sprue in man (Batt *et al.* 1983a).

Dietary Sensitivity (Hall 1994b)

It is well recognised that there is a group of intestinal and cutaneous diseases which respond to dietary modification. These diseases may reflect a diagnosis of a true dietary allergy, a food intolerance or an alteration in digestibility and fat content. There is a perception that many such diseases are truly immunological but there are many non-immunological mechanisms that operate. These include contamination by chemicals (preservatives), microbes and/or toxins, idiosyncratic responses due to enzyme deficiencies (e.g. hypolactasia), pharmacological effect (e.g. caffeine, tyramine), direct histamine release (e.g. strawberries, shellfish) and fermentation of unabsorbed solute (e.g. sorbitol).

True allergy is rarely identified as there are no clear diagnostic criteria or characteristic histological changes (Fig. 50.7). Gluten-sensitive enteropathy has been clearly identified in Irish setters, but any allergic nature has not been proved (Hall & Batt 1992). There are anecdotal reports of sensitivities to beef, pork, dairy products, soya, eggs etc. (Strombeck & Guilford 1991). It would appear that cutaneous signs are probably more common than intestinal signs, although intestinal permeability may detect

Table 50.14 Anthelminthics for canine intestinal parasites.

Generic drug	Spectrum	Trade name	Dosage (mg/kg per day)	Remarks
Febantel	Roundworms Hookworms Whipworm (Cestodes)	Drontal Plus	15	Can be given with food, combined with praziquantel and pyrantel
Fenbendazole	Roundworms Hookworms Whipworms Cestodes	Panacur	50 100	Three daily doses Single dose
Mebendazole	Roundworms Hookworms Whipworms Cestodes	Telmin KH	22	2 days for ascarids; 5 days for all worm species; hepatotoxicity?
Niclosamide	Cestodes	Yomesan	125	Fasting required
Nitroscanate	Roundworms Hookworms Cestodes	Lopatol	50	Tablet given whole with small amount of food
Oxfendazole	Roundworms Hookworms Whipworms Cestodes	Bandit	10	3 daily doses
Piperazine	Roundworms Hookworms	Various	100 200	Intestinal hypomotility Safe but not very effective
Praziquantel	Cestodes	Droncit (Drontal Plus)	5	Oral or injectable; good efficacy
Pyrantel	Roundworms	Strongid	5	Repeat for hookworms

All proprietary drug names are trademarks.

Table 50.15 Drugs used for the treatment of *Giardia*.

Generic drug	Trade name	Dosage (mg/kg per day)	Remarks
Metronidazole	Torgyl	50	Divided b.i.d. for 5 days, neurotoxicity at high dose
Furazolidone	Neftin*	8	Divided b.i.d. for 5 days, teratogenic
Fenbendazole	Panacur	20	For 5 days
		50	For 3 days
Albendazole	Valbazen*	50	Divided b.i.d. for 5 days
Ipronidazole	Ipropran*	126 mg/l	Added to drinking water
Tinidazole*		44	s.i.d. for 3 days, experimental
Quinacrine*		6.6	p.o. for 5 days GI side-effects common, teratogenic. Availability?

Barr *et al.* 1994
All proprietary drug names are trademarks.
* Not licensed for dogs in UK.

Box 50.2   Antibiotics used in small intestine disease (see page 62 for dosages).

Antibiotics should not be used routinely for non-specific small intestine disease because of adverse effects:

- selection of resistant strains and overgrowth of fungi and resistant organisms,
- diarrhoea caused by neomycin and ampicillin (pseudomembranous colitis),
- *Salmonella* carrier state,
- systemic toxicities, e.g. gentamicin.

Indications for use:

- systemic infection,
- specific bacterial infection,
- severe mucosal damage (i.e. ulceration and haemorrhage),
- neutropenia ($<3 \times 10^9$/l),
- small intestine bacterial overgrowth (SIBO).

Neomycin and some sulphonamides (e.g. sulphaguanidine) may be preferred because they are not absorbed from the intestine but their spectrum is often not ideal.

Campylobacter	erythromycin, enrofloxacin, tylosin, tetracyclines
Clostridium	ampicillin, cephalosporin, chloramphenicol, clindamycin, metronidazole
Salmonella	chloramphenicol, trimethoprim–sulphas, amoxycillin, enrofloxacin
Yersinia	tetracycline, streptomycin, kanamycin
Gastrointestinal aerobes	ampicillin, amoxycillin, cephalosporins, streptomycin, kanamycin, gentamicin, chloramphenicol
Gastrointestinal anaerobes	ampicillin, cephalosporins, chloramphenicol, clindamycin, lincomycin, metronidazole
Idiopathic SIBO	oxytetracycline, metronidazole, amoxycillin, tylosin

---

subclinical mucosal damage (Rutgers *et al.* 1995). Classical intradermal skin testing and radioaller gosorbent (RAST) IgE testing are of no clear value. The use of gastroscopic topical antigen testing is technically demanding and only identifies type 1 hypersensitivities (Elwood *et al.* 1994; Guilford *et al.* 1994a) and it is unclear if the results truly reflect a specific allergy. Definitive proof is by response to an exclusion diet and relapse on re-challenge (see Box 50.3). Once a diagnosis has been confirmed the disease can be managed by choosing a diet not containing offending antigen or agent. Rarely a dog will not eat the chosen diet and antihistamines and steroids can be used, but the success rate varies.

Inflammatory Bowel Disease (IBD)

This is characterised by a lymphocytic–plasmacytic, eosinophilic and granulomatous enteritis, which form the basis of a histological diagnosis (Fig. 50.8 and 50.9) related to the predominant cell type observed (Dibartola *et al.* 1982; Quigley & Henry 1983; Ochoa *et al.* 1984; Van der Gaag & Happé 1990; Jergens *et al.* 1992). It is presumed

that an immune response to luminal dietary, bacterial or self antigen produces mucosal damage, i.e. villus atrophy and inflammatory infiltrate with secondary release of inflammatory mediators (Batt & Hall 1989). There can be an increased leukocyte count and in some cases of eosinophilic gastroenteritis an eosinophilia may be seen. Laboratory tests are unremarkable but a decreased folate and cobalamin may be seen. Confirmation of diagnosis is by biopsy and the dominant infiltrate can be identified. There are varied inflammatory cells along with degrees of villus atrophy, villus fusion, necrosis and crypt abscessation. The treatment of inflammatory bowel disease is given in Box 50.4.

Lymphangiectasia

This is a rare disease of unknown aetiology (Suter *et al.* 1985; Flesjå & Yri 1977) where a dilatation of intestinal lymphatics causes leakage of lipoproteins and lymphocytes. The clinical signs are of a severe weight loss and diarrhoea which may lead to a protein losing enteropathy. Lymphopenia and hypoproteinaemia are characteristic (but diagnosis by intestinal biopsy is essential). The usual findings

Box 50.3 Dietary management of small intestine disease.

Dietary modification may either be a primary treatment in dietary sensitivities or a supportive measure in small intestine diseases such as SIBO, IBD, and lymphangiectasia (Hall 1996).

Characteristics of an 'ideal' intestinal diet:
- highly digestible
- not markedly hypertonic
- moderately low in fat (<15% DM) ± enriched in ω-3 unsaturated fatty acids for anti-inflammatory effect
- lactose-free in case of lactose intolerance
- derived from a single protein source ('hypoallergenic')
- moderately fermentable fibre (e.g. ispaghula, beet pulp)
- generous quantities of water and fat-soluble vitamins, and essential minerals
- good palatability
- nutritionally balanced.

Intestinal diets
e.g. Commercially prepared diets fulfil most of the above criteria, but home-cooked boiled chicken and rice or cottage cheese and rice are cheaper temporary alternatives.

Exclusion/elimination diets are used to diagnose dietary sensitivity and are chosen based on the dietary history of the patient:

- single protein source: e.g. chicken, fish, egg, cottage cheese, tofu, venison etc. Plus single carbohydrate source: rice, potato, tapioca
- feed for up to 3 weeks as sole food (up to 10 weeks for food allergic skin disease?)
- challenge with original diet to confirm sensitivity
- rescue with exclusion diet
- challenge with single proteins until relapse (up to 2 weeks) to determine sensitivity
- devise diet from commercial pet food avoiding identified sensitivities.

Additives
- Medium chain triglyceride oil.
  1–2 ml/kg introduced gradually, as initial tolerance is sometimes poor.
- Vitamin/mineral supplements. Use paediatric supplements in exclusion diet as they do not contain meat extracts.

Box 50.4 Management of inflammatory bowel disease.

Initial treatment

- Restricted antigen ('hypoallergenic') exclusion diet (see Box 50.3)
- Immunosuppressive drugs (see Box 50.5)
- ± antibiotics

Follow-up

- Withdraw drug therapy and attempt to maintain on diet
- Devise suitable maintenance diet based on results of exclusion
- repeat pharmacological intervention if relapse

include a normal villus height, but dilated lymphatics in all layers of small intestine. Dilated lacteals may be seen in IBD, but submucosal lymphatics are normal. The treatment is based upon a severely fat restricted fat-free diet but there is a requirement to satisfy the essential fatty acids by supplementing medium chain triglyceride oil which is absorbed directly into the portal blood. Anti-inflammatory drugs (prednisolone 0.5 mg/kg daily) are of unknown value. Overall the prognosis is very poor.

Neoplasia

There are two major forms of neoplasia in the small intestine epithelial (adenoma and adenocarcinoma) and lym-

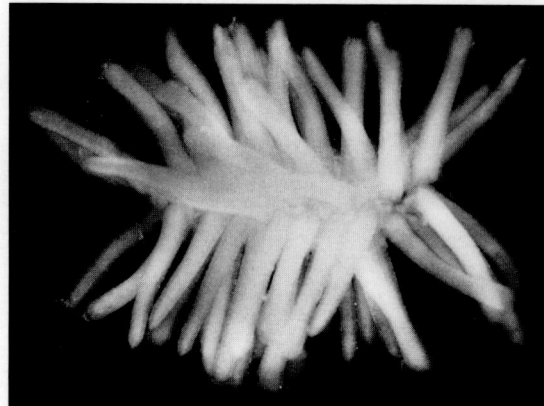

a

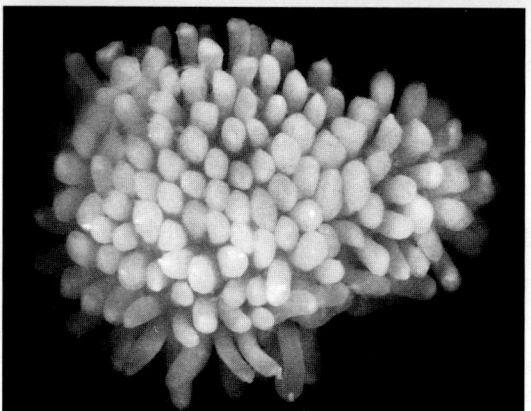

b

Fig. 50.7   Dissecting microscopic appearance of jejunal suction biopsy specimens from (a) a normal dog, showing long slender villi with fluffy appearance of surface glycocalyx and mucus, and (b) an Irish Setter with gluten-sensitive enteropathy showing partial villus atrophy.

phosarcoma. Other tumours such as smooth muscle tumours do occur either in the benign or malignant form.

Adenocarcinomas cause diarrhoea through mucosal infiltration, lymphatic obstruction, partial obstruction and secondary SIBO (Fig. 50.10). The clinical signs are variable but include vomiting, inappetence and weight loss; in some cases there is gastrointestinal perforation and the dogs present as an acute abdomen. Diagnosis is by palpation, imaging and often at laparotomy. Metastatic spread is via lymphatics locally and to mesenteric nodes. The treatment of these conditions is via resection of the affected portion of the small intestine. The site of the tumour dictates the extent and the involvement of the resection but single isolated adenomas or adenocarcinomas can successfully be treated.

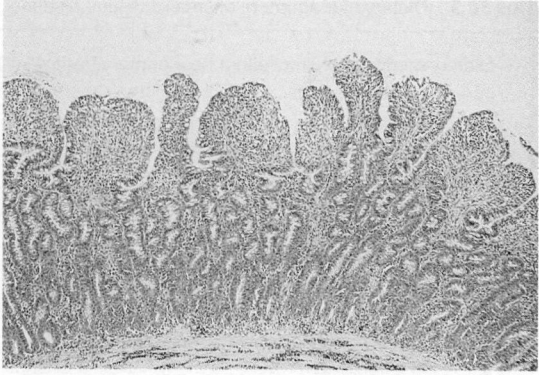

Fig. 50.8   Histological appearance of jejunal biopsy from a dog with lymphocytic–plasmacytic enteritis. Stunted, distorted villi are infiltrated with lymphocytes and plasma cells. (Haematoxylin and eosin.)

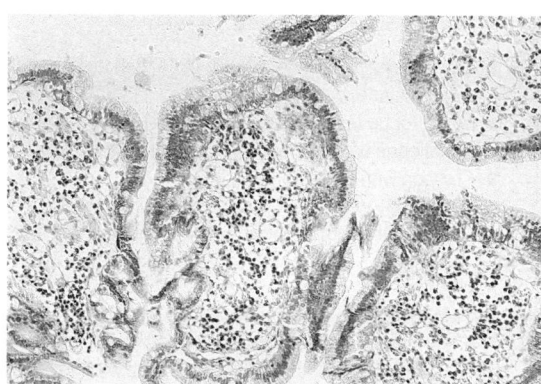

Fig. 50.9   Histological appearance of jejunal biopsy from a dog with eosinophilic enteritis. Partial villus atrophy and infiltration of the lamina propria with darkly staining eosinophils are seen, but unusually other inflammatory cells are sparse. (Toluidine blue.)

Lymphosarcoma (Fig. 50.11)

There are two forms of lymphoma that affect the small intestine, diffuse or solid. The former is characterised by a diffuse infiltration of mucosa by malignant lymphocytes, usually extending between submucosal layers, and sometimes involving Peyer's patches and mesenteric nodes. The mucosal surface may be ulcerated, and cause protein-losing enteropathy and/or melaena. There is usually inappetence, persistent diarrhoea and severe weight loss. Diagnosis is by biopsy, although it is sometimes difficult to differentiate

Box 50.5   Immunosuppressive drugs used in small intestine disease.

Corticosteroids

- Indications
  - □ inflammatory bowel disease – lymphocytic/plasmacytic and eosinophilic enteritis,
  - □ possibly in dietary sensitivity and lymphangiectasia,
  - □ often used in conjunction with hypoallergenic diet and antibiotic cover.
- Prednisolone
  - □ 2–4 mg/kg per day p.o. divided b.i.d. then gradual reduction to minimum dose necessary suggested protocol (modified from Strombeck & Guilford 1991):
  - □ 1–2 mg/kg every 12 h p.o. for 1–2 weeks until response (maximum 4 weeks)
    followed by 1–2 mg/kg every 24 h p.o. for 1–2 weeks
    followed by 0.5–1.0 mg/kg every 24 h p.o. for 4 weeks
    followed by 0.5–1.0 mg/kg every 48 h p.o. for 4 weeks
    followed by tapering withdrawal over 2 weeks
  - □ beneficial effect on brush border enzyme activities as well as anti-inflammatory/immunosuppressive action
  - □ potential for gastrointestinal bleeding
  - □ increased appetite often helpful although patient is in catabolic state.
- Dexamethasone or betamethasone less effective or even deleterious.

Azathioprine (Imuran)

- Initial loading dose, then reducing dose and frequency when response occurs e.g. 2 mg/kg per day p.o. for 5 days, then every other day
- Potent immunosuppressive that can permit 50% reduction in steroid dose (alternate day therapy)
- Monitor haematology for bone marrow suppression

Metronidazole

- 10 mg/kg p.o. t.i.d., reducing to b.i.d. or s.i.d.
- Reputed inhibition of cell-mediated immunity as well as antibacterial

---

lymphoma from inflammatory bowel disease with lymphocytic plasmacytic infiltrates. In the diffuse form the response to chemotherapy protocols is generally poor. In the few cases where there is an isolated single lymphoma mass resection before chemotherapy can meet with better success.

Protein-Losing Enteropathies

If small intestine mucosal disease is so severe that protein leakage into the gut lumen exceeds the protein synthetic abilities of the dog, hypoproteinaemia develops. Prolonged starvation is unlikely to produce clinically significant hypoproteinaemia. Typically in protein-losing enteropathy both albumin and globulin are lost, aiding differentiation from hepatic and renal causes of hypoproteinaemia (Fig.

50.12). Redistribution of body fluid will ultimately lead to ascites and oedema when albumin falls below 10–15 g/l.

Protein losing enteropathy is associated with a number of small intestine diseases:

- inflammatory bowel disease (lymphocytic–plasmacytic and eosinophilic enteritis),
- lymphangiectasia,
- lymphosarcoma.

Diagnosis by intestinal biopsy after ruling out hepatic and renal disease (Fig. 50.12). Hypoproteinaemia increases the risk of anaesthesia and wound dehiscence after surgery, and so peroral biopsy is preferred. Plasma transfusions may provide temporary relief during the peri-operative period, and diuretics may reduce ascites. Spironolactone (1–2 mg/kg b.i.d. p.o.) is preferred over frusemide (0.125–

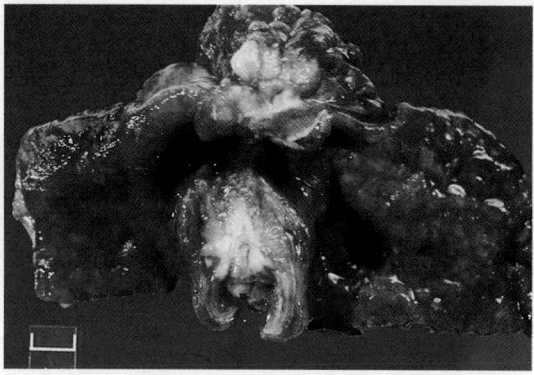

Fig. 50.10   Section through an annular adenocarcinoma arising in the proximal jejunum, demonstrating narrowing of the lumen and ulceration. This dog presented with chronic diarrhoea and microcytic anaemia, presumably secondary to partial obstruction and chronic low-grade bleeding. Bacterial overgrowth (1.2×10^8 organisms/ml) was documented in duodenal juice.

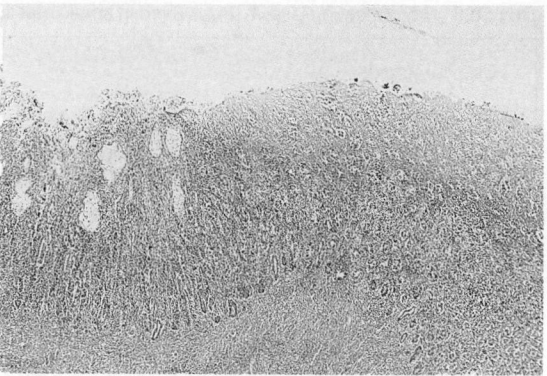

Fig. 50.11   Histological appearance of intestinal lymphosarcoma. Normal mucosal architecture has been destroyed by malignant lymphocyte infiltration, and the luminal surface is ulcerated. (Haematoxylin and eosin.)

Table 50.16   Differential diagnosis of melaena.

Generalised bleeding disorder
- thrombocytopenia
- clotting factor defect

Swallowed blood
- epistaxis
- oral bleeding
- haemoptysis

Oesophageal disease
- ulceration
- neoplasia

Pancreas
- acute pancreatitis

Liver
- neoplasia
- liver failure

Gastric disease
- widespread erosions or ulcers
  - NSAIDs, corticosteroids, uraemia, mastocytoma, liver failure, gastrinoma
- severe gastritis
- sharp foreign bodies
- neoplasia

Small intestine
- haemorrhagic (gastro)enteritis
- duodenal ulcers
  - NSAIDs, corticosteroids, mastocytoma, uraemia, liver failure, gastrinoma
- severe ulcerated inflammatory bowel disease (IBD)
- foreign bodies
- hookworms
- neoplasia
  - mast cell tumour
  - lymphosarcoma
  - adenocarcinoma
  - leiomyoma, leiomyosarcoma
- vascular
  - laceration
  - varices, aneurysm, arteriovenous (AV) fistula
  - polyarteritis
- ischaemia
  - hypovolaemic shock (Addison's)
  - intussusception
  - thrombosis/infarction
  - volvulus
  - mesenteric avulsion

0.25 mg/kg b.i.d. p.o.) as it is potassium-sparing. Paracentesis should be reserved for cases where respiratory embarrassment is severe, and only one-third of the fluid should be removed at one time. Ultimately, treatment of the underlying small intestine disease is essential.

MELAENA

The presence of dark, tarry, digested blood in faeces is termed melaena and reflects either swallowed blood, or gastrointestinal bleeding generally arising proximal to the large intestine (see also Chapter 36, page 281). Gastric bleeding is often accompanied by haematemesis. Melaena of small intestine origin may or may not be associated with diarrhoea depending on the cause. The differential diagnosis is listed in Table 50.16.

Melaena should be distinguished from oxidation of faecal pigments following prolonged exposure to air, and dark stool produced after certain medicaments, e.g. bismuth preparations, metronidazole and iron.

The presence of chronic low-grade bleeding, such as from a leiomyoma, that does not produce gross melaena may be suspected by finding a microcytic, iron-deficiency anaemia, and confirmed by testing for faecal occult blood. After ruling out swallowed blood and generalised bleeding, prolonged or profuse melaena should be investigated first by endoscopy and then by laparotomy if no gastric or duodenal lesions are found.

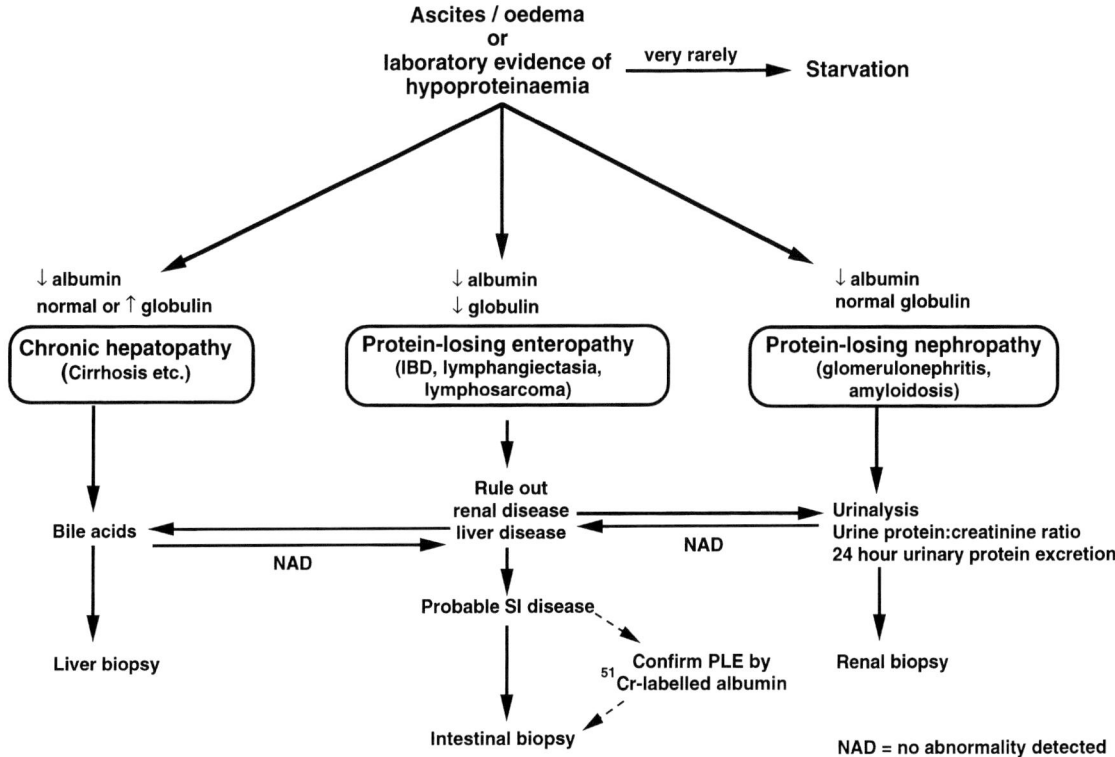

Fig. 50.12   Approach to a protein-losing enteropathy. Even prolonged starvation is a rare cause of hypoproteinaemia in dogs; for example, anaemia is seen in exocrine pancreatic insufficiency (EPI) before serum protein concentrations fall significantly. Hypoproteinaemia is usually a reflection of decreased hepatic protein synthesis or increased renal or intestinal loss, and their effects on albumin and globulin concentrations may give some clues as to the cause. Diarrhoea is common in protein-losing enteropathy (PLE), but its presence does not rule out the other possible causes. Confirmation of a PLE by ^{51}Cr-labelled albumin is not practical, and therefore liver and renal disease must be ruled out before a tentative diagnosis of PLE is made and intestinal biopsy can be justified.

SHORT BOWEL SYNDROME

Seen following extensive intestinal resection and has a
complex pathophysiology, including SIBO, gastric hypersecretion, malabsorption and malnutrition (Williams &
Burrows 1981). Intensive pharmacological treatment and
nutritional support with a low fat, highly digestible diet,
supplemented with medium chain triglyceride oil, elemen-
tal diets and vitamins/minerals are required, although the
prognosis is poor.

REFERENCES AND
FURTHER READING

Anderson, N.V., Sherding, R.G., Merritt, A.M. & Whitlock, R.H.
  (1992). *Veterinary Gastroenterology*, 2nd edn. Lea and Febiger,
  Philadelphia.

Barr, S.C., Boud, D.D. & Heeller, R.I. (1994). Efficiency of fenbendazole against giardiasis in dogs. *Amercian Journal of Veterinary
  Research*, 55, 988.

Batt, R.M. (1984). *Chronic Small Intestinal Disease in the Dog.*
  Proceeding of the 8th Kal Kan Symposium.

Batt, R.M. (1979). Techniques for single and multiple peroral
  jejunal biopsy in the dog. *Journal of Small Animal Practice*, 20,
  259–268.

Batt, R.M. (1992). Diagnosis and management of malabsorption in
  dogs. *Journal of Small Animal Practice*, 33, 161–166.

Batt, R.M. & Hall, E.J. (1989). Chronic enteropathies in the dog.
  Journal of Small Animal Practice, 30, 3–12.

Batt, R.M. & Morgan, J.O. (1982). Role of serum folate and
  vitamin B_{12} concentrations in the differentiation of small
  intestinal abnormalities in the dog. *Research in Veterinary
  Science*, 32, 17–22.

Batt, R.M., Bush, B.M. & Peters, T.J. (1983a). Subcellular biochemical studies of a naturally occurring enteropathy in the dog
  resembling chronic tropical sprue in human beings. *American
  Journal of Veterinary Research*, 44, 1492–1496.

Batt, R.M., Needham, J.R. & Carter, M.W. (1983b). Bacterial overgrowth associated with a naturally occurring enteropathy in the
  German shepherd dog. *Research in Veterinary Science*, 35, 42–46.

Batt, R.M., McLean, L. & Riley, J.E. (1988). Response of the
  jejunal mucosa of dogs with aerobic and anaerobic bacterial
  overgrowth to antibiotic therapy. *Gut*, 29, 473–482.

Batt, R.M., Barnes, A., Rutgers, H.C. & Carter, S.D. (1991).
  Relative IgA deficiency and small intestinal bactrial overgrowth
  in German shepherd dogs. *Research in Veterinary Science*, 50,
  106–111.

Batt, R.M., Hall, E.J., McLean, L., Simpson, K.W. & Morton,
  D.B. (1992). Small intestinal bacterial overgrowth and enhanced

intestinal permeability in clinically healthy Beagle dogs.
  American Journal of Veterinary Research, 53, 1935–1940.

Burrows, C.F., Batt, R.M. & Sherding, R.G. (1995). Diseases of
  the small intestine. In: *Textbook of Veterinary Internal Medicine.
  Diseases of the Dog and Cat*, (eds S.J. Ettinger & E.C. Feldman),
  5th edn. pp. 1169–1232. W.B. Saunders, Philadelphia.

DiBartola, S.P., Rogers, W.A., Boyce, J.T. & Grimm, J.P. (1982).
  Regional enteritis in two dogs. *Journal of the American
  Veterinary Medical Association*, 181, 904–908.

Elwood, C.M., Rutgers, H.C. & Batt, R.M. (1994). Gastroscopic
  food sensitivity testing in 17 dogs. *Journal of Small Animal
  Practice*, 35, 199–203.

Flesjå, K. & Yri, T. (1977). Protein-losing enteropathy in the
  Lundehund. *Journal of Small Animal Practice*, 18, 11–23.

Freeman, W.H. & Bracegirdle, B. (1966). *An Atlas of Histology.*
  Heinemann, Oxford.

Guilford, W.G. (1994a). What's new in gastrointestinal diagnosis?
  Gastroscopic food sensitivity testing and radiopaque markers.
  Proceedings of the 1994 BSAVA Congress, p. 41. BSAVA,
  Cheltenham.

Guilford, W.G. (1994b). New developments in dietary management of intestinal disease. *Journal of Small Animal Practice*, 35,
  620–624.

Guilford, W.G., Strombeck, D.R., Rogers, Q., Frick, O.L. &
  Lawoko, C. (1994). Development of gastroscopic food sensitivity testing in dogs. *Journal of Veterinary Internal Medicine*, 8,
  414–422.

Hall, E.J. (1994a). Small intestinal disease – is endoscopic biopsy
  the answer? *Journal of Small Animal Practice*, 35, 408–414.

Hall, E.J. (1994b). Gastrointestinal aspects of food allergy: a
  review. *Journal of Small Animal Practice*, 35, 145–152.

Hall, E.J. (1996). Gastrointestinal problems (dog and cat) In:
  BSAVA Manual of Small Animal Nutrition and Feeding, (eds
  J.M. Wills & N.C. Kelly), pp. 144–152. BSAVA, Cheltenham.

Hall, E.J. & Batt, R.M. (1990). Enhanced intestinal permeability to
  ^{51}Cr-labeled EDTA in dogs with small intestinal disease.
  Journal of the American Veterinary Medical Association, 196,
  91–95.

Hall, E.J. & Batt, R.M. (1991). Differential sugar absorption for
  the assessment of canine intestinal permeability: the cel-
  lobiose/mannitol test in gluten-sensitive enteropathy of Irish
  setters. *Research in Veterinary Science*, 51, 83–87.

Hall, E.J. & Batt, R.M. (1992). Dietary modulation of gluten sensitivity in a naturally occurring enteropathy of Irish setter dogs.
  Gut, 33, 198–205.

Hall, E.J. & Batt, R.M. (1996). Urinary excretion of intravenously
  administered simple sugars in dogs. *Research in Veterinary
  Science*, 60, 280–282.

Hayden, D.W. & Van Kruiningen, H.J. (1973). Eosinophilic gastroenteritis in German shepherd dogs and its relationship to visceral larva migrans. *Journal of the American Veterinary Medical
  Association*, 162, 379–384.

Jergens, A.E., Moore, F.M., Haynes, J.S. & Miles, K.G. (1992).
  Idiopathic inflammatory bowel disease in dogs and cats: 84

cases (1987–1990). *Journal of the American Veterinary Medical Association*, **201**, 1603–1608.

Jones, B. & Liska, W.D. (eds) (1986). *Canine and Feline Gastroenterology*. W.B. Saunders, Philadelphia.

Loth, L., Leib, M.S., Davenport, D.J. & Monroe, W.E. (1990). Comparisons between endoscopic and histologic evaluation of the gastrointestinal tract in dogs and cats: 75 cases (1984–1987). *Journal of the American Veterinary Medical Association*, **196**, 635–638.

Miller, M.E., Christensen, G.S. & Evans, H.E. (1964). *Anatomy of the Dog*. W.B. Saunders, Philadelphia.

Ochoa, R., Breitschwerdt, E.B. & Lincoln, K.L. (1984). Immunoproliferative small intestinal disease (IPSID) in Basenji dogs: Morphological observations. *American Journal of Veterinary Research*, **45**, 482–490.

Quigley, P.J. & Henry, K. (1983). Eosinophilic enteritis in the dog: a case report with a brief review of the literature. *Journal of Comparative Pathology*, **91**, 387–392.

Quigg, J., Brydon, G., Ferguson, A. & Simpson, J. (1993). Evaluation of canine small intestinal permeability using the lactulose/rhamnose urinary excretion test. *Research in Veterinary Science*, **55**, 326–332.

Rutgers, H.C., Batt, R.M. & Kelly, D.F. (1988). Lymphocytic-plasmacytic enteritis associated with bacterial overgrowth in a dog. *Journal of the American Veterinary Medical Association*, **192**, 1739–1742.

Rutgers, H.C., Batt, R.M., Hall, E.J., Sørensen, S.H. & Proud, F.J. (1995). Intestinal permeability testing in dogs with diet-responsive intestinal disease. *Journal of Small Animal Practice*, **36**, 295–301.

Rutgers, H.C., Batt, R.M., Elwood, C. & Lamport, A. (1996). Bacterial overgrowth in dogs with chronic intestinal disease. *Journal of the American Veterinary Medical Association*, **206**, 187–193.

Sancak, A.A., Rutgers, H.C., Molyneux, K., Hart, C.A. & Batt, R.M. (1995). A potential role for pathogenic *Escherichia coli* in acute and chronic diarrhoea in dogs. *Proceedings of the 1995 BSAVA Congress.*, p. 246. BSAVA, Cheltenham.

Simpson, K.W. (1996). Small intestinal disease. In: *BSAVA Manual of Canine and Feline Gastroenterology*, (eds J.W. Simpson & E.J. Hall), p. 143. BSAVA, Cheltenham.

Simpson, J.W. & Else, R.W. (1991). *Digestion Diseases in the Dog and Cat*. Blackwell Science, Oxford.

Sørensen, S.H., Proud, F.J., Adam, A., Rutgers, H.C. & Batt, R.M. (1994). A novel HPLC method for the simultaneous quantification of monosaccharides and disaccharides used in tests of intestinal permeability and function. *Clinica Chimica Acta*, **221**, 115–125.

Strombeck, D.R. & Guilford, W.G. (1991). *Small Animal Gastroenterology*, 2nd edn. Stonegate Publishing, Davis, California.

Suter, M.M., Palmer, D.G. & Schenk, H. (1985). Primary intestinal lymphangiectasia in three dogs: a morphological and immunopathological investigation. *Veterinary Pathology*, **22**, 123–130.

Van der Gaag, I. & Happé, R.P. (1990). Follow-up studies by peroral small intestinal biopsies and necropsy in dogs with chronic diarrhea. *Journal of Veterinary Medicine A*, **37**, 561–568.

Washabau, R.J., Strombeck, D.R., Buffington, C.A. & Harrold, D. (1986). Use of pulmonary hydrogen gas excretion to detect carbohydrate malabsorption in dogs. *Journal of the American Veterinary Medical Association*, **189**, 674–679.

Willard, M.D., Simpson, R.B., Fossum, T.W., *et al.* (1994). Characterisation of naturally developing small intestinal bacterial overgrowth in 16 German Shepherd Dogs. *Journal of the American Veterinary Medical Association*, **204**, 1201–1206.

Williams, D.A. (1987). New tests for pancreatic and small intestinal function. *Compendium on Continuing Education for the Practicing Veterinarian*, **9**, 1167–1175.

Williams, D.A. & Burrows, C.F. (1981). Short bowel syndrome – a case report in a dog and discussion of the pathophysiology of bowel resection. *Journal of Small Animal Practice*, **22**, 263–268.

Williams, D.A., Batt, R.M. & McLean, L. (1987). Bacterial overgrowth in the duodenum of dogs with exocrine pancreatic insufficiency. *Journal of the American Veterinary Medical Association*, **191**, 201–206.

Chapter 51

The Large Intestine

C. M. Elwood

INTRODUCTION

Signs of large intestinal disease are a common presentation in canine practice. An understanding of the normal and abnormal large intestine, a thorough clinical evaluation and a logical diagnostic approach, combined with technology that is becoming more readily available, means that many of these patients can be diagnosed and managed in general veterinary practice.

THE NORMAL CANINE LARGE INTESTINE

The large intestine is divided into the caecum, colon, rectum and anal canal (Fig. 51.11).

- The *caecum* is a short, spiral, blind-ending tube communicating with the colon at the caecocolic sphincter.
- The *ascending colon* begins at the ileocaecocolic junction in the right dorsal abdominal cavity and travels cranially to the right colic (or hepatic) flexure.
- The *transverse colon* travels from the right colic to the left colic (or splenic) flexure.
- The *descending colon* travels from the left colic flexure to the pelvic inlet where it becomes the rectum.
- The *rectum* runs in the pelvic canal to the anal canal.
- The *anal canal* is about 1 cm long and is surrounded by both smooth and striated anal sphincter muscles.

Arterial supply to the large intestine is via branches of the cranial and caudal mesenteric and the internal pudendal arteries. Venous drainage is to the hepatic portal vein via the caudal mesenteric vein, and to the caudal vena cava via the internal pudendal vein. Lymph drains to the right, middle and left colic lymph nodes. Nerve supply is from the spinal sympathetic outflow, via associated abdominal plexi (sympathetic) and from branches of the vagus and pelvic nerves (parasympathetic).

The wall of the large intestine is composed of eight layers (Fig. 51.1):

- The *epithelium* covers straight tubular glands (crypts of Lieberkühn), which extend through the mucosa, and contains goblet cells, epithelial cells and intra-epithelial lymphocytes.
- The *lamina propria* contains structural and immune cells, lymphatics and blood vessels.
- The *muscularis mucosa* is a thin, loose layer of smooth muscle.
- The *sub-mucosa* contains blood vessels, lymphatics and nerves.
- The longitudinal and circular *muscular coats* are composed of smooth muscle and allow both transverse and longitudinal contraction of the intestine.
- The *serosa* forms a loose visceral surface and is closely opposed to the visceral peritoneum.
- *Neural plexuses* lie in the sub-mucosa, between the circular and transverse muscle coats, and on the surface of the serosa.

FUNCTIONS OF THE LARGE INTESTINE

- *Absorption of faecal water* occurs predominantly in the proximal colon, and is achieved as water passes paracellularly following a transepithelial sodium and chloride gradient produced by active transcellular absorption. This process is extremely efficient; the large bowel absorbs 90% of the water presented to it, compared with approximately 75% in the ileum.

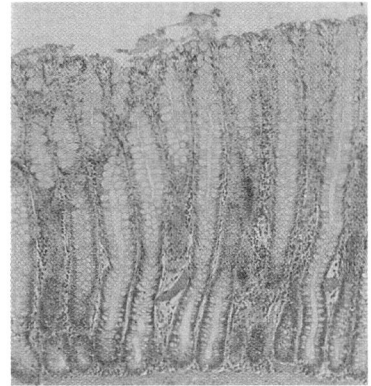

a

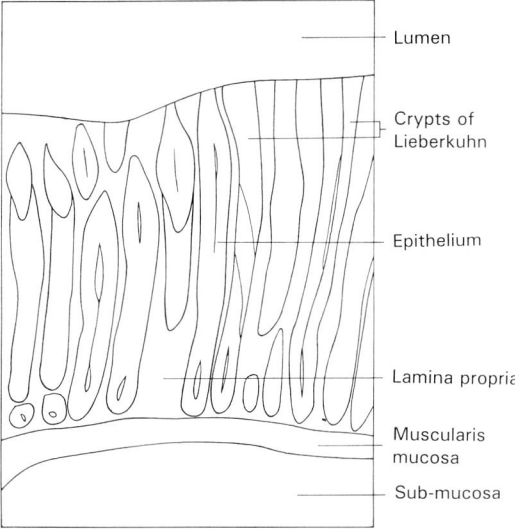

b

Fig. 51.1 (a) The histological appearance of the normal canine colonic mucosa. The epithelial layer is thrown into glands (crypts of Lieberkühn), which contain large numbers of goblet cells that produce copious lubricating mucus. The lamina propria contains blood vessels, lymphatics, structural elements and immune cells. (Haematoxylin and eosin (×100)) (b) Diagrammatic representation of (a), demonstrating the different regions within the large bowel wall.

In the diagram (b), the labelled regions are: Lumen, Crypts of Lieberkuhn, Epithelium, Lamina propria, Muscularis mucosa, Sub-mucosa.

- *Motility* of the proximal colon comprises segmental contractions to mix luminal contents, aiding dehydration of faecal matter, and propulsive contractions to move contents distally for voiding.
- *Storage* of faeces occurs predominantly in the descending colon and rectum.
- *Voiding* of faeces is a reflex activity under conscious control, occurring in response to signals from stretch receptors in the rectum and descending colon.

- Mucus production by epithelial goblet cells *lubricates* faeces.
- A combination of epithelial cell turnover, mucus production and tight junctions between epithelial cells *excludes* injurious luminal contents.
- Large intestinal lymphoid tissue allows *immune recognition* and response to luminal contents.

APPROACH TO THE PATIENT WITH LARGE INTESTINAL DISEASE

Signalment

When obtaining the signalment of the patient, the following may be considered:

- Age
  - Infectious diseases are more likely in young, immunocompromised or stressed individuals.
  - Foreign bodies and intussusceptions may be seen in all ages, but are more common in young dogs.
  - Inflammatory bowel diseases can present at any age.
  - Neoplasia is more common in older dogs.
- Breed
  - Histiocytic ulcerative colitis is reported in Boxer dogs and French Bulldogs.
- Sex
  - Male dogs have a higher incidence of colonic adenocarcinoma and lymphoma (Couto 1992).

History

The history should clarify the presenting clinical signs (Table 51.1 and Box 51.1). Where possible, diarrhoea

Table 51.1 The terms used to describe signs of large intestinal disease.

Clinical problem	Definition
Diarrhoea	Increased frequency or liquidity of faeces
Defecatory tenesmus	Straining to defecate
Dyschezia	Painful defecation
Constipation	Infrequent or difficult passage of stools
Haematochezia	Blood on the stool

Characteristic	Small intestinal Diarrhoea	Large intestinal Diarrhoea
Frequency of defecation	Approximately 3–4/day	Up to 10/day
Volume of stools	Increased	Small amounts, total volume normal or increased
Consistency of faeces	Soft to fluid	Soft
Straining to defecate	Rare	Usual
Vomiting	Occasional	Rare
Weight loss	Often	Rare
Inappetence	Variable	Rare
Blood on stool	Rare*	Frequent
Mucus on stool	Rare*	Frequent

Table 51.2 Clinical features that help to distinguish between large and small intestinal diarrhoea.

* Except with infectious causes.

Box 51.1 Clinical evaluation of the dog with large intestinal disease.

- Determine age, breed and sex.
- Determine spectrum of clinical signs and onset, progression and development of each.
- Determine responses to dietary or therapeutic intervention.
- Review history relating to the rest of the gastrointestinal tract and other body systems.
- Review medical history.
- Review husbandry, vaccination status, diet in the patient, and status of contact animals.
- Perform physical examination, with abdominal palpation in a relaxed patient.
- Perform rectal examination and collect required samples.
- Identify presenting clinical problems.
- Produce a differential diagnosis and plan.
- Use plan as a guide to a successful diagnostic or therapeutic conclusion.

should be classed as small or large bowel in origin (Table 51.2). Details should be obtained about the duration and progression of signs, response to medication or dietary changes and contact with potentially infectious animals, as well as the general medical history, other body systems, normal management and previous preventative medication. Signs are generally classified as chronic if they do not resolve after 3–4 weeks of therapy.

- Weight loss is more common with diseases involving the small intestine or with malignant neoplasia.

- Vomiting may indicate anterior abdominal, gastric or small intestinal involvement, or metabolic disease, but has been associated with up to 30% of cases of large bowel disease (Burrows 1992).
- Small intestinal signs may indicate that the large intestinal signs are secondary.
- Ribbon-shaped stools may be seen when there is rectal or anal narrowing or stricture.
- Haematochezia is associated with loss of mucosal integrity (inflammation, neoplasia, trauma), and with perianal disease.
- Previous trauma can be a cause of pelvic narrowing.

Physical Examination

A full physical examination should always be performed. Indications of systemic involvement (e.g. tachycardia and dry membranes indicative of dehydration or pyrexia) suggest metabolic, inflammatory, infectious or neoplastic disease. The colon and associated or related structures should be palpated, and *palpation* should be repeated as required, particularly if sedation or anaesthesia allows a more thorough examination. Loops of small bowel that feel thickened or full of fluid and/or gassy content suggest small bowel involvement or primary small intestinal disease. A palpable mass may be a faecal bolus, neoplasia, a foreign body, granulomatous disease, an intussusception or an inversion. Faeces are often palpably indentable. *Rectal examination* should also be performed in every case, to identify anatomic and/or rectal mucosal abnormalities and to obtain samples for faecal analysis and cytology. Physical examination *should* detect rectal, anal or perianal disease.

Diagnostic Tests

Following identification of large intestinal disease, useful diagnostic tests include:

- Faecal parasitological examinations and culture – to identify bacterial and parasitic infections.
- Faecal and rectal mucosal cytology – to identify inflammatory cells and clostridial spores.
- Haematology – to identify systemic responses to inflammation or infection and red cell indices to identify and classify anaemia.
- Serum biochemistry – to identify metabolic disease, consequences of large bowel disease and involvement of other organs. Hyponatraemia and hyperkalaemia have been seen consequent to trichuriasis and salmonellosis ('pseudoAddisonian' ratios), as well as to hypoadrenocorticism (DiBartola *et al.* 1985).
- Urinalysis – to rule out renal abnormalities and urinary changes associated with possible prostatic causes for tenesmus.
- Radiographic examinations – to identify masses, displacements, foreign bodies, mucosal thickening, organ enlargement, hernias and ruptures (Fig. 51.2).
- Ultrasound examination – to identify masses, mucosal thickening, anomalies, foreign bodies, and other organ involvement and sometimes to direct biopsy (Figs 51.3 & 51.4) (Lamb 1990).

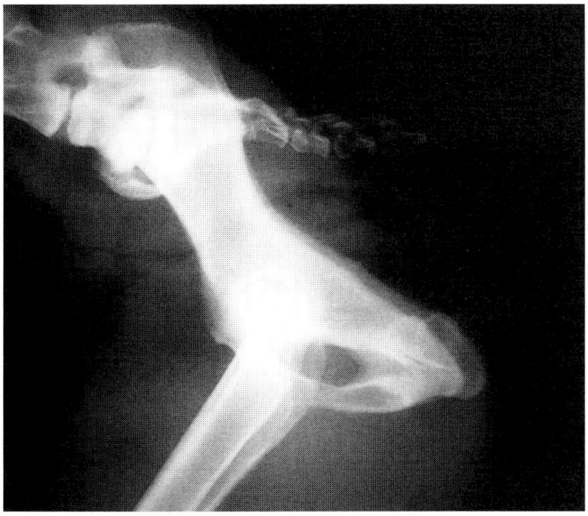

- Colonoscopy and proctoscopy – to visualise and biopsy the mucosa (Box 51.2).
- Intestinal biopsy and histopathology – to classify and identify inflammatory and neoplastic diseases, and to monitor therapy (Fig. 51.5).

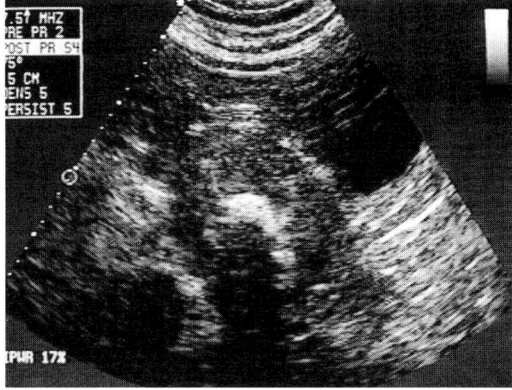

Fig. 51.3 A transverse image of a colonic adenocarcinoma in a 6-year-old Rough Collie, at the level of the bladder. The colonic wall is markedly thickened, with the normal, layered, mucosal pattern replaced by a relatively homogeneous, hypoechoic tissue. A small amount of gas or particulate matter in the lumen casts an acoustic shadow. This dog presented with haematochezia, tenesmus and dyschezia. (Courtesy of Mr C. R. Lamb.)

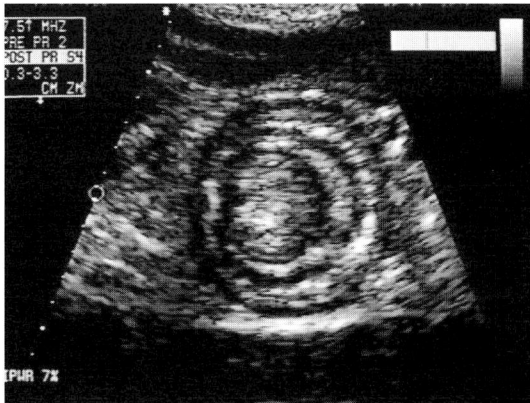

Fig. 51.4 The ultrasonographic appearance of an ileocolic intussusception in a 7-year-old Weimeraner bitch. The typical circular 'target' of the intussusception can be seen, and arises from the multiple layers in the lesion. This dog presented with mixed large and small intestinal diarrhoea. (Courtesy of Mr C. R. Lamb.)

Fig. 51.2 A plain lateral radiograph of the pelvic region of a dog with a perineal rupture. The area of rupture contains faeces and air and bulges beyond the normal perineal limits and is a potential cause of dyschezia and tenesmus. (Courtesy of Dr S. P. Gregory.)

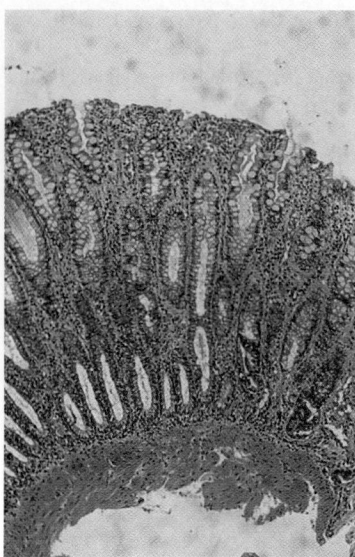

Fig. 51.5 Lymphoplasmacytic colitis in mucosal biopsies from a 4-year-old male Gordon Setter which presented with haematochezia. There is extensive infiltration of the lamina propria with lymphocytes and plasma cells, and superficial epithelial erosion. See also Fig. 51.16. (Haematoxylin and eosin (×100))

Table 51.3 Causes of large intestinal diarrhoea in the dog.

Acute colitis

Dietary hypersensitivity/intolerance/indiscretion

Bacterial colitis
  Campylobacteriosis
  Clostridium perfringens
  Colibacillosis
  Salmonellosis
  Yersiniosis

Parasitic colitis
  Giardiasis
  Trichuriasis

Fungal/algal/protozoal colitis

Idiopathic inflammatory bowel diseases
  Eosinophilic colitis
  Fibrinopurulent colitis
  Histiocytic ulcerative colitis
  Lymphoplasmacytic colitis
  Granulomatous colitis

Structural and anatomic abnormalities
  Caecal inversion
  Foreign body
  Ileo-colic intussusception

Neoplasia

Table 51.4 Causes of tenesmus and dyschezia in the dog.

Rectoanal disease
  Anal stricture
  Perianal fistula
  Anal sac abscessation
  Trauma
  Neoplasia

Extraluminal compression
  Intrapelvic mass
  Prostatic enlargement
  Pelvic narrowing

Intraluminal narrowing
  Stricture
  Neoplasia
  Foreign body
  Intussusception
  Caecal inversion

Musculoskeletal or abdominal pain

Large bowel diarrhoea unaccompanied by evidence of systemic involvement may often be managed by ruling out or treating parasite infestations, followed by dietary manipulations and non-specific treatment with metronidazole. Cases of chronic large bowel diarrhoea (longer than 3 weeks), or cases in which there is obvious systemic involvement merit a more aggressive diagnostic approach (Table 51.3 and Fig. 51.6).

Tenesmus may accompany large bowel diarrhoea, in which case the diagnostic approach should be similar. In cases of tenesmus or dyschezia where there is no diarrhoea, one should attempt to identify possible causes not associated with the large bowel (e.g. neuromuscular pain) from the history and physical examination. Systemic involvement should be identified as appropriate and a combination of rectal examination, diagnostic imaging, endoscopy and surgery used as necessary to define and treat the underlying problem (Table 51.4 & Fig. 51.7a).

Constipation is usually identified by the owner and may be confirmed by rectal and/or abdominal palpation of large, firm faecal boluses. Historical information relating to possible environmental, iatrogenic, or behavioural factors should be obtained. A full physical examination, including a digital rectal examination should be performed and should identify signs of systemic disease and of anal, rectal

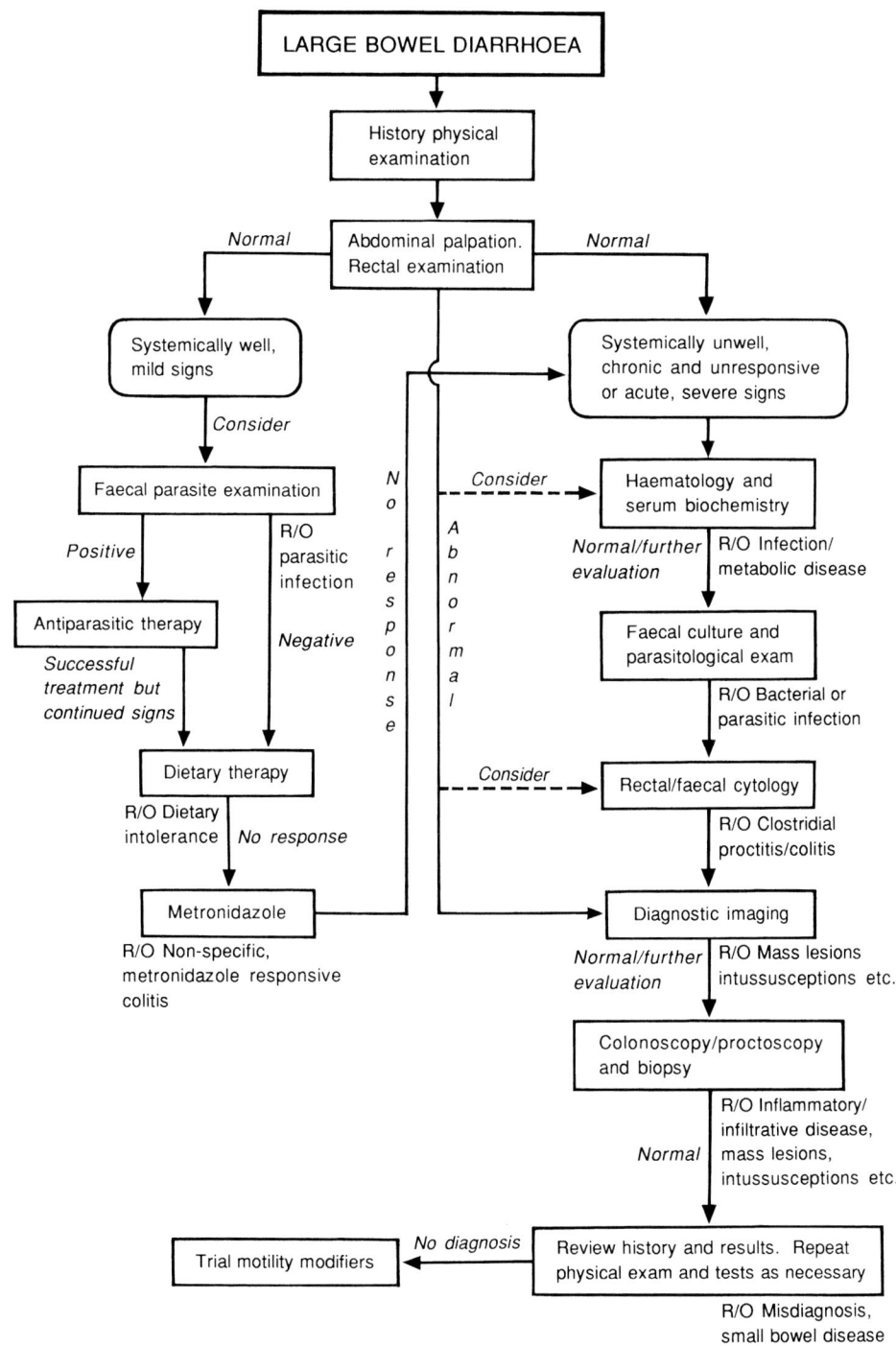

Fig. 51.6 An algorithm to guide the diagnostic process for large intestinal diarrhoea in the dog. Trial therapy may be appropriate for mild signs, but with evidence of more severe or chronic disease aggressive pursuit of a diagnosis, as well as definition of the extent of the disease process, is indicated. R/O, rule out.

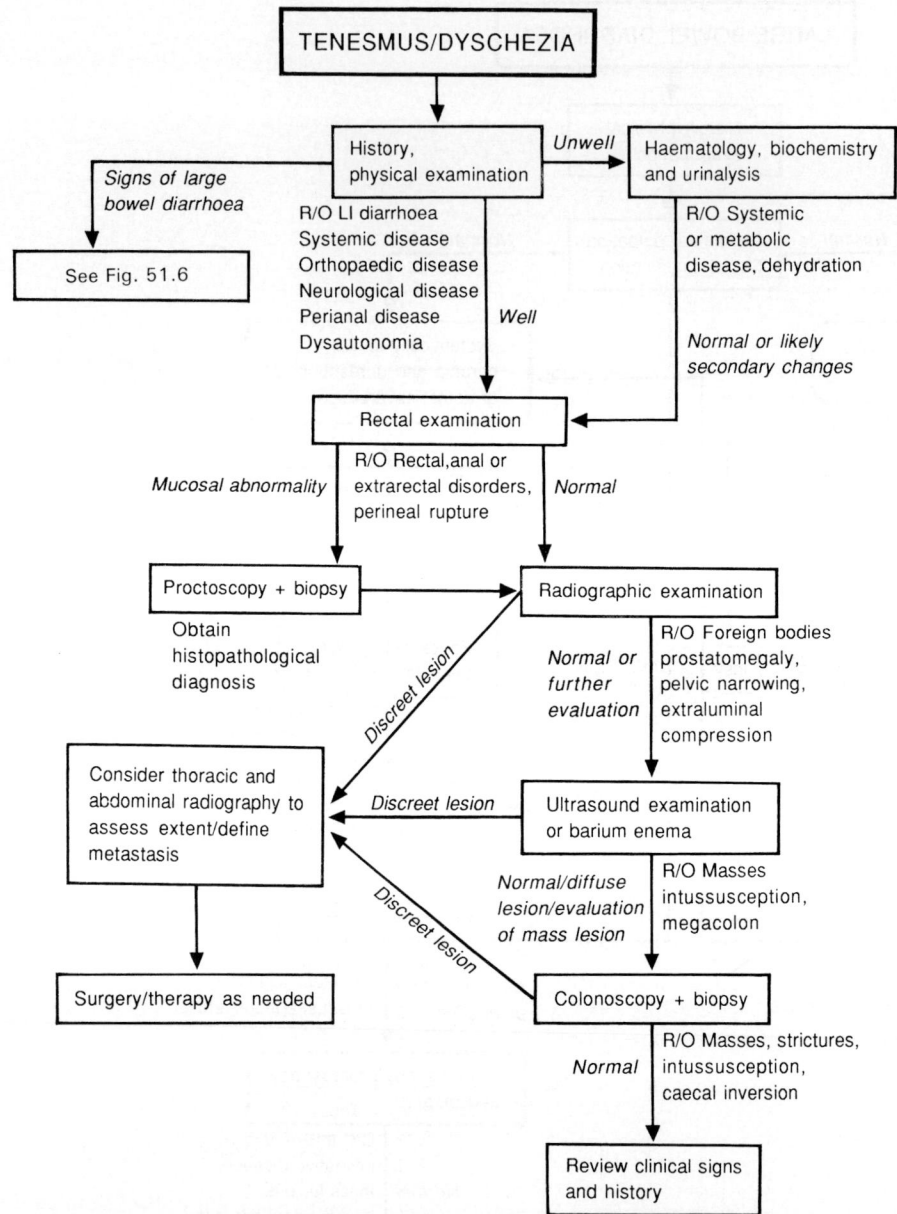

Fig. 51.7   (a) An algorithm to guide the diagnostic process for dyschezia or tenesmus in the dog. Possible causes of tenesmus/dyschezia that are not directly related to large intestinal disease should be ruled out by a thorough history and physical examination. Discovery of a discreet lesion, by whatever means, is an indication for further definition of the extent of the process and appropriate therapy. R/O, rule out.

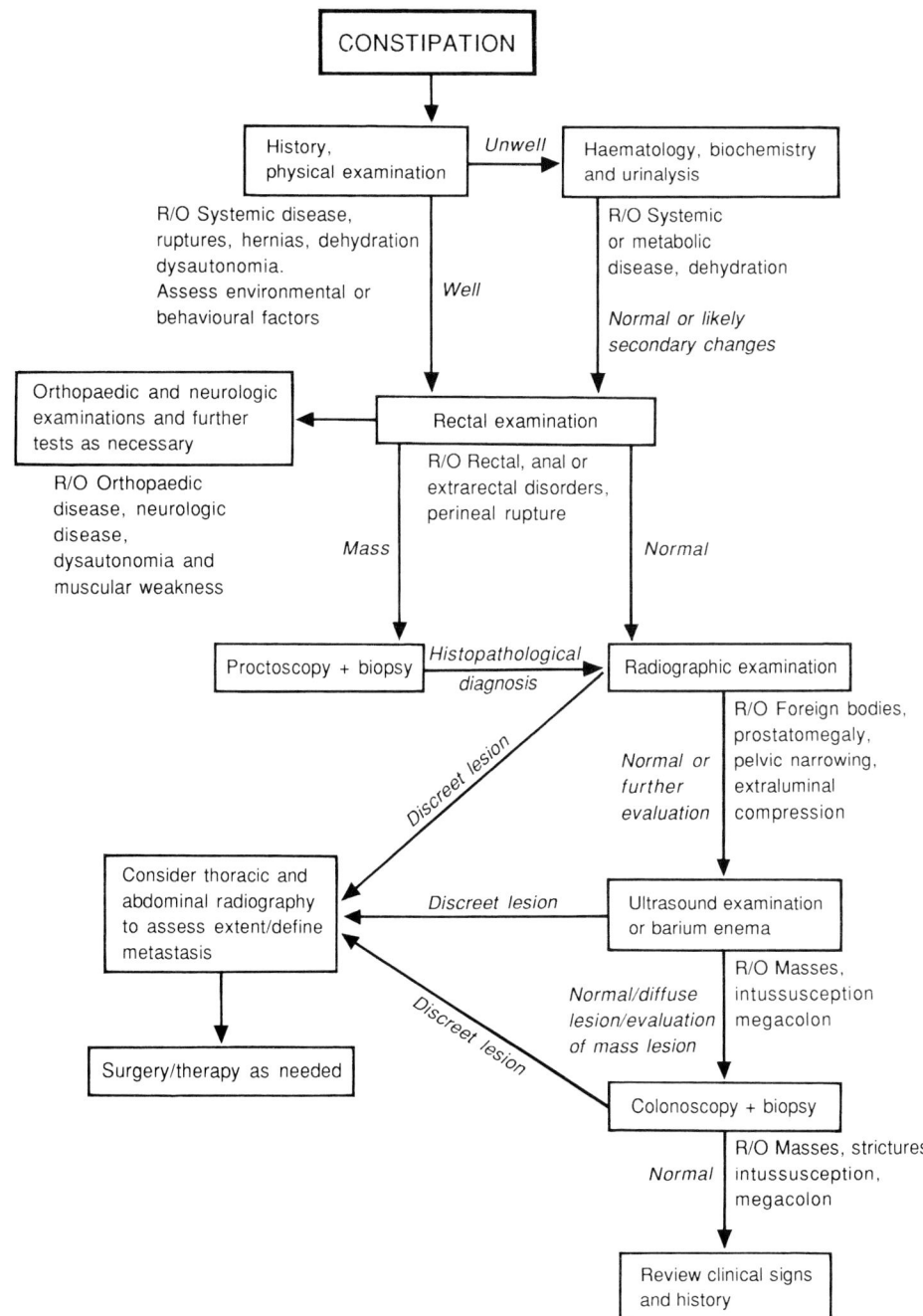

CONSTIPATION

History, physical examination → *Unwell* → Haematology, biochemistry and urinalysis

R/O Systemic disease, ruptures, hernias, dehydration dysautonomia.
Assess environmental or behavioural factors

R/O Systemic or metabolic disease, dehydration

Well

Normal or likely secondary changes

Orthopaedic and neurologic examinations and further tests as necessary ← Rectal examination

R/O Orthopaedic disease, neurologic disease, dysautonomia and muscular weakness

R/O Rectal, anal or extrarectal disorders, perineal rupture

Mass

Normal

Proctoscopy + biopsy → *Histopathological diagnosis* → Radiographic examination

Discreet lesion

R/O Foreign bodies, prostatomegaly, pelvic narrowing, extraluminal compression

Normal or further evaluation

Consider thoracic and abdominal radiography to assess extent/define metastasis ← *Discreet lesion* ← Ultrasound examination or barium enema

Discreet lesion

R/O Masses, intussusception megacolon

Normal/diffuse lesion/evaluation of mass lesion

Surgery/therapy as needed

Colonoscopy + biopsy

R/O Masses, strictures, intussusception, megacolon

Normal

Review clinical signs and history

b

Fig. 51.7 (b) An algorithm to guide the diagnostic process for constipation in the dog. Environmental and behavioural causes should be ruled out based upon a thorough history.

Physical examination should identify deydration, severe weakness, ruptures and hernias, and neuromuscular disease. R/O, rule out.

or pararectal disease. Neurological and/or orthopaedic examinations should be performed where indicated by history and general physical examination. Subsequent diagnostic testing is aimed at ruling out systemic and metabolic causes of constipation, with subsequent evaluation of the colon and rectum by appropriate use of diagnostic imaging and colonoscopy/proctoscopy (Table 51.5 and Fig. 51.7b).

Haematochezia can occur with both large and small bowel diarrhoea, in which case a diagnosis should be pursued as appropriate to these problems (Table 51.6 and

Table 51.5   Causes of constipation in the dog.

Diet and environmental
  Bone, hair, excess fibre or foreign body in colon
  Altered environment/routine

Painful defecation
  Anal sac disease
  Perianal fistula
  Rectoanal neoplasia
  Stricture
  Trauma

Inability to assume defecatory posture
  Orthopaedic or neuromuscular disease

Obstruction
  Extraluminal compression (pelvic narrowing, prostatic
    enlargement, mass)
  Intraluminal narrowing (foreign body, neoplasia,
    stricture)

Inability to raise intra-abdominal pressure
  Perineal hernia
  Inguinal hernia
  Diaphragmatic rupture
  Rupture of abdominal wall

Neuromuscular weakness
  Megacolon
  Dysautonomia
  Central and peripheral nerve damage
  Myopathy/Neuropathy
  Myasthenia gravis
  Metabolic disease (hypokalaemia, hypocalcaemia,
    hypercalcaemia)

Dehydration

Drug effects
  Opiates and opioids
  Diuretics
  Anti-cholinergics
  Sucralfate, kaolin

Table 51.6   Causes of haematochezia in the dog.

Anal or peri-anal disease
  Perianal fistula
  Anal gland abcess
  Anal or perianal neoplasia
  Anal or perianal trauma

Haemostatic abnormalities
  Disseminated intravascular coagulation
  Thrombocytopenia
  Coagulation defects

Vascular anomalies

Inflamed or eroded mucosa
  Caecal inversion
  Colonic ulceration (e.g. corticosteroid toxicity)
  Foreign bodies
  Idiopathic inflammatory bowel disease
  Ileo-colic intussusception
  Large intestinal neoplasia
  Trauma
  Viral, bacterial, fungal, protozoal or parasitic enteritides

Fig. 51.8). In the absence of these signs, the diagnostic approach is aimed at identifying abnormalities of the large intestinal mucosa (e.g inflammatory bowel disease, neoplasia, parasitism), the mucosal blood supply and the haemostatic system. The extent and type of any surgical disease should be defined using appropriate combinations of radiography, ultrasonography and endoscopy (Box 51.2).

DISEASES OF THE LARGE INTESTINE

Acute Colitis

Acute colitis is manifested by the sudden onset of large intestinal diarrhoea in an otherwise healthy animal. Acute colitis is a common presentation, with no apparent age or breed incidence. Signs are often self-limiting or respond to non-specific therapy. Following exclusion of faecal parasitism by faecal examination (and treatment if present), diagnosis is usually based upon response to therapy, which should include withholding of food for 24–48h, followed by feeding either a restricted protein or a high fibre diet for 3–4 days, then a gradual change to normal feeding. A short (5–7 days) course of metronidazole and/or fenbendazole can be considered in more severe cases. The prognosis is generally good, but if signs are not controlled, or relapse

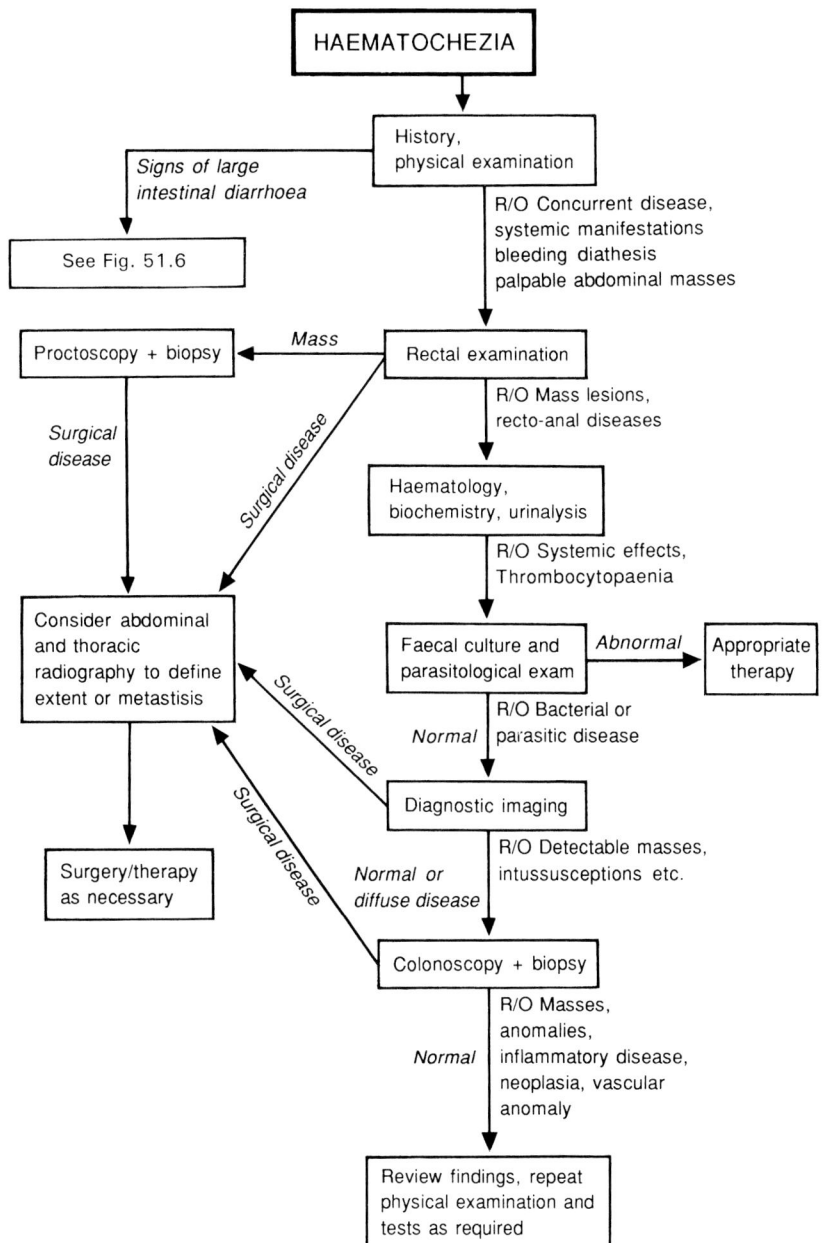

Fig. 51.8 An algorithm to guide the diagnostic process for haematochezia in the dog. After ruling out systemic or infectious disease, investigations should be directed to finding areas of loss of mucosal integrity. R/O, rule out.

Box 51.2 Colonoscopy and proctoscopy.

Applications

- Study of large intestinal or rectal disease.
- To sample rectal or large intestinal mucosa.
- Foreign body retrieval.

Contraindications

- Excessive friability of the mucosa with associated risk of perforation.
- Infectious diseases and zoonoses.
- Rectal or intestinal perforation.
- Severe stricture or obstruction.
- Severe haemorrhagic diatheses.

Equipment

- Human rigid proctoscopes are suitable for dogs (Fig. 51.9). Rigid forceps can obtain sizeable biopsies.
- Colonoscopy and biopsy can be performed using standard flexible equipment.

Patient preparation

- A clean endoscopic field is essential for effective endoscopy.
- Animals should be fasted for 24–36 h.
- A number (3+) of thorough warm water enemas should be administered, every 30 min to 1 h, up to 1 h before examination.
- Human colonic lavage solutions may also be used (Burrows 1989; Richter & Cleveland 1989).

Technique: rigid proctoscopy

- Animals should be sedated or anaesthetised and be standing, or in sternal or right lateral recumbency.
- Perform a digital rectal examination.
- Insert lubricated proctoscope with obdurator in place.
- Remove obdurator and close end port. Inflate the descending colon under visual inspection.
- Perform thorough visual examination of descending colon and rectum (Fig. 51.10).
- Obtain biopsies using rigid forceps, taking care not to biopsy deeper than the mobile mucosa. Sample three to four regions routinely and any areas of abnormality.

Technique: flexible colonoscopy

- Animals should be anaesthetised and placed in left lateral recumbency.
- Perform digital rectal examination.
- Insert 10–20 cm of endoscope into rectum/colon while insufflating before careful inflation of the colon and rectum.
- Negotiate splenic and hepatic flexures until the ileocaecocolic junction is seen (Fig. 51.11).
- In some cases it is possible to use biopsy forceps to negotiate passage of the ileocolic valve, allowing inspection and biopsy of the distal ileum (Fig. 51.11).
- Carefully examine caecum, colon and rectum while withdrawing endoscope. Obtain biopsies from the ileocaecocolic valve region, the transverse colon and descending colon (two to three per site), and from areas of obvious abnormality.

Endoscopic abnormalities

The normal colonic mucosa is pale pink, smooth, slightly glistening and with visible sub-mucosal vessels (Figs 51.12 & 51.13). Abnormal findings and possible causes are described in Table 51.7 and illustrated in Figs 51.14, 51.15, 51.16, 51.17, 51.18 & 51.19.

Sample handling

- Biopsies may be oriented on to card, mucosal side up, and placed in fixative for histology.
- Smears or brushings may identify inflammatory cells or organisms in certain circumstances but should not be relied upon as a sole means of diagnosis.

Table 51.7   Possible causes of typical colonoscopic and proctoscopic findings.

Endoscopic finding	Possible cause
Corrugated, thickened wall	Infiltrative disease (inflammation, infection, neoplasia)
Erythema	Inflammation (variable with anaesthesia, degree of distension etc.)
Excessive faecal matter	Inadequate preparation or elimination defect
Excessive mucus production	Inflammation or neoplasia
Increased mucosal friability	Inflammation or neoplasia
Increased rigidity to wall of bowel	Neoplasia, inflammatory disease, post-traumatic scarring
Luminal narrowing with normal mucosa	Benign stricture or extraluminal compression
Mucosal bleeding	Inflammation, bleeding diathesis, vascular anomaly or neoplasia
Mucosal mass lesions	Benign or malignant neoplasia, granuloma
Mucosal ulcers or erosions	Inflammation, abrasion, mucosal perfusion defect or neoplasia

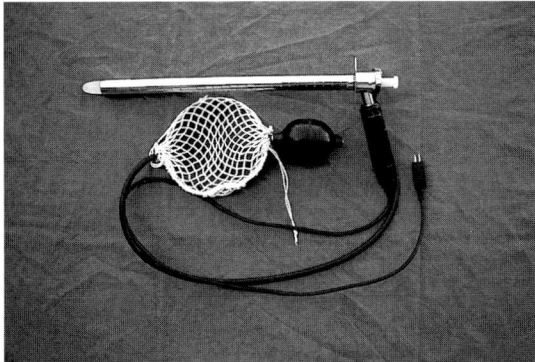

Fig. 51.9   A Welch-Allyn human proctoscope assembled with obdurator and inflation bulb in place. The working length is 25 cm and external diameter is 17 mm.

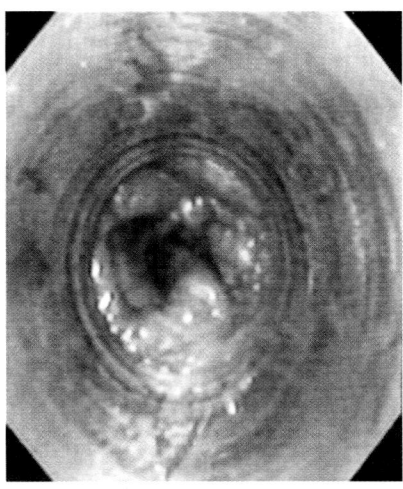

Fig. 51.10   A proctoscopic view of the (uninflated) normal canine colon (obtained by use of a flexible videoendoscope passed into the proctoscope).

upon withdrawal of therapy, further investigations should be considered (Fig. 51.6).

Dietary Hypersensitivity and Intolerance

Dietary hypersensitivity and intolerance can both cause signs of large intestinal disease (Strombeck & Guildford 1990). There are no reported breed incidences, but clinical experience suggests that Boxers and Golden Retrievers may be predisposed to hypersensitivity. All ages can potentially be affected. Dietary hypersensitivity/intolerance is characterised by large intestinal signs that respond to feeding a hypoallergenic diet (one comprising a restricted number of foodstuffs) and relapse upon re-challenge. Definitive diagnosis of dietary hypersensitivity relies upon demonstration of a true immunological mechanism, which is rarely achieved. Management of these conditions may

require the long-term feeding of an appropriate diet, but disease can be transient (see Box 51.3).

Bacterial Colitis

Campylobacteriosis

Campylobacter spp. can cause acute and chronic large intestinal diarrhoea in dogs. Disease is more common in stressed, kennelled or young animals. Diarrhoea is typically watery with mucus and blood; pyrexia and signs of gastroenteritis may be seen in acute infection (Fox *et al.* 1983). Diagnosis is by culture of microaerophilic organisms. Supportive and non-specific therapy should be administered as appropriate.

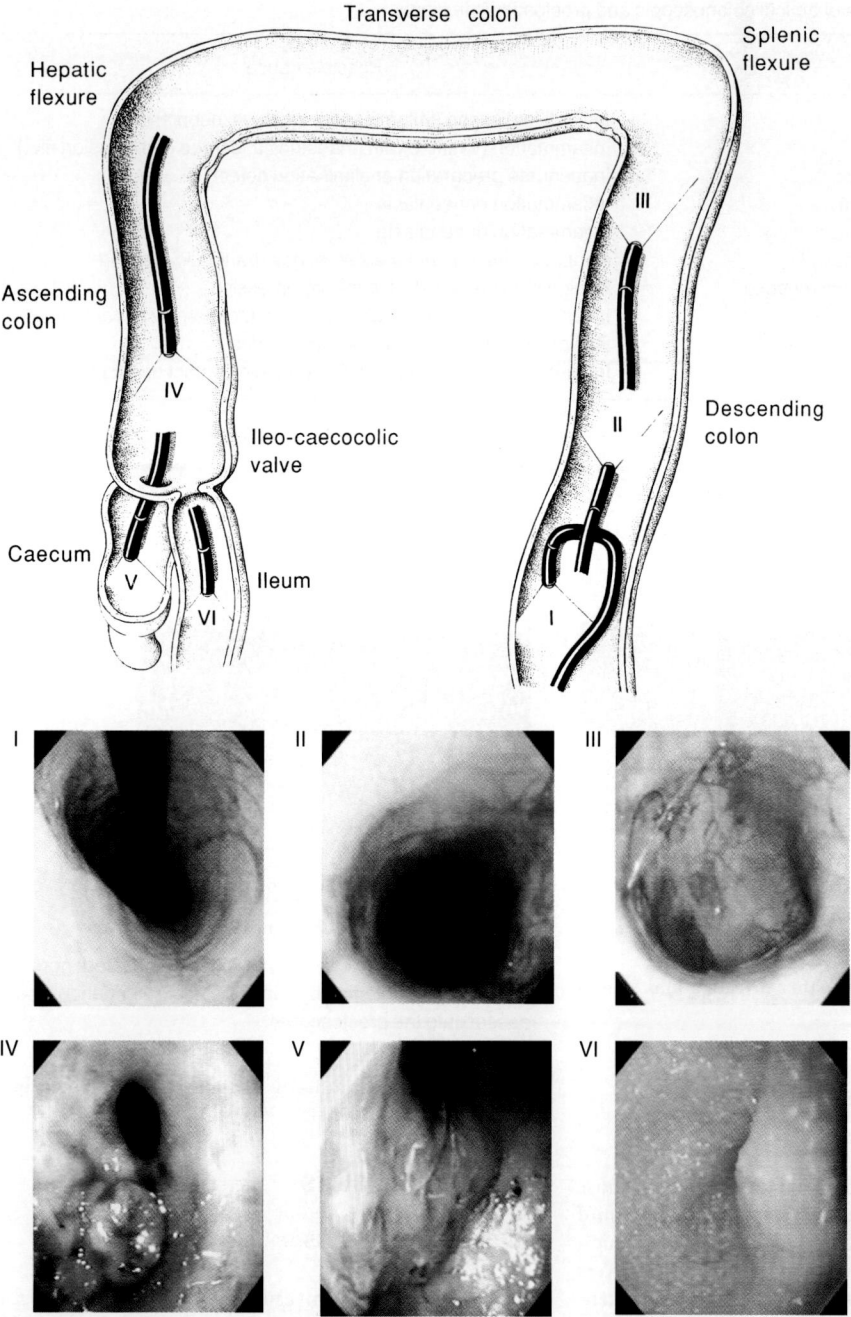

Fig. 51.11 A diagrammatic representation of the positions of a flexible endoscope when obtaining standard colonoscopic views; I, the endoscope is retroflexed to view the rectum; II, the descending colon; III, the splenic flexure; IV, the ileocaecocolic valve region; V, the caecum; VI, the ileum, which can sometimes be seen by passing the endoscope through the ileocolic valve using biopsy forceps as a guide.

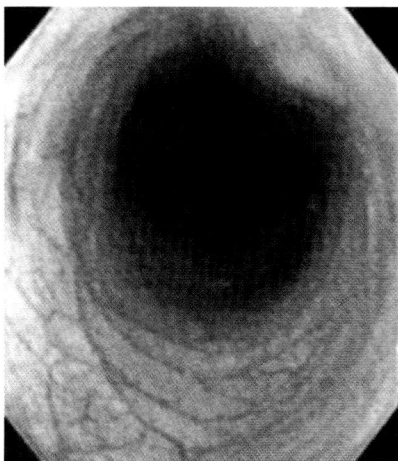

Fig. 51.12 The endoscopic appearance of the normal canine colon. The mucosa is pink and moist, and submucosal blood vessels can be seen.

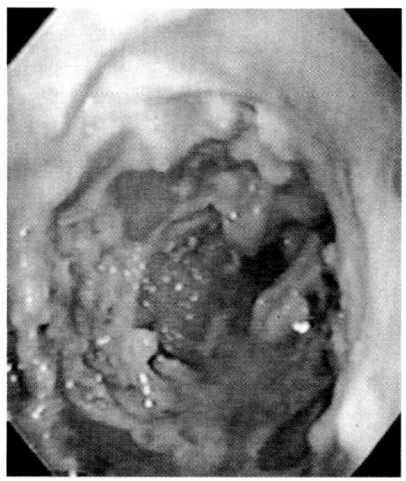

Fig. 51.14 The endoscopic appearance of excessive mucus production in a 3-year-old male Boxer with histiocytic ulcerative colitis.

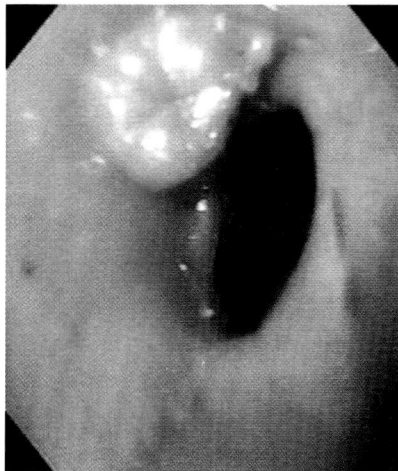

Fig. 51.13 The endoscopic appearance of the normal ileocaecocolic valve region. The ileocolic valve is a raised, tightly closed, 'button-like' projection, immediately adjacent to the open caecal sphincter. Small amounts of faeces are present, which can be difficult to eliminate using enemas alone.

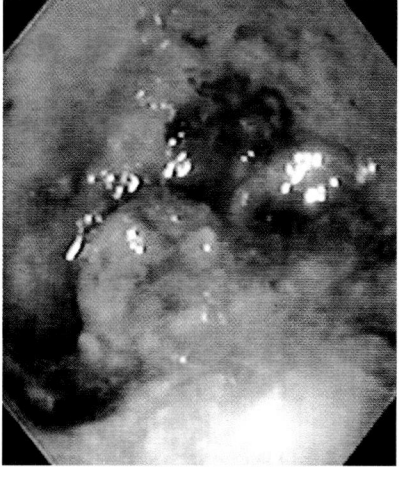

Fig. 51.15 The endoscopic appearance of the ileocolic valve region of the same dog as Fig. 51.14. The mucosa is roughened, friable and haemorrhagic, and there is plentiful mucus.

Campylobacter spp. are often sensitive to erythromycin, but specific therapy should be based upon culture and sensitivity. Because this infection is prevalent in the normal population, possible underlying disease should be considered as the cause of signs. This is a zoonosis.

Clostridiosis

Clostridium perfringens is a reported cause of large intestinal diarrhoea in dogs (Twedt 1992). Signs are believed to occur as a result of enterotoxin, released during sporulation,

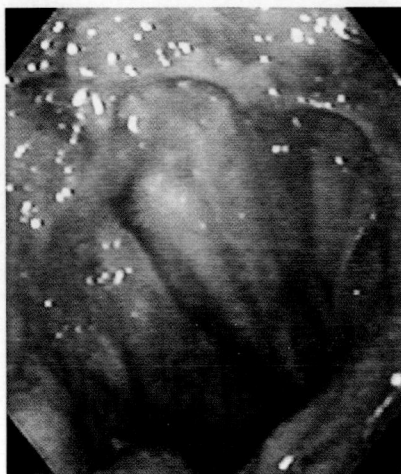

Fig. 51.16 The endoscopic appearance of lymphoplasmacytic colitis (see Fig. 51.5). There is mucosal oedema, erythema, erosion and excessive mucus.

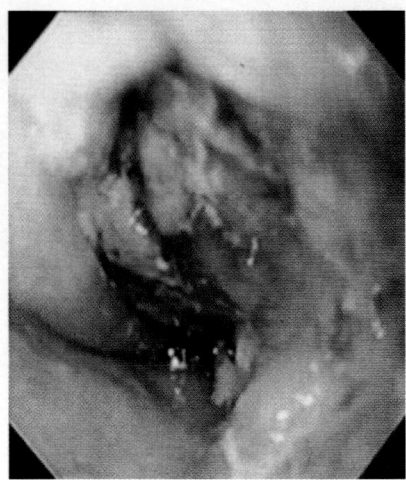

Fig. 51.18 The endoscopic appearance of an irregular, haemmorhagic intraluminal mass in a 5-year-old male Rough Collie that presented with haematochezia. Biopsy of the mass confirmed adenocarcinoma.

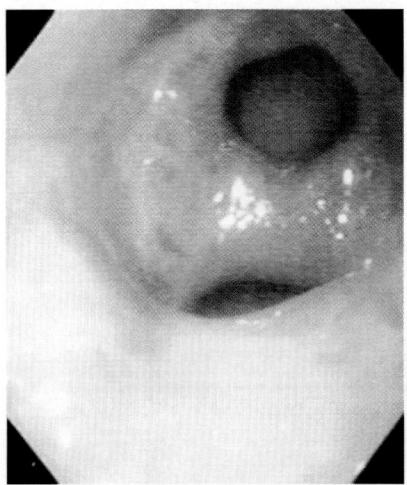

Fig. 51.17 The endoscopic appearance of the ileocaecocolic junction of an 8-year-old male castrated Springer Spaniel with a mucoid colonic adenocarcinoma. There is loss of the normal valvular appearance with mucosal thickening and an irregular mucosal surface. This dog presented with chronic defecatory tenesmus.

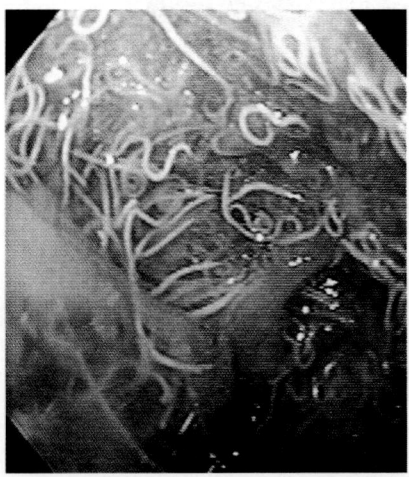

Fig. 51.19 The endoscopic appearance of the caecum of a 1-year-old male Greyhound that presented with large intestinal diarrhoea. Numerous long, thin writhing worms could be seen, which were confirmed as *Trichuris vulpis*.

causing direct mucosal damage. Alkaline faeces are thought to favour sporulation. Acute, large intestinal diarrhoea may be seen, sometimes with small bowel signs and vomiting. Fever is unusual. Diagnosis is by clinical suspicion, combined with demonstration of typical 'safety pin' like spores on faecal cytology, by culture of large numbers of organisms or by demonstration of high faecal entero-toxin levels. Therapy includes a high fibre diet and 5–7 days oral metronidazole or tylosin. Prognosis is generally good.

Box 51.3 Nutritional management of large intestinal disease.

High fibre diets
High fibre diets can aid the management of large intestinal disease. Both soluble (e.g. pectin) and insoluble (e.g. cellulose) fibre have beneficial actions upon motility, faecal water content, colonic bacterial load and epithelial function. Fibre can, however, worsen signs in some cases (e.g. by increasing faecal bulk where colonic hyperstimulation or stricture exist) and should therefore be used with caution. If fibre is to be added to a diet, it should be very thoroughly mixed before feeding.

Restricted protein diets
Oligoantigenic diets (diets restricted to a small number of protein sources, commonly referred to as hypoallergenic diets) can be effective in managing chronic colitis. Dietary antigens may be a stimulus for ongoing immune responses. A diet should be fed which is easily assimilated and should ideally contain foodstuffs that the animal has not encountered before. Protein sources for home-cooked diets include chicken, turkey, rabbit, egg and low fat cottage cheese, carbohydrate sources include rice, potato and pasta. These diets should be fed exclusively for a minimum of 4 weeks to evaluate responses, and for long-term use (more than 3 months) minerals and vitamins should be supplemented. Non-animal origin vitamin and mineral supplements may be obtained from some health food outlets. Proprietary hypoallergenic diets may help many cases and are nutritionally complete. Long-term use should be based upon relapse of signs after re-challenge with the original precipitating diet.

Low residue diets
Diets that are easily digested and produce a minimum faecal bulk (i.e. low fibre, high biological value) can be useful to manage cases where the colon is extremely sensitive to stimulation and frequent defecation remains a problem (e.g. severe, unremitting inflammatory bowel disease).

Dietary therapy is important in managing canine large intestinal disease. Different diets may need to be fed to determine what is most suitable for an individual case.

Colibacillosis

Escherichia coli is a common inhabitant of the canine gastrointestinal tract. Certain serotypes have been implicated as a cause of disease, signs of which have included large intestinal diarrhoea and haematochezia. Diagnosis requires demonstration of pathogenic strains in faeces, and is not routinely available. Little is known about the spectrum of clinical signs, or therapy. If suspected, a suitable antibiotic might be used (e.g. amoxycillin/clavulanic acid, enrofloxacin) for up to 6 weeks (Leib & Matz 1995).

Salmonellosis

Salmonella spp. can cause acute or chronic large intestinal diarrhoea, with associated fever, leucocytosis and systemic signs. Debilitated, immunosuppressed, young, old or stressed animals are at greater risk. Sources of infection include infected humans and animals, and uncooked meat. Diagnosis is by culture of organisms from faeces. Antibiotic therapy should be based upon sensitivity testing. Fluoroquinolones (e.g. enrofloxacin) are a suitable initial choice, and may eliminate intracellular carriage of bacteria,

preventing the chronic carrier state (Table 51.8). Non-specific therapy should be administered as appropriate. Prognosis is fair, with some cases becoming carriers. Because this infection is prevalent in the normal population, possible underlying disease should be considered as the cause of signs. The disease is a zoonosis.

Yersiniosis

Yersinia enterocolitica can cause acute and chronic large intestinal diarrhoea (Papageorges *et al.* 1983). Diagnosis is by isolation of the organism on faecal culture and antibiotic therapy should be based upon culture and sensitivity. The organism has been isolated from healthy dogs.

Parasitic colitis

Giardiasis

Giardia spp. can cause large intestinal diarrhoea and an ulcerative colitis (Watson 1980). It is more common in

Table 51.8   Therapeutic agents used in the management of large intestinal disease in the dog.

Drug/agent	Use	Dose rate	Side-effects
Hypoallergenic diet	Suspected dietary intolerance or hypersensitivity	To appetite	None
Low residue diet	Megacolon, colitis	To appetite	None
High fibre diet	Non-specific therapy of lower intestine disease, clostridiosis. Stool softening	To appetite	May worsen signs, and can potentially cause blockage and dehydration
Ispaghula husk (Isogel TM)	Increase faecal fibre content	1 tsp/10 kg per meal	May worsen signs by by increasing bulk
Lactulose syrup	Stool softener, laxative	0.5–1 ml/kg t.i.d. (to effect)	May cause diarrhoea and dehydration
Metronidazole	Non-specific immune modulator, antianaerobic bacteria (including clostridia).	10 mg/kg b.i.d. Giardiasis 25 mg/kg b.i.d.	Neurotoxicity at high doses
Albendazole (Valbazen™)	Giardiasis	25 mg/kg b.i.d. for 2 days	Blood dyscrasias at high doses Teratogenic
Fenbendazole (Panacur)	Trichuriasis, other intestinal nematodes and giardia	50 mg/kg p.o. s.i.d. for 3 days	None reported
Pyrantel/febantel/ praziquantel (Drontal Plus™)	Trichuriasis, other intestinal nematodes	As per directions	None reported
Sulphasalazine (Salazopyrin™)	Inflammatory colitis	10–30 mg/kg b.i.d.–t.i.d. p.o.	Keratoconjunctivitis sicca (KCS). Other immune-mediated disease
Olsalazine (Dipentum™)	Inflammatory colitis	100–500 mg per dog b.i.d. p.o.	KCS has been reported, but less than above
Mesalazine (Asacol™)	Inflammatory colitis	100–500 mg per dog b.i.d.–t.i.d. p.o.	Unknown
Prednisolone	Idiopathic inflammatory bowel diseases	2–4 mg/kg per day p.o., tapering off over 4–6 weeks	Immunosuppression, hyperadrenocorticism
Azathioprine	Idiopathic inflammatory bowel diseases	2 mg/kg s.i.d. p.o., for 5 days then 2 mg/kg every other day	Immunosuppression Bone marrow suppression. Pancreatitis
Enrofloxacin (Baytril™)	Sensitive bacterial infection (e.g. *Salmonella* spp.)	5 mg/kg s.i.d. p.o.	Cartilage damage in growing animals
Chloramphenicol	Sensitive bacterial infection (e.g. *Salmonella* spp.)	40–50 mg/kg t.i.d.–q.i.d. p.o.	Bone marrow suppression
Tylosin (Tylan™)	Idiopathic colitis	20–40 mg/kg per day with food	Nausea and vomiting has been reported
Erythromycin	Sensitive bacterial infection (e.g. *Campylobacter* spp.)	10–20 mg/kg b.i.d.–t.i.d. p.o.	Transient vomiting
Diphenoxylate (Lomotil™)	Intractable large bowel diarrhoea and faecal incontinence	0.05–0.2 mg/kg p.o. b.i.d./t.i.d.	Constipation, ileus

Table 51.8 *Continued.*

Drug/agent	Use	Dose rate	Side-effects
Dicyclomine (Merbentyl™)	Anti-cholinergic antispasmodic.	0.2 mg/kg b.i.d.–t.i.d. p.o.	Constipation, ileus
Loperamide	Intractable large bowel diarrhoea and faecal incontinence	0.1–0.2 mg/kg b.i.d.–t.i.d. p.o.	Constipation, ileus
Colonic lavage solution (Klean-Prep™)	Preparation for endoscopy	10–30 ml/kg twice, 12 h and 1 h beforehand.	Diarrhoea (transient) Abdominal cramping
Enemata	Preparation for endoscopy and treatment of constipation	Warm water to fill colon	Recto-colonic trauma

kennelled populations. Diagnosis is by demonstration of trophozoites in a direct faecal smear or faecal cysts by zinc sulphate flotation and three samples should be evaluated. Useful therapies include metronidazole and albendazole (Table 51.8).

Trichuriasis

Trichuris vulpis can cause acute, chronic or intermittent large intestinal diarrhoea in the dog. Infection in the UK is most commonly seen in kennelled dogs (e.g. greyhounds). Adult worms infest the caecum and large intestine, causing mucosal inflammation and thickening, sometimes with severe systemic effects (Malik *et al.* 1990). Diagnosis is by identification of typical bioperculated eggs in faeces; shedding may be intermittent, necessitating repeated examination in some cases. Endoscopy may demonstrate occult infections (Fig. 51.19). Trichuriasis has been associated with a syndrome of hyponatraemia and hyperkalaemia ('pseudoAddison's disease') (DiBartola *et al.* 1985) Antiparasitic therapy, e.g. fenbendazole or praziquantel/pyrantal/febantel, is generally successful in eliminating infection (Table 51.8). Eggs are long-lived and environmental cleaning, with regular faecal examination, has been recommended when re-infection is a problem.

Fungal/Algal/Protozoal Colitis

Various fungal, algal and protozoal conditions (e.g. entamoebiasis, protothecosis) can cause large intestinal diarrhoea, but have not been reported in the UK. Diagnosis is by demonstration of organisms in cytological and histopathological specimens and, in some cases (e.g. histoplasmosis), by serology.

Idiopathic Inflammatory Bowel Diseases

Idiopathic inflammatory bowel disease comprises a group of diseases characterised by histological infiltrate into the wall of the gut. This can often affect the entire gastrointestinal tract or may be regional affecting either the small or large intestine. In cases where signs compatable with inflammatory large intestinal disease fail to respond to treatment it is essential to rule out small intestinal disease.

Eosinophilic Colitis

This rare idiopathic inflammatory bowel disease is characterised by an eosinophilic infiltration in the large intestinal lamina propria (Johnson 1992). Signs include large intestinal diarrhoea and haematochezia. A circulating eosinophilia may be seen, and parasitic infestation should be ruled out by faecal analysis along with other causes of eosiniophilia such as Addison's disease. Diagnosis is based upon mucosal histopathology. Treatment should include elimination of parasites, a hypoallergenic diet and, initially, immunosuppressive doses of prednisolone, tapering over 4–6 weeks. Sulphasalazine, olsalazine or mesalazine may be used as anti-inflammatories, and azathioprine may prove to be effective in some cases. Eosinophilic infiltration may also be a manifestation of generalised disease. Prognosis is variable.

Histiocytic Ulcerative Colitis

This idiopathic condition has been reported to occur in young Boxer dogs and the French Bulldog (Kennedy & Cello 1966; van der Gaag *et al.* 1978; Hall *et al.* 1994). The disease is characterised by infiltration of the lamina propria and submucosa of the large intestine by periodic acid-Schiff (PAS) positive macrophages. Signs include large intestinal diarrhoea with watery faeces and weight loss. Colonoscopic findings include a friable mucosa, thickening and rigidity of the colonic wall, ulceration, excessive mucous production and haemorrhage (Figs 51.14 & 51.15). Diagnosis is based upon demonstration of PAS positive macrophages in biopsy material. Treatment may be attempted with non-specific therapy, corticosteroids and anti-inflammatory compounds, but the long-term prognosis is poor.

Granulomatous Colitis

A granulomatous enterocolitis has been described in which a mixed inflammatory cell population is associated with granuloma formation and mucosal thickening in the colon and ileum (DiBartola *et al*. 1982). No aetiologic agents have been detected, and no response to antibacterial agents is reported. A partial response to corticosteroids is seen in some cases, but the prognosis appears to be poor.

Lymphoplasmacytic Colitis

Lymphoplasmacytic colitis is an idiopathic inflammatory bowel disease of unknown aetiology (Richter 1992). No apparent breed or age predisposition exists. Signs include large intestinal diarrhoea, haematochezia and mucoid stools. Mucosal inflammation may be seen on endoscopic examination (Fig. 51.16). Diagnosis is based on characteristic mucosal histopathology and by ruling out possible infectious agents (Fig. 51.5). Useful therapies include dietary management, metronidazole, immunosuppressive doses of prednisolone tapering over 4–6 weeks, non-steroidal anti-inflammatory drugs (sulphasalazine, olsalazine, mesalazine) and, in refractory cases, immunosuppression with azathioprine (Table 51.8) (Nelson *et al*. 1988; Simpson *et al*. 1994). Tylosin has been reported as effective in some cases (van Kruiningen 1976). Human rectal infusion products for local administration of corticosteroid may be considered. Prognosis is generally good.

Panfibrinonecrotic Colitis

A single case report exists of a 8-year-old Terrier which had enteritis and colitis, with leucocytosis (Dvorak *et al*. 1991). No pathogens were isolated but a partial response to antibacterial therapy was seen. A subtotal colectomy was associated with a clinical cure.

STRUCTURAL AND ANATOMIC ABNORMALITIES

Caecal Inversion

This condition is rare, with no reported age, breed or sex incidence. Causes for inversion of the caecum into the ascending colon are unknown, although infestation with *Trichuris vulpis* has been implicated (Miller *et al*. 1984). Clinical features include haematochezia, abdominal pain, weight loss, diarrhoea, tenesmus, vomiting and soft stools. Mid-abdominal fluid densities may be seen on plain radiographs, and intraluminal filling defects of the ascending colon on contrast radiographs. The ultrasonographic appearance has not been described, but an intraluminal tissue mass would be expected. An intraluminal tissue mass may be seen upon endoscopy of the ascending colon. Surgical resection is expected to be curative.

Foreign Bodies

Solid or linear foreign bodies can be ingested and reach the large intestine or may be placed in the large bowel in situations of abuse; puppies may be at a higher risk of ingestion. Signs result from obstruction, irritation or abrasion and include large bowel diarrhoea, haematochezia, dyschezia, tenesmus, constipation and signs of intestinal obstruction. Diagnosis is by demonstration of a foreign object in the large intestine, using palpation, radiography, ultrasonography, endoscopy or exploratory surgery. The object should be removed endoscopically, surgically or by careful use of lubricants (e.g. liquid paraffin), with supportive care as necessary.

Ileo-Colic Intussusception

No breed or sex predisposition seems to exist. Most cases occur in animals less than 6 months of age, but any age can be affected (Weaver 1977). Proposed underlying causes include intestinal parasitism, linear foreign bodies and other systemic diseases (e.g. distemper). Vomiting, pain, faecal mucus, haematochezia, anorexia and tenesmus can all be seen; signs may be chronic or acute. A mass may be palpable in a relaxed animal. The intussusception may be demonstrated on plain or contrast radiographs, ultrasonographically or upon colonoscopy. Treatment is by surgical reduction and/or resection (Fig. 51.20). Prognosis is generally good.

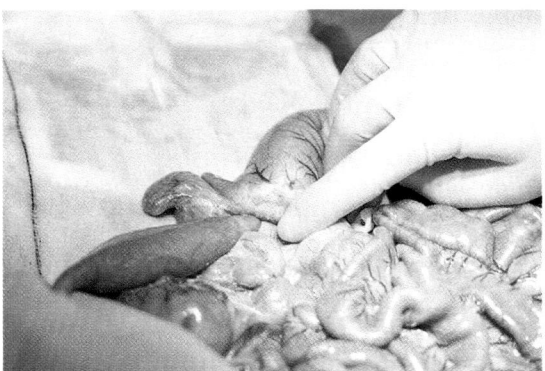

Fig. 51.20   An ileocolic intussusception as seen at surgery. The ileum can be seen to invaginate into the colon. The ileocaecocolic region can be recognised by the projecting caecum to the left of the surgeon's finger.

Short Colon

This congenital condition has been reported as a cause of lifelong tenesmus in a dog (Fluke *et al.* 1989). A low residue diet may help control signs.

Stricture

The aetiology of benign stricture is unknown, but previous trauma and scarring might be the cause; it has a sporadic incidence. Signs include tenesmus and dyschezia. Rectal strictures may be palpable per rectum. Obstruction to passage of faeces may be seen on plain radiographs and endoscopy will demonstrate the stricture. Sub-mucosal neoplasia should be excluded by appropriate use of ultrasonography, contrast radiography and surgery. Some strictures can be successfully managed using stool softeners alone; surgical resection or endoscopic balloon dilatation should be considered for more severe cases.

Trauma

Traumatic proctitis can occur iatrogenically or as a result of abuse. Non-specific therapy, stool softeners and antibiotics should be used as appropriate.

MALIGNANT NEOPLASMS

Malignant neoplasias of the large intestine include lymphosarcoma, adenocarcinoma, carcinoma, leimyosarcoma

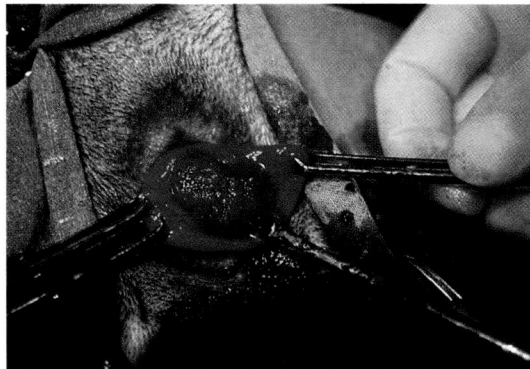

Fig. 51.21   Surgical resection of a rectal mass by a 'pull-through' technique. (Courtesy of Dr S. P. Gregory.)

and plasmacytoma. Benign tumours include polyps, adenomas and leimyomas. Signs include haematochezia, dyschezia and tenesmus; diarrhoea is less common. Perianal adenomas and anal sac adenocarcinomas which cause tenesmus should be detected on physical examination. Investigations should include haematology and biochemistry, thoracic radiography, abdominal ultrasonography, endoscopy (Figs 51.17 & 51.18) and biopsy to define the extent of the primary tumour and any metastases and any systemic complications. Diagnosis should be confirmed by histopathology. Stool softeners may provide some palliation, but, with the exception of lymphosarcoma, surgical resection is indicated where gross metastases are inapparent (Fig. 51.21). Endoscopic snare polypectomy may be used for benign lesions. Chemotherapy may be attempted for lymphosarcoma (Couto *et al.* 1989). Prognosis varies with the histologic type and extent of invasion and metastasis.

REFERENCES AND FURTHER READING

Burrows, C.F. (1989). Evaluation of a colonic lavage solution to prepare the colon of the dog for colonoscopy. *Journal of the American Veterinary Medical Association*, **195**, 1719–1721.

Burrows, C.F. (1992). Canine colitis, *Compendium on Continuing Education for the Practicing Veterinarian*, **14w**, 1347–1353.

Couto, C.G. (1992). Gastrointestinal neoplasia in dogs and cats. In: *Current Veterinary Therapy XI*, (eds R.W. Kirk & J.D. Bonagura), pp. 595–601. W.B. Saunders Company, Philadelphia.

Couto, G.C., Rutgers, H.C., Sherding, R.G. & Rojko, J. (1989). Gastrointestinal lymphoma in 20 dogs. *Journal of Veterinary Internal Medicine*, **3**, 73–78.

DiBartola, S.P., Rogers, W.A., Boyce, J.T. & Grimm, J.P. (1982). Regional enteritis in two dogs. *Journal of the American Veterinary Medical Association*, 181, 904–908.

DiBartola, S.P., Johnson, S.E., Davenport, D.J., Prueter, J.C., Chew, D.J. & Sherding, R.G. (1985). Clinicopathologic findings resembling hypoadrenocorticism in dogs with primary gastrointestinal disease. *Journal of the American Veterinary Medical Association*, 187, 60–63.

Dvorak, J., Willard, M.D. & Floyd, E. (1991). Panfibrinonecrotic colitis in a dog treated by subtotal colectomy. *Journal of the American Veterinary Medical Association*, 198, 264–266.

Fluke, M.H., Hawkins, E.C., Elliot, G.S. & Blevins, W.E. (1989). Short colon in two cats and a dog. *Journal of the American Veterinary Medical Association*, 195, 87–90.

Fox, J.G., Moore, R. & Ackerman, J.I. (1983). *Campylobacter jejuni*-associated diarrhoea in dogs. *Journal of the American Veterinary Medical Association*, 12, 1430–1433.

Gaag, I. van der, Toorenburg, J., van Voorhout, G., Happe, R.P. & Aalfs, R.H.G. (1978). Histiocytic ulcerative colitis in a French bulldog. *Journal of Small Animal Practice*, 19, 283–290.

Hall, E.J., Rutgers, H.C., Scholes, S.F.E., Middleton, D.J., *et al.* (1994). Histiocytic ulcerative colitis in boxer dogs in the UK. *Journal of Small Animal Practice*, 35, 509–515.

Johnson, S.E. (1992). Canine eosinophilic gastroenteritis. *Seminars in Veterinary Medicine and Surgery (Small Animal)*, 7, 145–152.

Kennedy, P.C. & Cello, R.M. (1966). Colitis of boxer dogs. *Gastroenterology*, 51, 926–931.

Kruiningen, H.J. van (1976). Clinical efficacy of tylosin in canine inflammatory bowel disease. *Journal of the American Animal Hospital Association*, 12, 498–501.

Lamb, C.R. (1990). Abdominal ultrasonography in small animals: Intestinal tract and mesentery, kidneys, adrenal glands, uterus and prostate. *Journal of Small Animal Practice*, 31, 295–304.

Leib, M.S. & Matz, M.E. (1995). Diseases of the large intestine. In: *Textbook of Veterinary Internal Medicine*, (eds S.J. Ettinger & E.C. Feldman), 4th edn. pp. 1233–1260. W.B. Saunders, Philadelphia.

Malik, R., Hunt, G.B., Hinchcliffe, J.M. & Church, D.B. (1990). Severe whipworm infection in the dog. *Journal of Small Animal Practice*, 31, 185–188.

Miller, W.W., Hathcock, J.T. & Dillon, A.R. (1984). Cecal inversion in eight dogs. *Journal of the American Animal Hospital Association*, 20, 1009–1013.

Nelson, R.W., Stookey, L.J. & Kazacos, E. (1988). Nutritional management of idiopathic chronic colitis in the dog. *Journal of Veterinary Internal Medicine*, 2, 133–137.

Papageorges, M., Higgins, R. & Gosselin, Y. (1983). *Yersinia enterocolitica* enteritis in two dogs. *Journal of the American Veterinary Medical Association*, 182, 618–619.

Richter, K.P. & Cleveland, M.V. (1989). Comparison of an orally administered gastrointestinal lavage solution with traditional enema administration as preparation for colonoscopy in dogs. *Journal of the American Veterinary Medical Association*, 195, 1727–1731.

Richter, K.P. (1992). Lymphocytic-plasmacytic enterocolitis in dogs. *Seminars in Veterinary Medicine and Surgery (Small Animal)*, 7, 134–144.

Simpson, J.W., Maskell, I.E. & Markwell, P.J. (1994). Use of a restricted antigen diet in the management of idiopathic canine colitis. *Journal of Small Animal Practice*, 35, 233–238.

Strombeck, D.R. & Guildford, W.G. (1990). Adverse reactions to food. In: *Small Animal Gastroenterology*, pp. 344–356. Stonegate Publishing, Davis, California.

Tams, T.R. (1990). *Small Animal Endoscopy*. C.V. Mosby, St. Louis.

Twedt, D.C. (1992). *Clostridium perfringens*-associated Enterotoxicosis in dogs. In: *Current Veterinary Therapy XI*, (eds R.W. Kirk & J.D. Bonagura) pp. 602–604. W.B. Saunders, Philadelphia.

Watson, A.D.J. (1980). Giardiasis and colitis in a dog. *Australian Veterinary Journal*, 56, 444–447.

Weaver, A.D. (1977). Canine intestinal intussusception. *Veterinary Record*, 100, 524–527.

Wills, J.M. & Simpson, K.W. (1994). *The Waltham Book of Clinical Nutrition of the Dog & Cat*. Pergamon Press, London.

Chapter 52

The Liver

E. Sevelius and L. Jönsson

INTRODUCTION

The liver is one of the most frequently injured organs and has an enormous reserve and regenerative capacity. It has been shown in experimental animals that removal of about 80% of the hepatocyte parenchyma is still compatible with normal liver function. Thus it requires severe and diffuse disease to deplete the functional reserve and cause liver failure. With the increasing use of screening tests, liver disease may be recognised earlier, and prognosis may be established better. Early recognition is important so that the disease can be correctly assessed and irreversible progression of the liver changes can be prevented or reduced.

ANATOMY AND FUNCTIONS

The liver has a dual blood supply consisting of the hepatic artery, and the portal vein. The portal vein is formed by the convergence of the splenic and mesenteric veins. These drain into the hepatic veins which in turn drain into the caudal vena cava. The hepatocyte has a wide variety of metabolic, synthetic, storage, catabolic and excretory functions.

(1) *Metabolic functions*. The liver is the central organ of glucose homeostasis, and responds rapidly to fluctuations in blood glucose. In the fed state excess blood glucose is shunted to the liver to be stored as glycogen whereas in the fasting state the liver maintains blood glucose levels by glycogenolysis and gluconeogenesis.

(2) *Synthetic functions*. Most serum proteins with the exception of the immunoglobulins, are synthesised in the liver. Albumin is the primary driver of oncotic pressure in plasma. A decrease in albumin causes oedema and ascites. Albumin is a negative acute phase protein, which decreases as a response to acute phase stimulation, implying that hypoalbuminaemia does not always indicate impaired liver function.

Most of the clotting factors, including prothrombin and fibrinogen, are synthesised by hepatocytes. Liver failure may thus lead to life threatening bleeding diathesis.

(3) *Storage functions*. The liver is an important storage site for glycogen, triglycerides, iron, copper and lipid-soluble vitamins. Severe liver disease can result from excessive storage for instance, copper in copper toxicosis and glycogen in the rare type II glycogenosis (Pompe's disease).

(4) *Catabolic functions*. Endogenous substances, including hormones and serum proteins, are catabolised by the liver in order to maintain a balance between their production and elimination. The liver is also the principal site for the detoxification of foreign compounds, such as drugs, chemicals, environmental contaminants and products of bacterial metabolism in the intestine.

(5) *Excretory functions*. The principal excretory product of the liver is bile, which provides a repository for the products of haem catabolism and also is vital for fat absorbtion in the small intestine.

DIAGNOSTIC APPROACH

Diagnosis of liver disease is not straightforward as the clinical manifestations of hepatic disease are often non-specific. The liver´s huge reserve capacity may delay recognition of liver disease, and disease processes in the liver may be secondary to multisystemic or extrahepatic diseases. It is important to keep in mind when approaching the patient with suspected liver disease that liver diseases may be acute or chronic primary or secondary. However with the aid of clinical history, a thorough clinical examination, appropriate laboratory tests and relevant complementary diagnostic procedures a correct diagnosis may be made in most cases. It is of major importance to rule out secondary disease processes (Fig. 52.1).

History and Clinical Findings

As in every patient, evaluation history is of great importance in the diagnostic procedure. Essential basic infor-

mation is breed, sex and age. Certain breeds are more prone to develop liver disease than others (Table 52.1). There are also some differences in disease incidence with respect to gender and sex. For example female Dobermann Pinschers are more prone to develop liver disease than are males. Dogs less than 1 year old may be suspected of having portosystemic shunts or hepatic fibrosis. In young unvaccinated puppies infectious canine hepatitis must be suspected.

Clinical signs and physical findings are often nonspecific and vary with the stage of the disease at presentation but are important in differentiating acute from chronic

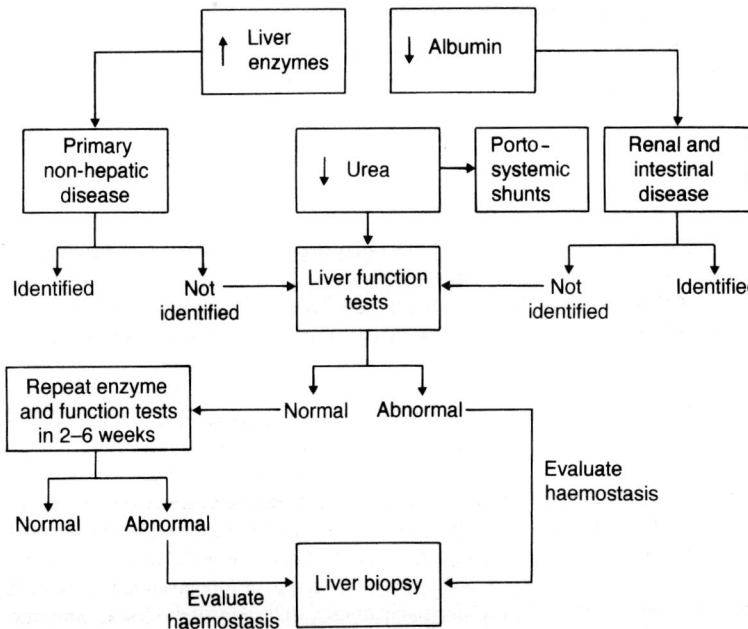

Fig. 52.1 Approach to the diagnosis of liver disease in the dog.

Table 52.1 Breeds predisposed to liver disease.

Bedlington Terrier	Copper associated toxicosis
West Highland White Terrier	Copper associated toxicosis
Dobermann Pinscher	Idiopathic chronic (active) hepatitis
English Cocker Spaniel	AAT-related chronic hepatitis /cirrhosis
American Cocker Spaniel	AAT-related chronic hepatitis /cirrhosis
	Idiopathic chronic hepatitis /cirrhosis
Skye Terrier	Idiopathic chronic hepatitis
German Shepherd	Idiopathic hepatic fibrosis
Standard Poodle	Lobular dissecting hepatitis
Irish Wolfhound	Portosystemic shunts
Yorkshire Terrier	Portosystemic shunts
Maltese Terrier	Vascular dysplasia

AAT, α-1-antitrypsin.

Acute hepatitis	Chronic hepatitis
Lethargy	Lethargy
Anorexia	Decreased appetite – anorexia
Vomiting/diarrhoea	Weight loss
Depression	Depression
Polydispia/polyuria	Nausea, vomiting diarrhoea
Icterus (consider pre- and post-hepatic causes as well)	Polydipsia/polyuria
Abdominal pain	Abdominal distention
Signs of hepatoencephalopathy (dementia, ataxia, circling, pacing, staggering, seizure, coma)	Ascites
	Bleeding tendency (haematemesis, melaena)
	Icterus
	Signs of hepatoencephalopathy

Table 52.2 History and clinical findings in acute and chronic liver disease.

liver disease (Table 52.2). In acute hepatic liver failure the history reveals sudden disease onset (hours to few days), in a previously healthy animal with no weight loss or ascites, which may be accompanied by depression, vomiting and icterus. Hepatomegaly, due to swelling of hepatocytes, cholestasis, and inflammation with increased synthesis of acute phase proteins, is commonly observed in acute disease, but may also be present in chronic liver disease. Chronic disease may also have a relatively short disease onset (days to few weeks), but is usually associated with weight loss.

The most common clinical findings in dogs with chronic liver disease are depression, weight loss and ascites (Table 52.2). Icterus is a less frequent finding and predominantly associated with cholangiohepatitis. Haemolytic anaemia must always be ruled out in icteric dogs. Abdominal distention caused by ascites suggests chronic disease rather than acute (Fig. 52.2). The relationship of clinical signs to food intake is important. Portosystemic shunts frequently cause encephalopathy, which may be precipitated by food ingestion. A history of taking any hepatotoxic drugs such as anthelmintic or anticonvulsant drugs may be suspected of causing liver disease. Possible exposure to specific poisons, like *Amanita* mushrooms, aflatoxins and blue-green algae should be investigated. Ascites is a common finding in chronic liver disease. Small livers are associated with chronic disease and found in liver cirrhosis and idiopathic hepatic fibrosis. In congenital portosystemic shunts small liver is often associated with renomegaly.

Clinical Findings

Jaundice

Jaundice, or icterus, is a yellow discoloration of the skin and sclerae that is produced by accumulation of bilirubin in the tissues and interstitial fluids. There are important pathophysiological differences between unconjugated and conjugated bilirubin. Unconjugated bilirubin is soluble in lipids and is tightly bound to albumin, in which form it cannot be excreted in the urine even when the blood levels are high. Diffusable unconjugated bilirubin in the blood may enter the tissues, particularly the brain, and produce toxic injury. In contrast, conjugated bilirubin is water soluble, non-toxic, and only loosely bound to albumin. Because of this conjugated bilirubin, when present in excess (as in obstructive jaundice), is excreted in the urine. Jaundice occurs when the equilibrium between the production and disposal of bilirubin is disturbed by one or more of the following mechanisms:

- excessive production by breakdown of red blood cells (*pre-hepatic* or haemolytic);
- impaired uptake and conjugation or secretion as a result of intrahepatic derangements (*hepatic* or hepatocellular);
- inhibition of bile outflow (*posthepatic* or obstructive).

It should be noted that more than one mechanism may be involved as for example in hepatocellular diseases such as

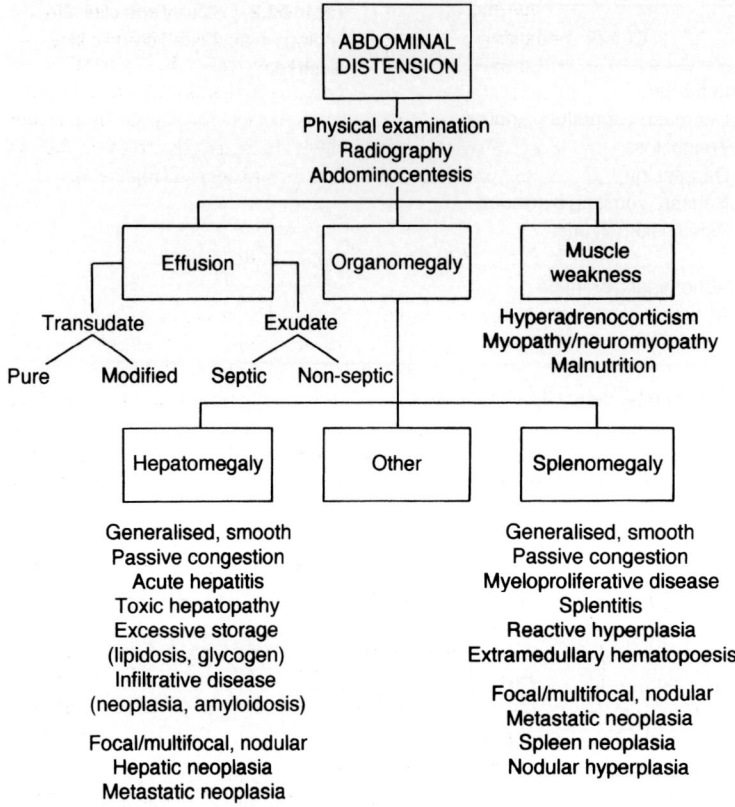

Fig. 52.2 Algorithm for initial evaluation of the dog with abdominal distention.

hepatitis and cirrhosis, in which there may be disruption of bilirubin uptake, conjugation and outflow into bile canaliculi. Disorders of bilirubin secretion or excretion are divided into intrahepatic and extrahepatic cholestasis. Various types of hepatitis and cirrhosis may act at several levels. Damage to the liver cells may impair the conjugation or secretory mechanisms, or the swelling and disorganisation of liver cells can compress and block the canaliculi. These disorders are intrahepatic causes of cholestasis. Extrahepatic cholestasis results from obstruction of the extrahepatic bile ducts. Tumours or inflammatory lesions strategically located at the outflow of the hepatic duct behave as extrahepatic obstructions. Prehepatic jaundice can occur in an acute haemolytic crisis from excessive production of unconjugated bilirubin, which exceeds the capacity of the liver to conjugate and excrete the bilirubin (Table 52.3).

Ascites

Ascites is the one most common clinical finding in chronic hepatitis predominantly associated with cirrhosis and chronic progressive hepatitis (Sevelius 1995). Paracentesis is consistent with a transudate (Table 52.4). Ascites often accompanies portal hypertension in animals with decompensated cirrhosis. The pathogenesis of ascites formation is complex and is shown in Fig. 52.3. It is thought that the increased formation of hepatic and interstitial fluid is important. Increased sinusoidal pressure results in an imbalance in Starling forces and drives serum proteins into the interstitial space. Eventually the protein-rich transudate weeps through the liver capsule into the peritoneal cavity. An increased renal retention of sodium and fluid, aggravates ascites formation and together with increased aldosterone release creates a vicious cycle. Hypoal-

Table 52.3   Differential diagnosis of jaundice.

Pre-hepatic jaundice
  Auto-immune haemolytic anaemia (AIHA)
  Incompatible blood transfusion
  Haemolytic bacteraemia
  Babesiosis
  Haemobartonellosis
  Toxic (zinc, anions)

Hepoatocellular jaundice
  Unspecific toxic hepatitis – drugs, endotoxin
  Infectious canine hepatitis
  Salomonellosis
  Toxoplasmosis
  Leptospirosis
  Chronic hepatitis
  Cirrhosis
  Primary or metastatic neoplasia

Obstructive jaundice
Intrahepatic
  Cirrhosis
  Neoplasia
  Cholestasis
  Cholangitis/cholangiohepatitis

Extrahepatic
  Acute and chronic pancreatitis
  Pancreatic carcinoma
  Bile duct carcinoma
  Duodenal neoplasia
  Cholecystitis/cholelithiasis
  Bile duct rupture

buminaemia also contributes to the formation of ascites because of decreased plasma oncotic pressure. Hypoalbuminaemia in liver disease may be reversible or irreversible. Reversible acute phase induced hypoalbuminaemia may contribute to ascites formation in chronic hepatitis. Ascites in these cases usually resolves fast as albumin concentrations return to normal (Fig. 52.3).

Hepatic Encephalopathy

The complex neurobehavioural signs referred to as hepatic encephalopathy develop in animals with severe acquired acute and chronic liver failure or congenital portosystemic shunts. Basically it is a metabolic disorder of the central nervous system and neuromuscular system. If the hepatic function can be restored, the encephalopathy is reversible without residual complications. The neurochemical basis of hepatic encephalopathy is caused by toxic compounds absorbed from the intestine that have escaped hepatic detoxification because of hepatocyte dysfunction or the existence of structural or functional vascular shunts (Table 52.5).

Hyperammonaemia is usually present in dogs with hepatic encephalopathy. Most of the ammonia is of intestinal origin, coming from production of ammonia, digestion of proteins in the small intestine and bacterial catabolism of dietary protein and urea secreted into the intestine.

The clinical signs of hepatic encephalopathy are variable and include anorexia, vomiting, (hypersalivation), bizarre behavioural changes, ataxia, staggering, head pressing, circling, aimless wandering, blindness, seizures and coma may be seen. The onset can be obvious and abrupt, or insidious and the clinical signs can be precipitated by

Table 52.4   Characteristics of abdominal effusions.

	Transudate	Modified transudate	Exudate
Parameter			
Total protein (g/l)	<25	25–50	>30
Number of cells (10^9/l)	<0.5	0.5–5.0	>5.0
Clinical diagnosis	Protein-losing enteropathy	Cardiac failure	Peritonitis
	Chronic liver disease	Hepatic disease	Pancreatitis
	Protein-losing nephropathy	Neoplasia	Haemorrhage
			Urinary tract rupture
			Biliary tract rupture
			Rupture of lymphatics

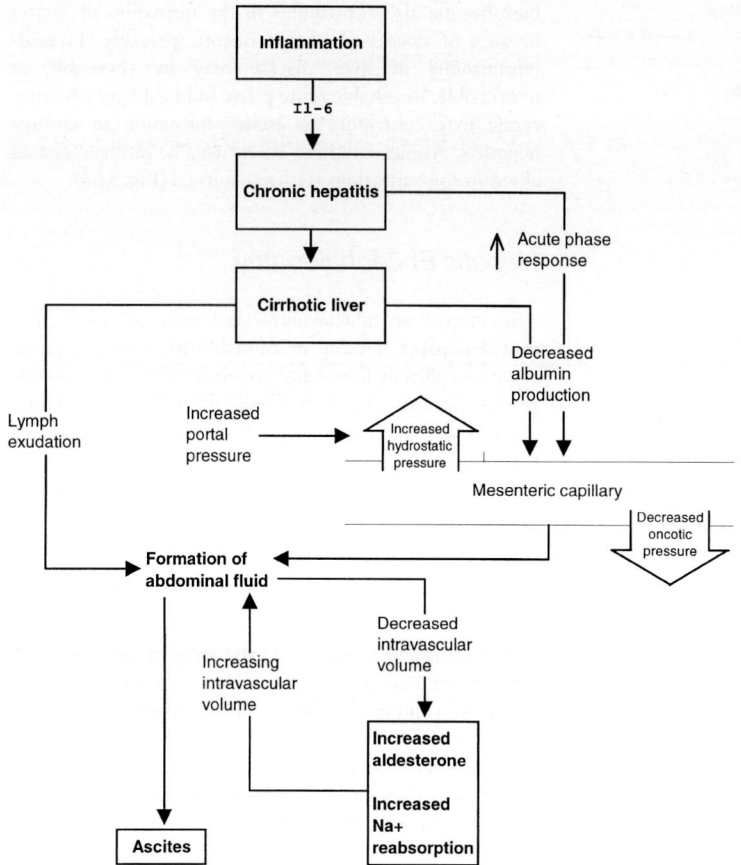

Fig. 52.3   Possible mechanisms of ascites formation in chronic hepatitis and cirrhosis.

Table 52.5   Possible mechanisms of hepatoencephalopathy.

- Impaired hepatic function blocks the degradation of ammonia to urea, and hyperammonaemia constitutes a neurotoxin.
- The combined actions of ammonia, mercaptans and short-chain fatty acids derange neuronal function or transmission of signals.
- Normal neurotransmitters, i.e. dopamine, are displaced by such false neurotransmitters as γ-aminobutyric acid (GABA) and octopamine.
- Elevated plasma levels of tryptophan and its metabolite, serotonin may be toxic to the brain or may lead to decreased production of excitatory neurotransmitters and increased production of weak neurotransmitters.

protein-rich meals. Many dogs appear normal between exacerbations, but some animals are chronically lethargic and mentally dull. Affected dogs may show intolerance to anaesthetics, sedatives, tranquillisers and anticonvulsant drugs. For management see Table 52.6.

Coagulopathy

The liver is important for maintaining normal clotting homeostasis. In acute or chronic liver disease the levels of clotting factors may be reduced due to decreased synthesis. Biliary obstruction may cause vitamin K deficiency, since bile is necessary for absorption of vitamin K. Thrombocytopenia owing to decreased synthesis or increased consumption may complicate the coagulation abnormality. Disseminated intravascular coagulopathy may follow acute

Table 52.6 Management of hepatic encephalopathy.

- Lactulose orally at a daily dosage of 5–20 ml, or as enema if severe encephalopathy or comatose.
- Neomycin should be administered at a dosage of 10–20 mg/kg p.o.
- Phenobarbitone is administered intravenously to dogs with seizures if hypoglycaemia is ruled out. Lactulose enema may also be beneficial for these patients.
- Correct alkalosis and hypokalaemia as they may potentiate encephalopathy.
- Dextrose solution is given intravenously to dogs with hypoglycaemia to prevent seizures
- Restricted dietary protein. If homemade diet is chosen, cottage cheese is recommended as a primary protein source. The daily protein intake should be maximum 2 g/kg. Supplementation of vitamins A, B, C, E and K is recommended.

Table 52.7 Routine screening tests for liver disease.

Alanine aminotransferase (ALT)
Alkaline phosphatase (ALP)
γ-Glutamyltransferase (GGT)
Fasting serum bile acids (SBA) (and postprandial when needed)
Total protein
Albumin
Scanning serum protein electrophoresis
(Total bilirubin, TB)
Isoelectric focusing for phenotyping of α-1-antitrypsin should be considered last as it is not widely available
Urinalysis – Biurate crystals

hepatic necrosis and is often seen with infectious canine hepatitis and neoplasia.

Laboratory Analysis

As the liver is affected in many disease processes it is essential to make a baseline haematological and biochemical profile to rule out these diseases. There are a number of well known enzymatic and functional tests available for diagnosing liver disease. However, none of these tests is specific for any one disease. Therefore it is necessary to combine various tests to achieve optimal diagnostic accuracy (Table 52.7). Liver biopsy is however necessary for a definitive diagnosis. Serum protein electrophoresis has been demonstrated to be a good prognostic marker of chronic liver disease (Sevelius & Andersson 1995).

Routine Haematology

Haematology is often normal but changes may include the development of anaemia, abnormal erythrocyte morphology and reduced platelet number or function. Poikilocytes, acanthocytes and target cells are abnormally shaped erythrocytes seen in dogs with serious liver disease. Erythrocyte microcytosis is associated with both acquired and congenital portosystemic shunts and fibrosis. A regenerative anaemia caused by blood loss associated with gastrointestinal ulceration and/or a coagulopathy is occasionally recognised. More commonly, anaemia is non-regenerative (normocytic, normochromic).

Routine Biochemical Profile

Increased serum levels of serum alanine aminotransferase (ALT) reflects hepatocellular damage. The magnitude of ALT elevation shows the extent of the hepatocyte damage but indicates neither prognosis nor reversibility. Increased ALT levels may persist for weeks during repair process in the liver. Elevation of ALT is seen with primary as well as secondary liver disease.

Aspartate aminotransferase (AST) is not liver specific but often parallels the ALT activity. It has no evident diagnostic advantage over ALT. Increased AST and creatine kinase (CK) levels suggest muscle damage rather than liver damage.

Alkaline phosphatase (ALP) is a membrane-bound enzyme found in hepatocytes and biliary epithelial cells. Increased activity of this enzyme reflects intra- or extrahepatic cholestasis or decreased bile flow and is mainly due to increased production but also to decreased clearance. The corticosteroid induced isoenzyme is easily separated from liver and bone isoenzymes by heating serum to 65°C. At this temperature these isoenzymes are inactivated while the steroid induced is not (Teske *et al.* 1986). Treatment with certain anticonvulsant drugs may lead to elevation of ALP concentrations as a consequence of either increased enzyme production or liver damage.

γ-glutamyltransferase (GGT) is another membrane bound enzyme (in biliary epithelial cells) which has been shown largely to parallel ALP in cholestasis. It is a very liver specific enzyme which remains elevated longer than the other enzymes during recovery from hepatobiliary disease.

Albumin concentration in serum may reflect the hepatic synthesis of the protein. Hypoalbuminaemia in liver disease may be reversible or irreversible. Irreversible hypoalbuminaemia reflects impaired liver function while reversible hypoalbuminaemia is caused by a switch in the protein production by the liver towards the synthesis of acute phase proteins and a concomitant decreased albumin synthesis (Eckersall & Connor 1988; Sevelius & Andersson 1995). It should be noted that 25–30% of normal liver function is considered enough to maintain sufficient concentrations of normal liver serum albumin. In a recent study reversible hypoalbuminaemia was associated with normal or increased α-globulins whereas irreversible hypoalbuminaemia in terminal liver disease was associated with almost abolished α-globulins (Sevelius & Andersson 1995).

Total bilirubin (TB) concentrations indicate the hepatic ability for uptake, conjugation and excretion of bilirubin. It is an insensitive test, indicating whether icterus is present or not rather than a marker of true liver function. The routine measurement of TB with conventional methods should be replaced or supplemented by other methods to permit the quantitation of non-protein-bound bilirubins in plasma (Rothuizen & van den Ingh 1988).

Liver Function Tests

Serum bile acids (SBA) are synthesised by hepatocytes from cholesterol. They are secreted into the biliary system and excreted into the intestine. Bile acids are almost completely reabsorbed in the ileum and returned to the liver with the portal blood, from which they are cleared efficiently by the liver (enterohepatic circulation) (Center et al. 1985). Increased fasting serum bile acid concentration in peripheral blood is associated with liver dysfunction and a consequence of impaired hepatic ability of extracting the bile acids from the circulation. The SBA test cannot be used for discriminating between different kinds of liver diseases or for prognostic purposes. The diagnostic accuracy increases with a combined fasting and 2 h postprandial test which is a particularly valuable test for diagnosing congenital or acquired portosystemic shunts.

Scanning protein electrophoresis has been found to be a helpful tool in evaluating liver function and also in determining prognosis of chronic liver disease (Sevelius & Andersson 1995). The fractions of importance, apart from albumin, are α-1-antitrypsin (AAT) also known as α-1-antiprotease or α-1-protease inhibitor, and haptoglobin, i.e. the α-globulins (Fig. 52.4) localised in the α-region. Haptoglobins and AAT are acute phase proteins increasing in serum concentration in acute as well as chronic disease. These acute phase proteins are synthesised in the liver, thus a decrease may reflect impaired liver function. AAT is an efficient inhibitor of leukocyte elastase protecting the tissue from proteolytic degradation. Apart from impaired liver function decreased AAT fractions in less severe liver disease may be associated with the I-phenotype of AAT (Pi I) (see 'Isoelectric focusing').

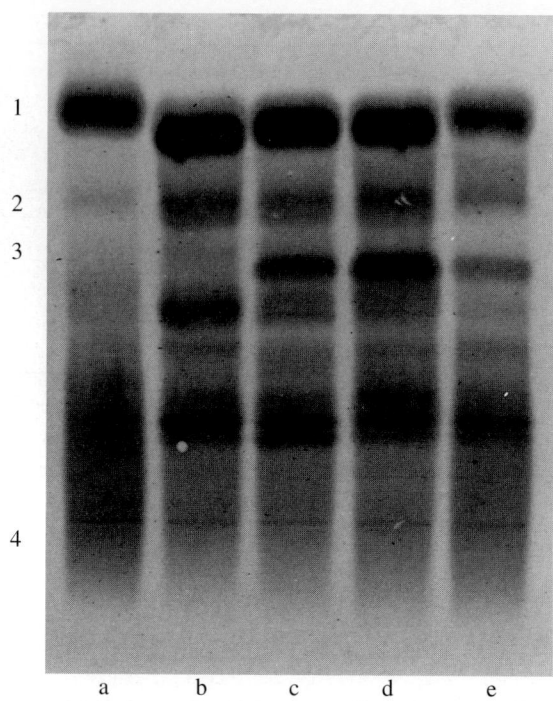

Fig. 52.4 Scanning electrophoresis of serum from five dogs: (a) Late stage cirrhosis. Pronounced decrease in albumin as well as α-1- and α-2-globulins. Increase in gamma globulin. Bad prognosis. (b) Healthy dog. Slight haemolysis at sampling causes a slower migrating haptoglobin (Hp), complexed with haemoglobin (Hb). (c) Chronic nonspecific hepatitis. (d) Chronic cholangiohepatits. Normal fractions of albumin and α-1-globulin. Hp increased. Good prognosis. (e) Chronic progressive hepatitis. Albumin is decreased, but α-1-fractions are only slightly decreased. Hp is slightly increased and gamma globulin significantly increased. Fairly good prognosis. 1 = albumin, 2 = α-1-antitrypsin, 3 = Hp, 4 = gamma globulin.

Isoelectric Focusing

With isoelectric focusing (pH gradient 4.2–4.8) three different phenotypes of canine AAT has been found so far. They are labelled PiF (Fast), PiI (Intermediate) and PiS (Slow) (Juneja et al. 1981; Sevelius et al. 1994). They appear in either homozygous forms, PiFF, PiII or PiSS or as heterozygotes PiFI, PiFS or PiIS (Fig. 52.5). AAT of the I-type has a tendency to accumulate in the hepatocytes leading to cell death and chronic hepatitis and/or cirrhosis. The I-type is most frequently found in healthy as well as diseased English Cocker Spaniels (Fig. 52.5).

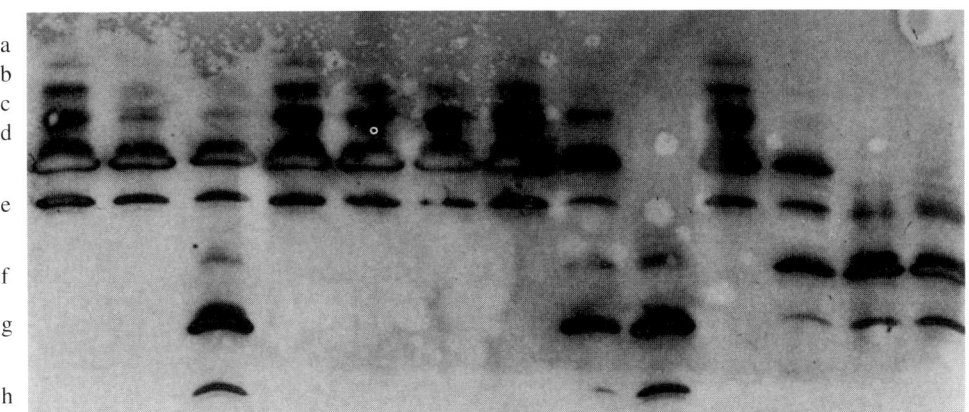

Fig. 52.5 Immunoprint pattern of canine AAT phenotypes after isoelectric focusing with a pH gradient of 4.2–4.8, anode at the top. (Samples 1–13; 'positions' a–h). Each AAT phenotype comprises several fractions with different amounts of sialic acid. The F (fast) type appears as five bands in the upper half of the immunoprint. The main fraction of the I (intermediate) type is seen at position f.

The S (slow) type appears as three fractions. Its major fraction has an isoelectric point equal to that of the slowest fraction of the I type, seen at position g. Sample 1, 2, 4, 5, 6, 7 and 10 are FF homozygotes; Samples 3 and 8 are FS heterozygotes; Sample 9 is an SS homozygote; 11 is an FI heterozygote and 12 and 13 are II homozygotes.

Diagnostic Imaging

Radiography

The diagnostic accuracy of radiography in hepatology is limited, but survey abdominal radiographs help in assessing size and shape of the liver. For differential diagnosis of hepatomegaly see Table 52.8. A small liver is usually a sign of chronic disease and is most commonly seen in dogs with cirrhosis and congenital portosystemic shunts. It must be noted that deep chested dogs have a liver that normally may appear as small. Renomegaly is commonly associated with portosystemic shunts. Renal or cystic calculi associated with shunts are rarely radiodense and need a contrast or ultrasonographic examination for detection. The shape of the liver may be affected by hepatic masses although liver tumours are seldom diagnosed radiographically.

Contrast Radiography
The administration of barium sulphate may be useful to demonstrate the position of the stomach and more readily demonstrate the size and form of the liver. Cholecystography to demonstrate gallstones and the biliary system has limited application in the dog. Angiography is com-

Table 52.8 Differential diagnosis of hepatomegaly.

Acute and chronic hepatitis
Neoplasia (hepatocellular carcinoma, bile duct carcinoma, lymphosarcoma)
Nodular hyperplasia
Amyloidosis
Lipidosis (diabetes mellitus)
Glycogen storage (Pompe´s disease)
Steroid hepatopathy
Severe anaemia – extra-medullary haematopoesis
Acute and chronic congestion

monly used for the identification of congenital vascular anomalies.

Ultrasonography

Ultrasonography is a valuable aid in evaluating focal liver disease. Objective criteria are lacking for evaluating liver size. Space occupying lesions like tumours, cysts, abscesses and granulomas can be observed. Ultrasonography is an excellent means of demonstrating radiolucent gallstones (Fig. 52.6) and represents a non-invasive way of diagnosing and localising portosystemic shunts in those cases where the vascular anomaly can be visualised. Ultrasonographic examination is a poor technique for demonstrating generalised or diffuse hepatocellular disease as the various echo patterns are hard to separate from each other (Lamb 1990) and should not be relied on as final diagnosis (Figs 52.7 and 52.8). Ultrasound-guided liver biopsy sampling is a safe and useful technique for focal as well as generalised liver changes.

Scintigraphy

Nuclear hepatic scintigraphy is a way of diagnosing neoplasia and shunts and accurately assessing the effect of surgical

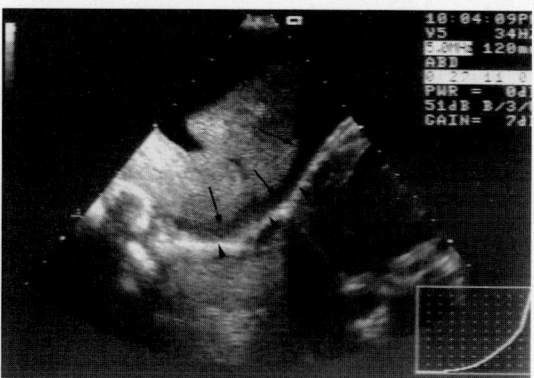

Fig. 52.8 Ultrasonogram of a liver with hepatic fibrosis. The small liver is surrounded by peritoneal effusion marked by arrows. Arrow heads mark diaphragm.

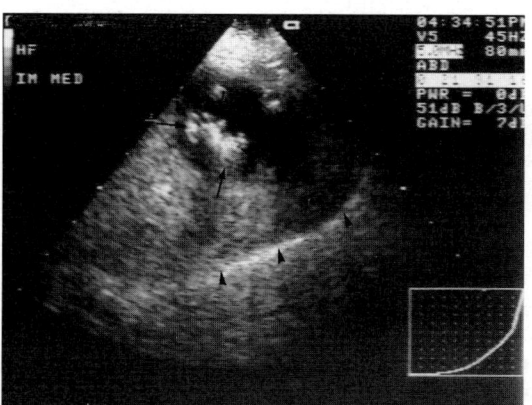

Fig. 52.6 Ultrasonogram of a liver with cholelithiasis. Arrows mark sludge and arrow heads mark diaphragm.

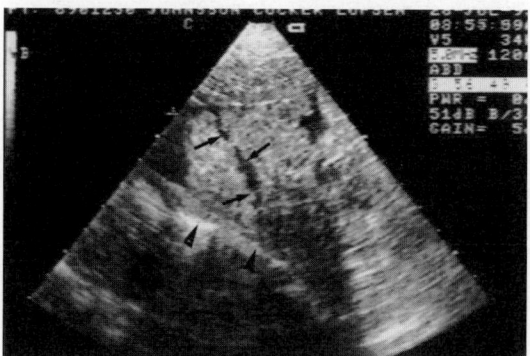

Fig. 52.7 Ultrasonogram of a liver with chronic progressive hepatitis. Arrows mark the irregular lining of the lobule and arrow heads mark diaphragm.

Table 52.9 Indications for liver biopsy.

- Persistent elevations of liver enzymes over a period of time from weeks to months
- Persistent abnormal liver function tests, increased bile acids or hypoalbuminaemia (which may include only hypoalbuminaemia)
- Minor enzyme elevations in dogs with the Pil or S phenotypes
- Unexplainable hepatic radiographic or ultrasonographic changes
- To evaluate response to treatment

correction of portosystemic shunts. Owing to the need for radioactive materials this technique cannot be widely used and is limited to research institutions.

Liver Biopsy

Histopathological examination of a liver biopsy is still the major diagnostic tool for establishing an aetiological diagnosis. For indications see Table 52.9. As far as possible hepatic manifestation of non-hepatic disease should be ruled out. There is no one best method for collection of liver biopsies. The method used depends on the preference and experience of the clinician and on the clinical manifestation of the liver disease. With abdominal effusion and small liver, laparotomy with full visualisation of the liver is recommended. With the laparoscopic and laparotomy techniques wedge biopsies can be taken. Otherwise most commonly a Tru-Cut or Menghini 1.2- or 1.4-mm needle is used (Table 52.10). The small sample obtained is a fundamental limitation of any method so at least two to three biopsies should be taken. Rare complications to biopsy are bile peritonitis and haemorrhage. The patient´s clotting function should be evaluated and if necessary corrected before biopsy. The minimal clotting assay should include activated clotting time (ACT) and platelet count. A more extended assessement of clotting includes prothrombin time (PT) and activated partial thromboplastin time (APTT) and mucosal bleeding time as well.

SPECIFIC DISEASES OF THE LIVER

Hepatic disease may be primary or secondary, acute or chronic, inflammatory or non-inflammatory (Table 52.11). For differential diagnosis see Table 52.12.

Table 52.10   Liver biopsy techniques.

Blind percutanous biopsy
Ultrasound-guided biopsy
At laparotomy with full visualisation of the liver
Keyhole technique
Laparoscopy

Table 52.11   Classification of canine liver disease.

Inflammatory

Infectious
Bacterial
- leptospirosis
- *Salmonella*
- *Helicobacter canis*
Virus (infectious canine hepatitis, herpes virus)

Non-infectious
Chronic hepatitis
Cirrhosis
Idiopathic fibrosis
Toxic liver degeneration

Non-inflammatory
  Portosystemic shunts / vascular dysplasia
  Hepatic fibrosis
  Nodular hyperplasia
  Neoplasia

Table 52.12   Differential diagnosis of secondary canine liver disease.

Hyperadrenocorticism
Diabetes mellitus
Pancreatitis
Chronic bowel disease
Severe bacterial infection/sepsis
Shock
Anaemia
Congestive heart failure
Trauma

Table 52.13   Aetiology of acute hepatitis (acute hepatic failure).

Hepatotoxins	
Drugs	Ketoconazole, mebendazole, oxibendazole, teracyclines, trimpethoprim–sulfadiazine, paracetamol
Toxic agents	Blue-green algae, *Amanita* mushrooms, heavy metals
Infections	
Virus	Infectious canine hepatitis, herpes virus
Bacteriae	Leptospirosis
Mycoses	Histoplasmosis
Protozoa	Toxoplasmosis
Systemic disorders	Acute pancreatitis, haemolytic anaemia
Hepatic injury	Trauma, hyperthermia, diaphragmatic hernia with liver entrapment, anaesthetic hypotension and hypoxia, liver lobe torsion

Acute Hepatic Failure

The clinical and laboratory features of acute hepatic failure are not specific, but reflect disruption of one or more major liver functions such as: metabolism of fat, carbohydrates and protein; synthesis of plasma proteins and coagulation factors; and detoxification and excretions of drugs, toxins and metabolites. For aetiology see Table 52.13.

Infectious Agents

Infectious canine hepatitis caused by canine adenovirus is rare today due to routine vaccination. In leptospirosis, salmonellosis and toxoplasmosis the liver is one of several organ systems involved. Extrahepatic bacterial infection associated with sepsis is an important cause of acute cholestatic hepatopathy. Non-specific bacterial invasion may occasionally occur due to ascending biliary infections.

Toxic Liver Disease

Many substances can damage the liver. The hepatic injury induced varies from mild to fulminant hepatic failure. Disease onset is often very acute with severe clinical signs (Table 52.2).

Diagnosis

Markedly elevated liver enzymes are common. Liver biopsy is useful to verify the diagnosis, but mostly not available in the acute phase of the disease. Hepatic degeneration and necrosis with only slight inflammatory reaction may be seen histologically.

Treatment

Specific therapy is rarely available and symptomatic supportive therapy is usually necessary (Table 52.14).

Chronic Hepatitis

Chronic hepatitis encompasses the majority of cases of canine liver disease. It is an aetiologically diverse group of

diseases, which have been classified in various ways over the years (Table 52.15). Various types of chronic hepatitis have a similar clinical manifestation and can all progress to more severe forms of hepatitis to finally end with liver cirrhosis independent of cause. Many studies over the past years have shown that certain breeds are predisposed to develop liver disease. Aetiology still remains unknown in many cases (Table 52.16).

Copper Associated Hepatitis

An important issue is whether accumulated copper in dogs with chronic hepatitis or cirrhosis is the cause rather than the consequence of the disease. Accumulation of copper may potentially occur secondary to any chronic liver disease with cholestasis that impedes the normal biliary excretion of copper. This is probably the case in various breeds with chronic hepatitis associated with cholestasis. Histochemical examination of liver tissue by special copper stains provide a semiquantative means of demonstrating increased hepatic copper accumulation. Normal hepatic copper concentration in the dog is below 400 ppm and hepatic damage in Bedlington Terriers occurs when copper content exceeds about 2000 ppm.

Copper-storager Hepatitis in Bedlington Terriers

Copper storage hepatitis, chronic progressive hepatitis in Bedlington Terriers, copper hepatoxicosis and copper toxicosis are different names for the inherited disease well known in Bedlington Terriers. The disease is characterised by massive accumulation of copper in hepatic lysosmes. Bedlington hepatitis is inherited in an autosomal recessive

Table 52.14   Treatment of acute hepatic failure.

Specific therapy	Antidotes, e.g. acetylcysteine for paracetamol (140 mg/kg p.o. or i.v. as a 20% solution repeated in 6 h)
Supportive therapy	Fluids and electrolytes. Ringer's solution or 0.9% NaCl with initial supplementation of potassium (20–30 mEq/l of administered fluid) and a bolus of glucose (10–25%)
Therapy for complications	*Hepatic encephalopathy*: Lactulose (5–20 ml t.i.d.–q.i.d., p.o.) Antibiotics (metronidazole 7.5 mg/kg b.i.d.–t.i.d., p.o., and neomycin 10-20 mg/kg t.i.d., p.o. *Ulceration / GI bleeding* Ranitidine (2–4 mg/kg b.i.d., s.c. or i.v.) Famotidine (0.5–1 mg/kg s.i.d.–b.i.d., p.o.) Sucralfate (1 g/25 kg t.i.d.–q.i.d., p.o.)
Prevention of bacteraemia	Cephalexin 15 mg/kg t.i.d., p.o., s.c. or i.m. or Enrofloxacin 2.5 mg/kg, b.i.d., p.o. or i.v.
Dietary management	See Chronic hepatitis

Primary hepatocellular	Intrahepatic cholestasis
Copper toxicosis	Chronic cholangitis
AAT-related chronic hepatitis	Chronic cholangiohepatitis
AAT-related cirrhosis	
Drug-induced chronic hepatits	
Idiopathic chronic non-specific hepatitis	
Idiopathic chronic progressive hepatits	
Virus-induced chronic hepatitis	
Immune-mediated chronic hepatitis?	
Systemic lupus erythaematosus	
Lobular dissecting hepatitis	
Fibrosing hepatopathies	

Table 52.15 Classification of chronic hepatitis.

AAT, α-1-antitrypsin.

Table 52.16 Aetiology of chronic hepatitis.

Metabolic
Primary hepatic copper accumulation (Bedlington Terrier, West Highland White Terrier)
Accumulation of α-1-antitrypsin (AAT) in hepatocytes

Drugs
Anticonvulsants (primidone, phenobarbital)
Antiparasitic (oxibendazole-diethylcarbamazine)

Infections
Infectious canine adenovirus associated hepatitis
Leptospirosis
Helicobacter canis

Idiopathic

manner and the disease is common and world-wide. In the United States, reported prevalence is as high as 66%. A recent Swedish study showed a prevalence of 49% and in the UK about 30% has been reported.

Clinical Signs and Diagnosis. The clinical signs and physical findings vary with the stage of the disease at presentation. There are three forms of copper toxicosis:

(1) *Asymptomatic form* – these dogs are identified when they are routinely checked by biopsy before mating or after routine biochemical screening. Increased serum ALT activity may or may not be present.
(2) *Acute form* – dogs can be presented with fulminant hepatic failure without a previous history of hepatic disease. Clinical signs are acute in onset and include depression, anorexia and vomiting. In some patients,

acute haemolytic anaemia with marked jaundice is present.

Biochemical abnormalities typical of hepatic disease often develop, with markedly increased ALT, ALP and GGT concentrations as well as increased SBA levels, hyperbilirubinaemia and abnormal haemostatic parameters such as PT and APTT. Histochemical staining of a liver biopsy for copper is necessary to confirm the diagnosis. However, it is important to initiate intensive supportive therapy immediately, as this form of the disease is life-threatening. Biopsy sampling should not be performed until the general condition has stabilised.

(3) *Chronic form* – clinical signs are usually observed in middle-aged dogs which exhibit varying degrees of vomiting, depression and weight loss. Icterus and ascites may or may not be present. The haemogram is usually normal. Serum ALT, ALP and GGT activities may be moderately elevated. Hypoalbuminaemia eventually develops. Some dogs do not show clinical signs until cirrhosis has developed. In these cases, ascites and hypoalbuminaemia are often present.

Therapy. Specific therapy in both asymptomatic dogs and in those with chronic disease is as follows.

(1) *Decoppering agents* – D-Penicillamine, 10–15 mg/kg b.i.d. p.o. on empty stomach. May cause vomiting and /or anorexia; if so, decrease the dosage or give trientine, 10–15 mg/kg b.i.d. p.o. Tetramine is related to trientine and appears to be safe, effective and more potent than the other chelators, but it is not available commercially. D-penicillamine and trientine are copper chelator drugs which bind copper and increase its urinary excretion.

Zinc gluconate, 3 mg/kg per day t.i.d. p.o., or zinc sulphate, 2 mg/kg per day t.i.d. p.o. in three doses, on an empty stomach. Zinc compounds decrease intestinal copper absorption rather than increase its excretion. Zinc therapy may be added to chelator therapy but should not be used alone in dogs with hepatitis.

(2) *Vitamins* – Vitamin E, 500 mg/day has an antioxidant effect that protects against lipid peroxidation.

(3) *Feeding* – A low copper diet will inhibit further copper accumulation, but not remove excess hepatic copper. A copper restricted diet is also important in asymptomatic dogs as it can prevent accumulation of copper to hepatotoxic levels.

Commercially made specific diets, low protein diets or a homemade diet based on cottage cheese, boiled egg and rice, supplemented with vegetable oil and balanced vitamin mineral supplement is fed (see Table 52.17).

Bedlingtons with Fulminant Disease. Dogs with fulminant disease need intensive supportive care with correction of fluid, electrolyte and acid–base imbalances:

- Administer half strength saline (0.45%) or Ringer's solution, which is limited in lactate content, to avoid conversion of lactate anions to bicarbonate. Calculate fluid volume needs by assessing rehydration, maintenance requirements and daily losses.
- Glucose supplementation at an initial dosage of 10%, or higher, reduced to 2.5–5% for maintenance.
- Potassium chloride supplementation is recommended (20–30 mEq/l fluid), until serum biochemical results are available.
- Add B complex vitamins (1 IU/l fluid).
- If concomitant signs of haemolytic anaemia are present, give trientine dihydrochloride, which may chelate copper during a haemolytic episode (not D-penicillamine).

Table 52.17 Home made diets for dogs with copper toxicosis

Rice (cooked)	170 ml
Cottage cheese	60 ml
Hard-boiled egg (large)	2
Animal fat	45 ml
Vegetable oil	15 ml
Bone meal	5 ml
Lo-salt	1.5 ml
Multi-vitamin and mineral tablet	1

Recipe can be kept in refrigerator or freezer.
Warm before feeding

Marks *et al.* (1994a & b)

For further management of the stabilised patient with chronic disease see 'Therapeutics' (page 552).

Prognosis
The prognosis is related to the form and stage of the disease at presentation. For dogs presented with the acute, fulminant form of copper storage hepatitis the prognosis is often poor. In the chronic form, the prognosis is fair for dogs presented before severe fibrosis and cirrhosis have developed.

Prevention
The importance of examining a liver biopsy for copper accumulation, before mating any Bedlington terrier must be stressed. To avoid a false-negative diagnosis the biopsy should be taken after 1 year of age.

Copper Associated Hepatitis in West Highland White Terriers
A different type of copper storage hepatitis has been described in West Highland White Terriers in the United States. This disease differs from the Bedlington hepatitis in that the copper accumulation does not progressively increase with age and the copper levels in the West Highland White Terrier do not reach the same height. These dogs can either be asymptomatic or presented with chronic hepatitis or cirrhosis.

Swedish studies have shown an increased incidence of chronic hepatitis and cirrhosis in the West Highland White Terrier, as well. However, only slightly elevated hepatic copper levels were found and were considered secondary to the chronic hepatitis or cirrhosis through decreased biliary excretion. This indicates differences in disease presentation, even in the same breed, between various countries.

Copper Accumulation in Other Breeds

Dobermann Pinschers. Dobermann Pinschers are affected by a chronic hepatitis, histologically resembling idiopathic chronic active hepatitis. Hepatic copper concentrations are often increased, but this has been considered secondary to chronic cholestasis. In the authors' experience there is no uniform histopathological appearance that seems to be related to the stage of the disease at which the dogs are presented. The majority of affected dogs are females and the mean age at presentation is 5 years. Clinical signs are typical of liver disease as described previously, with polydipsia, polyuria, weight loss, ascites, icterus, anorexia, depression, vomiting and diarrhoea. Polydipsia and polyuria are often reported in dogs that have only a few other clinical signs.

Biochemically, liver enzymes are usually markedly increased, in contrast to dogs with chronic progressive hepatitis. Liver biopsy with special copper staining is obligatory to reach a definitive diagnosis and prognosis. The lower copper content, and the periportal location of the copper, indicates that copper accumulation is secondary to cholestasis in Dobermann Pinscher hepatitis, and not primary as in copper toxicosis in the Bedlington Terrier.

Treatment and prognosis:

- Corticosteroids are recommended and reported beneficial in some cases.
- The use of copper chelators is controversial, but may reduce hepatic copper concentrations.
- Ursodeoxycholic acid therapy might be beneficial, but experience of this therapy is limited so far.

For further treatment see 'Therapeutics' (page 552).

Many affected dogs are presented in a late stage of liver disease and the prognosis is often poor. However dogs diagnosed in the early stage of the disease have a favourable prognosis. The longest survivor in one study has lived for more than 5 years.

Skye Terriers. Chronic liver disease associated with accumulation also occurs in Skye Terriers. It is estimated that disturbed biliary secretion of copper and consequent accumulation is caused by abnormal intracellular bile metabolism.

Other Breeds. There are American reports indicating that copper accumulation might be a potential problem in many breeds including Labrador Retrievers, Cocker Spaniels, German Shepherds, Pekingese and others. However, the role copper plays in the development of chronic liver disease in dogs is still debated. In both veterinary and human medicine it is a well established fact that copper accumulation occurs secondary to chronic liver disease. In Sweden we have not, so far, found evidence of primary copper storage disease in any breed other than the Bedlington Terrier. In other breeds, copper staining with rubeanic acid has demonstrated only small numbers of copper granules, mostly periportally, typical of accumulation secondary to liver disease breeds. Most of the diseased dogs had the I-phenotype in either homozygous or heterozygous forms (see 'Isoelectric focusing', page 540).

α-1-Antitrypsin (AAT) Related Hepatitis

Serum deficiency of AAT has long been known to cause chronic liver disease in humans. A corresponding canine disease was recently described (Sevelius & Jönsson 1993; Sevelius *et al.* 1994). Accumulated AAT detected on immunostaining was found in the periportal hepatocytes of dogs with chronic progressive hepatitis and cirrhosis, but

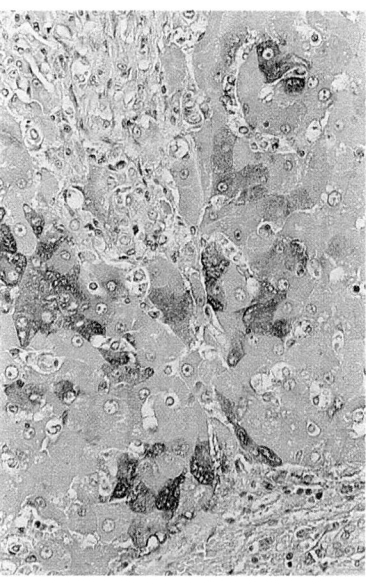

Fig. 52.9 Liver biopsy from an English Cocker Spaniel with chronic progressive hepatitis and the FI phenotype of α-l-antitrypsin (AAT). Accumulation of AAT as brownish globules in the hepatocytes in the periportal tract. (Haematoxylin and eosin.)

also with chronic non-specific hepatitis (Fig. 52.9). English cocker spaniels are predominantly affected, but the disease is also seen in American cocker spaniels and in various other breeds. Most of the diseased dogs have the PiI type homozygously or heterozygously (see 'Isoelectric focusing', page 540). Depending on the stage of the disease when the clinical signs develop the three forms of the disease were:

- non-specific chronic hepatitis,
- chronic progressive hepatitis,
- cirrhosis.

Clinical Signs and History

Dogs with AAT related chronic hepatitis are often presented in late stage of the disease as are also many dogs with other types of chronic hepatitis (Table 52.2). A few dogs have a concomitant haemolytic crisis, the mechanism of which is yet unknown.

Diagnosis

Combining biochemical findings, clinical signs and history with the known breed incidence aids in diagnosing the disease (Table 52.18). Liver biopsy examination with immunostaining for AT is mandatory for diagnosis. Diseased cocker spaniels should always have AAT related disease on the differential list as well as dogs with the PiI phenotype.

Table 52.18 Biochemical parameters in acute and chronic canine liver disease.

Laboratory test	Cirrhosis	Chronic progressive hepatitis*	Chronic non-specific hepatitis*	Acute and chronic cholangio-hepatitis*	Acute liver disease	Portosystemic shunts
ALT	↑	↑	↑↑	↑↑↑↑	↑↑↑↑	↑
ALP	↑↑↑	↑↑	↑↑	↑↑↑↑	↑↑	↑
GGT	↑↑	(↑)	ND	↑↑↑↑	ND	ND
Fasting SBA	↑↑↑	↑↑ (↑)	↔	↑↑↑↑	↑	↑↑
SBA post prandial	ND	ND	ND	ND	ND	↑↑↑↑
Albumin	↓(↓)	(↓)	↔	↔	↔	(↓)
AAT	↔	↔	↑	(↑)	↓	ND
Haptoglobin	↓	↑	↑	↑	(↑)	ND

(Sevelius & Andersson 1995).
* histopathological diagnosis.
ND, not determined in sufficient number of dogs for statistic evaluation; ALT, alanine aminotransferase; ALP, alkoline phosphatase; GGT, γ-glutamyltransferase; SBA, serum bile acids; AAT, γ-1-antitrypsin.

Specific Therapy

Corticosteroids (prednisolone) are given to prohibit further accumulation of AAT globules in the hepatocytes (see 'Therapeutics', page 552).

Prognosis and Disease Prevention

In dogs with early diagnosis and treatment of the disease prognosis is fair. With advanced disease prognosis is poor. Isoelectric focusing of serum from Cocker Spaniels used for breeding is recommended and an annual liver profile on individuals with the PiI should be performed. Even in cases with only minor elevations of liver enzymes a liver biopsy is performed with immunostaining for AAT. If AAT globules are present the dog should not be mated.

Anticonvulsant Drug Induced Chronic Hepatitis

The anticonvulsant drugs primidone and phenobarbitone cause liver enzyme induction, but they can also lead to severe chronic hepatitis and cirrhosis. To minimise the risks of developing liver disease the lowest possible dosage that controls seizures should be given. It is also wise to perform a liver profile and monitor phenobarbitone concentration (15–35 μg/ml) at regular intervals, every 6 months to once a year. If liver disease has developed it may be reversed by decreased dosage or change of drugs, when possible. Phenobarbitone supplemented with potassium bromide may allow dose reduction of phenobarbitone.

Idiopathic Chronic Hepatitis in the Dobermann Pinscher

Dobermanns are affected by a chronic hepatitis histologically resembling chronic active hepatitis in man (Johnson *et al.* 1982). Hepatic copper concentrations are often elevated, but this has been considered secondary to chronic cholestasis. Females are predominantly affected by this disease.

Clinical Signs

See Table 52.2.

Diagnosis

Liver enzymes are usually markedly elevated in contrast to dogs with other types of chronic hepatitis apart from cholangiohepatitis. Liver biopsy is necessary for a definitive diagnosis.

Specific Therapy

Corticosteroids (0.5–1 mg/kg prednisolone reducing to every other day on a long-term basis) are reported beneficial in some cases. The use of copper chelators may reduce hepatic copper concentrations. Ursedeoxycholic acid therapy may be beneficial (see 'Therapeutics', page 552).

Prognosis

Many affected dogs are presented in the late stage of the disease and the prognosis is often poor. Dogs diagnosed in an early stage of the disease have a favourable prognosis.

Cirrhosis

Liver cirrhosis is the end stage of any disease process that causes progressive inflammation, necrosis and fibrosis irrespective of cause.

Clinical Signs and History

Lethargy, anorexia and gastrointestinal signs are commonly reported. Maelena and haematemesis are more commonly seen in cirrhosis than in the other types of chronic liver disease. Ascites is by far the most common clinical finding, icterus is less commonly seen. According to one study 43% of diseased dogs were first presented in a cirrhotic stage showing the silent disease progression in many dogs (Sevelius 1995).

Diagnosis

In some cases liver enzymes as well as SBA concentrations may be normal. Hypoalbuminaemia is the most persistent laboratory finding. In the late stage of the disease the α-globulin fractions are usually markedly decreased on scanning electrophoresis. Ultrasound imaging shows a small nodular liver, but liver biopsy is necessary for a definitive diagnosis (see also Fig. 52.10).

Treatment and Prognosis

Treatment is discussed under 'Therapeutics' (page 552). Overall prognosis is poor, but with normal or increased α-globulins prognosis improves. On the other hand with decreased or almost abolished α-globulins prognosis is poor.

Chronic Cholangiohepatitis

Little is yet known about the aetiology of this disease. Ascending intestinal infections and association with chronic colitis are suggested causes. There is no breed or

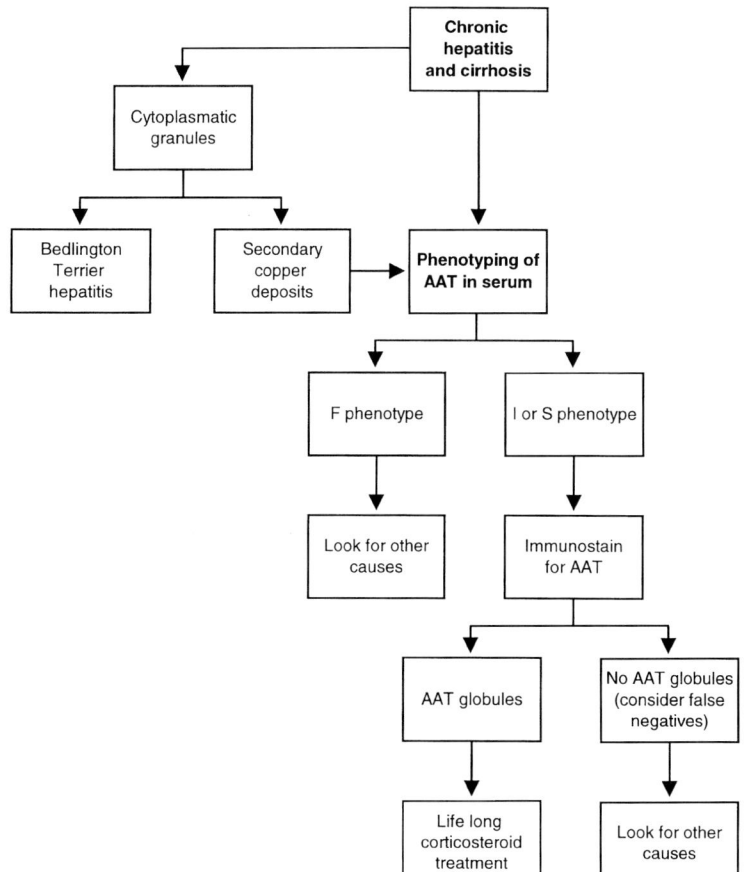

Fig. 52.10 Diagnostic approach to chronic hepatitis and cirrhosis in the dog.

sex predilection. Acute disease relapses are common and icterus is commonly present (Sevelius 1995).

Diagnosis

Marked elevation of liver enzymes and bile acids in combination with icterus are common findings (Table 52.18).

Specific Treatment

Antibiotics should be given in the initial management as infection from the gastrointestinal tract may be suspected (see 'Therapeutics', page 552).

Prognosis

Dogs surviving the initial phase of the disease outbreak have a favourable prognosis.

Lobular Dissecting Hepatitis

Juvenile and young dogs are affected by a disease morphologically similar to chronic progressive hepatitis. Histological features in this disease are fine collagen and reticulin fibres subdividing the lobular parenchyma, piecemeal necrosis and variable mononuclear or mixed cellular inflammatory infiltration. The aetiology for this disease is not known, but it has been described particularly in Rottweilers, Mastín Español and Standard Poodles although it may occur in dogs of various other breeds. The most striking difference from the other types of chronic hepatitis (except idiopathic hepatic fibrosis) is the young age at disease onset. The majority of affected dogs are presented at an age of 7 months or younger. More females than males are affected and many of the diseased dogs are related.

Clinical Signs

Historical complaints and clinical signs are similar to those described for chronic progressive hepatitis, with ascites and weight loss being the major features. Icterus is also commonly reported.

Treatment and Prognosis

Treatment is discussed under 'Therapeutics' (page 552). Most dogs are presented in an advanced stage of the disease and prognosis is reported to be poor.

Idiopathic Hepatic Fibrosis

Hepatic fibrosis is a non-inflammatory disease of unknown aetiology, characterised by increased accumulation of collagen and connective tissue in the liver, with ascites as the most common clinical finding. Red blood cell microcytosis is common on complete blood count. It has been described

in adolescent and young dogs with a predilection for German Shepherds (Rutgers *et al.* 1993).

Diagnosis

Microcytosis and hypoproteinaemia are frequently seen in these cases. Clinical biochemistry shows an increase in most liver enzymes but there are no specific changes. A liver biopsy is necessary to establish diagnosis.

Treatment

Prednisolone 0.5–1.0 mg/kg per day, but this has to be adjusted to meet the needs of each case. Colchicine 0.025 mg/kg is useful and other steps should be taken to minimise the clinical manifestation of hepatic encephalopathy.

Prognosis

Long-term survival is possible but prognosis should be guarded.

Portosystemic Shunts

Portosystemic shunts (PSS) are congenital or acquired vascular anomalies between the portal and systemic venous systems. A variety of shunts have been described. Acquired shunts may form in response to portal hypertension as a result of cirrhosis or chronic hepatitis, which opens up collateral vessels around the liver.

Any portosystemic shunt will lead to hepatic atrophy and the development of hepatic encephalopathy.

Clinical Signs

These are highly variable (see 'Hepatic encephalopathy', page 537).

Diagnosis

Liver enzymes may be slightly elevated in PSS. Plasma urea and creatinine are usually low and postprandial bile acids markedly elevated. Microcytosis of red blood cells are present in two-thirds of the cases. Biurate crystals in the urine are highly suspicious of PSS. The diagnosis is confirmed by contrast venoportography or when the shunt is visualised with ultrasonography.

Treatment

Surgery is the only successful method of treatment. Correction of extrahepatic shunts is more rewarding than correction of intrahepatic shunts. Several approaches to shunt correction are described (Hardy 1989). For presurgical medical treatment see Table 52.6.

Presurgical Management

- Restrict dietary protein, using commercial low protein diets. If a homemade diet is chosen, cottage cheese is recommended as a primary protein source. The daily protein intake should be a maximum 2 g/kg. Supplementation with vitamins A, B, C, E and K is recommended.

- Lactulose is given orally at a daily dosage of 5–20 ml.
- Neomycin should be administered at a dosage of 10–20 mg/kg p.o. s.i.d.
- Phenobarbitone is administered intravenously to dogs with seizures after hypoglycaemia has been ruled out. Lactulose enema may also be beneficial for these patients.
- 25% dextrose solution is given intravenously to dogs with seizures related to hypoglycaemia.

Surgical Treatment. The goal of surgery is to identify the shunting vessel(s) and to ligate it (them), with simultaneous measurement of portal vein pressure, (which should not exceed 20–23 cmH₂O). The ligature can be tied loosely, initially, then adjusted as necessary before the knot is locked. Monitoring heart rate, systemic blood pressure and observing the colour of viscera are important during surgery. Hypothermia should be prevented by using heating pads and warm intravenous fluids. The most serious postsurgical complication is life-threatening shock associated with severe portal hypertension.

While several approaches to intrahepatic shunt are described, correction of extrahepatic shunts is rewarding. It must be emphasised that surgical management should only be attempted by an experienced surgeon.

Postsurgical Management. Careful monitoring and the initial postsurgical period is critical to the outcome to surgery:

- Monitor body temperature, packed cell volume and blood glucose regularly every 1–4 h (the more frequently the better).
- Measure albumin concentration daily.
- Administer dextrose intravenously if hypoglycaemia is present.
- Fluids are given intravenously with supplementation of 2.5–5% dextrose and 20–30 mEq/l potassium per litre fluid when needed.
- Seizures are severe complications after surgery. Symptomatic treatment includes normalising blood glucose, electrolytes and acid–base balance as well as giving phenobarbitone intravenously. Occasionally, seizures, due to cerebral oedema, are a complication of surgical shunt ligation. Osmotic agents, such as mannitol, reduce intracranial pressure by decreasing brain water content. A 20% solution of mannitol is usually given (0.5–2 g/kg i.v.) every 4–6 h. Prognosis with this complication is poor.
- When needed, nutritional support should be given.

Cholelstasis

Cholestasis may be produced by intrinsic liver disease and is then called intrahepatic cholestasis, seen predominantly with cholangiohepatitis but also with other liver diseases such as cirrhosis, toxic secondary hepatitis and liver tumours. Extrahepatic cholestasis, which tends to be more severe, is caused by obstruction of the large bile ducts. It is most frequently caused by pancreatic tumours, but is also seen with duodenal tumours, inflammatory processes and biliary stones. In any event, cholestasis represents a defect in the transport of bile across the canalicular membrane.

Cholelithiasis

Choleliths (gallstones) may be incidental findings observed during imaging with ultrasonography or at necropsy. Aged, female, small-breed dogs appear to be at increased risk for the development of choleliths. Sometimes the gallstones are clinically silent, but they may be associated with cholecystitis and cause vomiting, anorexia, jaundice, fever and abdominal pain. Dogs develop cholesterol, bilirubin and mixed stones. The rarity of canine cholelithiasis, compared with man may be due to:

- decreased concentrations of cholesterol in canine bile;
- absorption of ionised calcium from the gall bladder, limiting the amount of free ionised calcium in bile.

Diagnosis
As choleliths are usually radiolucent, ultrasonography is an excellent method for diagnosis.

Treatment
Surgical removal is indicated in patients with choleliths associated with hepatobiliary disease.

Steroid Hepatopathy

This hepatic disorder is caused by either exogenous steroid administration or endogenous hyperadrenocorticism. Steroid hepatopathy should be considered in dogs with hepatomegaly, which is due to glycogen accumulation in the hepatocytes. The clinical signs are those of hypercorticism, including polyuria/polydipsia. Increased serum ALP activity is the most consistent biochemical abnormality. Serum albumin, bilirubin and blood ammonia concentrations are normal. Liver biopsy may be necessary to rule out other causes of liver disease and shows typical vacuolisation of the hepatocytes.

Steroid hepatopathy is reversible after withdrawal of exogenous cellucocorticoids or treatment of spontaneous hyperadrenocorticism. The length of time required for complete resolution is unpredictable, varying from weeks to months. In general, the greater the dose and duration of steroid therapy, the longer the time required for the hepatopathy to resolve.

Nodular Hyperplasia

Nodular hyperplasia of the liver is an age-related phenomenon. It is a common post-mortem finding in dogs over 8 years of age with no breed or sex predilection. No specific cause of nodular hyperplasia has been identified in dogs. The hyperplastic nodules are usually not associated with clinical signs but can cause moderate increases in serum ALT and marked increase in ALP activity.

The significance of nodular hyperplasia to the clinician is that when hepatic nodules are identified by ultrasonography, laparoscopy or surgery, benign nodular hyperplasia should be considered in the differential diagnosis. The hyperplastic nodules can become quite large and mimic hepatocellular adenoma or carcinoma. Histologically, it can be difficult to differentiate hyperplastic nodules from neoplasia by a small sample from a needle biopsy. Thus, a wedge biopsy obtained at surgery is usually necessary.

Liver Tumours

Hepatic neoplasia can be either primary or metastatic, the latter being far more common than the former. Primary tumours are hepatocellular carcinoma and bile duct carcinoma. Biochemical abnormalities are unspecific and variable and can mimic both extrahepatic disease and chronic hepatitis. Exploratory laparotomy in combination with histopathological evaluation is the best way to get a diagnosis. Benign nodular hyperplasia is common in dogs and should not be confused with hepatic tumours. Needle biopsy may provide a diagnosis particularly in cases with diffuse hepatic malignant lymphoma.

THERAPEUTICS

Acute Hepatitis

When a tentative diagnosis of acute hepatitis is made intensive initial therapy is often necessary. Removal of the causative agent is ideal but often impossible, therefore the goal is to support the dog until hepatic regeneration occurs. For this, intensive fluid therapy, management of hepatic encephalopathy and bleeding disorders as well as prevention of bacteriaemia are mandatory (Table 52.14).

The optimal therapy for chronic hepatitis includes removing the causative agent, stimulating hepatocellular regeneration and healing, limiting the inflammatory process, and supporting the patient by symptomatic therapy and by controlling complications such as hepatic encephalopathy and bleeding disorders. It is essential to follow up the effect of long-term treatment by repeated liver biopsy in 6–12 months.

Therapy for Chronic Hepatitis
(Table 52.19)

Supportive and Symptomatic

Fluid therapy is often needed in treating the initial episode of chronic hepatitis regardless of cause. Half strength saline (0.45%) with dextrose (2.5%) is the fluid of choice. Potassium levels should be monitored and potassium supplemented as indicated by serum potassium levels (20–25 mEq/l fluids). Rest is important in the initial management as it reduces pain and provides an increased hepatic blood flow facilitating hepatic cell regeneration.

Anti-Inflammatory and Antifibrotic

Anti-inflammatory treatment of chronic hepatitis seems to be beneficial in many cases although the use of corticosteroids is controversial and there are no controlled studies to prove their effect in dogs. Rationales for using corticosteroids are:

- to inhibit immune reactions found in many dogs with various types of chronic hepatitis (Andersson & Sevelius 1992);

Table 52.19 Therapeutic concerns in chronic hepatitis.

Removal of the causative agent
Specific – directed against a causative agent
Supportive and symptomatic
Anti-inflammatory and antifibrotic
Antioxidant therapy
Dietary management
Gastrointestinal ulceration
Reduction of hepatotoxic bile acids
Infection
Ascites
Coagulopathies
Hepatic encephalopathy

- to prohibit further accumulation of AAT globules in the hepatocytes, as corticosteroids are potent inhibitors of interleukin-1, interleukin-6 and tumour necrosis factor synthesis and may help in terminating the acute phase response;
- to inhibit the progression of fibrosis.

Prednisolone (0.5–1 mg/kg per day) is recommended initially, with the dose gradually tapering to 0.25 mg/kg every other day. The clinician must be aware of the risks including increasing severity and mortality in bacterial cholangiohepatitis and viral hepatitis. Corticosteroids may also worsen signs of hepatic encephalopathy. Colchicine inhibits collagen secretion and stimulates collagenase activity to break down fibrous tissue in the liver. Clinical improvement and increased long-term survival have been reported in man. Clinical trials of these beneficial effects in dogs are restricted to three single case reports. Recommended dosage is 0.03 mg/kg per day, p.o. is recommended for 6–30 months.

Antioxidant

Recent reports indicate that decreased levels of the antioxidant vitamin E in hepatocytes contributes to oxidant damage of the hepatocytes. For this reason treatment with high dosage of vitamin E (500 mg/day) may be beneficial in diminishing oxidant damage by protecting against lipid peroxidation.

Dietary

Nutritional support is important in the management of hepatic insufficiency. Good quality protein should be fed to minimise production of nitrogenous wastes. Protein intake must be restricted if there is impending or ongoing hepatic encephalopathy. If this is the case, the calorie deficit is made up by easily digestible, complex carbohydrates, such as rice and pasta. Fat intake should be restricted in dogs with severe obliterative liver disease or major bile duct obstruction. Frequent feeding of small meals will help minimise gluconeogenesis from muscle and breakdown of hepatic glycogen, and enhance protein and glucose tolerance. Addition of soluble dietary fibres is reported to be beneficial in forming a number of organic acids, which decrease colonic pH and consequently reduce ammonia production and absorption. Insoluble dietary fibres will help prevent constipation, which is an important risk factor for hepatic encephalopathy. Protein-restricted diets for the management of chronic renal failure can be fed, but are not ideal. A diet specifically designed to meet the complex nutritional requirements of dogs with liver disease is available.

Vitamins and Minerals

Vitamins B, C and E should be supplemented in most cases. Vitamin K may be indicated in rare patients with haemorrhagic tendencies associated with prolonged cholestasis, in which case parenteral administration may be required. Dietary zinc supplementation may be needed as deficiency is reported in hepatic disease, where it is associated with reduced ammonia tolerance. Zinc may also have an antifibrotic effect with reduced ammonia tolerance and may inhibit hepatic accumulation of copper. Intakes of sodium and copper should be restricted in dogs with ascites and hepatic copper accumulation, respectively.

Gastric Ulceration

Ranitidine or famotidine is indicated to prevent and treat gastrointestinal bleeding in patients with gastrointestinal ulceration or coagulopathy particularly when corticosteroids are given. Sucralfate is a local ulcer-protecting agent which is not absorbed. It can be given concurrently to other medication.

Reducing Hepatotoxic Bile Acids

Ursodeoxycholic acid (8–15 mg/kg, s.i.d.) is effective in reducing toxic bile acids which cause hepatocellular death and inflammation. Another beneficial effect of ursodeoxycholic acid may be related to immunomodulation by reducing the aberrant major histocompatibility complex class I. In humans it is reported to be effective predominantly in patients with severe cholestatic liver disease.

Infection or Sepsis

Amoxycillin (22 mg/kg b.i.d. p.o.) with metronidazole (7.5 mg/kg b.i.d.) is a good choice of antibiotic combination for initial treatment.

Ascites

Acute phase induced ascites usually resolves quickly without administration of diuretics. Patients with mild ascites may be treated with sodium restricted diet and cage rest. If this is insufficient to control ascites cautious diuretic treatment is initiated with spironolactone (1–2 mg/kg b.i.d.) or furosemide (1–2 mg/kg b.i.d.). Once ascites is reversed diuretics should be withdrawn.

Coagulopathy

Management of coagulopathy must be aggressive. Fresh whole blood or fresh plasma transfusion is necessary to provide clotting factors. Heparin (100 units/kg, i.v. or s.c. t.i.d.) therapy should be started in cases of disseminated intravascular coagulopathy with frequent monitoring of coagulation parameters. Prognosis is poor if reponse to treatment has not occurred within 24–48 h. Chronic cholestatic disease and bile duct obstruction can induce vitamin K deficiency. Injections of vitamin K1 (1 mg/kg per day i.m.) are given and will help reverse prothrombinaemia associated with bile duct obstruction.

Hepatic encephalopathy

See Table 52.6.

REFERENCES

Andersson, M. & Sevelius, E. (1992). Circulating autoantibodies in dogs with chronic liver disease. *Journal of Small Animal Practice*, **33**, 389–394.

Center, S.A., Baldwin, B.H., Erb, H.N. & Tennant, B.C. (1985). Bile acid concentrations in the diagnosis of hepatobiliary disease in the dog. *Journal of American Veterinary Medical Association*, **187**, 935–940.

Eckersall, P.D. & Conner, J.G. (1988). Bovine and canine acute phase proteins. *Veterinary Research Communications*, **12**, 169–178.

Hardy, R.M. (1989). Diseases of the liver and their treatment. In: *Textbook of Veterinary Internal Medicine*, (ed. S.J. Ettinger), 3rd edn. pp. 1479–1527. W.B. Saunders, Philadelphia.

Johnson, G.F., Zawie, D.A., Gilbertson, S.R. & Sternlieb, I. (1982). Chronic active hepatitis in Doberman pinschers. *Journal of American Veterinary Medical Association*, **180**, 1438–1442.

Juneja, R.K., Reetz, I., Christensen, K., Gahne, B. & Andresen, E. (1981). Two dimensional gel electrophoresis of dog plasma proteins. Genetic polymorphism of an alpha 1-protease inhibitor and another postalbumin. *Hereditas*, **95**, 225–233.

Lamb, C.R. (1990). Abdominal ultrasonography in small animals: Examination of the liver, spleen and pancreas. *Journal of Small Animal Practice*, **31**, 6–15.

Marks, S.L., Rogers, Q.R. & Strombeck, D.R. (1994a). Nutritional support in hepatic disease. Part 1 Metabolic alterations and nutritional considerations in dogs and cats. *Compendium on Continuing Education for the Practicing Veterinarian*, **16**, 971–979.

Marks, S.L., Rogers, Q.R. & Strombeck, D.R. (1994b). Nutritional support in hepatic disease. Part 2 Dietary management of common liver disorders in dogs and cats. *Compendium on Continuing Education for the Practicing Veterinarian*, **16**, 1287–1296.

Rothuizen, J. & van den Ingh, T. (1988). Covalently protein-bound bilirubin conjugates in cholestatic disease of dogs. *American Journal of Veterinary Research*, **49**, 702–704.

Rutgers, H.C., Haywood, S. & Kelly, D.F. (1993). Idiopathic hepatic fibrosis in 15 dogs. *Veterinary Record*, **133**, 115–118.

Sevelius, E. (1995). Diagnosis and prognosis of chronic hepatitis and cirrhosis in dogs. *Journal of Small Animal Practice*, **36**, 521–528.

Sevelius, E. & Andersson, M. (1995). Serum protein electrophoresis as a prognostic marker of chronic canine liver disease. *Veterinary Record*, **137**, 663–667.

Sevelius, E. & Jönsson, L. (1993). Some new pathogenic aspects of chronic liver disease in the dog. *Proceedings of the 11th Annual ACVIM Forum*, Washington DC. pp. 253–255. ACVIM, Blacksberg, Virginia.

Sevelius, E., Andersson, M. & Jönsson, L. (1994). Hepatic accumulation of alpha-1-antitrypsin in chronic liver disease in the Dog. *Journal of Comparative Pathology*, **111**, 401–412.

Teske, E., Rothuizen, J., De Bruijne, J.J. & Mol, A. (1986). Separation and heat stability of the coticosteroid-induced and hepatic alkaline phosphatase isoenzymes in canine plasma. *Journal of Chromatography*, **369**, 349–356.

FURTHER READING

Boer, H., Nelson, R.W. & Long, G.G. (1984). Colchicine therapy for hepatic fibrosis in a dog. *Journal of American Veterinary Medical Association*, **185**, 303–305.

Bunch, S.E. (1994). Specific and symptomatic medical management of diseases of the liver. In: *Textbook of Veterinary Internal Medicine*, (ed. S.J. Ettinger), 4th edn. pp. 1358–1371. W.B. Saunders, Philadelphia.

Center, S.A. (1994). Pathophysiology and laboratory diagnosis, and diseases of the liver. In: *Textbook of Veterinary Internal Medicine*, (ed. S.J. Ettinger), 4th edn. pp. 1261–1312. W.B. Saunders, Philadelphia.

Dayrell-Hart, B., Steinberg, S.A., Vanwinkle, T.J. & Farnbach, G.C. (1991). Hepatotoxicity of phenobarbital in dogs: 18 cases (1985–1989). *Journal of American Veterinary Medical Association*, **199**, 1060–1066.

Heinrich, P.C., Castell, I.V. & Andus, T. (1990). Interleukin 6 and the acute phase response. *Biochemical Journal*, **265**, 621–636.

Holt, D. (1994). Critical care management of the portosystemic shunt patient. *Compendium on Continuing Education for the Practicing Veterinarian*, **16**, 879–892.

Johnson, S.E. (1994). Diseases of the liver. In: *Textbook of Veterinary Internal Medicine*, (ed. S.J. Ettinger), 4th edn. pp. 1313–1357. W.B. Saunders, Philadelphia.

Meyer, D.J. & Thompson, M.B. (1993). Bile acids – Beyond their value as a liver function test. In: *Proceedings of the 11th ACVIM Forum*, Washington DC, 210–212.

Rutgers, H.C. & Harte, J.G. (1994). Hepatic disease. In: *The Waltham Book of Clinical Nutrition of the Dog and Cat*, (eds J.M. Wills & K.W. Simpson), pp. 239–276. Pergamon Press, Oxford.

Rutgers, H.C., Haywood, S. & Batt, R.M. (1990). Colchicine treatment in a dog with hepatic fibrosis. *Journal of Small Animal Practice*, **31**, 97–101.

Solter, P.F., Hoffman, W.E., Hungerford, L.L., Siegel, J.P., St. Denis, S.H. & Dorner, J.L. (1991). Haptoglobin and ceruloplasmin as determinants of inflammation in dogs. *American Journal of Veterinary Research*, **52**, 1738–1742.

Twedt, D. (1985). Cirrhosis: A consequence of chronic liver disease. *Veterinary Clinics of North America*, **15**(1), 151–176.

Weiss, D.J., Armstrong, P.J. & Mruthyunjaya, A. (1995). Anti-liver membrane protein antibodies in dogs with chronic hepatitis. *Journal of Internal Veterinary Medicine*, **9**, 267–271.

Woo, P. & Gorman, N.T. (1989). The acute-phase protein response and amyloidosis. In: *Veterinary Clinical Immunology*, (eds R.E.W. Halliwell & N.T. Gorman), pp. 97–106. W.B. Saunders, Philadelphia.

Chapter 53

Diseases of the Exocrine Pancreas

K. W. Simpson

The exocrine pancreas has a major role in the digestion of food. It secretes enzymes that are capable of digesting a wide variety of foodstuffs and bicarbonate-rich fluid which serves to solubilise secreted enzymes and neutralise gastric acid so that optimal enzyme activity is maintained. Pancreatic secretions have an important role in the absorption of cobalamin (vitamin B_{12}) and the regulation of the small intestinal bacterial flora and directly influence small intestinal function by modifying certain enzymes on the intestinal brush border and exerting trophic effects on the mucosa.

Disease of the exocrine pancreas is most often a consequence of inflammation (acute or chronic) or a reduction in pancreatic mass. Neoplasia and infection are less common causes of disease.

STRUCTURE AND FUNCTION OF THE EXOCRINE PANCREAS

Structure

The canine pancreas consists of a right and left lobe joined together by a central body and is situated in the cranial abdomen in close proximity to the stomach and duodenum. Pancreatic secretions are routed into the intestine via a duct system. In most dogs the duct system consists of a central duct which arises from both lobes of the pancreas and communicates within the pancreas. Secretions reach the intestine through two ducts which communicate with the central duct. These ducts terminate on intestinal papillae known as the major and minor duodenal papillae. The major duodenal papilla is shared with the common bile duct and is located a few centimetres proximal to the minor papilla.

Histologically the pancreas is composed of many secretory lobules which are made up of acinar cells. These secretory acini are drained by a branching duct system which is lined by a variety of epithelial cells. The acini and ducts are surrounded by a dense network of capillaries, nerves and lymphatics.

Function

Pancreatic acinar cells are responsible for the synthesis of digestive enzymes which can be broadly categorised according to their substrate as: proteolytic, e.g. trypsin, chymotrypsin, elastase, carboxypeptidase; amylolytic, e.g. amylase; lipolytic, e.g. lipase, phospholipase. Pancreatic duct cells secrete bicarbonate-rich fluid and pancreatic intrinsic factor. The site of production of bacteriocidal peptides and certain ill-defined trophic factors has not been clearly established.

Synthesis and Secretion of Enzymes

Digestive enzymes are synthesised in the endoplasmic reticulum and undergo modification in the Golgi apparatus (Fig. 53.1a). It is in the Golgi stacks that proteins destined for export are segregated from intracellular proteins and are packaged into condensing vacuoles which mature into zymogen granules. Zymogen granules migrate towards the luminal cell membrane where fusion with the cell membrane results in the discharge of their contents into the acinar ductal space. Zymogen granule membranes then appear to be endocytosed and recycled.

Many of the enzymes synthesised by the pancreas can injure cells and tissues. The pancreas is protected from autodigestion by several mechanisms: (1) potentially harmful digestive enzymes are secreted in an inactive form and are activated only on entry into the duodenum by trypsin following its activation by the brush border enzyme enterokinase; (2) between synthesis and secretion the

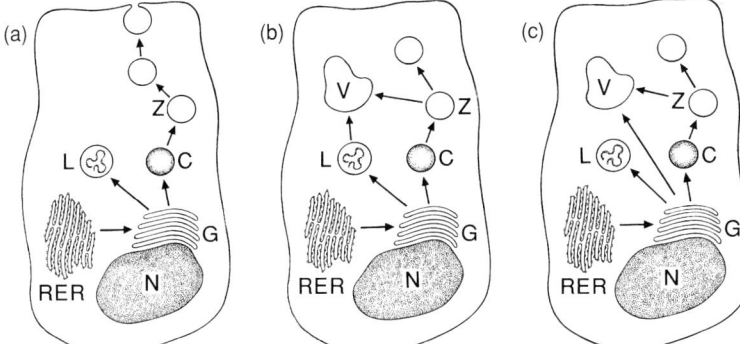

Fig. 53.1 Intracellular trafficking of digestive and lysosomal enzymes. Digestive and lysosomal enzymes are synthesised in the rough endoplasmic reticulum (RER) and transported to the Golgi apparatus (G) next to the nucleus (N).

(a). Normal separation of lysosomal and digestive enzymes. Digestive enzymes are concentrated in condensing vacuoles (C) and zymogen granules (Z) that fuse with the luminal plasma membrane and release their contents into the luminal space by exocytosis.

(b). A choline deficient ethionine supplemented diet blocks exocytosis and zymogen granules accumulate. The zymogen granules fuse with lysosomes (L) to form large vacuoles (V) which contain digestive and lysosomal enzymes.

(c). Hyperstimulation with cerulein results in co-segregation of lysosomal and digestive enzymes in large vacuoles. Mature zymogen granules also fuse with these vacuoles. Exocytosis at the luminal plasma membrane is blocked. (Adapted from Steer & Meldoplesi 1987)

enzymes are contained in membrane-bound zymogen granules; (3) potent enzyme inhibitors (e.g. pancreatic secretory trypsin inhibitor) are present within acinar cells and zymogen granules and serve to inactivate small amounts of prematurely activated enzymes.

Fluid and Electrolyte Secretion

The cells lining the duct system appear to be the major site of fluid and electrolyte secretion. Fluid composition changes according to the volume of secretion. At low rates of secretion the concentrations of chloride are higher than those of bicarbonate, whereas at higher rates the bicarbonate concentration is higher than chloride. Bicarbonate is responsible for solubilising zymogens within the pancreatic duct system and neutralising gastric acid in the duodenum to provide an optimal pH for pancreatic enzyme activity. Pancreatic duct cells also produce intrinsic factor (IF) which is a protein necessary for the absorption of cobalamin (vitamin B_{12}).

Regulation of Pancreatic Secretion

Phases of Secretion
Classically, pancreatic response to a meal has been divided into cephalic, gastric and intestinal phases. Under normal

feeding conditions these phases overlap and occur simultaneously, though the intestinal phase appears to be quantitatively the most important.

Stimulants of Secretion
The intestinal phase starts when chyme enters the duodenum. Protein digestion products such as peptides and amino acids (especially tryptophan and phenylalanine) and the products of fat digestion, long-chain fatty acids (>C8) and monoglycerides are potent stimulants of pancreatic enzyme secretion. Gastric acid entering the duodenum is a major stimulant of pancreatic fluid and electrolyte secretion.

Mediation of Secretion
The cephalic and gastric phases are mediated by the vagus nerve and the release of hormones such as gastrin. The intestinal phase is mediated by a variety of neuroendocrine mechanisms. Enteropancreatic, cholinergic and vagovagal systems seem to be important mediators of the enzyme response to low loads of amino acids and fatty acids. Hormones, particularly cholecystokinin (CCK: released from the intestine into the bloodstream), appear to be the major mediators of enzyme secretion in response to high loads of amino and fatty acids. Cholecystokinin is also the principle mediator of pancreatic intrinsic factor secretion in the dog. Secretin released by gastric acid is probably the most important physiological mediator of pancreatic bicar-

bonate secretion. There are synergistic effects of secretin and CCK on pancreatic fluid and electrolyte secretion. The pancreas not only secretes in response to a meal but secretes cyclically throughout the day. Peaks in interdigestive secretion are accompanied by an increase in biliary secretion and intestinal motility. These cycles are thought to be mediated by motilin and may serve as an intestinal housekeeper by flushing digestive products, cell debris and bacteria along the intestine.

Inhibition of exocrine pancreatic secretion has not been studied as extensively as stimulation. However it appears that glucagon and somatostatin decrease pancreatic secre-

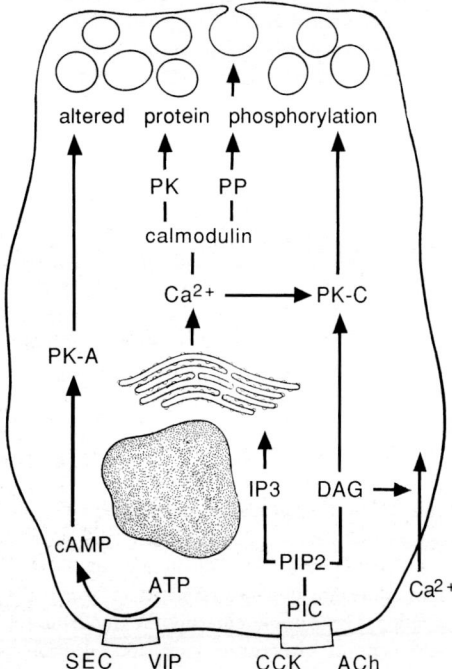

Fig. 53.2 Summary diagram of stimulus–secretion coupling of pancreatic acinar cell protein secretion. Cholecystokinin (CCK) and acetyl choline (ACh) act via the second messengers inositol triphosphate and diacylaglycerol, and secretin (SEC) and vasoactive intestinal peptide (VIP) via cyclic AMP (cAMP), to cause increases in intracellular calcium and protein kinases which result in altered phosphorylation of structural and regulatory proteins and acinar cell protein secretion. Abbreviations: PIP2, phosphatidylinositol-4,5-bisphosphate; IP3, inositol-1,4,5-triphosphate; DAG, diacylglycerol; PK-A, cyclic-AMP-activated protein kinase; PK, protein kinase; PP, protein phosphatase; PK-C, phospholipid-dependent protein kinase; PIC, phosphorolipase C. (Reproduced from Simpson 1993)

tion. Products of digestion and proteolytic enzymes may also have a role in inhibiting pancreatic secretion possibly by decreasing the release of mucosal CCK, though this has not been clearly demonstrated in the dog.

Stimulus Secretion Coupling

The major agonists of pancreatic secretion are CCK and acetylcholine for enzymes, and secretin for fluid and electrolytes. These substances bind to specific receptors located on the basal membranes of acinar and duct cells and stimulate the release of intracellular second messengers. This results in the alteration of protein phosphorylation and fusion and discharge of zymogen granule contents into the acino ductal space in acinar cells, and fluid secretion from ductal cells (Fig. 53.2). CCK receptors on pancreatic duct cells presumably mediate IF secretion.

Adaptation of Pancreatic Enzyme Secretion to Diet

In addition to their role in mediating secretion CCK, secretin and insulin, and their second messengers, regulate the synthesis of digestive enzymes. Adaptation to diets of different protein, fat and carbohydrate content has been clearly demonstrated in rats: increased synthesis of proteolytic enzymes occurs in response to increasing dietary protein, increased synthesis of lipase in response to triglyceride and increased synthesis of amylase in response to carbohydrate. These increases in synthesis appear to be mediated by CCK via phospholipase C for protein, secretin via adenylate cyclase for lipase and insulin, possibly via tyrosine kinase, for amylase. Increased enzyme synthesis is not accompanied by increased transcription of the appropriate mRNA when diets are fed for periods of up to 24h. However increases in mRNA can be measured when diets are fed for more prolonged periods. These observations suggest that the pancreas is well adapted to making short- and long-term changes in the synthesis of digestive enzymes in response to changing dietary intake.

PANCREATITIS

Inflammation of the pancreas can be broadly categorised as acute, recurrent acute or chronic. Acute and recurrent acute pancreatitis are characterised by sudden episodes of inflammation and appear to be the most frequent form of pancreatitis in the dog. Acute pancreatitis may resolve or may cause continued inflammation (chronic or recurrent acute) or necrosis which can be complicated by secondary infection and pseudocyst or abscess formation (Fig. 53.3). Chronic pancreatitis is characterised by low-grade or subclinical inflammation and may be a factor in the develop-

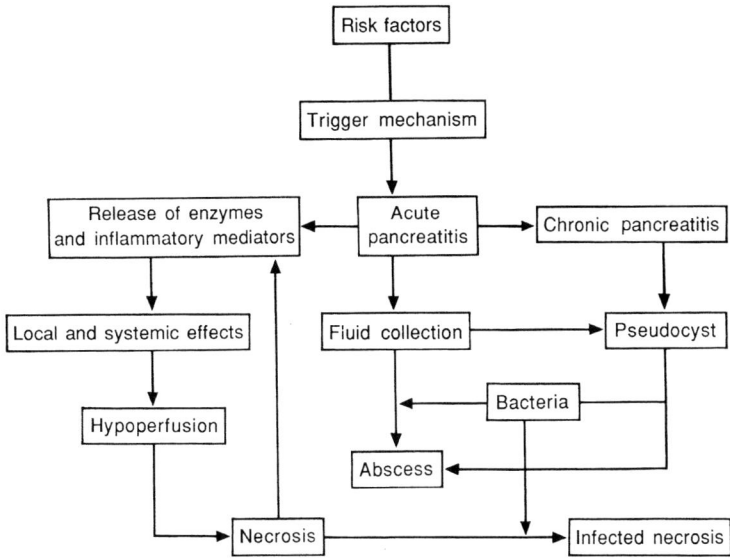

Fig. 53.3 Schematic diagram of the proposed progression of pancreatitis in dogs. (From Simpson & Lamb 1995)

ment of diabetes mellitus and exocrine pancreatic insufficiency (EPI) in dogs.

Pathogenesis

Although it is known that pancreatitis can occur following abdominal trauma (including surgical manipulation of the pancreas), the pathogenesis of spontaneous canine pancreatitis is poorly understood. Numerous potential aetiological factors have been linked to acute pancreatitis in dogs including hyperlipidaemia, obesity, high fat diet, glucocorticosteroids, hypercalcaemia, certain drugs and toxins and, possibly, a hereditary predisposition in Miniature Schnauzers.

Irrespective of the initiating cause pancreatitis is generally believed to occur when digestive enzymes are activated prematurely within the pancreas. Information on the cellular events that are associated with the development of pancreatitis has been provided by experimental models. Pancreatic hyperstimulation with CCK (or its analogue cerulein), dietary supplementation with ethionine, calcium infusion and obstruction of the pancreatic duct lead to the formation of large intracellular vacuoles in acinar cells (Fig. 53.1b & c, Fig. 53.4). Vacuole formation is thought to be a consequence of the uncoupling of exocytosis of zymogens and abnormal intracellular trafficking of digestive and lysosomal enzymes (Fig. 53.1b & c). These subcellular perturbations are thought to facilitate the intracellular activation of digestive enzymes.

Oedematous pancreatitis induced by CCK hyperstimulation in dogs is characterised by a rapidly developing but

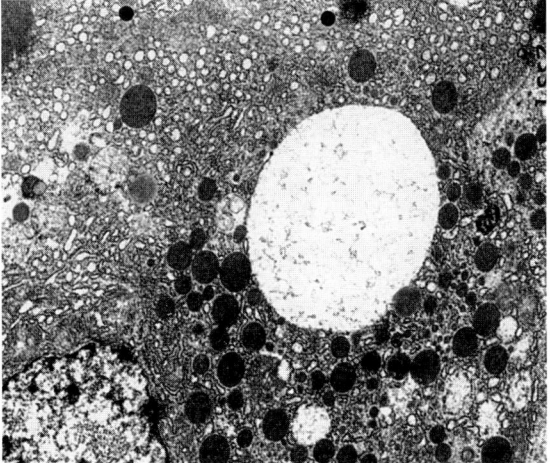

Fig. 53.4 Electron micrograph of a pancreatic acinar cell after cholecystokinin (CCK) infusion (10 µg/kg per hour for 6 h). Large intracytoplasmic vacuoles are evident which probably reflect a block on exocytosis and abnormal intracellular trafficking of digestive enzymes.

self-limiting burst of trypsinogen activation. This finding suggests an ability of the pancreas to regulate trypsinogen activation after it has been initiated and may explain why mild oedematous pancreatitis does not always progress to severe necrotising pancreatitis. Pancreatic hyperstimulation may also be of direct relevance to naturally occurring pancreatitis in dogs. CCK is normally released by cells in the duodenum in response to intraluminal fat and amino acids and co-ordinates and stimulates pancreatic secretion and gallbladder contraction during digestion. It is possible that high fat diets exert their effects via the excessive release of cholecystokinin and that hypercalcaemia, organophosphates and high levels of circulating glucocorticoids also facilitate or cause pancreatic hyperstimulation; however, this has not been proved.

Often pancreatic inflammation is a self-limiting process, but in some animals reduced pancreatic blood flow and leukocyte migration into the inflamed pancreas may cause progression of mild pancreatitis to pancreatic necrosis (Fig. 53.3). Secondary infection may arise by bacterial translocation from the intestine. Release of active pancreatic enzymes and inflammatory mediators into the systemic circulation adversely affect the function of many organs and cause derangements in fluid balance.

Further study of the cellular mechanisms governing enzyme secretion, activation and limitation of activation will hopefully provide information that will be useful in preventing and ameliorating acute pancreatitis in the patient population.

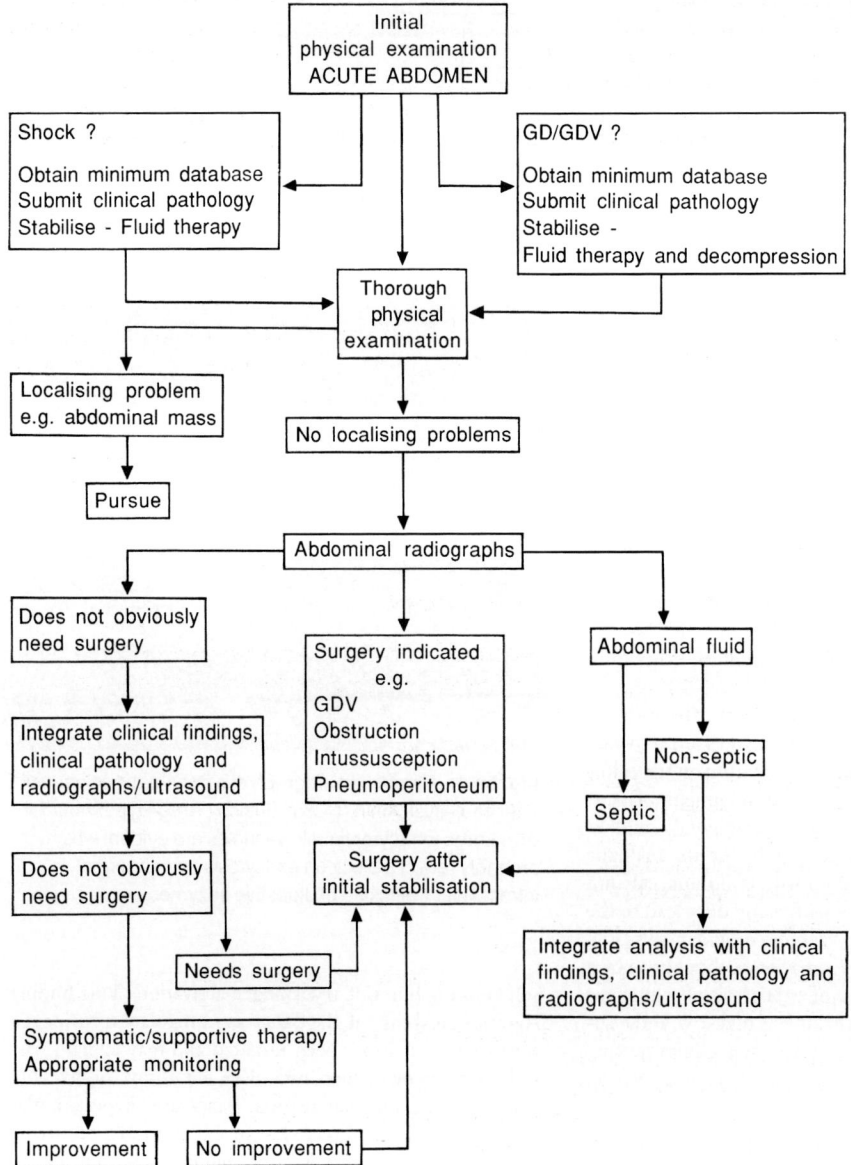

Fig. 53.5 Diagnostic approach to abdominal pain. GD/GDV, gastric dilation/gastric dilation and volvulus.

Diagnosis

There is currently no single specific test for pancreatitis in the dog and diagnosis is based on a combination of compatible clinical, clinicopathological and imaging findings.

Clinical Findings

History

The history may indicate potential risk factors associated with pancreatitis such as obesity, dietary indiscretion, high fat diet or exogenous glucocorticoid administration. Clinical signs often reported by owners of dogs with pancreatitis include lethargy, anorexia, hunched stance, vomiting, diarrhoea, increased respiratory rate and enlarged abdomen. Some dogs have a history of icterus preceded by vomiting.

Physical Examination

Physical findings in dogs with acute pancreatitis are highly variable and range from depression, to mild dehydration

with signs of abdominal pain, to acute abdominal crisis with shock (tachycardia, prolonged capillary refill time, tacky mucous membranes, hypothermia), petechiation, icterus and ascites. An abdominal mass is palpated in some dogs.

Diagnostic Approach and Differential Diagnosis

The diagnostic approach and selection of diagnostic tests intially depends on clinical findings. The differential diagnosis of acute pancreatitis is usually centred around the problems of vomiting and abdominal pain (Table 53.1). The diagnostic approach to vomiting is covered in more detail in Chapter 49, the diagnostic approach to abdominal pain is summarised in Fig. 53.5. A summary of the approach to a dog with vomiting and abdominal pain and suspected pancreatitis is presented in Fig. 53.6.

In vomiting dogs the initial approach is to distinguish self-limiting from more severe causes of vomiting on the basis of physical findings and a minimum database (e.g. packed cell volume, total protein, azostick, urinalysis, plasma concentrations of sodium and potassium). Where vomiting is associated with systemic signs of illness or is

Table 53.1 Differential diagnosis of pancreatitis.

Causes of abdominal pain	
Gastric	Dilatation/volvulus, ulceration,
Intestinal	Obstruction, intussusception, rupture, torsion, enteritis
Pancreatic	Pancreatitis
Hepatic	Acute hepatitis, ruptured bile duct, hepatic neoplasia
Splenic	Torsion, ruptured neoplasm
Urogenital	Nephritis, pyelonephritis, ruptured bladder, ureteral/urethral calculi, pyometra, prostatitis
Peritoneum	Primary or secondary peritonitis (e.g. chemical – bile and urine; septic – ruptured viscus)
Pseudoabdominal pain	Discospondylitis, prolapsed disc
Causes of vomiting	
Gastric	Gastritis, ulceration, neoplasia, outflow obstruction, foreign bodies, motility/functional disorders
Intestinal	Inflammatory bowel disease, neoplasia, foreign bodies, intussusception, torsion, rupture, bacterial overgrowth, functional disorders
Non-gastrointestinal	Pancreas – pancreatitis, pancreatic neoplasia
	Liver – Cholangiohepatitis, biliary obstruction
	Genitourinary – pyomertra, nephritis, nephrolithiasis,
	Urinary – obstruction, prostatitis peritonitis
Metabolic/endocrine	Uraemia, hypoadrenocorticism, Diabetic ketoacidosis, hepatic encephalopathy, hypercalcaemia, septicaemia
Drugs	Digoxin, erythromycin, chemotherapy, apomorphine, xylazine
Toxins	Strychnine, ethylene glycol, lead
Dietary	Indiscretion, intolerance, allergy
Neurological	Vestibular disease, encephalitis, neoplasia, raised intracranial pressure
Infectious	Distemper, parvovirus, infectious canine hepatitis, leptospirosis, *Salmonella*

- Obtain a minimum database: CV/TP/BUN/glucose/ urinalysis and Na/K.

- Detect or rule out: azotemia (renal or prerenal), anaemia, dehydration, hypoglycaemia, hypokalaemia, hyponatraemia.

- Submit blood for haematology, biochemistry (including amylase and lipase) before initiating treatment.

- Start symptomatic therapy based on clinical findings and results of minimum database e.g. lactated Ringer's with 14 mEq/500 ml KCl given at 2× maintenance to correct dehydration and hypokalaemia.

- Schedule further diagnostic tests.

- Perform abdominocentesis if radiography or ultrasound demonstrate fluid or loss of serosal detail, free gas, or if a ruptured viscus is suspected.

- Integrate clinical findings, clinical pathology, results of radiography and ultrasonography and centesis to try to establish a diagnosis.

Fig. 53.6 Diagnostic and therapeutic plan for a dog with vomiting and cranial abdominal pain suspected of having acute pancreatitis. TP, total protein; PCV, packed cell volume; TLI, trypsin-like immunoreactivity; BUN, blood urea nitrogen.

persistent the clinician has to differentiate metabolic, poly-systemic infectious, toxic and neurological causes from intra-abdominal causes. This is usually achieved on the basis of combined historical and clinical findings coupled with a minimum database and the evaluation of haematology and serum chemistry profile, urinalysis and abdominal radiography. Measurement of serum amylase or lipase is often reported on routine serum chemistry profile. Additional procedures such as ultrasonography, abdominal paracentesis or assay of trypsin-like immunoreactivity are usually performed on the basis of these initial test results and help to distinguish pancreatitis from other intra-abdominal causes of vomiting.

Where abdominal pain is the major finding, localising abnormalities such as abdominal distension are rapidly pursued with radiography, ultrasonography and paracentesis while providing supportive treatment on the basis of physical findings and a minimum database and awaiting the results of haematology, serum chemistry profile and urinalysis (Figs 53.5 and 53.6). Abdominal pain can arise from any intra-abdominal structure. Musculoskeletal disorders such as discospondylitis and prolapsed discs can sometimes be hard to distinguish from abdominal causes of pain.

It is noteworthy that diarrhoea, which was bloody in some cases, was a more frequent sign than vomiting in dogs with experimental acute pancreatitis. Acute pancreatitis and its complications (infection, pseudocyst or abscess for-

Table 53.2 Common clinicopathological abnormalities in dogs with acute pancreatitis.

Increased	Decreased	Variable
BUN/creatinine	Platelets	PCV
ALT/AST/ALP	Albumin, total protein	WBC count
Bilirubin	Calcium	Na, K, Cl
Cholesterol		Glucose

BUN, bloodurea nitrogen; ALT, alanine aminotransferase; AST, aspartate aminotransferase; ALP, alkaline phosphatase; PCV, packed cell volume; WBC, white blood cells.

mation) should also be considered in the differential diagnosis of icterus and pyrexia. Some dogs with pancreatitis show few localising clinical signs. Diagnosis in these animals requires a high index of suspicion and use of versatile diagnostic tests such as ultrasonography.

Clinicopathological Findings

Haematology

Haematological abnormalities in acute pancreatitis range from mild neutrophilia and slightly increased haematocrit, through marked leukocytosis with a left shift, to thrombo-cytopenia, anaemia and leukopenia with a degenerative left shift (Table 53.2). If thrombocytopenia is detected, blood clotting tests (OSPT – one-stage prothrombin times, APTT – activated prothrombin time, FDP – fibrin degra-dation products) are performed to determine if the patient has a disseminated intravascular coagulopathy (DIC). Where available the measurement of antithrombin III is useful in the early diagnosis of DIC.

Serum Biochemistry

Serum biochemical abnormalities in dogs with acute pan-creatitis include azotaemia (pre-renal and renal), increased liver enzymes (alanine aminotransferase (ALT), aspartate aminotransferase (AST), alkaline phosphatase (AP)), hyperbilirubinaemia, lipaemia, hyperglycaemia, hypopro-teinaemia, hypocalcaemia, metabolic acidosis and variable alterations (usually decreased) in sodium, potassium and chloride (Table 53.2). These abnormalities reflect pancre-atic damage, fluid depletion secondary to vomiting or peri-toneal effusion and the effects of pancreatic enzymes and inflammatory mediators on other organs.

Urinalysis

Evaluation of urine specific gravity usually enables azo-taemia to be characterised as renal or prerenal. Transient proteinuria occurs in some dogs with acute pancreatitis, possibly as a consequence of pancreatic enzyme-mediated glomerular damage. The absence of white cell casts or bac-teria helps to rule out pyelonephritis as a cause of abdomi-nal pain.

Pancreas Specific Enzymes

Classically, elevations in serum amylase and lipase activity have been used as indicators of pancreatic inflammation; however, these tests are not very accurate because some dogs with pancreatitis have normal results and others with non-pancreatic disorders may have elevated enzyme activ-ities. Both amylase and lipase are normally present in other organs and their serum activities may increase with non-pancreatic disorders including intestinal obstruction (amylase), corticosteroid administration (lipase) and renal disease (both enzymes).

These limitations have stimulated development of assays for enzymes thought to be solely of pancreatic origin. Trypsin–like immunoreactivity (TLI) is one candidate; in contrast to amylase and lipase, serum TLI is abolished by pancreatectomy (Fig. 53.7), high concentrations of TLI occur in dogs with acute pancreatitis (Fig. 53.8) and low concentrations occur in dogs with exocrine pan-creatic insufficiency. TLI is therefore a useful indicator of both pancreatic mass and inflammation; non-pancreatic diseases such as renal disease may however affect it. The time at which TLI is measured in relationship to the onset of pancreatitis may also have important effects on its utility to detect pancreatitis: TLI may not stay elevated throughout the course of the disease and may actually transiently decrease in dogs recovering from an acute bout of pancreatitis. Clinical use of the TLI assay for acute cases is hampered by the fact that it may take 3–7 days to get a result. For the time being, the widely available assays for amylase and lipase are likely to remain the most popular enzyme tests for the initial diagnosis of canine pancreatitis, though TLI is clearly the most specific.

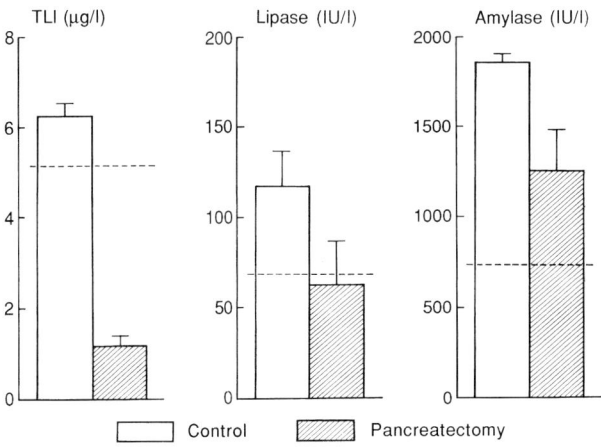

Fig. 53.7 The effects of pancreatectomy on circulating amylase, lipase and trypsin-like immunoreactivity (TLI). The horizontal dashed lines indicate the lower limit of the normal ranges in dogs. Only serum TLI is significantly reduced following pancreatectomy. (Graph drawn using data from Simpson *et al.* 1991)

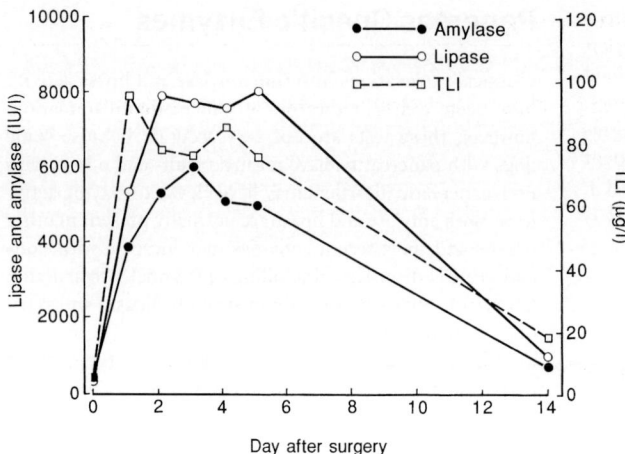

Fig. 53.8 Circulating activities of amylase (IU/l), lipase (IU/l) and concentrations of trypsin-like immunoreactivity (TLI µg/l) in dogs with acute pancreatitis. (From Simpson *et al.* 1989)

Abdominal Paracentesis

Examination of peritoneal fluid may aid detection of various causes of acute abdominal signs such as pancreatitis, gastrointestinal perforation or ruptured bile duct (Table 53.3). Suppurative, non-septic peritonitis sometimes occurs in animals with pancreatitis. Higher activities of amylase, lipase or concentrations of TLI in abdominal fluid than plasma are suggestive of pancreatitis, although difficulty in obtaining enough fluid may preclude analysis.

Diagnostic Imaging

Radiography

The pancreas is not normally visible on abdominal radiographs. Radiographic findings in dogs with acute pancreatitis may include loss of serosal detail and increased opacity in the right cranial quadrant of the abdomen, displacement of the duodenum ventrally and/or to the right, dilated hypomotile duodenum and caudal displacement of the transverse large intestine. Punctate calcification is occasionally identified in dogs with long-standing pancreatitis; it indicates saponification of mesenteric fat around the pancreas.

Although these signs often are absent, and are non-specific, radiography remains a useful diagnostic method for pancreatitis largely because it may enable detection of other abnormalities that can cause similar signs (e.g. gastric foreign body or intestinal obstruction). Radiography is a logical first choice imaging modality for animals with gastrointestinal signs. Negative or equivocal radiographic findings may be followed up with ultrasonography or an upper gastrointestinal contrast study.

Ultrasonography

Ultrasonography enables examination of the pancreas and other adjacent structures that are not normally visible on radiographs; therefore, ultrasonography is more sensitive than radiography for pancreatitis. Pancreatic ultrasonography in dogs requires a high resolution transducer and careful attention to transducer position. The left lobe of the pancreas may be visible adjacent to the greater curvature of the stomach from a ventral or left lateral approach. The right lobe may be visible dorsomedial to the duodenum and ventral to the liver and right kidney. The pancreas is normally hyperechoic compared with the liver. Practical difficulties that may prevent an optimal ultrasound examination in dogs with pancreatitis include excessive intestinal gas, excessive breath motion, obesity and inability to achieve the desired transducer position if the abdominal wall is splinted due to pain. Use of analgesia and/or sedation contributes greatly to the quality of pancreatic ultrasound scans by reducing breath motion and relaxing the abdominal wall.

Ultrasonographic findings in canine pancreatitis include enlarged, hypoechoic pancreas (Fig. 53.9), cavitary lesions such as abscess or pseudocyst (Fig. 53.10), dilated pancreatic duct, swollen hypomotile duodenum, biliary dilatation (Fig. 53.11) and peritoneal fluid. Ultrasonography enables some direct assessment of pancreatic morphology; however, it cannot reliably distinguish between pancreatic necrosis and oedema or between pancreatitis and pancreatic neoplasia. Dogs with either relatively severe pancreatitis or neoplasia may have ultrasonographic signs of enlarged hypoechoic pancreas, localised peritoneal fluid and local lymphadenopathy.

Ultrasound-guided fine needle aspirates of cavitary lesions can distinguish abscess from pseudocyst. Pancreatic

Table 53.3 Abdominocentesis and peritoneal lavage in cases of pancreatitis.

Abdominocentesis
A four quadrant or ultrasound-guided abdominal tap should performed to obtain abdominal fluid in patients with:
● Palpable or ultrasound demonstrated fluid
● Radiographs show loss of serosal detail or free gas
● Suspected rupture of viscus

Analysing abdominal fluid
Gross appearance
● e.g. Clear, cloudy, yellow, red, viscous, watery

PCV/protein/specific gravity
● Hemmorrhagic ? – compare fluid PCV with peripheral PCV
● Serosanguinous?
● Transudate, modified transudate, exudate

Cytology
● Cell count – white cells, red cells, other cells, bacteria, fungi

Biochemical evaluation
● BUN, creatinine – if suspect urinary tract rupture
● ± amylase, lipase, TLI if suspect pancreatitis
● Protein

Interpreting abdominal fluid analysis:

	Appearance	Nucleated cells	Protein	SG
Transudates				
Pure	Clear, colourless	<2 500/µl	<2.5 g/l	<1.016
Modified	Serosanguinous	<7 000/µl	2.5 g/l	1.010–1.031
Exudates				
Septic	Cloudy, red, dark yellow	>20 000/µl	2.5 g/l	1.020–1.031
Non-septic	Cloudy, red, dark yellow	<20 000/µl	2.5 g/l	1.017–1.031

● Increased neutrophils in peritonitis.
● Neutrophils + intracellular bacteria = perforation = surgery
● Gram stain aids antibacterial selection
● Neoplastic cells?
● Eythrophagacytosis suggests haemorrhage is not acute
● Bilirubin crystals suggests bile duct rupture

Diagnostic peritoneal lavage
Provides more consistent results than abdominocentesis where small amounts of fluid in abdomen.

● Infuse 22 ml/kg warm LRS into the peritoneal cavity, shake abdomen and collect fluid for analysis.
● Normal cell count is fewer than 500 WBC/mm^3.
● Presence of bacteria, vegetable matter or WBC >2000/mm^3 (especially if degenerate) suggests surgical intervention may be warranted.
● PCV ≥ 2% suggests haemorrhage.
● Can measure amylase, lipase, TLI, creatinine in lavage fluid.

PCV, packed cell volume; BUN, blood urea nitrogen; TLI, trypsin-like immunoreactivity; SG, specific gravity; WBC, white blood cells; LRS, lactated Ringers solution.

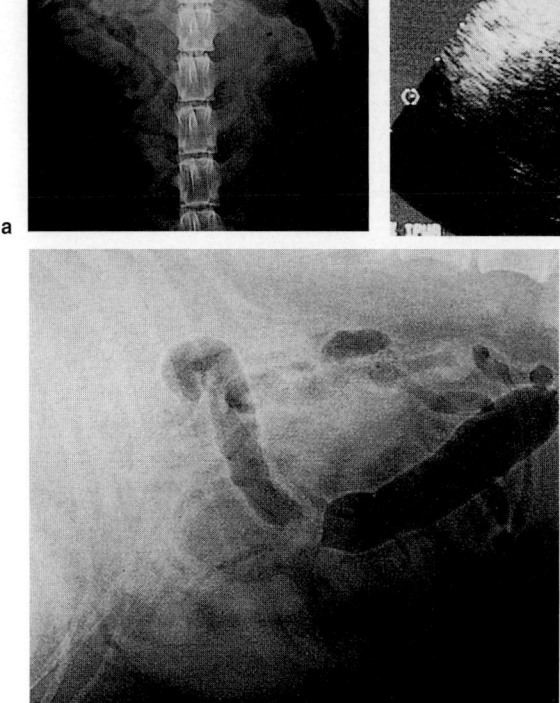

Fig. 53.9 Ultrasound findings in a Rottweiler with vomiting and signs of abdominal pain due to acute pancreatitis. (a),(b) Abdominal radiographs showed equivocal increased opacity and reduced serosal detail in the cranial abdomen. (c) Ultrasound image showing the enlarged right lobe of the pancreas as an irregular hypoechoic structure adjacent to the duodenum. (From Simpson & Lamb 1995)

abscesses contain exudate composed mainly of degenerate neutrophils whereas pseudocysts contain mucinous, often blood-stained, fluid that in some animals is viscous and resembles saliva in appearance. A high TLI in pseudocyst fluid confirms its pancreatic origin.

Assessment of Severity

Once a diagnosis of pancreatitis has been reached an attempt should be made to assess the severity of the disease because this determines the prognosis and influences the intensity of treatment required. The severity of pancreatitis is broadly correlated with the degree of pancreatic damage, ranging from mild with pancreatic oedema, through severe with pancreatic necrosis, to extremely severe with infected pancreatic necrosis.

Prognostic Indicators

Clinical and clinicopathological criteria are used to predict the severity of acute pancreatitis. The presence of shock or abnormalities such as oliguria, azotaemia, hypocalcaemia, hypoglycaemia, hypoproteinaemia, acidosis, leukocytosis, falling haematocrit, thrombocytopenia and DIC should be considered likely indicators of severe pancreatitis in the dog.

Single prognostic indicators include assay of trypsinogen activation peptide (TAP), trypsin complexed with inhibitors and phospholipase A_2. Trypsinogen activation peptide has been shown to accurately predict severity in humans with pancreatitis and is under evaluation in the dog. This peptide is released when trypsinogen, a pancreas-specific enzyme, is converted to its active form and rapidly accumulates in the urine and plasma of dogs with experi-

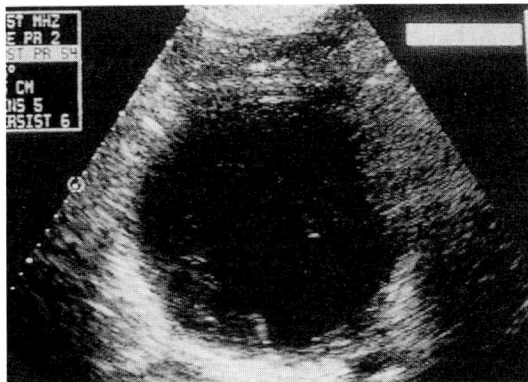

Fig. 53.10 Diagnostic images of a pancreatic pseudocyst. A lateral abdominal radiograph showed an ill-defined soft tissue mass in the mid-abdomen caudal to the stomach. Poor serosal detail of the mass was compatible with local peritoneal fluid and/or adhesions. Ultrasound image showing a 3-cm diameter cavitary lesion with a thin irregular wall and anechoic contents. Ultrasound-guided fine needle aspiration produced viscous, slightly blood-stained, clear fluid that had few cells and a high trypsin-like immunoreactivity (TLI). These findings are typical of pancreatic pseudocyst. (From Simpson & Lamb 1995)

mental acute pancreatitis. All of these prognostic indicators require further validation before clinical application.

Morphological assessment of severity is accomplished in humans by use of contrast enhanced computed tomography (CE-CT). Where lack of pancreatic perfusion is encountered, i.e necrosis, fine needle aspiration is used to distinguish infected from sterile necrosis. Substantially reduced mortality has been achieved by the detection and surgical treatment of patients with infected necrosis. The lack of availability of CT has restricted veterinary application to date, but the relative accessibility of the canine pancreas to ultrasound-guided needle aspiration holds the potential of the adoption of a similar approach.

Treatment

Medical treatment is based on maintaining or restoring adequate tissue perfusion and inhibiting inflammatory mediators and pancreatic enzymes; surgical treatment consists principally of removing infected necrotic pancreatic tissue.

Initial Therapy

The initial medical management of acute pancreatitis is usually started before the diagnosis is confirmed and is therefore based on the presenting clinical findings. Dogs with a history of vomiting who are mildly dehydrated are given crystalloids (usually lactated Ringer's solution) at a rate that will provide maintenance and replace both deficits and ongoing losses over a 24-h period. Dogs with signs of shock require more aggressive support. The volume deficit can be replaced with crystalloids at an initial rate of 60–90 ml/kg per hour, then tailored to maintain tissue perfusion and hydration. Colloid solutions can be used in shocked animals to reduce the amount of crystalloid required (e.g. degraded gelatine; Haemaccel™, at 10–20 ml/kg per day i.v.). Other colloids such as dextran 70 and hetastarch may also have antithrombotic effects that help maintain the microcirculation.

Other symptomatic therapy initially considered in the vomiting animal are nothing by mouth, and antiemetics or antacids when vomiting is persistent. Prophylactic antibiotic cover (e.g. cephalosporins, ampicillin) may be warranted in animals with shock. Analgesia can be provided using opioids (e.g. buprenorphine 0.0075–0.01 mg/kg i.m.).

Specific Therapy

Once a diagnosis of pancreatitis is confirmed fluid therapy is continued and more specific therapy may be employed. The majority of dogs with acute pancreatitis respond to fluid therapy and nothing by mouth for 48 h. Hence, specific therapy is usually reserved for dogs that do not respond to fluid therapy or those that have signs of DIC. No treatment regimens have been critically evaluated in dogs with naturally occurring pancreatitis.

Specific therapy in humans has developed along the lines of stopping further pancreatitis from occurring and limiting the local and systemic consequences of pancreatitis. Therapies aimed at inhibiting pancreatic secretion (e.g. glucagon, somatostatin) or the intracellular activation of proteases (e.g. gabexate mesilate) which have been of benefit in ameliorating the severity of experimental pancreatitis have shown little benefit in the treatment of clincal patients. This lack of success is probably related to the timing of therapy in relation to the development of pancreatitis; experimental therapy is usually initiated before or shortly after the induction of pancreatitis whereas most patients are not presented until 24–48 h after the onset of pancreatitis. This has led to increased emphasis on damage limitation; ameliorating the effects of inflammatory mediators or pancreatic enzymes and maintaining pancreatic perfusion. The systemic effects of pancreatitis may be ame-

liorated in experimental animals by maintaining an adequate protease:antiprotease balance. Natural protease
inhibitors contained in plasma help restore the
protease:antiprotease balance when administered in high
volumes. For this reason it may be beneficial to administer
fresh frozen plasma (10–20 ml/kg) to dogs with pancreatitis. The administration of fresh frozen plasma may also be
beneficial for management of DIC. Heparin administration
(75–150 IU/kg s.c. t.i.d.) may also be warranted in the early
stages of acute pancreatitis to delay the development of
DIC. Heparin may also clear lipaemic serum, a frequent
finding in acute pancreatitis, allowing a biochemical profile
to be run. Oral pancreatic enzyme extracts have been
reported to reduce pain in humans with chronic pancreatitis, but are less likely to be effective in dogs as they do not
appear to have a protease-mediated negative feedback
system.

Dietary Management

Maintaining adequate nutrition during a bout of pancreatitis is difficult. Oral intake is usually withheld for the initial
48 h then gradually re-introduced. The rationale for giving
nothing by mouth even when vomiting is absent is to 'rest
the pancreas' by decreasing pancreatic stimulation. As fats
and amino acids are potent stimulators of pancreatic
enzyme secretion their effects are initially avoided by
feeding a diet high in carbohydrate and then gradually
increasing fat and protein content during the recovery
period (the first and second weeks after the onset).
Alternative strategies of minimising pancreatic stimulation
include total parenteral nutrition and feeding distal to the
CCK-releasing part of the intestine via a jejunostomy tube
but these options require further investigation before widespread clinical application. Continued fat restriction is
usually recommended for dogs who have had pancreatitis
and is based on clinical and experimental studies that
suggest an association between high fat meals, hyperlipidaemia and a 'high plane' of nutrition and pancreatitis. The
protein content of the diet may also be important as dogs
fed a choline-deficient ethionine-supplemented diet, or a
protein-restricted high fat diet, develop pancreatitis.
However, more precise recommendations of the dietary
management of acute pancreatitis are hampered by the
absence of controlled studies of the dietary management of
acute pancreatitis in dogs.

Patient Monitoring

Dogs with suspected or confirmed pancreatitis should be
carefully monitored to enable early detection of shock or
other systemic abnormalities. Minimal monitoring for
stable patients includes regular assessment of vital signs
and fluid and electrolyte balance. In dogs with systemic
abnormalities, monitoring should be more aggressive and
may include vital signs, weight, haematocrit, total protein,
fluid intake and output, blood pressure (central venous and
arterial), electrolytes and glucose, acid–base status,
platelets and coagulation status.

Ultrasound-guided fine needle aspiration of the pancreas may enable infected pancreatic necrosis to be
detected. Ultrasonography may also enable detection of
delayed consequences of acute pancreatitis such as pancreatic abscessation, pseudocyst formation and biliary
obstruction.

Surgical Intervention

The diagnosis of pancreatitis is occasionally made after
surgical exploration of the abdomen. Dogs with non-
specific clinical signs, normal serum amylase or lipase activities and ultrasonographic signs of pancreatic mass may be
explored because of post-hepatic biliary obstruction or suspicion of pancreatic neoplasia (Fig. 53.11).

There have been no clinical studies in dogs with acute
pancreatitis to examine the efficacy of surgical treatment.
Surgery is indicated to remove devitalised tissue in dogs
with infected pancreatic necrosis and to investigate and
relieve persistent biliary obstruction. Resection or surgical
drainage of pancreatic pseudocysts is not always necessary
as these can resolve spontaneously or after percutaneous
drainage.

EXOCRINE PANCREATIC INSUFFICIENCY

Exocrine pancreatic insufficiency (EPI) is characterised by
a lack of effective pancreatic exocrine secretions in the
small intestine. The lack of effective exocrine secretion is
usually a consequence of the severe reduction in pancreatic
mass caused by pancreatic acinar atrophy or chronic pancreatitis, but may occur secondary to excessive secretion of
gastric acid (increased destruction and decreased activity of
pancreatic enzymes by acid) or severe protein malnutrition
(decreased synthesis of pancreatic enzymes). Pancreatic
hypoplasia and concomitant diabetes mellitus has also
been rarely documented in dogs.

Pancreatic acinar atrophy (PAA) is probably the most
common cause of exocrine pancreatic insufficiency (EPI) in
the dog. The precise cause of PAA has not yet been determined (Table 53.4). Pancreatic acinar atrophy has an
increased prevalence in German Shepherd Dogs and may

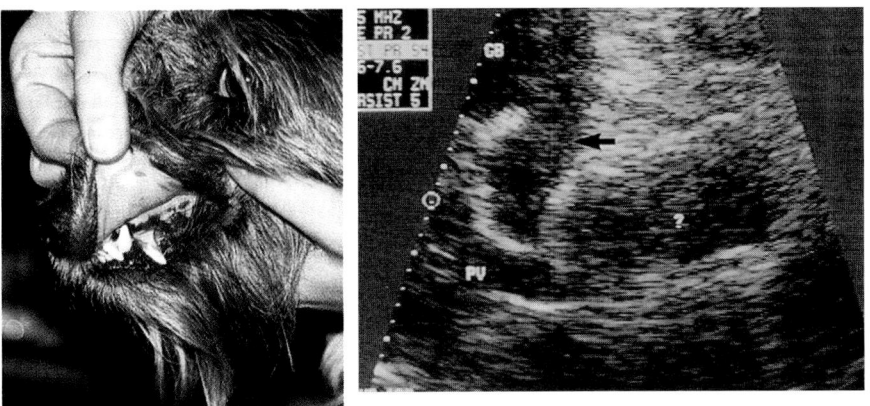

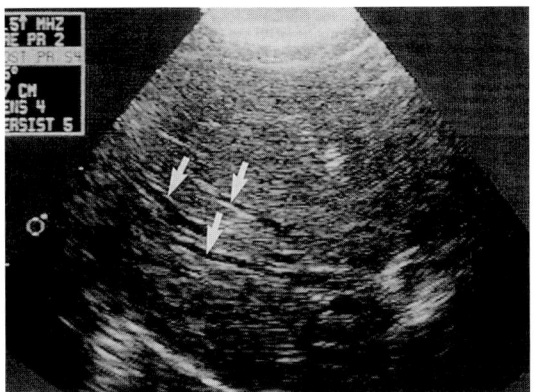

Fig. 53.11   Case example showing difficulties distinguishing pancreatitis from pancreatic neoplasia. (a) A 7-year-old female mixed breed dog had an acute onset of vomiting and inappetance; 4 days later jaundice developed. There was moderate neutrophilia and left shift, elevated serum bile acid, bilirubin, alanine aminotransferase (ALT) and alkaline phosphatase (ALP) and evidence of dehydration. Serum amylase and lipase activities were normal. (b) Thoracic and abdominal radiographs revealed no abnormalities; however, on ultrasonography there was a hypoechoic mass (?) adjacent to the portal vein (PV) and dilated cystic duct. (c) Other images showed evidence of intrahepatic biliary dilatation. The ultrasonographic diagnosis was probable biliary obstruction secondary to pancreatic mass. This was confirmed by exploratory laparotomy and a cholecystojejunostomy was performed. The surgeon was uncertain if the mass was inflammatory or neoplastic and a biopsy was obtained. After surgery the dog was treated using ampicillin and cimetidine and intravenous fluids. Histology showed pancreatic inflammation and fibrosis and necrosis of the surrounding fat. Vomiting resolved and the animal was given a low fat diet. Jaundice also gradually resolved and the dog returned home. (From Simpson & Lamb 1995.)

Table 53.4   Potential aetiologies of pancreatic acinar atrophy.

Hereditary	German Shepherd Dogs
	Collies, English Setters
Primary acinar problem	Pancreatic secretory trypsin inhibitor deficiency
Nutritional	Selective malabsorption
	Vitamin or mineral deficiency – E or B_{12} (cobalamin)
Decreased trophic stimuli	Abnormal CCK release
Immune destruction	Anti-pancreatic antibodies
Apoptosis	

be inherited as an autosomal recessive in this breed. A familial predisposition to PAA has also been reported in Collies and English Setters. Histologically, canine PAA closely resembles the pancreas of CBA/J mice in whom ultrastructural and biochemical studies suggested that pancreatic atrophy was a consequence of the premature activation of trypsinogen and chymotrypsinogen within the zymogen granule. A prospective study of the development of canine PAA is currently underway in German Shepherd Dogs. This study has demonstrated that subcellular pancreatic abnormalities (characterised by fusion of zymogen granules and proliferation of endoplasmic reticulum) and a decrease in TLI, preceded the development of gross pancreatic atrophy, reduced pancreatic protease secretion and diarrhoea in one dog. Other studies have examined the possibility that decreased CCK release or anti-pancreatic antibodies play a role in the genesis of PAA but have yielded no evidence to support their involvement in the development of PAA.

Pathophysiology

The extensive loss of exocrine pancreatic mass (approx. 90%), whether by atrophy or chronic inflammation, is required before signs of EPI are evident. The major signs of EPI, diarrhoea and weight loss, can be attributed to decreased intraduodenal concentrations of pancreatic enzymes, bicarbonate and various other factors with resultant malassimilation of fats, carbohydrates and proteins (Fig. 53.12). Abnormalities in the absorption of fat soluble vitamins and cobalamin, and changes in the number and composition of the small intestinal bacterial flora have also been documented in dogs with EPI and may contribute to their clinical condition. Other abnormalities encountered in dogs with EPI include alterations in glucose homeostasis (subclinical glucose intolerance), pancreatic and gastrointestinal regulatory peptides (e.g. vasoactive intestinal polypeptide, gastric inhibitory polypeptide) and the regulation of small intestinal mucosal growth, enzyme synthesis and enzyme degradation. The clinical significance of these abnormalities is unclear. The marked maldigestion of nutrients in EPI may lead to the development of protein calorie malnutrition which can further compromise residual pancreatic function, intestinal absorption and metabolic homeostasis.

Diagnosis

A diagnosis of exocrine pancreatic insufficiency is usually made on the basis of compatible clinical findings and by ruling out infectious, parasitic, metabolic and anatomic causes of small bowel diarrhoea (see Chapter 50) and demonstrating a subnormal circulating concentration of trypsin-like immunoreactivity (TLI $<2.5\,\mu g/l$).

Clinical Findings

Dogs with EPI usually present with a history of chronic small bowel diarrhoea (large volume, cowpat consistency)

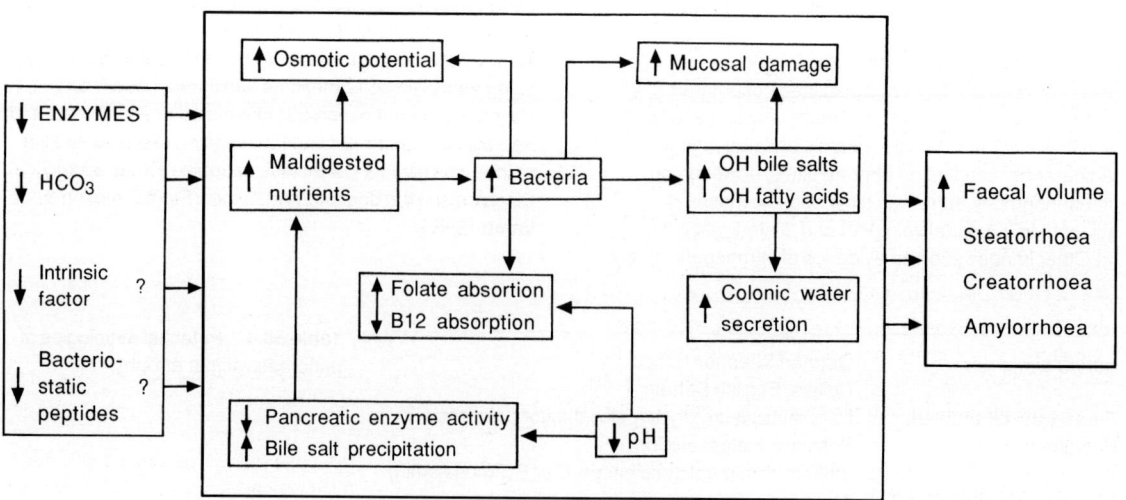

Summary of the luminal and intraluminal changes occurring in exocrine pancreatic insufficiency

Fig. 53.12   Pathophysiology of exocrine pancreatic insufficiency.

and weight loss (mild to extreme) which is often associated with a ravenous appetite. Poor haircoat and marked muscle loss are observed in some dogs. While pancreatic acinar atrophy is prevalent in young German Shepherd Dogs it is important to note that many other breeds are affected by EPI. Young dogs diagnosed with EPI are usually suspected to have pancreatic acinar atrophy whereas older dogs with EPI probably have a higher incidence of chronic pancreatitis.

Clinicopathological Tests

Routine haematology and biochemistry are usually unremarkable in dogs with EPI apart from small increases in alanine aminotransferase and a decrease in cholesterol. Serum concentrations of cobalamin and folate are often decreased or increased respectively in dogs with EPI. However these changes are unhelpful in localising the cause of these abnormalities as intestinal dysfunction, intestinal bacterial overgrowth and diet can cause similar changes. Serum concentrations of vitamin E are often markedly reduced in dogs with EPI.

Tests of Pancreatic Function or Mass

The analysis of faeces for proteolytic activity (film digestion, azocaesin assay) and the indirect estimation of intestinal chymotrypsin activity (N-benzoyl-L-tyrosol-p-aminobenzoic acid or BT-PABA test) for the diagnosis of EPI have been largely superseded by the development of an assay which determines the concentration of TLI in serum. Serum TLI is derived solely from the pancreas (Fig. 53.7) and can be used as an indicator of pancreatic mass or inflammation. In dogs with EPI caused by atrophy or chronic inflammation the amount of TLI that leaks from the pancreas into the circulation is reduced and a subnormal TLI concentration can be demonstrated. Healthy dogs usually have a fasting (overnight fast) TLI concentration greater than 5.0 µg/l whereas dogs with EPI caused by reduced pancreatic mass have fasting concentrations <2.5 µg/l. Where the TLI concentration is between 2.5 and 5.0 µg/l the test should be repeated after ensuring adequate fasting. If the test result is still in this intermediary range the dog may have partial EPI. Options in this situation are re-evaluating the TLI for progresion to complete EPI, trying to confirm a diagnosis of EPI using a BT-PABA test or faecal azocasein digest or performing a treatment trial. The BT-PABA test and faecal azocaesin digest test are likely to be the best means of diagnosing EPI which is secondary to the destruction of pancreatic enzymes by hypersecretion of gastric acid.

Treatment

Exogenous Pancreatic Enzymes

Powdered pancreatic extracts (0.25–0.4 g/kg body weight per meal or 2.5 g/300 g food) are better than enteric coated tablets, granules and capsules. Pre-incubating enzymes with food is not advantageous. Whole pancreas (1.5–3 g/kg body weight per meal) is an effective treatment when available and can be stored frozen for at least three months. In dogs who show a good response the dose of pancreatic extract or pancreas can be gradually decreased to the smallest amount that maintains remission.

Diet

In clinical practice a good response has been observed when dogs with EPI are fed either a normal maintenance diet or a highly digestible fat-restricted diet which is supplemented with pancreatic enzymes. The outcome in terms of survival of dogs with EPI is also reported to be similar in dogs with EPI fed maintenance diets and those fed modified diets.

Highly digestible fat-restricted diets are theoretically attractive owing to the limited digestive capabilities of dogs with EPI. Clinical studies have shown that highly digestible diets are beneficial in reducing faecal volume, borborygmi and flatulence but have no clear effects on faecal consistency, appetite or coprophagy. Studies in dogs with experimental EPI suggest that it is fat digestibility, rather than the amount of fat which is important and have demonstrated an inverse correlation between fat digestibility and faecal water content. However, further controlled trials are necessary to determine if feeding a fat-restricted highly digestible diet is warranted on a routine basis. Fat-restricted, highly digestible diets may be useful in the treatment of dogs with EPI that show poor weight gain in response to initial treatment – enzyme therapy and a maintenance diet. Dietary supplementation with medium chain triglyceride oil (2–4 ml/meal) may also be beneficial in these patients.

Vitamin Supplementation

Although the significance of subnormal concentrations of cobalamin and vitamin E in dogs with EPI is unclear, the provision of supplementary cobalamin (vitamin B_{12} 1 mg s.c. every month) and vitamin E (400–500 IU p.o. s.i.d. every month) may be prudent. A vitamin K responsive coagulopathy has been reported in cats with EPI and it seems sensible to examine the vitamin K status of dogs with EPI who have laboratory evidence of a coagulopathy.

Treatment Failures

Confirm EPI

Review the patient's history, physical examination and laboratory findings to ensure that EPI is a likely cause of the diarrhoea. TLI is like any other laboratory test: if the results don't fit the patient then re-submit the test.

Inadequate Enzyme Supplementation

Check the enzyme supplement is appropriate (non-enteric coated powder), current and being fed at the correct dose. A new batch, change of preparation or increased amounts may produce a response. If a response is not being achieved with a dose of 0.4g/kg of non-enteric coated powdered extract or 3g/kg body weight per meal whole pancreas, consider other reasons for treatment failure.

Hyperacidity

Lipase is the most acid-sensitive enzyme and its activity may be enhanced by decreasing gastric acid secretion. A treatment trial with cimetidine (5–10mg/kg p.o. b.i.d.) may reveal whether the enzyme supplement is being inactivated.

Bacterial Overgrowth

Many dogs with EPI have an abnormal flora in their duodenum. This abnormal flora is often of little consequence, but in some cases may cause a lack of response to pancreatic enzymes. The abnormal flora cannot be predicted accurately by serum concentrations of cobalamin and folate so a trial with an antibiotic such as oxytetracycline (20mg/kg p.o. t.i.d. 28 days) may be undertaken.

Small Intestinal Disease

Some dogs with EPI have small intestinal disease causing malabsorption despite adequate enzyme supplementation. Routine haematology and biochemistry are almost always normal in uncomplicated EPI, so abnormalities such as hypoproteinaemia (which may indicate a protein-losing enteropathy) should be pursued. Dogs with EPI that respond poorly to the above treatment modifications and have no evidence of extra-intestinal disorders usually require further investigation of small intestine.

TUMOURS OF THE EXOCRINE PANCREAS

Pancreatic adenocarcinomas can arise from the acinar or ductal cells of the pancreas and tend to arise in the central portion of the gland. As they enlarge they may obstruct the common bile duct, invade the duodenum or stomach and frequently metastasise to the liver. Widespread metastasis to the omentum, lymph nodes, lung and bone is also common. Pancreatic adenocarcinomas have usually metastasised at the time of diagnosis. Older animals tend to be affected and Airdale Terriers may be predisposed. Clinical signs are usually non-specific and may include weight loss, inappetence, vomiting, abdominal distension and icterus. Icterus is usually due to obstruction of the common bile duct or widespread metastasis to the liver.

Physical examination may reveal a cranial abdominal mass, abdominal pain or an abdominal effusion. Panniculitis has been reported in some dogs with pancreatic tumours.

Routine clinicopathological tests may reveal increases in alkaline phosphatase and bilirubin suggestive of cholestasis or biliary obstruction. Amylase and lipase may be variably affected. Where an effusion is detected paracentesis and cytological evaluation may provide supportive evidence for the diagnosis of carcinoma. Radiographs may reveal the presence of a cranial abdominal mass, loss of serosal detail or pulmonary metastases. Ultrasound is more useful than radiographs for diagnosing pancreatic masses and detecting metastasis. It can sometimes be difficult or impossible to distinguish pancreatitis or its sequelae from pancreatic neoplasia, and surgical biopsy of the pancreas is required to confirm a diagnosis.

There is no effective treatment for pancreatic adenocarcinomas and survival time has not exceeded a year.

REFERENCES AND SUGGESTED FURTHER READING

Pathogenesis of Pancreatic Disease

Leach, S.D., Gorelick, F.S. & Modlin, I.M. (1992). New perspectives on acute pancreatitis. *Scandinavian Journal of Gastroenterology, Supplement*, **192**, 29.

Simpson, K.W. (1993). Current concepts of the pathogenesis and pathophysiology of acute pancreatitis in the dog and cat. *Compendium on Continuing Education for the Practicing Veterinarian*, **15**, 247–253.

Simpson, K.W., Beechey-Newman, N. *et al.* (1995). Cholecystokinin-8 induces pancreatitis in dogs associated with short burst trypsinogen activation. *Digestive Diseases and Sciences*, **40**, 2152–2161.

Steer, M.L. & Meldoplesi, J. (1987). The cell biology of experimental pancreatitis. *New England Journal of Medicine*, **316**, 144–150.

Simpson, K.W. & Lamb, C.R. (1995). Pathogenesis, diagnosis and treatment of acute pancreatitis in the dog. *In Practice* (supplement to *Veterinary Record*), **17**, 328–337.

Westermarck, E., Batt, R.M., Vaillant, C. & Wibug, M. (1993). Sequential study of pancreatic structure and function during development of pancreatic acinar atrophy in a German shepherd dog. *American Journal of Veterinary Research*, **54**, 1088.

Diagnosis and Treatment of Acute Pancreatitis

Crane, S.W. (1986). Diagnostic peritoneal lavage. In: *Veterinary Therapy IX*, (ed. R.W. Kirk), p. 3. W.B. Saunders, Philadelphia.

Johnson, S.E. (1992). Fluid therapy for gastrointestinal, pancreatic, and hepatic disease. In: *Fluid Therapy in Small Animal Practice*, (ed. S.P. DiBartola), pp. 507–528. W.B. Saunders, Philadelphia.

Murtaugh, R.J. (1987). Acute pancreatitis: diagnostic dilemmas. *Seminars in Veterinary Medicine and Surgery Small Animal*, **2**, 282–295.

Macintire, D.K. (1988). The acute abdomen – differential diagnosis and management. *Seminars in Veterinary Medicine and Surgery Small Animal*, **3**, 302–310.

Salisbury, S.K., Lantz, G., Nelson, R.W. & Kazaros, E.R. (1988). Pancreatic abscess in dogs: six cases (1978–1986). *Journal of the American Veterinary Medical Association*, **193**, 1104.

Saunders, H.M. (1991). Ultrasonography of the pancreas. In: *Problems in Veterinary Medicine*, Vol. 3, *Ultrasound*, (ed. P.M. Kaplan), p. 583. W.B. Saunders, Philadelphia.

Simpson, K.W., Batt, R.M., McClean, L. & Morton, D.B. (1989). Circulating concentrations of trypsin-like immunoreactivity and activities of amylase and lipase after pancreatic duct ligation in dogs. *American Journal of Veterinary Research*, **50**, 629–632.

Simpson, K.W., Simpson, J.W., Lake, S., Morton, D.B. & Batt, R.M. (1991). Effect of pancreatectomy on plasma activities of amylase, isoamylase, lipase and trypsin-like immunoreactivity in dogs. *Research in Veterinary Science*, **51**, 78–82.

Steinberg, W.M. & Schlesselman, S.E. (1987). Treatment of acute pancreatitis: Comparison of animal and human studies. *Gastroenterlogy*, **93**, 1420–1426.

Williams, D.A. (1995). Exocrine pancreatic disease. In: *Textbook of Veterinary Internal Medicine*, (eds S.J. Ettinger & E.C. Feldman), 4th edn. pp. 1372–1392. W.B. Saunders, Philadelphia.

Diagnosis and Treatment of Exocrine Pancreatic Insufficiency

Boari, A., Williams, D.A., Famigli-Bergamini, P. (1994). Observations on exocrine pancreatic insufficiency in a family of English setter dogs. *Journal of Small Animal Practice*, **35**, 247–251.

Hall, E.J., Bond, P.M., Butt, R.M. & McLean, L. (1990). A survey of the diagnosis and treatment of canine exocrine pancreatic insufficiency. *Journal of Small Animal Practice*, **32**, 613–619.

Simpson, J.W., Maskell, I.E., Quigg, J. & Markwell, P.J. (1994). Long term management of canine exocrine pancreatic insufficiency. *Journal of Small Animal Practice*, **35**, 133–138.

Westermarck, E., Wilberg, A. & Juntilla, J. (1990). Role of feeding in the treatment of dogs with pancreatic degenerative atrophy. *Acta Veterinaria Scandinavica*, **31**, 325–331.

Williams, D.A. & Batt, R.M. (1988). Sensitivity and specificity of radioimmunoassay of serum trypsin-like immunoreactivity for the diagnosis of canine exocrine pancreatic insufficiency. *Journal of the American Veterinary Medical Association*, **192**, 195.

Williams, D.A., Batt, R.M. & McLean, L. (1987). Bacterial overgrowth in the duodenum of dogs with exocrine pancreatic insufficiency. *Journal of the American Veterinary Medical Association*, **191**, 201–206.

Neoplasia of the Pancreas

Brown, P.J., Mason, K.V., Merrett, D.J., Mirchandani, S. & Miller, R.I. (1994). Multifocal necrotising steatitis associated with pancreatic carcinoma in three dogs. *Journal of Small Animal Practice*, **35**, 129–132.

Johnson, S.E. (1989). Pancreatic APUDomas. *Seminars in Veterinary Medicine and Surgery Small Animals*, **14**, 202–212.

Lamb, C.R., Simpson, K.W., Boswood, A. & Mathewman, L.A. (1995). Ultrasonography of pancreatic neoplasia in the dog: a retrospective review of 16 cases. *Veterinary Record*, **137**, 65–68.

Withrow, S.J. (1989). Tumors of the gastrointestinal system: exocrine pancreas. In: *Clinical Veterinary Oncology*, (eds S.J. Withrow & E.G. MacEwen), p. 192. Lippincott, Philadelphia.

Section 7

Diseases of the Endocrine System

Edited by Michael E. Herrtage

INTRODUCTORY COMMENTS

The advances in our knowledge of endocrine disease over the last 10 years has meant that it is now impossible to cover the entire field of canine endocrinology in a textbook of this size. These chapters have been designed to provide a practical guide for veterinarians in practice by highlighting some of the problem areas in diagnosis and management of the different endocrine disorders. A brief overview of endocrine physiology is given in Chapter 54, which is necessary not only for a good understanding of the pathophysiology of endocrine disease, but also for understanding the rationale and limitations of endocrine function tests. Protocols for some of the more commonly used function tests are given in this chapter. Practical problems of diagnosis and management of specific endocrine diseases are detailed in Chapters 55–61.

Chapter 54

Endocrine Physiology and Function Testing

M. E. Herrtage

INTRODUCTION

The hypothalamus and pituitary form a complex functional unit that controls much of the endocrine system. The pituitary gland is a small ovoid structure which lies in a distinct fossa, the sella turcica, within the sphenoid bone just ventral to the hypothalamus. The pituitary consists of two functional and morphological parts which have separate origins; the anterior lobe of the pituitary or adenohypophysis develops from Rathke's pouch, which arises from the roof of the oral cavity and the posterior lobe of pituitary or neurohypophysis which is a ventral extension of the hypothalamus.

The hypothalamus is important in the regulation of anterior and posterior pituitary function. The release of hormones from the anterior lobe of the pituitary is controlled by hypothalamic peptides which are transported to the anterior pituitary by the capillaries of the hypothalamic–hypophyseal portal circulation (Table 54.1). The hypothalamus contains a number of autonomic centres that control thirst, satiety, body temperature, emotional reactions and sympathetic responses. It serves as an important link between the brain and the endocrine system.

The anterior lobe of the pituitary produces and releases a number of trophic hormones which control many of the endocrine glands (Fig. 54.1). The anterior lobe consists of three components: the pars distalis, the pars intermedia and the pars tuberalis. Three cell types can be identified: acidophils, basophils and chromophobes. The acidophils include somatotrophs which secrete growth hormone and lactotrophs which secrete prolactin; basophils include gonadotrophs which secrete follicle-stimulating hormone and luteinising hormone and thyrotrophs which secrete thyroid-stimulating hormone; chromophobes include corticotrophs which secrete adrenocorticotrophic hormone and cells which secrete melanocyte-stimulating hormone. The actions of these hormones are summarised in Table 54.2.

In the case of those hormones which control a specific endocrine gland, for example the thyroid and adrenal, there is a negative feedback mechanism whereby the hormone of the target gland affects the secretion of the relevant releasing factor from the hypothalamus and/or the trophic hormone from the anterior lobe of the pituitary (Figs 54.2 and 54.3).

In contrast, growth hormone, prolactin and MSH do not act through a target endocrine gland. Control of the release of these hormones is a balance of effects of the relevant stimulatory and inhibitory factors produced by the hypothalamus on the anterior lobe of the pituitary (Fig. 54.4).

PROTOCOLS FOR ENDOCRINE FUNCTION TESTS

Pituitary Function Testing

Anterior Lobe Function

Hypothalamic–pituitary–thyroid and adrenal testing are dealt with under thyroid function tests and adrenocortical function tests respectively.

Growth Hormone Stimulation Test

Indication

- Used to diagnose pituitary dwarfism (congenital hypopituitarism), acromegaly and to evaluate patients with adult-onset growth hormone-responsive alopecia.
- Basal concentrations of growth hormone (GH) are often difficult to interpret due to overlap between normal dogs and those with growth hormone deficiency. Therefore, provocative testing with an α_2-

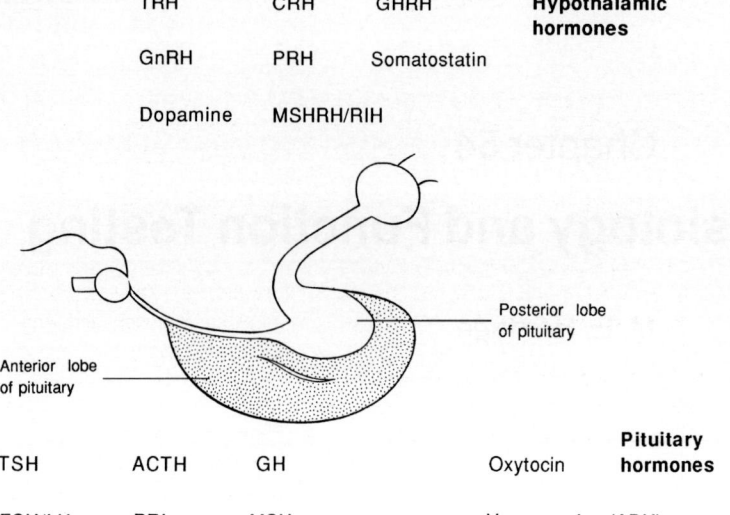

TRH   CRH   GHRH   **Hypothalamic hormones**

GnRH   PRH   Somatostatin

Dopamine MSHRH/RIH

Anterior lobe
of pituitary

Posterior lobe
of pituitary

TSH   ACTH   GH   Oxytocin   **Pituitary hormones**

FSH/LH   PRL   α MSH   Vasopressin (ADH)

Fig. 54.1 Hypothalamic–pituitary physiology.

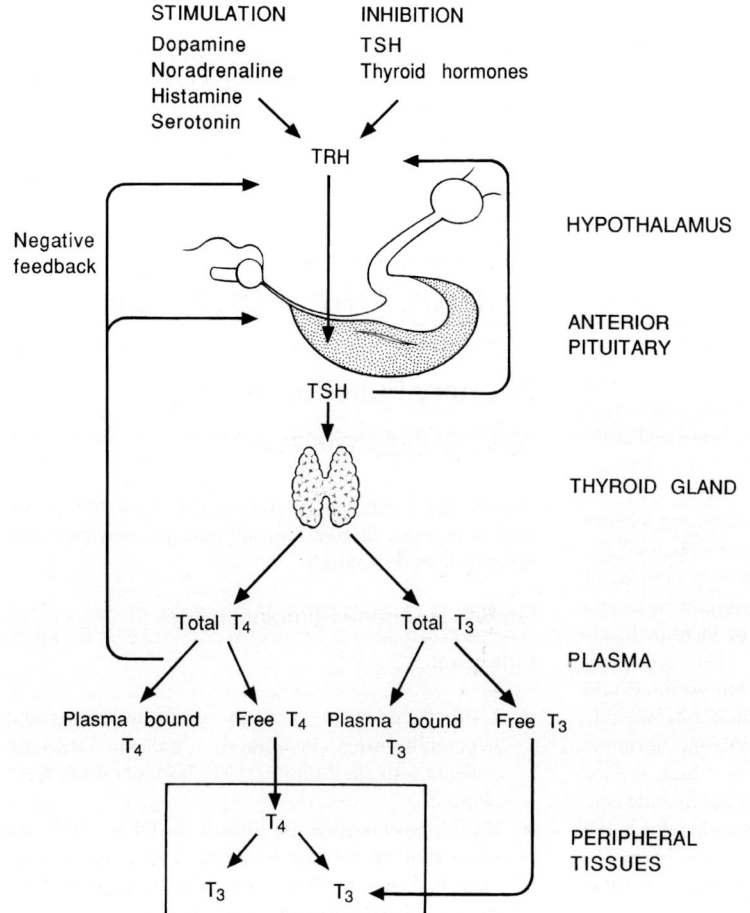

STIMULATION   INHIBITION
Dopamine   TSH
Noradrenaline   Thyroid hormones
Histamine
Serotonin

TRH

Negative
feedback

HYPOTHALAMUS

ANTERIOR
PITUITARY

TSH

THYROID GLAND

Total T_4 Total T_3

PLASMA

Plasma bound T_4 Free T_4 Plasma bound T_3 Free T_3

T_4

T_3 T_3 T_3

PERIPHERAL
TISSUES

Fig. 54.2 Regulation of thyroid function.

Table 54.1　Hypothalamic control of hormone release from the anterior lobe of the pituitary.

Anterior lobe hormone	Hypothalamic hormone (stimulatory)	Hypothalamic hormone (inhibitory)
TSH – thyroid-stimulating hormone	TRH – thyrotrophin releasing hormone	
ACTH – adrenocorticotrophic hormone	CRH – corticotrophin releasing hormone	
GH – growth hormone	GHRH – growth hormone releasing hormone (*somatocrinin*)	GHRIH – growth hormone release inhibitory hormone (*somatostatin*)
FSH – follicle-stimulating hormone	GnRH – gonadotrophin releasing hormone	
LH – luteinising hormone	GnRH – gonadotrophin releasing hormone	
PRL – prolactin	PRH – prolactin releasing hormone	PRIH – prolactin release inhibitory hormone (*dopamine*)
MSH – melanocyte-stimulating hormone	MSHRH – MSH releasing hormone	MSH-RIH – MSH release inhibitory hormone

Table 54.2　Actions of the hormones released from the anterior lobe of the pituitary.

TSH – thyroid stimulating hormone stimulates the biosynthesis of thyroid hormones and the release of thyroxine into the circulation.

ACTH – adrenocorticotrophic hormone maintains adrenocortical size and stimulates the adrenal to secrete glucocorticoids.

GH – growth hormone stimulates growth of the long bones provided the growth plates are open. It also enhances protein anabolism and has marked anti-insulin activity. It is diabetogenic in adults.

FSH – follicle-stimulating hormone stimulates ovarian follicular growth and maturation in the female. In the male, it stimulates testicular growth and spermatogenesis along with testosterone.

LH – luteinising hormone is required for ovulation and stimulates the formation of the corpus luteum. With FSH it stimulates maximum oestrogen secretion. In the male, LH (ICSH) stimulates the interstitial cells to produce testosterone.

PRL – prolactin, in conjunction with other hormones, induces mammary development and lactation. Prolactin also maintains lactation in the female. In the male it has a stimulatory effect on prostate growth.

MSH – melanocyte stimulating hormone is produced primarily in the pars intermedia as part of the prohormone pro-opiomelanocortin (POMC). MSH controls melanin formation in the melanocytes of the epidermis.

adrenergic agonist (such as clonidine or xylazine) is recommended.

Method

(1) Collect blood into EDTA, centrifuge immediately and store frozen (less than −20°C) for basal GH concentration.
(2) Inject either: clonidine (Catapres™) 10 μg/kg intravenously (maximum dose 300 μg) or xylazine (Rompun™) 100 μg/kg intravenously.
(3) Collect second blood sample into EDTA, centrifuge immediately and store frozen for GH concentration 20 min later.

Samples should be sent frozen to the Biochemical Laboratory, Department of Clinical Sciences of Companion Animals, Utrecht, The Netherlands.

Interpretation

- GH concentrations are generally reduced in pituitary dwarfism and show little or no response to stimulation with clonidine or xylazine.
- Reduced GH concentrations with little or no response to stimulation may be found in adult-onset growth hormone-responsive alopecia. However reduced responses may be found in dogs with hypothyroidism or hyperadrenocorticism and these more common disorders should be excluded first.
- Basal GH concentrations are generally elevated in acromegaly and are not usually further stimulated by clonidine or xylazine.

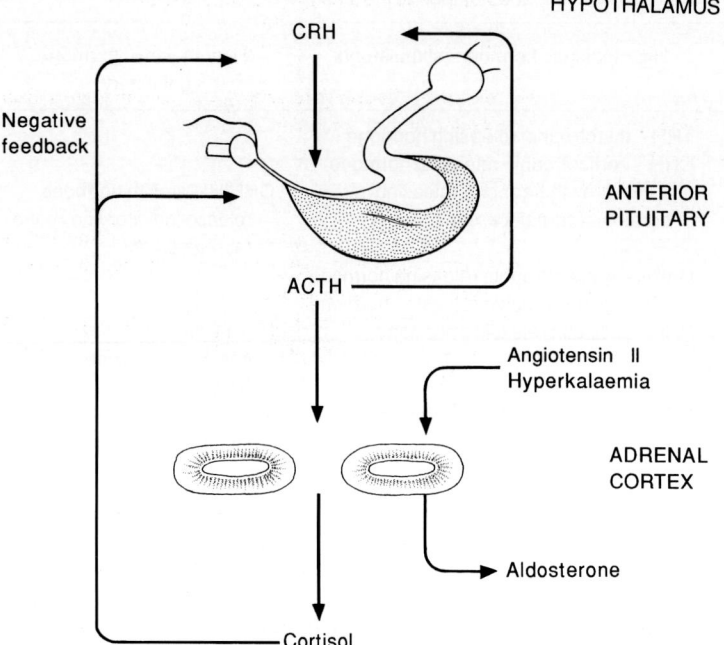

Fig. 54.3   Regulation of adrenal function.

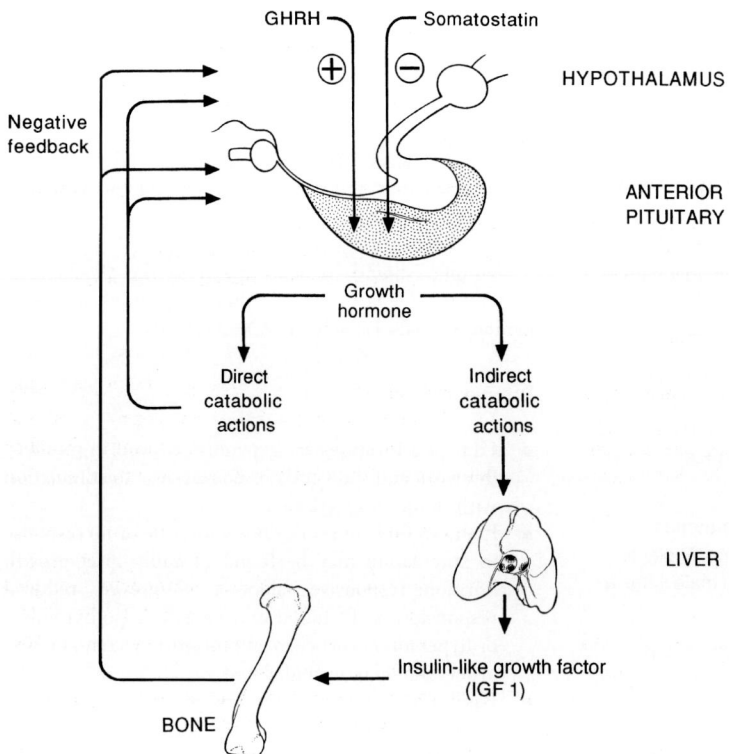

Fig. 54.4   Regulation of growth hormone release.

Basal Serum Insulin-Like Growth Factor 1 (IGF1)

Indication

- Used in the diagnosis of pituitary dwarfism and acromegaly. IGF1 concentration is regulated by GH and nutritional status and is less subject to fluctuation than GH. This makes a single determination more meaningful.

Interpretation

- Serum IGF1 concentrations are decreased in pituitary dwarfs. The sensitivity can be increased by comparing IGF1 concentrations with normal littermates. IGF1 may also be depressed in chronic debilitating disease.
- Elevated IGF1 concentrations are seen in dogs with acromegaly.

Posterior Lobe Function

Only indirect tests of vasopressin (ADH) release are commonly used in veterinary practice.

Water Deprivation Test

Indication

- Used in the diagnoses of diabetis insipidus.

Method

(1) Collect urine and plasma samples if osmolality is being measured. Only urine is required; if specific gravity is being measured.
(2) Weigh patient.
(3) Withhold all fluids and food.
(4) Collect urine and plasma after 8 h and then at 2 h intervals until the test is complete.
(5) Weigh patient each time urine and plasma is collected.
(6) Stop test if patient demonstrates adequate concentrating ability (specific gravity >1.020) or if patient becomes dehydrated and loses 5% of its body weight or more.

Interpretation

- Cases of central or nephrogenic diabetes insipidus fail to concentrate urine (specific gravity <1.010) and urine osmolality remains low and does not exceed that of plasma.
- This test does not always give conclusive results.

Vasopressin (ADH) Response Test

Indication

- Used to differentiate central diabetes insipidus from nephrogenic diabetes insipidus.

Method

(1) Collect urine and plasma samples if osmolality is being measured. Only urine is required if specific gravity is to be measured.
(2) Inject desmopressin (DDAVP™) intramuscularly. Use 2 μg for dogs less than 15 kg and 4 μg for dogs over 15 kg.
(3) Collect urine and plasma samples every 2 h.

Interpretation

- Dogs with nephrogenic diabetes insipidus will show very little for no response to vasopressin and the urine specific gravity and osmolality will remain low.
- Dogs with central diabetes insipidus will concentrate their urine (specific gravity >1.015) and the urine osmolality will rise by 50% or more and the urine osmolality will exceed the plasma osmolality.

Thyroid Function Tests

Basal Plasma or Serum Thyroxine (T_4)

Indication

- Used for initial screening for hypothyroidism or hyperthyroidism. T_4 is the main secretory product of the thyroid gland. May also be used for the therapeutic monitoring of thyroxine replacement therapy.

Method

- A plasma or serum sample is required and preferably, this should be separated before posting to the laboratory. For therapeutic monitoring, a sample is taken before and 4–6 h after treatment.

Interpretation

- Total T_4 concentration is the most commonly used measurement although the active, free T_4 concentration may be more accurate depending on the laboratory technique used.
- Dogs with T_4 concentrations in the mid to high normal range usually have normal thyroid function but T_4 concentrations below or in the low-normal range may be

normal, hypothyroid or suffering from non-thyroid illness (sick euthyroid syndrome). Age, breed, time of day and ambient temperature may affect T_4 concentrations. Certain non-thyroidal illnesses (e.g. chronic renal failure, hyperadrenocorticism, diabetes mellitus) and treatment with certain drugs (e.g. anticonvulsants, glucocorticoids, phenylbutazone) may be associated with reduced T_4 concentrations.

Basal Plasma or Serum Tri-iodothyronine (T_3)

Comment

- T_3 concentrations are less accurate than T_4 in distinguishing euthyroidism from hypothyroidism. Although T_3 is more active metabolically, most is produced by deiodination of T_4 within cells.

Thyroid Antibodies

Indication

- Antibodies to T_4 and T_3 should be considered in animals with spuriously high T_4 or T_3 concentrations and clinical signs of hypothyroidism.

Interpretation

- Antibodies to T_4 and T_3 are considered to be an indicator of active lymphocytic thyroiditis.

TSH Stimulation Test

Indication

- Used to diagnose hypothyroidism by evaluating the response of the thyroid gland to exogenous TSH. The test is limited by the expense and availability of TSH.

Method

(1) Collect plasma or serum sample for basal T_4 concentration.
(2) Administer bovine TSH intravenously at a dose rate of 0.1 IU/kg up to a maximum dose of 5 IU.
(3) Collect second sample for T_4 concentration 6 h later.

Interpretation

- A diagnosis of primary hypothyroidism can be confirmed if both the pre- and post-T_4 samples are below the reference range for basal T_4 concentration.
- In normal animals, the T_4 concentration should stimulate to well within or above the normal reference range for T_4. In most cases the T_4 concentration should increase by at least 1.5 times the basal concentration.

- Interpretation of intermediate results is more difficult and may occur in association with non-thyroid illness, treatment with certain drugs, secondary hypothyroidism or possibly in the early stages of primary hypothyroidism.

TRH Stimulation Test

Indication

- Used in the diagnosis of hypothyroidism to evaluate thyroid function. In humans, the test is used to evaluate TSH secretion by the pituitary gland.

Method

(1) Collect plasma or serum sample for basal T_4 concentration.
(2) Administer 200 μg/dog protirelin (TRH-Cambridge™) intravenously. Injection may cause salivation, vomiting, and tachycardia.
(3) Collect second sample for T_4 concentration 4 hours later.

Interpretation

- Similar to TSH stimulation test although stimulation of T_4 concentrations is less than with TSH and the response to TRH shows greater individual variation.

Endogenous TSH Concentration

Indication

- Used in the diagnosis of primary hypothyroidism.

Method

- A plasma or serum sample is required and this should be separated before posting to a laboratory using a validated canine TSH assay.

Interpretation

- Results are promising, but need further validation. A high TSH concentration in conjunction with a low T_4 concentration is highly suggestive of primary hypothyroidism.

Adrenocortical Function Tests

Basal Plasma or Serum Cortisol

A single resting or basal plasma or serum cortisol determination is of limited diagnostic value because of the overlap in cortisol concentrations obtained from normal and abnormal disease states. In particular:

- Stress associated with sample collection can result in higher than normal cortisol concentrations in samples from animals with normal hypothalamic–pituitary–adrenocortical axis (HPA) function.
- Recent administration of glucocorticoids such as hydrocortisone, prednisolone or prednisone may result in elevated cortisol concentrations due to cross-reactivity in many cortisol assays. For this reason glucocorticoids should be withheld for at least 24 h before testing. There is no cross-reactivity with dexamethasone.

ACTH Stimulation Test

Indication

- Used to screen for hyperadrenocorticism; to distinguish hyperadrenocorticism from iatrogenic Cushing's disease (secondary hypoadrenocorticism); to monitor the response to mitotane (o,p'-DDD; Lysodren™) therapy; and to diagnose primary hypoadrenocorticism (Addison's disease).

Method

(1) Collect plasma or serum sample for basal cortisol concentration (see note above about withholding glucocorticoids).
(2) Inject 0.25 mg of synthetic ACTH (tetracosactrin; Synacthen™) intravenously to dogs over 5 kg. Use only 0.125 mg in dogs less than 5 kg.
(3) Collect a second sample for cortisol concentration 30–60 min later.

Interpretation

- In normal dogs, pre-ACTH cortisol concentrations are usually between 20 and 250 nmol/l with post-ACTH cortisol concentrations between 250 and 550 nmol/l.
- An exaggerated response (post-ACTH cortisol concentrations greater than 660 nmol/l) are expected in hyperadrenocorticism. The ACTH stimulation test reliably identifies more than 50% of dogs with adrenal-dependent hyperadrenocorticism and about 85% of dogs with pituitary-dependent hyperadrenocorticism. Exaggerated responses to ACTH may also be seen in chronic illness, for example uncontrolled diabetes mellitus.
- The ACTH stimulation test is the best screening test for distinguishing spontaneous hyperadrenocorticism from iatrogenic Cushing's disease where reduced responses to ACTH are recorded due to adrenocortical suppression as a result of glucocorticoid administration.
- Reduced responses to ACTH are also seen in hypoadrenocorticism (Addison's disease). Usually both pre- and post-ACTH cortisol concentrations are less than 15 nmol/l.
- A flat response to ACTH is seen in mitotane-treated cases of hyperadrenocorticism. The post-ACTH cortisol concentration should not exceed 125 nmol/l if the disease is well controlled. At concentrations above 250 nmol/l clinical signs of hyperadrenocorticism are likely to be present.
- Disadvantages of the ACTH stimulation test are that it does not reliably differentiate adrenal-dependent from pituitary-dependent hyperadrenocorticism and that a diagnosis of hyperadrenocorticism cannot be excluded on the basis of a normal ACTH response. If the clinical signs are compatible with hyperadrenocorticism, a low-dose dexamethasone suppression test would then be recommended.

Low-dose Dexamethasone Suppression Test (LDDST)

Indication

- Used to screen for hyperadrenocorticism.

Method

(1) Collect plasma or serum for cortisol determination.
(2) Inject 0.01 mg/kg of dexamethasone intravenously.
(3) Collect a second sample for cortisol concentration 4 h later and a third sample 8 h after dexamethasone administration.

Interpretation

- A plasma or serum cortisol concentration exceeding 40 nmol/l at 8 h is regarded as diagnostic for hyperadrenocorticism. The LDDST reliably identifies all dogs with adrenal-dependent hyperadrenocorticism and about 90% with pituitary-dependent hyperadrenocorticism. However stress during therapy may cause animals without hyperadrenocorticism to break the suppressive effect of dexamethasone.
- The cortisol concentrations at 0 and 4 h are not required for the diagnosis of hyperadrenocorticism but may be informative in the differential diagnosis. Suppression of the cortisol concentration to less than 30 nmol/l at 4 h with a rebound escape of suppression at 8 h would be suggestive of pituitary-dependent hyperadrenocorticism.

High-dose Dexamethasone Suppression Test (HDDST)

Indication

- Used to differentiate pituitary-dependent hyperadrenocorticism from adrenal-dependent hyperadrenocorticism. It cannot be used as a screening test for hyperadrenocorticism.

Method

(1) Collect serum or plasma for cortisol determination.
(2) Inject 0.1 or 1.0 mg/kg of dexamethasone intravenously.
(3) Collect two post-dexamethasone samples, one at 4 h and a second at 8 h after the dexamethasone.

Interpretation

- A plasma cortisol concentration that declines by more than 50% from the pre-dexamethasone value at either 4 or 8 h post-dexamethasone is consistent with pituitary-dependent hyperadrenocorticism. A decrease of less than 50% can be due to an adrenocortical tumour or to pituitary-dependent hyperadrenocorticism. About 15–20% of dogs with pituitary-dependent hyperadrenocorticism fail to suppress adequately to high doses of dexamethasone.

Plasma Endogenous ACTH Concentration

Indication

- Used to differentiate pituitary-dependent hyperadrenocorticism from adrenal tumour and to distinguish primary from secondary hypoadrenocorticism.

Method

- Blood is collected into a cooled plastic EDTA tube and centrifuged at 4°C immediately. Plasma should then be harvested and stored frozen (less than −20°C) in a plastic tube. Samples should be transported frozen to the laboratory from the assay. Stringent sample handling is crucial since hormone activity in the plasma will reduce rapidly resulting in falsely low values.

Interpretation

- Endogenous ACTH concentrations in normal dogs range from 10 to 70 pg/ml. Dogs with adrenal tumours have very low endogenous ACTH concentrations (<20 pg/ml) whereas cases with pituitary-dependent hyperadrenocorticism tend to have high-normal to high concentrations (>40 pg/ml).
- Dogs with primary hypoadrenocorticism have very high endogenous ACTH concentrations (>500 pg/ml).

Endocrine Pancreatic Function Tests

Serum Insulin

Indication

- Used to diagnose insulin secreting pancreatic tumours (insulinomas).

Method

- A serum sample is collected. The animal is usually fasted although serial serum insulin concentrations may be measured during an intravenous glucose tolerance test.
- A blood glucose concentration must be determined at the same time in order to evaluate the significance of the serum insulin concentration.

Interpretation

- Serum insulin concentrations in normal fasting dogs are between 5 and 20 mIU/l with a normal blood glucose (3.5–5.0 mmol/l). A serum insulin concentration of greater than 20 mIU/l with a low blood glucose (<3.0 mmol/l) is consistent with an insulinoma.
- If normal insulin concentrations are found in a hypoglycaemic dog then an insulinoma is still possible, but if the serum insulin is low, this diagnosis is unlikely.
- The insulin:glucose ratio has proved useful in making a diagnosis of insulinoma in some cases. A ratio of more than 4.2 U/mol is consistent with an insulinoma.

Chapter 55

Management of Pituitary Disorders

M. E. Herrtage

CONGENITAL HYPOPITUITARISM

Congenital hypopituitarism results in inadequate secretion of growth hormone with resultant retardation of growth (pituitary dwarfism). This rare condition has been reported in a number of breeds of dog, but is most commonly seen in German Shepherd Dogs, where it has been shown to be inherited as an autosomal recessive trait (Andresen & Willeberg 1976). Pituitary dwarfism is most commonly associated with cystic dilatation of Rathke's pouch which causes pressure atrophy of the anterior pituitary.

Although affected animals appear normal at birth, retarded growth is usually evident from weaning onwards. A deficiency of growth hormone produces proportionate dwarfism. The degree of stunting is variable and probably depends on the extent of pituitary damage. Although delayed growth plate closure and dental eruption have been reported, in most cases these delays appear to be minimal.

Growth hormone is required to produce a normal adult hair coat; in pituitary dwarfism the fine puppy coat is retained and becomes woolly in appearance. The hair coat is slowly lost over the trunk, leading to bilaterally symmetrical, non-pruritic alopecia developing over the areas of friction by a year of age. The head and feet are generally spared and affected dogs retain the facial characteristics of a puppy. The skin becomes hyperpigmented in the areas of alopecia.

The function of other endocrine systems controlled by the anterior lobe of the pituitary usually remains normal or near normal. More severe cases, however, may develop signs of secondary hypothyroidism and/or secondary hypoadrenocorticism. Gonadal involvement may result in testicular atrophy in the male and abnormal oestrus cycles in the bitch.

The differential diagnosis of stunting is given in Table 55.1. The diagnosis of congenital hypopituitarism can be made by measurement of growth hormone concentrations.

Since basal growth hormone concentrations may be low in healthy animals, a stimulation test using clonidine and xylazine should be performed (Eigenmann et al. 1984a). Growth hormone concentration can be assessed indirectly by assaying for insulin-like growth factor (IGF-1). Pituitary dwarfs also have abnormally low IGF-1 concentrations (Eigenmann et al. 1984a).

Thyroid function tests and adrenal function tests should be performed to assess thyroidal and adrenal function.

Canine growth hormone is not available for therapeutic use, but bovine, porcine and human growth hormone have been used for treatment. The diagnosis is usually made too late in development to gain much in growth and affected animals will remain permanent dwarfs. Growth hormone administration, however, has been effective in producing regrowth of the hair coat at a dose of 0.1 IU/kg subcutaneously three times a week for 4–6 weeks. Treatment with exogenous growth hormone can be associated with the development of antibodies, which could possibly interfere with its action (van Herpen et al. 1994). Growth hormone is expensive and its repeated use may result in diabetes mellitus.

Thyroid hormone replacement should be used in cases of secondary hypothyroidism (see Chapter 56). Thyroid hormone therapy has also been used to stimulate hair growth in pituitary dwarfs with normal thyroid function with variable success. Half the normal replacement dose of thyroxine may need to be administered for several months to produce a response.

GROWTH HORMONE-RESPONSIVE ALOPECIA IN MATURE DOGS

An endocrine alopecia which responds to exogenous growth hormone administration has been described, however the aetiology of this condition remains unclear and

water and may become anorexic and lose weight. Despite their increased thirst, these dogs remain mildly to moderately dehydrated. Central nervous signs may be noted, particularly diabetes insipidus is associated with a pituitary tumour.

Table 55.3 Differential diagnosis of polydipsia/polyuria.

Polyuria with compensatory polydipsia
  Osmotic diuresis
    Diabetes mellitus
    Primary renal glycosuria/Fanconi's syndrome
    Polyuric renal failure/post-obstructive diuresis
  Interference with ADH release and/or renal response to
    ADH
    Chronic renal failure
    Glomerulopathy/nephrotic syndrome
    Pyelonephritis
    Pyometra
    Hyperadrenocorticism
    Chronic liver disease
    Hypercalcaemia
    Hypoadrenocorticism
    Central diabetes insipidus
    Nephrogenic diabetes insipidus
    Hypokalaemia
    Hyperthyroidism
    Drugs/diet

Primary polydipsia
  Psychogenic polydipsia

ADH, vasopressin.

Routine haematological, biochemical and electrolyte profiles are generally unremarkable in dogs with central or primary nephrogenic diabetes insipidus. When abnormalities are present, they are usually secondary to dehydration. Very dilute urine of low specific gravity, usually between 1.001 and 1.005, is the most significant finding. The urine specific gravity is almost invariably less than glomerular filtrate, that is <1.010, indicating good renal tubular function with resorption of solute in excess of water. Urine osmolality is also low and is typically less than that of plasma, which is often mildly or moderately raised due to the concomitant dehydration (Table 55.4). In psychogenic polydipsia, the plasma osmolality is usually decreased due to the overhydration.

A carefully monitored water deprivation test will confirm the dog's inability to concentrate its urine in diabetes insipidus, despite becoming dehydrated. Renal function must be assessed before carrying out this test and the test should always be discontinued if the patient loses more than 5% of its body weight. Urine and plasma osmolality measurements provide more definitive information than urine specific gravity alone (Table 55.4).

The vasopressin response test is used to distinguish central diabetes insipidus from nephrogenic diabetes insipidus. Dogs with central diabetes insipidus will concentrate their urine in response to the administration of exogenous ADH whereas dogs with nephrogenic diabetes insipidus will show no response.

Successful treatment of central diabetes insipidus requires long-term replacement therapy using desmopressin, a vasopressin analogue. Desmopressin is available as an injection and as nasal drops, which provide antidiuretic activity for about 8 h. One to four drops of the nasal preparation placed in the conjunctival sac twice daily will

Table 55.4 Differentiation of central diabetes insipidus (CDI), nephrogenic diabetes insipidus (NDI) and psychogenic polydipsia (PP).

Parameter	Before water deprivation	After water deprivation		
		CDI	NDI	PP
Urine (U)				
U specific gravity	<1.010	<1.010	<1.010	<1.025
U osmolality	<300	<300	<300	<700
Plasma (P)				
P osmolality	>300 CDI or NDI <295 PP	>310	>310	±310
U:P osmolality	<1.0	<1.0	<1.0	2–3
ADH response	<1.0	>1.0	<1.0	>1.0

Osmolality measured in mOsm/kg. ADH, vasopressin.

control the polydipsia and polyuria in most dogs with central diabetes insipidus.

Chlorpropamide, an oral sulphonylurea hypoglycaemic agent, potentiates the effects of ADH on the renal tubules and therefore requires the presence of at least some endogenous ADH. Although chlorpropamide has been shown to be effective in partial central diabetes insipidus in man, the results in dogs have been inconsistent and variable. It may take several weeks to obtain an effect and hypoglycaemia is a potential side-effect. A dose of 10–40 mg/kg orally once daily has been suggested in dogs.

Thiazide diuretics such as hydrochlorothiazide and chlorothiazide have a paradoxical effect in both central and nephrogenic diabetes insipidus. Urine output may be decreased by up to 50%, although the urine is still not isosthenuric. The suggested doses for hydrochlorothiazide and chlorothiazide are 2–4 mg/kg twice daily and 20–40 mg/kg twice daily respectively. The precise dose should be tailored individually to each patient and the effect may be enhanced by concurrent use of a sodium-restricted diet. Patients should be monitored periodically for electrolyte disturbances, particularly hypokalaemia.

Idiopathic central diabetes has a favourable prognosis with treatment. Animals with an expanding hypothalamic or pituitary tumour have a guarded prognosis, especially if neurological signs are present. Central diabetes insipidus following head trauma carries a variable prognosis; spontaneous remission may occur within a few days or weeks in some cases, but in others the damage is permanent. Nephrogenic diabetes insipidus has a more guarded prognosis.

REFERENCES

Andresen, E. & Willeberg, P. (1976). Pituitary dwarfism in German Shepherd dogs: Additional evidence of simple autosomal recessive inheritance. *Nordisk Veterinaer Medicin*, **28**, 481–486.

Eigenmann, J.E. (1981). Diabetes mellitus in elderly female dogs: recent findings on pathogenesis and clinical implications. *Journal of the American Animal Hospital Association*, **17**, 805–812.

Eigenmann, J.E., Zanesco, S., Arnold, U. & Froesch, E.R. (1984a). Growth hormone and insulin-like growth factor 1 in German Shepherd dwarf dogs. *Acta Endocrinologica*, **105**, 289–293.

Eigenmann, J.E., Patterson, D.F., Zapf, J. & Froesch, E.R. (1984b). Insulin-like growth factor 1 in the dog: a study in different dog breeds and in dogs with growth hormone elevation. *Acta Endocrinologica*, **105**, 294–301.

van Herpen, H., Rinjberk, A. & Mol, J.A. (1994). Production of antibodies to biosynthetic human growth hormone in the dog. *Veterinary Record*, **134**, 171.

Rijnberk, A., van Herpen, H., Mol, J.A. & Rutteman, G.R. (1993). Disturbed release of growth hormone in mature dogs: a comparison with congenital growth hormone deficiency. *Veterinary Record*, **133**, 542–545.

Schmeitzel, L.P. & Lothrop, C.D. (1990). Hormonal abnormalities in Pomeranians with normal coat and in Pomeranians with growth hormone-responsive dermatosis. *Journal of the American Veterinary Medical Association*, **197**, 1333–1341.

Selman, P.J., Mol, J.A., Rutteman, G.R., Van Garderen, E. & Rijnberk, A. (1994). Progestin-induced growth hormone excess in the dog originates in the mammary gland. *Endocrinology*, **134**, 287–292.

Chapter 56

Diagnosis of Hypothyroidism

C. Scott-Moncrieff

Hypothyroidism results in decreased production of thyroid hormones thyroxine (T_4) and triiodothyronine (T_3) from the thyroid gland. It is a common disease in dogs but is very rare in the cat (Rand *et al.* 1993).

CAUSES OF HYPOTHYROIDISM

More than 95% of cases of canine hypothyroidism are believed to be due to acquired primary hypothyroidism. Destruction of the thyroid gland can result from lymphocytic thyroiditis, idiopathic thyroid atrophy, or rarely neoplastic invasion. Secondary hypothyroidism (deficiency of thyroid stimulating hormone (TSH)) is well described in humans but uncommonly recognised in the dog, probably because a validated assay for canine TSH has been unavailable until recently. Causes of acquired secondary hypothyroidism in the dog include pituitary neoplasia and pituitary malformations such as cystic Rathke's pouch. Tertiary hypothyroidism (deficiency of thyrotrophin releasing hormone (TRH)) has not been documented in dogs.

Congenital hypothyroidism (cretinism) occurs in dogs, but is rarely diagnosed because it usually results in early puppy death. Causes of congenital hypothyroidism include thyroid agenesis, dysgenesis and dyshormonogenesis. Juvenile onset hypothyroidism has been reported in a family of Giant Schnauzers and in a Boxer. In both cases secondary hypothyroidism was suspected because of improved T_4 secretion after repeated administration of TSH (Greco *et al.* 1991; Mooney & Anderson 1993).

SIGNALMENT

Any breed may develop hypothyroidism, however some breeds such as the Golden Retriever and the Doberman Pinscher have been reported to be at higher risk in several studies (Nesbitt *et al.* 1980; Milne & Hayes 1981; Panciera 1994). Other breeds which are suspected to have a predisposition for hypothyroidism are shown in Table 56.1.

Middle aged dogs are at increased risk of hypothyroidism. In a recent study mean age at diagnosis was 7.2 years with a range of 0.5–15 years (Panciera 1994). Spayed females and neutered male dogs are at increased risk for developing hypothyroidism compared with sexually intact animals (Panciera 1994).

CLINICAL SIGNS

Thyroid hormone deficiency affects all organ systems causing a decrease in the basal metabolic rate. The clinical signs tend to be vague, diffuse and insidious in onset and are usually not pathognomonic for the disease. The most common clinical signs are metabolic and dermatological abnormalities (Table 56.2). Clinical signs such as obesity and unwillingness to exercise are often attributed to ageing. Although 41% of hypothyroid dogs are reported to be obese (Panciera 1994) most cases of obesity are due to overfeeding not hypothyroidism.

The alopecia observed in hypothyroidism is usually bilaterally symmetrical, although hair loss in areas undergoing friction is also common. The lateral trunk and the tail are usually the first areas to be affected. In many cases the hair is brittle and easily epilated. Loss of primary guard hairs may result in a puppy like hair coat.

The reproductive system may also be adversely affected in hypothyroidism (Table 56.3). It should be noted however that two studies have failed to demonstrate a correlation between breeding performance and thyroid status in experimental male beagles or in a large group of racing male and female greyhounds (Beale *et al.* 1992; Johnson *et al.* 1995). Other organ systems which may be affected by

Table 56.1 Breeds suspected of a predisposition for hypothyroidism.

Golden Retriever	Dachshund
Doberman Pinscher	Irish Setter
Great Dane	Miniature Schnauzer
Shetland Sheepdog	Poodle
Cocker Spaniel	Boxer
Airedale	Pomeranian

Table 56.2 Common clinical signs of hypothyroidism.

Effects on metabolic rate
Lethargy
Dullness
Unwillingness to exercise
Cold intolerance
Weight gain

Skin and hair coat
Dry scaly skin
Hyperkeratosis
Hyperpigmentation
Seborrhoea
Myxoedema
Superficial pyoderma
Coarse dull hair coat
Alopecia
Change in coat colour
Hypertrichosis

Table 56.3 Reproductive abnormalities associated with hypothyroidism.

Reproductive organs (female)
Prolonged inter-oestrus intervals
Failure to cycle
Infertility
Weak or still born puppies

Reproductive organs (male)
Low libido
Testicular atrophy
Infertility
Hypospermia
Azospermia

hypothyroidism include the eyes, heart and peripheral and central nervous systems (Table 56.4).

Although less common than the typical clinical signs discussed above, it is important to be aware of the neurological manifestations of hypothyroidism, because affected dogs may not show the more characteristic clinical signs until later in the course of the disease. Lower motor neuron dysfunction is the best documented neurological manifestation of hypothyroidism (Indrieri *et al.* 1987; Jaggy *et al.* 1994). In some reported cases, clinical signs were consistent with a peripheral neuropathy, whereas in other cases it was not possible to establish whether a neuropathy, myopathy, or both was the cause of clinical signs. Affected dogs had weakness, ataxia, quadriparesis or paralysis and in some cases decreased spinal reflexes. Lameness with no detectable neurological signs has also been reported associated with hypothyroidism (Budsberg *et al.* 1993).

Abnormalities consistent with intracranial disease such as cranial nerve dysfunction, abnormal postural reactions and gait deficits may also occur in canine hypothyroidism (Table 56.4) (Bichsel *et al.* 1988; Jaggy *et al.* 1994). Clinical

Table 56.4 Less common clinical signs of hypothyroidism.

Eyes
Corneal lipid deposits
Corneal ulceration
Uveitis
Keratoconjunctivitis

Heart
Bradycardia
Weak apex beat
Low voltage R waves

Neuromuscular system
Lower motor neuron paresis/paralysis
Decreased spinal reflexes

Central nervous system
Circling
Head tilt
Strabismus
Facial nerve paralysis
Decreased facial sensation
Hemiparesis, ataxia
Depression, irritability
Seizures

Skeletal system (congenital hypothyroidism)
Disproportionate dwarfism
Short broad skull
Epiphyseal dysgenesis

signs resolve after thyroid hormone supplementation. Dogs with myxoedema coma, which is a very rare manifestation of hypothyroidism in dogs, may demonstrate mental dullness, severe depression and inappetence.

Although hypothyroidism has also been associated with idiopathic facial nerve paralysis, megaoesophagus and laryngeal paralysis, a causal relationship has not been established. Thyroid supplementation alone does not appear to consistently reverse the clinical signs in these disorders.

Congenital or juvenile onset hypothyroidism may result in stunted disproportionate growth, epiphyseal dysgenesis and mental retardation. Affected dogs have a large broad head, short limbs, a dull mental state and a puppy-type hair coat. Most severely affected puppies die in the first few weeks of life.

DIAGNOSIS

A clinical suspicion of hypothyroidism may be obtained by evaluation of the signalment, history and physical examination, results of a haematology, biochemistry and urinalysis and measurement of basal thyroid hormone concentrations. Tests that may be utilised to confirm the diagnosis include provocative thyroid function tests, measurement of endogenous TSH concentration and response to thyroid hormone supplementation.

Laboratory Findings

Clinicopathological changes that are commonly observed in dogs with hypothyroidism are a normocytic normochromic non-regenerative anaemia, fasting hypertriglyceridaemia and hypercholesterolaemia (Table 56.5). Changes that are less common include increased concentrations of leptocytes (target cells) and mild to moderate increases in alanine transaminase (ALT), aspartate aminotransferase (AST), alkaline phosphatase (ALP) and creatine kinase (CK). These changes are all non-specific, however their presence may be supportive evidence for a diagnosis of hypothyroidism.

Table 56.5 Common clinicopathological changes observed in canine hypothyroidism.

Normocytic normochromic anaemia
Hypertriglyceridaemia
Hypercholesterolaemia

Basal Thyroid Hormone Concentrations

The two most important thyroid hormones secreted by the thyroid gland are thyroxine (T_4) and 3,5,3′ triiodothyronine (T_3). Thyroxine is the predominant secretory product of the thyroid gland, while the majority of serum T_3 is derived from the extrathyroidal deiodination of T_4. Both T_3 and T_4 are highly protein bound to serum carrier proteins such as thyroglobulin, transthyretin and albumin. Only unbound (free) hormone penetrates cell membranes, binds to receptors and has biological activity. Protein-bound hormone acts as a reservoir and buffer to maintain a steady concentration of free hormone in the plasma despite rapid alterations in release and metabolism of T_3 and T_4 and changes in plasma protein concentrations.

Free T_4 is mono-deiodinated within cells to T_3 which binds to receptors and induces the cellular effects of thyroid hormone. Serum concentrations of T_4 are thought to be the main determinant of feedback control of TRH and TSH secretion.

Total T_4 Concentration

Total T_4 concentration is the most commonly performed static thyroid hormone measurement and is a good initial screening test for canine hypothyroidism. In general a dog with a normal T_4 concentration may be assumed to have normal thyroid function, however a basal T_4 concentration below the normal range is not diagnostic for hypothyroidism. In this case the animal may be normal, hypothyroid, or suffering from a non-thyroidal illness with a secondary decrease in the basal T_4 concentration (sick euthyroid syndrome). Factors such as time of day, age, breed and ambient temperature, may affect the total T_4 concentration without altering metabolically active free thyroid hormone concentrations. In one study, 50–60% of normal dogs had a low serum total T_4 at some time during the day. Oestrus, pregnancy, obesity, malnutrition, exogenous glucocorticoids and drugs such as trimethoprim–sulfamethoxazole, anticonvulsants, salicylates and phenylbutazone may also change the basal T_4 concentration. Systemic illnesses that are particularly likely to decrease basal T_4 concentrations include hyperadrenocorticism, diabetes mellitus, hypoadrenocorticism, renal failure, hepatic failure and infection. Changes in protein binding, decreased conversion of T_4 to T_3, inhibition of TSH secretion and inhibition of thyroid hormone synthesis by the thyroid gland are potential mechanisms for decreased total T_4 concentrations in euthyroid dogs.

Free T₄ Concentration

Since only the unbound fraction of serum T_4 is biologically active, measurement of free T_4 has been hypothesised to be useful in differentiating euthyroid dogs from hypothyroid dogs. Despite the usefulness of free T_4 assays in humans, most commercial assays for free T_4 do not appear to add additional diagnostic information in the dog (Nelson *et al.* 1991). This may be due to the use of single stage solid phase (analogue) radioimmunoassays for free T_4 developed for humans, which may not be ideal for measuring free T_4 in the dog owing to differences in serum binding proteins. A commercial direct free T_4 assay which utilises an equilibrium dialysis step had better accuracy than the analogue methods in dogs (Scott-Moncrieff *et al.* 1994). This assay had an accuracy of 97% compared with an accuracy of 79% for total T_4.

Basal T₃ Concentration

T_3 concentrations are less accurate in distinguishing euthyroid from hypothyroid dogs since T_3 concentrations tend to fluctuate in and out of the normal range even more than T_4 concentrations in euthyroid dogs (Miller *et al.* 1992). Spurious T_3 measurements may also occur due to the presence of anti-T_3 antibodies which interfere with commercial assays for T_3. In most antibody specific techniques, anti-T_3 antibodies result in spuriously high values for T_3. Anti-T_3 antibodies are considered to be an indicator of lymphocytic thyroiditis in dogs and can be identified in up to 50% of dogs with hypothyroidism (Beale *et al.* 1990). Since 18% of euthyroid dogs also have anti-T_3 antibodies however, their presence is not diagnostic for hypothyroidism. Anti-T_4 antibodies have also been reported although they occur less commonly. Theoretically these antibodies could increase a low T_4 concentration into the normal range and result in a false diagnosis of euthyroidism. Anti-thyroid antibodies do not interfere with response to thyroid supplementation in dogs with hypothyroidism.

TSH Stimulation Test

The TSH stimulation test evaluates the responsiveness of the thyroid gland to exogenously administered TSH and is a test of thyroid reserve. It is an accurate test of thyroid function in dogs but its use is limited by the expense and limited availability of TSH. The cost of the TSH stimulation test may be decreased by storing reconstituted TSH either refrigerated for up to 1 month or frozen at −20°C for up to 3 months. The most reliable protocol requires collection of a serum sample for measurement of a basal T_4 fol-

lowed by administration of bovine TSH intravenously at a dose of 0.1 units/kg (maximum dose 5 units). A second sample for measurement of T_4 is collected 6 h later. Results may reveal a normal response, a blunted response (sick euthyroid syndrome) or no response (hypothyroidism). Various criteria have been used to interpret the TSH stimulation test. A diagnosis of hypothyroidism can be confirmed if both the pre- and the post-T_4 samples are below the reference range for basal total T_4 concentration. A euthyroid state is confirmed if the post-T_4 concentration is above the reference range for basal T_4. Interpretation of intermediate results is more difficult and should take into consideration the clinical signs and severity of concurrent systemic disease (Fig. 56.1). The TSH stimulation test is not useful for evaluation of thyroid function in dogs already receiving thyroid supplementation, since exogenous thyroid hormone will suppress the synthesis and release of TSH and result in thyroid atrophy. Exogenous supplementation must therefore be withdrawn 6–8 weeks before TSH testing.

TRH Stimulation Test

This test was designed for use in people to evaluate TSH secretion by the pituitary gland after administration of TRH. In dogs the test has been used to evaluate the thyroid by measurement of T_4 production after TRH administration. Unfortunately the change in serum T_4 after TRH administration is not as large as after TSH administration and some dogs with normal thyroid function have decreased response to TRH. For this reason the test is of limited clinical utility. Various protocols have been reported

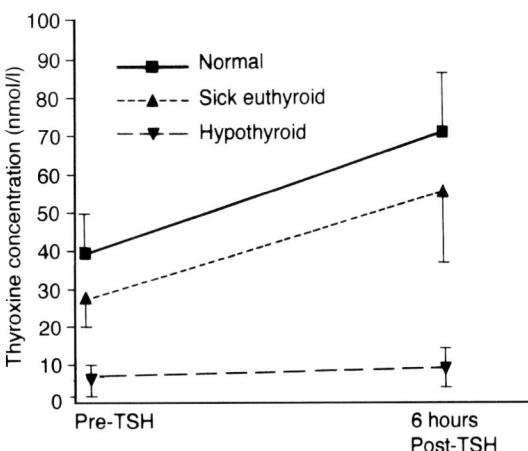

Fig. 56.1 Interpretation of the TSH stimulation test.

with the most commonly used dose being 0.1 mg/kg of TRH administered intravenously with samples collected before and 6 h after TRH administration. Side-effects such as salivation, vomiting, urination, defecation, miosis, tachycardia and tachypnoea may be observed at this dose. Recent studies have suggested that a lower fixed dose of 100–600 μg TRH intravenously, with samples collected at 0 and 4 h, is as reliable as the higher dose and less likely to result in side effects (Sparkes *et al.* 1995).

Endogenous TSH Concentration

A new assay for endogenous canine TSH has recently become available. Early validation studies in dogs with experimentally induced hypothyroidism have been encouraging, but the assay has yet to be validated in large numbers of clinical cases. Preliminary studies suggest that a low total T_4 concentration in conjunction with an increased TSH concentration is highly supportive of hypothyroidism.

Therapeutic Trial

In some cases the most practical approach to confirming the diagnosis of hypothyroidism is to perform a therapeutic trial. This is an acceptable practice providing the following guidelines are followed. Every attempt should be made to rule out non-thyroidal illness before starting a therapeutic trial. There is no evidence that thyroid supplementation is beneficial in sick euthyroid dogs and may be detrimental. Thyroxine supplementation should be initiated using a veterinary licensed product at the appropriate dose and frequency (see below). Objective criteria should be used to assess response to treatment.

If a positive response to treatment occurs, the clinician should be prepared to withdraw therapy to confirm that clinical signs return. This will ensure that dogs with thyroid responsive diseases do not remain on thyroid supplementation for life. Dogs with thyroid responsive diseases are those dogs in which the clinical signs improve due to the non-specific effects of thyroid hormone or unrelated to therapy. If therapy is unsuccessful, therapeutic monitoring should be performed to identify the cause of treatment failure (see below). Since an incorrect diagnosis is the most common cause of treatment failure, the clinician should be prepared to withdraw therapy and pursue other diagnoses.

TREATMENT

Synthetic thyroid hormone products are preferable to those of animal origin since synthetic products (salts of T_3 or T_4)

are more stable and better standardised for potency. Sodium levothyroxine (synthetic T_4) is the initial thyroid supplement of choice. Levothyroxine has a serum half-life of 12–16 h and peak concentrations are achieved at 4–12 h after administration. Recommendations for initiation of therapy are to administer a veterinary licensed product at a dose of 20 μg/kg twice a day. Some dogs will ultimately only require supplementation once a day. Once a clinical response is achieved, a trial with once a day therapy can be instituted. Some authors recommend dosing based on body surface area (0.5 mg/m²). In animals with concurrent heart disease a sudden increase in the basal metabolic rate due to initiation of therapy can lead to cardiac destabilisation. These animals should be started on 50% of the recommended starting dose for thyroxine and the dose then adjusted using therapeutic monitoring.

Synthetic triiodothyronine administration is only indicated in those few situations when T_4 supplementation has failed to achieve a response in a dog with confirmed hypothyroidism. This may occur due to impaired T_4 absorption from the gastrointestinal tract. T_3 supplementation is not recommended for initial therapy because only serum T_3 concentrations are normalised while T_4 levels remain low. Dogs receiving T_3 supplementation may be more susceptible to iatrogenic thyrotoxicosis since serum T_4 concentrations are important in the feedback regulation of the hypothalamic–pituitary–thyroid axis. Combination products that contain both T_3 and T_4 should be avoided for similar reasons. The plasma half-life of synthetic T_3 is 5–6 h so it needs to be administered three times a day. The initial starting dose is 4–6 μg/kg every 8 h.

Response to Therapy

Clinical improvement should be observed in 4–6 weeks from initiation of therapy although an improvement in the patient's activity level may occur within 1 week. Dermatological abnormalities may take several months to completely resolve and initially the appearance of the hair coat may worsen as old hair is shed. Reproductive and clinicopathological abnormalities are usually the last to resolve. If the response to therapy is being used to confirm the diagnosis, treatment should be withdrawn after a complete response is achieved. If clinical signs recur the diagnosis is confirmed and treatment can be reinstituted. If no recurrence of clinical signs is observed, a thyroid responsive disease should be suspected and thyroid supplementation should not be continued.

Poor Response to Therapy

An absent or inadequate response to therapy may be due to incorrect diagnosis, poor owner compliance, inadequate dose of thyroid supplementation, poor oral absorption of thyroid supplement, or use of thyroid supplements of animal origin. Defective conversion of T_4 to T_3 and resistance of peripheral tissues to the action of thyroid hormone are theoretical causes of treatment failure that have not been well documented in dogs.

Therapeutic Monitoring

Monitoring of serum T_4 and T_3 concentrations will allow the clinician to identify the reason for failure to respond to thyroid supplementation and allow individualisation of the dose and dosing frequency. Measurement of serum T_3 and T_4 concentrations should be performed after at least one month of therapy. A serum sample is taken before and 4–6 h after treatment and submitted for measurement of T_4 concentrations. Dosage and frequency of thyroid supplementation can then be adjusted appropriately. Both T_4 measurements should be in the normal reference range and ideally the T_3 concentration should also normalise. In some cases the T_3 may remain below the reference range. This does not usually indicate a problem in the conversion of T_4 to T_3 and is not necessarily an indication to switch to T_3 supplementation.

REFERENCES

Beale, K.M., Halliwell, R.E.W. & Chen, C.L. (1990). Prevalence of antithyroglobulin antibodies detected by enxyme-linked immunosorbent assay of canine serum. *Journal of the American Veterinary Medical Association*, **196**, 745–748.

Beale, K.M., Bloomberg, M.S., Van Gilder, J., Wolfson, B.B. & Keisling, K. (1992). Correlation of racing and reproductive performance in greyhounds with response to thyroid function testing. *Journal of the American Animal Hospital Association*, **28**, 263–269.

Bischel, P., Jacobs, G. & Oliver, J.E. (1988). Neurological manifestations associated with hypothyroidism in four dogs. *Journal of the American Veterinary Medical Association*, **192**, 1745–1747.

Budsberg, S.C., Moore, G.E. & Klappenbach, K. (1993). Thyroxine-responsive unilateral forelimb lameness and generalized neuromuscular disease in four hypothyroid dogs. *Journal of the American Veterinary Medical Association*, **202**, 1859–1860.

Greco, D.S., Feldman, E.C., Peterson, M.E., Turner, J.L., Hodges, C.M. & Shipman, L.W. (1991). Congenital hypothyroid dwarfism in a family of giant schnauzers. *Journal of Veterinary Internal Medicine*, **5**, 57–65.

Indrieri, R.J., Whalen, L.R., Cardinet, G.H. & Holliday, T.A. (1987). Neuromuscular abnormalities associated with hypothyroidism and lymphocytic thyroiditis in three dogs. *Journal of the American Veterinary Medical Association*, **190**, 544–548.

Jaggy, A., Oliver, J.E., Ferguson, D.C., Mahaffey, E.A. & Glaus, T. (1994). Neurological manifestations of hypothyroidism: a retrospective study of 29 dogs. *Journal of Veterinary Internal Medicine*, **8**, 328–336.

Johnson, C.A., Nachreiner, R.F. & Mullaney, T.P. (1995). Effects of hypothyroidism on canine reproduction. *Proceedings of the American College of Veterinary Internal Medicine*, 990 (Abstract).

Miller, A.B., Nelson, R.W., Scott-Moncrieff, J.C., Neal, L. & Bottoms, G.D. (1992). Serial thyroid hormone concentrations in healthy euthyroid dogs, dogs with hypothyroidism, and euthyroid dogs with atopic dermatitis. *British Veterinary Journal*, **148**, 451–458.

Milne, K.L. & Hayes, H.M. (1981). Epidemiologic features of canine hypothyroidism. *Cornell Veterinarian*, **71**, 3–14.

Mooney, C.T. & Anderson, T.J. (1993). Congenital hypothyroidism in a boxer dog. *Journal of Small Animal Practice*, **34**, 31–35.

Nelson, R.W., Ihle, S.L., Feldman, E.C. & Bottoms, G.D. (1991). Serum free thyroxine concentrations in healthy dogs, dogs with hypothyroidism, and euthyroid dogs with concurrent illness. *Journal of the American Veterinary Medical Association*, **198**, 1401–1407.

Nesbit, G. H., Izzo, J., Peterson, L. & Wilkins, R.J. (1980). Canine hypothyroidism: a retrospective study of 108 cases. *Journal of the American Veterinary Medical Association*, **177**, 1117–1122.

Panciera, D.L. (1994). Hypothyroidism in dogs: 66 cases (1987–1992). *Journal of the American Veterinary Medical Association*, **204**, 761–767.

Rand, J.S., Levine, J., Best, S.J. & Parker, W. (1993). Spontaneous adult-onset hypothyroidism in a cat. *Journal of Veterinary Internal Medicine*, **7**, 272–276.

Sparkes, A.H., Gruffydd-Jones, T.J., Wotton, P.R., Gleadhill, A., Evans, H. & Walker, M.J. (1995). Assessment of dose and time responses to TRH and thyrotropin in healthy dogs. *Journal of Small Animal Practice*, **36**, 245–251.

Scott-Moncrieff, J.C., Nelson, R., Ferguson, D. & Neal, L. (1994). Measurement of serum free thyroxine by modified equilibrium dialysis in dogs. *Proceedings of the American College of Veterinary Internal Medicine*, 990 (Abstract).

Chapter 57

Disorders of Calcium Metabolism

F. P. Gaschen

Calcium is involved in many body functions. Muscle contraction, neural excitability, blood coagulation and many subcellular functions all require the presence of calcium. It is also of central importance for maintenance of homeostasis. About 99% of total body calcium is stored in the inorganic matrix of the bone. Extracellular fluids contain only minute amounts of the mineral. Routinely performed laboratory tests measure total calcium in the serum. Ionised calcium is the biologically active form and accounts for approximately 50% of total serum calcium, 40% of serum calcium is bound to albumin, and 10% circulates in the form of calcium complexes (Rosol *et al.* 1995). Disorders of calcium metabolism are relatively frequently diagnosed in canine medicine. Among dogs affected with such disorders, hypercalcaemia is much more prevalent than hypocalcaemia.

HYPERCALCAEMIA

Aetiology

The differential diagnoses of hypercalcaemia in dogs are listed in Table 57.1. Over a period of 12 months, malignancy associated hypercalcaemia was the most frequent diagnosis among hypercalcaemic dogs presented to the University of Berne Clinic for Companion Animals. This was followed by chronic renal failure, hypoadrenocorticism and primary hyperparathyroidism (Fig. 57.1). These four diseases are generally considered the most common differential diagnoses of hypercalcaemia in dogs (Elliott *et al.* 1991). Ingestion of specific houseplants and intoxication with cholecalciferol-containing rodenticides have been reported to cause hypervitaminosis D with resultant hypercalcaemia in the dog (Dougherty *et al.* 1990).

Malignancy Associated Hypercalcaemia (MAH)

In dogs, hypercalcaemia is often secondary to remote effects of cancer. Malignant tumours such as canine lymphoma (10–40% of cases), multiple myeloma (10–15% of cases), and apocrine cell adenocarcinomas of the anal sacs (approximately 80% of cases) can produce humoral or local factors leading to osteoclastic bone resorption and hypercalcaemia. Plasma ionised calcium levels are generally increased in such paraneoplastic hypercalcaemia. A detailed description of MAH can be found in Chapter 35, page 265.

Chronic Renal Failure (CRF)

Dogs affected with CRF and secondary renal hyperparathyroidism are mostly normocalcaemic or even hypocalcaemic. However hypercalcaemia has been reported to occur in 10–20% of dogs with CRF. Despite the increase in total serum calcium, the concentration of ionised calcium remains normal or even decreased. Factors involved in the pathogenesis of hypercalcaemia in these animals include parathormone-mediated increased bone resorption, decreased renal calcium excretion due to decreased glomerular and tubular function, as well as increased intestinal calcium absorption and increased calcium complexing with anions (Kruger & Osborne 1994a). Renal failure may also be a complication of hypercalcaemia caused by extrarenal mechanisms. Measurements of plasma levels of ionised calcium and serum parathormone (PTH) may help differentiate between primary and secondary hypercalcaemia in patients with renal failure (Fig. 57.2).

Table 57.1   Common differential diagnoses of canine hypercalcaemia.

Paraneoplastic syndrome:
  Ectopic:
    Lymphoma
    Multiple myeloma
    Apocrine cell adenocarcinoma of the anal sacs
    Other carcinomas such as squamous cell carcinoma
    Mammary adenocarcinoma
  Topic:
    Primary hyperparathyroidism

Chronic renal failure

Hypoadrenocorticism

Vitamin D intoxication

Granulomatous diseases such as systemic mycoses

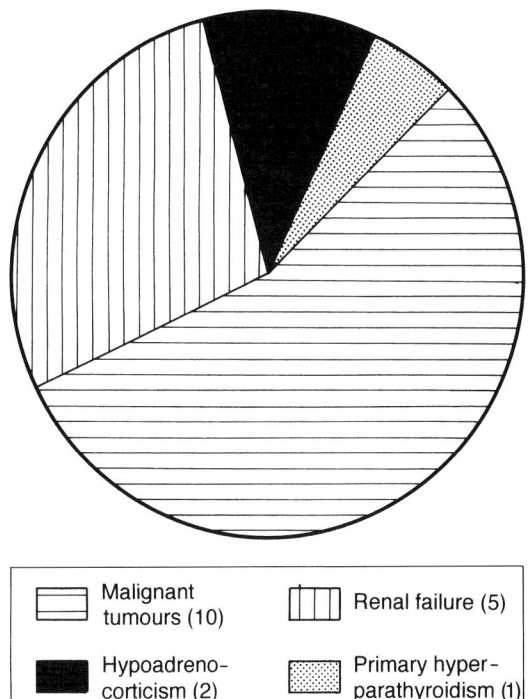

Malignant tumours (10)
Hypoadreno-corticism (2)
Renal failure (5)
Primary hyper-parathyroidism (1)

Fig. 57.1   Final diagnosis in 18 hypercalcaemic dogs with classifiable disease seen at the University of Berne Clinic for Companion Animals between November 1994 and October 1995. Causes of malignancy-associated hypercalcaemia were: malignant lymphoma ($n = 7$), mammary adenocarcinoma ($n = 2$), squamous cell carcinoma ($n = 1$).

Hypoadrenocorticism

Mild to moderate hypercalcaemia is quite prevalent in dogs with hypoadrenocorticism with up to 45% of cases affected. Plasma ionised calcium levels remain normal in these patients. The increase in total serum calcium may be secondary to severe haemoconcentration and reduced renal clearance of calcium. Glucocorticoid deficiency may also encourage enhanced intestinal absorption of calcium.

Primary Hyperparathyroidism

Primary hyperparathyroidism occurs typically in older dogs. There does not appear to be any breed predisposition. Parathyroid adenoma has been reported more frequently than adenocarcinoma. PTH-mediated effects include increased bone resorption and mobilisation of calcium by the osteoclasts. Hypercalcaemia is associated with increased levels of ionised calcium as a consequence of increased PTH secretion (Feldman 1994).

Clinical Signs

The clinical signs attributable to hypercalcaemia are summarised in Table 57.2. Other signs related to the underlying cause or to the dramatic consequences of hypercalcaemia may dominate the clinical picture (for example persistent vomiting and dehydration associated with renal failure). Polyuria occurs secondary to interference by increased calcium concentrations on the action of antidiuretic hormone on the distal renal tubules. This is followed by compensatory polydipsia. Gastrointestinal signs are also frequently observed and are mainly due to decreased excitability of gastrointestinal smooth muscle and soft tissue mineralisation. Alterations in membrane excitability are responsible for neuromuscular signs ranging from generalised weakness to rare seizure activity. Cardiovascular manifestations such as ECG changes and cardiac arrhythmias are uncommon in dogs.

Table 57.2   Clinical signs frequently associated with hypercalcaemia in dogs.

Polyuria/polydipsia
Lethargy
Inappetence/anorexia
Muscle weakness
Vomiting
Diarrhoea or constipation
Signs of lower urinary tract inflammation

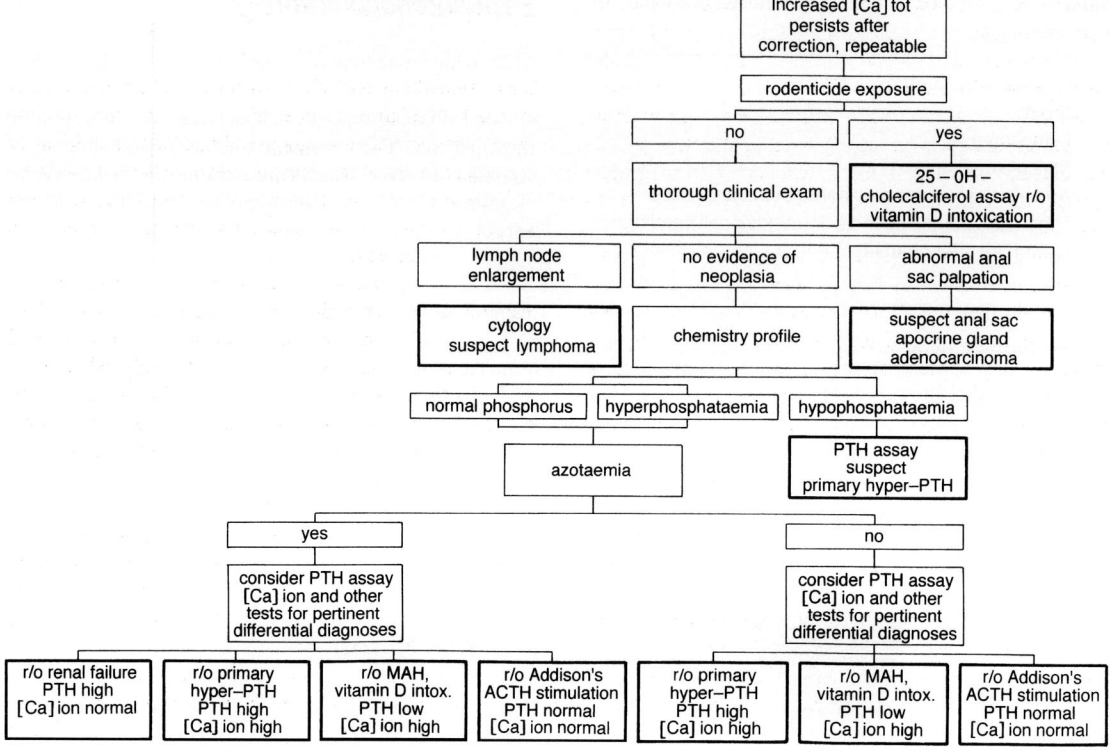

Fig. 57.2   Algorithm for the diagnostic approach to the hypercalcaemic dog. Abbreviations: [Ca] tot, serum total calcium; [Ca] ion, serum ionised calcium; PTH, parathyroid hormone; hyper-PTH, hyperparathyroidism; MAH, malignancy associated hypercalcaemia.

Diagnostic Approach (Fig. 57.2)

Laboratory error should always be suspected in case of a single increase in total serum calcium. Growing dogs have higher normal values for serum calcium concentrations than adult dogs. If the increase is confirmed, adjustment of total serum calcium proportionally to serum albumin should be calculated according to the following formula:

$$\text{Corrected Ca (mmol/l)} = \text{Measured total Ca (mmol/l)} + 1/40 \times \left[35 - \text{albumin (g/l)} \right]$$

This equation has been established to adjust calcium concentrations in patients with hypoalbuminaemia. In the author's experience, it is also applicable to haemoconcentrated dogs. This reflects the fact that alterations in serum albumin may influence total serum calcium but do not affect the ionised calcium concentrations.

Patients with corrected total serum calcium concentrations above 3.5 mmol/l and/or product of serum calcium and phosphorus concentrations higher than 5.6 are at risk of developing soft tissue mineralisation and subsequent complications. Severe increases in serum calcium levels warrant an aggressive diagnostic and therapeutic approach.

Laboratory investigations in hypercalcaemic dogs should include a complete blood count and serum biochemistry profile as well as urinalysis. Haematological abnormalities are related to the underlying disorder. A decreased Na/K ratio may be present in cases of hypoadrenocorticism. Renal azotaemia is a common finding in hypercalcaemic dogs. Reversible hypercalcaemia-mediated changes in renal haemodynamics are dominated by vasoconstriction and may lead to reduced glomerular filtration rate (GFR). Persistent hypercalcaemia may be followed by irreversible damage to renal tissue caused by vasoconstriction and nephrocalcinosis. Phosphate levels may be normal to increased in hypercalcaemic azotaemic patients. Primary hyperparathyroidism is classically associated with hypo-phosphataemia since PTH decreases the renal tubular reabsorption of phosphorus (Feldman 1994). Urinalysis consistently reveals isosthenuria. This and other factors may predispose hypercalcaemic dogs to develop urinary tract infections. Calcium phosphate or calcium oxalate crystals or urolith formation may also occur due to hypercalciuria.

Newer diagnostic tests such as determination of plasma ionised calcium and serum parathormone concentrations (intact molecule assay) are now available at many laboratories, and make the diagnostic work up of the hypercalcaemic dog easier. However, a thorough clinical examination followed by simple ancillary tests remains crucial and these newer tests should be used with discrimination by the astute clinician.

Diagnostic imaging rarely allows a definitive diagnosis in hypercalcaemic dogs. Radiographs are not very sensitive for demonstrating soft tissue mineralisation (for example in the kidneys) or alterations in bone density. Ultrasonographic examination of the kidneys may help documenting the presence of irreversible parenchymatous damage but remains of little help in differentiating between renal or extrarenal origin for hypercalcaemia. Detection of a hyperechogenic band at the corticomedullary junction is compatible with hypercalcaemic nephropathy but has also been reported in other renal diseases. Thorough ultrasonographic scanning of the ventral neck may allow visualisation of parathyroid nodules in cases of primary hyperparathyroidism (Fig. 57.3) and justify surgical exploration of the thyroid area (Fig. 57.4).

Symptomatic Therapy

Correction of the underlying disorder leading to hypercalcaemia is the ultimate goal of treatment. However, the short-term objective is to correct hypercalcaemia in order to reduce the risk of irreversible consequences such as mineralisation of the renal parenchyma. Drugs used in the immediate treatment of hypercalcaemia and their dosages are listed in Table 57.3.

Mild to moderate increases in serum calcium may respond to simple rehydration and diuresis with physiological saline solution, leading to enhanced natriuresis and associated calciuresis. Once the dog is fully rehydrated, further calciuresis may be promoted by the administration of the loop diuretic frusemide. Avoid using thiazide diuretics as they lead to increased renal calcium reabsorption. Some animals may require frequent, high doses of frusemide to lower the serum calcium concentration. Glucocorticoids have some calcium lowering effects and are mainly effective in dogs with lymphoma and paraneoplastic hypercalcaemia. They alter the appearance of neoplastic lymphoid cells and therefore should only be used after the cause of hypercalcaemia has been identified.

If the first line therapy remains unsuccessful, the use of calcium lowering agents that inhibit bone resorption such as bisphosphonates (Kruger & Osborne 1994b; Petrie 1996), salmon calcitonin (Dougherty et al. 1990) and mithramycin (Rosol et al. 1994) may be considered. These substances are not approved for use in dogs and may have serious side-effects. The reader is advised to consult the available literature before using them in patients.

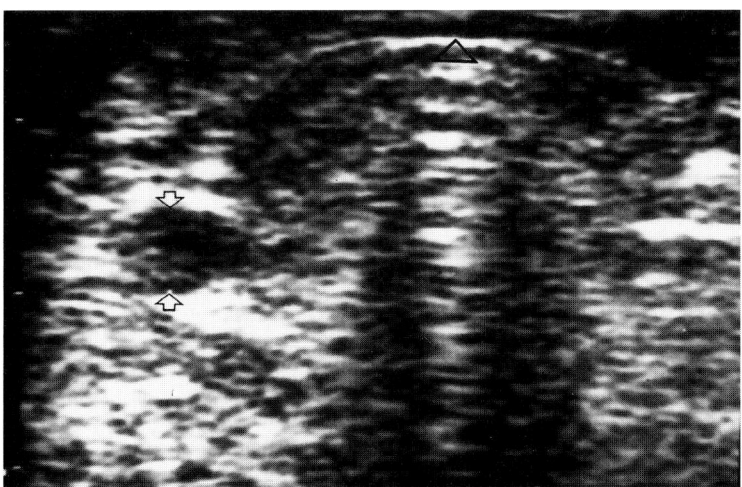

Fig. 57.3 Ultrasound picture of the ventral neck in a 10-year-old Daschund with hypercalcaemia. The white arrows show the edges of a hypoechoic nodule in the right thyroid lobe with a diameter of approximately 5 mm, the arrow head points to the ventral aspect of the trachea. The serum parathyroid hormone concentration was increased. A parathyroid adenoma was diagnosed histologically.

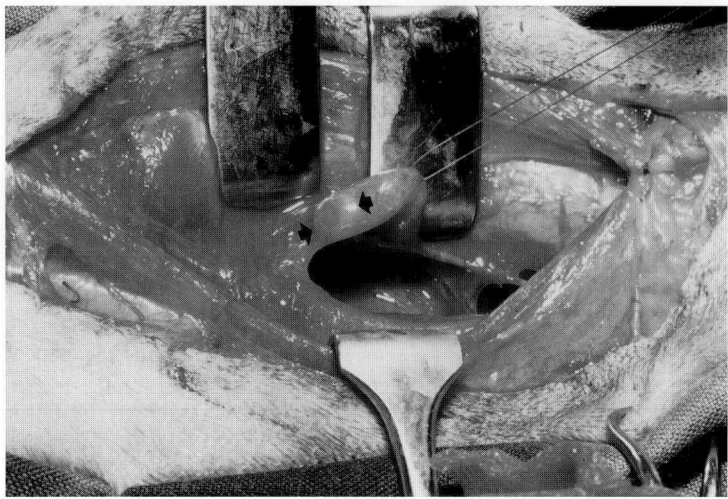

Fig. 57.4   Picture of the ventral neck of a dog with primary hyperparathyroidism. The enlarged parathyroid gland is delineated by the black arrows. Courtesy of Dr U. Weber, Berne, Switzerland.

Table 57.3   Drugs used in the symptomatic treatment of hypercalcaemia.

Drug	Recommended dosage
0.9% NaCl solution	Replace total fluid deficits, induce diuresis using double maintenance infusion rate
Frusemide	5 mg/kg i.v. bolus followed by repeat injections of the same dosage every 1 to 8 h and possibly as constant rate infusion depending on severity of hypercalcaemia and response. Full rehydration is a prerequisite. Maintain hydration and electrolyte balance with appropriate infusion of 0.9% saline solution with KCl added. Monitor serum potassium carefully.
Prednisolone	1-2 mg/kg p.o. once to twice daily
Mithramycin (plicamycin, Mithracin™)	25 mg/kg i.v., maximum effect approximately 2 days post-injection. (Mithramycin is currently withdrawn from the market in some European countries)
Bisphosphonates Etidronate (Didronel™) Pamidronate (Aredia™) Clodronate (Bonefos™)	(Delayed effect) 5 mg/kg p.o. once daily No canine dose published 20–25 mg/kg diluted in 500 ml 0.9% saline as a single infusion over 4 h
Salmon calcitonin (Miacalcic™)	(Immediate effect) 4–6 IU s.c. every 8–12 h. Start with lower dose and closely monitor serum calcium

Treatment of Primary Hyperparathyroidism

Surgical resection of the parathyroid nodule results in disappearance of hypercalcaemia. In a retrospective study of numerous cases of canine hyperparathyroidism (Feldman 1994), dogs with presurgical serum calcium concentrations below 3.5 mmol/l had a lower risk of developing postsurgical hypocalcaemia. Prophylactic vitamin D and calcium therapy immediately following recovery from surgery is recommended in patients with presurgical serum calcium higher than 3.5 mmol/l in order to prevent the occurrence of hypocalcaemia.

Prognosis

The prognosis of hypercalcaemia depends on the underlying disorder and the severity of the secondary changes. Primary hyperparathyroidism carries a good prognosis. Malignancy-associated hypercalcaemia resolves rapidly after successful treatment of the underlying tumour, however the involved malignancies typically have a guarded to poor long-term prognosis. The presence of chronic renal failure as a cause or a complication of hypercalcaemia warrants a guarded prognosis depending on the severity of renal damage.

HYPOCALCAEMIA
Aetiology

Decreased total serum calcium in dogs is most frequently associated with hypoalbuminaemia and decreased protein bound calcium fraction. Few hypocalcaemias are confirmed after calculating the corrected value for serum calcium (see equation above). Puerperal tetany and hypoparathyroidism are the two diseases causing severe and symptomatic hypocalcaemia. Renal failure, acute pancreatitis, critical illness may cause mild to moderate hypocalcaemia usually without related clinical signs.

Puerperal Tetany or Eclampsia

This condition is most often observed in small breed bitches with large litters and typically occurs at the time of maximal milk production, 2–4 weeks postpartum. However, it has been reported in a variety of breeds and may also occur antepartum. Although the exact pathogenesis has not been elucidated, calcium entering the extracellu-lar space is not sufficient to match the losses occurring through mammary secretion. PTH has not been directly implicated in the pathogenesis of eclampsia. Recent theories in cows affected with a similar condition focus on the insufficient stimulation of osteoclast numbers at the bone surface in hypocalcaemic animals.

Hypoparathyroidism

Primary hypoparathyroidism is a rare condition in dogs. It results from the immune-mediated destruction of the parathyroid glands and leads to insufficient production of PTH and hypocalcaemia affecting the ionised calcium levels.

It is possibly more frequent in middle aged female dogs. Secondary hypoparathyroidism may occur following excision of parathyroid tumours as the remaining parathyroid glands are temporarily suppressed and non-functional (see the preceding section on treatment of parathyroid tumours under hypercalcaemia).

Clinical Signs

Severe hypocalcaemia is associated with clinical signs in most cases (Table 57.4). The predominant signs result from increased excitability of neuromuscular membranes.

Table 57.4   Clinical signs associated with hypocalcaemia.

Neuromuscular:
   Muscle tremors, twitching
   Muscle cramps and spasms
   Stiff gait
   Ataxia
   Weakness
   Seizures

Behavioural :
   Restlessness
   Panting
   Facial rubbing
   Aggressiveness
   Hypersensitivity to exogenous stimuli
   Disorientation

Other:
   Hyperthermia
   Inappetence
   Tachy- or brady-arrhythmias
   Polyuria/polydipsia

Seizure activity was a common feature in a retrospective study of dogs with primary hypoparathyroidism (Feldman 1994). Behavioural changes are also frequently noticed. Hyperthermia results from exaggerated muscle activity.

Diagnostic Approach

A thorough physical examination as well as laboratory investigations such as complete blood count, serum biochemistry profile and urinalysis can be helpful in identifying the cause of hypocalcaemia. The possibility of laboratory error should be considered in the absence of compatible clinical signs or underlying diseases. Correction of calcium concentration relative to albumin should be calculated (see equation in hypercalcaemia section). Clinically affected dogs have low corrected total serum calcium concentrations (less than 1.6 mmol/l). Hyperphosphataemia is a feature of hypoparathyroidism. Small breed bitches with puerperal tetany may have concurrent hypoglycaemia. Other abnormalities may give some information on an underlying disorder. Electrocardiographic changes may be noticed in severe forms with bradycardia, prolongation of ST and QT segments, and deep, wide T waves.

Symptomatic Treatment (Table 57.5)

Hypocalcaemia may represent a medical emergency in the dog and demand prompt action by the clinician. Immediate therapy for tetany consists of intravenous administration of calcium gluconate. Calcium chloride is very irritating to tissues and its use is not recommended. Side-effects associated with rapid intravenous administration or overdosage

of calcium include shortening of QT interval followed by ventricular tachyarrhythmias or possibly bradycardia which may be detected by ECG monitoring of the dog during calcium injection. The injection should be given slowly and temporarily interrupted if complications occur.

As response to oral medication with vitamin D is often delayed, the post-tetany hypocalcaemic dog should be supported with subcutaneous injections of diluted calcium gluconate for a period of 1–4 days after initiation of long-term treatment. Frequent monitoring of total serum calcium concentration is recommended during this period. The puppies of bitches with puerperal tetany should be kept away from their mother for at least 24 h. Recurrent hypocalcaemic crises may dictate early weaning.

Oral administration of substances with vitamin D activity to promote intestinal calcium absorption and oral supplementation with calcium are the cornerstone of long-term treatment. Bitches affected with puerperal tetany are treated orally with calcium and possibly vitamin D for the duration of lactation. Life-long continuation of oral vitamin D and in some instances calcium therapy is necessary in dogs affected with primary hypoparathyroidism. Daily determinations followed by weekly determinations of total serum calcium are required for fine tuning treatment. If iatrogenic hypercalcaemia occurs, both vitamin D and calcium therapy should be temporarily discontinued. The delay before relief of toxicity after discontinuation of treatment is approximately 1–3 weeks for dihydrotachysterol and 1–14 days for calcitriol. Gradual withdrawal of long-term therapy is generally possible in dogs with secondary hypoparathyroidism. The entire process may take 3–4 months and con-

Table 57.5 Drugs used in the symptomatic treatment of hypocalcaemia.

Drug	Recommended dosage
Calcium gluconate (10%) (diverse formulations)	*Tetany*: 5–15 mg/kg elemental calcium (corresponds to 0.5–1.5 ml/kg solution) slowly i.v. over 10–30 min, administer solution at body temperature, adapt dose to patient response *Post-tetanic support*: same as above diluted 1 : 1 with 0.9% saline solution and administered s.c.
Oral calcium (diverse formulations)	*Maintenance*: 1–4 g total or 25–50 mg/kg elemental calcium daily in 2–4 doses p.o.
Dihydrotachysterol (AT 10™)	0.03 mg/kg p.o. daily during first 2 days or until effect demonstrated, then 0.02 mg/kg p.o. daily during following 2 days, finally 0.01 mg/kg p.o. daily as maintenance
Calcitriol (Rocaltrol™)	0.03–0.06 mg/kg p.o. daily

siderable variation in individual response has been reported (Feldman 1994).

Prognosis

The prognosis for primary hypoparathyroidism is good for dogs with owners committed to life-long treatment and regular estimations of serum calcium concentrations. Eventual recovery of parathyroid function is common in secondary hyperparathyroidism. Recurrence has been observed in bitches with puerperal tetany during subsequent lactations. The prognosis of other conditions associated with hypocalcaemia may be found in the sections discussing those disorders.

REFERENCES

Dougherty, S.A., Center, S.A. & Dzanis, D.A. (1990). Salmon calcitonin as adjunct treatment for vitamin D toxicosis in a dog. *Journal of the American Veterinary Medical Association*, **196**, 1269–1272.

Elliott, J., Dobson, J.M., Dunn, J.K., Herrtage, M.E. & Jackson, K.F. (1991). Hypercalcaemia in the dog: a study of 40 cases. *Journal of Small Animal Practice*, **32**, 564–571.

Feldman, E.C. (1994). Disorders of the parathyroid glands. In: *Textbook of Veterinary Internal Medicine*, (eds S.J. Ettinger & E.C. Feldman), 4th edn. pp. 1437–1465. W.B. Saunders, London.

Kruger, J.M. & Osborne, C.A. (1994a). Canine and feline hypercalcemic nephropathy. Part I. Causes and consequences. *Compendium on Continuing Education for the Practicing Veterinarian*, **16**, 1299–1315.

Kruger, J.M. & Osborne, C.A. (1994b). Canine and feline hypercalcemic nephropathy. Part II. Detection, cure and control. *Compendium on Continuing Education for the Practicing Veterinarian*, **16**, 1445–1458.

Petrie, G. (1996). Management of hypercalcaemia using dichloromethylene bisphosphorate (clodronate). *Proceedings of the Sixth Annual Congress of the European Society of Veterinary Internal Medicine*, p. 80.

Rosol, T.J., Chew, D.J., Hammer, A.S., *et al.* (1994). Effect of mithramycin on hypercalcemia in dogs. *Journal of the American Animal Hospital Association*, **30**, 244–250.

Rosol, T.J., Chew, D.J., Nagode, L.A., *et al.* (1995). Pathophysiology of calcium metabolism. *Veterinary Clinical Pathology*, **24**, 49–63.

Chapter 58

Management of Hyperadrenocorticism

P. P. Kintzer and M. E. Peterson

Hyperadrenocorticism is a relatively common endocrine disorder of middle- to old-aged dogs. Pituitary-dependent hyperadrenocorticism accounts for 85–90% of cases, while adrenocortical neoplasia is responsible for the remainder. The clinical signs of hyperadrenocorticism and routine laboratory findings are summarised in Tables 58.1 and 58.2. The radiological signs found in hyperadrenocorticism are given in Table 58.3. The diagnosis of hyperadrenocorticism can be confirmed using the low-dose dexamethasone test or adrenocorticotrophic hormone (ACTH) stimulation test with the high-dose dexamethasone suppression test or endogenous plasma ACTH concentrations used to differentiate pituitary-dependent hyperadrenocorticism from adrenocortical neoplasia (see Chapter 54). Ultrasound, computed tomography and magnetic resonance imaging may also be used to distinguish pituitary-dependent hyperadrenocorticism from adrenocortical neoplasia. The choice of treatment for a given dog with hyperadrenocorticism depends on several factors including cause, severity of disease, presence of malignancy, available treatment options, and clinician and client preferences.

PITUITARY-DEPENDENT HYPERADRENOCORTICISM

Medical Treatment with Mitotane

Mitotane (*o,p'*-DDD, Lysodren™) is the drug most frequently used for the treatment of dogs with pituitary-dependent hyperadrenocorticism. Mitotane is an adrenocorticolytic agent with a direct cytotoxic effect on the adrenal cortex, resulting in selective, progressive necrosis and atrophy.

Since mitotane is a fat-soluble drug, its absorption is poor when administered orally to fasted dogs (Watson *et al.* 1987). Therefore, mitotane should be administered with meals.

Induction Dosage

The initial recommended treatment protocol is as follows:

- Mitotane: 40–50 mg/kg per day p.o. administered for 7–10 days.
- Prednisone or prednisolone: 0.2 mg/kg per day p.o. administered concurrently with daily mitotane. Glucocorticoid supplementation will reduce the prevalence of adverse effects associated with the circulating cortisol concentration rapidly falling into the normal or subnormal range during initial treatment.

Monitoring Induction Dosage

The efficacy of the initial 7–10-day induction period is determined by an ACTH (tetracosactrin) stimulation test. Daily glucocorticoid administration must be withheld on the morning of ACTH stimulation testing, because prednisone and prednisolone both cross-react in most cortisol assays, resulting in a falsely high serum cortisol concentration. To ensure adequate control of hyperadrenocorticism, both the basal and post-ACTH serum cortisol concentrations must be lowered into the basal reference range (approximately 25–125 nmol/l). The length of daily treatment needed to adequately reduce adrenal reserve varies and can range from 5 days to 2 months. The initial 7–10-day induction treatment is sufficient in most dogs.

In dogs still responding to exogenous ACTH with serum cortisol concentration above the basal reference range, daily mitotane administration should be continued and ACTH stimulation tests repeated at 7–10-day intervals until the serum cortisol concentration falls into the basal reference range. On the other hand, if low basal or post-ACTH cortisol concentration develops after the initial treatment period, mitotane should be withheld and glucocorticoid continued until the cortisol value rises to within

Table 58.1 Clinical signs of hyperadrenocorticism in approximate decreasing order of frequency.

Polydipsia and polyuria
Polyphagia
Abdominal distension
Liver enlargement
Muscle wasting/weakness
Lethargy, poor exercise tolerance
Skin changes
Alopecia
Persistent anoestrus or testicular atrophy
Calcinosis cutis
Myotonia
Neurological signs

the basal reference range. This usually takes 2–6 weeks but can take up to 12–18 months in rare instances.

Maintenance Dosage

Maintenance mitotane at a dosage of 50 mg/kg per week in two to three divided doses is instituted once the induction treatment has successfully reduced adrenal reserve. While routine glucocorticoid supplementation is rarely necessary during maintenance mitotane treatment, an appropriate dosage of glucocorticoid should be administered during periods of stress.

Monitoring Maintenance Dosage

An ACTH stimulation test is performed after 1, 3, and 6 months of treatment and every 6 months thereafter to evaluate the efficacy of maintenance mitotane administration. If the basal or post-ACTH serum cortisol concentration increases above the basal reference range, indicating a relapse, daily mitotane is re-instituted at 40–50 mg/kg for at least 5 days; the weekly maintenance dosage is subsequently increased by approximately 50% after adrenal reserve has been appropriately reduced.

Relapses are common during maintenance mitotane administration, occurring in about one-half of dogs during the first year of treatment. Because of repeated relapse, maintenance dosages as high as 300 mg/kg per week may be necessary to control signs of hyperadrenocorticism in some dogs. Several factors may contribute to relapse in these dogs. One important factor under control of the clinician is the administration of an initial weekly maintenance dosage of at least 50 mg/kg. Fewer than 25% of dogs can be maintained long-term with less than 50 mg/kg per week, and very few with less than 40 mg/kg per week.

Adverse Effects

Side-effects (i.e., lethargy, weakness, anorexia, vomiting, diarrhoea, and ataxia) are relatively common during mitotane administration, and clients should be advised of

Table 58.2 Routine laboratory findings in hyperadrenocorticism.

Haematology
  Lymphopenia ($<1.5 \times 10^9$/l)
  Eosinopenia ($< 0.2 \times 10^9$/l)
  Neutrophilia
  Monocytosis
  Erythrocytosis
Biochemistry
  Increased alkaline phosphatase (often markedly
    elevated)
  Increased ALT
  High normal fasting blood glucose. Rarely diabetic.
  Decreased blood urea
  Increased cholesterol (>8 mmol/l)
  Lipaemia
  Increased bile salts
Urinalysis
  Urine specific gravity <1.015
  Glycosuria (<10% of cases)
  Urinary tract infection
Other findings
  Low T_4 levels
  Subnormal response to TSH

ALT, alanine amino transferase; TSH, thyroid stimulating hormone.

Table 58.3 Radiological signs of hyperadrenocorticism.

Abdominal radiographs
  Liver enlargement
  Good radiographic contrast
  Pot-bellied appearance
  Calcinosis cutis/soft tissue mineralisation
  Distended bladder
  Cystic calculi
  Adrenal enlargement/calcification
  Osteopenia
Thoracic radiographs
  Tracheal and bronchial wall calcification
  Pulmonary metastasis from adrenocortical carcinoma
  Osteopenia
  Congestive heart failure (rare)
  Pulmonary thromboembolism (rare)

their occurrence. During the daily induction period, approximately one-quarter of dogs develop one or more of these adverse reactions; however, they are relatively mild in most dogs and usually resolve quickly when mitotane is discontinued and glucocorticoid supplementation is increased. Similarly, if side-effects develop during maintenance mitotane administration, the drug is discontinued and glucocorticoid supplementation given. If adverse clinical signs continue for longer than a few hours after cessation of mitotane and administration of glucocorticoid, the dog should be evaluated and an ACTH stimulation test performed as soon as possible to exclude other disorders including mineralocorticoid insufficiency. If the adverse clinical signs were caused by a low circulating cortisol concentration, maintenance dosages of mitotane can usually be restarted in 2–4 weeks.

Hypoadrenocorticism with complete glucocorticoid and mineralocorticoid insufficiency (Addison's disease) develops in about 5% of dogs during maintenance mitotane administration, usually during the first year of treatment, although it can occur at anytime. It is not possible to predict which dogs will develop Addison's disease. In the authors' experience, dogs developing iatrogenic Addison's disease need glucocorticoid and mineralocorticoid replacement administration for the remainder of their lives and additional mitotane administration is not required.

Medical Treatment with *L*-deprenyl

L-deprenyl (selegiline hydrochloride) is a monoamine oxidase inhibitor that inhibits ACTH secretion by increasing dopaminergic tone to the hypothalamic–pituitary axis. The use of *L*-deprenyl for treatment of hyperadrenocorticism has been evaluated in dogs. Although the effectiveness of treatment is variable, one major advantage of *L*-deprenyl is the lack of any severe side-effects, including iatrogenic hypoadrenocorticism. A veterinary formulation (Anipryl™) is available in Canada and is currently undergoing review by the Food and Drug Administration in the United States. A human product is also available (Eldepryl™) but is very expensive.

Current Recommendations

Treatment is initiated at a dosage of 1 mg/kg daily. If an inadequate response is seen after 2 months, the dosage is increased to 2 mg/kg per day. If this dosage also proves ineffective, alternative treatment is necessary. If effective, daily treatment is continued for the remainder of the dog's life.

Monitoring Response

Response to treatment is evaluated by clinical signs. Up to 50% of dogs may fail to adequately respond to treatment.

Contraindications

L-deprenyl appears to be a safe and effective treatment alternative in most dogs with hyperadrenocorticism. However, *L*-deprenyl is not currently recommended for treatment of pituitary-dependent hyperadrenocorticism in dogs with concurrent diabetes mellitus, pancreatitis, heart failure, renal disease or other severe illness. The drug should not be administered concurrently with other monoamine oxidase inhibitors, opioids, tricyclic and related antidepressants, or selective serotonin reuptake inhibitors and related antidepressants, because severe adverse drug interactions have been reported in humans.

Medical Treatment with Ketoconazole

Ketoconazole is an imidazole antifungal drug that lowers the circulating cortisol concentration by enzymatic inhibition of steroid biosynthesis. It has minimal effect on mineralocorticoid production. Ketoconazole can be used to effectively control hyperadrenocorticism in dogs. Unfortunately, ketoconazole is not completely efficacious in many dogs. In the authors' experience, one-third to one-half of dogs fail to adequately respond to treatment.

Initial Dosage

The initial recommended dosage of ketoconazole is 10 mg/kg b.i.d. for 14 days. Alternatively, treatment is initiated at 5 mg/kg b.i.d. for the first 7 days to assess drug tolerance, then increased to 10 mg/kg.

Monitoring Induction Dosage

The efficacy of the initial 14-day course of treatment is determined by an ACTH stimulation test. To ensure adequate control of hyperadrenocorticism, both the basal and post-ACTH serum cortisol concentrations must be lowered into the basal reference range. If the serum cortisol concentrations remain above this range, the dosage is increased to 15 mg/kg b.i.d., and an ACTH response test repeated in 14 days.

Dosages of up to 20 mg/kg b.i.d. are occasionally necessary. Such higher dosages are associated with a higher incidence of adverse effects. Twice daily administration is then continued at the effective dosage, and ACTH response testing should be performed at 3–6-month intervals during long-term treatment to ensure that basal and post-ACTH serum cortisol concentrations remain in the basal reference range.

Adverse Effects

Adverse effects seen in dogs receiving ketoconazole are relatively uncommon. They include vomiting, anorexia, diarrhoea and hepatotoxicity. Such drug intolerance may, however, necessitate permanent discontinuation of ketoconazole.

In addition, clinical signs associated with glucocorticoid deficiency can occur during ketoconazole administration. Discontinuation of ketoconazole and glucocorticoid supplementation usually results in rapid resolution of signs. Ketoconazole is re-instituted at a lower dosage in these dogs, once clinical signs have resolved and serum cortisol concentrations have risen. The occurrence of mineralocorticoid deficiency associated with ketoconazole administration has not been reported in dogs.

Disadvantages of Ketoconazole Compared with Mitotane

Disadvantages of ketoconazole administration to treat hyperadrenocorticism include the following:

- expense of the drug, which may be prohibitive for some clients;
- adverse effects caused by drug intolerance, requiring discontinuation of treatment;
- substantial subset of dogs that fail to adequately respond;
- twice daily administration, which must be maintained for the remainder of the animal's life.

Currently, ketoconazole is used in rare dogs unable to tolerate mitotane and, occasionally, on an interim basis in dogs undergoing radiotherapy to control serum cortisol concentrations until the full effects of the radiotherapy on pituitary ACTH production are manifest.

Radiotherapy

Radiotherapy for hyperadrenocorticism is currently indicated in dogs that have pituitary macrotumours ($\geq$1 cm in diameter), with or without concomitant neurological signs, and dogs with smaller pituitary tumours causing neurological signs or impinging on adjacent structures. The role of radiotherapy in dogs with small, neurologically 'silent', non-invasive pituitary tumours remains to be determined.

Clinical Signs Associated with Pituitary Macrotumours

Neurological signs associated with pituitary macrotumours vary considerably in severity and include lethargy, anorexia, depression, pacing, head pressing, circling, aggression, behaviour changes, paresis, cranial nerve deficits, seizures, stupor and coma. Although dogs with larger tumours tend to have more severe deficits, clinical signs do not necessarily correlate with tumour size in the individual patient.

The most important prognostic factor associated with response to treatment and survival time is the severity of neurological signs. The prognosis in dogs with large tumours and severe neurological signs is poor to grave.

Protocol

Radiotherapy is administered with megavoltage irradiation. Most treatment protocols involve the administration of 45–50 Gy in 3–4 Gy fractions. Computerised systems to plan treatment protocols are recommended to facilitate the delivery of the desired dose of radiation to the tumour while minimising the dose received by surrounding normal tissues. Side-effects of radiotherapy include otitis externa, skin changes, alopecia, deafness, and neurological toxicity.

Monitoring

Dogs undergoing radiotherapy should be closely monitored. In some dogs, neurological signs improve markedly in a few weeks, while in others improvement is slow or absent. Reduction of ACTH secretion by the tumour is not predictable, and if it occurs it may not be evident for 6–12 months after therapy. Therefore, during this time, medical treatment with mitotane or an alternative agent may be indicated.

Periodic examination and endocrinological evaluation is necessary to determine the occurrence of side-effects and the necessity for continued medical treatment of hyper-adrenocorticism. Median survival time is approximately 2 years.

ADRENOCORTICAL TUMOURS

Medical Therapy with Mitotane

Mitotane is an effective and relatively safe therapeutic alternative for dogs with cortisol-secreting adrenocortical tumours and is the treatment of choice for dogs with non-resectable or recurrent adrenocortical carcinoma (Kintzer & Peterson 1994). In these dogs, mitotane is used as a true chemotherapeutic agent with the therapeutic goal of destroying all tumour tissue. Although complete destruction of an adrenal adenoma may not be necessary, most dogs have either known adrenal carcinoma or have not been surgically explored, so histological examination of the tumour has not been performed. Unfortunately, the development of direct mitotane toxicity limits the dosage of mitotane that can be given and prevents the induction of complete adrenocortical insufficiency in many dogs.

Induction Dosage

Dogs with adrenal tumours require higher daily induction dosages of mitotane than those generally required by dogs with pituitary-dependent hyperadrenocorticism. More importantly, a longer period of induction (more than 2 weeks) is necessary in about half of the dogs to satisfactorily decrease serum cortisol concentrations.

Mitotane administration is initiated at a dosage of 50–75 mg/kg daily for 10–14 days. Concurrent prednisone supplementation (0.2 mg/kg per day) is given throughout the period of mitotane administration. Serum cortisol determinations (both basal and ACTH-stimulated) are a practical and relatively reliable means of assessing response to treatment, although they do not correlate with tumour response in all dogs.

Monitoring Induction Dosage

The therapeutic goal is to decrease serum cortisol to low or undetectable concentrations. If the ACTH-stimulated serum cortisol concentration falls but remains within or above the basal reference range, mitotane is continued at the dosage of 50–75 mg/kg per day, and ACTH response testing is repeated every 10–14 days until serum cortisol concentrations fall below normal.

If this initial daily dosage is ineffective, with little to no decrease in serum cortisol concentrations, the daily dosage of mitotane should be increased by increments of 50 mg/kg every 10–14 days until some decrease in serum cortisol concentrations is seen or drug intolerance occurs. Daily mitotane is then continued at the dosage at which some response was seen or at the highest tolerated dosage, and ACTH stimulation testing is continued at 10–14-day intervals until the circulating cortisol concentration falls below the basal reference range.

Maintenance Dosage

An initial maintenance mitotane dosage of 75–100 mg/kg per week in divided doses, together with daily maintenance glucocorticoid supplementation, is initiated once undetectable to low-normal serum cortisol concentrations are documented.

Monitoring Maintenance Dosage

An ACTH stimulation test should be repeated 1–2 months after initiation of the maintenance dosage. This maintenance dosage is continued if the ACTH-stimulated serum cortisol concentration remains low to undetectable. If the cortisol concentration rises into the basal reference range, the weekly maintenance dosage should be increased by 50%. If the serum cortisol concentration rises above the basal reference range, daily mitotane treatment should be re-instituted until the cortisol concentration falls to a low or undetectable value; the weekly maintenance dosage should then be increased by 50%. Subsequent dosage adjustments are based on periodic ACTH stimulation tests at 3–6-month intervals as well as the dog's tolerance of the medication itself.

Relapses are not uncommon, occurring in one-half to two-thirds of dogs during maintenance therapy. Reasons include too low an initial mitotane dosage, continued adrenal tumour growth or metastasis, or both. Dogs with known metastatic disease are more difficult to control on a long-term basis, presumably because of progression of disease.

In general, dogs with adrenal tumours require a maintenance dosage of mitotane twice that needed by dogs with pituitary-dependent hyperadrenocorticism. About a quarter of dogs with adrenal tumours can be expected to need a maintenance dosage of greater than 150 mg/kg per week. In some dogs, adverse reactions prevent the administration of even higher dosages of mitotane in an attempt to control clinical signs or tumour growth. On the other hand, 15–20% of dogs can be treated successfully with the protocol recommended for pituitary-dependent hyperadreno-corticism (i.e. an induction dosage of 40–50 mg/kg per day for 7–10 days, followed by maintenance dosage of 50 mg/kg per week). Such dogs probably have either an adenoma or small carcinoma without widespread metastasis. A small percentage of dogs still succumb to tumour progression despite a decrease of serum cortisol concentrations into or below the normal resting range, presumably because of drug-resistant, non-functional tumour cells.

Adverse Effects

Adverse effects, including anorexia, lethargy, weakness and diarrhoea, are seen in about 60% of dogs. While adverse reactions are caused by low circulating cortisol concentrations in some dogs, direct drug toxicity causes these adverse reactions in about half, independent of mitotane's effect on cortisol secretion.

If severe side-effects occur, mitotane is discontinued, glucocorticoid supplementation continued, and the dog re-evaluated as soon as possible to exclude glucocorticoid and mineralocorticoid deficiency. If serum electrolyte concentrations are normal but serum cortisol concentrations sub-normal, glucocorticoid supplementation is increased to 0.4 mg/kg per day to exclude cortisol deficiency. If adverse side-effects recur when maintenance mitotane is re-instituted despite such an increase in daily glucocorticoid dosage, direct drug toxicity is likely. Management of such toxicity involves re-instituting mitotane at a 25–50% lower dosage once signs of toxicity have resolved. Consequently, cortisol concentrations will usually rise to within or above the basal reference range. The resting and post–ACTH cortisol concentrations must, however, be kept in the normal resting range to prevent recurrence of signs of hyper-adrenocorticism. Restitution of the higher weekly mainte-nance dosage can be attempted at a later date, but recurrence of side-effects is likely.

Hypoadrenocorticism with complete glucocorticoid and mineralocorticoid deficiency (Addison's disease) rarely develops. If iatrogenic Addison's disease occurs, mitotane is discontinued and appropriate supplementation with glucocorticoid and fludrocortisone acetate instituted. Additional mitotane is not necessary unless hypoadreno-corticism resolves and cortisol concentrations again increase into or above normal resting range. Iatrogenic hypoadrenocorticism is not undesirable and, in fact, may enhance the dog's long-term prognosis, since all functional neoplastic adrenocortical tissue (as well as any remaining normal adrenal tissue) has probably been destroyed.

Surgical Treatment

Adrenalectomy is often an appropriate and effective treat-ment for hyperadrenocorticism caused by adrenal tumours

and is the treatment of choice for a dog with an adrenal adenoma or small carcinoma. Preoperative staging should include a thoracic radiograph and abdominal ultrasound (if not previously performed) to evaluate for the presence of metastatic disease or vascular invasion. The authors recom-mend administration of ketoconazole to attempt to control hyperadrenocorticism, as evidenced by basal and post–ACTH serum cortisol concentrations in the basal reference range, for 3–4 weeks before surgery in order to diminish the anaesthetic and surgical risks associated with cortisol excess.

Technique

The technique of adrenalectomy in the dog has been well described, including the advantages and disadvantages of the ventral midline and retroperitoneal approaches. The ventral midline approach is preferred in most animals for several reasons:

- Both adrenal glands can be readily examined.
- The abdomen can be thoroughly explored for metasta-tic lesions.
- Anaesthesia time is not substantially lengthened when compared with the retroperitoneal approach (especially in dogs in which preoperative lateralisation of the tumour was inconclusive).
- Wound healing and dehiscence are rare.

Regardless of the approach chosen, careful tissue dissec-tion and meticulous haemostasis are extremely important. A thorough exploration of the abdomen should be undertaken in all dogs, including evaluation of the con-tralateral adrenal gland and a careful search for metastatic disease.

Intra-operative Management

Close intra-operative monitoring, including temperature, electrocardiogram, blood pressure, fluid balance and tissue perfusion is imperative. An isotonic electrolyte solution such as lactated Ringer's is administered at 10 ml/kg per hour throughout anaesthesia and surgery.

Because the contralateral adrenal gland is atrophied, adrenocortical insufficiency rapidly ensues after successful adrenalectomy unless large doses of glucocorticoids are administered during and after surgery. Dexamethasone (0.1–0.2 mg/kg) is administered intravenously just before adrenalectomy, again at the completion of surgery, and then every 6–8 h in the immediate postoperative period. Alternatively, dexamethasone at a dosage of

0.02–0.04 mg/kg is added to intravenous fluids and infused over 4–6 h starting immediately before adrenalectomy.

Postoperative Complications

Complications may include poor anaesthetic recovery with cardiac arrest, pulmonary thromboembolism, acute renal failure, pneumonia, pancreatitis, and acute adrenal insufficiency. Intensive postoperative monitoring is necessary to prevent, recognise, and treat these potential complications.

Postoperative Monitoring

To evaluate adrenal reserve and exclude occult metastasis or incomplete resection, an ACTH stimulation test is performed on the first postoperative day. After completion of the test, prednisone should be administered at a dosage of 0.5 mg/kg b.i.d. for 3–4 days.

In dogs with adrenal insufficiency, this dosage is tapered over 10–14 days to a daily maintenance dosage of 0.2 mg/kg and is continued until the remaining adrenal gland has regained function. Prednisone can usually be discontinued within 2 months (as determined by ACTH stimulation testing). Glucocorticoid supplementation is discontinued if the postoperative ACTH stimulation test demonstrates residual tumour, indicated by a normal to exaggerated post-ACTH serum cortisol concentration.

REFERENCES AND FURTHER READING

Bruyette, D.S., Ruel, W.W., Entriken, T., Griffin, D. & Darling, L.A. (1997). Management of canine pituitary-dependent hyperadrenocorticism with *L*-deprenyl (Anipryl). *Veterinary Clinics of North America (Small Animal Practice)*, **27**, 278–280.

Kintzer, P.P. & Peterson, M.E. (1991). Mitotane (o,p'-DDD) treatment of 200 dogs with pituitary hyperadrenocorticism. *Journal of Veterinary Internal Medicine*, **5**, 182–190.

Kintzer, P.P. & Peterson, M.E. (1994). Mitotane (o,p'-DDD) treatment of dogs with adrenocortical neoplasia: 32 cases (1980–1992). *Journal of the American Veterinary Medical Association*, **205**, 54–61.

Feldman, E.C. & Nelson, R.W. (1992). Use of ketoconazole for control of canine hyperadrenocorticism. In: *Current Veterinary Therapy XI*, pp. 349–352. W.B. Saunders, Philadelphia.

LaRue, S.M. (1995). Radiation therapy for pituitary tumors. In: *Current Veterinary Therapy XII*, pp. 356–360. W.B. Saunders, Philadelphia.

Peterson, M.E. (1982). O,p'-DDD (mitotane) treatment of canine pituitary-dependent hyperadrenocorticism. *Journal of the American Veterinary Medical Association*, **182**, 527–528.

Peterson, M.E. & Kintzer, P.P. (1994). Medical treatment of pituitary-dependent hyperadrenocorticism in dogs. *Seminars in Veterinary Medicine and Surgery (Small Animal)*, **9**, 127–131.

Watson, A.D.J., Rijnberk, A. & Moolenaar, A.J. (1987). Systemic availability of o,p'-DDD in normal dogs, fasted and fed and in dogs with hyperadrenocorticism. *Research in Veterinary Science*, **43**, 160–165.

Chapter 59

Diagnosis of Hypoadrenocorticism

M. E. Peterson and P. P. Kintzer

CAUSES OF HYPOADRENOCORTICISM

Primary Hypoadrenocorticism

Naturally-occurring, primary hypoadrenocorticism is an uncommon endocrinopathy caused by atrophy or destruction of the adrenal cortices (Addison's disease). This type of hypoadrenocorticism almost always results in subnormal glucocorticoid and mineralocorticoid secretion and, in the vast majority of cases, is thought to be the end result of an immune-mediated process.

A few dogs with primary hypoadrenocorticism have normal serum electrolyte concentration (so-called atypical hypoadrenocorticism). In these dogs, it has been hypothesised that the progression of the disorder is a gradual process in which glucocorticoid secretion becomes subnormal before mineralocorticoid secretion is substantially affected. In other dogs, previous therapeutic intervention may have obscured abnormalities in serum electrolytes, or serial testing may be necessary to demonstrate abnormalities.

Primary adrenocortical insufficiency can also occur secondary to the administration of the adrenocorticolytic drug mitotane (o,p'-DDD), or, very rarely, secondary to infiltrative disease processes such as systemic fungal infection or metastatic neoplasia.

Secondary Hypoadrenocorticism

Naturally-occurring, secondary hypoadrenocorticism is very rare; however, iatrogenic secondary hypoadrenocorticism, induced by glucocorticoid administration, is common. In dogs with secondary adrenal insufficiency, deficient pituitary adrenocorticotrophic hormone (ACTH) secretion results in inadequate glucocorticoid production, while mineralocorticoid secretion is usually preserved because ACTH has little trophic effect on mineralocorticoid production.

SIGNALMENT

Spontaneous primary hypoadrenocorticism is typically a disorder of young to middle-aged female dogs; in the authors' series of 220 cases 70% were female. In this study, some breeds (Great Dane, Portuguese Water Dog, Rottweiler, Standard Poodle, West Highland White Terrier and Wheaton Terrier) had a significantly higher risk of developing primary hypoadrenocorticism than other breeds. Because of the rarity of the disorder, similar data are not available for spontaneous secondary hypoadrenocorticism.

HISTORICAL AND CLINICAL ABNORMALITIES

Historical and clinical findings in dogs with primary hypoadrenocorticism and their approximate rate of occurrence as a percentage are shown in Table 59.1.

The severity and duration of historical and clinical abnormalities varies greatly between dogs as does the occurrence of any given clinical finding. The typical clinical picture is that of a dog with chronic, often progressive clinical signs that have been present for up to a year. Some dogs, however, have acute addisonian crisis on examination, a true medical emergency. In these dogs, a thorough history usually uncovers that clinical findings consistent with hypoadrenocorticism have been present for weeks or months before the crisis.

Table 59.1 Historical and clinical findings in dogs with primary hypoadrenocorticism.

Findings	Percentage occurrence
Lethargy/depression	95
Anorexia	90
Vomiting	75
Weakness	75
Weight loss	50
Dehydration	45
Diarrhoea	40
Waxing/waning course	40
Collapse	35
Previous response to therapy	35
Hypothermia	35
Slow capillary refill time	30
Shaking	27
Polyuria/polydipsia	25
Melaena	20
Weak pulse	20
Bradycardia (<60 bpm)	18

Table 59.2 Percentage occurrence of clinicopathological abnormalities in dogs with primary hypoadrenocorticism.

Clinicopathological abnormalities	Percentage occurrence
Hyperkalaemia	95
Hyponatraemia	80
Low Na : K ratio (<27)	95
Hypochloraemia	40
Hypercalcaemia	30
Azotaemia	85
Decreased total CO_2 (metabolic acidosis)	40
High alanine aminotrasferase	30
Hyperbilirubinaemia	20
Hypoglycaemia	17
Anaemia	25
Eosinophilia	20
Lymphocytosis	10

There is no single historical or clinical finding or set of clinical signs that is pathognomonic for hypoadrenocorticism. Furthermore, clinical findings consistent with spontaneous canine hypoadrenocorticism are commonly seen in a wide variety of more prevalent diseases. Therefore, it is important for the clinician to maintain a high index of suspicion for the disorder. Important diagnostic clues are:

- a waxing waning course of illness (intermittent signs),
- exacerbation of clinical signs by stress,
- response to non-specific treatment and supportive care.

ROUTINE LABORATORY FINDINGS

Common clinicopathological abnormalities found in dogs with primary hypoadrenocorticism and their approximate rate of occurrence as a percentage are listed in Table 59.2.

Serum biochemical abnormalities classically associated with primary hypoadrenocorticism are hyperkalaemia, hyponatraemia, azotaemia and mild to moderate metabolic acidosis. In addition, hypercalcemia may be seen in up to 30% of cases. Electrolyte disturbances cannot be relied upon for the definitive diagnosis of hypoadrenocorticism, however. Hyperkalaemia has been reported in a variety of other diseases including:

- trichuriasis
- ascariasis
- salmonellosis
- parvovirus
- severe diarrhoea
- malabsorption syndromes
- gastric torsion
- duodenal perforation
- severe chronic hepatic failure
- acute renal failure
- chronic renal failure
- urethral obstruction
- uroabdomen
- chronic heart failure
- ascites
- pericardial effusion
- acidosis
- severe tissue destruction
- primary polydipsia.

Azotaemia is usually prerenal in origin and resolves with adequate fluid therapy. Continuing azotaemia should prompt consideration of (1) inadequate fluid administration, or (2) ischemic renal damage resulting in acute renal failure.

On urinalysis, over 50% of dogs can be expected to demonstrate an impaired ability to concentrate their urine (specific gravity <1.030 in the presence of high serum urea and creatinine concentrations). This abnormality is probably the result of medullary washout and sluggish medullary blood flow and can make the confirmation of prerenal azotaemia more difficult.

ELECTROCARDIOGRAPHIC FINDINGS IN HYPOADRENOCORTICISM

An electrocardiogram is recommended in all dogs with bradycardia and those with marked hyperkalaemia (>6.5 mmol/l), because abnormalities of cardiac conduction may be life threatening in some dogs with hypoadrenocorticism. The classic electrocardiographic findings seen in animals with hyperkalaemia are as follows:

- QRS prolongation,
- low R wave amplitude,
- high T wave amplitude,
- P-R interval prolongation,
- absence of P waves (sinoatrial standstill).

Because of the influence of other electrolyte abnormalities, metabolic acidosis, and impaired tissue perfusion, electrocardiographic findings may not correlate well with serum potassium concentration in many dogs.

RADIOGRAPHIC FINDINGS IN HYPOADRENOCORTICISM

Radiographs may demonstrate abnormalities associated with volume depletion and decreased tissue perfusion including:

- microcardia,
- a narrowed caudal vena cava or descending aorta,
- underperfusion of lung fields,
- microhepatica.

Megaoesophagus is a very rare manifestation of hypoadrenocorticism; the authors have seen one dog that had a radiographically demonstrable megaoesophagus that resolved with treatment of adrenocortical insufficiency.

DIAGNOSTIC TESTS FOR HYPOADRENOCORTICISM

Definitive diagnosis of hypoadrenocorticism requires demonstration of inadequate adrenal reserve as evidenced by a low basal serum (or plasma) cortisol concentration with a subnormal or absent response to exogenous ACTH administration. The protocol for ACTH stimulation testing is as follows:

- Synthetic ACTH solution (tetracosactrin, Synacthen™) – blood sample for serum cortisol determination is drawn before and 30–60 min after the intravenous or intramuscular injection of 0.25 mg.

Several caveats regarding ACTH stimulation testing in animals with suspected adrenocortical insufficiency should be kept in mind.

- If acute adrenocortical insufficiency is suspected, the ACTH stimulation test can be done immediately or, alternatively, delayed until the patient has been stabilised with parenteral fluid and glucocorticoid administration.
- ACTH stimulation testing should be performed using synthetic ACTH administered intravenously, because in dogs with hypovolaemia or severe dehydration, impaired tissue perfusion may impede absorption of the ACTH injection resulting in inaccurate and misleading data.
- Many glucocorticoid preparations including prednisone, prednisolone and cortisone cross-react with serum cortisol assays falsely elevating results, and therefore they should not be administered until after ACTH stimulation testing is complete.
- Dexamethasone sodium phosphate is a rapid-acting glucocorticoid that does not interfere with cortisol assays and is recommended for the initial treatment of acute adrenocortical insufficiency.
- If the patient has received prednisone, prednisolone, hydrocortisone or cortisone, treatment must be switched to dexamethasone for at least 24 h before an ACTH response test can be performed.

DISTINGUISHING PRIMARY AND SECONDARY HYPOADRENOCORTICISM

Hyperkalaemia coupled with an inadequate adrenal reserve indicates primary hypoadrenocorticism. It must be remembered, however, that hyponatraemia can develop in some dogs with secondary hypoadrenocorticism.

Plasma ACTH determination is necessary to differentiate primary from secondary adrenal insufficiency in dogs with normal electrolyte concentrations. Plasma ACTH concentrations are high in dogs with primary hypoadrenocorticism as a consequence of the loss of negative feedback of cortisol on the pituitary gland, but they are undetectable to low in dogs with secondary hypoadrenocorticism. Plasma samples for ACTH concentration should ideally be drawn before corticosteroid administration and must be appropriately handled to ensure accurate results.

FURTHER READING

Feldman, E.C. & Peterson, M.E. (1986). Hypoadrenocorticism. *Veterinary Clinics of North America*, **14**, 751–766.

Kintzer, P.P. & Peterson, M.E. (1994). Diagnosis and management of primary spontaneous hypoadrenocorticism (Addison's disease) in dogs. *Seminars in Veterinary Medicine and Surgery (Small Animal)*, **9**, 148–152.

Hardy, R.M. (1995). Hypoadrenal gland disease. In: *Textbook of Veterinary Internal Medicine*, pp. 1579–1593. W.B. Saunders, Philadelphia.

Kintzer, P.P. & Peterson, M.E. (1995). Hypoadrenocorticism in dogs. In: *Current Veterinary Therapy XII*, pp. 425–429. W.B. Saunders, Philadelphia.

Peterson, M.E. & Kintzer, P.P. (1996). Pretreatment clinical and laboratory findings in dogs with hypoadrenocorticism: 225 cases (1979–1993). *Journal of the American Veterinary Medical Association*, **208**, 85–91.

Chapter 60

Management of Diabetes Mellitus

M. E. Herrtage

Diabetes mellitus is a heterogeneous condition in the dog rather than a single disease entity. It is characterised by a relative or absolute deficiency of insulin secretion by the beta cells of the islets of Langerhans in the pancreas. Carbohydrate metabolism and in particular blood glucose concentration is controlled by the balance between the action of catabolic hormones, for example glucagon, cortisol, catecholamines and growth hormone on the one hand, and the principal anabolic hormone, insulin, on the other. A relative or absolute deficiency of insulin results in decreased utilisation of glucose, amino acids and fatty acids by peripheral tissues, particularly liver, muscle and adipose tissue. Failure of glucose uptake by these cells leads to hyperglycaemia. Once the renal threshold for glucose reabsorption is exceeded, an osmotic diuresis ensues with loss of glucose, electrolytes and water in the urine. A compensatory polydipsia prevents the animal becoming dehydrated. The loss of glucose leads to catabolism of the body's reserves especially of fats. Excessive fat catabolism leads to the production and accumulation of ketone bodies and the onset of diabetic ketoacidosis (Fig. 60.1). In diabetic ketoacidosis, the dog is unable to maintain an adequate fluid intake and becomes rapidly dehydrated due to the uncontrolled osmotic diuresis. The dehydration and acidosis requires emergency care if the animal is to survive.

In man, diabetes is classified as type I, insulin-dependent diabetes mellitus (IDDM) and type II, non-insulin-dependent diabetes mellitus (NIDDM). This classification has not proved very useful in veterinary medicine since nearly all dogs with diabetes mellitus require insulin therapy regardless of the underlying aetiology. Classifying diabetes mellitus into primary and secondary causes is of more use clinically in the dog (Table 60.1). In secondary diabetes which is caused by peripheral insulin resistance there is initially a compensatory increase in insulin secretion, but after a period of time the islets cells become exhausted, the beta cells are destroyed and their function is permanently lost.

SIGNALMENT AND CLINICAL SIGNS

Diabetes mellitus is a disease of middle-aged dogs with a peak incidence around 8 years of age. Genetic predisposition to diabetes has been found in Keeshunds and Samoyeds. Cairn Terriers, Poodles and Dachshunds may also be over-represented. Entire females are more frequently affected than males and this is due mainly to the induction of growth hormone by progesterone or progestagens.

Polyuria, polydipsia, increased appetite and weight loss develop over a few weeks in uncomplicated cases. In entire bitches, this usually occurs in the metoestrus phase of the oestrus cycle.

Hepatomegaly, muscle wasting and infections of the urinary or respiratory tracts may be noted on clinical examination. Ulcerative skin lesions and cutaneous xanthomata have occasionally been reported. If the diabetes remains uncontrolled, an accumulation of ketone bodies may occur which causes metabolic acidosis and leads to depression, anorexia, vomiting, rapid dehydration. Coma and death may result from severe hypovolaemia and circulatory collapse.

DIAGNOSIS

Urine analysis reveals persistent glycosuria and often ketonuria. Despite the high solute load in the urine which would tend to increase the specific gravity of the urine, many older dogs may have impaired renal concentrating power and thus the specific gravity of the urine is variable, typically between 1.015 and 1.045. Bacterial cystitis is

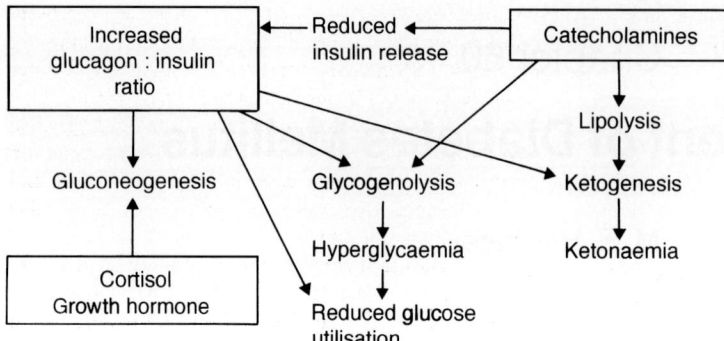

Fig. 60.1 Pathogenesis of diabetic ketoacidosis.

Table 60.1 Aetiology of diabetes mellitus in the dog.

Primary islet cell degeneration
  Islet cell destruction (?auto-immune)
  Chronic pancreatitis
Secondary diabetes mellitus
  Obesity – causing down-regulation of insulin receptors
  Antagonism to insulin
    By counter-regulating hormones
      Progesterone-induced growth hormone excess
      Particularly entire bitches in metoestrus
      Hyperadrenocorticism
    By drug therapy
      Glucocorticoids
      Progestagens

common and occasionally may involve gas-producing organisms which can cause emphysematous cystitis.

Plasma biochemistry reveals hyperglycaemia (>9 mmol/l) and hyperlipidaemia. In some patients the blood will be lactescent due to lipaemia. Liver enzymes are usually raised and liver function tests such as bile acid concentrations may be abnormal. In cases where diabetes is associated with pancreatitis, amylase and lipase concentrations may be elevated.

In diabetic ketoacidosis, there are serious derangements in fluid, electrolyte and acid–base status. The most frequent abnormalities are prerenal azotaemia, hyponatraemia and acidosis.

TREATMENT

Treatment can be divided into the acute management of diabetic ketoacidosis and the stabilisation of the uncompli-

cated diabetic. The ketoacidotic dog can be stabilised as for the uncomplicated case, once it has started to feed normally.

Management of Diabetic Ketoacidosis

Although the healthy ketotic diabetic can usually be managed conservatively without fluid therapy or intensive care, diabetic ketoacidosis characterised by hyperglycaemia, ketonaemia, metabolic acidosis, dehydration and electrolyte imbalance is a medical emergency that is associated with a high mortality (Macintire 1993). Treatment should consist of replacement of fluid and electrolytes, reduction of blood glucose concentration, correction of acidosis and identification of precipitating causes. A treatment protocol is given in Table 60.2.

Fluid Therapy

Intravenous replacement of fluid and electrolytes is essential to the successful management of diabetic ketoacidosis. Unless serum electrolytes suggest otherwise, 0.9% sodium chloride is the initial fluid of choice. The fluid deficit is usually about 10% of body weight and this should be replaced over a period of 24–48 h.

Sodium chloride may be alternated with lactated Ringer's solution or, if the blood glucose falls below 10 mmol/l, a solution containing 0.18% sodium chloride and 4% glucose. Urine output should be measured and if possible, a central venous catheter used to monitor central venous pressure during fluid therapy.

Insulin Therapy

Soluble insulin should be used in the treatment of diabetic ketoacidosis. Although intermittent administration using

Table 60.2 Treatment protocol for diabetic ketoacidosis in the dog.

---

(1) *Intravenous fluid and electrolyte replacement*
  0.9% sodium chloride initially then alternate with lactated Ringer's solution.
  Monitor urine output and if possible, central venous pressure.

(2) *Insulin therapy*
  (a) Low-dose insulin infusion – add 5 units soluble insulin to 500 ml lactated Ringer's solution and infuse at a rate of 0.1 units/kg per hour through a separate intravenous catheter. Use of an infusion pump or paediatric burette is helpful in controlling the rate of infusion. Monitor blood glucose concentration every 2 h.
  (b) Soluble insulin injection – a dose of 1 unit/kg is divided and a quarter of the dose given intravenously and three-quarters intramuscularly. The dose is repeated every 4–6 h. Monitor blood glucose concentration every 2 h.

(3) *Continue intravenous fluid and electrolyte replacement*
  Continue alternating 0.9% sodium chloride with lactated Ringer's solution while blood glucose remains above 10 mmol/l.
  Use 0.18% sodium chloride with 4% glucose solution when blood glucose falls <10 mmol/l.

(4) *Potassium supplementation*
  Ideally supplementation with potassium should be based on serum potassium concentrations. In the absence of serum potassium measurements, add 20 mmol/l of potassium chloride to each 500 ml bag of intravenous fluid solution. This will be safe providing the dog has adequate urine production.

(5) *Phosphate supplementation*
  Phosphate shifts in the same way as potassium. Hypophoshataemia is only likely to occur in severe diabetic ketoacidosis, but can be severe (<0.5 mmol/l). Dose of 0.01–0.03 mmol/kg per hour of potassium phosphate in calcium free fluid e.g. normal saline is required if hypophosphataemia is suspected.

(6) *Correction of acidosis*
  Bicarbonate therapy is not necessary provided renal function has been re-established. It is only indicated in life-threatening acidosis and only one-third of the calculated replacement dose should be used to prevent excessive plasma bicarbonate concentrations.

(7) *Antibiotic therapy*

---

the intravenous and intramuscular routes has been used, low dose intravenous insulin infusions using 0.1 units/kg per hour are effective and appear to be associated with fewer side-effects such as hypokalaemia and hypoglycaemia. Low dose intravenous insulin infusion provides a steady, gradual reduction of blood glucose and ketone concentrations and is less likely to cause increases in glucagon, cortisol and growth hormone that can occur with intermittent bolus administration of insulin.

Blood glucose should be monitored every 2 h. Glucose containing fluids should be introduced when the blood glucose concentration falls below 10 mmol/l and the insulin infusion should be stopped when the blood glucose reaches 6 mmol/l. Once the insulin infusion is halted, blood glucose concentrations will increase so that further infusion of insulin may be required if the patient is not eating or a longer acting insulin preparation may be introduced if its appetite has returned.

Potassium Supplementation

A deficit in total body potassium is usually masked by the acidosis which causes potassium to move extracellularly. Serum potassium concentration can decrease rapidly as renal function improves and as insulin therapy causes potassium to move back into the cells. Although hypokalaemia is less likely to occur with low-dose insulin infusion, replacement therapy should be started within a few hours of instigating fluid and insulin therapy.

In the absence of serum potassium measurements, 20 mmol of potassium chloride should be added to every 500 ml of intravenous fluid solution given after insulin therapy has commenced.

Phosphate Supplementation

Phosphate moves between the intracellular and extracellular compartments in the same way as potassium. Hypophosphataemia can cause haemolytic anaemia, weakness, ataxia and seizures. Phosphate supplementation is only usually required in dogs with severe diabetic ketoacidosis. Potassium phosphate at a dose of 0.01–0.03 mmol/kg per hour intravenously is recommended to correct hypophosphataemia.

Bicarbonate Therapy

The use of sodium bicarbonate to correct the acidosis in diabetic ketoacidosis is controversial. Rapid correction of the acidosis with bicarbonate can lead to metabolic alkalosis, tissue anoxia due to a shift to the left of the haemoglobin–oxygen dissociation curve and paradoxical cerebral acidosis because CO_2 crosses the blood–brain barrier more rapidly than HCO_3^- ions. For these reasons bicarbonate should be used only in life-threatening acidosis (arterial pH < 7.0). Provided normal renal function is restored and adequate fluid therapy is given, the acidosis will resolve without bicarbonate administration.

Antibiotic Therapy

Broad spectrum antibiotic therapy is required because bacterial infection is often a common precipitating factor for diabetic ketoacidosis and the use of intravenous and urinary catheters may predispose the patient to infection.

Other common concurrent illnesses in the dog with diabetic ketoacidosis include pancreatitis, renal failure, congestive heart failure, hyperadrenocorticism and pyometra. Entire bitches may be resistant to insulin therapy due to the metoestrus phase of their oestrus cycle.

Management of Uncomplicated Diabetes Mellitus

The primary goal of diabetes therapy is to maintain normoglycaemia and thereby control the signs that occur secondary to hyperglycaemia and glycosuria which result in the development of complications (Table 60.3). The essentials of good stabilisation of diabetes mellitus in the dog require understanding by the owner, and adherence to a regular daily routine that involves diet, insulin administration and regular, controlled exercise.

Stabilisation can be carried out satisfactorily at home, but particularly if the dog is ketotic, it may be preferable to hospitalise the animal during stabilisation since it is easier to monitor blood glucose more closely.

Table 60.3 Complications associated with canine diabetes mellitus.

Hypoglycaemia
Ketoacidosis
Cataract formation
Hepatic lipidosis
Pancreatitis
Infections
Retinopathy ⎫
Diabetic nephropathy ⎬ Rare
Diabetic neuropathy ⎪
Skin disease ⎭

Most diabetic dogs are presented with severe islet cell degeneration and atrophy. Therefore diabetes mellitus in dogs is insulin-dependent. Rarely, bitches may be presented during the metoestrus phase of the oestrus cycle before islet cell exhaustion has occurred. If ovariohysterectomy is performed immediately the signs of diabetes become apparent in these patients, there may be complete remission of clinical signs. However, in the majority of bitches this opportunity is missed or goes unnoticed and permanent damage to the islet cells occurs.

Dietary Therapy

Appropriate dietary therapy is an essential part of the management of diabetes. The diet must be well-balanced and constant in both composition and amount fed at each meal. It is therefore most convenient to use a commercial diet. Canned or dry foods which contain digestible complex carbohydrates should be fed as slow digestion minimises the fluctuations in postprandial blood glucose concentrations. Semi-moist foods which contain a predominance of easily assimilated carbohydrates in the form of disaccharides and propylene glycol should be avoided because of marked postprandial hyperglycaemia (Holste *et al.* 1989). There is evidence that diets with high fibre content improve glycaemic control by delaying starch hydrolysis and glucose absorption thereby reducing post-prandial fluctuations in blood glucose (Nelson *et al.* 1991). High fibre diets are also beneficial in correcting obesity. However, there may be disadvantages in using high fibre diets such as reduced palatability and the fact that low caloric density may cause the patient to lose excessive weight or fail to gain weight in those patients already below ideal body weight. The author tends to reserve high fibre diets for those patients that are difficult to stabilise and/or are obese.

Finally, the feeding schedule should be designed to enhance the action of insulin and minimise postprandial hyperglycaemia. The daily caloric intake should occur when insulin is present in the circulation and capable of handling glucose absorbed from the intestine. Several small meals are preferable to one large feed as these will help minimise post-prandial hyperglycaemia and thus help to control fluctuations in blood glucose. The author routinely recommends two equal meals fed at times to coincide with insulin activity. In cases that prove difficult to stabilise three to four smaller meals are fed during the day.

Titbits and scavenging must be avoided as they tend to destabilise diabetic patients.

Insulin Therapy

For routine stabilisation in the dog insulin zinc suspension (lente) which contains a mixture of 30% insulin zinc suspension (amorphous) and 70% insulin zinc suspension (crystalline) is the preparation of choice. When given by subcutaneous injection, it is an intermediate acting insulin with an onset of activity at 1–2 h, peak activity around 6–12 h and a duration of action of between 18 h and 26 h in the dog. The times for peak activity and duration of action vary with the individual, but in most dogs once daily administration is adequate.

Lente insulin is usually given as a single morning injection at the same time or just before the first meal, with the second meal given 6–8 h later to coincide with peak insulin activity. An initial dose of between 0.5–1.0 unit/kg is used. Insulin is probably best dosed on body surface area rather than a simple weight basis. Thus small dogs (<15 kg) tend to require 1.0 unit/kg and larger dogs (>25 kg) receive 0.5 unit/kg. Although the subcutaneous route is ideal for long-term use, the intramuscular route may be used initially, especially in moderately dehydrated or ketotic animals, because absorption from subcutaneous depots in these patients may be slow and erratic.

Insulin should be administered using specific 0.5 ml or 1.0 ml syringes calibrated in units (100 units/ml). Insulin preparations should be stored in a refrigerator at 2–8°C because they are adversely affected by heat or freezing. Preparations should be rolled gently to re-suspend the particles before use.

A dog will usually take 2–4 days to respond fully to a dose of insulin or a change in preparation. It is important to avoid increasing the dose too quickly before equilibration has occurred as this can lead to a sudden and precipitous fall in blood glucose due to overdosage with insulin. In most cases, adjustments in the insulin dose should be made in small changes of not more than 2–4 units per injection.

The type of preparation and frequency of administration may require alteration in those patients that prove difficult to stabilise with this standard routine. However, it is good for the clinician to become familiar with one type of insulin preparation and only change from that preparation if the insulin is the cause of the instability.

The standard routine:

8.00 a.m.	Give lente insulin injection subcutaneously.
8.30 a.m.	Feed half of the measured daily ration.
2.30 p.m.	Feed second half of the daily ration.

Keep daily routine constant including exercise.
Avoid titbits and scavenging.

Monitoring Therapy

Ideally monitoring should consist of serial blood glucose concentrations as tighter diabetic control can be gained than with urine glucose estimations. Initially at least two blood glucose estimations should be made, one before insulin is administered and the second just before the second feed. Once the dog appears fairly stable more frequent blood samples should be taken throughout the day to assess the degree of stabilisation. An assessment of daily water intake can also provide useful information about the degree of diabetic control.

Blood glucose concentrations should ideally be maintained between 5 and 9 mmol/l (Fig. 60.2). The blood glucose concentration will usually be highest in the morning before insulin is administered and lowest just before the second feed. A trace of glucose in the morning urine sample may be acceptable but the urine should be negative at other times in the day. However, it is important to remember that urine glucose may not reflect the blood glucose concentration at the same point in time and if the urine glucose is negative, the blood glucose concentration could be hypoglycaemic (<3.0 mmol/l), normoglycaemic or hyperglycaemic (>5.5 mmol/l).

Although the author's clients monitor urine for glucose and ketones regularly, he does not advocate adjusting daily insulin dosages on the basis of morning urine glucose mea-

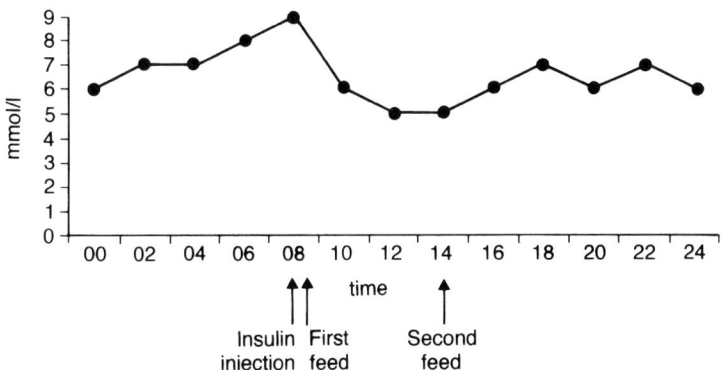

Fig. 60.2 Ideal diabetic control of blood glucose.

surements. Instead, he prefers to continue with a fixed insulin dosage unless the patient remains unstable for more than several days.

Measurement of glycated proteins such as fructosamine and glycosylated haemoglobin, are used increasingly in the dog to monitor the response to treatment. The irreversible, non-enzymatic glycation process occurs throughout the life span of the protein, mainly albumin in the case of fructosamine, and is proportional to the glucose concentration over that time. These measurements reflect the average blood glucose concentration over the preceding 1–2 weeks in the case of serum fructosamine and 2–3 months in the case of glycosylated haemoglobin (Jensen 1995). Fructosamine concentrations less than 400 mmol/l indicate good glycaemic control whereas concentrations above 500 mmol/l are found in newly diagnosed or poorly controlled diabetics (Reusch *et al.* 1993). Glycosylated haemoglobin is less routinely available as an assay. Well controlled diabetic dogs have between 4% and 6% glycosylated haemoglobin, whereas poorly controlled diabetics have concentrations greater than 7% (Nelson 1995).

Diabetic records (Fig. 60.3) should be kept by the owner for each patient as alterations to stability can be assessed more easily over a period of time. Insulin requirements will be increased by infection, oestrus particularly the metoestrus phase to the cycle, pregnancy and ketoacidosis. It is recommended that entire bitches should undergo ovariohysterectomy to avoid insulin resistance at subsequent seasons.

Investigation of Instability

If a dog appears to be poorly stabilised at home despite repeated attempts to provide adequate glycaemic control,

check the diabetic record and examine the patient for signs of disease that could cause insulin resistance, for example infection, oestrus, pregnancy, ketoacidosis or hyperadrenocorticism. Go through the daily routine with the owner to make sure that the diet is constant and measured and that there is no access to titbits or scavenging. Check the insulin preparation for type, expiry date and storage and the ability of the owner to administer insulin (adequate mixing, correct dosage and injection technique).

If an obvious cause cannot be determined, the dog should be hospitalised on its daily routine and serial blood glucose determinations made every 1–2 h throughout the day. Determinations made with glucose reagent strips and a glucose meter are simple, fast and sufficiently accurate for this purpose. The results should then be plotted on a graph against time, although it is important to realise that precise glucose curves may vary from day to day in any diabetic patient.

Three major causes of instability can be determined from the graph of serial blood glucose determinations. The first is insulin-induced hyperglycaemia also called the Somogyi overswing, where excessive insulin dosage leads to paradoxical hyperglycaemia (Fig. 60.4). The blood glucose concentration is high in the morning before insulin is given, but falls sharply to hypoglycaemic concentrations (<3.5 mmol/l) after insulin administration. The hypoglycaemic period is short in duration and is not associated with signs of hypoglycaemia. In fact, the nadir can easily be missed if frequent sampling is not performed. The low blood glucose concentration stimulates the release of hormones antagonistic to insulin, such as glucagon, cortisol and catecholamines, and these cause the glucose concentration to rebound quickly to high levels. If blood glucose and/or urine glucose concentrations were measured only before insulin and before the second feed, the concentra-

DIABETIC RECORD

Date	Urine exam	Insulin time and dose	Food	Drink	Body weight	Blood results	Notes
12 Oct	am glucose –ve ketones –ve	14 units lente insulin s.c. 8.00 am	3/4 tin Doggo 8.30 am 2.30 am	1.2 l	28 kg	2.00 pm Blood glucose 4.8 mmol/l	Bright

Fig. 60.3   Diabetic record.

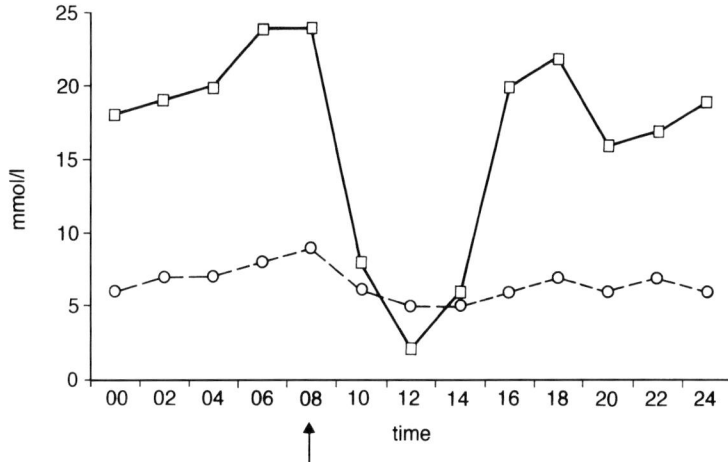

Fig. 60.4 Blood glucose curve in insulin-induced hyperglycaemia. The ideal blood glucose curve is represented by the dashed line. The arrow denoted the timing of the insulin injection.

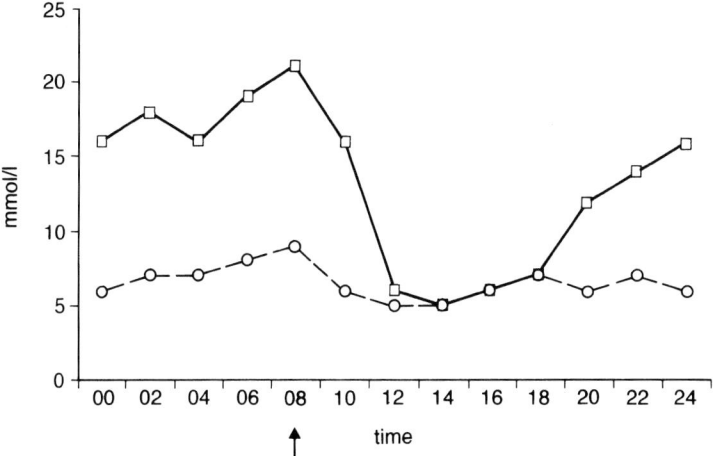

Fig. 60.5 Blood glucose curve in rapid metabolism of insulin. The ideal blood glucose curve is represented by the dashed line. The arrow denotes the timing of the insulin injection.

tions would be high and this could easily be misinterpreted as a reason for increasing the daily insulin dose, when in fact, the dog is already being overdosed. The treatment for insulin-induced hyperglycaemia is to reduce the daily dose of insulin to prevent the hypoglycaemia that causes the dramatic swing in blood glucose concentrations.

The second cause of instability is due to rapid metabolism of insulin which means that an intermediate acting insulin preparation does not last for a full 24 h (Fig. 60.5). In such cases, the blood glucose concentration is high in the morning before insulin is given, but falls to normal concentrations for much of the day. However after the second feed the blood glucose concentration rises and remains high for

the remainder of the day. This results in a considerable period of hyperglycaemia and results in glycosuria in the morning and often nocturnal polydipsia and polyuria. The treatment of rapid insulin metabolism is either to try a longer acting insulin preparation, for example protamine zinc insulin or ultralente, or to administer two doses of lente insulin 12 h apart with four small meals given approximately at 6-h intervals.

The third cause of instability is associated with insulin resistance. In these cases, the animal remains persistently hyperglycaemic despite an insulin dosage of more than 2.2 units/kg per day (Fig. 60.6). Although some patients can be stabilised satisfactorily at doses higher than this, peripheral

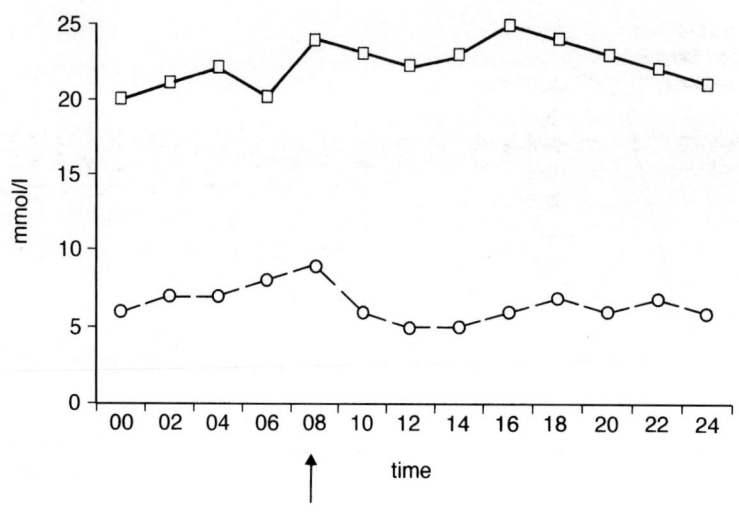

Fig. 60.6 Blood glucose curve in insulin resistance. The ideal blood glucose curve is represented by the dashed line. The arrow denotes the timing of the insulin injection.

Table 60.4 Causes of insulin resistance in the dog.

Obesity
Hyperadrenocorticism
Exogenous glucocorticoid administration
Metoestrus phase of the oestrus cycle
Exogenous progestagen administration
Acromegaly
Hypothyroidism
Impaired absorption of insulin
Excessive insulin antibody formation
Phaeochromocytoma
Glucagonoma

antagonism to insulin activity is likely to be present. In those cases where adequate stabilisation is not possible, thorough investigation of the patient is required to try and identify the precise cause of insulin resistance. Some of the causes of insulin resistance are listed in Table 60.4. Correction or treatment of the underlying cause will usually enable the patient to be stabilised at a lower dose of insulin with improved glycaemic control.

REFERENCES

Holste, L.C., Nelson, R.W., Feldman, E.C. & Bottoms, G.D. (1989). Effect of dry, soft moist, and canned dog food on post-prandial blood glucose and insulin concentrations in healthy dogs. *American Journal of Veterinary Research*, **50**, 984–989.

Jensen, A.L. (1995). Glycated blood proteins in canine diabetes mellitus. *Veterinary Record*, **137**, 401–405.

Macintire, D.K. (1993). Treatment of diabetic ketoacidosis in dogs by continuous low-dose intravenous infusion of insulin. *Journal of the American Veterinary Medical Association*, **202**, 1266–1272.

Nelson, R.W. (1995). Diabetes mellitus. In: *Textbook of Veterinary Internal Medicine*, (eds S.J. Ettinger & E.C. Feldman), 4th edn. pp. 1529–1530. W.B. Saunders, Philadelphia.

Nelson, R.W., Ihle, S.L., Lewis, L.D., Salisbury, S.K., Miller, T., Bergdall, V. & Bottoms G.D. (1991). Effects of dietary fibre supplementation on glycemic control in dogs with alloxan-induced diabetes mellitus. *American Journal of Veterinary Research*, **52**, 2060–2066.

Reusch, C.E., Liehs, M.R., Hoyer, M. & Vochezer, R. (1993). Fructosamine: a new parameter for diagnosis and metabolic control in diabetic dogs and cats. *Journal of Veterinary Internal Medicine*, **7**, 177–182.

Chapter 61

Diagnosis of Insulinoma

M. E. Herrtage

Functional islet cell tumours (insulinomas) are the most frequently occurring tumours of the endocrine pancreas in dogs. Most insulin-secreting tumours are malignant islet cell carcinomas which metastasise to regional lymph nodes and/or the liver. Early diagnosis is important as dogs with metastases have significantly reduced survival times.

PATHOPHYSIOLOGY

Insulinomas are composed of neoplastic β-cells which continue to release insulin despite the presence of hypoglycaemia. Hypoglycaemia is normally the major inhibitory stimulus for insulin secretion. As a result of hyperinsulinism, tissue utilisation of glucose continues, the hypoglycaemia worsens and ultimately clinical signs develop. The onset and severity of clinical signs is determined by the degree of hypoglycaemia and the rate at which the plasma concentration of glucose falls. A rapid decline in plasma glucose concentration may occur with fasting, exercise or excitement in dogs with insulinomas.

The brain is an obligate consumer of glucose. Cerebral cells have limited stores of glycogen and a limited ability to utilise protein and amino acids for energy. These cells will be the first affected by hypoglycaemia. Prolonged and profound hypoglycaemia causes ischaemic neuronal cell damage identical to that caused by cerebral hypoxia.

Hypoglycaemia is a potent stimulus for the release of hormones that have an antagonistic action to insulin. These include glucagon, growth hormone, glucocorticoids, catecholamines and possibly thyroid hormones. These hormones act in concert to raise the plasma glucose concentration. Some of the clinical manifestations of hypoglycaemia such as muscle tremors, nervousness, restlessness and hunger may result from stimulation of the sympathetic nervous system and increased levels of circulating catecholamines.

CLINICAL SIGNS

Insulinomas usually occur in middle-aged to older dogs (mean age of 9.0 years) of any breed, although medium to large breeds appear to be predisposed (Dunn et al. 1993). No sex predisposition has been reported.

A tentative diagnosis of hyperinsulinism is generally based on fulfilment of the criteria from Whipple's triad: (1) the presence of neurological signs typical of hypoglycaemia, which may be precipitated by exercise or excitement, (2) hypoglycaemia (plasma glucose less than 3 mmol/l) at the time of the clinical signs, and (3) resolution of clinical signs following feeding or administration of glucose.

Clinical signs associated with hypoglycaemia include fatigue, generalised weakness, collapse, muscle tremors, altered behaviour, confusion/disorientation, apparent blindness, ataxia, inco-ordination, stupor and seizures. The differential diagnosis of episodic weakness and collapse is given in Table 61.1. These signs are usually episodic in nature and may occur with fasting, exercise or excitement in dogs with insulinomas. Provocative stimuli such as the intravenous administration of glucagon or glucose, results in excessive secretion of insulin from neoplastic β-cells. This response may be even greater if glucose is administered orally since a number of intestinal hormones (glucagon, secretin, cholecystokinin, gastrin and gastric inhibitory peptide) are secreted in response to oral glucose and these in turn increase insulin secretion. It is by this mechanism that feeding has been reported to initiate clinical signs in dogs with insulinomas.

Seizure activity is one of the most common clinical manifestations of hypoglycaemia. The seizures may be grand mal or focal in nature and are normally self-limiting, lasting between 30 s and 5 min. Peripheral neuropathy with nerve degeneration and demyelination has also been associated with canine insulinoma in a few cases (Schrauwen 1991).

Table 61.1 Differential diagnosis of episodic weakness in the dog, including seizures.

Cardiovascular disorders	Neurological disorders
Bradyarrhythmia	Congenital or acquired spinal disorders including
Tachyarrhythmia	Wobbler syndrome
Congenital heart disease e.g. aortic or pulmonic	Epilepsy (various causes)
stenosis, tetralogy of Fallot, reverse shunting PDA	Vestibular disease
Acquired heart disease e.g. valvular, myocardial,	Cerebellar disorders
pericardial	Thiamine deficiency
Heartworm disease (dirofilariasis, angiostrongylosis)	Congenital disorders e.g. hydrocephalus
Vasovagal syncope	Acquired disorders e.g. old dog encephalitis, CVA,
Vasodilation	tumours
(Aortic) thromboembolism	Lysosomal storage diseases
	Giant axonal neuropathy
Respiratory disorders	Progressive axonopathy – Boxer
Laryngeal paralysis	Tetanus
Brachycephalic airway disease	Botulism
Tracheal collapse	Narcolepsy/cataplexy – Doberman Pinscher, Poodle,
Severe coughing	Labrador Retriever
Filaroides osleri	Generalised tremor
Pulmonary disease	Jack Russell ataxia
Pleural effusions	Scottie cramp – also in the Norwich and Jack Russell
Thoracic masses	Terrier, Dalmatian
	Episodic falling in the Cavalier King Charles Spaniel
Haematological disorders	
Anaemia	*Metabolic disorders*
Myeloproliferative disorders	Hepatic encephalopathy
Polycythaemia	Uraemic encephalopathy
Hyperviscosity syndrome	Hyperglycaemia
Haemoglobinopathies	Hypoglycaemia
Pyrexia of unknown origin	Hyponatraemia
	Hyperkalaemia
Orthopaedic disorders	Hypokalaemia
Degenerative joint disease particularly hips or stifles	Hypercalcaemia
Polyarthritis – various types	Hypocalcaemia
	Hypermagnesaemia
Neuromuscular disorders	Hypomagnesaemia
Myasthenia gravis	Acidosis
Polymyositis	Hyperthermia (heatstroke)
Hereditary myopathy of Labrador Retrievers	Hypoxia
Sex-linked muscular dystrophy – Irish Terriers, Golden	Shock
Retrievers	
Myotonia in Chow Chows, Staffordshire Terriers	*Endocrine disorders*
Malignant hyperthermia	Insulinoma
Mitochondrial myopathies	Hyperadrenocorticism – myotonia
Exertional myopathy (rhabdomyolysis)	Hypoadrenocorticism
	Hypoparathyroidism
	Hypothyroidism
	Phaeochromocytoma
	Diabetic ketoacidosis

PDA, patent ductus arteriosus.
CVA, cerebrovascular accident.

Insulinomas are generally small tumours and do not lead to malignant cachexia. Thus weight loss is not a feature of this disease.

LABORATORY FINDINGS

A presumptive diagnosis of insulinoma is based on the presence of typical clinical signs in association with persistent hypoglycaemia and an inappropriately high plasma insulin concentration.

A fasting plasma glucose concentration of 3 mmol/l or less is found in most cases. Some dogs with insulinoma show no clinical signs despite having extremely low blood glucose concentrations (<2 mmol/l) because they are able to adapt to these low concentrations over a prolonged period of time. Differential diagnosis of hypoglycaemia in adult dogs includes insulinoma, liver disease, extra-pancreatic neoplasia, septicaemia and hypoadrenocorticism (Table 61.2).

Plasma insulin concentrations greater than 20 mU/l in association with hypoglycaemia are inappropriate and an insulin glucose ratio greater than 4.2 U/mol are considered diagnostic (Dunn *et al.* 1992). In normal dogs, insulin levels fall as glucose concentrations decrease, however, in animals with insulinomas, insulin secretion generally remains high despite hypoglycaemia.

In borderline cases, an intravenous glucose tolerance test using 0.5 g glucose/kg body weight has proved useful. Insulin secreting tumours retain a degree of responsiveness to the glucose challenge and a glucose half-life of less than 20 min and/or a fractional clearance rate of more than 3%/minute is highly suggestive of insulinoma in the dog.

Table 61.2 Differential diagnosis of hypoglycaemia in adult dogs.

Incorrect anticoagulant/delayed separation of serum from red blood cells
Functional islet cell tumour (insulinoma)
Excessive insulin administration
Extra-pancreatic tumours, particularly hepatic tumours
Liver disease
Septicaemic or endotoxic shock
Hypoadrenocorticism
Idiopathic in working dogs
Severe polycythaemia

Although hypoalbuminaemia, hypokalaemia and increases in alkaline phosphatase and alanine aminotransferase have occasionally been reported in cases of insulinoma, these findings are not specific or helpful in achieving a definitive diagnosis.

ULTRASONOGRAPHY

Abdominal ultrasonography using a high quality diagnostic ultrasound machine has been used to examine the pancreas of dogs with suspected insulinomas. In one study a pancreatic mass was identified as a spherical or lobular hypoechoic nodule in 75% of dogs with insulinomas (Lamb *et al.* 1995). Tumours as small as 7 mm have been identified in the pancreas. However, ultrasonography has proved less sensitive for the detection of hepatic or lymphatic metastases.

PATHOLOGY

Insulinomas may be located in the left lobe (44%), right lobe (35%) or body (14%) of the pancreas. Tumours are usually solitary but multiple masses may occur. Rarely, there is a diffuse islet cell tumour with no discrete nodule. There does not appear to be a difference in survival in relation to tumour location within the pancreas, but there is a suggestion that tumours with a high mitotic count carry a worse prognosis.

Insulinomas in dogs are highly malignant and there is often gross evidence of metastasis at the time of diagnosis.

MANAGEMENT

Management of insulinomas should be directed at specific treatment of the tumour, reduction of insulin secretion and correction of hypoglycaemia.

Surgical resection of the pancreatic tumour and metastatic tumour masses should be the first approach to therapy. Postoperative recovery is routine in many cases, but complications including pancreatitis, hyperglycaemia, overt diabetes mellitus and hypoglycaemia occur. In all cases, hypoglycaemia will eventually recur due to metastases.

Table 61.3 Medical management of insulinoma (chronic hypoglycaemia).

Dietary therapy	Small frequent meals
	Composition high in protein, fat and complex carbohydrates
Prednisolone	0.5–1.0 mg/kg p.o. daily in divided doses
Diazoxide	10 mg/kg p.o. daily in divided doses increasing up to 60 mg/kg daily if required to control clinical signs
Octreotide	10–20 µg b.i.d. or t.i.d.
	Patients must be carefully monitored since octreotide may increase the depth and duration of the hypoglycaemia

Medical management should be used if widespread metastasis is present or if hypoglycaemia recurs after surgery. This should consist of dietary control (frequent small meals of a diet high in proteins, fats and complex carbohydrates), the use of prednisolone which inhibits insulin and stimulates glycogenolysis, and diazoxide, a non-diuretic, benzothiazine antihypertensive drug which inhibits insulin secretion (Table 61.3). Octreotide, a somatostatin analogue which inhibits insulin synthesis and secretion, has also been used and has been shown to be effective in some cases (Simpson *et al.* 1995).

PROGNOSIS

The prognosis is guarded due to the malignant nature of the disease. However, many dogs do well with medical and surgical management. The median time to recurrence of clinical signs after surgery was 12 months (range 4–16 months) and the median postoperative survival time was 14 months (range 10–33 months) in one study (Dunn *et al.* 1993).

REFERENCES

Dunn, J.K., Heath, M.F., Herrtage, M.E., Jackson, K.F. & Walker, M.J. (1992). Diagnosis of insulinoma in the dog: a study of 11 cases. *Journal of Small Animal Practice*, **33**, 514–520.

Dunn, J.K., Bostock, D.E., Herrtage, M.E., Jackson, K.F. & Walker, M.J. (1993). Insulin-secreting tumours of the canine pancreas: clinical and pathological features of 11 cases. *Journal of Small Animal Practice*, **34**, 325–331.

Lamb, C.R., Simpson, K.W., Boswood, A. & Matthewman, L.A. (1995). Ultrasonography of pancreatic neoplasia in the dog: a review of 16 cases. *Veterinary Record*, **137**, 65–68.

Simpson, K.W., Stepien, R.L., Elwood, C.M., Boswood, A. & Vailliant, C.R. (1995). Evaluation of the long-standing somatostatin analogue Octreotide in the management of insulinoma in three dogs. *Journal of Small Animal Practice*, **36**, 161–165.

Schrauwen, E. (1991). Clinical peripheral polyneuropathy associated with canine insulinoma in the dog. *Veterinary Record*, **128**, 211–212.

Section 8

Urology

Edited by Jonathan Elliott and Neil T. Gorman

Chapter 62

Renal Failure

R. A. Squires, J. Elliott and S. Brown

INTRODUCTION

Renal disease is a common and important condition in veterinary clinical practice. The purpose of this chapter is to:

(1) define the pathophysiology of renal failure,
(2) describe the management of acute renal failure,
(3) describe the management of chronic renal failure.

For clarity the following definitions will be used:

- *Renal disease* – Damage or functional impairment of the kidneys. Can vary in severity from very mild, to severe enough to cause uraemia.
- *Renal insufficiency* – Renal functional impairment not severe enough to cause azotaemia, but sufficient to cause loss of renal reserve. Urine concentrating ability is usually diminished.
- *Azotaemia* – An abnormal increase in the concentration of non-protein nitrogenous wastes (such as creatinine and urea nitrogen) in blood.
- *Renal failure* – Renal functional impairment sufficient to cause azotaemia. Urine concentrating ability is usually impaired.
- *Uraemia* – Literally means urine in the blood – may be defined as the constellation of adverse clinical signs caused by advanced renal failure, or (occasionally) other causes of severe azotaemia.

Chronic renal failure is the most common cause of uraemia. However, other conditions such as acute renal failure, lower urinary tract obstruction and rupture of the urinary tract occasionally cause uraemia. Regardless of its cause, a profound reduction in urinary excretory function leads inevitably to a characteristic clinical syndrome, with disturbed function of many organ systems. Uraemia is not caused solely by the accumulation of metabolic waste products. Impairment of other important metabolic and endocrine renal functions contributes substantially to the observed clinical signs. Table 62.1 lists typical clinical features of uraemia.

Uraemia should be distinguished from azotaemia. Azotaemia is defined biochemically as an increase in the concentrations of creatinine and urea nitrogen (BUN) in blood which are used to assess renal excretory function. Azotaemia may arise as a consequence of:

- inadequate renal blood perfusion (prerenal azotaemia),
- intrinsic renal failure (renal azotaemia), or
- postrenal obstruction or rupture of the urinary tract (postrenal azotaemia).

All uraemic patients are azotaemic. Mildly azotaemic patients do not have sufficient renal impairment to show signs of uraemia. For example, it is very unusual for uncomplicated prerenal azotaemia to be sufficiently severe to cause uraemia. The severity of uraemia depends not only upon the degree of renal impairment, but also on the rate of deterioration. Rapid deterioration to a given degree of renal impairment will cause more intense clinical signs than gradual progression.

Causes of uraemia are legion. The clinician must seek to determine a specific diagnosis to guide therapy and to increase the accuracy of prognosis. The first requirement is to determine whether uraemia is due to intrinsic renal failure or some other cause, such as postrenal obstruction. Most uraemic patients have intrinsic renal failure. If intrinsic renal failure is present, the second step is to determine whether it is acute or chronic. Historical findings, physical examination and simple screening diagnostic tests are helpful in this regard. Once the cause of uraemia has been categorised as acute renal failure (ARF), chronic renal failure (CRF) or postrenal disease, the range of differential diagnoses is substantially narrowed and a specific diagnosis is much

Table 62.1 Clinical features typical of uraemic patients.

Fluid, electrolyte and serum biochemical disturbances
   Polyuria/polydipsia
   Dehydration
   Azotaemia
   Metabolic acidosis
   Hyperphosphataemia
   Hyperkalaemia or hypokalaemia – not in every case
   Hypercalcaemia or hypocalcaemia – not in every case

Gastrointestinal disturbances
   Anorexia
   Vomiting
   Halitosis
   Oral ulceration/stomatitis
   Gastropathy, gastritis and gastric ulceration
   Gastrointestinal bleeding

Haematological disturbances
   Normocytic, normochromic, non-regenerative anaemia
      (lack of erythropoeitin)
   Platelet function defect/bleeding tendency
   Non-infectious acquired immunodeficiency –
      lymphopenia and neutrophilia (with
      hypersegmentation)

Endocrine and metabolic disturbances
   Negative nitrogen balance, with tissue protein
      catabolism and weight loss
   Secondary hyperparathyroidism, calcitriol deficiency and
      osteodystrophy
   Peripheral insulin resistance and glucose intolerance
   Hypertriglyceridaemia
   Low triiodothyronine (T_3)
   Normal or slightly increased plasma cortisol and ACTH
      levels

Cardiovascular and pulmonary disturbances
   Systemic arterial hypertension
   Uraemic pneumonitis

Neuromuscular disturbances
   Weakness
   Lethargy
   Depression
   Uraemic encephalopathy – seen in people, not usually in
      dogs
   Peripheral polyneuropathy – seen in people, not usually
      in dogs

ACTH, adrenocorticotrophic hormone.

more easily made. The frequently encountered pathways that lead to uraemia are:

- acute renal failure
  - renal ischaemia
  - nephrotoxins
  - upper urinary tract infections (acute pyelonephritis)
- urinary tract obstruction
  - trauma
  - neoplasia
  - urinary calculi
- chronic renal failure
  - renal degeneration
  - immune-mediated disease
  - upper urinary tract infection (chronic pyelonephritis)
  - neoplasia

Table 62.2 lists a selection of differential diagnoses for uraemia using the popular 'DAMNIT' classification scheme.

Pathophysiology of the Uraemic Syndrome

The primary role of the kidneys is to maintain fluid and electrolyte homeostasis and to excrete nitrogenous wastes and excess acid. A normal animal has substantially more nephrons than are necessary to achieve this. The number of functional nephrons and the glomerular filtration rate (GFR) must fall below one-third of normal before urine concentrating ability is substantially impaired. If the GFR declines to less than 25% of normal, azotaemia develops. Uraemic patients frequently have a GFR that is less than 10% of that of a normal animal. The ability to concentrate urine normally is compromised when approximately two-thirds of the functional nephrons have been impaired and becomes particularly marked in the early stages of renal failure.

The clinical syndrome of uraemia results from:

- accumulation of many substances due to excretory failure (see Table 62.3);
- increased secretion of substances in an attempt to compensate for renal failure (e.g. parathyroid hormone (PTH) secretion occurs in response to renal phosphate retention (Nagode & Chew 1992));
- lack of production of regulatory substances by the kidney (e.g. calcitriol (active vitamin D) and erythropoietin leading to disordered calcium and phosphate metabolism and non-regenerative anaemia respectively).

Table 62.2 Examples of possible causes of uraemia categorised according to the 'DAMNIT' scheme.

Degenerative	Advanced chronic interstitial nephritis → CRF
	Renal infarcts → CRF
	Congestive heart failure → CRF
Developmental	Familial nephropathy → CRF
Autoimmune	Anti-glomerular basement membrane antibodies → glomerulonephritis → CRF
Allergic	Anaphylactic shock → ARF
Metabolic	Addison's disease → hypovolaemic shock → ARF
	Hypercalcaemia → CRF
	Metabolic disease → urolith formation → urinary outflow obstruction
Neoplastic	Bilateral renal lymphoma or carcinomas → CRF
	Urethral or bladder neck transitional cell carcinoma → urinary outflow obstruction
Iatrogenic	Excessive vitamin D supplementation → hypervitaminosis D → hypercalcaemia → renal failure
	Deep anaesthesia → arterial hypotension → renal ischaemia → acute renal failure
	Relative or absolute overdose of nephrotoxic drugs (e.g. aminoglycosides, cisplatin, amphotericin B) → renal failure
	Surgical e.g. ligation of ureters during OVH → urinary outflow obstruction
Idiopathic	Renal amyloidosis → CRF
	Most forms of glomerulonephritis → CRF
Infectious	Pyelonephritis → CRF
	Lyme (borreliosis) nephropathy → CRF
	Leptospirosis → ARF
	Septic shock → ARF
Immune-mediated	Immune complex-mediated glomerulonephritis → CRF
Toxic	Ethylene glycol ingestion → ARF
Traumatic	Ruptured bladder, avulsed or ruptured ureters or urethra → urine retention
	Fractured kidneys or haemorrhagic shock → ARF

OVH, ovariohysterectomy.
CRF, chronic renal failure.
ARF, acute renal failure.

Clinical Approach to the Azotaemic Patient

When presented with an animal that has biochemical evidence of azotaemia, a logical approach is required to provide appropriate management and prognosis for the case. Fig. 62.1 summarises the approach to the diagnosis of suspected uraemia. The initial investigation should be directed at determining whether the case constitutes one of ARF or CRF.

ACUTE RENAL FAILURE

Signs of Acute Renal Failure

The clinical signs of ARF are the same whatever the cause and consist of non-specific signs such as vomiting, anorexia, lethargy and dehydration. In some, but by no means all cases, halitosis and oral ulceration will be noted. An underlying cause may or may not be obvious from the history or physical examination. Prompt diagnosis is essential in the management of an acute azotaemic crisis to give the maximum chance of survival. Laboratory tests will show sudden elevations of serum urea, creatinine, phosphate and often potassium concentrations and should be used to confirm the diagnosis. A sudden 50–100% increase in serum urea and creatinine concentration, by definition, consititutes ARF. In most cases, serum concentrations of urea and creatinine before the onset of the problem will not be available. Oliguria (production of less than 0.5 ml* of urine per kg per hour) was thought to be the hallmark of ARF but more recently non-oliguric ARF has been recognised as being relatively common and, if recognised and treated, this type carries a better prognosis than oliguric ARF (Polzin *et al.* 1989).

*In an animal which has been fully rehydrated, urine production should exceed 1 ml/kg per hour.

Table 62.3   Substances that accumulate in uraemia and are thought to contribute to the clinical syndrome.

Accumulating substance	Proposed adverse effects
Urea	Weakness, anorexia, vomiting, glucose intolerance, bleeding disorder

Guanidino compounds:
  guanidine
  (di)methylguanidine
  creatinine
  creatine
  guanidinoacetic acid
	Weight loss, platelet function defect

guanidinosuccinic acid	Guanidinosuccinic acid is thought to interfere with platelet factor III release

Aliphatic amines:
  dimethylamine
  trimethylamine
	Uraemic breath odour, encephalopathy

Polyamines:
  spermine
  spermidine
	Spermine reduces erythropoiesis

'Middle molecules' – poorly-defined middle-sized molecules, (MW 500 to 2000; i.e. larger than amines and guanidino compounds)	Uncertain, speculative role, many adverse effects have been hypothesised
Peptides & polypeptide hormones	Accumulate due to reduced excretion or increased secretion occurs as a compensating response to renal failure
parathyroid hormone	Osteodystrophy, nephrotoxicity, impaired erythropoiesis, cardiotoxicity
insulin	Hyperinsulinism may lead eventually to islet exhaustion and diabetes mellitus
glucagon	Insulin resistance/glucose intolerance
growth hormone	Insulin resistance/glucose intolerance
gastrin	Hypergastrinaemia contributes to gastritis
Myoinositol	Neuropathy
Ribonuclease	Impaired erythropoiesis, decreased cellular proliferation
Cyclic adenosine monophosphate (cAMP)	Abnormal platelet function

Derivatives of aromatic amino acids:
  tryptophan
  tyrosine
  phenylalanine
	Anorexia

Causes of Acute Renal Failure

It is useful to divide the causes of ARF into four categories (see Table 62.4) and to try to identify the category into which the animal falls, at the start of the treatment, as this will affect both the prognosis and the management of the case.

Prerenal and Intrinsic Primary Renal Causes of ARF

Prerenal ARF is caused by factors that decrease the blood flow to the kidneys including all causes of circulatory shock. The physiological response of the kidney under these circumstances is to reduce urine output, retaining

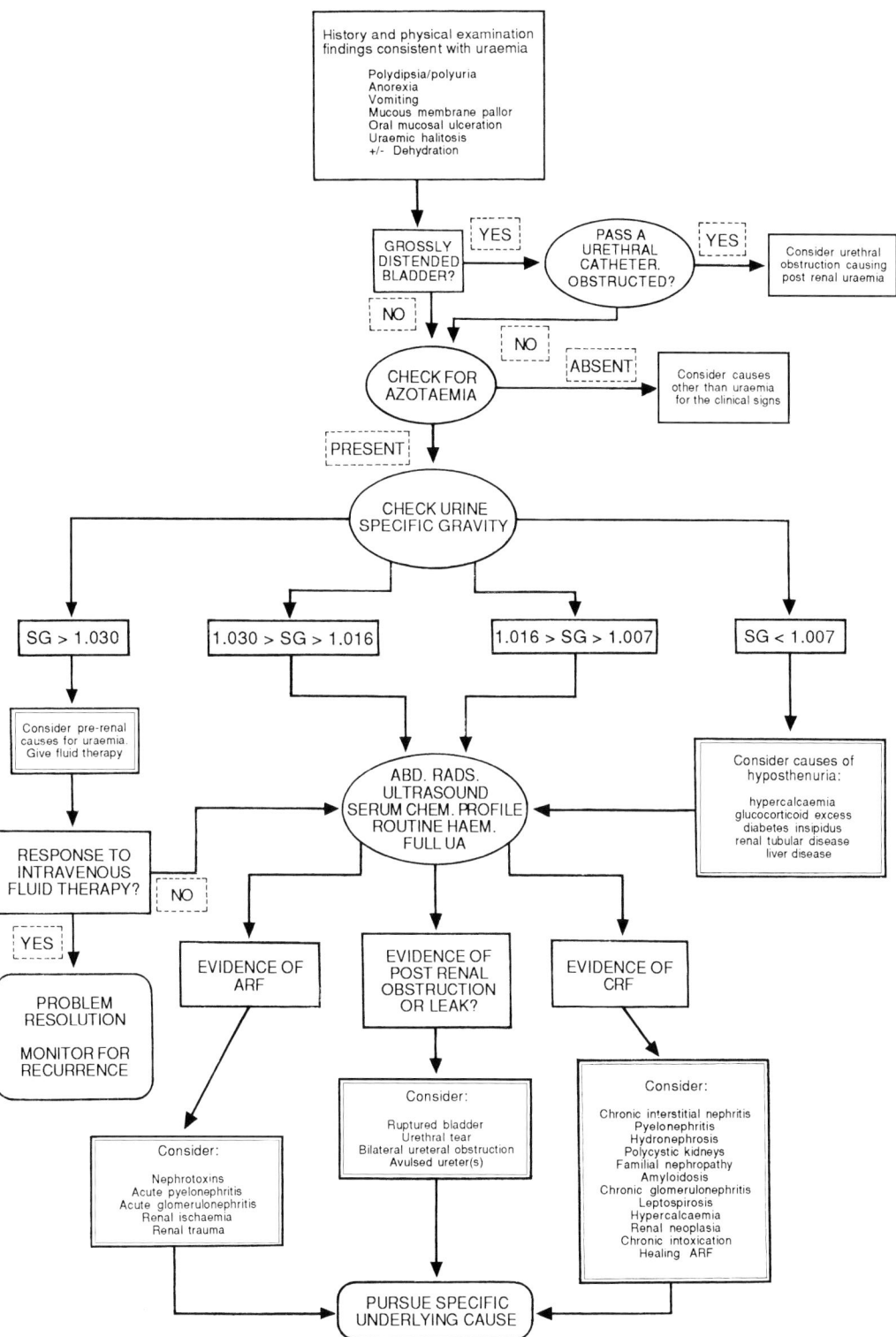

Fig. 62.1 An algorithm for the initial approach to diagnosis of suspected uraemia. SG, specific gravity; Abd. Rads., abdominal radiographs; serum chem. profile, serum chemistry profile; routine haem., routine haematological examination; UA, urine analysis; ARF, acute renal failure; CRF, chronic renal failure.

Table 62.4 Causes of acute renal failure.

Category	Prognosis
Prerenal failure	Good, if underlying cause is treatable and recognised early – return of normal renal function can occur
Primary intrinsic renal failure	Guarded – may require prolonged and intensive support to allow time for return of normal renal function in some cases
Postrenal failure	Good, if underlying cause is treatable and recognised early – return of normal renal function can occur
Decompensated chronic renal failure	Very poor prognosis

Table 62.5 Nephrotoxic substances associated with acute intrinsic renal failure.

Therapeutic agents:	**Other causes:**

Antimicrobials
  aminoglycosides
  amphotericin B
  cephaloridine
  sulphonamides
  tetracyclines*
  polymixin B
  colistin
	Glycols
	  ethylene glycol, diethylene glycol
	
	Hypercalcaemia
	  hypercalcaemia of maligancy
	  hypervitaminosis D (rodenticides)
	
	Hypokalaemia

Cancer chemotherapy agents
  cisplatin
  high-dose methotrexate
  high-dose cyclophosphamide
  (tumour lysis syndrome)
	Heavy metals
	  zinc, arsenic, mercury, thallium, lead, bismuth
	
	Organic solvents
	  carbon tetrachloride
	  chloroform

Gaseous anaesthetics
  methoxyflurane
  enflurane
	Other agents
	  haemoglobin/myoglobin
	  snake bite/bee sting
	  i.v. radiocontrast agents
	  paraquat

Other agents
  cyclosporin
  ethylenediaminetetraacetic acid (EDTA)
  mannitol (high dose)
  non-steroidal anti-inflammatory drugs	

* Probably because of impurities in out-of-date products.

sodium and water to support the circulation. Renal blood flow is supported during such hypotensive states by local production of prostaglandins. Non-steroidal anti-inflammatory drugs, even at therapeutic doses, may inhibit the protective effects of these prostaglandins resulting in damaging renal ischaemia (Rubin 1986). If renal ischaemia is maintained for any length of time, acute tubular necrosis and intrinsic renal failure will follow. Early recognition of prerenal ARF with prompt, effective support of the circu-

lation and treatment of the underlying cause will prevent this progression.

Primary intrinsic acute renal failure can be related to abnormalities of the glomeruli, tubules, intersitium or vessels and results from a wide range of aetiologies (Osborne & Polzin 1983). The pathophysiology in primary intrinsic ARF remains uncertain in many cases. The most common precipitating factors are nephrotoxins (see Table 62.5) and renal ischaemia leading to acute tubular necrosis.

Some patients, however, have few or no lesions that are visible on light microscopy yet exhibit severe excretory renal failure. A better understanding of the pathogenesis of such processes might lead to the development of therapies designed to halt the progression of the process in its early stages.

Differentiation between Prerenal and Primary Intrinsic ARF

This is sometimes possible from the history and clinical signs but often laboratory tests are required, particularly as there is a tendency for prerenal failure to progress to acute tubular necrosis. Examination of a urine sample before the administration of fluid therapy is most important in this respect (see Table 62.6). Leakage of excessive amounts of protein into the urine would indicate a primary glomerular lesion and identification of haemoglobinuria or myoglobinuria would suggest pigment damage as the primary cause of ARF.

Important exceptions to these principles include:

- contrast media-induced ARF and pigment injury where urine sodium concentration may be low despite the intrinsic renal damage;
- Addison's disease, where the animal has prerenal azotaemia, USG is usually below 1.030, due to the wasting of sodium (as a result of hypoaldosteronism) and consequent loss of the hypertonic medullary gradient;
- hypercalcaemic dogs often have low USG in the face of dehydration – hypercalcaemia antagonises the actions of anti-diuretic hormone in the kidney (hypercalcaemia, if left untreated, can lead to primary intrinsic renal failure by causing structural damage to the renal tubules);

- prior administration of diuretic or glucocorticoid therapy will reduce renal concentrating ability in animals with normal excretory function;

NB USG of <1.007, (hyposthenuria) is evidence of active dilution of the glomerular filtrate by the renal tubules, and is not typical of renal failure or uraemia (may occur with hypercalcaemia, diuretic or glucocorticoid therapy and is observed frequently in certain familial nephropathies such as in the Lhasa Apso).

Differentiation of ARF from Chronic End-Stage Renal Disease

This is an important distinction to make at the start of the management of a uraemic crisis as the prognosis in chronic end stage disease is extremely poor. The factors which help make this distinction are presented in Table 62.7.

The ultimate diagnostic test and prognostic indicator is renal biopsy which would differentiate ARF from chronic decompensated renal disease and may provide an aetiological diagnosis. However, renal biopsy, which is usually carried out percutaneously under ultrasound guidance, is an invasive procedure that is not without risk. Biopsy can, however, provide an assessment of the reversibility of the renal pathology and be a useful diagnostic tool.

Postrenal Causes of ARF

Postrenal causes of ARF are either obstructive or traumatic and are often associated with complete anuria. A careful history and physical examination may reveal evidence of

Table 62.6 Differentiation between pre-renal and intrinsic acute renal failure.

Parameter	Prerenal	Intrinsic renal
Urine [Na+]	<10 mmol/l	>20 mmol/l
FE$_{Na}$*	<1%	>2%
Urine osmolality	>500 mosmol/l	<350 mosmol/l
Urine specific gravity (USG)	>1.030	1.007 to 1.015
Urine to serum creatinine ratio	>40	<20
Urine to serum urea ratio	>8	<3
Urine microscopy	Benign sediment	Active sediment (tubular casts, red cells, white cells)

$$* \, FE_{Na}(\%) = \frac{Urine\,[Na] \times Plasma\,[Creatinine]}{Urine\,[Creatinine] \times Plasma\,[Na]} \times 100\%$$

Table 62.7   Clinical features that help distinguish between acute and chronic renal failure.

Parameter	Acute	Chronic
History	Perfectly healthy until very recently. May have been recently anaesthetised or exposed to a toxin or nephrotoxic drug	Weeks to months of polyuria/polydipsia, weight loss and low grade vomiting (several times a week)
Physical exam	Good body condition. Extremely depressed relative to the degree of azotaemia	May be cachectic. Tolerates severe azotaemia rather well (like a drug addict, it is used to the toxins)
Kidney size	Normal-sized or large (swollen) – may be painful.	Usually small and non-painful. Some chronic diseases can cause renal enlargement: • Renal neoplasia – lymphoma (bilateral), adenocarcinoma (unilateral) • Polycystic kidneys • Hydronephrosis
Laboratory tests Packed cell volume	Anaemia is not usually present, unless acute gastrointestinal haemorrhage occurs.	Non-regenerative anaemia is often a feature, especially after rehydration
Potassium, phosphate and acid/base	Hyperkalaemia, hyperphosphataemia and metabolic acidosis are often present. Hypokalaemia is a feature of polyuric ARF	Hyperkalaemia is absent until terminal acute exacerbation occurs. Animals may be hypokalaemic. Hyperphosphataemia is common. Metabolic acidosis is mild
Urinalysis	Sediment is often contained – casts, cells, debris etc. coming from the kidneys. Urine specific gravity low despite the presence of dehydration (unhelpful)	Urine sediment is inactive Urine specific gravity low despite the presence of dehydration (unhelpful)
Urine production	Often anuric or oliguric. Can have polyuric ARF (e.g. aminoglycoside toxicity)	Polyuric until the very terminal stages
Response to therapy	Often reversible, if the patient can be supported through the crisis.	Irreversible, although correction of any prerenal component may reduce the degree of azotaemia.

NB None of the laboratory tests can be used definitively in this differentiation as elevations in the same parameters are seen in both situations.

trauma or urinary obstruction, signs of which are particularly evident when the lower urinary tract disease is involved. Radiography (both plain and contrast studies) and ultrasonography are extremely useful techniques in the diagnosis of rupture or obstruction of the urinary tract at any level. Emergency management of the metabolic consequences resulting from ARF are considered below.

Management of Acute Renal Failure

Management of the ARF patient is directed at correcting the fluid and electrolyte imbalances and promoting urine output and excretion of waste products. The goals in the management of ARF are presented in Table 62.8 in the order in which they should be addressed.

Hyperkalaemia

This is the most life-threatening complication of ARF and in some circumstances requires immediate emergency therapy. High extracellular K^+ concentration leads to muscle weakness and conduction disturbances in excitable tissues. The ECG changes which result are spiking of the T wave and a decreased QT interval, a widening of the QRS complex, flattening of the P wave, an increased PR interval and eventually loss of the P wave with atrial standstill. At concentrations >8.0 mmol/l, sinoventricular rhythms, ventricular tachycardia or asystole can occur. Emergency therapies for hyperkalaemia are presented in Table 62.9.

Table 62.8 Goals in the management of the acute renal failure patient (in order of priority).

Correct life-threatening hyperkalaemia
Correct life-threatening metabolic acidosis
Rehydrate the animal, maintain fluid and electrolyte
   balance
Promote urine output if still anuric but do not over-hydrate
Dialyse to remove excess fluid and waste products if still
   anuric
Alleviate vomiting
Provide nutritional support

These treatments are applicable when serious ECG abnormalities are present. Calcium gluconate is the most rapidly acting therapy but the one with the shortest duration of action. If subsequent therapy described below promotes urine output to increase, control of serum K^+ concentration can be achieved by judicious fluid therapy. Chronic hyperkalaemia may result if the animal remains oliguric. An ion exchange resin can be administered orally or as a retention enema in such cases (sodium polystyrene sulphonate 2 g/kg, divided three times daily). Peritoneal dialysis will also reduce plasma potassium ion concentration. It should be remembered that, in animals with ARF which are polyuric (e.g. postobstructive polyuric phase of renal failure and polyuric intrinsic ARF caused by aminoglycoside toxicity), excessive loss of potassium ions can occur and hypokalaemia can rapidly result.

Close monitoring of blood potassium concentration is therefore necessary as both hyperkalaemia and hypokalaemia can occur. In-house, laboratory monitoring of blood potassium should ideally be available to allow measurement every 6 h initially, to ensure the correct fluid therapy is administered (see below). Thereafter, measurement on a once daily basis will assist in the management of the case. In the absence of in-house laboratory testing for potassium, serial ECG recordings can be used as an indicator of extracellular fluid K^+ concentration with the QT interval increasing as the plasma K^+ concentration falls.

Table 62.9 Emergency management of life threatening hyperkalaemia.

Treatment	Mechanism and speed of action	Possible adverse effects
10% calcium gluconate (0.5–1 ml/kg)	Protects the myocardium against the toxic effects of potassium. Works immediately but effects are short lived	Administer i.v. slowly, while monitoring the ECG. Overdosage can lead to rhythm disturbances
Sodium bicarbonate (1–2 mmol/kg)	Corrects the metabolic acidosis and so drives potassium ions back into the cells, thus lowering the plasma [K^+]. Takes 15–30 min to work	Over correction of the acidosis can lead to hypocalcaemia, tissue hypoxia, paradoxical CSF acidosis. Some renal failure patients can be hypocalcaemic on presentation – glucose infusions may be preferable
Glucose ± insulin 2 g of glucose ± 1 unit of soluble insulin per kg (Infuse glucose as a hypertonic solution (20%) into a large vein)	Glucose stimulates endogenous insulin release. Insulin stimulates the uptake of both glucose and K^+ into cells, lowering plasma [K^+]. Takes 15–30 min to work	There is controversy as to whether exogenous insulin is required – glucose alone may be just as effective. Insulin infusions may be dangerous in cases of Addison's disease

Metabolic Acidosis

Metabolic acidosis is another potentially life-threatening electrolyte disturbance which occurs in ARF and which may require specific emergency therapy. Catabolism of protein continues to produce metabolic acid which the kidney fails to excrete. Should the blood pH fall below 7.1, the consequences can be very serious and decreased force of cardiac contractility, ventricular arrhythmias and CNS disturbances (coma) can result. Alkalinisation therapy should begin if the blood pH is <7.2. The dose of sodium bicarbonate required is calculated from the formula:

$$\text{Dose (mmol)} = 0.3 \times \text{body weight (kg)} \times (24\text{-measured bicarbonate})$$

Half of this dose should be given by slow intravenous injection and the rest should be added to the fluids over the next 6–8h (rapid correction can lead to hypertonicity). Over-correction of metabolic acidosis with sodium bicarbonate can result in hypocalcaemia, hypokalaemia, a shift in the haemoglobin dissociation curve and volume overload of the extracellular fluid (see Chapter 2).

Many practices do not have the ability to assess the acid–base status of their critically ill patients in-house. Some clinical laboratories will offer total venous CO_2 on chemistry panels. In addition, this measurement can be made, in house, on 100 μl of venous blood using the Harleco micro CO_2 system (Lam & Tan 1978).

Fluid Therapy in Acute Renal Failure

Most patients with ARF of whatever cause will initially be suffering from a degree of dehydration which should be assessed from the history and on physical examination before fluid replacement therapy is administered.

- The fluid deficit should be rapidly replaced (over 6–8h) and fluids for maintenance should be added to the volume given, as should an estimate of ongoing losses.
- A potassium-free replacement fluid (0.9% sodium chloride) would be chosen in the first instance if the serum K^+ concentration is elevated.
- Monitor body weight and clinical state of hydration.
- Monitor PCV, total proteins, serum electrolytes, urea and creatinine.
- Monitor urine output (timed collection).
- Monitor central venous pressure (if you are concerned about overhydration).

Flow charts in the patient's record assist in accurately recording the response to fluid therapy and in deciding what adjustments should be made.

Should urine output be restored by fluid therapy to 2 ml/kg per hour or greater, fluid therapy should be continued to:

- correct any remaining dehydration,
- replace insensible and urinary losses (measured by urine collection).

Most animals will enter a polyuric phase following resumption of urine flow. Fluid therapy should keep up with insensible losses and urine output so that dehydration does not hinder the recovery of renal function. Addition of potassium to the fluids will be necessary as losses of potassium via the kidney will be heavy and anorexia usually persists. Hypokalaemia causes muscle weakness, anorexia and vomiting and retards the recovery of the renal concentrating mechanism. Potassium supplementation of the fluids may be necessary in the polyuric stage but should not exceed 0.5 mmol/kg per hour.

When supporting an animal in renal failure on intravenous fluids for several days, once rehydration has been fully accomplished, the concentration of sodium in the fluids should be reduced in the maintenance phase (0.45% NaCl and 2.5% dextrose with added potassium may prove suitable). These animals are incapable of excreting fluid and electrolyes supplied in excess of their requirements just as they are incapable of surviving fluid and electrolyte deficiencies by reducing losses through their kidneys. Thus, fluid and electrolyte balance requires close attention to detail to avoid over-hydration and overload with sodium, while at the same time preventing excessive losses of fluid leading to dehydration and subsequent deterioration in the animal's condition.

Fluid therapy should continue until the serum urea and creatinine levels return to normal or stabilise (remain the same for 3 consecutive days) at an elevated level and the animal is able to take water and food by mouth. Fluid therapy should never be stopped abruptly in an azotaemic patient. A gradual tapering of the daily fluid volume coupled with close monitoring will ensure the animal remains well hydrated. If the azotaemia worsens and the patient deteriorates, intravenous fluid therapy should be re-instituted. In some cases, subcutaneous rather than intravenous fluids may be used and administered at home by the owners. If the animal shows no clinical improvement and remains severely azotaemic despite intensive well controlled supportive fluid therapy, and dialysis is not considered an option, euthanasia should be considered after 5–7 days. Peritoneal dialysis will lessen the azotaemia and control the metabolic and electrolyte disturbances, allowing more time for healing of acute renal lesions to occur. Biopsy results are useful to help decide whether or not to undertake the considerable effort and expense involved in peritoneal dialysis.

Conversion of Oliguria to Non-Oliguria

If oliguria persists once rehydration has been accomplished, an attempt should be made to increase the urine volume (see Table 62.10).

Given that the animal has to be 5% dehydrated before the dehydration is clinically detectable, it is suggested that a fluid load which represents 3–5% of body weight should be administered to ensure full rehydration has been accomplished. Slight over-hydration may be preferable to ongoing dehydration (Polzin *et al.* 1989). If oliguria still persists once this volume of fluid has been administered, fluid therapy should be reduced until other measures have successfully increased urine output.

Diuretic therapy is used in the persistently oliguric patient in an attempt to promote urine output. The loop diuretic, frusemide, is commonly used alone or in combination with mannitol or dopamine. Mannitol has theoretical advantages over frusemide. Its osmotic properties may minimise renal tubular cell swelling and so improve renal function, it exerts its effects throughout the nephron and it may expand the extracellular fluid volume and inhibit renin secretion. Measures to enhance renal blood flow would seem logical in cases of renal ischaemia. Dopamine dilates renal arterioles by acting at specific dopamine (DA-1) receptors. In addition, dopamine receptors on proximal renal tubules inhibit absorption of sodium and therefore

water, increasing tubular fluid flow. Unlike other drugs which decrease renal vascular resistance, dopamine does not reduce peripheral vascular resistance or arterial blood pressure to any great extent, when given at low doses (see Table 62.10 for dose rates). Dopamine has effects on α- and β-adrenoceptors when administered at higher doses which may give rise to undesirable effects. If the urine flow does not increase in the first few hours, the infusion should be discontinued. Fenoldopam is a highly selective DA-1 agonist which lacks the adrenoceptor mediated side-effects of dopamine and which is active after oral administration (Brooks *et al.* 1990) and so shows great potential for the future. Oliguric renal failure that has not responded to mannitol or frusemide may respond to a combined infusion of dopamine and frusemide which are synergistic.

Peritoneal Dialysis

In patients that remain oliguric with severe intractable hyperkalaemia, metabolic acidosis and azotaemia, peritoneal dialysis should be considered, particularly for patients with primary intrinsic ARF with no pre-existing renal disease. The time demands of this procedure and the in-house monitoring and nursing care required are great often limiting its use to specialist centres. It is most effective when initiated before the onset of severe uraemic complica-

Table 62.10 Therapy of the oliguric acute renal failure patient.

Treatment	Dosage and route of administration	Comments
Fluid challenge (replacement fluid)	30–50 ml/kg i.v. at a rate of 6 ml/kg per hour	Closely monitor patient for signs of over-hydration (CVP)
Frusemide	2 mg/kg, i.v.; double or triple this dose can be given if no response is seen within 60 min	Can be combined with other diuretics. Very high doses can cause permanent deafness
Mannitol	0.25–0.5 g/kg i.v. over 3–5 min – should see a response in 20–30 min	Total daily dose of mannitol should not exceed 2 g/kg. If no response seen in 60 min, stop infusion
	Maintain with an infusion of 2–5 m/min of a 5–10% solution	Mannitol should not be used in animals which are already over- hydrated
Dopamine	2–5 µg/kg per minute as a continuous infusion (combine with frusemide at 1 mg/kg every hour)	Use an infusion pump (or a micro-giving set) to ensure accurate administration
	Dilute in 0.9% saline adding 30 mg per 500 ml (60 µg/ml)*	Monitor ECG for evidence of tachycardia or arrhythmias
	Stop if there is no improvement in 6 h	Dopamine and frusemide have been shown to be synergistic

* If the drug is administered using a micro-giving set with a biuret, which delivers 60 drops per ml, each drop contains 1 µg, making calculation of the infusion rate simple.

tions so the decision to use dialysis should be made as early as possible.

The principles of peritoneal dialysis are relatively simple:

- The peritoneal membrane is used as a dialysing membrane. Fluid of a carefully considered composition is instilled into the peritoneal cavity and left in place for a variable time (the dwell time).
- During the dwell time, equilibration of nitrogenous waste products, electrolytes and water occurs across the peritoneal membrane
- Fluid is drained from the peritoneal cavity, thus removing the waste products from the animal's body.
- The process is repeated continuously, replacing the peritoneal fluid that has been drained with a fresh batch of dialysate.

In addition to the management of oliguric primary intrinsic ARF, peritoneal dialysis may also be useful in the early treatment of some acute toxicities, to remove the toxin from the animal (e.g. ethylene glycol poisoning, barbiturate poisoning).

A detailed description of the practicalities of peritoneal dialysis is not appropriate for this text and the reader is referred to an excellent review and a retrospective study (Crisp *et al.* 1989; Chew *et al.* 1992). There is little point initiating dialysis in patients with moderate azotaemia (urea 15–30 mmol/l, creatinine 300–500 μmol/l) unless a rapid deterioration is expected. These levels of azotaemia are the expected levels which can be maintained in an anuric animal on peritoneal dialysis until recovery of renal function occurs (Chew *et al.* 1992).

Management of Vomiting in ARF Patients

Frequent vomiting is often a problem in ARF patients which adds to fluid losses and patient discomfort. Vomiting may be due to central effects of uraemic toxins and to gastric ulceration. Intravenous fluid therapy, if successful, should reduce the levels of uraemia and hence the central stimulation of the chemoreceptor trigger zone. Nevertheless, additional treatment may be necessary. Hypergastrinaemia contributes to gastric hyperacidity and ulceration of uraemia. Gastrointestinal ulceration may prove a significant source of blood loss in ARF patients, particularly as blood vessel fragility increases and platelet function is reduced in uraemia. Blockade of gastric histamine receptors by H_2-receptor antagonists such as cimetidine or ranitidine reduces the severity and frequency of vomiting in ARF patients (Chew 1990). Other potentially useful anti-emetics are presented in Table 62.11.

No controlled clinical studies have been undertaken to identify the most effective and safest anti-emetic in ARF patients. A logical approach is to use an H_2 antagonist initially and to add metoclopramide if control is not achieved by the H_2 antagonist alone.

Table 62.11   Anti-emetic therapy for acute renal failure patients.

Drug treatment	Comments
H_2 antagonists 　Cimetidine 5 mg/kg i.v. b.i.d 　Ranitidine 2 mg/kg i.v. s.i.d. or b.i.d.	Note reduced dosing frequency in renal failure. CNS toxicity has been reported in human patients with renal disease
Ulcer healing agents 　Sucralfate 1 g to large dogs, 0.5 g to small dogs (all given p.o. t.i.d.)	If given with H_2 blockers should be administered 30 min before these drugs. Can enhance the absorption of aluminium salts – potential for aluminium toxicity
Anti-emetics 　Metoclopramide 0.2–0.4 mg/kg t.i.d or q.i.d. by s.c. injection or 1–2 mg/kg per day added to i.v. fluids if vomiting is intractable	Metoclopramide is a dopamine receptor antagonist so should not be combined with dopamine infusions
Phenothiazines (Chlorpromazine 0.5 mg/kg up to four times daily (i.m.))	Phenothiazines are α-adrenoceptor antagonists and will potentiate hypotension in dehydrated patients. They are also dopamine receptor antagonists and should not be combined with dopamine infusions.

Nutrition of the ARF Patient

Catabolism of the tissues will inevitably occur in a sick anorexic animal, to provide the energy required for basic cellular functions and for repair of damaged tissues. Breakdown of tissue stores will produce nitrogenous waste products, release potassium, hydrogen and phosphate ions and so contribute to the load with which the damaged kidneys have to cope. Thus, provision of nutritional support is indicated for any patient with protracted ARF. Sufficient non-protein calories should be provided so that dietary protein is not broken down to provide energy. Protein should be of high quality but limited quantity. Ideally, if vomiting is controlled, feeding can be achieved via the enteral route using a nasogastric tube and feeding a liquidised commercially available clinical diet, until the animal will take food by mouth. Frequent small meals should be administered in this way. Parenteral nutrition is complicated in ARF patients because of their susceptibility to over-hydration. Calories should be supplied by the infusion of 20–25% dextrose (administered via a jugular catheter). The exact nutritional requirements for dogs in ARF have not been studied. Basal energy expenditure (BEE) can be calculated from the formula:

$$BEE = (30 \times \text{weight in kg}) + 70 \text{ kcal/day}$$
$$(\text{for patients weighing} > 2 \text{ kg})$$

Energy requirements during illness increase by 1.5- to 2-fold (see Lippert & Buffington 1992). A solution of 25% dextrose provides 0.85 kcal/ml. For parenteral nutritional support 0.3 g/kg per day of a balanced amino acid solution has been recommended in addition to dextrose (Finco & Barsanti 1983).

Specific Therapy for Primary Intrinsic ARF

In many cases of primary intrinsic ARF, the initiating cause is unknown. If diagnostic tests do suggest the initiating cause once the animal is showing clinical signs of ARF it may be too late to administer specific therapy, which would have been appropriate in the initiating stages. For example, dimercaprol, a chelator of heavy metals, is indicated in the early stages of arsenic poisoning. The dimercaprol–arsenic complexes formed are excreted via the kidneys and so this treatment is of no use once ARF has become established.

If, at the time of presentation, nephrotoxins are present in high concentrations, peritoneal dialysis should be considered to remove them rapidly and prevent further damage. This approach would be applicable for a case of ethylene glycol poisoning that had been diagnosed early.

Ethylene glycol produces its nephrotoxic effects following its metabolism to glyoxalate and oxalate (Grauer & Thrall 1986). The first step in its metabolism is catalysed by the liver enzyme, alcohol dehydrogenase. Strategies to prevent ethylene glycol metabolism can be employed if the condition is recognised and diagnosed early (within 6–12 h of ingestion). Competitive inhibition of metabolism can be achieved by the administration of ethanol. Alternatively, potent inhibition of alcohol dehydrogenase can be accomplished using 4-methylpyrazole (free base obtained from Aldrich Chemical Company, dissolved in sterile water to form a 5% solution and filtered with a 0.22 μm filter before use). This drug has been shown to be effective in the management of ethylene glycol poisoning in the dog (Dial *et al.* 1989). Treatment protocols are presented in Table 62.12.

CHRONIC RENAL FAILURE (CRF)

By definition, patients with CRF have been azotaemic for more than 2 weeks and may well, over time, start to show other features of the uraemic syndrome described above. The clinical and laboratory features which allow a distinction to be made between animals with ARF and acute exacerbations of CRF have been dealt with (see pages 635–636). Dogs with CRF do not always present in an acute metabolic crisis. The clinical features which may characterise uraemia are summarised in Table 62.13 and the most common historical and physical problems which should suggest CRF as a possible diagnosis are:

Table 62.12 Treatment protocols for the management of ethylene glycol toxicity.

Ethanol – 5.5 ml of 20% ethanol per kg administered i.v. every 4 h for five treatments and then every 6 h for five more treatments

Many animals will become comatosed. Ethanol enhances diuresis and so increases fluid requirements

4-methylpyrazole – 20 mg/kg of a 5% solution given i.v. initially, followed by 15 mg/kg at 12 and 24 h, and 5 mg/kg 36 h after presentation

No toxic effects have been seen in the dog. 4-methylpyrazole does not contribute to CNS or renal concentrating disorders (unlike ethanol)

Table 62.13 A problem-specific database for small
animal patients suspected of being uraemic.

Screening tests
  History
  Physical examination (including retinal examination)
  Urine analysis
  Serum chemistry profile
  Routine haematological examination
  Abdominal radiographs
  Arterial blood pressure measurement

*Additional tests that may be indicated, depending on the
     results of screening tests*
  Urine bacterial or fungal culture
  Abdominal ultrasonographic examination
  Excretory urography
  Chest radiographs
  Renal biopsy
  Screen for various infectious agents: *Leptospira* spp.
  Urine protein : urine creatinine ratio
  Serum parathyroid hormone and ionised calcium
  Endogenous creatinine clearance or other means of
     measuring glomerular filtration rate

- polyuria/polydipsia;
- weight loss/failure to thrive (loss of muscle mass), poor hair coat;
- anorexia with vomiting (usually on an empty stomach and sometimes containing changed blood);
- weakness, lethargy and depression;
- pallor and dryness of mucous membranes, oral ulceration.

These problems tend to progressively worsen over a period of weeks. As the signs are non-specific, each with a number of possible diagnoses, a minimum database should be collected for each patient where uraemia is suspected. This is summarised in Table 62.13.

Age, Breed and Sex

Although male and female dogs of all ages and breeds may develop uraemia, consideration of the age, breed and sex of a uraemic patient can be instructive when attempting to determine the underlying cause of the problem. Certain canine breeds are prone to inherited, familial nephropathies, which can cause proteinuria or uraemia, or both (Davenport *et al.* 1986; see Table 62.14 for examples). In most familial nephropathies, the kidneys are thought to

be normal at birth, with progressive deterioration in structure and function over the first months to years of life. Thus patients with familial nephropathy tend to be relatively young when renal failure and uraemia ensue (although this is not always the case). In contrast, patients with uraemia caused by various degenerative and neoplastic renal disorders tend to be middle-aged or older.

Laboratory Evaluation

The history and physical examination may provide presumptive evidence that uraemia is present. Further diagnostic tests are required to confirm the presence of uraemia, determine its severity, and discover its underlying cause. In patients suspected of being uraemic, it is particularly important to obtain samples of blood and urine before the initiation of fluid therapy. Samples obtained later will not accurately reflect the urine concentrating ability or the degree of azotaemia.

Urinalysis

The use of urine concentration in animals that are azotaemic in distinguishing between prerenal azotaemia and intrinsic primary renal failure is discussed above (see Table 62.6). Apart from the essential SG measurement, a full urinalysis is recommended for patients suspected to be uraemic. Urine dipstick and sediment examination may reveal a cause of uraemia. Evidence of bacteria or unexplained high numbers of white cells in the sediment would be indications for urine culture. Casts (cylindrical moulds of renal tubular lumina) generally suggest an active cause of renal damage.

Serum Biochemistry Profile

When the serum chemistry profile results become available, the most important parameters to evaluate and the interpretation of abnormal findings are presented in Table 62.15.

Routine Haematology

CRF is frequently associated with a moderately severe, normocytic, normochromic, non-regenerative anaemia (King *et al.* 1992). The anaemia of CRF is primarily due to failure of red blood cell production and may take weeks to months to develop. Although the packed cell volume (PCV) of a patient with chronic uraemia may be normal at the time

Table 62.14 Some breeds affected by familial nephropathies.

Breed	Nature of the nephropathy*
Basenji	Fanconi syndrome. Usually presented at 1–5 years of age for PU/PD. May be seen with glucosuria and aminoaciduria before azotaemia develops. May develop acute renal failure or pyelonephritis
Beagle	Unilateral renal agenesis. Predisposes to the development of uraemia, if function of the solitary kidney is compromised
Bull Terrier	(1) Polycystic kidney disease associated with valvular heart disease. May present with haematuria and recurrent UTIs, rather than uraemia, at 6–15 months of age. Alternatively, may present with cardiac disease and renal lesions found incidentally. (2) Progressive nephropathy, possibly inherited by an autosomal dominant gene. Variable rate of progression – usually present with signs of uraemia between 1 and 5 years of age
Cairn Terrier	Congenital polycystic renal and hepatic disease. Usually presented at about 6 weeks of age for abdominal distension due to hepatomegaly and renomegaly, rather than for uraemia
Chinese Shar-Pei	Renal amyloidosis. Usually presented for signs of renal failure or uraemia. Renal medulla and sometimes glomeruli are infiltrated
Cocker Spaniel	Progressive nephropathy. Usually presented at 6 months to 2 years of age for signs of uraemia. Proteinuria of glomerular origin is an early feature of the disease
Doberman Pinscher	Probably a form of familial glomerulonephritis. Usually are presented at 1–2 years of age for signs of uraemia. May also manifest signs of nephrotic syndrome due to proteinuria
Lhasa Apso and Shih Tzu	Progressive nephropathy. Usually presented at about 1–2 years of age for signs of early renal failure or uraemia. Rate of progression of disease is very variable
Norwegian Elkhound	Glomerulopathy with interstitial fibrosis. Usually are presented at 8 months to 5 years of age for signs of uraemia. May be glucosuric, despite normal blood glucose concentration
Samoyed	Progressive nephropathy. More common and more severe in males than females. Males are usually presented for signs of uraemia at less than 1 year of age; females for mild renal failure at about 5 years. Proteinuria occurs early in this disease due to glomerular pathology
Soft Coated Wheaten Terrier	Disorder of renal maturation with thin cortices and cortical cysts. Usually presented at 5–30 months for signs of renal failure. Some may be presented for signs of protein losing nephropathy and nephrotic syndrome, without uraemia
Standard Poodle	Cystic glomerular atrophy with immature glomeruli and tubular dilation/atrophy. Presented at 3 months to 2 years of age for signs of renal failure. Significant proteinuria is usually found

* For more details concerning these disorders, see Davenport *et al.* 1986.
PU/PD, polyuria/polydipsia; PLN, protein-losing nephropathy; UTI, urinary tract infection.

of initial presentation, it frequently declines into the low range after correction of any dehydration. Assessment of the total plasma protein (TPP) at the same time as the PCV will allow early recognition of anaemia in dehydrated patients. The lymphopenia and mild neutrophilia seen in some uraemic patients are not useful in discriminating different causes of uraemia. Moderate to severe neutrophilia may indicate an upper urinary tract infection or urosepsis.

Table 62.15   Important serum chemistry parameters to assess in chronic renal failure patients.

Parameter	Comments/Interpretation
Creatinine	Rate of excretion depends on GFR (produced at a constant daily rate). In CRF, tubular secretion of creatinine may occur in male dogs. Cachectic animals produce less creatinine per day due to reduced muscle mass. More accurate clinical chemistry indicator of GFR than urea but nevertheless, GFR has to fall by 75% before rise in plasma creatinine is detectable
Urea	Produced by the liver from ammonia and excreted by the kidney, roughly in proportion to GFR. Factors other than renal function affect blood urea: Increased: • after high protein meals • after gastrointestinal haemorrhage • in dehydrated patients (reabsorbed by the tubules) Decreased: • in liver failure • after prolonged fasting. Urea is less reliable than creatinine as an indicator of renal function
Phosphate	Hyperphosphataemia can be a feature of all forms of azotaemia
Potassium	Hyperkalaemia is a feature of oliguric ARF but can occur in the terminal phases of end stage CRF. Hypokalaemia is present in some CRF patients and may reduce renal function further
Calcium	A serum total calcium concentration over 3.3 mmol/l in a uraemic patient warrants further investigation, (hypercalcaemia can be the cause, rather than a consequence of renal failure)

GFR, glomerular filtration rate; CRF, chronic renal failure; ARF, acute renal failure.

Imaging Studies

Abdominal radiography and/or abdominal ultrasonography is indicated in the investigation of all patients suspected of being uraemic. Important findings have been covered in Table 62.7. Radiographs of the abdomen should be scrutinised for the presence of radio-opaque urinary calculi. Cystic calculi are not usually associated with uraemia in dogs, but bilateral ureteral calculi occasionally cause hydroureter, urinary outflow obstruction and postrenal azotaemia. Renal calculi may be associated with pyelonephritis. Radiolucent urinary calculi can be imaged by ultrasound or positive contrast excretory urography.

Screening for Infectious Diseases

Several serovars of *Leptospira interrogans* have recently been implicated as the cause of subacute renal failure in dogs (Rentko *et al.* 1992). Affected patients had no icterus, or other evidence of hepatic involvement. Glucosuria occurred in more than half of the dogs, sug-

gesting renal tubular damage. Leptospirosis should be considered in the differential diagnosis of all canine patients with acute and subacute renal failure. Appropriate precautions should be taken in handling the urine from these animals. Serological testing and dark field microscopic examination of urine samples are indicated. However negative dark field microscopic findings do not rule out leptospirosis.

Glomerulonephritis

Glomerulonephritis is covered in detail in Chapter 65 on proteinuria but for completeness it is important to introduce it within this section on chronic renal failure. Glomerular inflammation causes two important clinical syndromes in dogs. First, by causing glomerular injury, glomerulonephritis can lead to progressive losses of GFR that can lead to chronic renal failure, thereby producing azotaemia and/or uraemia. Second, marked proteinuria can result in hypoalbuminaemia and, if severe, oedema and/or ascites. This latter constellation of abnormalities is referred to as the nephrotic syndrome.

Management of CRF

CRF is associated with irreversible, usually progressive renal damage, so the prognosis for improvement of renal function is poor. Despite this, medical management of CRF can substantially reduce the severity of uraemia and improve length and quality of life. There is often a substantial prerenal component to the azotaemia in newly-presented CRF patients, so rehydration may help. CRF reduces the ability to excrete salt and water loads and over-zealous fluid therapy in an attempt to reduce the azotaemia may cause complications (e.g. exacerbate hypertension). Identification and treatment of any complicating factors (such as urinary tract infection) is important and will improve the long-term prognosis. Recent advances in therapy of CRF have occurred in the following areas:

- progression of chronic renal disease,
- systemic arterial hypertension,
- renal secondary hyperparathyroidism,
- modification of dietary intake,
- anaemia of chronic renal disease.

In animals with CRF, the overall aims of therapy are to:

- enhance the quality of life by reducing the prevalence and severity of associated complications,
- extend the duration of life by reducing mortality from complications and preventing the progression of renal disease.

Progressive Renal Dysfunction

Pathophysiology and Treatment Goals

Dogs with CRF frequently exhibit progressive loss of renal function that is characterised by progressive decrements of GFR. This has at least two important consequences:

(1) The disease is inherently unstable and frequent re-evaluations and adjustments in therapy are required.
(2) Efforts designed to slow the rate of progression of renal disease are particularly important in veterinary medicine (dialysis and transplantation are not true practical options).

Not all animals exhibit evidence of progressive decrements of renal function over time. In some animals with experimentally-induced chronic renal disease, renal function is stable for a prolonged period of time (Brown *et al.* 1991a & b). In others, renal function (GFR) actually increases for months to years following the diagnosis of renal failure. This is particularly common in animals that

Table 62.16 Possible causes of progressive renal disease in dogs.

Primary renal disease
  Tubulointerstitial disease (e.g. pyelonephritis)
  Glomerular disease (e.g. hereditary glomerulopathy)
  Vascular disease (e.g. systemic hypertension)

Altered homeostasis
  Hyperphosphataemia
  Hyperparathyroidism
  Hyperlipidaemia
  Systemic hypertension
  Metabolic acidosis

Adaptive changes in nephron structure and function
  Glomerular hyperfiltration
  Glomerular hypertension
  Glomerular hypertrophy

survive ARF. The causes of progression of renal disease in dogs are incompletely understood (see Table 62.16).

Progressive decrements of GFR may result from the primary disease process which has not been controlled. For example, an animal with an inflammatory glomerular disease may suffer decrements of GFR over time as a result of continued glomerular injury. However, many animals suffering from progressive decrements of renal function do not exhibit an apparent cause of progression. In these animals, the disruption of homeostasis which results from CRF or the adaptive response of the kidney to injury may perpetuate renal injury (see Table 62.16). Experimental models of CRF using inbred strains of rats (Hostetter *et al.* 1981; Brenner *et al.* 1982) have been used to extrapolate to the clinical management of dogs. It is likely that a genetically heterogeneous set of dogs will respond to CRF in a somewhat different manner and recommendations based on information obtained from canine studies should be more reliable.

Management of Progressive Renal Dysfunction

If a primary disease which is damaging the kidneys can be identified, this should be treated. If a dog with CRF suffers from progressive renal dysfunction that cannot be attributed to a primary renal disease, careful evaluation of the patient for possible causes of progression is in order (see Table 62.17).

Generally the screening tests detailed in Table 62.13 are indicated. Other diagnostic tests of utility are listed in

Table 62.17 Management of a patient with progressive renal disease.

Abnormality	Diagnostic tests	Management therapy
Hyperphosphataemia	Plasma phosphate concentration	Dietary phosphate restriction and or intestinal phosphate binders
Hyperparathyroidism	Plasma PTH concentration (Fractional excretion of phosphate if PTH unavailable)	Dietary phosphate restriction and/or intestinal phosphate binders and/or oral calcitriol therapy
Hyperlipidaemia	Plasma cholesterol concentration	Low fat and or dietary omega-3 fatty acid supplementation
Systemic hypertension	Blood pressure determination	Antihypertensive therapy
Metabolic acidosis	Plasma bicarbonate concentration	Dietary alkalinisation
Glomerular hypertension	No clinical test available	ACE inhibition and/or dietary protein restriction
Glomerular hypertrophy	Renal biopsy	ACE inhibition and/or dietary protein restriction

ACE, angiotensin-converting enzyme; PTH, parathyroid hormone.

Table 62.17 together with possible therapies. Management of systemic and glomerular hypertension, hyperparathyroidism and anaemia will be discussed in detail below.

Monitoring Success of Therapy for Progressive Renal Dysfunction

- Progressive renal dysfunction is generally monitored by sequential measurement of plasma creatinine concentration.
- Plasma urea concentration has considerably less utility in dogs with CRF, in which changes in dietary protein intake are frequent (see Table 62.15).
- In some animals, the increase in plasma creatinine concentration is not linear with time, making it difficult to discern modest changes in the rate of progression of chronic renal disease.
- Changes in muscle mass and the amount of creatinine secreted by the functioning nephrons may confound the use of sequential measurements of plasma creatinine concentration to assess GFR (see Table 62.15).

Systemic and Glomerular Hypertension

Pathophysiology and Treatment Goals

Frequently, dogs with CRF exhibit elevations of systemic arterial pressure (Cowgill & Kallet 1983; Ross 1989). Renal failure can cause alterations in body fluid and electrolyte balance, leading to systemic hypertension. Alternatively, systemic hypertension can lead to renal injury in rats (Bidani *et al.* 1990; Bidani *et al.* 1987). Studies to determine the importance of systemic hypertension in the progression of renal disease in dogs have yet to be reported. Glomerular hypertension, hypertrophy and hyperfiltration are thought to be maladaptive changes which do occur in dog models of CRF where renal mass has been reduced (Brown *et al.* 1990).

Management of Systemic Hypertension

Antihypertensive therapy should be instituted only if systemic blood pressure can be reliably measured. The oscillometric and Doppler ultrasound methods can be employed to assess blood pressure but their reliable use requires considerable attention to detail. Blood pressure measurement generally requires handling of the animal by unfamiliar personnel in a strange environment, conditions which are likely to activate the sympathetic nervous system and elevate blood pressure. It has been suggested that results obtained in dogs with heart rates >90 beats per minute be considered unreliable (Bovee *et al.* 1993). If an animal with progressive renal disease shows complications of systemic hypertension (e.g. hypertensive retinopathy, unexplained epistaxis or seizures, left ventricular hypertrophy), then antihypertensive therapy is indicated. If no clear evidence of hypertensive end-organ damage is present only marked systemic hypertension (systolic arterial pressure

Table 62.18 Antihypertensive therapy in chronic renal failure.

Class of agent	Dose rate	Comments
Reduced sodium diet	<0.3% sodium on dry matter basis*	Considered the first stage of antihypertensive therapy. May lower blood pressure through contraction of extracellular fluid volume. Animals with renal dysfunction adapt slowly to changes in sodium intake – dietary adjustments should be made gradually, over 10–14 days.
Diuretics chlorothiazide hydrochlorothiazide frusemide	 20–40 mg/kg every 12–24 h 2–4 mg/kg every 12–24 h 2–4 mg/kg every 12–24 h	Further reduce extracellular fluid volume. Not used routinely in CRF because: • Overzealous use of either dietary sodium restriction or diuretic therapy in an animal with renal failure may lead to a vicious circle of dehydration, declining renal function and reduced fluid intake. • Animals with CRF and systemic hypertension are refractory to diuretic therapy.
β-adrenoceptor antagonists propranolol atenolol	 5–20 mg every 8–12 h* 2 mg/kg every 24 h†	Lower blood pressure mainly through their ability to reduce cardiac output. However, in CRF, the reduction of pressure within the glomerulus may be more important than lowering systemic arterial pressure. The effects of β-adrenoceptor inhibitors on glomerular pressure in dogs have not been examined.
Vasodilators ACE inhibitors captopril enalapril lisinopril benazepril	 0.5–2.0 mg/kg every 8–12 h‡ 0.5–1.0 mg/kg every 12–24 h§ 0.4–2.0 mg/kg every 24 h† 0.5 mg/kg every 24 h	Lower systemic blood pressure by reducing the generation of angiotensin II (vasoconstrictor agent) Chronic administration of an ACE inhibitor preferentially lowers intraglomerular pressure and thus, appears to be appropriate therapy for dogs with CRF
α-antagonists prazosin	 0.25–2.0 mg/kg every 8–12 h*	May produce systemic hypotension upon initial administration – hospitalise for observation during the initial 1–2 days of therapy.
calcium antagonists verapamil diltiazem dihydropyridine type: nifedipine amlodipine	 0.5–1.0 mg/kg every 8 h* 0.5–1.25 mg/kg every 8 h Not determined Not determined	Have little effect on intraglomerular pressure in experimental models of glomerular hypertension (led to enhanced renal injury). Until further information is available in dogs with CRF, use cautiously and only when necessary to control markedly hypertensive animals.

* Cowgill 1986.
† Littman 1992.
‡ Ross & Labato 1989.
§ DeLellis & Kittleson 1992.
ACE, angiotensin-converting enzyme.

>200 mmHg, mean arterial pressure >140 mmHg, and/or diastolic pressure >110 mmHg) justifies therapy. A variety of anti-hypertensive agents can be considered in dogs with progressive, chronic renal disease (see Table 62.18).

Unfortunately, little objective information regarding efficacy is available, making it difficult to offer recommendations. In all patients, assessment of the efficacy of anti-hypertensive therapy should be based upon measurements of blood pressure. If an antihypertensive agent is ineffective after 2–4 weeks of use, dosage can be increased or a new class of antihypertensive agent employed. In some cases, combination therapy is appropriate (e.g. diuretic plus adrenergic inhibitor or ACE inhibitor plus calcium channel antagonist).

Management of Glomerular Hypertension

ACE inhibitors have been shown to limit glomerular capillary hypertension and hypertrophy in an experimental model of diabetic nephropathy in dogs (Brown *et al.* 1993). Efforts to lower glomerular hypertension might prove beneficial in dogs with CRF and trial therapy with an ACE inhibitor could be considered. At the present time however, we do not know if the beneficial effects of antihypertensive therapy outweigh the potential risks in patients where there is no evidence of systemic hypertension. In addition it should be emphasised that a reduction in glomerular pressure would be expected to lower GFR, perhaps exacerbating the extent of azotaemia. If antihypertensive therapy is used to lower glomerular pressure, care should be taken to avoid systemic hypotension by measuring systemic arterial blood pressure (ABP) at regular intervals (every 2 weeks initially).

Renal Secondary Hyperparathyroidism

Pathophysiology and Treatment Goals

Animals with CRF frequently exhibit renal secondary hyperparathyroidism. This is generally attributed to phosphate retention and/or inadequate renal conversion of 25-hydroxycholecalciferol to 1,25-dihydroxycholecalciferol (calcitriol), the activated form of vitamin D.

Renal secondary hyperparathyroidism has a variety of effects on the animal. An important consideration is the deleterious effects of excess parathyroid hormone (PTH) secretion on bone metabolism, termed renal osteodystrophy. This may result in bone pain or severe osteomalacia ('rubber jaw'). However, the former is not commonly appreciated in dogs with renal disease and the latter is an uncommon complication of severe, long-standing renal

Table 62.19 Possible effects of renal secondary hyperparathyroidism.

(1) Progression of renal disease
(2) Uraemic complications:
  ● Metabolic
     glucose intolerance
     hyperlipidaemia
  ● Haematolgical
     non-regenerative anaemia
     immunosuppression
  ● Musculoskeletal
     osteodystrophy
     arthritis
     myopathy
  ● Cutaneous
     ulceration
     calcification
     pruritis
  ● Other
     pancreatitis
     encephalopathy
     cardiomyopathy
     soft-tissue calcification

failure. Recently, studies have implicated PTH in a wide variety of manifestations of the uraemic syndrome, such as the anaemia of renal failure and uraemic encephalopathy (see Table 62.19; Massry 1989; Brown & Finco 1994).

Thus the two principal arguments for the suppression of renal secondary hyperparathyroidism are to reduce uraemic signs and to slow the progression of renal failure. The importance of PTH as a uraemic toxin or as a cause of progressive renal failure is, however, controversial.

Management of Renal Secondary Hyperparathyroidism

Any approach to therapeutic management must include a careful documentation of the animal's problems. A staged approach is appropriate to this problem in all azotaemic animals.

(1) In hyperphosphataemic animals attempt to reduce plasma phosphate into the normal range:
  ● Feed a low phosphate diet (<0.5% phosphate on a dry matter basis).
  ● If still hyperphosphataemic after 2–4 weeks mix intestinal phosphate binders with diet.

- Start at 60 mg/kg per day for 2–4 weeks, increase sequentially to 100–150 mg/kg per day.
- Use aluminium rather than calcium salts if calcitriol therapy is to be given.

(2) If normophosphataemic (or phosphate restriction has resulted in a stable plasma phosphate):
- Measure plasma PTH concentration by an intact molecule or N-terminal assay.
- If plasma PTH concentration is elevated, consider starting calcitriol therapy, particularly if the animal has signs attributable to high PTH or CRF is progressing (see Table 62.19).
- Check plasma calcium concentration – calcitriol should not be given if plasma ionised calcium is high.
- Administer calcitriol at an initial dose of 1.5–3.5 ng/kg per day (Chew & Nagode 1992) or 6.6 ng/kg per day (Brown & Finco 1994) given separately from food.
- Measure plasma phosphate and calcium every 2 weeks and PTH after 4–6 weeks.
- If no reduction in PTH, continue dosing for 4–6 weeks and reassess. If still no effect, stop dosing unless ionised calcium can be measured when dose can be increased to a maximum of 10 ng/kg per day (assess ionised calcium twice weekly on this dose).
- If calcitriol lowers PTH, continue therapy long term only if a benefit of reducing PTH has been detected.
  NB Calcitriol is an experimental therapy and owners should be appraised of this fact.

Monitoring Success of Therapy for Renal Secondary Hyperparathyroidism

The success of therapy for renal secondary hyperparathyroidism should be judged by the effect of therapy on the uraemic complications and/or the progression of CRF and it is these complications which ultimately should be monitored in each patient. To ensure the therapy has any chance of achieving success, it is necessary to document control of PTH secretion by assay of plasma PTH concentration sequentially. Achievement of such control does not, however, guarantee benefit to the patient in all cases.

Dietary Therapy

Pathophysiology and Treatment Goals

A wide variety of recommendations have been made for dietary therapy in animals with CRF. These have generally been to modify or control dietary intake of energy, phosphate, protein, or fat. The rationale for these dietary modifications is based upon two potential benefits:

- reduce clinical signs (i.e. control uraemia),
- slow the progression of renal failure.

Dietary therapy for animals with CRF should be individualised as no two animals will respond identically to a dietary intervention. In addition, little is known about the effects of renal failure on dietary requirements of animals. For these and other reasons, an approach to dietary management of renal failure that relies solely on the use of a special commercial diet is flawed. Adjustments will be required in all animals and should be made on the basis of serial evaluations of the patient.

Dietary Modification in Uraemic Animals

Some animals exhibit clinical signs that may be attributable to the effects of uraemic toxins. In these animals, modification of dietary intake attempts to modify the extent and severity of these abnormalities as indicated in Table 62.20.

Animals with CRF frequently exhibit weight loss and other signs of malnutrition, due to inadequate intake of calories. Some dogs will find special diets unpalatable. If a pet ingests less of a reduced protein diet, then malnutrition will ensue. To generate required energy, body protein stores will be catabolised, resulting in the counterproductive liberation of nitrogenous wastes with consequent enhanced production of uraemic toxins. Consequently, a variety of modified protein diets should be offered to a uraemic pet to determine if one particular product is appealing to it.

Dietary Modification in Non-Uraemic Animals

The rationale for the use of dietary modification in animals that are not suffering from clinical abnormalities of uraemia is to slow the progression of renal failure, either by modifying the homeostatic consequences of CRF or by preventing maladaptive changes of surviving nephrons (glomerular hyperfiltration, hypertension and hypertrophy). Little is known about the mechanisms of progression of renal disease in dogs. Experimental studies have suggested that dietary phosphate restriction reduces morphological or functional progression of renal disease in dogs (Brown *et al.* 1991a; Finco *et al.* 1992a & b). However, dietary protein restriction is of uncertain benefit in dogs with early renal disease (Polzin *et al.* 1984; Robertson *et al.* 1986; Finco *et al.* 1992b) where the degree of azotaemia is

Table 62.20 Dietary modification of the uraemic chronic renal failure patient.

Dietary modification	Beneficial effects	Guidelines
Dietary phosphate restriction	Slows the rate of progression of renal failure. Reduces renal secondary hyperparathyroidism	See section on management of renal secondary hyperparathyroidism
Dietary protein restriction	Limits the extent of azotaemia and the toxic effects of nonprotein nitrogen compounds. Slows rate of progression of renal disease (controversial)	Level of protein restriction employed to limit the extent of uraemia should be adjusted depending upon the clinical response. Initial dietary protein level of about 20% (dry matter) might be used (diets as low as 9% protein on a dry matter basis are available)
Dietary alkalinisation	Controls metabolic acidosis	Sodium bicarbonate, potassium citrate, or calcium carbonate will effectively control acidosis at a dose of 1–3 mEq of base/kg per day (3–9 mEq/kg per day are required if a renal tubular acidification defect exists)

not leading to clinical signs. Clearly, dietary protein restriction does not prevent glomerular hypertension or hypertrophy in dogs following marked reduction in renal mass (Brown *et al.* 1991b).

Monitoring Success of Dietary Therapy

The appropriate method for monitoring therapy depends upon the rationale for dietary modification. Accordingly, clinical signs, biochemical changes, and/or rate of change of GFR (i.e. plasma creatinine concentration) should be carefully monitored.

Anaemia of Renal Failure

Pathophysiology and Treatment Goals

Many animals with CRF exhibit a normocytic normochromic non-regenerative anaemia which has been attributed to two general causes:

- a lack of erythropoietin production,
- depressing effects of the uraemic environment on red cell production and life span.

A relative or absolute lack or erythropoietin (EPO) is an important causative factor in the anaemia of CRF in dogs (King *et al.* 1992). Recently, the use of recombinant EPO therapy has made it possible to restore a normal haematocrit in many animals with CRF. In so doing, it has become

apparent that some of the clinical signs present in these animals, such as lethargy and inappetance, are attributable to the effects of anaemia. These clinical abnormalities will wholly or partially resolve upon improvement of the patient's haematocrit (Cowgill 1992; King *et al.* 1992).

Management of the Anaemia of Renal Failure

Although relative or absolute lack of EPO is primarily responsible for most cases of anaemia present in animals with CRF, one should rule out other possible factors:

- blood loss (e.g. hookworm or flea infestation, haematuria),
- nutritional imbalances associated with renal failure may limit erythropoietic potential.

These abnormalities should be corrected, where possible. Approximately 50% of dogs with anaemia of CRF exhibit laboratory evidence of iron deficiency (i.e. reduced serum iron concentration of reduced transferrin saturation; Cowgill 1992). These animals should receive iron supplementation.

Therapy with Human Recombinant EPO (r-HuEPO)

This product is available in the United Kingom on prescription from a pharmacist. The following are published guidelines (Cowgill 1992):

- Reserve r-HuEPO for animals with a haematocrit of <20%.
- Give an initial dosage of 50–100 U/kg per day injected subcutaneously three times weekly.
- A noticeable increase in haematocrit should be seen within 5–10 days often accompanied by an increase in appetite and activity.
- Check haematocrit twice weekly and adjust dose accordingly to avoid life-threatening polycythaemia – aim for a haematocrit just below normal (individual variation occurs in dose required).
- If animal is refractory to r-HuEPO from the start of treatment – suspect iron deficiency.
- If patient responds and then becomes refractory – often due to anti-r-HuEPO antibody formation which is usually reversible when r-HuEPO therapy is discontinued.
- Uncommon, potential adverse effects of r-HuEPO include vomiting, skin reactions, seizures, systemic hypertension, arthralgia, mucocutaneous reactions, and fever.
- Iron supplementation (100–300 mg $FeSO_4$/day) if required.

Because many animals eventually develop antibodies and become refractory to r-HuEPO therapy, it is unwise to initiate therapy too early in an individual animal with evidence of progressive renal failure and anaemia.

Alternative Management Options for the Anaemia of Renal Failure

Other treatments, such as androgenic steroid therapy or calcitriol to suppress PTH secretion, can be considered in the anaemic patient. However, these manoeuvres can generally be expected to produce only a small increment in haematocrit.

REFERENCES

Bidani, A.K., Schwartz, M.M. & Lewis, E.J. (1987). Renal autoregulation and vulnerability to hypertensive injury in remnant kidney. *American Journal of Physiology*, **252**, F1003–F1110.

Bidani, A., Mitchell, K., Schwartz, M.M., Navar, L.G. & Lewis, E.J. (1990). Absence of glomerular injury or nephron loss in a normotensive rat remnant kidney model. *Kidney International*, **38**, 28–38.

Bovee, K.C., Buranakari, C. & Watanabe, T. (1993). Comparison of direct arterial blood pressure between repeated short interval measurements and continuous 24-hour recording in genetically hypertensive dogs. *Proceedings, 11th Annual Meeting of the American College of Veterinary Internal Medicine*, Washington. p. 936. ACVIM, Blacksberg, Virginia.

Brenner, B.M., Meyer, T.W. & Hostetter, T.H. (1982). Dietary protein intake and the progressive nature of renal disease: The role of hemodynamically mediated glomerular injury in the pathogenesis of progressive glomerular sclerosis in aging, renal ablation, and intrinsic renal disease. *New England Journal of Medicine*, **307**, 652–659.

Brooks, D.P., Depalma, P.D. & Cyronak, M.J. (1990). Identification of fenoldopam prodrugs with prolonged renal vasodilator activity. *Journal of Pharmacology and Experimental Therapeutics*, **254**, 1084–1089.

Brown, S.A. & Finco, D.R. (1994). Reassessment of the use of calcitriol in chronic renal failure. In: *Current Veterinary Therapy XII*, (eds R. Kirk & J. Bonagura). W.B. Saunders, Philadelphia.

Brown, S.A., Finco, D.R., Crowell, W.A., Choat, D.C. & Navar, L.G. (1990). Single-nephron adaptations to partial renal ablation in the dog. *American Journal of Physiology*, **258**, F495–F503.

Brown, S.A., Crowell, W.A., Barsanti, J.A., White, J.V. & Finco, D.R. (1991a). Beneficial effects of dietary mineral restriction in dogs with marked reduction of functional renal mass. *Journal of the American Society of Nephrology*, **1**, 1169–1179.

Brown, S.A., Finco, D.R., Crowell, W.A. & Navar, L.G. (1991b). Dietary protein intake and the glomerular adaptations to partial nephrectomy in dogs. *Journal of Nutrition*, **121**, S125–S127.

Brown, S.A. Walton, C., Crawford, P. & Bakris, G. (1993). Long-term effects of antihypertensive regimens on renal hemodynamics and proteinuria. *Kidney International*, **43**, 1210–1218.

Chew, D.J. (1990). Acute intrinsic renal failure. *Proceedings of the 14th Kal Kan Symposium*, pp. 69–92.

Chew D.J. & Nagode, L.A. (1992). Calcitriol in the treatment of chronic renal failure. In: *Current Veterinary Therapy XI*, (eds R.W. Kirk & J.D. Bonagura). W.B. Saunders, Philadelphia.

Chew, D.J., Dibartola, S.P. & Crisp, M.S. (1992). Peritoneal dialysis. In: *Fluid Therapy in Small Animal Practice*, (ed. S.P. DiBartola), pp. 573–597. W.B. Saunders, Philadelphia.

Cowgill, L.D. (1986). Systemic hypertension. In: *Current Veterinary Therapy IX*, (ed. R.W. Kirk). W.B. Saunders, Philadelphia.

Cowgill, L.D. (1992). Pathophysiology and management of anemia in chronic renal progressive renal failure. *Seminars in Veterinary Medicine and Surgery*, **7**, 175–182.

Cowgill, L.D. & Kallet, A.J. (1983). Recognition and management of hypertension in the dog. In: *Current Veterinary Therapy VIII*, (ed. R.W. Kirk). W.B. Saunders, Philadelphia.

Crisp, M.S., Chew, D.J., Dibartola, S.P. & Birchard, S.J. (1989). Peritoneal dialysis in dogs and cats: 27 cases (1976–1987). *Journal of the American Veterinary Medical Association*, **195**, 1262–1266.

Davenport, D.J., Dibartola, S.P. & Chew, D.J. (1986). Familial renal disease in the dog and cat. In: *Contemporary Issues in Small Animal Practice, Vol. 4 Nephrology and Urology*, (ed. E.B. Breitschwerdt). Churchill Livingstone, New York.

Dial, S.M., Thrall, M.A. & Hamar, D.W. (1989). 4-Methylpyrazole as treatment for naturally acquired ethylene glycol intoxication. *Journal of the American Veterinary Medical Association*, **195**, 73–76.

DeLellis, L.A. & Kittleson, M.D. (1992). Current uses and hazards of vasodilator therapy in heart failure. In: *Current Veterinary Therapy XI*, (eds R.W. Kirk & J.D. Bonagura). W.B. Saunders, Philadelphia.

Finco, D.R. & Barsanti, J.A. (1983). Parenteral nutrition during a uraemic crisis. In: *Current Veterinary Therapy VIII*, (ed. R.W. Kirk), pp. 994–996. W.B. Saunders Company, Philadelphia.

Finco, D.R., Brown, S.A., Crowell, W.A., Duncan, R.J., Barsanti, J.A. & Bennett, S.E. (1992a). Effects of dietary phosphorus and protein in dogs with chronic renal failure. *American Journal of Veterinary Research*, **53**, 2264–2271.

Finco, D.R., Brown, S.A., Crowell, W.A., Groves, C.A., Duncan, J.R. & Barsanti, J.A. (1992b). Effects of phosphorous/calcium-restricted and phosphorous/calcium-replete 32% protein diets in dogs with chronic renal failure. *American Journal of Veterinary Research*, **53**, 157–163.

Grauer, G.F. & Thrall, M.A. (1986). Ethylene glycol (antifreeze) poisoning. In: *Current Veterinary Therapy IX*, (ed. R.W. Kirk), pp. 206–212. W.B. Saunders, Philadelphia.

Hostetter, T.H., Olson, J.L., Rennke, H.G., Venkatachalam, M.A. & Brenner, B.M. (1981). Hyperfiltration in remnant nephrons: A potentially adverse response to renal ablation. *American Journal of Physiology*, **241**, F85–F93.

King, L.G., Giger, U., Diserens, D. & Nagode, L.A. (1992). Anemia of chronic renal failure in dogs. *Journal of Veterinary Internal Medicine*, **6**, 264–270.

Lam, C.W.K. & Tan, I.K. (1978). Evaluation of the Harleco micro CO_2 system for the measurement of total CO_2 in serum or plasma. *Clinical Chemistry*, **24**, 143–145.

Lippert, A.C. & Buffington, C.A. (1992). Parenteral nutrition. In: *Fluid Therapy in Small Animal Practice*, (ed. S.P. DiBartola), pp. 384–418. W.B. Saunders, Philadelphia.

Littman, M. (1992). Update: Treatment of hypertension in dogs and cats. In: *Current Veterinary Therapy XI*, (eds R.W. Kirk & J.D. Bonagura). W.B. Saunders, Philadelphia.

Massry, S.G. (1989). Parathyroid hormone: A uremic toxin. *Adv. Exp. Med. Biol.*, **223**, 1–17.

Nagode, L.A. & Chew, D.J. (1992). Nephrocalcinosis caused by hyperparathyroidism in progression of renal failure: treatment with calcitriol. *Seminars in Veterinary Medicine and Surgery (Small Animal)*, **7**, 202–220.

Osborne, C.A. & Polzin, D.J. (1983). Azotaemia: A review of what's old and what's new. Part II Localisation. *Compendium on Continuing Education for the Practicing Veterinarian*, **7**, 561–574.

Pion, P.D. (1992). Current uses and hazards of calcium channel blocking agents. In: *Current Veterinary Therapy XI*, (eds R.W. Kirk & J.D. Bonagura). W.B. Saunders, Philadelphia.

Polzin, D.J., Osborne, C.A., Hayden, D.W. & Stevens, J.B. (1984). Influence of reduced protein diets on morbidity, mortality, and renal function in dogs with induced chronic renal failure. *American Journal of Veterinary Research*, **45**, 506–517.

Polzin, D., Osbourne, C.A. & O'Brien, T. (1989). Disease of the kidneys and ureters. In: *Textbook of Veterinary Internal Medicine*, Vol. 2, (ed. S.J. Ettinger), 3rd edn. pp. 1962–2046. W.B. Saunders, Philadelphia.

Rentko, V.T., Clark, N., Russ, L.A. & Shelling, S.H. (1992). Canine leptospirosis. A retrospective study of 17 cases. *Journal of Veterinary Internal Medicine*, **6**, 235.

Robertson, J.L., Goldschmidt, M., Kronfeld, D.S., Tomaszewski, J.E., Hill, G.S. & Bovee, K.C. (1986). Long-term renal responses to high dietary protein in dogs with 75% nephrectomy. *Kidney International*, **29**, 511–519.

Ross, L.A. (1989). Hypertensive diseases. In: *Textbook of Veterinary Internal Medicine*, (ed. S. Ettinger). W.B. Saunders, Philadelphia.

Ross, L.A. & Labato, M.A. (1989). Use of drugs to control hypertension in renal failure. In: *Current Veterinary Therapy X*, (eds R.W. Kirk & J.D. Bonagura). W.B. Saunders, Philadelphia.

Rubin, S.I. (1986). Non-steroidal antiinflammatory drugs, prostaglandins and the kidney. *Journal of the American Veterinary Medical Association*, **188**, 1065–1068.

Chapter 63

Enlarged Kidneys

A. G. Torrance

INTRODUCTION

Kidney enlargement (renomegaly) is an uncommon condition in the dog and usually arises from pathological changes. Congenital unilateral renal agenesis induces compensatory physiological hypertrophy of the remaining kidney, but unilateral renomegaly when both kidneys are present is pathological. Bilateral compensatory renal hypertrophy is sometimes seen in animals with portosystemic shunts, but in most other cases bilateral renomegaly implies renal pathology. The causes of renomegaly (Table 63.1) are:

- hydronephrosis,
- acute nephrosis,
- acute pyelonephritis,
- idiopathic polycystic kidney disease,
- renal neoplasms,
- acromegaly.

Signs of renal failure coupled with the finding of bilateral renomegaly is suggestive of acute renal failure in dogs.

Hydronephrosis

Obstruction of urine flow causes a progressive dilatation of the renal pelvis. In bilateral ureteric or urethral obstruction, the patient will die from acute postrenal renal failure before significant atrophy of renal parenchyma occurs, but in cases of unilateral ureteric obstruction compensation by the unobstructed kidney will allow the development of gross hydronephrosis. The renal pelvis progressively dilates causing pressure atrophy of the renal parenchyma and eventually the kidney becomes a distended, fibrous, fluid-filled sac. In the early stages, the distension of the renal capsule will induce signs of renal pain, but in many cases the first indication of hydronephrosis is progressive abdominal enlargement due to a large, unilateral, abdominal mass. Obstructive lesions may be congenital or acquired. Congenital obstructions include; ureteral atresia, stenosis, torsion and ureterocoele. These abnormalities may be seen in association with ectopic ureters. Acquired causes of obstruction include: neoplasms, blood clots, uroliths, trauma, inflammatory masses and inadvertent ureteral ligation.

Acute Nephrosis

Affected kidneys are normal sized or enlarged unless there is pre-existing chronic renal failure. The diagnosis and management of these cases is dealt with in detail in Chapter 62.

Pyelonephritis

Pyelonephritis is interstitial inflammation of the kidney associated with bacterial infection. In acute cases, one or both kidneys may be enlarged. Chronic pyelonephritis causes structural damage, fibrosis and scarring and is associated with reduced renal size. Most cases are caused by ascending urinary tract infection. Signs of acute pyelonephritis may be quite vague but include: mild renomegaly, renal pain, fever, anorexia, dehydration, weight loss, polyuria/polydipsia and vomiting. Neutrophilic leukocytosis and pyuria may be present. Renal concentrating ability is often impaired. Persistently dilute urine with a positive urine culture, even in the absence of azotaemia, is suggestive of pyelonephritis. The source of urinary tract infection may be difficult to localise but the presence of white blood cell casts confirms the presence of inflammation in the upper urinary tract. Unfortunately, the absence of white cell casts does not rule out pyelonephritis.

Polycystic Renal Disease

Polycystic renal disease occurs in Cairn Terriers where it appears to be a familial problem (Polzin *et al.* 1989). Affected animals develop abdominal enlargement due to renomegaly at 2–6 weeks of age and the progressive replacement of renal parenchyma by the expanding cysts leads to renal failure and death from uraemia. There is no effective treatment and most cases progress to end stage renal failure and death. The development of multiple cysts in affected kidneys is usually ascribed to obstruction of renal tubules by debris or fibrosis, but a recent microdissection study of human polycystic kidneys suggested that acquired cystic disease is the result of hyperplasia and dilatation of the remaining nephrons rather than the result of obstruction or fibrosis (Vandeursen *et al.* 1991).

Renal Neoplasia

Tumours are an important cause of unilateral renomegaly in the dog. Primary renal malignancies such as renal cell carcinoma and transitional cell carcinoma, are relatively rare and vary in their behaviour. Some tumours are highly invasive locally and cause erosion of the renal artery and vein while others are quite static. Some metastasise early

Table 63.1 Causes of pathological renomegaly in the dog.

Disease	Bilateral or unilateral	Signs of renal failure*	Prognosis
Renal lymphoma†	Bilateral (usually)	+/–	Very poor

Hydronephrosis
Acquired:
    neoplasia, trauma, uroliths,
        iatrogenic ligation
Congenital:
    ureteral agenesis, torsion
        or stenosis, ureterocoele
        (often associated with
        ectopic ureters)
	Unilateral or bilateral	+/–	Guarded if unilateral
			
			Very poor if bilateral unless
			    obstruction can be relieved

Acute nephrosis (toxic, ischaemic
    or infections)
	Bilateral	+	Guarded, can resolve with
			    appropriate treatment

Acute pyelonephritis	Unilateral or bilateral	+/– (fail to
		    concentrate
		    urine if bilateral)
			Guarded, can resolve with
			    appropriate treatment

Portosystemic shunts†	Bilateral	–	Can be good – depends on site of the shunt
Polycystic renal disease	Bilateral	+	Poor
Primary renal neoplasms	Unilateral	–	Guarded
Metastatic disseminated neoplasia†	Bilateral or unilateral	+/–	Very poor

Acromegaly†	Bilateral	+/– (PU/PD due to
		    glucosuria)
			Good in the dog if induced by
			    progesterone

PU/PD, polyuria/polydipsia.
* (+) Clinical and laboratory signs of acute or chronic renal failure are usually present. (+/–) These signs are usually present but the animal can also show no signs of renal disease. (–) signs of renal disease are usually absent.
† These diseases are likely to involve other organ systems. The remainder are organ-specific diseases.

whereas others are curable by excision. The presence of an irregular mass involving part or all of one kidney should always prompt careful evaluation for local and distant metastasis. German Shepherd Dogs have an hereditary predisposition for nodular dermatofibrosis combined with renal cystadenocarcinomas (Cosenza & Seely 1986). Such animals present with skin nodules particularly affecting the limbs and palpable mid-abdominal masses.

HISTORY AND PHYSICAL EXAMINATION

A careful history should be taken and a complete physical examination should be performed as this will allow the con-struction of a relevant problem list which underpins the success of further diagnostic testing.

Organomegaly should be identified during systematic palpation of the abdomen and the following questions addressed:

(1) Is it renomegaly?
(2) Is renomegaly unilateral or bilateral?
(3) Are the renal contours smooth or irregular?
(4) Are other abdominal masses present?
(5) Is there renal or sub-lumbar pain?

Other physical findings which may be relevant to the diagnosis are presented in Table 63.2.

Table 63.2 Physical findings of diagnostic importance in animals presenting with renomegaly.

Historical and physical finding	Possible diagnostic implication
Signs of renal failure (see Chapter 62) Buccal ulceration, uraemic breath, dehydration, poor concentrating ability and oliguria/polyuria (acute or decompensated chronic)	Many possible causes – acute nephrosis (ischaemic, toxic, infectious), bilateral pyelonephritis, bilateral hydronephrosis
Pallor and emaciation (additional findings which suggest a chronic problem)	Polycystic renal disease, renal lymphoma, metastatic neoplasms
Neurologic/encephalopathic signs	Portosystemic shunt Lymphoma
Haematuria (no dysuria)	Renal neoplasia
Dysuria and haematuria	Hydronephrosis (urinary calculi, renal trauma) Pyelonephritis (with lower urinary tract infection)
Urinary calculi	Hydronephrosis (renal calculi) Portosystemic shunt (urate crystals)
Urinary incontinence with urine scalding	Congenital anatomical defect causing incontinence leading to hydronephrosis
Microhepatica	Portosystemic shunt
Hepatomegaly	Acute tubular nephrosis (leptospirosis)
Signs of acromegaly – enlargement of the skull, mandible (prognathia inferior) and tongue	Acromegaly
Signs of systemic sepsis – fever, depression, tachycardia, vomiting, petechiation	Acute tubular nephrosis (leptospirosis) Acute pyelonephritis (sepsis)
Skin nodules	Renal cystadenocarcinoma (in German Shepherd Dog, associated with dermatofibrosis)

FURTHER DIAGNOSTIC TESTS

Renomegaly is very unlikely to be a trivial finding. Careful diagnostic enquiry is always indicated. This should begin with a database of information without which it is impossible to proceed logically and be sure that significant factors have not been overlooked. A suitable database for a patient with renomegaly should include:

- complete blood count including platelets,
- biochemical profile including electrolytes,
- urinalysis (collected by cystocentesis or a voided sample),
- survey radiographs of the abdomen and thorax.

Urinalysis findings consistent with urinary tract inflammation or infection (>3 white blood cells per high power field) should be followed with an aerobic urine culture. The presence of white blood cell casts is strongly suggestive of pyelonephritis.

Diagnostic imaging is the next important step and both ultrasound and intravenous urography are very helpful. Of the two techniques, ultrasound evaluation is preferable because it is less invasive, does not necessarily require general anaesthesia, and allows assessment of renal size without the problems of magnification. In addition, having assessed the internal structure of an enlarged kidney, an ultrasound-guided biopsy can be obtained immediately. Parameters have been devised for assessing renal size from contrast radiographs (Feeney et al. 1982) and ultrasound images (Barr et al. 1990; Lamb 1990).

Excretory Urogram in the Ventrodorsal View

In dogs:

Kidney length : Length of L2 vertebral body
= 2.5–3.5

Maximal Saggital Dimension on Ultrasound

In the dog kidney length is directly proportional to body weight. See Table 63.3 (Barr et al. 1990).

Renal ultrasound can reliably distinguish between polycystic renal disease, hydronephrosis, lymphoma, mass lesions and sub-capsular fluid or infiltration (Lamb 1995). Changes in echogenicity are also associated with certain diseases. Ultrasonographic findings in acute pyelonephritis are variable. There may be dilatation of the renal pelvis, an hyperechoic mucosal line within the renal pelvis, focal hypoechoic areas in the medulla and focal hyper- or hypo-echoic cortical lesions.

The diagnosis of idiopathic polycystic disease and hydronephrosis can be established with the minimum data-

Weight range (kg)	Number of kidneys examined	Renal length (cm)		
		Range	Mean	s.d.
0–4	2	3.2–3.3	3.2	0.09
5–9	16	3.2–5.2	4.4	0.5
10–14	10	4.8–6.4	5.6	0.6
15–19	20	5.0–6.7	6.0	0.4
20–24	20	5.2–8.0	6.5	0.72
25–29	44	5.3–7.8	6.9	0.58
30–34	32	6.1–8.7	7.2	0.6
35–39	24	6.6–9.3	7.6	0.72
40–44	12	6.3–8.4	7.6	0.54
45–49	8	7.6–9.1	8.5	0.46
50–59	6	7.5–10.6	9.1	1.27
60–69	4	8.3–9.8	9.0	0.63
90–99	2	8.6–10.1	9.4	1.06

s.d., standard deviction.

Table 63.3 The relationship between kidney length and body weight in dogs.

base and diagnostic ultrasound or intravenous urogram. Other causes of renomegaly require more specific diagnostic information. Pyelonephritis can be diagnosed by the minimum database, ultrasound and urine culture (if there are white blood cell casts). In cases where the infection cannot be specifically localised to the kidney, a renal biopsy may be necessary. Acute tubular nephrosis and localised and disseminated malignancies are diagnosed by renal biopsy and histopathology. Acromegaly may be strongly suspected on clinical signs and the presence of diabetes mellitus but should be confirmed by insulin-like growth factor 1 (IGF1) assay.

A cluster of signs of portosystemic shunts is often identified on the minimum database: microhepatica; microcytosis; non-regenerative anaemia; hypoproteinaemia; low blood urea with normal creatinine; hypoglycaemia; urinary urate crystals; and renomegaly. Compromised liver function must be identified with fasting and postprandial bile acids and the diagnosis confirmed by radiographic contrast studies.

Portosystemic shunts can also be identified quite reliably by skilled abdominal ultrasonographers (Lamb & Mahoney 1994).

PROGNOSIS

Refer to Table 63.1.

REFERENCES

Barr, F.J., Holt, P.E. & Gibbs, C. (1990). Ultrasonographic measurement of normal renal parameters. *Journal of Small Animal Practice*, **31**, 180–184.

Cosenza, S.F. & Seely, J.C. (1986). Generalised nodular dermatofibrosis and renal cystadenocarcinomas in a German shepherd dog. *Journal of the American Veterinary Medical Association*, **189**, 1587–1590.

Feeney, D.A., Barber, D.L. & Johnston, G.R. (1982). The excretory urogram: techniques, normal radiographic appearance, and misinterpretation. *Compendium on Continuing Education for the Practicing Veterinarian*, **4**, 233–240.

Lamb, C.R. (1990). Abdominal ultrasonography in small animals: intestinal tract and mesentery, kidneys, adrenal glands, uterus and prostate. *Journal of Small Animal Practice*, **31**, 295–304.

Lamb, C.R. & Mahoney, P.N. (1994) Comparison of three methods for Calculating portal blood flow velocity in dogs using duplex – Doppler ultrasonography. *Veterinary Radiology and Ultrasound*, **35**, 190–194.

Lamb, C.R. (1995). Abdominal ultrasonography in small animals. In: *Veterinary Ultrasonography*, (ed. P. Goddard), CAB pp. 21–25. International, Wallingford, Oxon.

Polzin, D., Osborne, C. & O'Brien, T. (1989). Diseases of the kidneys and ureters. In: *Textbook of Veterinary Internal Medicine*, Vol. 2, (ed. S.J. Ettinger), 3rd edn. W.B. Saunders, Philadelphia.

Vandeursen, H., Van-Damme, B., Baert, J. *et al.* (1991). Acquired cystic disease of the kidney analysed by microdissection. *Journal of Urology*, **146**, 1168–1172.

Chapter 64

Haematuria

A. G. Torrance

INTRODUCTION

Haematuria is the presence of blood in the urine. This may have arisen from blood loss in the renal parenchyma, discontinuity of the endothelial/epithelial barrier at any anatomical position in the urine collecting system from renal pelvis to urethral orifice, or shedding of blood into the urine from the genital or accessory sex organs. A single transient episode of mild haematuria may be clinically insignificant, but persistent or heavy haematuria is always an indication for diagnostic investigation because the underlying cause can be very serious.

The urinary tract is an important site of bleeding in animals with systemic coagulopathies and, in unexplained haematuria, investigation of haemostasis should never be overlooked. Haematuria may first be observed as brown or red discoloration of the urine (macroscopic haematuria) or it may be discovered during urinalysis performed for another reason (microscopic haematuria). The first objective for the clinician investigating brown or red discoloration of the urine is to distinguish between haematuria and haemoglobinuria or other pigmentary sources of discoloration. The second objective is to determine the source of haematuria and this problem lends itself well to methodical diagnostic investigation.

CAUSES AND DISTINGUISHING FEATURES OF HAEMATURIA

The causes of haematuria and those historical, physical or laboratory features which can be used to distinguish these are presented in Table 64.1.

History

Haematuria can be a manifestation of systemic diseases and therefore, as with all internal medicine cases, a full medical history must be obtained. Issues of importance include breed and family history of coagulopathy, presence or absence of bleeding from other systems, access to toxins such as rodenticides, history of trauma or hyperthermia, the nature of trauma and the presence or absence of systemic signs of disease such as weakness or weight loss. In road accident victims there should always be a high level of suspicion of urinary tract trauma.

The timing of haematuria within the urine stream is an important criterion for localising the source, but can be over-interpreted due to the difficulties of observation.

- The shedding of blood from external genitalia in between urinations is consistent with a urethral or genital source of bleeding.
- The presence of blood throughout the urine stream is consistent with a renal parenchymal source, generalised bladder disease, coagulopathies, severe prostatic disease or proximal urethral disease.
- The appearance of haematuria at the end of urination is associated with localised lesions within the bladder, especially of the ventral bladder wall.

The presence or absence of dysuria is very important and should be confirmed after history taking by direct observation of urination. The chronicity of the problem can be established by asking when the last normal urination occurred and precise details of voiding behaviour can be obtained by asking the client to describe the most recent voiding episode.

Physical Examination

A complete physical examination must be performed before focusing on the urogenital system. Meticulous palpation of the abdomen can help to localise the source of haematuria.

Table 64.1 Causes and features of haematuria.

Category of haematuria	Possible source/cause	History/clinical features	Laboratory findings
Renal parenchymal haematuria	Idiopathic Polycystic disease Glomerulopathies Tubulo/interstitial inflammation Renal tumours (except lymphoma) Trauma Renal infarction Vascular anomalies	Haematuria without dysuria Blood present throughout urination	Red cell casts Proteinuria which is disproportionate for the degree of haematuria
Lower urinary tract haematuria	Urinary tract infection Neoplasia Toxic drugs (cyclophosphamide) Trauma Anatomical lesions (polyps/ diverticuli) Calculi	Haematuria is usually associated with dysuria If the lesion is localised, haematuria is noted at the end of urination (especially ventral bladder wall)	Infection or inflammation is associated with pyuria
Genital haematuria	Prostate Uterus Vagina (neoplasia, trauma, inflammation)	Shedding of blood can occur between urinations (can also be seen with urethral disease)	Compare voided sample with urine obtained by cystocentesis – haematuria confined to the voided sample suggests genital tract or distal urethra as source
Haematuria secondary to systemic disease	Thrombocytopenia Von Willebrand's disease Coagulopathies Hyperthermia Strenuous exercise	Bleeding noted from other sites in the body Breed or family history may indicate an inherited defect History of poisoning	Platelet number reduced *or* Bleeding time prolonged *or* Prothrombin time and/or activated partial thromboplastin time prolonged

- The kidneys should be assessed for size, symmetry and presence or absence of pain.
- The bladder, prostate and urethra can be investigated by the combined approach of abdominal and rectal palpation.
- Rectal palpation must always be performed.
- The presence of static masses, crepitus, movable cystic or urethral calculi, pain, distension, or displacement can all be assessed by palpation.
- Observation of urination is an important extension of the physical examination and is necessary in many cases.

Urinalysis – Defining the Problem of Haematuria

The actual presenting problem in cases investigated for haematuria is likely to be urine discoloration or some other urinary tract sign such as dysuria. Haematuria is a problem that can only be identified on urinalysis (Table 64.2). In cases with urine discoloration, haematuria must be distinguished from other causes of pigmenturia such as haemoglobinuria, myoglobinuria and bilirubinuria, by the combined approach of urine biochemistry and sediment analysis. Urine dipstick biochemistry tests for occult blood do not differentiate haematuria, haemoglobinuria and myoglobinuria. Haematuria may produce a more stippled appearance of the dye in the reagent pad, but this finding should not be relied upon. The presence of large concentrations of formaldehyde or ascorbic acid in urine can give false positives for occult blood.

A simple laboratory method for distinguishing haemoglobinuria, myoglobinuria and haematuria was described by Chew & DiBartola (1986).

- Centrifuge the reddish-brown urine sample.
- If the pellet is red and the supernatant clear, it suggests haematuria.
- If the supernatant remains red, add 2.8 g of ammonium sulphate to 5 ml sample and centrifuge again.
- If the supernatant is clear and the pellet dark brown, it suggests haemoglobinuria.
- If the supernatant remains brown, it suggests myoglobinuria.

Urinalysis – Localising the Source of Haematuria

The presence of dysuria usually implies a lower urinary tract source unless renal haemorrhage is sufficiently severe to cause lower urinary tract obstruction by blood clots. Comparing urinalysis of a voided sample with urine obtained by cystocentesis is helpful in ruling out blood contamination from the genital tract and distal urethra. In males, haemorrhage from the prostate gland can enter urine stored in the bladder as well as voided urine. The presence of significant proteinuria and haematuria in the absence of pyuria suggests that the haematuria may be due to a glomerulopathy. The localising value of proteinuria disappears if there is concomitant pyuria because haematuria, pyuria and proteinuria will all occur in inflammation or infection at any location within the urinary tract. Bleeding into the urinary tract will induce some proteinuria, but haematuria associated with a glomerular lesion will be accompanied by proteinuria which is disproportionate for pure blood loss alone. The magnitude of proteinuria must be assessed in cases where a glomerular lesion is suspected. This can be done by measuring 24-h protein loss or more conveniently by calculating the protein:creatinine ratio on a single urine sample.

Table 64.2 Urinalysis findings and their significance in the patient with haematuria.

Test	Finding	Interpretation
Urine dipstick	Occult blood positive Protein positive	Red cells, haemoglobin or myoglobin could give positive result – check urine sediment
Urine sediment examination	Red cell casts White cell casts	Indicate a renal problem with or without active inflammation
	Clumps of epithelial cells with neoplastic features	Transitional cell carcinoma†
	Red cells: >8 / hpf (voided) >5 / hpf (catheterised) >3 / hpf (cystocentesis)*	Significant haematuria investigate cause
	White blood cells	Indicates inflammatory disease leading to haematuria
	No red cells seen despite occult blood positive on dipstick	Sample haemolysed – check for red cell ghosts (particularly if urine dilute) or haemoglobinuria or myoglobinuria
Urine protein to creatinine ratio	>3 in the absence of pyuria	Suggests significant glomerular disease

* The number of red cells seen in a cystocentesis sample depends on the quality of the technique – therefore this figure can be misleading as microscopic haematuria can be induced by cystocentesis.
† Not a consistent finding in neoplasitic diseases of the lower urinary tract. Similar clumps of cells can occasionally be observed in cases of inflammatory bladder disease.
hpf, high-power field.

The following formula is used to calculate the protein : creatinine ratio using SI units:

$$\left(\frac{\text{urine protein concentration (g/l)}}{\text{urine creatinine concentration (}\mu\text{mol/l)}} \right) \times 8840$$

Values of the ratio >3 suggest that there is significant (glomerular) proteinuria (see Chapter 65 on proteinuria).

Diagnostic Imaging of the Urinary Tract

In most cases diagnostic imaging is necessary in evaluating haematuria. The following points are worthy of note:

- Plain abdominal radiographs are a good starting point for identifying masses, anatomical abnormalities and radio-opaque calculi.
- Neoplasms of the urinary tract frequently metastasise and so in most cases thoracic radiographs are also justified.
- Intravenous urography provides good visualisation of both kidneys and a qualitative estimate of renal perfusion and function. The anatomy and filling of the ureters can be assessed. As the contrast enters the bladder, transurethral injection of gas will produce a double contrast cystogram which reveals the details of the anatomy of the bladder wall and the presence of calculi or masses.
- Positive and negative contrast studies are of great value, the intravenous urogram (IVU) combined with a double contrast cystogram is invaluable.
- The urethra is evaluated by contrast urethrogram, or vagino-urethrogram in the female.
- Contrast urethrography will delineate urethral masses or calculi and leakage of contrast into the prostate can be an indicator of significant prostatic disease.

Ultrasound imaging can also be used to good effect in the investigation of haematuria. Ultrasound is best used in conjunction with contrast studies to provide ancillary information about the renal parenchyma, radiolucent stones, the prostate and the bladder wall. Ultrasound guided biopsy of the urogenital tract is an extremely useful and relatively non-invasive method for making the definitive diagnosis.

Cystoscopy

Cystoscopy in small animal medicine was the subject of reviews (McCarthy & McDermaid 1990; Senior 1992). The advantages of cystoscopy over radiography are direct visu-alisation of lesions and use of endoscopic instruments to obtain diagnostic material.

- Direct examination of the urethral opening, urethra, bladder and ureteral openings achievable with the cystoscope is superior to surgical exposure because of the magnification of the scope and the excellent lighting.
- Most female dogs can be evaluated transurethrally with rigid human cystoscopes, while males can be investigated using flexible bronchoscopes or arthroscopes by prepubic percutaneous cystoscopy. The transurethral approach is the least invasive technique.
- In prepubic percutaneous cystoscopy, the bladder is filled with saline and the endoscope is introduced directly using a percutaneous approach and a sharp trochar. Distension of the bladder is maintained by saline flow until the internal structure of the bladder wall has been fully examined. At the end of the procedure, the bladder is drained and the instrument removed. In some cases, the bladder is maintained by catheterisation for 48–72 h to ensure that the puncture site seals. The procedure is described in detail by McCarthy & McDermaid (1990).

Urinary tract pathology, which can be assessed by cystoscopy, is limited to luminal and mucosal lesions. A modified cystoscopic technique has been described which allows visualisation of the submucosa and deeper tissues by ultrasound. Use of this technique in small animals has been described in detail (McCarthy & McDermaid 1990), the main problem with using it for the investigation of haematuria is reduced visibility in cases with severe, ongoing, bleeding.

Exploratory Surgery

In most cases the source of haematuria can be identified non-invasively. Surgery should be employed in a curative rather than diagnostic capacity. Indications for exploratory surgery are relatively few and include:

- individual catheterisation of ureters to establish which kidney is the source of haemorrhage;
- determination of the source of severe, life threatening, haemorrhage when haemostatic parameters are normal;
- investigation of the traumatised urinary tract for small ruptures which cannot be clearly identified by imaging.

Haematuria originating from the prostate or female genital tract can be difficult to differentiate from haematuria of urinary tract origin. Manual palpation, radiography, contrast radiography, ultrasonography and direct visualisation by vaginoscopy can be used to investigate the female genital tract. In the male, prostatic bleeding can be identified by obtaining an ejaculate or performing a prostatic wash. Rectal examination, plain radiographs and ultrasound are particularly useful in evaluating prostatic diseases, while contrast radiography has limited usefulness (see Chapter 73 on prostatic diseases).

PROGNOSIS

Many of the causes of haematuria, e.g. urolithiasis, urinary tract infections, idiopathic renal haematuria, trauma, benign prostatic hypertrophy and prostatitis are amenable to treatment and have quite a good prognosis. Coagulopathies, idiopathic renal haematuria, chemical cystitis and trauma can produce life-threatening haemorrhage which may require emergency treatment. Idiopathic renal haematuria is interesting in this respect, often it is unilateral and nephrectomy of the affected side is curative, but cases have been described where the second kidney became involved with ultimately fatal consequences (Jennings *et al.* 1992).

The outlook for animals with renal or lower urinary tract tumours is not so encouraging. In respect of renal neoplasms it is generally agreed that nephrectomy is the treatment of choice for renal haemangiomas and meets with success. In cases of renal carcinomas nephrectomy can only be viewed as palliative. There have been some recent publications of surveys of urogenital neoplasia which have provided useful prognostic information. In a study of 115 dogs with neoplasms of the lower urinary tract (Norris *et al.* 1992):

- 97% of the tumours were epithelial in origin and malignant.
- Lower urinary tract tumours were most common in older dogs weighing more than 10 kg.
- Haematuria and inflammatory urine sediments were the most frequently reported problems and cases had neoplastic cells in the urine sediment.
- Contrast cystography was the most useful investigative technique, 96% of the dogs had a mass or filling defect in the lower urinary tract.
- Regional or distant metastases were common (37%) at initial diagnosis and distant metastasis was evident in 51% at necropsy.
- Prognosis was poor, only 16% of treated dogs had a survival time of 1 year or more.

   ○ Tumours that involved either the bladder or the urethra had a better prognosis than those that involved both.
   ○ Tumours that were amenable to complete surgical excision had the best prognosis.
   ○ Partial resection with radiation therapy or chemotherapy was not very effective.

In a study of 41 female dogs with infiltrative urethral disease (Moroff *et al.* 1991):

- 71% had epithelial neoplasia.
- 24% had chronic active urethritis and 5% had leiomyoma.
- Stranguria and haematuria were the most common problems.
- The prognosis for chronic active urethritis was better than that for epithelial neoplasia.

Most of the dogs with urethral neoplasia were euthanased at the time of diagnosis or shortly thereafter, whereas the dogs with chronic active urethritis were treated with antibiotics, prednisolone and cyclophosphamide. Responses to treatment were quite good and completely resolved the signs in 50% of the cases.

REFERENCES

Bagley, R.S., Center, S.A., Lewis, R.M., *et al.* (1991). The effect of experimental cystitis and iatrogenic blood contamination on the urine protein/creatinine ratio in the dog. *Journal of Veterinary Internal Medicine*, **5**, 66–70.

Chew, D.J. & Dibartola, S.P. (1986). *Manual of Small Animal Nephrology and Urology*. Churchill Livingstone, New York.

Jennings, P.B., Mathey, W.S., Okerberg, C.V., *et al.* (1992). Idiopathic renal hematuria in a military working dog. *Military Medicine*, **157**, 561–564.

McCarthy, T.C. & McDermaid, S.L. (1990). Cystoscopy, *Veterinary Clinics of North America: Small Animal Practice*, **20**, 1315–1340.

Moroff, S.D., Brown, B.A., Matthiesen, D.T., *et al.* (1991). Infiltrative urethral disease in female dogs: 41 cases (1980–1987). *Journal of the American Veterinary Medical Association*, **199**, 247–251.

Norris, A.M., Laing, E.J., Valli, V.E.O., *et al.* (1992). Canine bladder and urethral tumors: a retrospective study of 115 cases (1980–1985). *Journal of Veterinary Internal Medicine*, **6**, 145–153.

Senior, D.F. (1992). Use of cystoscopy, In: *Current Veterinary Therapy X.1*, (eds R.W. Kirk & J.D. Bonagura). W.B. Saunders, Philadelphia.

Chapter 65

Proteinuria

P. J. Barber

INTRODUCTION

Proteinuria is defined as an abnormally high concentration of protein in the urine. It is a relatively common laboratory finding, usually detected using urine dipstick reagent test strips.

Proteinuric disorders may be classified as prerenal, renal and postrenal (see Table 65.1).

NORMAL PHYSIOLOGY

Normal Urine Protein Content

A small amount of protein is normally present in the urine of healthy animals and urine protein excretion of up to 30 mg/kg/day may be considered normal. Functional proteinuria is recognised and characterised by excess urinary protein excretion in the absence of renal disease, is transient and reversible in nature and usually mild and non-pathological. The primary mechanism is unclear, but thought to be related to renal vasoconstriction or changes in glomerular capillary permeability and may occur during strenuous exercise (McCaw *et al.* 1985), pyrexia, exposure to extremes of temperature, stress and congestive cardiac failure. Functional proteinuria has been well characterised in man, but is not well understood in dogs.

Normal Urine Protein is from Three Sources

Filtered by the Glomerulus

- Urine is an ultrafiltrate of plasma.
- Proteins of low molecular weight (<7000 kDa) are freely filtered by the renal glomerulus.

- Albumin
  - has a molecular weight of about 69 000 kDa, close to the cut off for glomerular filtration;
  - in plasma is negatively charged, so although it is present in relatively high concentrations, it appears in low concentrations in the ultrafiltrate;
  - is incompletely resorbed (see below) and so is the major urinary protein.
- Other relatively small proteins, such as haemoglobin, circulate bound to larger plasma proteins and so are not readily filtered.
- The composition of the glomerular filtrate is modified on passage through the proximal tubule, most of the filtered protein being reabsorbed to prevent protein wastage.
- Tubular protein reabsorption is energy dependent, proteins being taken up into the tubular cells by pinocytosis and degraded to their constituent amino acids.

Active Secretion into the Renal Tubule

Epithelial cells of the renal tubules secrete small quantities of protein into the tubular lumen. Tamm–Horsfall protein (also known as uromucoid) is a mucoprotein which is synthesised by the epithelial cells and thought to possess anti-viral activity. Urokinase and secretory immunoglobulin A are also secreted into the tubule.

Derived from the Lower Urogenital Tract

A small amount of protein enters the urine both from the genital tract and during passage through the lower urinary tract.

PATHOPHYSIOLOGY OF PROTEINURIA

Classification of proteinuria is usually based on the anatomical site at which the excess protein enters the urinary tract (see Table 65.1).

Table 65.1   Causes of proteinuria.

Category	Pathophysiology	Disease	Major protein lost
Prerenal	A high concentration of low molecular weight protein is present in the blood such that the filtered load exceeds the resorptive capacity of the tubule	Multiple myeloma	Immunoglobulin* (Bence-Jones proteins)
		Paraproteinaemias Lymphoma Leukaemia Chronic infections	Immunoglobulin*
		Haemolytic anaemia	Haemoglobin
		Rhabdomyolysis	Myoglobin
Renal	(1) Glomerular proteinuria (damage to glomerular filtration barrier) (2) Defective tubular reabsorption	Renal amyloidosis Glomerulonephritis Acute tubular necrosis Acute/chronic renal failure Polycystic renal disease Fanconi's syndrome	Mainly albumin Mainly albumin Enzymes, Polypeptide hormones Immunoglobulin fragments Fibrin degradation products Retinol binding protein α_1 microglobulin β_2 microglobulin
	(3) Renal parenchymal inflammation	Pyelonephritis	Inflammatory exudate (white cell casts)
Postrenal	Inflammation of the ureters, and lower urinary tract	Urinary tract infection (urethrocystitis) Urolithiasis Urinary tract trauma Prostatitis Vaginitis	Inflammatory exudate
	Neoplasia of the lower urinary tract	Tumours of the urethra and bladder	Degenerative cells and inflammatory exudate

* Loss of albumin will occur as the disease progresses and damage to the glomerular membrane occurs due to the high filtered load of immunoglobulin.

Prerenal Proteinuria

Prerenal proteinuria (overload proteinuria) occurs when:

- an abnormally high concentration of a low molecular weight protein is present in the blood;
- a reduction or relative deficiency in plasma protein binding sites, leads to increased free protein molecules available for filtration.

For example: Excess haemoglobin in the circulation occurs as a result of various causes of intravascular haemolysis (e.g. immune-mediated haemolytic anaemia) and may exceed the binding capacity of haptoglobin. Free haemo-globin is filtered at the glomerulus and is then present in such high concentrations in the filtrate that the resorptive capacity of the tubules is exceeded producing haemoglobinuria.

Prerenal proteinuria occurs in a number of diseases, the clinical signs of which are not related to urine protein loss. Detection of proteinuria and determination of the type of protein being excreted may aid in the diagnosis of these diseases. Examples are shown in Table 65.1.

Renal Proteinuria

The occurrence of proteinuria associated with primary renal disease may be explained by three mechanisms.

Alteration of Selective Permeability of Glomerular Filtration Barrier (Glomerular Proteinuria)

Proteinuria results from damage to the glomerular filtration barrier, allowing serum proteins to pass more easily and in greater quantities into the filtrate. The damage may involve an increase in 'pore' size and/or a change in the electrical charge. The two most common causes of this type of damage are renal amyliodosis and glomerulonephritis.

Renal Amyliodosis
Renal amyliodosis is characterised by the extracellular deposition of fibrillar proteins arranged in a beta-pleated sheet configuration. This configuration gives these proteins their properties of insolubility and resistance to proteolysis, as well as their specific staining characteristics. There are a number of classes of amyloidosis defined in man, but only reactive systemic amyloidosis is of significance in small animal medicine.

Reactive Systemic Amyloidosis

- This occurs secondary to inflammatory, neoplastic and chronic infectious disease.
- Amyloid deposits are amino terminal fragments of serum amyloid A protein, which is present in increased concentrations in chronic inflammatory conditions.
- Only a small percentage of patients with such inflammatory disease develop amyloid deposits and it is thought that these individuals have an impaired ability to degrade this acute phase reactant.

Amyliodosis is rare in the dog although is recognised as a familial disease in Chinese Shar-Pei dogs (DiBartola *et al.* 1990). Severe proteinuria occurs when amyloid deposits cause glomerular damage. However, up to 36% of Shar-Pei dogs with familial amyloidosis have medullary amyloid deposits without significant glomerular deposits. Medullary deposition may result in fibrosis and interference with the blood supply to the inner portion of the medulla causing papillary necrosis. In such cases of medullary amyliodosis, proteinuria may be mild or absent, although the deposits will interfere with renal concentrating ability.

Glomerulonephritis
Glomerular inflammation causes two important clinical syndromes in dogs:

- By causing glomerular injury, glomerulonephritis can lead to progressive losses of glomerular filtration rate, thereby producing azotaemia and/or uraemia.

- Marked proteinuria can result in hypoalbuminaemia and, if severe, oedema and/or ascites. This latter constellation of abnormalities is referred to as the nephrotic syndrome.

Filtration failure and nephrotic syndrome can occur independently or simultaneously in animals with glomerulonephritis. Interestingly, most dogs with glomerular disease exhibit azotaemia (Kurtz *et al.* 1972; Murray & Wright 1974; Wright *et al.* 1981; Jeraj *et al.* 1984; Jaenke & Allen 1986; MacDougall *et al.* 1986; Center *et al.* 1987; DiBartola *et al.* 1980). In contrast, many cats develop oedema and ascites without elevations of urea or creatinine in the plasma (Nash *et al.* 1979; Wright *et al.* 1981).

Glomerulonephritis is a condition caused by an immune-mediated mechanism. Antibody–antigen complexes present in the glomerulus activate complement and lead to glomerular damage. This can occur in three ways:

- pre-formed circulating antigen-antibody complexes may become trapped in the glomerulus;
- *in situ* immune complex formation may occur due to antigens of non-glomerular origin becoming trapped on the glomerular membrane;
- antibodies directed against components of the glomerular basement membrane (not confirmed in the dog).

Glomerulonephritis may be further classified morphologically into membranous, proliferative, membranoproliferatve and sclerotic. In man, this classification is used to aid the formulation of therapy and prognosis, but such correlations have not been validated in the dog.

Glomerulonephritis may be found in association with any chronic antigenic stimulus, including infectious, inflammatory and neoplastic diseases. Metabolic disorders (such as diabetes mellitus and hyperadrenocorticism) and administration of various drugs and vaccines may also lead to glomerulonephritis (see Grauer 1992).

The main features of glomerular proteinuria are summarised in Box 65.1.

Defective Tubular Resorption (Tubular Proteinuria)

Primary tubular proteinuria is characterised by incomplete tubular resorption of proteins in the presence of normal glomerular permeability. Proteinuria in this situation is due to low molecular weight proteins that normally pass the glomerular filtration barrier. These include enzymes (e.g. lysozyme, ribonuclease, alanine aminopeptidase), polypeptide hormones (e.g. calcitonin, glucagon, insulin, prolactin,

Box 65.1   Summary of glomerular proteinuria.

Glomerular proteinuria, whether caused by glomerulonephritis or amyliodosis, has the following features:

- Characteristically massive
- In many cases may lead to clinical signs related to protein loss:
  - Weight loss
  - Lethargy
  - Nephrotic syndrome – plasma colloid osmotic pressure is lowered sufficiently to lead to oedema formation. Ascites, pleural effusion and pitting oedema of dependent peripheral tissues may result.
  - In some animals with glomerular proteinuria, clinical signs caused by thromboembolism can occur, in part due to antithrombin III deficiency (Grauer 1992).
- Initially, proteinuria may be the sole clinical finding, however the glomerulonephritis or amyloidosis will eventually lead to renal damage and, if unresolved, to renal failure and the uraemic syndrome.

parathyroid hormone), immunoglobulin fragments, fibrin and fibrin split products, retinol-binding protein, α_1-microglobulin, β_2-microglobulin and amino acids.

Tubular proteinuria is:

- relatively rare,
- typically mild,
- found in some cases of acute tubular necrosis, acute and chronic renal failure, polycystic kidney disease and Fanconi's syndrome.

Mixed tubular and glomerular proteinuria is thought to be relatively common and may pose diagnostic difficulties. Fanconi's syndrome represents a group of metabolic abnormalities, associated with proximal tubular resorptive defects which cause loss of glucose, amino acids, calcium, phosphate, sodium and other solutes (Bovée *et al.* 1979).

Fanconi's syndrome has the following features:

- It may be hereditary (as in Basenjis).
- It may be acquired (aminoglycoside and heavy metal toxicity).
- Clinical signs are dependent on the severity of the tubular defect.

- Generally the losses of glucose and amino acids are not detrimental but polyuria and polydipsia frequently result and progression to renal failure is common.

Renal Parenchymal Inflammation

Any cause of inflammation within the kidney parenchyma (pyelonephritis) will lead to exudation of inflammatory proteins into the filtrate and hence proteinuria. Causes include infections, toxins, immunological disorders and drug reactions.

Postrenal Proteinuria

Postrenal proteinuria is caused by inflammatory and degenerative lesions of the urogenital tract distal to the kidneys. Proteinuria is usually mild to moderate and associated with an active urine sediment. Diagnosis is rarely a problem as clinical signs are usually directly attributable to the lower urinary tract (see Chapters 64 and 66). The lesions may affect the ureters, bladder, prostate, or urethra and include cystitis, prostatitis, urolithiasis, neoplasia of the urogenital tract, especially transitional cell carcinomas, and vaginitis.

DIAGNOSTIC APPROACH TO PROTEINURIA

Proteinuria is usually detected by qualitative screening tests, such as urine dipstick reagent strips. On documenting proteinuria, the diagnostic approach should attempt to answer the following:

- Is protein persistently present in the urine?
- Is the amount of protein in the urine significant?
- What is the source of the protein loss? (Identifying the nature of the protein may help to localise the source of protein loss.)

As there are many conditions that may induce proteinuria, generalisations regarding a diagnostic approach are difficult. An outline approach is illustrated in Fig. 65.1. Animals may have more than one pathological process leading to proteinuria.

History

A complete medical history should be taken, however particular emphasis should be placed on the following aspects

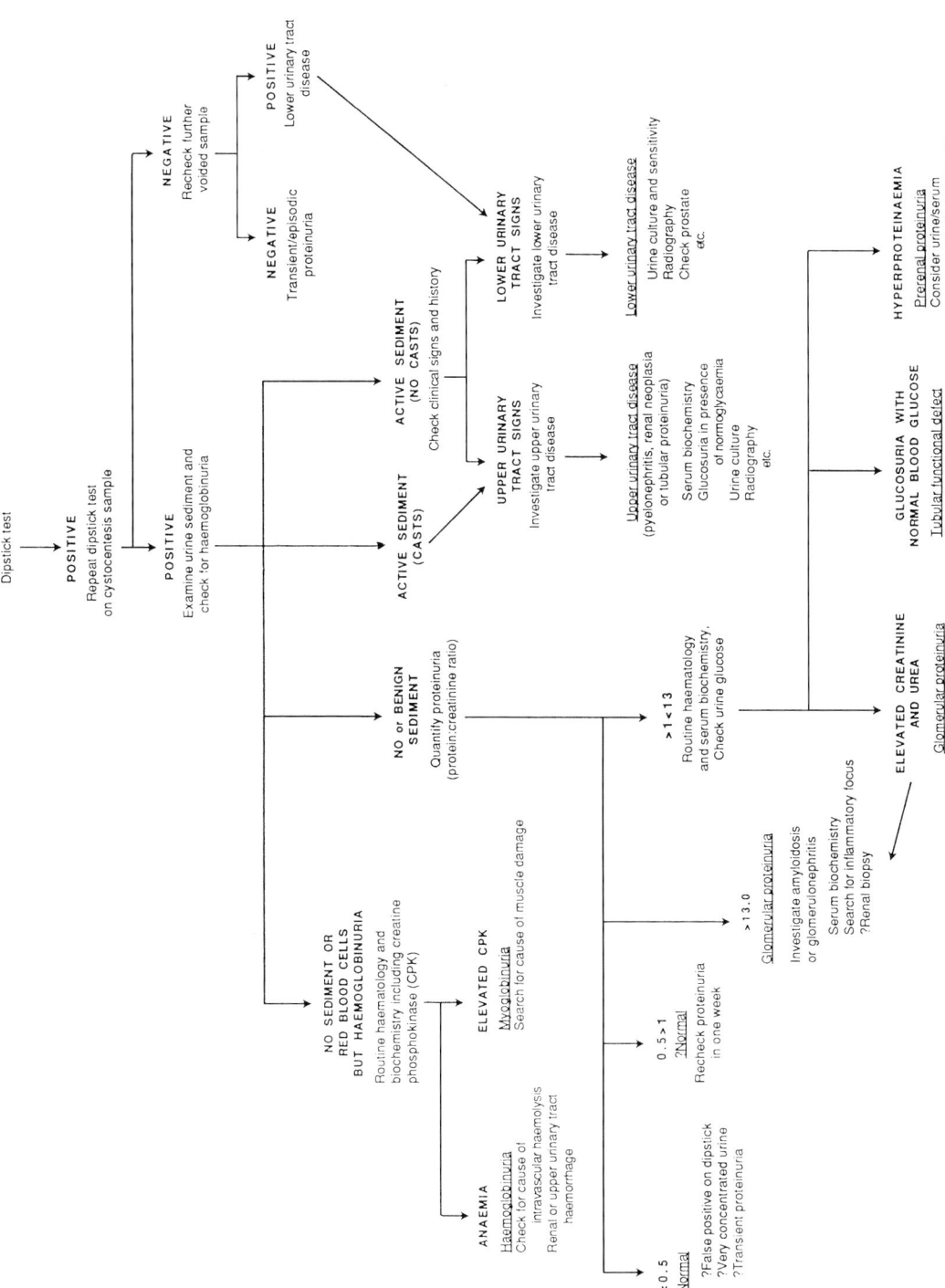

Fig. 65.1 Schematic diagram on approach to the diagnosis of proteinuria in the dog. (Adapted from Barber, P.J. (1996) Proteinuria. In: *Manual of Canine and Feline Nephrology and Urology* (eds J.G. Bainbridge & J. Elliott), pp. 75–84. BSAVA, Cheltenham.)

which may aid the clinician in reaching a diagnosis: signalment, signs of lower urinary tract disease, evidence of systemic disease and previous medical history.

Physical Examination

A complete physical examination is necessary, although frequently unrewarding in many conditions associated with proteinuria. A source of chronic inflammation or neoplasia is occasionally found in association with glomerulonephritis or amyliodosis. Non-specific systemic signs of emaciation, poor hair coat and depression may be related to the presence of renal failure. Particular attention should be paid to the urogenital system including palpation of both kidneys, bladder and prostate where possible. An ophthalmoscopic examination may reveal evidence of hypertension. Dilatation and tortuosity of retinal blood vessels, retinal haemorrhages, retinal detachments and hyphaema can occur with severe systemic hypertension (Dukes 1992). Ocular lesions have also been reported to occur in cases of prerenal proteinuria where the high level of circulating protein leads to hyperviscosity of the blood (Kirscher *et al.* 1988).

Table 65.2 summarises the important historical, physical and routine laboratory findings which may point to the underlying disease and suggests further diagnostic tests which would be appropriate in such cases.

Table 65.2   Concurrent historical, physical and laboratory findings and their significance in proteinuric animals.

Historical, physical and *laboratory findings*	Likely disease syndrome	Possible causes	Confirmatory tests
Weakness, pallor, jaundice, red discoloration of the urine	Immune-mediated haemolytic anaemia (intravascular haemolysis)	Auto-immune haemolytic anaemia	Auto-agglutination Coombs' test
Regenerative anaemia, haemolysed plasma, haemoglobinuria		Secondary immune-mediated haemolytic anaemia (malignant lymphoma, SLE, drugs)	Diagnose secondary disorder Stop drug therapy
Pyrexia (unknown origin) Neurological signs Ocular lesions	Paraproteinaemias leading to hyperviscosity syndrome	Multiple myeloma Lymphoma Leukaemia	Serum and urine protein electrophoresis Bone marrow aspirate for a tissue diagnosis
Hyperproteinaemia (polyclonal or monoclonal gammopathy) Many haematological abnormalities possible			
Peripheral oedema Abdominal distension (ascites – transudate) Dyspnoea (pleural effusion – transudate)	Nephrotic syndrome	Glomerulonephritis } Amyloidosis }	Urine protein : creatinine ratio >13, very few cells seen in sediment Renal biopsy
Hypoalbuminaemia Hypercholesterolaemia (Hypergammaglobulinaemia indicative of an inflammatory focus)			
Blindness, (retinal detachment, tortuous vessels, haemorrhage) Hyphaema	Hypertension*	Glomerulonephritis Amyloidosis	Urine protein : creatinine ratio >13, very few cells seen in sediment Renal biopsy

Table 65.2 *Continued.*

Historical, physical and *laboratory findings*	Likely disease syndrome	Possible causes	Confirmatory tests
Pyrexia (unknown origin) Shifting lameness Skin problems *Anaemia, leucopenia, thrombocytopenia*	Immune-mediated multisystemic disease	SLE Drug reaction (e.g. potentiated sulphonamides)	Anti-nuclear antibody test Coombs' test Stop drug therapy
Acute depression, weakness and vomiting *Elevated urea, creatinine, phosphate, and potassium*	Acute renal failure	Acute tubular necrosis (toxic, ischaemic or infections)	Tubular casts, signs of inflammation in urine sediment Renal biopsy
Chronic weight loss, anorexia, vomiting, PU/PD and pallor *Elevated urea, creatinine and phosphate*	Chronic renal failure	Chronic pyelonephritis Glomerulonephritis } Amyloidosis } Polycystic renal disease	Urine culture Renal imaging (IVU, US) Urine protein : creatinine ratio >13, very few cells seen in sediment Renal biopsy Renal imaging (IVU, US)
Dysuria, haematuria, pollakiuria, stranguria *Red cells, white cells and bacteria may be present in urine sediment*	Lower urinary tract disease	Urinary tract infection Urolithiasis Bladder/urethral neoplasia Prostatitis/vaginitis	Culture urine/prostatic fluid Radiography (double contrast cystogram) Ultrasound (bladder, prostate) Biopsy tissue, sample and analyse calculi

* Hypertension can occur in chronic renal failure, and glomerular hypertension may lead to increased protein leakage across the glomerulus. The degree of proteinuria in such cases is much less than with primary glomerular disease
SLE, systemic lupuserythematosus; PU/PD, polyuria/polydipsia; IVU, intravenous urogram; US, ultrasound.

Urinalysis

- For screening purposes, a voided sample is acceptable.
- The first urine voided in the morning should be collected (mid-stream) as this will be the most concentrated.
- If proteinuria is discovered on a screening test:
  - Ensure the problem is persistent by examining subsequent samples (obtain by cystocentesis).
  - Interpret qualitative tests (dipstick tests) with care taking into account urine concentration (estimated by specific gravity; Table 65.3) and microscopic sediment examination.
  - A trace positive reaction is more likely to be significant in dilute than in concentrated urine.
  - If there is an active urine sediment, this should be investigated whatever the protein concentration. Performing a urine protein:creatinine ratio on such a sample is unnecessary.
- A second sample, preferably obtained by cystocentesis, will confirm the persistence of proteinuria and may aid in anatomical localisation of the source of the protein.
- A negative result implies transient proteinuria or a disease distal to the bladder.
- It should be noted that cystocentesis samples may still contain elements from the proximal urethra and prostate due to reflux of urine into the bladder.

Table 65.3 Significance of proteinuria: effect of urine concentration.

Normal urine protein concentration: <20 to 30 mg/kg per day		
Urine protein concentration	Urine specific gravity	Comments
Negative	Any specific gravity	Normal Unless main protein is not albumin such as Bence-Jones proteins, globulins etc.
<0.65 g/l	Any specific gravity	Normal
0.65–2.0 g/l	>1.030	Questionable result, repeat screen in future

A number of semi-quantitative dipstick tests for urine protein assessment have been developed, and all have limitations. Most dipstick tests are based on buffered tetrabromophenol blue reagent, which is extremely sensitive to albumin but relatively insensitive to a number of pathological urinary proteins, producing false negative results in the presence of globulin, Bence-Jones proteins and other non-albumin proteins. False positives occur in samples contaminated with chlorhexidine or quaternary ammonium based disinfectants. Urine samples should not be taken in the 24 h following the use of radiographic contrast media, as these may cause transient proteinuria and can also produce false positive results in a number of tests (Feeney *et al.* 1986).

Proteinuria as a result of inflammatory exudate may be identified by microscopic examination of the urine sediment. An active urine sediment (pyuria and haematuria) is generally associated with postglomerular proteinuria. These changes could occur in upper or lower urinary tract neoplasia and inflammatory diseases. Haematuria alone without pyuria may be associated with urinary tract infections, trauma, neoplasia, urolithiasis and nephrolithiasis, glomerulonephritis and polycystic kidney disease (by erosion of vessels). The presence of leucocyte or red blood cell casts would confirm renal involvement, however these casts tend to disintegrate in dilute urine and so are difficult to find. Physical examination and historical information usually aid the differentiation of upper and lower urinary tract disease (Lees & Rogers 1986).

The presence of significant proteinuria with very few cells in the sediment suggests diseases that do not involve active inflammation of the urinary tract. In this situation, evaluation of a protein:creatinine ratio to quantify the urinary protein loss will be useful in determining the significance and the site of protein loss.

Urine Protein : Creatinine Ratio

Quantitative laboratory evaluation of urine protein concentration depends not only on the amount of protein filtered but also the degree of concentration of the filtrate by the renal tubules, therefore total 24-h protein excretion is more useful in quantifying protein losses. Collection of urine output for 24 h is impractical for veterinary practice. The excretion of creatinine is constant given a stable glomerular filtration rate. If the protein loss is also constant, then relating urine protein concentration to urine creatinine concentration eliminates variation in urine volume (the tubular concentration of urine increasing both protein and creatinine concentrations equally). The urine protein:creatinine ratio is calculated by dividing the urine protein concentration by the urine creatinine concentration. Before this calculation can be made, both concentrations must be converted to the same units (see Table 65.4).

It has been shown that the urine protein:creatinine ratio in a randomly collected urine sample correlates well with measured 24-h urinary protein excretion with and without proteinuria (White *et al.* 1984; Center *et al.* 1985; Grauer *et al.* 1985). Samples submitted for laboratory evaluation of protein and creatinine concentrations should be centrifuged to remove particulate and cellular matter. Time of sampling and feeding do not affect the predictive value of the ratio (McCaw *et al.* 1985; Jergens *et al.* 1987).

Interpretation of the Urine Protein : Creatinine Ratio

Although the magnitude of proteinuria can be used to predict the site of protein loss, there is great variability in ratios with different diseases. The values in Table 65.5 should only be considered as guidelines.

Routine Haematology and Serum Biochemistry

Results of routine haematology and serum biochemistry tests may be helpful in cases of prerenal and renal proteinuria. Examples are given in Table 65.2.

Table 65.4   Measurement of urine protein : creatinine ratio.

$$\text{Urine protein : creatinine ratio} = \frac{\text{Urine protein concentration (mg/dl)}}{\text{Urine creatinine concentration (mg/dl)}}$$

Conversion factors: total protein from g/l to mg/dl   multiply by 100
                                            creatinine from μmol/l to mg/dl   divide by 88.4

Protein : creatinine ratio only correlates to 24-h protein excretion in cases where:

(1) Glomerular filtration rate is stable.
     Therefore may be inaccurate in acute renal failure.
(2) Protein loss during a 24-h period is constant.
(3) Glomerular filtration and tubular concentration of urine affect creatinine and protein in a similar manner.
(4) There is no significant urinary tract inflammatory disease or urine sediment (probably still valid in sediment showing
     5–20 red blood cells per high power field (Bagley *et al.* 1991)).
(5) Protein : creatinine ratio is less than 1. The predictive value of the ratio decreases as the ratio exceeds the normal
     range and in these cases it should be used only as an estimate of 24-h protein excretion.

Table 65.5   Summary of urine protein : creatinine ratio.

Ratio	Significance
<0.5	Normal
>0.5 <1.0	May be normal but suspicious of mild disease
>1.0 <5.0	Mild protein loss – suggests prerenal disease
>5.0 <13.0	Mild to moderate protein loss – postrenal disease
	Glomerular lesions can give ratios in this range
>13.0	Severe protein loss – commonly seen in glomerular proteinuria
	(animals with amyloidosis tend to have the highest ratios).
	(Center *et al.* 1985; Lulich & Osborne 1990)

The presence of a hyperproteinaemia or evidence of haemolysis or leukaemia may suggest a prerenal cause.

An elevated protein:creatinine ratio with a very few cells in the urine sediment and no hyperproteinaemia is strong evidence of a glomerular problem. Plasma protein concentration in glomerular disease is variable, hypoalbuminaemia occurring if the protein loss is severe but conversely hyperglobulinaemia may be associated with the chronic inflammatory focus initiating the lesion. Nephrotic syndrome is characterised by massive proteinuria, hypoalbuminaemia (leading to subcutaneous oedema, ascites or pleural effusion) and hyperlipidaemia. The pathophysiology of the hyperlipidaemia is not fully understood. The severity of protein loss required to produce the nephrotic syndrome only occurs in renal amyloidosis or glomerulonephritis.

Biochemistry screens also allow the assessment of renal function which may well be significantly reduced, leading to elevations in urea, creatinine and phosphate in a number of renal causes of proteinuria.

Further Diagnostic Procedures

- Urine culture.
- Urinary tract contrast radiography.
- Ultrasound provides useful information in many situations.
- Protein electrophoresis allows the quantitative estimation of the proteins in the urine and comparison with serum electrophoresis may be used to confirm the presence of a prerenal proteinuria.
- Assay of proteins such as lysozyme and ribonuclease in the urine would confirm diagnosis of specific tubular proteinuria.

- Immunological assays to assess immune-mediated glomerular disease.

Renal Biopsy

Renal biopsy is not a diagnostic test to be undertaken lightly. Ultrasound-guided percutaneous biopsy is the method of choice, but carries significant risks. The main indication for renal biopsy in animals with proteinuria, is to distinguish between renal amyliodosis and glomerulonephritis and to gain information that will affect therapeutic decisions and prognosis. However, recent work in man has shown that biopsy-tailored therapy has no advantages over empirical therapy in cases of nephrotic syndrome (Levey *et al.* 1987). Renal biopsy is unnecessary in animals already showing a degree of renal failure, as this is unlikely to be reversible and carries a poor prognosis, whatever the underlying cause.

PROGNOSIS AND MANAGEMENT

Management of Prerenal and Postrenal Proteinuria

The prognosis in cases of proteinuria is extremely variable depending on the aetiology. Prerenal or postrenal proteinuria is usually readily reversible with specific therapy unless the aetiology involves a neoplastic lesion.

Management of Glomerular Inflammation

It is important to be certain of the diagnosis of glomerular inflammation (glomerulonephritis) before commencing therapy. Unfortunately, little objective information is avail-

Table 65.6 Management of glomerular inflammation.

Therapy	Recommended drug or diet and dose	Comments
Diuresis	Frusemide; 2–4 mg/kg every 8 to 24 h (dogs)	Reduces fluid accumulation in cases of oedema
Dietary salt restriction	<0.3% sodium on a dry matter basis	Reduces fluid accumulation in cases of oedema
Antithrombotic therapy	Aspirin; 0.5 mg/kg every 12 h	Used if: Antithrombin III levels <70% of normal Plasma albumin < 10 g/l Plasma fibrinogen > 3 g/l
Angiotensin converting enzyme inhibition	Enalapril; 0.5 mg/kg every 12 h Captopril; 1 mg/kg every 8 to 24 h Benazepril; 0.25–0.5 mg/kg every 24 h	Slow progression of renal disease and reduces proteinuria in rodent models of glomerulonephritis (GN) and in spontaneous GN in people. Avoid hypotension – monitor blood pressure
Dietary protein restriction	14–18% protein on a dry matter basis	Slow progression of renal disease and reduces proteinuria in rodent models of GN and in spontaneous GN in people. Protein restriction may limit hepatic production of albumin
Anti-inflammatory therapy	(1) Prednisolone; 1–4 mg/kg per day (2) Cyclophosphamide; 2.2 mg/kg per day for 3 days, discontinue for 4 days, then repeat cycle (3) Eicosapentaenoic acid; 0.5–5 g daily with food	These therapies have not been established to be effective – some animals may worsen during therapy
Antihypertensive therapy	See Chapter 62	Avoid hypotension, monitor arterial blood pressure at regular intervals

able upon which to base therapeutic choices, even if the diagnosis is based on a renal biopsy and the type of lesion has been carefully characterised. Glomerulonephritis often exhibits a waxing and waning clinical course which means that a minimum of two determinations for each of the baseline values for plasma concentrations of creatinine and albumin and the degree of proteinuria (quantitation of 24-h urinary protein excretion or determination of the urine protein:creatinine ratio) should be obtained before the institution of therapy; additional determinations will be necessary in unstable patients. Details of possible therapies are presented in Table 65.6.

Dogs with the nephrotic syndrome are often in a hypercoagulable state and anticoagulation therapy, such as aspirin is appropriate, particularly if one or more of the three conditions in Table 65.6 applies.

Anti-inflammatory or immunosuppressive therapy may prove beneficial in some patients. It should be emphasised, however, that these therapies have not yet been established to be effective and some animals may actually worsen during a trial. Consequently, all treated patients should be carefully monitored – baseline values for creatinine, albumin, and the extent of proteinuria should be recorded and the effect of therapy must be measured by sequential re-evaluation of these parameters. Possible anti-inflammatory treatment regimes are given in Table 65.6.

Monitoring Success of Therapy for Glomerular Inflammation

The specific goals in the management of glomerular inflammation are generally to slow the rate of progression of renal disease and to reduce the extent of proteinuria in order to prevent the development of, or reduce the extent of, the nephrotic syndrome. The former goal can best be assessed by sequential determinations of serum creatinine (initially every 2–4 weeks; less frequently in stable patients). Proteinuria (24-h urinary protein excretion or urine protein:creatinine ratio) should be assessed at each evaluation.

Animals with glomerular inflammation may exhibit systemic arterial hypertension and appropriate therapy (see Chapter 62) is indicated. If antihypertensive therapy is employed, care should be taken to avoid systemic hypotension by measuring systemic arterial blood pressure at regular intervals (initially every 2 weeks; less frequently in stable patients).

Prognosis of Cases with Glomerular Inflammation

It is clear that cases of glomerular inflammation can be managed as described in the section above. The prognosis in cases of immune-mediated, renal proteinuria depends on the localisation of an antigenic source. In some cases, treatment of an infection, removal of a neoplastic mass or discontinuing drug therapy may lead to complete resolution of the proteinuria. However, in the majority of cases, the underlying disease is not found and the lesion termed idiopathic. Spontaneous resolution of the proteinuria has been reported but most cases will develop significant renal damage. As renal damage is almost inevitable in cases of amyliodosis or glomerulonephritis, it is important that in those cases presented before the onset of renal failure, vigorous attempts are made to localise and eradicate the underlying cause. Cases presenting in, or progressing to, frank renal failure carry a poor prognosis.

Occasionally mild transient proteinuria of no apparent cause occurs. This does not require full investigation unless renal function is impaired or serum biochemistry or urine sediment abnormalities are present. Follow-up screening to confirm the transient (rather than recurrent) nature of the proteinuria, is advisable.

REFERENCES

Bagley, R.S., Center, S.A., Lewis, R.M., *et al.* (1991). The effect of experimental cystitis and iatrogenic blood contamination on the urine protein/creatinine ratio in the dog. *Journal of Veterinary Internal Medicine*, 5, 66–70.

Bovée, K.C., Joyce, T., Blazer-Yost, B., Goldschmidt, M.S. & Segal, S. (1979). Characterization of renal defects in dogs with a syndrome similar to the Fanconi syndrome in man. *Journal of the American Veterinary Medical Association*, 174, 1094–1099.

Center, S.A., Wilkinson, E., Smith, C.A., Erb, H. & Lewis, R.M. (1985). 24-hour urine protein/creatinine ratio in dogs with protein-losing nephropathies. *Journal of the American Veterinary Medical Association*, 187, 820–824.

Center, S., Smith, C., Wilkinson, E., Erb, H. & Lewis, R. (1987). Clinicopathologic, renal immunofluorescent, and light microscopic features of glomerulonephritis in the dog: 41 cases (1975–1985). *Journal of the American Veterinary Medical Association*, 190, 81–90.

DiBartola, S.P., Spaulding, G., Chew, D. & Lewis, R. (1980). Urinary protein excretion and immunopathologic findings in dogs with glomerular disease. *Journal of the American Veterinary Medical Association*, 177, 73–77.

DiBartola, S.P., Tarr, M.J., Webb, D.M. & Giger, U. (1990). Familial renal amyloidosis in Chinese Shar Pei dogs. *Journal of the American Veterinary Medical Association*, 197, 483–487.

Dukes, J. (1992). Hypertension: A review of the mechanisms, manifestations and management. *Journal of Small Animal Practice*, 33, 119–129.

Feeney, D.A., Walter, P.A. & Johnston, G.R. (1986). The effect of radiographic contrast media on the urinalysis. In: *Current Veterinary Therapy IX*, (ed. R.W. Kirk). W.B. Saunders, Philadelphia.

Grauer, G.F. (1992). Glomerulonephritis. *Seminars in Veterinary Medicine and Surgery (Small Animal)*, **7**, 187–197.

Grauer, G.F., Thomas, C.B. & Eicker, S.W. (1985). Estimation of quantitative proteinuria in the dog, using the urine protein-to-creatinine ratio from a random, voided sample. *American Journal of Veterinary Research*, **46**, 2116–2119.

Jaenke, R. & Allen, T. (1986). Membranous nephropathy in the dog. *Veterinary Pathology*, **23**, 718–733.

Jeraj, K.P., Vernier, R.L., Polzin, D., *et al.* (1984). Idiopathic immune complex glomerulonephritis in dogs with multisystem involvement. *American Journal of Veterinary Research*, **45**, 1699–1705.

Jergens, A.E., McCaw, D.L. & Hewett, J.E. (1987). Effects of collection time and food consumption on the urine protein/creatinine ratio in the dog. *American Journal of Veterinary Research*, **48**, 1106–1109.

Kirschner, S.E., Niyo, Y., Hill, B.L. & Betts, D.M. (1988). Blindness in a dog with IgA-forming myeloma. *Journal of the American Veterinary Medical Association*, **193**, 349–350.

Kurtz, J.M., Russell, S.W., Slauson, D.O. & Schrecter, R.D. (1972). Naturally occurring canine glomerulonephritis. *American Journal of Pathology*, **67**, 471–482.

Lees, G.E. & Rogers, K.S. (1986). Diagnosis and localization of urinary tract infection. In: *Current Veterinary Therapy IX*, (ed. R.W. Kirk). W.B. Saunders, Philadelphia.

Levey, A.S., Lau, J., Pauker, S.G. & Kassirer, J.P. (1987). Idiopathic nephrotic syndrome. Puncturing the biopsy myth. *Annals of Internal Medicine*, **107**, 697–713.

Lulich, J.P. & Osborne, C.A. (1990). Interpretation of urine protein–creatinine ratios in dogs with glomerular and non-glomerular disorders. *Compendium on Continuing Education for the Practicing Veterinarian*, **12**, 59–73.

MacDougall, D.F., Cook, T., Steward, A.P. & Cattell, V. (1986). Canine chronic renal disease: Prevalence and types of glomerulonephritis in the dog. *Kidney International*, **29**, 1144–1157.

McCaw, D.L., Knapp, D.W. & Hewett, J.E. (1985). Effect of collection time and exercise restriction on the prediction of urine protein excretion, using urine protein/creatinine ratio in dogs. *American Journal of Veterinary Research*, **46**, 1665–1669.

Murray, M. & Wright, N. (1974). A morphological study of canine glomerulonephritis. *Laboratory Investigation*, **30**, 213–221.

Nash, A.S., Wright, N., Spencer, A., Thompson, H. & Fisher, E.Y. (1979). Membrane nephropathy in the cat: a clinical and pathological study. *Veterinary Record*, **105**, 71–77.

White, J.V., Olivier, N.B., Reimann, K. & Johnson, C. (1984). Use of protein-to-creatinine ratio in a single urine specimen for quantitative estimation of canine proteinuria. *Journal of the American Veterinary Medical Association*, **185**, 882–885.

Wright, N., Nash, A., Thompson, H. & Fisher, E. (1981). Membranous nephropathy in the cat and dog. *Laboratory Investigation*, **45**, 269–277.

Chapter 66

Dysuria

J. C. R. Scott-Moncrieff

INTRODUCTION

Dysuria is defined as painful or difficult urination. Dysuria is usually accompanied by stranguria (straining, or hesitancy before, during, or after urination) and pollakiuria (increased frequency of urination). Dysuria, stranguria and pollakiuria are clinical signs of lower urinary tract (bladder, urethra) disease, and may be caused by inflammation and/or partial urinary tract obstruction. Disorders of the upper urinary tract (kidneys, ureters) do not cause signs of dysuria unless there is concomitant involvement of the lower urinary tract. A list of aetiologies for dysuria in dogs is shown in Table 66.1.

The most common cause of dysuria in dogs is bacterial cystitis/urethritis (Barsanti & Finco 1979). Organisms, commonly isolated, include *Escherichia coli*, *Staphylococcus* spp., *Proteus* spp., *Klebsiella* spp., and *Streptococcus* spp. Factors thought to predispose to urinary tract infection are shown in Table 66.2 (see also Chapter 67). Other common causes of dysuria in dogs include urolithiasis, and neoplasia of the bladder, urethra or prostate.

It is possible for two or more causes of dysuria to coexist (e.g. diseases that cause urinary tract inflammation such as neoplasia and urolithiasis may predispose to secondary bacterial tract infection). Conversely, urinary tract infection by urease producing organisms (*Staphylococcus* spp. *Proteus* spp.) may predispose to struvite urolith formation due to alkalinisation of the urine and increased availability of ammonium ions (Osborne *et al.* 1981).

HISTORY

Obtaining a thorough history is always essential for the diagnosis of dysuria. The clinician's approach to a case of dysuria will depend on whether they are dealing with a first-time event or a recurrent problem.

Important historical facts to be established concerning urination in dysuric animals are:

- Increased or decreased frequency?
- Increased or decreased volume?
- Stranguria present?
- Haematuria present?
- Interrupted or weak urine stream?
- Inappropriate location of urination? (Urination in the house may indicate pollakiuria but should be distinguished from incontinence, polyuria, and behavioural problems.)
- Is the urine foul-smelling?
- Perineal, vulval or penile licking?
- Duration of clinical signs?
- If previous treatment given, what was the response?

Questions about the presence of systemic signs of disease are important since clinical signs such as polyuria, polydipsia, anorexia, weight loss, vomiting and diarrhoea should alert the clinician to the possibility of urinary tract rupture or obstruction, metabolic disorders that predispose to urinary tract infection (hyperadrenocorticism, diabetes mellitus), or disorders that may be associated with urolith formation (hypercalcaemia, hepatic encephalopathy). Other important historical information includes the duration of clinical signs, occurrence of previous episodes, and their response to treatment. If stranguria is the presenting complaint, the clinician should be careful to establish that straining is due to urinary tract disease rather than to disorders of the gastrointestinal or reproductive tract.

PHYSICAL EXAMINATION

Although a thorough physical examination of all body systems is obviously important in a patient with dysuria, special attention should be paid to the urinary and reproductive tract as outlined below (Table 66.3).

Table 66.1   Differential diagnosis of dysuria in dogs.

Aetiology	Possible causes
Infectious agents	Bacteria Yeast (*Candida albicans*) Mycoplasma Parasitic (*Capillaria plica*; *Dioctophyma renale*)
Chemical agents	Cyclophosphamide
Immune mediated	Granulomatous urethritis
Trauma	Foreign body Iatrogenic Ureteral laceration/rupture
Neurogenic	Reflex dyssynergia
Metabolic (including nutritional)	Urolithiasis
Iatrogenic	Urethral catheters (in-dwelling or used for back flushing) Urethrostomy
Anatomical abnormalities	Urachal anomalies Ureterocoele Urethral stricture Phimosis Urethral prolapse
Neoplasia	Transitional cell carcinoma Papilloma Undifferentiated carcinoma Squamous cell carcinoma Adenocarcinoma Fibroma Leiomyoma Other
Other structures compressing urinary tract	Prostate, uterus

- Observe micturition.
- Carefully palpate the bladder before and after voiding.
- Perform a rectal examination.
- Examine external genitalia.
- Perform a neurological examination.

DIAGNOSTIC APPROACH

It is important to have a clear and logical approach to the dysuric patient. There are routine laboratory (Table 66.4) and diagnostic imaging tests (Table 66.5) which are applicable to most cases. The results of these routine tests may require that uroliths be collected for specific analysis or that tissue from the lower urinary tract be sampled for histopathological examination. If the history and physical examination suggest that there has been or is obstruction to urine flow, the metabolic status of the patient should be assessed and if required immediate action taken before any further diagnostic procedures. Of particular importance is complete obstruction of the urethra which leads to acute renal failure and the reader is referred to Chapter 62 for management of such a case.

Table 66.2 Predisposing causes for urinary tract infection in gods.

Mechanical disruption	Urolithiasis
	Neoplasia
	Foreign body
	Urethral catheters
Polyuric states	Hyperadrenocorticism
	Renal failure
Systemic diseases causing immunosuppression	Hyperadrenocorticism
	Diabetes mellitus
Anatomical abnormalities	Urachal diverticuli
Incomplete voiding	Detrusor atony
	Lower motor neuron bladder
Outflow obstruction	Neoplasia
	Urolithiasis
Iatrogenic	Perineal urethrostomy

Diagnostic Imaging

Radiography and ultrasonography should be undertaken in dogs where a urinary tract infection has been ruled out as the primary cause of the dysuria (see Fig. 66.1). Such studies help to establish the presence of urolithiasis, neoplasia or other less common causes of dysuria. Diagnostic imaging should also be performed in dogs with recurrent or persistent urinary tract infections. A summary of the important imaging techniques and the information they provide is presented in Table 66.5.

Collection of Uroliths

Where the presence of uroliths has been confirmed, it is essential to analyse a representative sample so that appropriate medical, dietary or surgical therapy be given. Treatment based solely on the type of crystals found in the urine can lead to mismanagement. Large uroliths are gener-

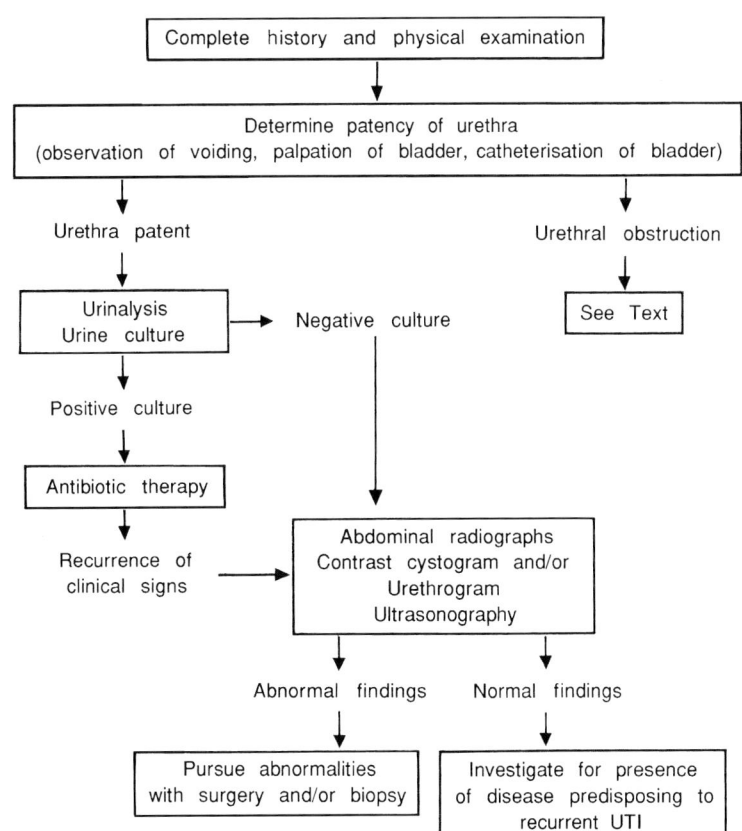

Fig. 66.1 Algorithm outlining the approach to dysuria in the dog.

Table 66.3 Important examinations which should be performed in the dysuric animal.

Examination	Finding	Significance
Observe micturition	Normal stream	Urethral patency established
	Non-productive straining	Suspect uretheral obstruction, attempt to pass a urinary catheter
Pass urinary catheter if dog unable to void urine unassisted	Unable to pass catheter	Physical obstruction of urethra (such as tumour or urolith)
	Catheter passes easily	Functional obstruction such as dyssynergia
Bladder palpation	Small thickened bladder (urgency caused by cystitis leads to frequent voiding)	Cystitis
	Gentle palpation of bladder may readily elicit voiding	
	Large bladder that does not easily express (care when palpating such a bladder – may rupture)	Uretheral obstruction that may require immediate medical and surgical therapy
	Large bladder, easily expressed (disruption of tight junctions following chronic distension – e.g. neurological disease)	Bladder atony
	Irregular hard masses	Uroliths
	Soft tissue masses	Neoplasia
	No palpable baldder	Recent voiding or suspect rupture of the bladder
Rectal palpation	Masses on the pelvic floor	Prostatomegaly – male
		Vagina/cervix abnormalities – female
		Urethral/bladder neck tumour
		Urethral urolith
	Masses dorsal to rectum	Sub-lumbar lymph nodes
Genital examination	Inflammation or discharge	Evidence of repeated attempts to urinate, local infection
Neurological examination	Neurological deficits	Suspect neurological cause of dysuria. Normal neurological examination does not rule out neurological disease of the bladder

ally collected by cystotomy but there are now alternative methods of obtaining representative samples, which include voiding hydropulsion and catheter assisted retrieval (see Chapter 68).

Non-Surgical Techniques to Obtain Tissue for Cytological or Histopathological Examination

If masses are identified within the bladder, prostate or urethra, and surgical resection is not considered feasible or warranted due to extent of disease or financial restraints, tissue for cytological and/or histopathological examination may sometimes be obtained by non-surgical techniques.

In patients with palpable soft tissue masses within the lumen of the bladder, fine needle aspiration may be used to obtain tissue for cytological evaluation. Cytological specimens may also sometimes be obtained by lavaging the bladder with 50–100 ml of sterile isotonic saline. Specimens may also be obtained by forceful aspiration through a urethral catheter with the tip placed at the level of the lesion (Melhoff & Osborne 1977). In some cases, if a mass can be visualised ultrasonographically, tissue samples can be obtained from the bladder or prostate using a needle biopsy instrument under direct ultrasonographic guidance.

Table 66.4 Diagnostic laboratory tests used in dysuric animals.

Test	Indication	Finding	Diagnostic value
Complete urinalysis (Dipstick plus urine microscopy) (If suspect urethral disease – compare voided and cystocentesis samples)	Routine	Pyuria Haematuria Proteinuria Bacteriuria Epithelial cells Alkaline urine (pH > 8.5), Crystalluria Malignant cells	Indicative of a urinary tract infection or inflammation (absence of pyuria does eliminate urinary tract infection) Indicates presence of urease producing organism Supportive of urolithiasis (normal for some animals) Evidence of urinary tract neoplasia (absence does not rule out malignancy)
Urine culture (sample obtained by cystocentesis)	Routine	Can get false negatives if urine stored for 24 h at 4°C or false positives if remains at room temperature for more than 30 min. Quantitative cultures are not absolutely necessary	Indicative of bacterial infection
Urine culture (sample obtained by free catch or catheter)	Used if not possible to obtain a sample by cystocentesis	Should culture quantitatively. Untreated dogs can have >100 000 colonies per ml (catheterised sample)	Low numbers of bacteria (<1000 per ml) would indicate contamination of sample, higher numbers (>10 000 per ml) confirm bacterial infection
Haematology and biochemistry	Routine depending on history and physical findings	Changes compatible with hyperadrenocorticism, renal failure or diabetes mellitus Changes compatible with hepatic diseases and diseases leading to hypercalcaemia	Evidence of diseases which predispose to urinary tract infection Evidence of diseases which predispose to urate and oxalate urolithiasis

Table 66.5 Diagnostic imaging in cases of dysuria.

Technique	Information obtained
Plain radiographs	Determines adequacy of patient preparation for contrast studies Detects radio-opaque calculi, emphysematous cystitis
Double contrast cystogram	Determines the size, shape, location and integrity of the urinary bladder Detects intraluminal (uroliths or blood clots), mural or intramural lesions (neoplasia, polypoid cystitis). Congenital abnormalities may be found
Positive contrast cystogram using water soluble contrast agent	Indicated when rupture, herniation or displacement of the bladder is suspected
Intravenous excretory urography concurrent cystography	Used to evaluate the upper urinary tract to detect pyelonephritis, renoliths or ureteroliths
Urethrography (retrograde in males, voiding urethrogram in bitches)	Detection of urethral disease – care should be taken to differentiate urethral spasm and urethral stricture
Ultrasonography bladder	Non-invasive, does not require anaesthesia. Kindneys can be examined. Relatively sensitive in the detection of pyelonephritis

Cystoscopy using either a rigid or fibre-optic cystoscope may also be used to visualise and biopsy masses within the bladder or urethra. Samples suitable for histopathological evaluation may be obtained by this method. Techniques for cystoscopic evaluation of the urethra and bladder of both male and female dogs have been reported, but availability of suitable equipment and expertise is limited (Brearley & Cooper 1987; Senior 1992; McCarthy & McDermaid 1986).

PROGNOSIS

There are many causes of dysuria and the prognosis depends very much on the primary cause. A logical approach to patients with dysuria, as outlined in this chapter, will allow a specific diagnosis of the underlying disease process and hence an accurate prognosis.

REFERENCES

Barsanti, J.A. & Finco, D.R. (1979). Laboratory findings in urinary tract infections. *Veterinary Clinics of North America*, **9**, 729–748.

Brearley, M.J. & Cooper, J.E. (1987). The diagnosis of bladder disease in dogs by cystoscopy. *Journal of Small Animal Practice*, **28**, 75–85.

McCarthy, T.C. & McDermaid, S.L. (1986). Prepubic percutaneous cystoscopy in the dog and cat. *Journal of the American Animal Hospital Association*, **22**, 213–219.

Melhoff, T. & Osborne, C.A. (1977). Catheter biopsy of the urethra, urinary bladder, and prostate gland. In: *Current Veterinary Therapy VI*, (ed. R.W. Kirk). W.B. Saunders, Philadelphia.

Osborne, C.A., Klausner, J.S., Krawiec, D.R. & Griffith, D.P. (1981). Canine struvite urolithiasis: problems and their dissolution. *Journal of the American Veterinary Medical Association*, **179**, 239–244.

Senior, D.F. (1992). Use of cystoscopy. In: *Current Veterinary Therapy XI*, (ed. R.W. Kirk and J.D. Bonagura). W.B. Saunders, Philadelphia.

Chapter 67

Management of Bacterial Urinary Tract Infections

J. Elliott

INTRODUCTION

Bacterial infections of the urinary tract are a major cause of haematuria, pollakiuria and dysuria in the dog. However, it is important to recognise that some infections can exist without these typical clinical signs. This chapter will concentrate on the pathophysiology of urinary tract infections, treatment strategies and monitoring the response to therapy.

NORMAL DEFENCE MECHANISMS IN THE URINARY TRACT

It is difficult to induce a bacterial infection of the lower urinary tract experimentally in a normal animal. Although the distal urethra, vagina and prepuce has a normal bacterial flora, the proximal urethra and bladder are sterile. The factors that are important in preventing colonisation of the proximal urethra and bladder and examples of diseases which might compromise the normal defence mechanisms are presented in Table 67.1.

Bacteria will grow in urine, particularly if the osmolality and pH are not too high or too low. The physical flushing action of urine flowing in the ureters and urethra and regular emptying of the bladder are important means of removing any bacteria that have ascended from the distal urethra. In addition, anatomical and functional features, which ensure unidirectional urine flow, inhibit bacteria moving up the urinary tract. In order to colonise the proximal urethra and bladder, bacteria need to adhere to the mucosal surface. Mucopolysaccharide (glycosaminogly-

cans) produced by the uroepithelium is an important protective layer preventing bacterial adherence. Secretory IgA molecules in urine and cervicovaginal mucus will also inhibit bacterial adhesion to mucosal surfaces.

PATHOPHYSIOLOGY OF BACTERIAL URINARY TRACT INFECTIONS

Urinary tract infections are usually classified as:

- simple or uncomplicated (resolve with antibacterial treatment);
- recurrent or complicated (signs return within a variable time of stopping treatment):
  - re-infections – implies re-colonisation of the urinary tract after a bacteriological cure,
  - relapsing infections – implies clinical but not bacteriological cure was achieved.

With many first-time, uncomplicated urinary tract infections in bitches, the animal often responds well to treatment, makes a complete recovery and the problem does not recur once treatment stops. Whatever compromises the urinary tract defences of animals with simple bacterial urinary tract infections, would appear to be transient and resolves spontaneously. Efforts to identify the predisposing cause are unnecessary and often fruitless in such cases. The same can not be said of animals with recurrent urinary tract infections. In such cases, every effort should be made to identify the problem that predisposes to urinary tract infections so that this can be addressed in the treatment strategy. Where this is possible, therapeutic success is more likely to be achieved.

Table 67.1   Normal defence mechanisms of the lower urinary tract and factors that may predispose to urinary tract infections.

Defence mechanism	Examples of conditions that may compromise defence mechanism
Mechanical washout of the tract by repeated voiding (flushing action to remove bacteria)	Diseases causing residual urine volume* • atonic bladder (neurological problem) • anatomic abnormality (local stasis) • urolithiasis or tumours preventing emptying
Uni-directional flow of urine inhibiting ascending bacterial invasion • urethral high pressure zone (sphincter) • urethral peristalsis • ureterovesical flap valves and peristalsis	Reduced flushing or turbulent/retrograde flow may assist invasion • in-dwelling urinary catheter • ectopic ureter (partially obstructed)
Composition of urine • extremes of osmolality (particularly in cats) • extremes of pH	Reduced ability to produce concentrated or dilute urine • chronic renal failure • diabetes mellitus • hyperadrenocorticism • corticosteroid therapy
Maintenance of a non-adhesive surface of the uroepithelium • secretion of glycosaminoglycan layer (prevents adhesion of bacteria)	Damage to the uroepithelium • iatrogenic trauma (catheterisation) • urolithiasis • tumours Defective production of glycosaminoglycans?
Secretory IgA in urine and cervicovaginal mucus opsonising bacteria • enhances phagocyte function	Diseases causing immunosuppression – reduced phagocyte function • hyperadrenocorticism • corticosteroid therapy • diabetes mellitus
Normal length of urethra	Females more susceptible than males Perineal urethrostomy
Normal flora of distal urethra prevent adherence and invasion by uropathogens	Deficient/abnormal flora of distal urethra?

* Prolonged periods between voiding may occur in house-trained pets not given regular opportunities to urinate.

Bacteria that Cause Lower Urinary Tract Infections

A knowledge of the likely causative organism is a key factor in determining the type of therapy required for any infection.

• Uropathogens usually ascend via the urethra to the bladder and beyond. In order to achieve this, these bacteria need to adhere to the uroepithelium.
• Many are present in the normal faecal or skin flora but only certain serotypes are capable of ascending the urethra.

• In human medicine, most urinary tract infections are caused by *Escherichia coli*. There are many serotypes of *Escherichia coli* known to occur but only five have been identified which are capable of invading the urinary tract in man.
• Serotyping of uropathogens is not routinely carried out in veterinary medicine so we do not have such an accurate picture.

Simple Urinary Tract Infections

• Simple (uncomplicated) urinary tract infections may localise to the lower urinary tract (urethra and bladder).

- Clinical signs include haematuria, dysuria and pollakiuria.
- Upper urinary tract (ureters and kidneys) have clinical signs of fever, lumbar pain, lethargy, anorexia, vomiting and polyuria.
- Infections ascend from the distal urethra.
- Upper urinary tract infections are usually accompanied by infection of the lower urinary tract, this may be clinical or sub-clinical.
- Clinical lower urinary tract infections are often accompanied by sub-clinical renal infections.
- Uncomplicated urinary tract infections have no obvious predisposing factors but are primarily found to occur in bitches possibly due to their much shorter urethra when compared with the male dog.

Complicated Urinary Tract Infections

- A complicated urinary tract infection is secondary to an abnormality in the defence mechanisms of the urinary tract.
- This does not resolve spontaneously, and leads to a relapse or re-infection when antibacterial treatment stops.
- Multiple episodes of urinary tract infection occur.
- Re-infection with a different species or serotype of bacteria appears to occur more frequently than relapses (where the same strain of bacterium is responsible and was never eradicated completely).
- If re-infections occur once or twice a year, these should be treated as described for simple urinary tract infections.
- When re-infections occur three or more times a year, longer term antibacterial therapy may be necessary in an attempt to prevent re-infection if the underlying defect in host defence mechanism is undetectable or untreatable.

DIAGNOSTIC APPROACH

Confirmation of Bacterial Infection

Examination of a urine sample is central to the investigation of an animal suspected of having a urinary tract infection. Samples must be analysed before therapy is instituted. The following is a summary of important points which should be considered:

- Obtain urine sample by cystocentesis if possible.
- Examine urine microscopically as soon as possible after collection.

- Direct examination of an air-dried Gram-stained drop of urine can be a specific and sensitive indicator of bacteriuria (Allen *et al*. 1987).
- Presence of red, white and epithelial cells in urine sediment confirms the presence of inflammation of the urinary tract.
- Do not rely on strip tests to indicate the presence of white cells.
- The absence of white cells does not rule out infection.
- The presence of white cell casts suggests renal involvement.
- High urine pH (>8) is indicative of the presence of urease producing bacteria.

The ultimate diagnostic test which confirms the presence of bacterial infection of the urine is bacterial culture. Urine should ideally be cultured within 6 h of collection. If this is not possible a sample should be collected into a tube containing 1% boric acid as a preservative. Quantitative cultures are necessary for samples obtained by catheterisation and free-catch but not for those obtained by cystocentesis. Contamination of the sample by bacteria normally resident in the distal urethra complicates the diagnosis when samples are collected by these means. However, if >100 000 bacteria per millilitre of urine are found in a voided sample, or >10 000 bacteria per millilitre of urine are found in a catheterised sample, the diagnosis of significant bactiuria is confirmed (Polzin 1994).

- The necessity for confirmation of the diagnosis by urine culture for uncomplicated first-time urinary tract infections is debatable.
- If bacteria are detected microscopically in the urine and their morphology determined, a logical choice of antibacterial agent can be made on this information.
- Provided the patient is closely monitored for response to therapy, a successful outcome can often be achieved.

Localisation of the Infection within the Urinary Tract

It is often difficult to determine the extent of the infection within the urinary tract. In many cases (but not all), clinical signs will be indicative of a urethrocystitis but signs of pyelonephritis are more subtle and often subclinical. Pyelonephritis is a serious form of urinary tract infection which is more difficult to treat successfully. Those cases showing clinical signs or with laboratory findings suggestive of pyelonephritis, should be investigated further by diagnostic imaging techniques. Other cases are treated as urethrocystitis and the diagnosis reviewed on the basis of response to treatment. Entire male dogs with significant bactiuria should be assumed to have infected prostate glands and should be managed accordingly.

THERAPEUTIC APPROACH

Therapy for Simple Urinary Tract Infections

- If this is the first episode of urinary tract infection and the animal has not been treated with antibacterial drugs in recent months, *the susceptibility of uropathogens is reasonably predictable.*
- This is particularly true of the Gram-positive organisms.
- Sensitivity testing is not usually considered necessary in such cases.

Selection of Antibacterial Drug Therapy

Many antibacterial drugs are concentrated by the kidney such that urine concentrations are 10–300 times higher than plasma concentrations. For example, penicillins are freely filtered, not reabsorbed and actively secreted by proximal convoluted tubule cells into the glomerular filtrate and urine concentrations are up to 300 times higher than plasma concentrations. In addition, once the drug is present in the urine, it will remain there until the animal urinates. Ideally, the animal should be allowed to urinate just before the next dose. If, however, the dog has been treated with antibacterial drugs for some other reason within the last few weeks, antibacterial susceptibility of the

uropathogens will be much less predictable (particularly if Gram-negative organisms are involved) and sensitivity testing is advisable. If more than one organism is involved in the infection, sensitivity testing is recommended to assist in the logical choice of antibacterial agent.

Antibacterial therapy recommended in Table 67.2 for first-time urinary tract infections is based on successful clinical trials (see Ling 1993). Although no peer reviewed clinical trials have been undertaken using baquiloprim–sulphadimethoxine combinations, data from the company would suggest similar efficacy to trimethoprim–sulphadiazine against uropathogens. All bacteria listed, except *Pseudomonas aeruginosa*, would also be susceptible to clavulanate potentiated amoxicillin (11 mg/kg t.i.d. p.o.). Enrofloxacin (2.5 mg/kg b.i.d. p.o.) would be effective against all organisms (particularly Gram negatives). It could be argued, however, that these two most effective antibacterial drugs should be reserved for treatment of cases which recur rather than as first line drugs for routine use in simple urinary tract infections. These recommendations do not apply to cases where pyelonephritis or prostatitis are suspected as the concentration of antibacterial drug reaching the infected renal or prostatic tissue will be lower than that present in the urine.

Antibacterial Sensitivity Testing for Urinary Tract Infections

Standard bacterial disc sensitivity tests will underestimate the efficacy of many antibacterial drugs against uropath-

Table 67.2 Bacteria associated with lower urinary tract infections in the dog.

Bacteria*	% Frequency (1979)†	% Frequency (1990)‡	Recommended therapy§
Escherichia coli	37.8	42.0	trimethoprim–sulphadiazine (15 mg/kg b.i.d. p.o.)
Staphylococcus spp.	14.5	6	ampicillin (11 mg/kg t.i.d. p.o.) amoxicillin (11 mg/kg t.i.d. p.o.)
Streptococcus spp.	12.6	9.6	ampicillin (11 mg/kg t.i.d. p.o.) amoxicillin (11 mg/kg t.i.d. p.o.)
Proteus mirabilis	12.4	9.3	ampicillin (11 mg/kg t.i.d. p.o.) amoxicillin (11 mg/kg t.i.d. p.o.)
Klebsiella pneumoniae	8.1	8.3	cephalexin (10 mg/kg t.i.d. p.o.)
Pseudomonas aeruginosa	3.4	5.0	tetracycline (18 mg/kg t.i.d. p.o.)
Enterobacter	2.6	–	trimethoprim–sulphadiazine (15 mg/kg b.i.d. p.o.)

* Most cases of urinary tract infection are caused by a single organism. In 18% of cases two or more species of bacteria may be involved.
† Data from Ling *et al.* (1979), a study involving 1400 cases.
‡ Data from Aucoin (1990), mean frequency from three laboratories involving >4500 cases.
§ Empirical therapy based on knowledge of the species of causative organism in a simple, first-time urinary tract infection – success rate 80% (Gram-negative spp.) to 100% (Gram-positive spp.). Data from Ling (1993).

ogens. This is because the amount of antibacterial drug included in these discs is sufficient to produce drug concentrations within the culture medium around the disc which are close to the plasma concentrations achieved by therapeutic dosing. However, urine concentrations of most antibacterial drugs will exceed their plasma concentration, sometimes by as much as 300 times. If disc sensitivity tests are used, discs made specifically for urinary infections should be used. A test that provides more information is the broth dilution method, which enables the laboratory to quote a minimum inhibitory concentration (MIC) for each drug tested for the bacteria isolated. Broth dilution methods are not suitable for in-house testing and are not offered on a routine basis by many commercial laboratories.

Duration of Therapy and Monitoring Response to Therapy

No controlled studies have been undertaken in veterinary medicine to determine the most appropriate duration of antibacterial therapy for simple urinary tract infections. In human medicine, very short duration therapy is sometimes recommended. This would seem inappropriate for our species, probably because the problem is diagnosed at a later stage in dogs. Empirically, most authors recommend a course of 10–14 days of treatment. The clinical signs, if present, usually resolve relatively quickly (in the first 2–4 days). The reason for continuing therapy this far beyond a clinical cure is to allow time for the defences of the urinary tract to recover and so to prevent re-infection. A urine sample should ideally be obtained by cystocentesis 4–7 days after the start of treatment for bacterial culture, which should be negative if the correct therapy has been chosen. An alternative is to examine the urine sediment at this stage for the presence of bacteria and signs of inflammation. Follow-up culture of urine obtained by cystocentesis is strongly recommended 4–7 days after the course of treatment has been completed. The aim of antibacterial therapy is to effect a bacteriological cure – culture of urine obtained by cystocentesis is the most sensitive way of assessing whether or not this aim has been achieved. If the culture results are positive at this stage, a re-infection or a relapse has occurred and the infection is now a complicated infection and should be managed accordingly (see below). It is important to recognise that many bacterial urinary tract infections can be sub-clinical and that post-treatment culture is the only way to ensure a bacteriological cure has been achieved.

If pyelonephritis is suspected, the empirical recommended duration of therapy is 3–4 weeks and it is essential that a post-treatment follow-up bacterial culture is undertaken 2 and 6 weeks after the completion of therapy (Allen

& Jaenke 1985). Some cases of pyelonephritis only come to light when cases of bacterial urethrocystitis recur following appropriate treatment. In entire male dogs, infection of the prostate gland should be assumed when there is evidence of a urinary tract infection. Beta-lactam antibiotics penetrate poorly into prostatic fluid and antibacterials which would reach effective levels in the prostate gland and the urine include potentiated sulphonamides and enrofloxacin. Recommended duration of therapy for bacterial infection of the prostate gland is at least one month (Lees & Forrester 1992).

Identification of Factors Predisposing to Multiple Urinary Tract Infections

Examples of disease states predisposing animals to urinary tract infections are presented in Table 67.1. A more complete diagnostic investigation is warranted in patients with multiple episodes of urinary tract infection. Concomitant problems identified in the history or on physical examination may suggest the most appropriate tests to confirm the diagnosis. A minimum database for such a case should include:

- full routine haematology and plasma biochemistry screen,
- complete urinalysis including careful microscopic examination,
- urine culture and antibacterial sensitivity testing of bacterial isolates,
- survey abdominal radiographs.

More sophisticated diagnostic tests should be considered, depending on the information gathered in the minimum database. For example, if the pattern of disease suggests that bacteriological cure is not achieved and multiple episodes represent relapses rather than re-infection, despite correct antibacterial selection initially, one should consider the presence of an abscess or other nidus of infection into which drugs are unable to penetrate. These might include:

- pyelonephritis with pockets of infection in renal tissue,
- chronic bacterial prostatitis,
- deep-seated cystitis or polypoid cystitis,
- infected urolith.

The further diagnostic tests which should be considered include:

- urethrography, double contrast cystography and ultrasound examination to rule out urolithiasis, neoplasia

and structural abnormalities of the lower urinary tract;
- intravenous urography and ultrasound examination to rule out involvement of the upper urinary tract;
- examination and culture of a prostatic wash or ejaculate;
- low dose dexamethasone suppression test or adreno-corticotrophic hormone (ACTH) stimulation test to rule out hyperadrenocorticism.

Therapy for Recurrent Urinary Tract Infections

Selection of Antibacterial Drug

- It is imperative that some form of sensitivity testing is undertaken in these complicated cases.
- The choice of antibacterial drug for the treatment of recurrent urinary tract infection should always be based on culture of the organism and sensitivity testing.
- The most appropriate sensitivity test is the broth dilution method which determines the MIC value for each antibacterial drug.
- Antibacterial drug therapy should be based on sound pharmokinetic principles (see Table 67.3).
- An antibacterial drug, which has been shown to achieve a urine concentration that is at least 4 times the MIC value of the organism isolated, should be chosen (Polzin 1994).
- If disc sensitivity testing is used, the choice of antibacterial drug is based on less precise information.

If further investigations reveal a deep-seated renal or prostatic infection, the efficacy of antibacterial therapy will depend more on the plasma concentrations of the antibacterial drugs than their urine concentrations. The prostate gland represents a barrier to diffusion of drugs and if chronic prostatitis is thought to be a problem, drugs that penetrate this barrier should be chosen.

Duration of Therapy and Monitoring Response to Therapy

Having chosen the most appropriate antibacterial drug, the following protocol should be followed for complicated urinary tract infections:

- Collect a urine sample by cystocentesis for culture 5 days after starting therapy.
- If urine is sterile – continue therapy, if bacterial growth occurs – re-evaluate treatment.
- Continue treatment for 6 weeks (empirical).
- Daily doses should be administered after the animal has been allowed to urinate.
- Collect urine by cystocentesis for culture:
  - immediately before therapy due to stop,
  - 7–10 days after therapy has ceased,
  - 1, 2, 3 and 6 months after therapy has stopped.

This longer duration of therapy may be sufficient to eradicate the infection and allow time for the defence mechanisms to recover. It is important that the urethra and bladder of these animals are catheterised as infrequently as possible. Passing a urinary catheter will risk the introduction of bacteria and re-infection of these compromised patients.

Table 67.3 Mean urinary concentrations of antibacterial drugs used to treat canine urinary tract infections.

Antibacterial drug	Dosage and route of administration	Mean (± 1 s.d.) urine concentration (µg/ml)	Reference
Amoxycillin	11 mg/kg t.i.d. p.o.	202 ± 93	Ling *et al.* 1980a
Ampicillin	25 mg/kg t.i.d. p.o.	309 ± 55	Ling *et al.* 1980a
Cephalexin	10 mg/kg t.i.d. p.o.	805 ± 421	Ling 1993
Enrofloxacin	2.5 mg/kg b.i.d. p.o.	40	Polzin 1994
Gentamicin	2 mg/kg t.i.d. s.c.	107 ± 33	Ling *et al.* 1981
Marbofloxacin	2 mg/kg s.i.d. p.o.	41 ± 9.3	Univet, data on file
Nitrofurantoin	4.4 mg/kg t.i.d. p.o.	100	Barsanti & Johnson 1990
Sulfizoxazole	22 mg/kg t.i.d. p.o.	1466 ± 832	Ling *et al.* 1980b
Tetracycline	18 mg/kg t.i.d. p.o.	137 ± 64	Ling *et al.* 1980b
Trimethoprim-sulphadiazine	15 mg/kg b.i.d. p.o.	55 ± 19*	Sigel *et al.* 1981

* Based on the trimethoprim fraction.

Management of Animals that Become Re-Infected

- If re-infection continues to occur in animals where a predisposing cause cannot be identified at a frequency of three times a year or more, long-term low-dose antimicrobial therapy may be necessary.
- This situation arises in some bitches and presumably represents an unidentifiable defect in urinary defence mechanisms such as defective glycosaminoglycans layer.
- The urine should be sterile before long-term therapy commences.
- Antibacterial drugs are administered at one-third of the normal therapeutic daily dose, just before the animal is confined for the night (after it has urinated).
- The drugs which are recommended for this prophylactic treatment include trimethoprim–sulphadiazine, cephalexin or nitrofurantoin (Barsanti & Johnson 1990).
- Bimonthly urine cultures should be undertaken to ensure the urine remains sterile and colonisation with resistant bacteria does not occur.
- If such colonisation does occur, treatment of the new infection should be undertaken as described above.
- After 6 months of urine free of bacteria, long-term therapy can be stopped and many patients will remain free of infection thereafter.

Disadvantages of such prophylactic drug therapy include the selection of resistant bacteria and chronic drug toxicity. If trimethoprim is administered for periods of longer than 6 weeks, folate supplementation should be provided. Research continues into novel approaches for the management of animals who suffer from recurrent bacterial infections. Methods of increasing glycosaminoglycans production by mucosal surfaces is one line of research (see Senior 1985). Urinary antiseptics, such as hexamine (methenamine) hippurate may be used in place of antibacterial drugs in cases of frequent recurrent urinary tract infections. This drug is converted to formaldehyde in acidic urine (pH 5.5 – usually given with a urinary acidifier) and is safe provided renal function is normal. High doses are required, however, and its efficacy is controversial.

REFERENCES

Allen, T.A. & Jaenke, R.S. (1985). Pyelonephritis in the dog. *Compendium on Continuing Education for the Practicing Veterinarian*, 7, 421–431.

Allen, T.A., Jones, R.L. & Purvance, J. (1987). Microbiologic evaluation of canine urine: Direct microscopic examination and preservation of specimen quality for culture. *Journal of the American Veterinary Medical Association*, 190, 1289–1291.

Aucoin, D.P. (1990). Rational approaches to the treatment of first time, relapsing and recurrent urinary tract infections. *Problems in Veterinary Medicine*, 2, 290–297.

Barsanti, J.A. & Johnson, C.A. (1990). Genitourinary infections. In: *Infectious Disease of the Dog and Cat*, (ed. C.E. Greene), 2nd edn. W.B. Saunders, Philadelphia.

Lees, G.E. (1984). Epidemiology of naturally occurring feline bacterial urinary tract infections. *Veterinary Clinics North America Small Animal Practice*, 14, 471–479.

Lees, G.E. & Forrester, S.D. (1992). Update: Bacterial urinary tract infections. In: *Current Veterinary Therapy XI*, (ed. R.W. Kirk). W.B. Saunders, Philadelphia.

Ling, G.V. (1993). Urinary tract infections. In: *Antimicrobial Therapy in Veterinary Medicine*, (eds J.F. Prescott & J.D. Baggot), 2nd edn. Iowa State University Press, Ames.

Ling, G.V., Biberstein, E.L. & Hirsh, D.C. (1979). Bacterial pathogens associated with urinary tract infections. *Veterinary Clinics North America Small Animal Practice*, 9, 617–630.

Ling, G.V., Conzelman, G.M., Franti, C.E. & Ruby A.L. (1980a). Urine concentrations of five penicillins after oral administration to healthy adult dogs. *American Journal of Veterinary Research*, 41, 1123–1125.

Ling, G.V., Conzelman, G.M., Franti, C.E. & Ruby, A.L. (1980b). Urine concentrations of chloramphenicol, tetracycline and sulfisoxazole after oral administration to healthy adult dogs. *American Journal of Veterinary Research*, 41, 950–952.

Ling, G.V., Conzelman, G.M., Franti, C.E. & Ruby A.L. (1981). Urine concentrations of gentamicin, tobramycin, amikacin and kanamycin after subcutaneous administration to healthy adult dogs. *American Journal of Veterinary Research*, 42, 1792–1794.

Polzin, D.J. (1994). Management of recurrent bacterial urinary tract infections. *Compendium on Continuing Education for the Practicing Veterinarian*, 16, 1565–1571.

Senior, D.F. (1985). Bacterial urinary tract infections: invasion, host defenses, and new approaches to prevention. *Compendium on Continuing Education for the Practicing Veterinarian*, 7, 334.

Chapter 68

Canine Urolithiasis

D. F. Senior and J. Elliott

PATHOPHYSIOLOGY OF FORMATION OF UROLITHS

A urolith results from the crystallisation of lithogenic crystalloids in the urinary tract. Uroliths can form either in the kidney (renoliths) or more commonly in the bladder (urocystoliths). The key feature in the formation of a urolith is the formation of a crystal nidus. Such a nidus cannot form if the urine is undersaturated for the constituent solutes.

- Canine urine is usually supersaturated with respect to several mineral components.
- Crystals spontaneously precipitate when urine is above critical supersaturation as shown in Fig. 68.1.
- Even though spontaneous precipitation will not occur in the metastable range, already formed crystalline particles can continue to grow. On the other hand, crystal particles only dissolve when urine is undersaturated with respect to their mineral composition.

Clearly there are a number of mechanisms that can promote the formation of a clinially important urolith. These include:

- increased filtration of the lithogenic cystalloid (e.g. hypercalciuria, cystinuria);
- dehydration causing the urinary concentration of lithogenic crystalloids to increase;
- alteration in the urine pH which promotes urinary crystallisation (most commonly associated with urease produced by bacteria which hydrolyses urea to form ammonia and carbon dioxide resulting in an alkaline urine pH);
- reduced amounts of inhibitors of crystallisation and/ or crystal aggregation

  - glycosaminoglycans,
  - pyrophosphates,
  - nephrocalcin.

TYPES OF UROLITH

Various types of urolith are found in the dog, reflecting the different minerals that are supersaturated in canine urine (Bovee & Maguire 1984; Senior 1986; Escolar 1990; Senior 1996). The types of urocystolith are shown in Table 68.1 along with some of their characterisitics.

DIAGNOSIS

Clinical Signs

The clinical presentation of canine urocystoliths includes:

- signs of lower urinary tract disease
  - dysuria,
  - haematuria,
  - incontinence;
- urinary tract infection, often recurrent;
- some urocystoliths can be palpated in the bladder;
- some urocystoliths cause blockage of the urethra, particularly in the male dog at pelvic flexure of the urethra and at the base of the os penis, clinical signs of acute postrenal renal failure ensue (see Chapter 62);
- protracted cases can also give rise to ascending infections of the ureters and contribute to the development of pyelonephritis and ureteral blockage.

The evaluation of the clinical problems cited above have been dealt with in Chapters 64–67. Dogs with renoliths are

Table 68.1 Summary of information on canine uroliths.

Mineral	Predisposing factors	Urine pH predisposing to formation	Radiopacity	Crystal appearance	Breed predisposition
Magnesium ammonium phosphate $MgNH_4PO_4.6H_2O$ (struvite)	Supersaturation of urine with magnesium ammonium phosphate Urinary tract infection particularly urease producing bacteria Diet Anatomical abnormalities such as bladder diverticula Genetic predisposition	Alkaline	+ to ++++	Colourless prism	Miniature Schnauzer, Bichon Frisé, Cocker Spaniel
Calcium oxalate	Normocalcaemic hypercalciuria Diet Genetic predisposition	Can form at any pH but urine is usually acidic	++ to ++++	Dihydrate salt, colourless envelope or octahedral shape: monohydrate salt spindles	Miniature Schnauzer, Lhasa Apso, Yorkshire Terrier, Miniature Poodle, Shih Tzu, Bichon Frise
Calcium phosphate	Normocalcaemic hypercalcaiuria Diet Genetic predisposition Hypercalcaemia	Alkaline to neutral	++ to ++++	Amorphous or long thin prisms	Yorkshire Terrier, Miniature Schnauzer, Cocker Spaniel
Urate (ammonium urate and sodium acid urate)	In Dalmatians there is a defect in uric acid metabolism due to failure to convert uric acid to soluble salts along with impaired transport of urate acorss the hepatocyte membrane In non-Dalmatians all urate formed from degradation of purine nucleotides is metabolised by hepatic uricase to allantoin which is excreted by the kidneys In patients with hepatic portal shunts there is increased secretion of ammonia and uric acid into the urine forming ammonium urate crystals	Acid to neutral	0 to ++	Yellow brown amorphous shapes or sphericals	Dalmatian, English Bulldog, Miniature Schnauzer, Yorkshire Terrier
Cystine	In normal dogs cystine is freely filtered by the renal tubules and approximately 100% of the filtered load is reabsorbed in the proximal tubules In dogs predisposed to cystine uroliths only 80–90% is reabsorbed so that 10–20% comes out in the urine Cystine is very insoluble in an acid urine There is a genetic predisposition in certain breeds and lines within a breed	Acid to neutral	+ to +++	Flat colourless hexagonal plates	English Bulldog, Daschund, Basset Hound
Silica		Acid to neutral	++ to ++++	None observed	German Shepherd, Golden Retriever, Labrador Retriever, Miniature Schnauzer

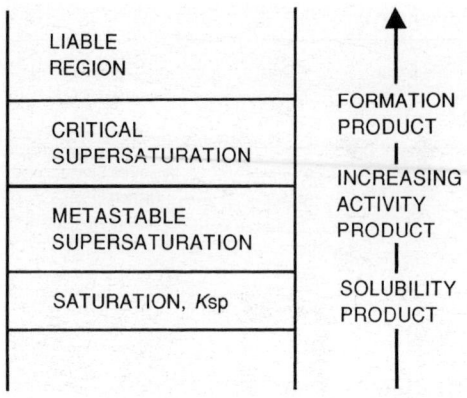

Fig. 68.1 Diagram to show the effect of increasing active product on solution saturation. (From Nancollas 1976.)

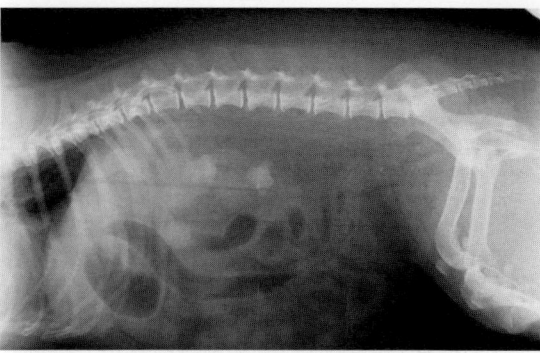

Fig. 68.2 Lateral abdominal radiograph of a dog demonstrating calcium oxalate renal calculi. (Courtesy of Dr F. Barr, University of Bristol, Department of Clinical Veterinary Science.)

often without overt clinical signs and may only be detected serendipitously upon imaging of the abdomen. Renoliths can cause renal colic and ureteral pain although this is rarely recognised. Single renoliths may have no impact on the overall renal function of the dog but the total functional mass will be reduced. In contrast, bilateral renoliths can lead to a progressive loss of renal functional mass with the accompanying loss of renal function and development of chronic renal failure.

Radiographic Appearance and Ultrasonographic Appearance

Radiographic analysis of the anatomical location and radio-density of urocystoliths is helpful because:

- Calcium salt and struvite urocystoliths are the most radiopaque.
- In male dogs, about 60% of radio-opaque urocystoliths are composed of calcium salts (mostly calcium oxalate).
- 20% are pure struvite.
- In female dogs, around 50% of radio-opaque nephro-liths are composed of struvite.
- Around 40% are composed of calcium salts.
- Cystine and ammonium urate urocystoliths tend to be more radiolucent and may require positive and double contrast studies for detection.
- Ultrasonographic evaluation allows location of radio-lucent urocystoliths when a contrast study is deemed to be too time consuming or yields equivocal results (see Figs 68.2–68.8).

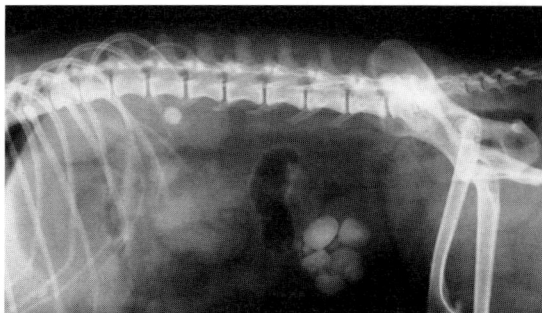

Fig. 68.3 Lateral abdominal radiograph of a dog showing calcium phosphate renal calculi and cystouroliths. (Courtesy of Dr F. Barr, University of Bristol, Department of Clinical Veterinary Science.)

Urinalysis

Urinalysis should be performed to determine urine pH, the presence or absence of infection and the mineral composition of crystals. Other important points include:

- If the urinalysis indicates the presence of urinary tract infection, a bacterial culture and sensitivity test should be performed.
- Crystals in the urine sediment usually match the mineral composition of the urolith.
- Patients with non-struvite urocystoliths can develop urinary tract infection with a urease-producing organism so that struvite crystals appear in the urine sediment.

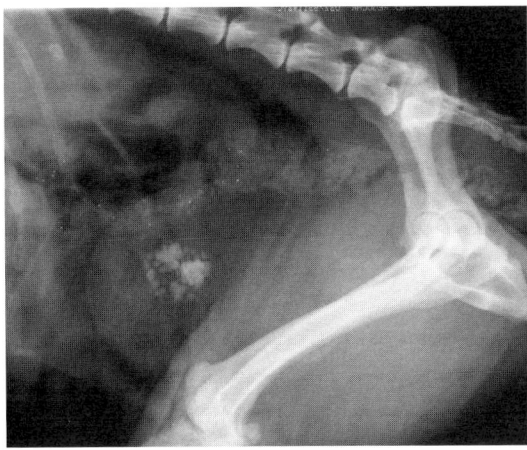

Fig. 68.4 Lateral abdominal radiograph of a dog showing renal struvite urolilths and struvite cystouroliths. (Courtesy of Dr F. Barr, University of Bristol, Department of Clinical Veterinary Science.)

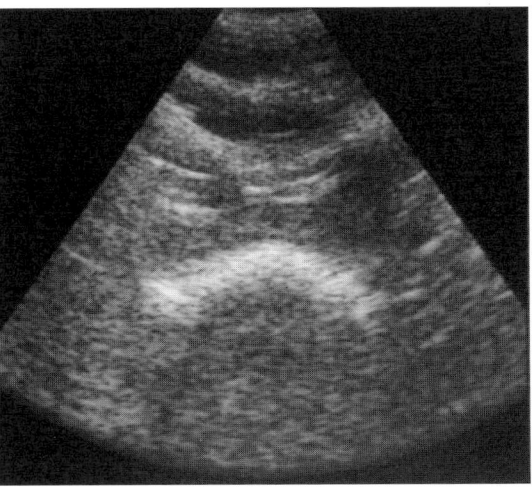

Fig. 68.6 Ultrasound of a renal struvite urolith and associated pyelonephritis. (Courtesy of Dr F. Barr, University of Bristol, Department of Clinical Veterinary Science.)

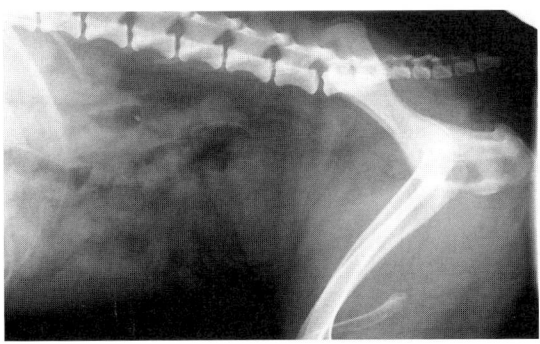

Fig. 68.5 Lateral abdominal radiograph showing the presence of weakly radiodense urate cystouroliths secondary to a hepatic-portal shunt. (Courtesy of Dr F. Barr, University of Bristol, Department of Clinical Veterinary Science.)

- Cystine crystalluria is definitive evidence that the patient has a renal reabsorption defect for cystine.

Examination of urine sediment should be made on fresh urine as soon as possible after collection because precipitation can develop in urine left at room temperature or refrigerated for a prolonged period. Such crystal formation may be irrelevant to the mineral composition of urocystoliths.

Haematology and Biochemistry

Haematological and biochemical evaluation can be a useful aid in the management of some cases of urolithiasis. The measurement of serum calcium levels in cases of calcium oxalate and calcium phosphate uroliths should be undertaken to rule out hypercalcaemia as a potential cause. In cases where urate uroliths are suspected it is appropriate to consider liver function tests including bile acids. In general it is advisable to monitor blood urea and creatinine and to assess glomerular function. The acid–base balance of the patient also has an effect on calciuresis and chronic acidaemia may lead to a gradual demineralisation of bone with enhanced calciuria. Two causes have been proposed to explain this effect, absorptive hypercalciuria and renal leak hypercalciuria. The former is associated with an increased intestinal absorption of calcium which suppresses parathyroid hormone activity and promotes calciuresis. The latter arises from a failure of the proximal renal tubules to reabsorb calcium from the filtrate and as a result leads to a hypercalciuria. These two causes can be distinguished from each other as fasting has no effect on calciuresis in the renal tubular leak form whereas it has a dramatic effect on calciuresis in the increased intestinal absorption form.

In cases where there is a partial blockage of the urethra, biochemical changes compatible with postrenal obstruction, notably azotaemia and metabolic acidosis, are seen. Where bilateral renoliths have destroyed renal mass, with or without infection, biochemical parameters compatible

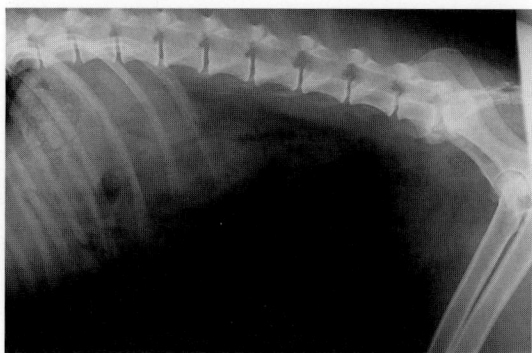

a

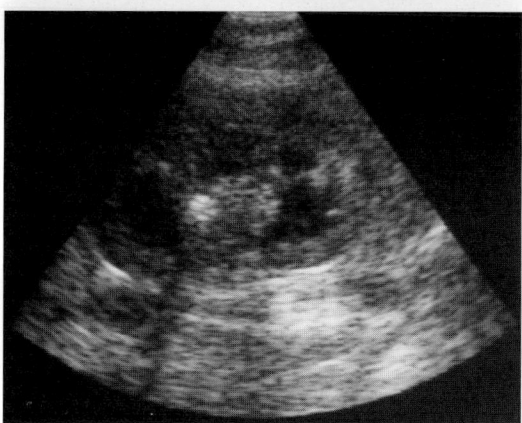

b

Fig. 68.7   (a) Lateral abdominal radiographic showing no evidence of uroliths. (Courtesy of Dr F. Barr, University of Bristol, Department of Clinical Veterinary Science.) (b) Ultrasound of the dog in 68.7(a) showing the presence of urate uroliths. (Courtesy of Dr F. Barr University of Bristol, Department of Clinical Veterinary Science.)

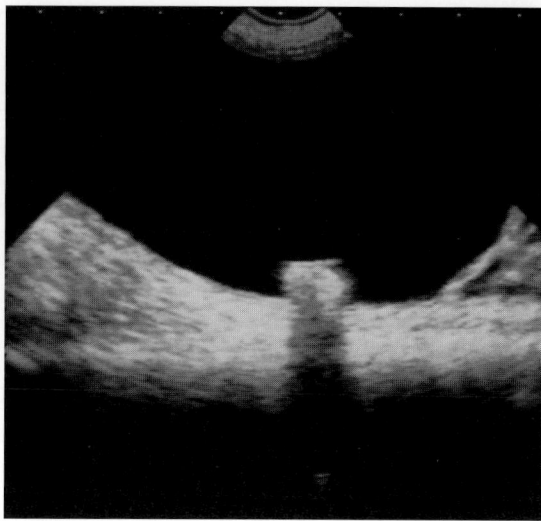

Fig. 68.8   Ultrasound of a bladder showing the presence of a struvite urolith. (Courtesy of Dr F. Barr, University of Bristol, Department of Clinical Veterinary Science.)

with chronic renal failure will be found. If cystine urocystoliths are suspected then measurement of urinary cystine may be helpful.

TREATMENT OF UROCYSTOLITHS

General comments

Accurate assessment of the mineral composition of urocystoliths is essential because the appropriate dietary and medical strategy for dissolution and prevention varies by mineral type.

- A strategy for dissolution and prevention of the wrong mineral may predispose to formation of urocystoliths composed of other minerals.
- The most accurate assessment of mineral composition is direct analysis of a urolith that has been passed spontaneously or recovered by a surgical or non-surgical removal procedure.
- Quantitative analysis such as crystallographic analysis, infrared spectroscopy, and X-ray diffraction are more accurate than chemical analysis for determination of mineral composition.
- Crystallographic analysis is capable of determining the composition of most urocystoliths but infrared spectroscopy or X-ray diffraction are necessary in some instances, e.g. to distinguish between urate and xanthine urocystoliths.

This evaluation should allow a decision concerning appropriate management options which may include surgical removal, urethrohydropropulsion, lithotripsy via cystoscopy, dietary/medical dissolution or vigilant observation. More importantly, the information should allow determination of the mineral composition of urocystoliths so that appropriate strategies may be adopted for dissolution and subsequent prevention of reformation of urocystoliths once they are removed. The management of urocystoliths is a balance between surgical intervention and medical management, the two are not mutually exclusive.

- Where there is a clear predisposing factor, such as urinary tract infection, the key route to success is not the simple removal of the urocystoliths by surgery but the adequate and long-term successful management of the urinary tract infection (see Chapter 67).
- Where there is a genetic predisposing factor, such as defective uric acid metabolism in the Dalmatian, then appropriate steps must be taken to circumvent this problem, repeated surgery is not the answer and medical alternatives must be used (Bartges *et al.* 1994).

Medical Management

The medical management can be considered in two parts, removal of predisposing factors such as infection and alterations in diet to decrease the saturation of crystals in the urine. The management of infections has been dealt with in detail in Chapter 67.

- Dietary manipulation has been successfully used in the dissolution and long-term prevention of the formation of some uroliths.
- The success of this approach is dependent upon modifying the urine so that it becomes undersaturated for the calculogenic crystalloid and produces a urinary pH that minimises the risk of insoluble salts forming.
- This approach has had a profound effect on the struvite urocystoliths and dissolution of the struvite urocystolith can be achieved with the appropriate diet. Once the struvite urocystolith has been dissolved, continued dietary management can be used to maintain urine that is undersaturated with calculogenic crystalloid, the key factor being maintenance of an acidic pH.

Diet alone is seldom effective in the dissolution of urate cystoliths and never effective in cystine uroliths. Allopurinol (15 mg/kg p.o. b.i.d.) is useful in the management of urate urocystoliths as it is an inhibitor of xanthine oxidase which is the enzyme responsible for catalysing the conversion of hypoxanthine and xanthine to uric acid (see Fig. 68.9). As a result increased hypoxanthine and xanthine are excreted in the urine. Hypoxanthine is highly soluble in urine whereas xanthine and urate are less so. The goal of this treatment is to increase the urinary xanthine concentration and reduce that of urate. In the case of cystine, 2-mercaptopropionylgylcine (15 mg/kg p.o. b.i.d.) is required as it forms soluble cystine complexes and avoids crystal precipitation. D-Penicillamine (15 mg/kg p.o. b.i.d.) has been used but this causes anorexia and vomiting in most dogs.

The dietary objectives and other medical considerations are summarised in Table 68.2.

Non-Surgical Removal

Catheter-Assisted Retrieval of Urocystoliths

If the size or shape of urocystoliths preclude their removal by voiding urohydropulsion, smaller urocystoliths that usually accompany larger ones may be obtained for quantitative analysis by aspiration through a transurethral catheter (Lulich & Osborne 1992). A urethral catheter is passed into the bladder, the bladder is palpated per abdomen, and if necessary it is moderately distended by injection of sterile isotonic saline. During aspiration of urine and saline solution into a syringe, an assistant should vigorously move the patient's abdomen up and down. This

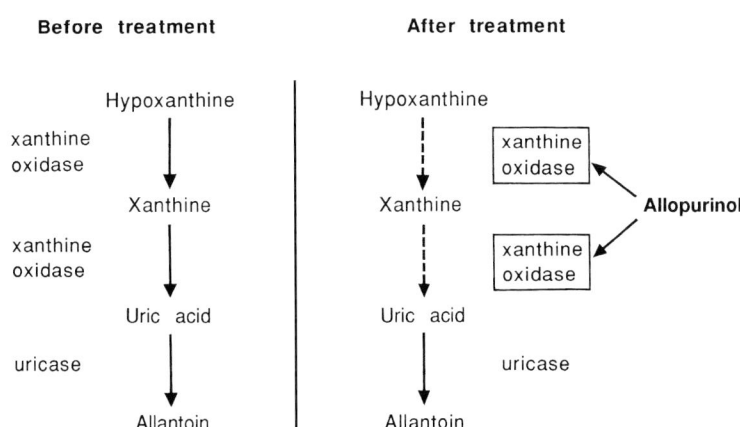

Fig. 68.9 Diagram to demonstrate the normal and abnormal xanthine oxidase pathway.

Table 68.2 Summary of treatment and management of canine uroliths.

Urocystolith	Aim	Objectives	Dietary Characterisitcs	Other management	Comments
Magnesium ammonium phosphate $MgNH_4PO_4.6H_2O$ (struvite)	Dissolution of urocystolith by increasing the solubility of crystalloids in the urine Decreasing the quantity and concentration of calculogenic crystalloids in the urine	Urine pH ≤ 6 SG < 1.015 Low urinary urea, magnesium and phosphorus	Low level of high quality protein, Low magnesium and phosphate High sodium to promote diuresis	It is essential to treat concurrent urinary tract infection	Should not be given to patients with heart failure, hypertension or to growing dogs
Magnesium ammonium phosphate (struvite)	Prevention of urocystolith	Urine pH < 6.5	Low magnesium, low phophorus Mild to moderate protein restriction	It is essential to treat concurrent urinary tract infection	
Calcium oxalate	Prevention of urocystolith formation after surgery	Urine pH 7.0–7.5 Reduce calcium excretion	Avoid excessive consumption of calcium and oxalate Restrict endogenous oxalate production by restricting protein There should be low sodium to avoid increased renal excretion of calcium Added potassium citrate to promote calcium citrate formation in the urine and an alkaline urine	It is essential to treat concurrent urinary tract infection	Nearly always require surgery to remove urocystolith, dietary considerations required to help minimise risk of recurrence
Calcium phopshate Calcium hydroxyapatitie Calcium hydrogen phophate dihydrate Calcium carbonate apatite	Prevention of urocystolith formation following surgery	Urine pH 7.0–7.5 Reduce calcium excretion	Avoid excessive absorption of calcium by feeding a low protein There should be moderate sodium to avoid increased renal excretion of calcium Added potassium citrate to promote calcium citrate formation in the urine and an alkaline urine		Nearly always require surgery to remove urocystolith Dietary considerations required to help minimise risk of recurrence
Urate	Dissolution of urocystolith Prevention of urocystolith formation following surgery	Urine pH 7.0–7.5 Reduce ammonium and urate excretion	Low level of protein to reduce the intake of purines Sodium bicarbonate or potassium citrate to prevent renal tubular production of ammonia	Treat with allopurinol 15 mg/kg p.o. b.i.d. Increase water consumption	Can be dissolved Many require voiding hydropulsion or surgery to remove urate urocystolith Dietary considerations required to help minimise risk of recurrence after surgery Always check to ensure urate crystals are not associated with portosystemic shunt

Table 68.2 *Continued.*

Urocystolith	Aim	Objectives	Dietary Characterisitcs	Other management	Comments
Cystine	Dissolution of urocystolith Prevention following surgical removal	Urine pH > 7.5 Reduce cystinuria	A protein source low in cystine or one that reduces cystinuria Alkalinise urine by adding sodium bicarbonate or potassium citrate to the diet may help	2-mercaptopropionyglycine (15 mg/kg b.i.d.) which forms a soluble cystine complex Increase water consumption	Complications of vomiting and chelation of divalent cations are noted when using D-penicillamine and this should be used with caution Voiding hydropulsion or surgery can be used to remove small cystine urocystoliths
Silicate	Surgical removal		Avoid soil eating to reduce intake of silicates	Increase water consumption	

will cause uroliths to disperse throughout the fluid in the bladder lumen. Small uroliths may then be aspirated into the catheter and collected for quantitative analysis. Identification of the type of urocystolith present will allow a decision to be made as to whether medical dissolution or surgical removal is appropriate. Antibiotic therapy before and after this procedure should be considered.

The limitation with this technique is that only small urocystoliths can be removed but it is an appropriate technique for obtaining small urocystoliths for subsequent analysis. This has a great bearing on the medical management that will be instituted.

Voiding Urohydropulsion

Non-surgical removal of small urocystoliths by voiding urohydropulsion has been described in dogs (Lulich *et al.* 1993). In this technique the patient is either anaesthetised or heavily sedated, the bladder is palpated, and if not distended with urine, it is moderately distended using isotonic saline injected through a transurethral catheter. The catheter is withdrawn, the patient is then positioned so that the vertebral column is approximately vertical, and the urinary bladder is gently agitated to promote movement of urocystoliths into the neck of the bladder. By applying steady pressure to the bladder, urine and uroliths are then manually expressed through the urethra into a cup. This procedure can be repeated until all urocystoliths identified by radiographic or ultrasound investigation have been accounted for. If uroliths are too numerous to count, the procedure is repeated until uroliths are no longer observed

in the expelled saline solution. Radiographic or ultrasound investigation can then performed to ensure that all urocystoliths have been removed. Medical and dietary management will be required following this procedure to minimise the risk of recurrence.

Patients should be selected carefully for urohydropulsion. The relationship of the size and shape of the urocystoliths to the diameter of the urethra should be considered. Urocystoliths of up to 4 mm diameter pass readily through the undilated urethra, however, urethral dilation allows passage of much larger urocystoliths. Uroliths larger than the smallest diameter of any portion of the distended urethral lumen, or those already lodged in the urethral lumen are unlikely to be voided. The urethral lumen can be further dilated with a urethral balloon dilation catheter. Side-effects of urohydropulsion include haematuria, bacterial infection of the urinary tract, and lodging of urocystoliths in the urethral lumen. Haematuria is transient and less severe than that observed following cystotomy, and uroliths lodged in the urethra can easily be flushed back into the bladder. Antibiotic therapy before and after this procedure should be considered since animals with uroliths may already have, or are predisposed to, catheter-induced bacterial urinary tract infections (Lulich & Osborne 1992). Contraindications to this technique include situations in which the bladder integrity is compromised, such as neoplasia of the bladder wall or immediately following cystotomy. Excessive force should not be used to compress the bladder since this may induce vesicoureteral reflux or cause bladder rupture. Lulich *et al.* (1993) reported that urocystoliths were completely removed from 15 of 21 animals in which the technique was attempted.

Surgical Removal

Surgical removal of multiple tiny urocystoliths is often required to relieve and prevent urethral obstruction. Complete removal of all urocystolith particles is often impossible. Where feasible such patients should undergo a full dissolution protocol for at least 6 weeks after surgery before conversion to a prevention protocol.

There are many occasions where surgical removal of urocystoliths for the relief of urethral obstruction is by far the most appropriate course of action. This is particularly so in cases of oxalate, phosphate and silicate urocystoliths for which there are no suitable dissolution dietary protocols. It is essential that appropriate postoperative treatment be given comprising both dietary and medical treatments as the surgery *does not affect the underlying processes that cause the urocystolith(s) to form.* Details of the surgical removal of urocystoliths from the bladder can be found in Waldron (1993). There are occasions when the urocystoliths become trapped behind the caudal aspect of the os penis or at the urethral flexure at the brim of the pelvis. In these circumstances every effort should be made to retropulse the offending urolith(s) back into the bladder so as to avoid urethral surgery. There are however times when this proves impossible and a penile or perineal urethrostomy has to be performed. Details of these surgical procedures can be found in Waldron (1993).

MANAGEMENT OF RENOLITHS

The same prinicples outlined above for the management of urocystoliths apply to the management of renoliths. Where there is diagnostic confirmation or a high index of suspicion that the mineral composition of the renolith is struvite then medical management is a route of treatment. However it should be remembered that patients with bilateral struvite nephroliths are in some degree of renal failure and dietary dissolution with a high sodium, low protein diet can lead to a medical crisis. In cases where the renolith is either calcium oxalate or calcium phosphate, surgical manage-

ment has to be considered and a decision on the procedure made. The choice is nephrotomy, pyelolithotomy or in extreme cases nephrectomy. Where there are bilateral nephroliths the surgeon has to make a decision on which kidney to do first and if it is to be a staged procedure. This is covered in detail by Christie & Bjorling (1993) and the reader is referred there for more complete information.

REFERENCES

Bartges, J.W., Osborne, C.A., Koeler, L., *et al.* (1994). An algorithmic approach to canine urate uroliths. *Proceedings 12th ACVIM Forum*, San Francisco, pp. 476–477.

Bovee, K.C. & Maguire, T.G.T. (1984). Qualitative and quantitative analysis of uroliths in dogs: Definitive determination of chemical type. *Journal of the American Veterinary Medical Association*, **185**, 983–987.

Christie, B.A. & Bjorling, D.E. (1993). Kidneys. In: *Textbook of Small Animal Surgery*, 2nd edn, (ed. D.H. Slatter), pp. 1428–1442. W.B. Saunders, Philadelphia

Escolar, E. (1990). Structure and composition of canine urinary calculi. *Journal of Veterinary Research*, **49**, 327–333.

Lulich, J.P. & Osborne, C.A. (1992). Catheter assisted retrieval of urocystoliths from dogs and cats. *Journal of the American Veterinary Medical Association*, **201**, 111–113.

Lulich, J.P., Osborne, C.A., Carlson, M., *et al.* (1993). Nonsurgical removal of urocystoliths in dogs and cats by voiding urohydropulsion. *Journal of the American Veterinary Medical Association*, **203**, 660–663.

Nancollas, G.H. (1976). The kinetics of crystal growth and renal stone formation. In: *Urolithiasis Research*, (eds H. Fleisch, W.G. Robertson, L.H. Smith, *et al.*), pp. 5–23. Plenum Press, New York.

Senior, D.F. (1986). Canine urolithiasis. In: *Nephrology and Urology*, (ed. E. Breitschwerdt), pp. 1–24. Churchill Livingstone, Edinburgh.

Senior, D.F. (1996). Urolithiasis – a nutritional perspective. In: *BSAVA Manual of Companion Animal Nutrition and Feeding*, pp. 188–197. BSAVA Publications, Cheltenham.

Waldron, D.R. (1993). Urinary bladder. In: *Textbook of Small Animal Surgery*, pp. 1450–1462. W.B. Saunders, Philadelphia.

Chapter 69

Urinary Incontinence

S. P. Gregory

INTRODUCTION

Urinary incontinence is defined as the involuntary passage of urine and is a common presenting sign which mainly affects bitches. A wide variety of conditions may result in urinary incontinence in the dog (see Table 69.1).

Incontinent animals may be presented as juveniles with congenital incontinence or as mature animals with acquired incontinence. In juvenile dogs the commonest causes of urinary incontinence are:

- ureteral ectopia,
- congenital sphincter mechanism incompetence,
- bladder hypoplasia,
- intersexuality,
- pervious urachus,
- developmental neurological abnormalities.

The common causes of acquired incontinence in the dog are urethral sphincter mechanism incompetence (SMI), prostatic disease, bladder neoplasia, ureterovaginal fistula, acquired neurological conditions, urinary retention with overflow and detrusor instability. It is essential to appreciate that several different abnormalities, all potentially causing/contributing to the incontinence, may co-exist within the same animal, so a careful diagnostic plan should be followed. For optimum treatment and prognostic advice, it is essential that all contributory factors are recognised and considered, so that (if necessary), a staged treatment plan can be discussed and agreed with owners, and a realistic prognosis given before sometimes lengthy and costly treatment begins.

PATHOPHYSIOLOGY

The bladder is a unique organ composed of smooth muscle (lined by the urothelium) which stores urine until an appropriate time and place is found by the animal for voluntary elimination. The normal bladder must be a highly compliant organ (i.e. be able to store a large volume with very little change in intravesical and detrusor pressure). The bladder is confluent with the urethra which is also composed predominantly of smooth muscle with a urothelial lining. Contrary to popular belief, there is no discrete urinary sphincter, urethral closure being maintained by a series of complex interacting factors. During the storage phase the urethra is not a patent tube and continence is maintained by resting urethral pressure exceeding the resting intravesical pressure. Factors important in maintaining this closed tube are the resting urethral smooth muscle tone, peri-urethral striated muscle tone, the effect of intra-abdominal pressure acting concomitantly on the proximal urethra as well as the bladder and the 'fleshiness' of the interlocking folds of urethral urothelium. Resting urethral tone may be augmented during times of physical stress by the reflex contraction of striated muscle around the caudal half of the urethra. Anatomical factors which are of particular importance in maintaining continence in the normal animal include normal ureterovesical terminations, a urethra of 'normal length' for the size of the animal and an intra-abdominal bladder neck.

In the normal animal, the processes regulating the filling and emptying cycles of the bladder are complex and rely on the interaction of central, somatic and autonomic nervous systems. The autonomic nervous system is respon-

Table 69.1   Causes of urinary incontinence in the dog (Holt 1990a).

Juvenile dogs	Adult dogs
Ureteral ectopia	Urethral sphincter mechanism incompetence
	Prostatic disease
Congenital sphincter mechanism incompetence	Bladder neoplasia
Bladder hypoplasia	Ureterovaginal fistula
Intersexuality	Neurological disease
Pervious urachus	Detrusor instability
	Cystitis
Developmental neurological abnormalities	Vaginal neoplasia
	Pelvic masses
Combinations of above	Vesicovaginal fistula
	Perineal rupture
	Combinations of above

Table 69.2   Summary of the autonomic and somatic innervation of the bladder.

		Nerves	Spinal segment	Neurotransmitter and receptor at bladder (effect of stimulation)
Autonomic nervous system (Involuntary, smooth muscle)	Parasympathetic	Pelvic	S1–S3	Acetylcholine – muscarinic (contraction of detrusor muscle)
	Sympathetic	Hypogastric	L1–L4 (dogs)	Noradrenaline α- trigone (contraction of urethral smooth muscle) β-body (relaxation of detrusor)
Somatic nervous system (Voluntary, striated muscle)	Pelvic muscles	Pudendal	S1–S3	Acetylcholine – nicotinic (contraction of peri-urethral striated muscle)
	Abdominal muscles	Segmental spinal nerves	Lumbar	Acetylcholine – nicotinic (contraction of abdominal muscles which raises intra-abdominal pressure)

sible for allowing urine storage during filling and urine elimination when the storage system has reached capacity. The somatic and central nervous systems allow the animal voluntarily to control storage and elimination and provide the 'fine tuning' of the system. The actions of the parasympathetic, sympathetic and somatic nervous systems in the control of bladder function are shown in Fig. 69.1. A simplified summary of the autonomic and somatic innervation of the bladder is presented in Table 69.2.

Predisposing Factors

Breed

Golden Retrievers and Skye Terriers appear particularly prone to ectopic ureters strongly suggesting an inherited predisposition (Holt, personal communication).

Urethral sphincter mechanism incompetence affects predominantly large/medium breeds of dog (Holt 1985a)

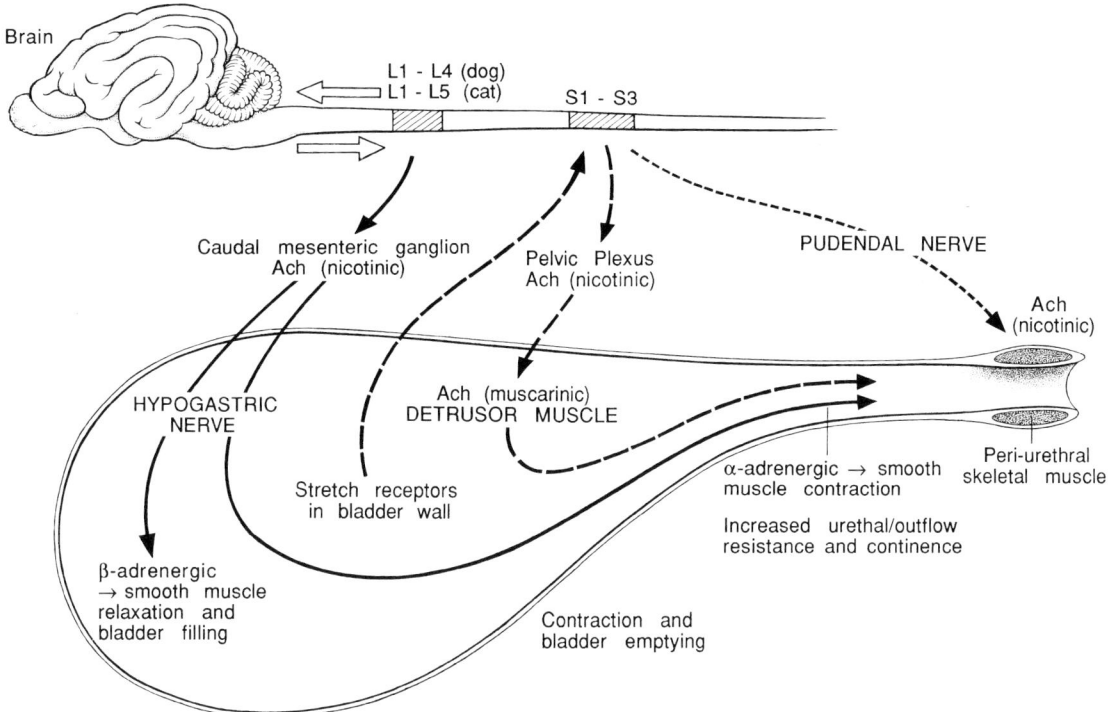

Fig. 69.1 The parasympathetic system is primarily involved with bladder emptying which is mediated via the pelvic nerve. Acetylcholine (Ach) released from the postganglionic parasympathetic nerve endings stimulates muscarinic receptors on the detrusor muscle to cause contraction of the bladder. The sympathetic system is primarily involved with bladder filling and storage and is mediated via the hypogastric nerve. Postganglionic sympathetic nerve fibres when stimulated release noradrenaline which acts on β-adrenergic receptors throughout the detrusor muscle (which mediate smooth muscle relaxation) and α-adrenergic receptors in the urethral smooth muscle and bladder trigone (which cause smooth muscle contraction and maintain urethral pressure above intravesicular pressure). The somatic nervous system affects peri-urethral striated muscle via the pudendal nerve. Somatic efferent nerves release acetylcholine which acts on nicotinic acetylcholine receptors to cause the skeletal muscle surrounding the urethra to contract, thus raising urethral pressure and maintaining urinary continence.

and in particular the Old English Sheep Dog, Rottweiler, Dobermann Pinscher, Weimaraner, Springer Spaniel, Irish Setter and Rough Collie (Holt & Thrusfield 1993).

Neutering

Urethral SMI is seen most commonly (but not exclusively) in neutered bitches (Holt 1985a; Thrusfield 1985; Arnold *et al.* 1989a; Krawiec 1989; Holt & Thrusfield 1993) and neutered male dogs. The mechanism is unclear, however possible explanations include neurological, vascular and hormonal changes following surgical removal of the reproductive tract in the bitch (Gregory 1994).

Docking

Recent work suggests a link between docking and urethral sphincter mechanism incompetence in the bitch. The reason is unclear but may reflect differences in pelvic musculature or urethral nerve supply between docked and undocked breeds.

Body Position

Most bitches suffering from urethral sphincter mechanism incompetence leak during recumbency. It has been shown that intravesical pressure is higher when the animal is recumbent than when it is standing. It is thought that in bitches with caudal bladder necks, the simultaneous transmission of increases in intra-abdominal pressure, to the bladder and proximal urethra, does not occur, resulting in a pressure gradient and the passive leakage of urine.

Obesity

Clinical observations reveal that some obese bitches suffering from urethral sphincter mechanism incompetence spontaneously improve following weight loss. This, together with the observation that incontinent bitches frequently have large amounts of fat surrounding the bladder neck has lead to the yet unproved hypothesis that the fat may shield the bladder neck and proximal urethra from intra-abdominal pressure changes.

Pathophysiology of Incontinence

Urinary incontinence may occur as the result of many pathophysiological processes which are often categorised to aid the understanding of the disease process. Incontinence can be subdivided and classified as neurogenic incontinence, non-neurogenic incontinence (normal anatomy) and non-neurogenic incontinence (abnormal anatomy) see Table 69.3. However, other methods have been suggested which divide or subdivide causes of incontinence into those

that occur due to a failure of storage or those that occur due to a failure of elimination.

Neurogenic Incontinence

Neurogenic incontinence may result from lesions affecting the central or peripheral nervous system and is a common sequel to a wide range of neurological and in particular traumatic lesions in the dog. There is some argument over how neurological lesions affecting bladder function should be classified but they are usually divided into upper motor neurone (UMN) lesions and lower motor neurone (LMN) lesions. Although the following are what is normally expected with UMN and LMN lesions, the signs seen in individual animals may vary and are dependent upon the site and extent of the neurological lesion.

UMN Lesions Affect the Brain → L7

- Cerebral lesions such as brain tumours:
  - These lesions are most likely to affect learned behaviour and therefore result in loss of voluntary control of urination.
- Brain stem and spinal lesions above L7:
  - A loss of voluntary control is caused.
  - In severe injuries to the spinal cord a state of spinal shock may occur where spinal reflexes are temporarily abolished.

Table 69.3 Pathophysiological categorisation of incontinence.

Category	Sub-category	Examples (not comprehensive)
Abnormal neurological examination	Upper motor neurone disorders Lower motor neurone disorders	Thoracolumbar disc lesion Trauma to the pelvic nerves following a RTA

Normal neurological examination	Abnormal anatomy	Congenital
		  Ectopic ureter
		  Persistent urachus
		  Intersex
		Acquired*
		  urethral SMI (caudal position of bladder neck) with
		    relatively short urethras
		  ureterovaginal fistula
		  masses or calculi affecting bladder or urethra

	Normal anatomy but abnormal bladder function	urethral SMI (reduced urethral tone) bladder atony following urinary obstruction detrusor instability (inflammatory or neoplastic disease)

RTA, road traffic accident; SMI, sphincter mechanism incompetence.
* In some cases (e.g. adult bitches suffering from urethral sphincter mechanism incompetence and a caudally positioned bladder neck), it may be unclear whether the abnormality is acquired or congenital.

○ The local reflex arc can remain intact and an increase in intravesical pressure may result in bladder emptying after a variable period of time, usually 4–38 days.

○ Bladder emptying is unconscious and frequently incomplete with high residual volumes.

○ Unconscious urine leakage may still occur if the intravesical pressure exceeds the intra-urethral pressure before the detrusor stretch receptors respond reflexly.

○ There may also be hypertonicity of the striated peri-urethral muscles as a result of lack of higher control and therefore in these animals, while still leaking passively, there may be extreme difficulty in emptying the bladder by manual compression.

- Lesions above L4 may additionally affect sympathetic innervation.
- Anal and perineal reflexes are generally intact.

LMN Lesions Affect The Sacral Cord, Cauda Equina and Pudendal Nerves

- LMN lesions interrupt the sacral reflex arc and therefore are most likely to affect the autonomic and somatic innervation to the bladder and peri-urethral muscle.
- The commonest presenting signs are passive leakage when intravesical pressure exceeds intra-urethral pressure. This may be once the bladder is full or may be precipitated by recumbency or some other external force raising intra-abdominal pressure.
- As the peri-urethral striated muscle is affected manual expression of the bladder is generally easy.
- Anal and perineal reflexes are usually absent.

Reflex Dyssynergia

- This type of incontinence results from a lack of co-ordination between normal detrusor function and hyperactive peri-urethral striated muscle tone. The affected animal's stream of urine may be jerky or tend to dribble or stop soon after initiation.
- It can occur with some upper motor neurone lesions, particularly partial or healing spinal cord lesions, or in neurologically intact dogs following painful pelvic stimulation.

HISTORY

A good history is vital and should enable the clinician to formulate a differential diagnosis list. It is important to allow time to get a full history from the owner and to establish from the owner's description, if:

- the dog is really incontinent and not suffering from dysuria, polyuria, nocturia or a behavioural problem;
- the dog is polydipsic as resulting polyuria may have precipitated the incontinence;
- the dog is able to walk normally;
- the defacation and urination position are normal.

Important historical information which should be obtained in cases of incontinence is summarised in Table 69.4. In addition to these pertinent facts, it is also important to establish if the signs have been treated previously and, if so, with what response.

PHYSICAL EXAMINATION

Thorough physical examination is important but the clinician should be aware that examination of incontinent animals, especially those with SMI, is frequently unremarkable. Other findings on the physical examination may suggest an underlying disease resulting in polyuria which may have precipitated the incontinence. Particular attention should be paid to the following areas when examining an incontinent animal.

External Genitalia

- Are the external genitalia wet or dry? Visible leakage of urine confirms incontinence. Is the discharge urine or some other fluid?
- Are the genitalia sore or inflamed? This provides information about severity of incontinence and owners' ability to cope with the problem.
- Are the genitalia normal in appearance and sited normally? Intersex dogs frequently have a vulva/prepuce which is ambiguous in appearance.
- Proper examination in some long haired animals may require coat clipping. (Ask owners' permission and warn them before you do this.)

Perineum

- Check the perineum for abnormal orifices and evidence of inflammation/soiling.

Abdominal Palpation

- Is the bladder palpable? If so, is it large or small, can any masses be felt? Before drawing any conclusions the owners should be asked when the animal last urinated.

Table 69.4 Important historical features of incontinence.

Age at onset

Since a puppy
- Suspect congenital anatomical abnormalities (ectopic ureters, intersexuality)
- May be first noticed when house training the pet

Over 6 months of age
- Suspect acquired abnormalities
- A possible pre-disposing factor may be identified from the history

Breed
- Breeds known to be prone to ectopic ureters include Golden Retriever, Skye Terrier
- Medium to large breeds are more prone to developing urethral sphincter mechanism incompetence (SMI), especially, the Dobermann, Old English Sheepdog and Rottweiler

Sex

Entire
- Bitches may occasionally suffer from urethral SMI
- Incontinence in entire male dogs is most commonly secondary to prostatic disease
- Bitches are more likely to have an ectopic ureter than male dogs

Neutered
- Most bitches with acquired urethral SMI develop signs within the first year post-spaying
- Continual incontinence post-neutering (days to weeks) – consider acquired ectopic ureter
- Urethral SMI is more likely to affect castrated than entire male dogs

Leakage

Where from?
- Leakage/urination from an inappropriate orifice in animals with congenital abnormalities, e.g. pervious urachus – leak from the umbilicus; intersex – leak from external genitalia or abnormal perineal orifice

When does leakage occur?
- When recumbent, or sleeping – typical of animals with urethral SMI
- Continual urine leakage is suggestive of an ectopic ureter
- Post-micturition dribble suggests an anatomical abnormality allowing urine to collect during urination with subsequent passive leakage (residual uterus masculinus in some intersex animals)

What is leaking?
- Leakage of fluids other than urine may suggest underlying causes or concomitant diseases, e.g. pus may leak from a prostatic abscess; blood may leak from lower urinary tract for a number of reasons (see Chapter 64)

How often does leakage occur?
- Continually – typical of some congenital anatomical abnormalities
- Intermittent (good days and bad) – animals with SMI frequently leak intermittently and have periods of deterioration and spontaneous improvement
- Need to establish this in order that response to therapy can be accurately assessed

How long has the animal shown signs?
- Useful information – gives you an indication of the owner's ability to cope with the problem

Urination (observe where possible)

Normal between episodes of leakage
- Bladder is able to fill and store some urine and the animal has some degree of voluntary control

Increased frequency, straining and haematuria
- Indicates that there may be an underlying or concomitant disease of the lower urinary tract, e.g. urinary tract infection, urolithiasis, urethral or bladder neoplasia (see Chapters 64 and 66)

Stream of urine intermittent
- Underlying cause of incontinence may also be producing partial obstruction of urination, e.g. bladder or urethral masses, reflex dyssynergia

Which orifice does the animal urinate from?
- This information will help in localising some anatomical abnormalities and gives you some indication as to how well the owners observe their animal

Neurological Examination

- Gross neurological deficits such as paraplegia are usually obvious, examination should be tailored to pick up more subtle defects.
- Anal tone – anus should be closed and tone should be felt on digital rectal examination.
- Bulbo-urethral reflex – manual compression of the vulva or bulbus glandis stimulates contraction of the rectum via the pudendal nerve.
- Perineal reflex – perineal stimulation should cause retroflexion of the tail and contraction of the anal sphincter.
- Normal bulbo–urethral and perineal reflexes suggest normal function of the sacral reflex arc.
- Pelvic limb proprioception.

Rectal/Vaginal Examination

- Urethral/prostatic palpation. Assess presence/absence of (1) urethral thickening, (2) prostatic enlargement and asymmetry and (3) pelvic masses.
- Check for a vestibulo-vaginal stricture.
- May be able to palpate caudal or displaced bladder.
- Check for perineal rupture especially if suspect prostatic disease.

Observe Urination

- Can the animal urinate normally?
- Is the stream continuous or intermittent?
- Does the animal initiate urination normally or is there straining?

DIAGNOSTIC TESTS

Urine Tests

Urine should always be collected for routine urinalysis plus bacteriology and sensitivity. In incontinent animals the bladder is frequently empty and therefore hard to palpate making cystocentesis difficult without ultrasound guidance.

Catheterise Urethra and Residual Volume Measurement

This is often done to obtain a urine sample. Can a catheter be passed easily? If so this tends to rule out urethral obstructive lesions. In bitches with SMI the urethra is more easily catheterised than normal bitches and in those with an ectopic ureter, the catheter often preferentially enters the ectopic ureter.

- A catheter placed inadvertently in an ectopic ureter can usually be passed further cranially than would normally be expected, may have a feeling of slight resistance to passage compared with a catheter in the urethra/bladder and urine flow will be small and, if carefully observed, may be peristaltic.
- If ureteral catheterisation is suspected, collect a urine sample for bacteriology as the results may differ from urine within the bladder and can provide useful data to take into account when considering the medical and surgical management of the affected animal.
- Measurement of residual volume can provide useful information particularly if an underlying neurological or obstructive lesion is suspected.
- The gold standard for measuring residual urine is catheterisation immediately post-micturition; however abdominal palpation, radiographic or ultrasonographic examinations may also be a useful subjective measure. Normal bitches should have a residual urine measurement less than 0.2–0.4 ml/kg or <10 ml (O'Brien 1988).

Plain Abdominal Radiograph

These are often unhelpful but can be a useful screen to rule out gross lesions such as calculi. Bladder neck position cannot be accurately assessed from either a plain film or a pneumocystogram. If you plan to follow the plain examination with a contrast study *remember* to give the animal an enema before the study begins. Taking a plain radiograph before the bladder is catheterised is helpful as it gives an indication of the volume of urine retained in the bladder.

Contrast Radiographic Examination

Intravenous urography (IVU) and retrograde vaginourethrography or urethrocystography are important diagnostic techniques. These have been discussed previously but there are several points worth re-emphasising.

- Ensure *all* animals are given an enema before the study as it is very difficult to see ureterovesical junctions if there is a lot of faecal material in the descending colon.
- Contrast medium affects the laboratory investigation of urine, collect samples *before* contrast is injected.
- The injection of ~1 ml/kg of air into the urinary bladder before the i.v. injection of contrast enhances visualisation of uretero-vesical emptying.

- The following film sequence provides the maximum information with the minimum number of films when performing a high concentration, low volume (bolus) IVU:
  - ○ e.g. Urograffin 370™, 700 mg of iodine per kg injected as a bolus (warm first)
  - ○ 0 min VD (ventrodorsal), centred at level of kidneys → nephrogram phase
  - ○ 5 min VD, centred at level of kidneys → pyelogram phase
  - ○ 10 min RLR (right lateral recumbency), centred over the mid abdomen
  - ○ 15 min RLR, centred ~2 cm in front of the hip, this view should include the whole pelvis.
- Ureters empty by peristalsis and it is normal not to see opacification of the whole ureteral length. Complete opacification may suggest an ascending urinary tract infection.
- Vagino-urethrocystography is very useful for confirming the presence of an ectopic ureter. The contrast appears more dense and therefore this examination should be performed after the intravenous urogram to avoid difficulty in assessing the ureterovesical terminations. Care should be taken *not* to inadvertently occlude the external orifice with the Foley catheter tip and in small dogs it will help to cut the end short. The other end may also be modified to allow attachment with a Luer tip syringe if a suitable connector is unavailable. Vaginal filling means that a VD view is usually unhelpful. The dose of contrast required to fill vagina before urethral filling occurs in bitches not under the influence of reproductive hormones is approximately 1 ml/kg (Holt 1989).

Ultrasound Examination of Ureteric Emptying

Despite contrast radiographic examination it can be difficult in some dogs, particularly those with urethral SMI, where the main differential diagnosis is an ectopic ureter, to see both ureters entering the bladder. This is because the ureters empty by peristalsis and, therefore, unless abdominal compression is applied do not normally contain contrast throughout their length. This difficulty observing the ureterovesical junctions on contrast radiography is often compounded in dogs with caudally positioned bladders (owing to superimposition by the pelvis). In cases when it is unclear if ureterovesical emptying is normal, ultrasound examination of the bladder is helpful (Lamb & Gregory 1994).

- The bladder is emptied of contrast medium/gas and moderately filled with sterile saline. The bladder trigone is then imaged and ureteric jets observed.

- The ureteral jets can be seen because of the differing specific gravity of the saline within the bladder and the urine entering the bladder via the ureters.
- No ureteric jet is seen on the affected side.
- If distended, an ectopic ureter may be seen bypassing the bladder neck.
- In dogs with very caudal bladders imaging of ureteric jets may be facilitated by a finger placed per rectum, pushing the bladder neck cranially.

Urodynamic Investigation

Despite there being many significant differences between urethral pressure profiles obtained from anaesthetised continent bitches and incontinent bitches with urethral SMI, the technique is not able to distinguish accurately between incontinent animals and those that are normal on an individual basis.

Detailed Neurological Evaluation

In some animals with neurological signs further more detailed investigation, such as myelography or electromyography, may be indicated.

Test Treatment

The response to trial treatment with a sympathomimetic agent such as phenylpropanolamine or exogenous oestrogens (see later) in cases of suspected urethral SMI, can often provide useful information to support the presumptive diagnosis made from the history and clinical examination.

TREATMENT OF URINARY INCONTINENCE

It is essential for the management of urinary incontinence that a thorough investigation is conducted and a definitive diagnosis has been reached. Details of surgical procedures are not included in this text and the reader is referred to surgical texts for further details.

Ureteral Ectopia

Ureteral ectopia occurs when a ureter bypasses the bladder and opens into the proximal urethra, vagina or uterus. These abnormalities are usually congenital but they can be acquired, most often iatrogenically and typically as a complication of ovariohysterectomy.

- Either sex can be affected but ectopic ureters are more common in females (Holt *et al.* 1982; Hayes 1984; Holt 1990a), and are the commonest cause of juvenile incontinence in bitches (Holt 1990a).
- Ectopic ureters may be unilateral or bilateral and the ureteric openings may be single, double or elongated (troughs) (Stone & Mason 1990).
- They often attach to the external surface of the bladder in the normal position and run, intramurally within the bladder wall, before opening into the proximal urethra (Stone & Mason 1990).
- They can be inherited in certain dog breeds within the United Kingdom (particularly Golden Retrievers and Skye Terriers) (Holt, personal communication).
- They may be associated with other abnormalities of the urinary tract, in particular hydroureter (Mason *et al.* 1990), hydronephrosis, bladder hypoplasia, urethral SMI, ureterocoele, urinary tract infection and vestibulovulval abnormalities (Holt *et al.* 1982; Dean *et al.* 1988).

The aim of treatment is to redirect the flow of urine from the ureter into the bladder by creating a new ureterovesicular stoma or in the case of severe and irreversible renal/ureteric disease to remove the ectopic ureter and associated kidney. The following options are available:

- ureteronephrectomy;
- re-implantation either by;
  - ○ ureteral excision and re-anastomosis via a tunnelling technique, or
  - ○ creation of a new stoma between an intramural ectopic ureter and the bladder lumen;
- if there is concomitant urethral SMI, surgical or medical treatment for this condition will be indicated.

The indications, methods and post-operative care are discussed in detailed surgical texts.

Uretheral Sphincter Mechanism Incompetence (SMI)

Classically the disease affects middle aged, neutered female bitches of medium to large breeds but may also occur in small dogs, entire females, juveniles and male dogs (Holt 1985a). Incontinence is often intermittent and may vary in severity but usually becomes worse with time. In 75% of neutered bitches the clinical signs develop within 3 years of neutering (Holt 1985a; Arnold *et al.* 1989a). SMI may also occur in juvenile bitches before the first season and in these dogs is the second most common cause of urinary incontinence after ureteral ectopia (Holt 1990a). In approximately 50% of these bitches the incontinence will spontaneously improve after the first season (Pearson *et al.* 1965; Holt 1985a, 1990a). In male dogs the disease has not been widely discussed in the literature but is most commonly seen in castrated adults. SMI may also be seen in animals suffering from intersexuality. In summary, compared with continent bitches, affected bitches:

- have shorter urethras (both anatomically and functionally);
- have lower urethral tone;
- have a more caudally positioned bladder neck;
- are usually neutered (mechanism unclear).

The main aim when treating SMI is to restore continence by increasing urethral tone. This may be achieved medically or surgically.

Medical Management

Exogenous oestrogens and sympathomimetic drugs are the two classes of drug usually used to treat SMI. Both classes of drug increase urethral tone.

Oestrogens

- Oestrogens achieve this by improving smooth muscle contractility and elasticity as well as sensitising the urethra to α-adrenergic stimulation, preventing atrophy of the mucous membrane and maintaining turgor of the blood vessels within the urethral wall (Creed 1983).
- The most common problem with oestrogens is that animals become refractory to treatment unless progressively higher doses are given.
- Specific side-effects of oestrogens at high dose rates are bone marrow suppression and aplastic anaemia, thrombocytopenia and leukopenia in the dog.
- They may also cause the dog to become attractive to other dogs or result in enlargement of the vulva, side-effects which are unacceptable to many owners.
- Exogenous oestrogens should *not* be used in entire bitches with juvenile SMI.
- There is a good chance (see above) that a significant number of bitches will spontaneously recover after the first season, which may be delayed or upset if exogenous oestrogens are given. Treatment of choice would be phenylpropanolamine.

Sympathomimetic Drugs

- Sympathomimetic drugs such as ephedrine and phenylpropanolamine act on the α-receptors within urethral smooth muscle resulting in increased urethral tone. They are however, non-selective in their actions and can affect other adrenoceptors in the body.

- The main problem associated with the sympathomimetic drugs is that incontinence is not adequately controlled in a proportion of dogs. However, some owners have reported behavioural changes ranging from lethargy to aggression and hyperactivity following treatment with phenylpropanolamine. The development of other side-effects related to an increase in blood pressure (which, theoretically might be expected to occur) have not, so far, been reported.

Drug Treatment

Drugs used in the treatment of SMI, their dose rates and comments are detailed in Table 69.5. Additional comments relating to medical management of incontinence are:

- Medical treatment usually means life-long treatment. In young animals the implications of long-term medical treatment versus surgical treatment, both in terms of possible side-effects and potential costs, should be discussed with the owner.
- In cases of long-term medical management owners should be encouraged to try to find the lowest dose of a drug which maintains continence to reduce potential adverse effects. In some animals with intermittent incontinence due to SMI, tactical treatment as required is advised.
- Animals refractory to treatment with oestrogens and sympathomimetic agents alone, might respond to a combination of exogenous oestrogens and a sympathomimetic agent.
- SMI in the male dog can be difficult to treat but in the author's opinion phenylpropanolamine is the drug of first choice.
- Overweight animals should be managed such that they regain their normal weight.

- Concomitant urinary tract infections or polyuria/polydipsia should be investigated and treated appropriately.
- Current medicine regulations require that drugs licensed for veterinary use, if available, should be the first choice.

The long-term efficacy of both classes of drugs in large numbers of bitches suffering from SMI is not documented. While it would seem that both types of drug are effective in many incontinent dogs, there are a proportion for whom medical treatment is unsuccessful either in the short or long term. This may be because of unacceptable side-effects, poor owner compliance or recurrence of incontinence.

Surgical Management

The lack of response of some bitches to medical treatment of SMI has prompted a search for surgical solutions to the problem. A number of techniques, many modelled on human surgical treatments for stress incontinence, have been described. These include:

- colposuspension (Holt 1985b, 1990b);
- injections of Teflon and collagen around the bladder neck (Arnold *et al.* 1989b, 1996);
- cysto-urethropexy (Massat *et al.* 1993);
- sling urethroplasties (Bushby & Hankes 1980; Hobson & Bushby 1985; Muir *et al.* 1994);
- the creation of an artificial sphincter (Dean *et al.* 1989).

Intersexuality and Developmental Abnormalities

Intersexuality is uncommon in the dog and not all animals with ambivalent genitalia will be incontinent. However, some are and can provide the clinician with interesting

Table 69.5 Drugs suitable for treating urethral sphincter mechanism incompetence in the dog.

Drug	Dose	Comments
Phenylpropanolamine	1–2 mg/kg 2–3 × daily p.o.	Veterinary licensed product
Testosterone propionate*	0.5–1 mg/kg, 2–3 × per week, s.c./i.m.	Veterinary licensed product
Oestradiol benzoate	1 mg daily for 3 days, then reduce to 1 mg every third day	Veterinary licensed product Injectable 5 mg/ml
Ephedrine hydrochloride	5–15 mg/kg t.i.d. p.o.	Non-veterinary licensed product
Diethylstilbestrol	0.1–1.0 mg/kg daily for 3–5 days, then reduce to 1.0 mg once weekly	Non-veterinary licensed product 1 mg tablets
Ethinyloestradiol	Dose not reported? half diethylstilboestrol dose	Non-veterinary licensed product 10 µg, 20 µg, 50 µg, 1 mg tablets

* Males only.

problems to be solved. Incontinence may be secondary to urethral sphincter incompetence or, more commonly, secondary to anatomical abnormalities which may provide a reservoir for urine to pool following urination and dribble from the vulva or prepuce later. These animals may have a variety of arrangements of genito-urinary anatomy (Holt *et al.* 1983) and in general terms it must be determined whether the problem is secondary to an anatomical or functional defect. These cases should be investigated thoroughly as for any other incontinent animal. Animals with anatomical defects may have other important abnormalities and an effort should be made to rule out all other defects. Having established the internal anatomy, cases with suspected SMI may be treated as described above and animals with obvious anatomical abnormalities (e.g. pervious urachus, uterus masculinus) should be surgically corrected if possible.

Detrusor Instability

In human medicine detrusor instability (DI), is an important differential diagnosis in the investigation of stress incontinence and is typically characterised by urgency, frequency and the inability to store normal volumes of urine within the bladder. The bladder is 'hyperactive' and on cystometric investigation is associated with poor compliance (low volume with high pressure) and waves of detrusor contractions. It would seem that some dogs suffer a similar type of incontinence (Holt 1990a), although there are no reports of this being supported objectively, with detailed cystometric studies in a series of clinical cases. In animals, signs of DI are commonly an adjunct to cystitis or some other bladder irritant. However, signs of DI may be reported in animals that are presented with incontinence where detailed investigation has failed to reveal an obvious cause. In these cases, particularly if they have failed to respond to conventional medical treatment, it is worth trying a short course of an anticholinergic drug (see Table 69.6). These products are unlicensed for use in the dog, are

not specific to detrusor muscle and often have antimuscarinic side effects (e.g. dry mouth, constipation, tachycardia). Clinicians should discuss proposed treatments with the owner before prescribing such drugs.

PROGNOSIS

The prognosis for an animal with urinary incontinence depends on the cause of the incontinence and thus can only be established once a case has been fully investigated and a definitive diagnosis reached. The ability to give a prognosis is therefore often dependent upon the owner's willingness to pay for a thorough work up. In the case of incontinence that is managed medically (e.g. urethral SMI in a bitch) owners should be made aware that treatment may be required for the rest of the animal's life. In some incontinent animals medical treatment may be unsuccessful either because the animal becomes refractory to the drug and dose prescribed or suffers from unacceptable drug side-effects. Anatomical abnormalities may be readily amenable to surgical correction and therefore in general provide an optimistic prognosis, however, it is important to remember that some anatomical abnormalities may require several surgical procedures to correct them (e.g. bilateral ectopic ureters) or may exist in combination with other anatomical abnormalities (e.g. an intra-pelvic bladder neck), and therefore, merit a less favourable prognosis.

In general the prognoses for incontinence are:

- Abnormal anatomy, infection or function, which can realistically be treated medically or surgically, carries a good prognosis.
- Abnormal anatomy in which there is a compromise in restoring normal anatomy carries a guarded prognosis.
- Functional abnormalities responsive to medical treatment carry an optimistic guarded prognosis, provided

Table 69.6 Drugs suitable for treating detrusor instability in the dog.

Drug	Dose	Formulation
Oxybutynin hydrochloride; (Ditropan™)	5 mg b.i.d. – t.i.d.	2.5 & 5.0 mg tablets
Flavoxate hydrochloride; (Urispas™)	100–200 mg b.i.d. – q.i.d.	100 mg tablets
Propantheline bromide; (Pro-Banthine™)	7.5–30 mg u.i.d. – t.i.d., start low	15 mg tablets
Dicyclomine hydrochloride; (Merbentyl™)	10 mg b.i.d. – q.i.d.	10 mg & 20 mg tablets, 10 mg/5 ml syrup

All these drugs are muscarinic receptor antagonists and may cause side-effects, including tachycardia. Dicyclomine is selective for the M_1-receptor and so should cause fewer cardiac side-effects. None of them have a veterinary product licence. Their use should be restricted to animals which have been thoroughly investigated and the pros and cons of treatment discussed with the owners.

medical treatment is maintained, if necessary, long term.

- A neoplastic bladder or urethral mass carries a poor long-term prognosis unless the mass is benign.
- Neurological abnormalities which may not respond to surgical management, often carry a poor prognosis.

REFERENCES

Arnold, S., Arnold, P., Hubler, M., Casal, M. & Rüsch, P. (1989a). Urinary incontinence in spayed bitches: prevalence and breed disposition. *Schweizer Archiv für Tierheilkunde*, **131**, 259–263.

Arnold, S., Jäger, P., Dibartola, S.P., *et al.* (1989b). Treatment of urinary incontinence in dogs by endoscopic injection of teflon. *Journal of the American Veterinary Medical Association*, **195**, 1369–1374.

Arnold, S., Hubler, M., Lott-Stolz, G. & Rusch, P. (1996). Treatment of urinary incontinence in bitches by endoscopic injection of gluteraldehyde cross-linked collagen. *Journal of Small Animal Practice*, **37**, 163–168.

Bushby, P.A. & Hankes, G.H. (1980). Sling urethroplasty for the correction of urethral dilation and urinary incontinence. *Journal of the American Animal Hospital Association*, **16**, 115–118.

Creed, K.E. (1983). Effect of hormones on urethral sensitivity to phenylephrine in normal and incontinent dogs. *Research in Veterinary Science*, **34**, 177–181.

Dean, P.W., Bojrab, M.J. & Constantinescu, G.M. (1988). Canine ectopic ureter. *Compendium on Continuing Education for the Practicing Veterinarian*, **10**, 146–158

Dean, P.W., Novotny, M.J. & O'Brien, D.P. (1989). Prosthetic sphincter for urinary incontinence: results in three cases. *Journal of the American Animal Hospital Association*, **25**, 447–454.

Gregory, S.P. (1994). Developments in the understanding of urethral sphincter mechanism incompetence in the bitch. *British Veterinary Journal*, **150**, 135–150.

Hayes, H.M. (1984). Breed associations of canine ectopic ureter: a study of 217 female cases. *Journal of Small Animal Practice*, **25**, 501–504.

Hobson, H.P. & Bushby, P. (1985). Surgery of the bladder. In: *Textbook of Small Animal Surgery*, (ed. D.H. Slatter), pp. 1786–1799. W.B. Saunders, Philadelphia.

Holt, P.E. (1985a). Urinary incontinence in the bitch due to sphincter mechanism incompetence: prevalence in referred dogs and retrospective analysis of sixty cases. *Journal of Small Animal Practice*, **26**, 181–190.

Holt, P.E. (1985b). Urinary incontinence in the bitch due to

sphincter mechanism incompetence: Surgical treatment. *Journal of Small Animal Practice*, **26**, 237–246.

Holt, P.E. (1989). Positive contrast vaginourethrography for diagnosis of lower urinary tract disease. In: *Current Veterinary Therapy X. Small Animal Practice*, (ed. R.W. Kirk), pp. 1142–1145. W.B. Saunders, Philadelphia.

Holt, P.E. (1990a). Urinary incontinence in dogs and cats. *Veterinary Record*, **127**, 347–350.

Holt, P.E. (1990b). Longterm evaluation of colposuspension in the treatment of urinary incontinence due to incompetence of the urethral sphincter mechanism in the bitch. *Veterinary Record*, **127**, 537–542.

Holt, P.E. & Thrusfield, M.V. (1993). Association in bitches between breed, size, neutering and docking and acquired urinary incontinence due to incompetence of the urethral sphincter mechanism. *Veterinary Record*, **133**, 177.

Holt, P.E., Gibbs, C. & Pearson, H. (1982). Canine ectopic ureter – a review of twenty-nine cases. *Journal of Small Animal Practice*, **23**, 195–208.

Holt, P.E., Long, S.E. & Gibbs, C. (1983). Disorders of urination associated with canine intersexuality. *Journal of Small Animal Practice*, **24**, 475–487.

Krawiec, D.R. (1989). Diagnosis and treatment of acquired canine urinary incontinence. *Companion Animal Practice*, **19**, 12.

Lamb, C.R. & Gregory, S.P. (1994). Ultrasonography of the ureteriovesicular junction in the dog: a preliminary report. *Veterinary Record*, **134**, 36.

Mason, K.L., Stone, E.A., Biery, D.N., Robertson, I. & Thrall, D.E. (1990). Surgery of ectopic ureters; pre and post operative radiographic morphology. *Journal of the American Animal Hospital Association*, **26**, 73–79.

Massat, B.J., Gregory, C.R., Ling, G.V., Cardinet, G.H. & Lewis, E.L. (1993). Cystourethropexy to correct refractory urinary incontinence due to urethral sphincter mechanism incompetence. Preliminary results in ten bitches. *Veterinary Surgery*, **22**, 260–268.

Muir, P., Goldsmid, S.E. & Bellenger, C.R. (1994). Management of urinary incontinence in five bitches with incompetence of the urethral sphincter mechanism by colposuspension and a modified sling urethroplasty. *Veterinary Record*, **134**, 38–41.

O'Brien, D. (1988). Neurogenic disorders of micturition. *Veterinary Clinics of North America: Small Animal Practice*, **18**, 529–538.

Pearson, H., Gibbs, C. & Hillson, J.M. (1965). Some abnormalities of the canine urinary tract. *Veterinary Record*, **77**, 775–781.

Stone, E.A. & Mason, K.L. (1990). Surgery of ectopic ureters, methods of correction and post operative results. *Journal of the American Animal Hospital Association*, **26**, 81–88.

Thrusfield, M.V. (1985). Association between urinary incontinence and spaying in bitches. *Veterinary Record*, **116**, 695.

Section 9

Reproductive Disorders

Edited by Jonathan Elliott and Neil T. Gorman

Chapter 70

Vaginal Discharge

H. K. Dreier

INTRODUCTION

Vaginal discharge can originate in the uterus, the vagina, vestibulum or the bladder. A vaginal flow from the genital tract can vary in quantity, colour, consistency and odour. It can be detected in the presence or absence of diseases of the genital organs, and also in ovariohysterectomised bitches. The causes can be many and varied.

CLINICAL DIAGNOSIS OF NORMAL OR DISEASED GENITAL TRACT WITH VAGINAL DISCHARGE

In every case of vaginal discharge, a clinical gynaecological examination must be carried out at the beginning. The gynaecological examination procedure consists of:

- history,
- clinical examination,
- inspection of the labia and surrounding structures, and of the abdomen,
- examination of genital irritation,
- inspection of the vestibulum, the vagina and the cervix,
- vaginal cytology, and
- palpation of the uterus and the mammary glands.

If necessary, supplementary examinations are carried out, such as:

- haematological investigations,
- hormone assay,
- radiological examination,
- ultrasound examination,
- microbiological and serological investigations,
- chromosomal examination.

In spite of effective investigative techniques such as X-rays and ultrasound, the clinical gynaecological examination should take precedence. Diagnosis of pregnancy in the bitch can be made very easily by abdominal palpation of the uterus between the 25th and 30th day postcoitus in approximately 95% of cases. An ultrasound examination should therefore be used to supplement palpation, and not undertaken as the sole diagnostic procedure.

Equipment Required

A range of vaginal specula is required for different sizes of bitch, with handles fitted with an integral light source or connected to a cold light source. If an endoscope is available, the examiner is better able to assess the genital mucosa with the improved light and magnification. A video camera and monitor enable the findings to be investigated and discussed in a group.

A wire loop with a long handle for the collection of material from the cranial vaginal area, and microscope slides are also needed.

History

The following should be recorded:

- age,
- breed,
- previous diseases,
- vaccinations,
- type of accommodation (house, kennel),
- first oestrus cycle,
- interval between oestrus cycles,
- duration and intensity of previous oestrus cycles,

- any hormonal treatment,
- mating behaviour,
- artificial insemination (AI),
- pseudopregnancy,
- progress of pregnancy,
- number of births,
- progress of parturition and puerperium,
- size of litter,
- previous epsiodes of eclampsia,
- relationship of bitch with neonates, and number of puppies delivered.

Inspection of the Labia and Surrounding Structures and the Abdomen

(Tables 70.1 & 70.2)

In assessing the labia and surrounding structures, the following should be noted:

- size,
- oedema,

Table 70.1 Appearance of the vulva with vaginal discharge: possible physiological and pathological causes.

High-grade oedema	Moderate oedema	Low-grade oedema	Oedema + inflammation	Non-oedematous
Pro-oestrus	Oestrus	Silent oestrus cycle without ovulation	Juvenile vaginitis	Puberty
Prolonged pro-oestrus	Silent oestrus	Metoestrus	Vaginitis	Anoestrus
Granulosa cell tumour	1st week of metoestrus	Closed pyometra	Open pyometra	Cystic glandular endometrial hyperplasia
Vaginal prolapse	Cycle without ovulation	Endometritis	Stump pyometra	Prolonged anoestrus
Residual ovary	Vaginal prolapse	Hydrometra	Foreign body	Endometritis
Accessory ovaries	Accessory ovaries	Mucometra	Endometritis	Vaginal tumour
Parturition	Residual ovary	Fetal maceration	(Pseudo)hermaphroditism	Subinvolution of placental sites
Uterine inertia	Pregnancy	No or insufficient cervical dilatation		
Torsion of the uterus	Hypoluteoidism	Delayed uterine involution		
Uterine prolapse	Abortion	Postpartum period infection		
Retained placenta	Hemorrhage due to pregnancy	Oestrogen therapy		
(Pseudo)hermaphroditism	Uterine prolapse			
Mating injury	Postpartum period Necrosis of placental sites			
Oestrogen therapy	(Pseudo)hermaphroditism Mating injury Oestrogentherapy			

Table 70.2 Abdomen: possible physiological and pathological reproductive conditions which cause changes in abdominal shape.

Marked enlargement	Slight enlargement	Hollow abdomen
Pregnancy >35–40 days	Pregnancy 25–35 days	Early postpartum period
Late abortion	Hypoluteoidism	Retained placenta
Fetal maceration/mummification	Small number of fetuses	
Haemorrhage due to pregnancy	Single fetus pregnancy	
Insufficient cervical dilatation	Insufficient cervical dilatation	
Torsion of the uterus	Retained placenta	
Closed pyometra	Delayed uterine involution	
Uterine tumour	Necrosis of placental sites	
	Open pyometra	
	Granulosa cell tumour	
	Uterine tumour	
	Hydrometra	
	Mucometra	

Table 70.3 Resistance to introduction of the vaginal speculum in cases of vaginal discharge under physiological and pathological conditions.

Introduction impossible	High resistance	Moderate resistance	Smoothly introducible
Remnants of hymen	Oestrous	Late pro-oestrus	All other cases
Vaginal cords (remnants of Müllerian ducts)	Vaginal tumour	Prolonged pro-oestrus	
Vaginal tumour	Oestrogen therapy	Granulosa cell tumour	
		Vaginal tumour	
		Oestrogen therapy	

- vaginal discharge,
- closure of the rima vulvae,
- extent of covering of vulva by the perineum,
- perilabial inflammation,
- necrosis,
- abscesses,
- new growth,
- prolapse of the vaginal mucosa.

Female Tail Deviation Reflex

Before introducing the vaginal speculum, the female tail deviation reflex should be tested by gently stroking the skin dorsal and lateral of the vulva with the finger. Flexing and raising of the tail and lifting of the vulva will occur if the bitch is in oestrus, pro-oestrus, or in a pathological state of hyperoestrogenism, or has a granulosa cell tumour or vaginal prolapse.

Inspection of the Vestibulum

The vestibule with the clitoris lying in the clitoral fossa can be assessed by parting the labia.

Inspection of the Vagina and Cervix

Vaginal Speculum

After introduction of the vaginal speculum, the vagina and cervix are made accessible for examination. The vaginal speculum is moistened with water warmed to body heat, and introduced almost vertically into the steeply sloping vestibule up to the hymen. Care should be taken to avoid introducing the vaginal speculum in the immediate vicinity of the clitoris (it is unpleasant and painful for the patient). The speculum is tilted by about 90° cranially, and in this position it is pushed further into the long vagina with a slightly twisting motion. Ensure that the instrument can be easily introduced (Table 70.3). During oestrus the vaginal speculum will remain in the vaginal and vestibular region without being held.

The tip of the vaginal speculum is withdrawn and rolled on to absorbent white paper in order better to assess the discharge. Then the colour, profile and abnormalities of the mucosa are examined through the vaginal speculum, together with the quantity, colour and consistency of the discharge (Tables 70.4 & 70.5). The examination should not last too long, so that not too much air enters the vagina, where it can change the profile of the mucosa.

Combined Vaginal Speculum and Endoscope

The endoscope is introduced through, and protected by the vaginal speculum. The good light and additional magnification afforded by the endoscope enable detailed information to be collected which could not be obtained with the naked eye alone. This applies above all in small and dwarf breeds where only a very small vaginal speculum can be used with a very restricted field of vision. The gross findings found in such cases are listed in Tables 70.6 and 70.7.

Table 70.4 Inspection of the vagina and cervix in the non-pregnant bitch.

Physiological or pathological state	Vaginoscopy findings
Anoestrus	Colour: rosy pink, no mucosal profile, dorsal vaginal fold
Postpartum period	Colour: rosy pink, no mucosal profile, dorsal vaginal fold
Pro-oestrus	Colour: pale pink, high-grade oedema, deep folds, bloody discharge
Oestrus	Colour: anaemic, increased folding, pale serosanguineous discharge
Metoestrus	Colour: rosy pink, longitudinal folds, greyish white discharge
Juvenile vaginitis	Colour: red, no mucosal profile, grey-green/ yellow discharge
Vaginitis	Colour: red, no mucosal profile, grey-green/ yellow discharge
Glandular endometrial hyperplasia	Colour: pale pink, no mucosal profile, greyish white discharge
Hydrometra	Colour: pale pink, no mucosal profile, watery discharge
Mucometra	Colour: pale pink, no mucosal profile, greyish white discharge
Pyometra with closed cervix	Colour: rosy pink, longitudinal folds, greyish white discharge
Pyometra with open cervix	Colour: pale pink or cyanotic, no mucosal profile, brown-red or greyish green-yellow discharge
Acute endometritis	Colour of cervix: red, colour of vagina: rosy pink, longitudinal folds greyish green-yellow discharge
Suboestrus	Colour: pale pink, low-grade oedema, small folds, bloody discharge
Prolonged pro-oestrus	Colour: anaemic, constricted vaginal lumen, bloody discharge (contains clots)
Granulosa cell tumour	Colour: anaemic, constricted vaginal lumen, bloody discharge
Vaginal prolapse	Colour: pale pink or anaemic, high-grade oedema, deep folds or increased folding Bloody or pale serosanguineous discharge
Urovagina	Colour: red, vagina tilted craniovertrally, pool of liquid in cranial vagina
Mating injury: vagina	Colour: anaemic, perforation of the vagina in the cranial area: red wound, wall of urinary bladder and/or mesometrium visible, bloody discharge (contains coagula)
Mating injury: clitoris	Rupture of the clitoris, high grade bloody discharge (contains coagula)
Foreign body	Colour: rosy pink, grey-green yellow discharge, foreign body sometimes visible

Table 70.5 Inspection of the vagina and cervix in pregnancy, parturition and in the postpartum period.

Physiological or pathological state	Vaginoscopy findings
Pregnancy	Colour: pale pink, oedema, greyish white or yellow discharge
Hypoluteoidism	Colour: pale pink, oedema, bloody red-brown discharge (contains coagula)
Abortion	Colour: red, oedema, open cervix, disagreeably coloured placenta + fetus, black and green partly brown discharge
Fetal maceration	Colour: red, oedema, open cervix, disagreeably coloured placenta + fetus, bloody or red-brown discharge
Fetal mummification	Colour: pale pink, oedema, greyish white or yellow discharge
No or insufficient dilatation of cervix	Colour: pale pink, closed cervix, green discharge
Parturition	Colour: pale pink, high-grade oedema, open cervix, fetal sac, fetus, green discharge
Uterine torsion	Colour: red, open cervix, violent contractions, no fetal sac or fetus, bloody discharge
Uterine inertia	Colour: pale pink, oedema, open cervix, flabby fetal sac, fetus and placenta, green discharge
Retained placenta	Colour: pale pink, oedema, open cervix, flabby fetal sac, fetus and placenta, green discharge
Uterine prolapse	Colour: grey red, violent contractions, bloody discharge, partial prolapse of the uterus into the vagina or complete prolapse of both horns, mucosal necrosis
Postpartum period	Colour: pale pink, numerous petechiae and haematomas, bloody brown-red discharge + tissue detritus
Delayed involution of uterus	Colour: pale pink, cyanotic, greyish red-brown discharge
Necrosis of placental sites	Colour: pale pink, cyanotic, greyish red-brown discharge
Postpartum infection	Colour: pale pink, cyanotic, greyish red-brown discharge
Postpartum intoxication	Colour: pale pink, cyanotic, greyish red-brown discharge
Haemorrhage due to pregnancy	Colour: pale pink, bloody discharge (contains coagula)
Subinvolution of placental sites	Colour: pale pink, bloody discharge

LABORATORY INVESTIGATION

Vaginal Cytology

Vaginal cytology permits a more exact assessment of the cycle and helps to confirm, extend and also to correct the clinical findings. Physiological and pathological conditions of the hormone balance can be inferred from the results of smears taken from the vaginal epithelium.

Obtaining Samples for Vaginal Cytology

Samples can be taken either blind from the vestibule by parting the labia, or from the vagina by looking down a vaginal speculum. The material for investigation is taken from the dorsal or lateral area of the vagina in a cranial to caudal direction using gentle pressure with a wire loop, and is transferred onto a degreased microscope slide and distributed as thinly and evenly as possible using a circular motion. A rough assessment of the smear can be made as it is being spread out – whether it is liquiform-bloody, greyish-matt or mucous, and whether it contains mucosal remnants. Obtaining cellular material with a cotton wool swab is not as successful as with the loop, because fragments of cotton wool can affect the smear. The prepared smears are all fixed in a mixture of ether and 96% alcohol for 20–30 min, or with a fixing spray, or air dried for 12–24 h, or passed over a flame two or three times (heat fixing). The smears are either Papanicolaou or Gram stained. In practice rapid staining can be done with Diff Quik™.

Cytological Assessment

When obtaining results, the following sequence should be followed. The prepared slide is first examined under

Table 70.6 Colours of vaginal discharge in the non-pregnant bitch under physiological and pathological conditions.

Bloody	Pale serosanguineous	Red-brown	Greyish white	Brown-red	Grey-green/yellow	Watery
Pro-oestrus (l)	Oestrus (l)	Abortion (m)	Metoestrus (m)	Open pyometra (l, m)	Juvenile vaginitis (m)	Urovagina (l)
Suboestrus (m)	Accessory ovaries (l)	Metoestrus (1st week) (m)	Vaginal tumour (m)	Stump pyometra (l, m)*	Vaginitis (m)	Cystic endometrial hyperplasia
Mating injury (c)	Residual ovary (l)	Prolonged pro-oestrus (l)	Pseudopregnancy (m)		Open pyometra (m)*	Hypertrophy of clitoris
Prolonged pro-oestrus (c)	Oestrogen therapy (l)	Suboestrus (m)	Mucometra (m)		Endometritis (m)	hyperplasia (l)
Granulosa cell tumour		Accessory ovaries (l)	Stump tumour (m)		Stump pyometra (m)	Hydrometra (l)
Stump haemorrhage (c)		Residual ovary (l)	Accessory ovaries (m)		Foreign body (m)	
Accessory ovaries (l)		Oestrogen therapy (l)	Residual ovary (m)			
Residual ovary (l)			Cystic endometrial hyperplasia (m)			
Oestrogen therapy (l)						

* Putrid odour.
Consistency is indicated by the following letters: l, liquiform; m, mucoid; c, contains coagula.

Table 70.7 Colours and consistency of vaginal discharge in pregnancy, parturition and in the postpartum bitch under physiological and pathological conditions.

Greyish-white-(yellowish)	Bloody or red-brown	Black and green, partly brown	Vitreous + greyish-white flakes	Green	Grey and red-brown (in)
Pregnancy (m)	Hypoluteoidism (l, m, c)	Abortion (l, m)	Onset of delivery (l, m)	Parturition (l, m)	Delayed uterine involution (l)
Fetal mummification (m)	Fetal maceration (m, d)*				Insufficient cervical dilatation (l, m)
	Haemorrhage due to pregnancy (l, m, c)				Necrosis of placental sites (d)*
	Parturition (l)				Uterine inertia (l)
	Torsion of the uterus (l)				Postpartum infection (l, m)
	Postpartum haemorrhage (m)				Retained placenta (l)
	Subinvolution of placental sites (m)				

* Putrid odour.
(in) indicates heterogeneous colouring. Consistency is indicated by the following letters: l, liquiform; m, mucoid; d, contains detritus; c, coagula.

100× magnification to assess the quality of the smear, cell distribution and the type of cell stain, then the whole of the smear is looked at randomly, and at least 100 cells from several fields of vision examined for diagnosis. Cellular elements present in a smear can include epithelial cells, erythrocytes, leucocytes, embryonic cells and sperm. Differentiation of the epithelial cells is significant (Tables 70.8 & 70.9).

Palpation of the Uterus and Mammary Gland

The examination begins with the identification of the cervix and ends with the horns of the uterus, or, rarely,

with the clearly enlarged ovaries. Palpation should proceed with no preconceptions. Primary evidence of a normal large uterus is sought, so that deviations from the norm can be detected. Except in very excitable or overweight bitches, abdominal palpation reveals a clear dimensional ratio between the cervix and the body and horns of the uterus. The ovaries usually escape palpation unless they are tumorous or have undergone high grade cystic changes. Ideal conditions for palpation are afforded by the stretched abdominal wall immediately after parturition.

Examination of the mammary glands is carried out with the patient in a supine position. In assessing the mammary tissue, note should be taken of the number and symmetry of the mammary glands, size, inflammation, necrosis, abscesses and tumours.

Table 70.8 Summary of vaginal epithelial cell cytology.

Basal cells:	Cells measuring 10–20 µm, cylindrical shape with the nucleus at the base, basophilic stain
Parabasal cells:	Cells measuring 15–25 µm, round shape, nucleus in the middle, basophilic stain. Intermediate cells: 20–30 µm, elongated or elliptical shape, acidophilic stain, nucleus in most cases on the periphery
Lower superficial cells:	35–60 µm, polygonal appearance, nucleus has a clear chromatin structure like the basal, parabasal and intermediate cells, stain is either basophilic or acidophilic
Upper superficial cells:	Like lower superficial cells in size and shape; the cell edges are raised to varying degrees; the nucleus is altered by pyknosis, karyorrhexis or karyolysis
Flakes:	Anuclear cells, like the superficial cells in size and shape

Table 70.9 Cell content of vaginal smear under different physiological and pathological conditions.

	BC	PBC	IMC	SFC	AC	RBC	WBC	BAC	CD	MUC	BAS	ACI	DIS	SP
Anoestrus	+	+	+	−	−	−	+	−	−	(+)	+	−	−	−
Pro-oestrus, early	−	+	+	−	−	++	(+)	−	−	(+)	+	−	−	(+)
Pro-oestrus, late	−	−	(+)	+	+	+	−	(+)	(+)	−	−	+	−	(+)
Oestrus	−	−	−	+	+	(+)	−	(+)	(+)	−	−	+	−	(+)
Silent oestrus	−	−	−	+	+	−/(+)	−	(+)	(+)	−	−	+	−	(+)
Metoestrus	+	+	+	−	−	−	+	−	−	+	+	−	−	(+)
Pregnancy	+	+	+	−	−	−	+	−	−	+	+	−	−	−
Prolonged pro-oestrus	−	−	−	+	+	+	−	+	+	−	−	−	+	−
Granulosa cell tumour	−	−	−	+	+	+	−	+	+	−	−	−	+	−
Endometritis	−	+	+	+	+	+	+	+	+	+	+	+	+	−
Pyometra, closed	+	+	+	−	−	−	+	−	−	+	+	−	−	−
Pyometra, open	−	+	+	(+)	−	+	+	+	+	+	+	−	+	−

++, high numbers present; +, present; (+), sometimes present; −, absent.
BC, basal cells; PBC, parabasal cells; IMC, intermediate cells; SFC, superficial cells; AC, anuclear cells; RBC, red blood cells; WBC, white blood cells; BAC, bacteria; CD, cell detritus; MUC, mucus; BAS, basophilic cells; ACI, acidophilic cells; DIS, discoloured cells; SP, sperm.

Haematological Investigations

Haematology is of questionable value in the diagnosis of gynaecological pathology. Even with pyometra, the blood parameters are often only changed to an insignificant degree, or not at all. They are therefore predominantly of supplementary importance to the clinically and gynaecologically determined diagnosis. Their particular value is in the formulation of a prognosis and the selection of therapy (Table 70.10).

Hormone Assay in Serum/Plasma

Hormone analysis in the blood is another way of further explaining physiological and pathological reproductive processes. Using radioimmmunoassays (RIA), oestrogen, progesterone, luteinising hormone (LH) and follicle stimulating hormone (FSH) can be quantitatively detected. The semiquantitative detection of progesterone is of particular significance in practice (Premate™, Target Canine Ovulating Timing Test™), as it can be carried out quickly, and the test kits are readily available (Table 70.11).

Table 70.10 Altered blood parameters in diseases of the genital organs with vaginal discharge.

Blood sedimentation rate-increased	Neutrophilia	Monocytosis	Lymphopenia	Eosinopenia
Prolonged pro-oestrus Endometritis Pyometra Pregnancy Fetal maceration Fetal mumification Postpartum infection Necrosis of placental sites	Cystic glandular endometrial hyperplasia Prolonged pro-oestrus Endometritis Pyometra Fetal maceration Fetal mummification Postpartum infection Necrosis of placental sites	Cystic glandular endometrial hyperplasia Prolonged pro-oestrus Endometritis Pyometra Fetal maceration Fetal mummification Postpartum infection Necrosis of placental ites	Cystic glandular endometrial hyperplasia	Prolonged pro-oestrus Endometritis

Hematocrit decreased	Creatinine and BUN increased
Prolonged pro-oestrus Granulosa cell tumour Endometritis Pyometra with haemorrhage Pregnancy Fetal maceration Fetal mummification Postpartum period Postpartum infection Necrosis of placental sites	Endometritis Pyometra Fetal maceration Fetal mummification Postpartum infection Necrosis of placental sites

BUN, blood urea nitrogen.

Decreased oestrogen	Increased oestrogen	Decreased progesterone
Suboestrus	Pro-oestrus	Oestrus without ovulation
	Hyperoestrogenism	Hypoluteoidism
	Oestrus	Abortion
	Prolonged pro-oestrus	Fetal maceration
	Granulosa cell tumour	Fetal mummification
	Pregnancy	

Table 70.11   Altered blood hormone levels in physiological states and diseases of the genital organs with vaginal discharge.

Microbiological and Serological Examination

In the conservative treatment of gynaecological pathology, and in the context of the care of breeding bitches, microbiological culture and antibiotic sensitivity testing are necessary. In suspicious cases, serological investigation for *Brucella canis* and *Toxoplasma gondii* is indicated.

DIAGNOSTIC IMAGING
Ultrasound

Ultrasound examination of the abdomen is carried out with a 5, 7.5 or, for larger breeds in rare cases, a 3.5 MHz transducer.

The patient is shaved and fasted, and is examined with a full bladder in a dorsal or slightly inclined lateral position. Starting from the urinary bladder, the uterus is examined. Any changes in organs can be recognised by an increased accumulation of fluid. In diseases like cystic endometrial hyperplasia, endometritis, pyometra, hydrometra and mucometra, the size, thickness of the walls, diameter of the lumen and amount of cells in the fluid can be assessed. Pregnancy can be established with certainty from the 25th day. Determination of the number of fetuses is not possible.

Radiographic Examination

The patient is placed in the lateral position and well stretched out. Emptying the bowel before examination is recommended, but emptying the bladder is unnecessary, as often a narrow uterine shadow can be seen better in the homogeneous soft tissue shadow of the bladder when it is fuller. Depending on the clinical findings, where there are alterations in the hypogastrium and the pelvis, better information on the changes in size and position of the dense abdominal organs can be obtained on X-ray by a contrasting presentation of the rectum and bladder. In addition, those organs attached by a short mesentery, like the ovary and the body and horns of the uterus, can be well defined with the help of a pneumoperitoneum. The ovaries and uterus can sometimes only be detected on X-ray when there has already been a considerable change in size. As with palpation, it is best to look for the area between the rectum and the urinary bladder and carefully examine the region around the apex of the bladder. The uterine bifurcation can generally be defined here. The horns of the uterus first bend slightly towards the cranioventral, then rise upwards. After that they are lost in the convolutions of the small intestine. A physiologically large uterus is rarely seen in young bitches. In older animals the uterus is sometimes seen in metoestrus as a sharply defined homogeneous soft tissue shadow, particularly if a low density fat deposit is present in front of the apex of the urinary bladder. The width and density of the horns is like that of the empty tonic coils of the jejunum, which can extend into the pelvic cavity. It is easy to confuse the two if the bifurcation cannot be defined.

Pregnancy can be recognised with certainty from the 50th day when the fetal skeleton can be detected. An exact determination of the number of fetuses is possible from the 55th day if the number is not too high.

DISEASES OF THE GENITAL ORGANS CAUSING VAGINAL DISCHARGE IN THE NON-PREGNANT BITCH

In the non-pregnant bitch coming into oestrus once or twice a year, the period when most diseases of the genital organs with vaginal discharge occur can be restricted to

Table 70.12 Diseases of the genital organs with vaginal discharge in the non-pregnant bitch.

Ovaries	Uterus	Vagina	Vestibulum
Suboestrus	Cystic glandular	Juvenile vaginitis	Mating injury
Hyperoestrogenism	endometrial hyperplasia	Mating injury	Clitoral hypertrophy
Prolonged pro-oestrus	Hydrometra	Vaginal prolapse	
Granulosa cell tumour	Mucometra	Vaginal tumour	
Accessory ovaries	Endometritis	Foreign body	
Residual ovary	Pyometra with closed cervix	Urovagina	
	Pyometra with open cervix		
	Stump pyometra		
	Uterine tumour		
	Stump haemorrhage		

about 2.5 months of the sexual cycle Table 70.12. This includes the period of ovarian activity with pro-oestrus, oestrus and metoestrus.

Diseases of the Ovary

Suboestrus

See Chapter 71 on female and male infertility.

Hyperoestrogenism

Normal Oestrus Cycle with Hyperoestrogenaemia
An apparently physiological oestrus cycle can cause hyperoestrogenaemia, which can have various effects on patients (Dreier *et al.* 1987).

High Grade Oestrous Bleeding
Many oestrus cycles are accompanied by such intensive bleeding that the haematocrit is clearly reduced or even reaches life-threatening levels. Most affected are breeds that also display pronounced vulval oedema, like Boxers, Dobermanns, Bulldogs, Mastiffs and others.

Changes in the Skin and Coat
Hyperoestrogenaemia in a bitch with a normal cycle can lead to changes in the coat and skin. The dermatological changes are: dull and shaggy coat; at first localised and later more widespread loss of hair; varying degrees of hyperkeratosis and pigmentation. At first the changes occur laterally from the spinal column, above the kidneys and ovaries and, as the disease continues, they extend to the start of the tail, the perineum, inner thighs and lower abdomen. In anoestrus these changes are reversible, and the bald patches disappear or become smaller. With each further stage in the cycle (pro-oestrus, oestrus, metoestrus) the bald areas become larger, and hyperkeratosis and pigmentation increase.

Prolonged Pro-oestrus

A prolonged pro-oestrus is present when labial oedema, vaginal discharge and altered behaviour persist beyond the physiological duration of pro-oestrus, or are observed again after a short pause (Arbeiter 1971; Dreier *et al.* 1987). Prolonged pro-oestrus is subdivided into types A, B and C.

Type A
Pro-oestrous phenomena do not subside, or else they recur after 8–14 days. Signs are: enlarged labia of a doughy oedematous consistency; swollen pale pinky red vaginal mucosa; and flesh coloured to brown-red vaginal discharge with coagula. Because of the excessively long oestrogenic effect, the vaginal smear usually shows a rise in organisms leading to discoloration (greyish red, grey, grey-blue) and an increase in cell detritus. The uterus is thickened and rounded, and the ovaries contain follicles or cysts. The average age is from 1 to 2 years.

Type B
About 3–4 weeks after a less pronounced pro-oestrus, symptoms reappear. There are various degrees of indurate labia and vestibular wall; hyperplastic thickened anaemic vaginal mucosa which narrow the vaginal passage; and a whitish discharge which gives the mucous membrane a mother-of-pearl sheen. Vaginal cytological findings are as in type A. The cervix is bulbous and thickened; and the ovaries are hardened and cystic. The average age is 5–6 years.

Type C

Following a normal pro-oestrus and pseudopregnancy, symptoms of pro-oestrus recur. Signs are: indurate labia and genital mucus; different vaginal discharge according to the hormonal influence (oestrogen, progesterone). The cervix is bulbous and enlarged; and the ovaries are thickened and round. Follicles and corpora lutea are present on the ovaries. Lactation is established. The average age is 3–4 years.

Therapy
Types A + B

- Hormone treatment: check red blood cell count before starting hormones. Warn owner about possible relapse after a future pro-oestrus, and give antibiotics for one week.
- Proligestone (Delvosteron™) in a dosage of 10–30 mg/kg bodyweight subcutaneously. In some circumstances a second treatment with half the dose is necessary after 10–14 days (Arbeiter & Lorin 1981).
- Ovariohysterectomy: with a severe anaemia, after unsuccessful hormone treatment or if the owner wishes it.

Type C

- Ovariohysterectomy

Granulosa Cell Tumour

This can occur on one side (more commonly) or on both sides, and become quite large. It can produce oestrogens which have the effect of causing massive indurative changes to the entire genital tract, as with a prolonged pro-oestrus of type B. Endometritis or pyometra can also occur. Depending on how long the tumour has existed, the patient will display loss of appetite, polydipsia, polyuria, emaciation, enlarged pear-shaped abdomen, high-grade changes in the coat and skin in the form of seborrhoea, hyperkeratosis and hyperpigmentation. Diagnosis is easily made on the basis of changes in the genital organs, X-ray, and ultrasonography results.

Therapy

- Ovariohysterectomy.
- Unilateral oophorectomy to retain the breeding capability of the bitch if the owner so wishes. The wisdom of this procedure should be discussed with the owner.

Residual Ovary

An oestrus cycle is observed again after ovariohysterectomy if an ovary or part or parts of an ovary (residual ovary) are left behind after surgery.

Therapy
Surgical removal of the germinative tissue.

Diseases of the Uterus

Cystic Glandular Endometrial Hyperplasia

Low-grade to moderate cystic glandular endometrial hyperplasia is usually only an incidental finding in the context of ovariohysterectomy or section. If high-grade cystic changes in the endometrial mucosa are present, firm enlarged labia, pale pink to anaemic vaginal mucosa and a cloudy mucous discharge are evident. There is a dense covering of vesicles, from miliary to pea-sized (Arbeiter 1966). In extreme cases the uterus can be several finger-breadths wide.

Therapy
Ovariohysterectomy.

Hydrometra

Very often a chance finding. The patient is in good general health, and is presented when varying quantities of a watery vaginal discharge are noticed. The vulva shows low-grade oedema, the vaginal mucosa is pale pink and has no profile. The uterus is thin-walled and can be up to several finger-breadths wide.

Therapy
Ovariohysterectomy.

Mucometra

This is also usually a chance finding. The patient displays no unusual behaviour and is presented because of a grey-white mucous vaginal discharge. The vulva shows low-grade oedema, the vaginal mucosa is pale pink and has no profile. The wall of the uterus is thin and the uterus can be up to several fingerbreadths wide.

Therapy
Ovariohysterectomy.

Endometritis

Acute Purulent Endometritis

In acute purulent endometritis, a discharge of pus is observed approximately 2–4 weeks after the end of the oestrus cycle. Patients are presented with high-grade exhaustion, loss of appetite and an increased internal body temperature. The mucosae are dry and reddened. The episcleral vessels show high-grade injection. The cervix is very reddened ('glaring red' is the pathognomonic), and yellow pus is discharging through the opened cervix. Palpation is painful and reveals a low-grade enlargement and solidity of the uterus.

Therapy

- Antibiotics and, if necessary, prostaglandin $F_{2\alpha}$: 50–250 µg/kg dinoprost s.c., b.i.d. over 5 days, with clinical and ultrasound checks.
- Ovariohysterectomy with intensive fluid therapy.

Chronic Purulent Endometritis

Chronic purulent endometritis is the final stage in a spontaneously degenerating pyometra. The sustained duration of the disease leads to exhaustion, loss of appetite, pale mucosa and a shaggy coat. Low-grade mucous/purulent discharge and low-grade enlargement and thickening of the uterus are evident.

Therapy

- Antibiotics and, if necessary, prostaglandin $F_{2\alpha}$: 50–150 µg/kg dinoprost s.c., b.i.d. over 5 days, with clinical and ultrasound checks.
- Ovariohysterectomy with intensive infusion therapy.

Pyometra

Pyometra is an inflammation of the uterus which causes an accumulation of pus in that organ. Progesterone closes the cervix and the pus cannot escape. Usually both horns of the uterus are affected, rarely only a single horn. The body of the uterus is usually of a solid consistency and almost never enlarged to the same extent as the horns.

Where there is a moderate accumulation of pus, the horns of the uterus have segment-shaped adhesions. In high-grade accumulations, the wall of the uterus becomes atrophic due to pressure and thin. In extreme cases, pus enters the abdominal cavity via the oviducts (pus pertubation) or via rupture of the wall of the uterus. Uterine rupture can occur as a result of trauma, jumping or merely by lifting the patient on to the examining or operating table, for example. The consequence is peritonitis. The patient has no appetite, a high fever, is vomiting, breathing heavily, has reddened, dry mucosae, high-grade injected episcleral vessels, a rapid pulse and a poorly filled vessel, draws the back up high and is dehydrated. Palpation of the abdomen only causes pain in the acute phase from 1–2 days, and there are no findings on palpation.

Reabsorption of toxins causes toxaemia and damage to various organs, like the bone marrow, liver etc. Middle-aged and elderly bitches are predisposed to this disorder. However, it can occur rarely in younger bitches after one of the first oestrus cycles (juvenile pyometra with closed or open cervix).

After either a very pronounced or a very slight oestrus cycle, there is increasing lassitude, loss of appetite, polydipsia and polyuria. According to Arbeiter (1966), these symptoms can be detected 8–10 weeks after the last oestrus, and according to Dow (1959), just 5–10 days after. The timing of the first symptoms of disease varies between two and several weeks after the end of the oestrus (Schoon *et al.* 1992); this tallies with the author's own observations.

Motor disorders in the area of the hind limbs can occur with no changes in general health, so that confusion can occur with intervertebral disc disorders. The labia show low-grade to moderate swelling and there is a genital discharge of varying quantity and colour (yellow-green to chocolate brown). The vaginal and cervical mucosa is pale pink or greyish red, the cervix is closed like a scar, or slightly open. The uterus is either distended in the ampullae (ampullary pyometra with closed cervix), thin and distended into a tube shape (typical pyometra with closed cervix) or thickened, of a solid consistency (involutional pyometra with open cervix).

Pyometra and inguinal hernia: the uterus with high-grade inflammatory changes shifts into the processus vaginalis. The rupture is usually unilateral. As the uterus increases in size, the hernia also becomes larger and therefore visible to the owner.

Pyometra is accompanied by leucocytosis with left shift. Information on the red blood count varies in the literature. Arnold (1994) describes an unchanged red blood count, whereas Sokolowski (1986) and Johnson (1989) report occasional anaemia. Stone *et al.* (1988) give the proportion of dogs with anaemia as 22%, and de Schepper *et al.* (1986) as high as 65%. Suter (1989) writes of the development of hypoplastic or symptomatic non-regenerative anaemia as a result of toxins which become active in pyometra.

Therapy

- The quicker an ovariohysterectomy can be carried out with accompanying fluid and antibiotic therapy, the more advantageous it is for the patient.
- If an inguinal hernia is present, the uterus is displaced backwards into the abdominal cavity. Ovariohysterec-

tomy. Closure of the breach. Intravenous fluid and antibiotic therapy.
- In the case of peritonitis, an immediate ovariohysterectomy is indicated with intensive fluid therapy, antibiotics and peritoneal lavage.
- The use of antibiotics and prostaglandin $F_{2\alpha}$: 50–250 µg/kg dinoprost s.c., b.i.d. 5–8 days, with clinical and ultrasound checks should only be considered in exceptional cases, with valuable breeding bitches, for example.

Stump Pyometra

In most cases stump pyometra is recognisable, by a purulent vaginal discharge and poor general health, within a year of the ovariohysterectomy being carried out. The residual organ is bulbous and thickened as in involutional pyometra, of a solid consistency and subject to inflammatory changes.

Therapy

- Conservative treatment: antibiotics
- Surgical treatment: Operative technique: laparotomy. Careful dissection of the altered uterine stump. The stump is removed between two clamps after placing a ligature in the vaginal area. The mucosa is excised and the remaining stump touched with povidone-iodine solution or similar.

Stump Bleeding

This is observed between the eighth and 14th day after an ovariohysterectomy. It occurs most rapidly when the indications for operation were hyperoestrogenaemia (prolonged pro-oestrus and granulosa cell tumour) or a difficult parturition. The uterine stump which, like the removed organ, is greatly influenced by the effects of oestrogen and pregnancy, is subject to particular degradation and reconstruction processes at this time, and is therefore easily irritated by excessive movement, causing tissue tears and ruptured vessels. Massive vaginal bleeding can ensue with significant blood clots being present in the early phase.

Therapy

The vagina is plugged with gauze for 24 h to stem the blood flow. About 5–15 m of 5-cm wide gauze, according to the size of the patient, is used to stem the blood in the cranial(!) vault of the vagina. The tampon is stitched to the vulva so that the patient cannot pull it out. Haemostatic drug treatment is indicated at the same time, and antibiotics because of the irritation to the vaginal mucosa by the tampon. The gauze is removed after 24 h to a maximum of 48 h.

Uterine Tumour

Uterine tumours are mostly leiomyomas or adenomas and are very often associated with a pyometra or endometritis. The inflammatory process predominates here, and so the tumour is not recognised. Uterine tumours can attain a considerable weight, for example 10 kg in a 36 kg German Shepherd.

Therapy
Ovariohysterectomy.

Diseases of the Vagina

Vaginitis

Juvenile Vaginitis
Juvenile vaginitis is understood to mean an inflammatory disease restricted to the vagina which occurs in young animals that have not reached sexual maturity. It recurs in individual kennels and is found in several puppies in the same litter. The hairs in the vulval region are stuck together by the purulent mucous discharge, and itching and sliding around on the vulval/perineal region can occur ('sledging'). When the labia are parted, the mucosa is oedematous, reddened and covered with purulent mucous discharge. After carefully introducing a very small vaginal speculum, a glaring red mucosa can be seen when there is high-grade vaginitis.

Therapy. Only high-grade vaginitis is treated with antibiotics. Low-grade and moderate cases are not treated so as not to overload the young organism with drugs unnecessarily. When sexual maturity is attained, inflammatory reactions subside.

Vaginitis
Vaginitis is rare inflammation of the vagina in the spayed or unspayed bitch.

Therapy. Antibiotics.

Mating Injury

During copulation, injuries can occur in the region of the hymen and the caudal vaginal area, but more often in the cranial vaginal passage, which is almost always accompanied by perforation of the wall of the vagina and simultaneous opening of the abdominal cavity. During mating the bitch shows she is in pain (yelping) and afterwards colours up again unusually deeply. Rarely, a bitch will allow mating during anoestrus; mating injuries are always the result.

On vaginal examination the red edges of the wound are in clear contrast to the anaemic mucosa during oestrus. Sometimes the site of perforation is so large that omentum, mesometrium, bladder and/or a loop of intestine can prolapse into the vagina. Abdominal palpation can be painful. Radiographic examination reveals a varying degree of pnueomoperitoneum (Figs 70.1 & 70.2).

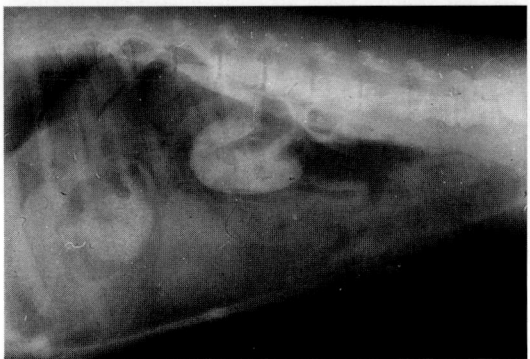

Fig. 70.1 Lateral abdominal radiograph demonstrating pneumoperitoneum following a vaginal injury sustained during mating.

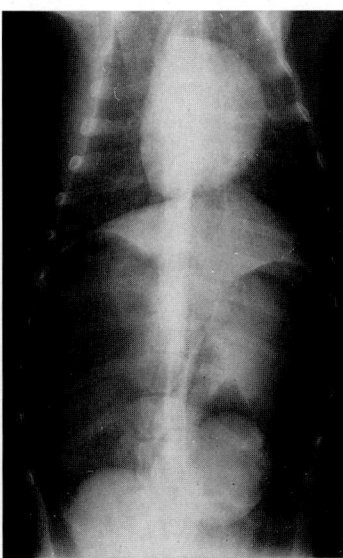

Fig. 70.2 Ventrodorsal abdominal radiograph demonstrating pneumoperitoneum following a vaginal injury sustained during mating.

Therapy

- Antibiotics
- Laparotomy: suture of the site of rupture with catgut and peritoneal lavage at laparotomy.

Vaginal Prolapse

Vaginal prolapse is predominantly observed during the first oestrus cycles, but isolated cases also occur later. It occurs more often in the Boxer, Dobermann and in Bulldog-type breeds. The excessively oedematous and hypertrophied vaginal mucosa prolapses either incompletely (trilobal, ventral and lateral portions of the mucosa, (Fig. 70.3) or completely (Fig. 70.4) between the labia. Lesions and necrosis of the mucosa occur because of the frequent licking and drying out of the surface of the prolapse, and also because the bitch slides on it. The prolabial vaginal mucosa can actually be bitten off because of excessive

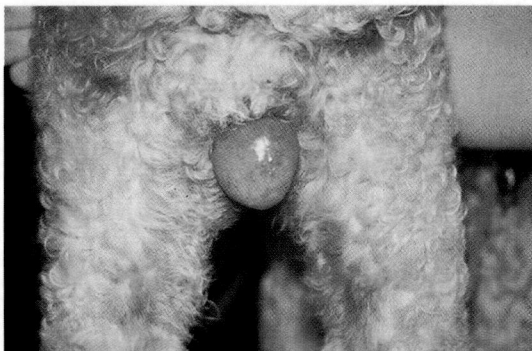

Fig. 70.3 Incomplete vaginal prolapse.

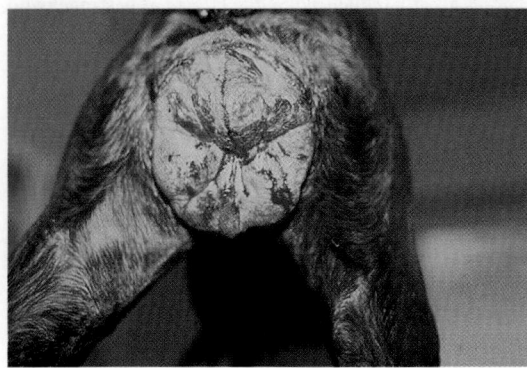

Fig. 70.4 Complete vaginal prolapse.

cleanliness (self-mutilation). This causes high-grade haemorrhage. Copulation cannot be completely achieved during mating and conception cannot be expected because of the high-grade presence of infective organisms. These animals should be withdrawn from breeding because of the considerable management required.

Therapy
Operative removal of the prolapsed vaginal tissue is successful.

Positioning the Patient. The patient can be placed in the dorsal position with the hind limbs tied well forward. In this way the pelvis with the external genital area is brought to the operating table almost horizontally.

Repair of an Incomplete (Trilobal) Vaginal Prolapse. After the introduction of a rigid urethral catheter (to locate and to protect the urethra), the prolapsed vaginal tissue is positioned as far forward as possible. The middle and the two lateral lobes are fixed one after the other with artery clamps. About 3–4 mm above the clamps, the hypertrophied mucosa is separated by stages with the scalpel, and the edges of the wound are brought together, again in stages, and stitched with close catgut stitches above the clamp which is fixing the remaining vaginal tissue and preventing bleeding. After the almost complete mobilisation of the three lobes of mucosa, a fourth part of the mucosa is removed from the side of the urethral opening in the same way. Altogether a maple-leaf shaped portion of the mucosa is completely removed.

Repair of a Complete Vaginal Prolapse. A rigid urethral catheter is introduced to locate and to protect the urethra. First, a deep incision is made between two strong clamps into the prolapsed vaginal tissue in the longitudinal direction of the vaginal passage, to enable the complete removal of the hypertrophied mucosa. One of the two clamps is moved by 90° to the deepest part of the incision. The excess vaginal mucosa is dissected away in a circular fashion in stages, as described above, and sutured with close stitches.

Vaginal Tumour

Vaginal tumours are detected significantly more often than ovarian or uterine tumours. They can become quite large and affect the passage of urine or faeces. They cause a grey-white mucoid vaginal discharge, often mixed with blood. The overwhelming majority of vaginal tumours are benign such as polyps, leiomyomas, fibromas, lipomas or lipofibromas. Malignant tumours do occur albeit rarely and include fibrosarcomas, spindle cell sarcomas or transmissible venereal tumours.

Therapy
The tumour is removed with the help of an episiotomy to expose the surgical site. The operative technique is described below.

Episiotomy. Two strong clamps are placed lateral to the raphe while pulling on the ventral commissure of the vulva. The perineum is separated up to the hymen with the scalpel between the two clamps. The episiotomy wound is closed using vertical, reabsorbable U-stitches (without stretching; catgut, polyglycolic acid, polyglactin 910) which achieve the bringing together of a wide area of wound surface. The surgical knots lie towards the vagina. The canthus of the dorsal commissure is brought together with one suture. The skin is dealt with intracutaneously with a continuous stitch or with sutures. Antibiotic spray and liquid wound dressing are applied.

Tumour Removal

- If the tumour is easily removable, such as a polyp, a clamp can be applied beneath the mass at the level of the mucosa, the neoplasm is dissected away above the clamp with a scalpel. The edges of the wound are sutured with catgut stitches above the clamp.
- If the tumour cannot be mobilised or is submucosal, either an oval incision is made around it, or the thin mucosa over the neoplasm is incised in order to be able to remove the whole tumour. The edges of the wound are brought together with catgut stitches.

Foreign Body

Both in the non-ovariohysterectomised bitch and in the spayed animal, a foreign body can cause a vaginitis or stump pyometra in the cranial area of the vaginal tissue (in Austria wall barley (*Hordeum murinum*), a wild grass species which grows beside paths, is a very commonly encountered foreign body).

Therapy
Removal of the foreign body by endoscope or surgical removal (laparotomy).

Urovagina

In dogs with a vagina which hangs down towards the cranioventral, urine can remain in the vaginal area and lead to inflammatory changes. The English Bulldog is a predisposed breed.

Therapy
There is no specific treatment.

Remnants of Hymen

A persisting hymen is rarely seen in the bitch and is not described in the literature. The author has seen a persistent hymen in two 6-month-old Boxer bitches (from the same litter) and a 7-month-old Poodle bitch. All three bitches were in oestrus for the first time and were straining painfully. A vaginal speculum could only be introduced into the vestibulum. The hymen was clearly domed in the bitches.

Therapy
Operative technique: an incision is first made in the hymen and it is then removed in a circular shape close to the mucosa. Because of the dammed up secretions vaginitis is present, and additional antibiotic treatment is necessary.

Diseases of the Vestibulum

Mating Injury

Rupture of the clitoris can occur during mating but is very rare; it is an absolute emergency because of the high-grade haemorrhage, and rapid action is indicated.

Therapy
Surgical intervention: the clitoris is sutured or removed.

Hypertrophy of the Clitoris

Clitoral hypertrophy is mainly seen in hermaphrodites (pseudohermaphroditismus masculinus externus). It causes local irritation, as the enlarged clitoris protrudes between the mostly hypoplastic labia. Because of the constant irritation by the surrounding hair, the passage of urine and licking, the enlarged clitoris is painful, showing inflammatory changes and there is a grey-yellowish-greenish discharge.

Therapy
Clitorisectomy. An oval incision is made around the clitoral fossa. The clitoris is dissected away with its corpus clitorides and the two crura clitorides which are attached to the arcus ischiadicus. The resultant cavity is made smaller with catgut gathering sutures, and the mucosae of the vestibule are brought together with catgut stitches.

DISEASES OF THE GENITAL ORGANS CAUSING VAGINAL DISCHARGE IN THE PREGNANT BITCH

Diseases of the Ovary

Hypoluteidism

See Chapter 71 on female and male infertility.

Diseases of the Uterus

Abortion

Abortion can be precipitated by trauma, hormonal disturbances or infection (*Brucella canis*, *E. coli*, *Streptococcus* spp., canine herpes virus, *Salmonella* spp., mycoplasmas, *Toxoplasma* and others). In abortion caused by infection, a green to black-green vaginal discharge commences between about the 40th and 50th day, with the passage of fetuses enclosed in membranes which have undergone pathological changes. Maceration and the commencement of mummification can be present.

Therapy

- Antibiotics and prostaglandin $F_{2\alpha}$ (dinoprost) at a dosage of 150 µg/kg s.c., b.i.d. over 5–8 days, antibiotics, with clinical and ultrasound checks.
- Ovariohysterectomy and antibiotics.

Fetal Maceration

The fetuses succumb to an intrauterine infection, after which they are subject to emphysematous decomposition.

The mother displays severe illness: loss of appetite, fever, lassitude, reddened/washed out mucosa and dehydration. Varying amounts of a foul smelling discharge flow from the vagina. Discoloured placentas and fetuses can be passed. Abdominal palpation is painful.

Therapy

Ovariohysterectomy. Antibiotics.

Fetal Mummification

Can be caused by a canine herpes virus infection (Carmichael & Greene 1990).

Therapy

- Ovariohysterectomy is the method of choice.
- Attempts to treat with prostaglandin $F_{2\alpha}$ (dinoprost) do not guarantee success.

Haemorrhage Due to Pregnancy

In the last third of pregnancy, haemorrhages of varying degree can occur. The probable cause is placentitis, which leads to detachment of the placenta and haemorrhage.

Therapy

Ovariohysterectomy is the method of choice.

Pregnancy and Inguinal Hernia

The gravid uterus is displaced into the processus vaginalis. As the length of the pregnancy increases, the hernia, which is usually unilateral, becomes larger.

Therapy

- If the puppies are wanted: laparotomy – replacement of the uterus and the ampullae in the abdomen, and repair of the hernia. Discuss genetic implications with the owner.
- If the litter is not wanted: ovariohysterectomy.

Dystocia (Table 70.13)

Before parturition there is further oedema of the vulva and perineum. The mucus of pregnancy is clear, interspersed with grey/whitish flakes. The cervix is closed and surrounded by copious amounts of mucus (Fig. 70.5). The opening of the cervix can take up to 24h, and the fetal sac is visible vaginoscopically (Fig. 70.6). If parturition is progressing normally, uterine activity is clearly recognis-

Table 70.13 Overview of dystocia in the bitch.

Type	Clinical findings	Treatment
Primary uterine inertia	No uterine activity can be recognised from the onset. There is mucoid amniotic fluid of various degrees of colour, and vaginoscopically the fetal sac is seen to be flaccid (Fig. 70.7)	There are always pauses during parturition. If no puppies have been born within 2h, treatment to stimulate the uterus is necessary to avoid too great a number of stillborn puppies. Subcutaneous or intramuscular administration of a uterine stimulant in a weight-dependent dosage in the following composition: 0.1–0.5IU oxytocin (Syntocinon™) + 10–50mg of the uterine spasmolytic vetrabutine hydrochloride (Monzaldon™). It can happen that a uterine stimulant is given for each fetus. This is only done when living puppies are being born. A repeat administration is possible after an interval of 2h if there is no rise in internal temperature and the amniotic fluid is physiologically normal. If no puppies are born after the second uterine stimulant, a section must be carried out. If parturition is very protracted, energy-giving supplements can be of benefit, e.g. glucose. A spasmolytic is given to optimise the effect of oxytocin, and to avoid uterine tetanus. Possible effects of oxytocin overdose are haemorrhages in the wall of the uterus and mesometrium, uterine tetanus with interruption of parturition, and rupture of the uterus.
		If only the last fetus remains, an obstetric forceps can be carefully inserted, protecting the soft birth canal.

Table 70.13 *Continued.*

Type	Clinical findings	Treatment
Secondary uterine inertia	After the birth of one or more fetuses, uterine activity ceases. There is mucoid amniotic fluid of various degrees of colour, and vaginoscopically the fetal sac is seen to be flaccid	As above provided there is no other cause
Dry birth canal	If parturition lasts a long time and the amniotic fluid drains away, the birth canal is dry. The puppies cannot be fully born and become stuck in the birth canal. Usually only the head and forelimbs, or the pelvis and hind limbs have emerged.	After applying a lubricant (liquid paraffin) in the birth canal, the puppies are extracted by gently pulling on skin folds over the limbs
Narrowed pelvis	After fracture of the pelvis, callus formation can lead to pelvic narrowing which can impede the passage of the fetuses	Conservative caesarean
Non-dilatation of the cervix	The cause of non-dilatation of the cervix is unknown where the litter size is physiologically normal	Conservative caesarean
Unicornual pregnancy	In a unicornual pregnancy the possibility exists that the cervix will not open. A smaller number of fetuses probably results in a deficit of fetal hormone, which is necessary to initiate parturition	Conservative caesarean
Single fetus	In the case of a single fetus, the rather rare impediment of too large a fetus can occur	Conservative caesarean
Simultaneous entry of two puppies into the birth canal	The simultaneous entry of two puppies into the birth canal hinders or stops the birth process with usually strong uterine action	Conservative caesarean
Malposition of the fetus	Malposition (head-breast and head-flank positions) transverse lie and malformations (hydrocephalus, anasarca, conjoined fetuses) can impede the birth process	Conservative caesarean
Rupture of the uterus	Rupture of the uterus is caused by trauma or an overdose of oxytocin, and can be detected on X-ray or ultrasound examination	Conservative caesarean

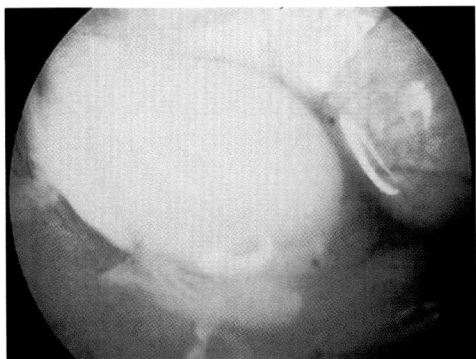

Fig. 70.5 Antepartum findings: severely oedematous mucosa, pregnancy mucus liquifies.

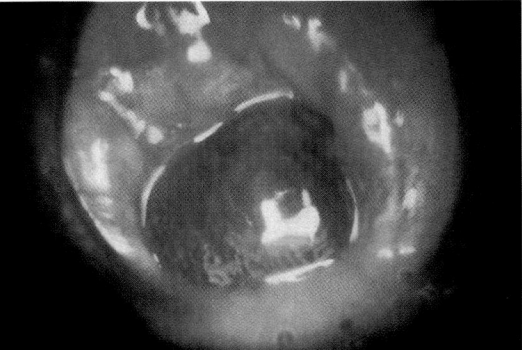

Fig. 70.6 Sub partu findings: the cervix is widened by the amniotic sac.

able and the fetal membranes are bulging into the birth canal.

The mucus that is passed before parturition, if labour has not started, must be neither green, red, brown, nor any variation of these colours (indication of pathological birth process). The internal body temperature is within the normal range before and during parturition. Any increase in temperature indicates a pathological process. Information from the breeder is very significant.

Assisted parturition is only required in 5–8% of cases. The birth can deviate from the physiologically normal for a variety of reasons, so this can increase the chance of survival of the mother and the puppies.

Torsion of the Uterus

This condition is very rare. One horn of the uterus is twisted once or more around the longitudinal axis near the

bifurcation of the uterus, and thus displaces the other horn, or there is a torsion between the bifurcation and the tip of the horn (Fig. 70.8). The puppies remaining *in utero* are dead due to lack of oxygen and shock. In general, animals giving birth are emergency cases. An animal in labour with torsion of the uterus is an absolute emergency.

- The bitch has already delivered one or more puppies and has strong contractions without delivering any more puppies.
- She presents with strong contractions and a bloody or red–brown vaginal discharge.
- The abdomen is more enlarged on one side.
- On vaginal examination, introduction of the vaginal speculum into the body of the uterus is impossible because of the fold of the torsion.
- Further investigations by X-ray or ultrasound are unnecessary – rapid treatment is more important.

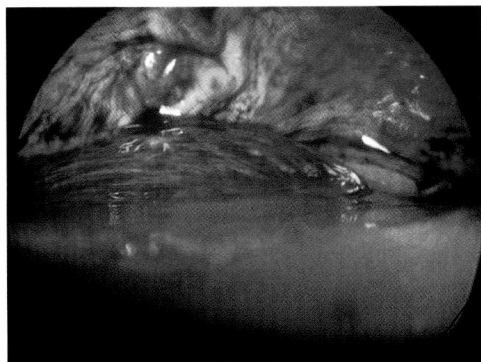

Fig. 70.7 Sub partu findings: a uterine inertia is characterised by a flabby fetal sac.

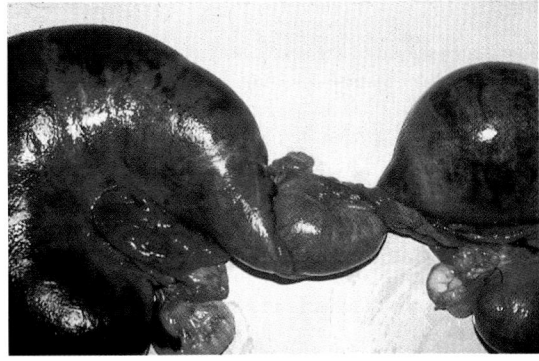

Fig. 70.8 Torsion of the uterus: 360°.

Therapy

Despite rapid surgery, the changes in the uterus are usually so severe that ovariohysterectomy (Porro section) can rarely be avoided.

Postpartum Uterine Inversion and Prolapse

Prolapse of the uterus can be observed after an easy, rapid birth, or, more rarely, after a long and difficult parturition. It can be complete or incomplete. The incomplete prolapse has a cylindrical appearance, and the complete uterine prolapse looks Y-shaped. If the prolapse exists for a long time postpartum, the surface dries out, and necrosis occurs.

Therapy

- *Conservative treatment*: Only indicated in fresh cases. Except in very calm patients, repositioning is carried out under heavy sedation and/or epidural anaesthesia. The prolapsed uterus is replaced up to the ends of the horns with the tip of a vaginal speculum, as used in the bitch. This process is controlled by palpating the abdomen.
- *Surgical method*: Laparotomy. The mesovarium is more tense and the ovaries are displaced caudally according to the degree of the prolapse. After bilateral ovariectomy the mesometrium is separated.
- The prolapsed parts of the uterus can be replaced in the abdominal cavity by gently pulling on the non-prolapsed uterus while simultaneously aiding repositioning with the tip of a vaginal speculum via the vagina. Hysterectomy is carried out using a catgut stump ligature.

Retained Placenta

The larger the litter, the more likely is the placenta to be retained. Older animals are more likely to retain the placenta than younger mothers. Retention of the membranes can result in postpartum atonia of the uterus, placentitis or placental necrosis. The evidence of retained placenta can be obtained both by vaginal examination (Figs 70.9 and 70.10) and by abdominal palpation. Dark black-green, sometimes friable, vaginal discharge is seen. The vaginal speculum shows dark green, sometimes friable membranes in the cervical canal and in the body and horns of the uterus, and large quantities of dark black-green watery lochia. On palpation, characteristic soft, bulbous uterine enlargement is detectable. Retained fetuses must be considered by differ-

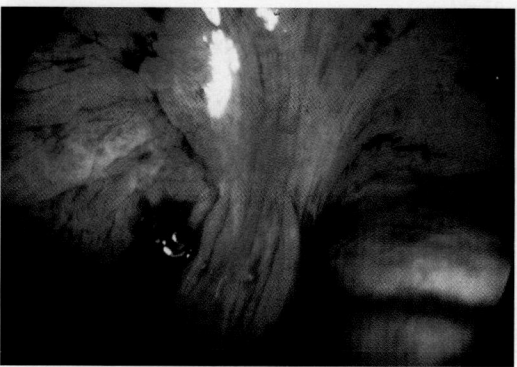

Fig. 70.9   Retained placenta: the septum intercornuale is clearly seen. In the right uterus horn is a retained placenta.

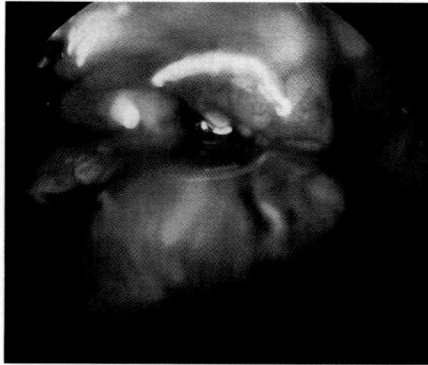

Fig. 70.10   Retained placenta.

ential diagnosis, and are recognised as solid cylindrical structures.

Therapy

- Timely removal, i.e. not many hours after the presumed end of the birth, of the retained placenta(s) with a forceps via an inserted vaginal speculum. If all the placentas have been removed, both horns of the uterus are easily recognisable on palpation.
- According to the size of the animal, 1–4 IU oxytocin are given subcutaneously or intramuscularly (not intravenously) 1–2 times a day to contract the uterus.

Postpartum Haemorrhage

Postpartum haemorrhage is caused by birth injuries and placental necrosis, or develops from subinvolution of the placental sites (Beck & McEntee 1966; Arbeiter 1976). Bleeding can vary in its intensity, and can be detected by clinical-gynaecological examination methods. Low-grade haemorrhages are characterised by a periodically occurring red to brown-red mucous discharge postpartum, which can last up to 10 weeks and longer. The mucosa is slightly anaemic, but general health is unaffected. With moderate haemorrhage the discharge is red-watery to mucous, interspersed with isolated clots. The mucosa is moderately anaemic. Severe haemorrhage occurs immediately after parturition, or between the first and fifth postpartum days. It is characterised by the gradual loss of red, watery discharge with large numbers of clots, severe anaemia and exhaustion.

Therapy

According to the degree of haemorrhage, the following treatments are available:

Low Grade Haemorrhage

- 1–4 IU oxytocin (Syntocinon™) subcutaneously 2–3 times a day
- 0.10–0.25 g chininum hydrochloricum orally per animal per day over 10–14 days
- Haemostatics (e.g. Reptilase™, i.a.) subcutaneously.

Moderate Haemorrhage

- 25–50 mg progestagens (e.g. medroxyprogesterone (Perlutex™), proligesterone (Delvosterone™)) subcutaneously
- Haemostatics (e.g. Reptilase™).

High Grade Haemorrhage

- 25–50 mg progestagens (e.g. medroxyprogesterone (Perlutex™), proligesterone (Delvosterone™)) subcutaneously
- Immediate ovariohysterectomy and blood transfusion.

Delayed Involution of the Uterus

The most commonly occurring pathology of the puerperium is postpartum atony of the uterus. It prepares the way for a series of other disorders of the postpartum phase. The causes are a long birth, overstretching of the wall of the uterus by a large number of fetuses (superfetation, hyperfetation), increased age, overweight mother, and disease in the mother before or during parturition.

Therapy

- 1–4 IU oxytocin (Syntocinon™) subcutaneously 2–3 times a day.

Postpartum Intoxication and Infection

General puerperal intoxication arises from the reabsorption of toxins from the dammed up contents of the uterus. It is usually chronic, manifests itself clinically most commonly around the third postpartum day, and lasts over several days. The disease is characterised by lassitude, loss of appetite, dehydration, low-grade rise in temperature, uneven skin temperature distribution, increased cardiac activity, weak rapid pulse, cyanosis of the mucosa and increased injection of the episcleral vessels. The lochia are mucous, a greyish red-brown colour, and have an unpleasant sweetish odour. On palpation, a poorly contracted uterus is detected. In contrast to intoxication, the progress of general puerperal infection is more stormy. The symptoms are exhaustion, loss of appetite, dehydration, high-grade increased body temperature, increased cardiac activity, small frequent pulse, reddened mucosa, increased epigastric tension, vomiting and complete suppression of lactation. The lochia are abundant, as in puerperal intoxication, greyish red-brown, of a mucous consistency and with an unpleasant sweetish smell.

Therapy
Antibiotics, fluid therapy, puppies reared on formula milk.

Necrosis of Placental Sites

One particular form of puerperal infection is placental necrosis. The causes are uterine infection, dead emphysematous fetuses and placentas which have remained too long in the uterus and which can lead to necrotic changes at the placental sites and rupture into the abdominal cavity. Clinically the symptoms are recognisable as those of a rapid onset septicaemia. The bitch declines very quickly. The low-grade to moderate lochia are yellow-brown and friable.

Therapy
Immediate ovariohysterectomy, intensive fluid therapy, peritoneal lavage and administration of antibiotics.

Subinvolution of Placental Sites

Subinvolution of the placental areas (Beck & McEntee 1966; Dreier 1980; Arbeiter & Dickie 1993; Dickie &

Table 70.14 Cervical and vaginal causes of dystocia not covered elswhere.

	Clinical findings	Treatment
Cervix		
No dilatation of the cervix	The bitch presents at the expected date with no uterine activity and a green vaginal discharge. The vaginal mucosa is pale pink, the cervix is closed, and the cervical mucus is various shades of green	Caesarian section
Insufficient dilatation of the cervix	The bitch presents at the expected date with uterine activity and green vaginal discharge	Caesarian section
Vagina		
Vaginal cords, remnants of Müllerian ducts	Vaginal cords are persistent Müllerian ducts, and are mainly found in the caudal area of the vagina. They can appear either at clinical vaginal examination or at mating or parturition as an obstruction	Operative technique: sedation is not normally required. Operative removal can be carried out with the patient in a standing position. Using a vaginal speculum and a long hook, the tissue is brought forward in front of the labia. Anaesthesia of the superficial mucosa is of benefit (lignocaine as Novesin™ 1% or Xylocaine™ spray). The cords are dissected out between two ligatures (catgut, Dexon™, Vicryl™).

Arbeiter 1993) is recognisable on colposcopy as a low-grade bright red to red-brown vaginal discharge, and on palpation by the ampullary uterine swellings, from the size of a pigeon's egg to that of a hen's egg, in the area of the placental sites. The patients have mildly anaemic mucosa and very largely unimpaired general health.

Therapy
Ovariohysterectomy.

REFERENCES AND FURTHER READING

Arbeiter, K. (1966). Klinische Diagnostik der Pyometraerkrankung der Hündin. *Wiener Tierärztliche Monatsschrift*, **5**, 346–350.

Arbeiter, K. (1971). Hormonal bedingte Genitalerkrankungen bei der Hündin. *Kleintierpraxis*, **16**, 129–168.

Arbeiter, K. (1976). Postpartale Metrorrhagien bei der Hündin. *Kleintierpraxis*, **21**, 5–7.

Arbeiter, K. & Lorin, D. (1981). Organ- und Blutbefunde bei hormonal bedingten Gynäkopathien der Hündin. *Wiener Tierärztliche Monatsschrift*, **68**, 191–196.

Arbeiter, K. & Dickie, M.B. (1993). Mögliche Folgen von SIPS auf die Fruchtbarkeit der Hündin. *Tierärztliche Umschau*, **48**, 420–424.

Arnold, S. (1994). Weiblicher Geschlechtsapparat. In: *Praktikum der Hundeklinik*, (eds H.G. Niemand & P.F. Suter), 8th edn. pp. 612–656. Blackwell, Berlin.

Beck, A.M. & McEntee (1966). Subinvolution of placental sites in the post partum bitch – a case report. *Cornell Veterinarian*, **56**, 269–277.

Carmichael, L.E. & Greene, C.E. (1990). Canine herpesvirus infection. In: *Infectious Diseases of the Dog and Cat*, (ed. C.E. Greene), pp. 252–258. W.B. Saunders, Philadelphia.

De Schepper, J., Stock, J., van der & Capiau, E. (1986). The morphological and biochemical blood profile in different forms of endometritis post oestrum (pyometra) in the dog. A study of 96 cases. *Vlaams Diergeneeskundig Tijdschrift*, **55**, 153–162.

Dickie, M.B. & Arbeiter, K. (1993). Diagnosis and therapy of the subinvolution of placental sites in the bitch. *Journal of Reproduction and Fertility Supplement*, **47**, 471–475.

Dow, C. (1959). The cystic hyperplasia-pyometra complex in the bitch. *Journal of Comparative Pathology*, **69**, 237–250.

Dreier, H.K. (1980). Physiologisches und patholgisches Puerperium bei der Hündin. *Tierärztliche Praxis*, **8**, 367–374.

Dreier, H.K., Coreth, H. & Kopschitz, M.M. (1987). Progesteron- und Östrogenbestimmung bei der Hündin im Verlauf des Normo- und Pathozyklus. *Kleintierpraxis*, **32**, 337–342.

Johnson, C.A. (1989). Vulvar dischanges. In: *Current Veterinary Therapy X*, (ed. R.W. Kirk), pp. 1310–1312. W.B. Saunders, Philadelphia.

Johnston, G.R., Feeney, D.A., Rivers, B. & Watter, P.A. (1991). Diagnostic imaging of the male canine reproductive organs. *Veterinary Clinics of North America*, **21**, 553–590.

Schoon, H.A., Schoon, D. & Nolte, I. (1992). Untersuchungen zur Pathogenese des Endometritis-Pyometra-Komplexes der Hündin. *Journal of Veterinary Medicine, Series A*, **39**, 43–56.

Sokolowski, J.H. (1986). Metritis, Pyometritis. In: *Small Animal Reproduction and Infertility*, (ed. T.J. Burke), pp. 279–283. Lea & Febiger, Philadelphia.

Stone, E.A. *et al.* (1988). Renal dysfunction in dogs with pyometra. *Journal of the American Veterinary Medical Association*, **193**, 457–464.

Suter, P. (1989). Anämien, hämorrhagische Diatesen. In: *Praktikum der Hundeklinik*, (eds H.G. Niemand & P.F. Suter), pp. 429–454. Paul Parey, Berlin.

Chapter 71

Canine Infertility

H. K. Dreier

Fertility is assured in genitally healthy adult animals with normal sexual behaviour. Reduced reproductive outcome can be the fault of both the bitch and the dog. Factors that can adversely affect fertility are to be found either in the hypothalamic–pituitary–gonadal axis or in the area of the other genital organs. Fertility is also influenced by sexual behaviour, stress, feeding, and by general diseases of the breeding animal (Table 71.1).

It is important that breeders be encouraged to keep exact records on their breeding dogs and bitches. Among other things, these should contain detailed information on the duration and intensity of, and intervals between, previous oestrus cycles, mating behaviour, course of pregnancy, number and progress of past parturitions, etc. (see Chapter 70 on vaginal discharge).

NORMAL CANINE OESTRUS CYCLE

The sexual cycle of the bitch is divided into pro-oestrus (6–8 days), oestrus (4–8 days), metoestrus (50–55 days) and anoestrus or resting phase (2–10 months).

Hormonal Profile of the Normal Oestrus Cycle

The secretion of gonadotrophin by the anterior lobe of the pituitary controls the sexual cycle. The hormonal situation at the time of ovulation was investigated by Phemister *et al.* (1972). In addition to histological examination of the ovaries and oviducts, blood concentrations of oestrogen, progesterone and luteinising hormone were measured. The authors established that in most bitches, ovulation occurs on the second or third day of oestrus, after a luteinising hormone peak is detected at the beginning of

oestrus. In 1973, Jones *et al.* reported on the results of hormone analysis in three Beagle bitches during ovarian activity. According to their report, the oestradiol-17β concentration increases during pro-oestrus. The level is highest (50–100 pg/ml) one day before the luteinising hormone peak. The highest concentration of luteinising hormone was detected on the first or second day of oestrus. Progesterone increases during oestrus and achieves its highest level during metoestrus (approx. 16 ng/ml). The authors are of the opinion that the release of luteinising hormone is dependent on the oestrogen rise during pro-oestrus. In recent years many hormonal analyses have been carried out on animals with normal oestrus cycles, with similar results. There are differing reports on the serum or plasma concentrations of luteinising hormone. The reasons for this are probably associated with different hormone preparations in the assays (Christie *et al.* 1971; Smith & McDonald 1974; Nett *et al.* 1975; Edquist *et al.* 1975; Concannon & Hansel 1975; Concannon *et al.* 1977; Austad *et al.* 1976; Wildt *et al.* 1978, 1979; Olson *et al.* 1982; Chakraborty 1987). Luteinising hormone is released in a pulsatory fashion, the intervals varying from less than 1 h to more than 7 h. The beginning of increased secretion was often associated with early pro-oestrus, or with the last 1–2 weeks of anoestrus. This luteinising hormone secretion should be regarded as the wave-like stimulation responsible for follicle development (Concannon *et al.* 1986). Luteinising hormone has a luteotrophic action. The primary secretion of luteinising hormone is necessary for progesterone release (Concannon 1980; Concannon *et al.* 1987).

Follicle stimulating hormone achieves levels of 260 ± 30 ng/ml during anoestrus, and falls to about 140 ng/ml during pro-oestrus (Olson *et al.* 1982). This drop in follicle stimulating hormone is caused by an oestrogen-linked negative feedback. In the pre-ovulatory phase, luteinising hormone and follicle stimulating hormone increase simultaneously. In contrast to luteinising hormone, follicle stimulating hormone shows two to four increases which are 1–2

Table 71.1 Overview of causes of infertility.

Ovaries	Testes	Uterus vagina vestibule	Penis prepuce	Mating time	Mating behaviour – bitch	Mating behaviour – dog	General disease
Anoestrus	Hypoplasia	See Chapter 70	See Chapter 72	Incorrect mating time	Inexperience		
Suboestrus	Aplaisa				Anaphrodisia	Inexperience	Infections
Silent heat	tumour				Aggressiveness	Lack of libido	Stress
Anovulatory cycle					Antipathy	Antipathy	Hypothyroidism
Hyperoestrogenism					Nymphomania	Aggressiveness	Hyperadrenocorticism
Hypoluteidism					Animal–human relationship	Animal–human relationship	

days longer than for luteinising hormone (Reimers *et al.* 1978).

Christie *et al.* (1971) determined the progesterone concentration in the blood of 16 Beagle bitches. This was 1–3 ng/ml during pro-oestrus, approximately 15 ng/ml during oestrus and up to 20.3 ng/ml in metoestrus. During anoestrus they found levels of about 2 ng/ml.

In 30 bitches of various breeds (Rottweiler, German Shepherd, Boxer, Dachshund, Poodle), with reference to cyclical changes in the vaginal mucosa, showed that oestradiol-17β achieves its highest level on the fifth day of the cycle pro-oestrus with an average of 110 pg/ml, and progesterone can be detected with a mean value of 3 ng/ml. At the pro-oestrus oestrus transition (around the tenth day of the cycle), oestradiol-17β reached 90 pg/ml and progesterone 15 ng/ml. At the end of oestrus the average oestradiol levels were 50 pg/ml, with progesterone values at 28 ng/ml. The highest progesterone concentrations (40 ng/ml) were determined during metoestrus (around the 30th day of the cycle). From this point, blood progesterone dropped continuously: 15 ng/ml on the 50th day of the cycle, 8 ng/ml on the 60th, 4 ng/ml on the 70th and 2 ng/ml on the 80th. Oestradiol-17β could still be detected on the 50th day of the cycle on average, with levels of 4 pg/ml (Dreier *et al.* 1987).

Blood prolactin only fluctuates slightly during pro-oestrus, oestrus and before implantation (Reimers *et al.* 1978; Olson *et al.* 1982). In the second half of pregnancy luteinising hormone rises slightly, and approximately ten increases in prolactin were recorded, whereas in the non-pregnant bitches only one to three increases were established (Graf 1978; DeCoster *et al.* 1983; Fernandez *et al.* 1987). The highest prolactin levels of 12 ng/ml and 3 ng/ml were observed in pregnant and non-pregnant bitches between the 55th and 60th day after peak luteinising hormone (McCann *et al.* 1987).

Androgens were detected both during the follicular period and the luteal phase in the bitch. During anoestrus serum testosterone is always less than 0.2 ng/ml; it rises slightly during pro-oestrus (0.3–1.0 ng/ml), falls off again during the luteal period and then remains low. Serum androsterone achieves levels of 0.6–2.3 ng/ml during pro-oestrus. These values remain high during metoestrus and then fall abruptly at the time of parturition (Concannon & Castracane 1982; Olson *et al.* 1984; Concannon 1985).

CLINICAL SIGNS OF THE CANINE OESTRUS CYCLE

The period of ovarian activity includes the follicular phases of pro-oestrus and oestrus with a combined duration of 10 to 16 days, and the luteal period with metoestrus lasting 50–55 days. Oestradiol-17β (E_2) is produced in the follicle wall causing, in addition to behavioural changes, oedema of the genitalia, proliferation of the mucosa and an increase in the permeability of blood vessel walls with associated diapedesis, vaginal bleeding. The corpora lutea are recognisable either by a slight swelling on the ovary or by being obviously raised up from the ovary; they secrete progesterone (P_4), activating the secretory phase. Of 1000 bitches of very different breeds which were followed up, the great majority were in heat twice a year (92.5%). When taking the history, those bitches having only one oestrus cycle (5.0%), or three cycles (2.5%) were rare. Any interval between oestrus cycles should be regarded as normal if it occurs regularly. A clinical gynaecological examination should be carried out to establish the cycle diagnosis (see Chapter 70, page 717).

Very Early Pro-oestrus

Very early pro-oestrus is characterised by oedematous labia and high-grade oedematous vaginal mucosa with marked rugae. The transparent discharge is mucus to liquid with no, or only very slight traces of blood. Obtaining material for a smear, and preparing the smear are very easy: the smear is fluid and mucus. There are many basophilic parabasal and intermediary cells, mucus, abundant leucocytes and isolated erythrocytes. Progesterone levels are <2 ng.

Pro-oestrus – Early

Enlarged oedematous labia with a smooth surface are typical; the discharge is bloody; vestibular mucosae are pale pink with a moist and glistening surface; insertion of the vaginal speculum is smooth and easy; there is high-grade oedematous pale pink to pinky red vaginal mucosa with the particularly characteristic longitudinal and transverse folds (Fig. 71.1) and bloody secretion in the deep folds; oedematous pale pink portio vaginalis uteri are observed and frequently cannot be distinguished from the rest of the vaginal vault; the cervix is slightly opened; the tonic uterus is tube-like. Obtaining material for a smear and the production of the smear are easy: the smear is fluid, red and glistening; there are many basophilic parabasal and intermediary cells, large quantities of erythrocytes and isolated leucocytes. Progesterone levels are <2 ng.

Pro-oestrus – Late

The oedematous labia display low-grade wrinkling on the surface; there is slight resistance to the introduction of the vaginal speculum; the colour of the vaginal mucosa is pale pink to anaemic, and the surface is beginning to show the formation of soft secondary folds (Fig. 71.2), secretions are watery and bloody; the uterus is tube-like. The smear is bright red when produced, and rather matt; under the microscope, mainly intermediary and superficial cells and a few erythrocytes are detectable. The acidophilic index (Ia), i.e. the percentage of acidophil-stained epithelial cells, is over 50%. Progesterone levels are <5 ng.

Pro-oestrus/Oestrus

The oedematous labia display a low-grade wrinkling on the surface; there is moderate resistance to the introduction of the vaginal speculum; the colour of the mucosa is anaemic and the surface shows the formation of soft secondary folds (Fig. 71.3). Secretions are flesh coloured; the uterus is tube-like. The smear is matt when produced; under the microscope mainly intermediary and superficial cells and few erythrocytes are to be seen. The acidophilic index (Ia) is more than 50%. Progesterone levels are <5 ng.

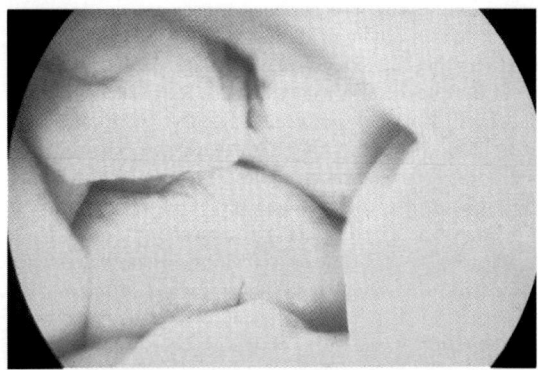

Fig. 71.2   Vaginal findings: late pro-oestrus.

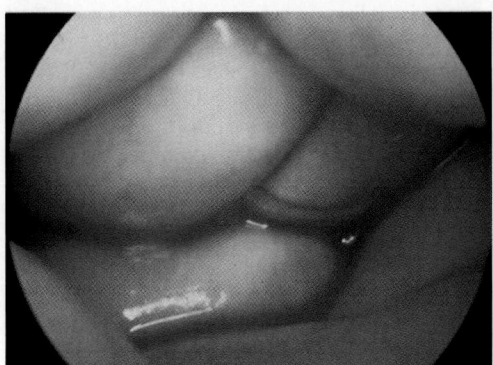

Fig. 71.1   Vaginal findings: early pro-oestrus.

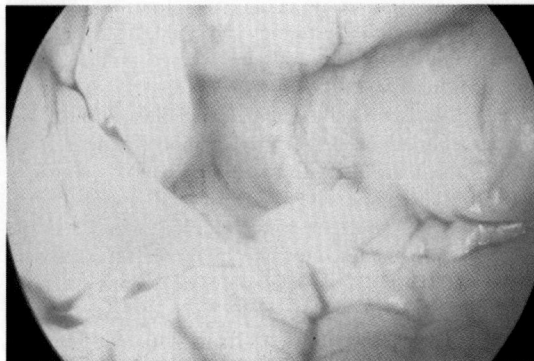

Fig. 71.3   Vaginal findings: pro-oestrus/oestrus.

Oestrus

Because of the obvious increase in progesterone, the swollen condition of the genitalia is subsiding, i.e. labia show obvious folds; there is strong resistance to the introduction of the vaginal speculum; the mucosa is dry, anaemic and folded (Fig. 71.4); there is a small amount of flesh coloured discharge; palpation of the uterus reveals a solid pipe-like cord; the vaginal smear is light, grainy and matt; microscopic investigation reveals: exclusively upper superficial cells and scales, acidophilic stain, few or no erythrocytes. The acidophilic index (Ia) is 100%. Progesterone levels are ≥5 ng.

Metoestrus – Early (First Week)

The labia are shrunken; mucosae are anaemic to pale pink; the cervix is open; the low-grade mucous secretions are brown-red or greyish-white/transparent (Fig. 71.5); the uterus is tube-like. Obtaining vaginal cytological material is easy, but the production of a thin smear is difficult because of the mucous character of the material for investigation; there are few superficial cells and mainly intermediary cells, numerous parabasal cells, abundant leucocytes and isolated erythrocytes in the smear. The acidophilic index (Ia) is about 0%. Progesterone levels are >10 ng.

Metoestrus

The labia are small and shrunken; mucosa are pale pink to pinky red with low grade cyanosis; the cervix is open to closed; mucous secretions are mainly grey/greyish-white/transparent (Fig. 71.6), but can also be yellow/yellowish-green; the uterus has subsided bilaterally. The vaginal cytological material presents difficulties in preparing a thin smear because of its high viscosity: numerous intermediary and parabasal cells, large numbers of leucocytes, abundant mucus and many mucous cells. The acidophilic index (Ia) is 0%. Progesterone levels are >10 ng.

Anoestrus

The labia are small and completely shrunken; the vagina is smooth with no profile, and the dorsal fold (Fig. 71.7) that ends in the cervix can be clearly recognised in the cranial dorsal area; the mucosa is pale pink; the uterus has subsided bilaterally. It is difficult to obtain vaginal cytological material and prepare a smear: there are few parabasal and basal cells, some mucus and isolated leucocytes. The acidophilic index is 0%. Progesterone levels are 0 ng.

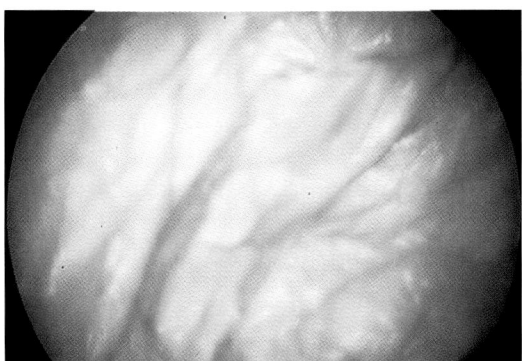

Fig. 71.4   Vaginal findings: oestrus.

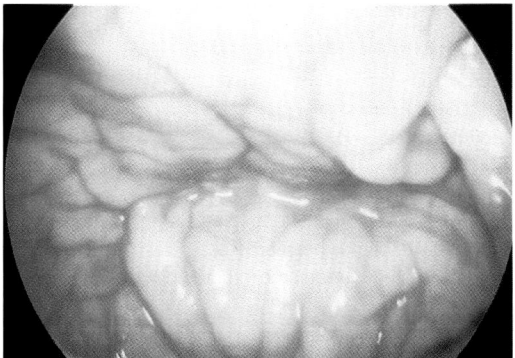

Fig. 71.5   Vaginal findings: early metoestrus.

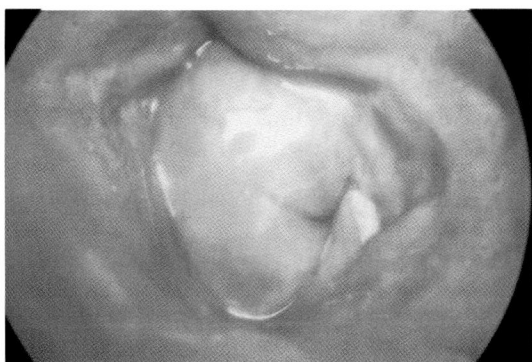

Fig. 71.6   Vaginal findings: metoestrus.

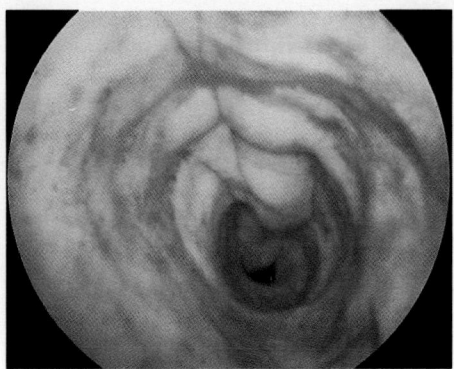

Fig. 71.7   Vaginal findings: anoestrus.

DETERMINATION OF TIME OF MATING

A clinical gynaecological examination with vaginal cytological findings and determination of blood progesterone concentration every 2 days are required to establish the optimum period for mating. The first examination should take place if possible between the third and sixth day of heat so that any necessary treatment can be started while there is still time. Also, owners repeatedly fail to recognise the beginning of heat in time.

The 2-day intervals in the clinical gynaecological examinations are therefore consistently maintained, so as to pinpoint the transition from pro-oestrus to oestrus as exactly as possible. This has occurred when the following observations can be made:

- labia with obvious fold formation on the surface;
- flesh coloured secretions;
- high-grade resistance to introduction of vaginal speculum ('adhesive resistance');
- rugae, anaemic vaginal mucosa with numerous secondary folds;
- tube-like uterus;
- vaginal cytological material easily obtained and spread; it is light, grainy and matt in appearance;
- superficial cells in almost all cases;
- acidophilic index is 100% of the nuclear pyknotic index;
- progesterone level $(P_4) \geq 5$ ng/ml.

If all these criteria are fulfilled for the first time, with the great majority of breeding bitches the first mating can wait for a further 4 days (extreme limits: 2–6 days). Any exceptions to this can only be recognised with intuition and expe-

rience. Thus with older animals it is better not to wait for 4 days and, according to the author's observations, with the English Bulldog there are hardly any superficial cells or scales (Dreier 1978).

FEMALE INFERTILITY

If infertility is suspected, it is in theory better to exclude first any mistaken observations by the breeder and any incorrect clinical gynaecological interpretations of the cycle by the veterinarian; only then should possible hormone therapy be considered. There are three broad groups to consider: abnormal mating behaviour, disorders of the oestrus cycle and disorders of pregnancy as shown in Table 71.2.

Mating Behaviour

The oestrus cycle causes behavioural changes characterised by increased licking of the external genitalia by the bitch, frequent passage of small quantities of urine (marking), less obedience, straying, and seeking contact with the male.

Table 71.2   Causes of infertility: behaviour, oestrus cycle and pregnancy.

Mating behaviour
   Incorrect mating time
   Inexperience
   Anaphirodisia
   Nymphomania
   Antipathy
   Animal–owner relationship

Oestrus cycle
   Anoestrus
   Suboestrus
   Silent heat
   Anovulatory cycle $P_4 < 2$ ng/ml
   Prolonged pro-oestrus >25 days
   Hyperoestrogenaemia
   Hyperoestrogenaemia after mating
   Subclinical bacterial infection
   Mycoplasma and ureplasma infections

Pregnancy
   Hypoluteinism
   Abortion

During pro-oestrus she will actually encourage the male, but, with a very few exceptions, will not permit mating. She is only ready for mating during oestrus. When the male smells at the genitalia of the bitch, she turns her tail to the side, or lifts it up, bringing the vulva into a horizontal position (presentation of the vulva); she allows the male to mount and hold her, and introduce his not yet fully erect penis into her vagina. If the penis is fully erect, the male changes position and emits the main fraction of his semen. While still tied, which can last up to 60 min, the final secretion is discharged. The normal mating act can be affected by various factors, which are discussed below.

Incorrect Mating Time

The most frequent reason for a bitch not accepting a dog, or a dog being uninterested in a bitch is that the time of mating has been incorrectly chosen.

Therapy
Determination of mating time (see page 738).

Inexperience

If one or even both sexual partners are mated for the first time, problems can occur during the act of mating because of inexperience.

Therapy
If possible, both partners should not be experiencing mating for the first time. If it is only the male who is inexperienced, a single artificial collection can be enough to stimulate the dog to mate the following day.

Anaphrodisia

The external signs of oestrus are either normal, slightly underdeveloped or completely absent. The bitch will not accept the dog.

Therapy
Artificial transfer of semen: this is carried out while the pelvis of the bitch is maintained in a raised position. Using a single-use syringe, the rubber connection from an infusion apparatus and a PVC inseminette, the main fraction of the semen is drawn up and slowly introduced without pressure precervically via a vaginal speculum. To prevent the semen flowing back out of the vagina, the bitch remains with the pelvis raised for 10 minutes or longer. In general, it should be pointed out that the semen must be examined before every insemination, and all apparatus used for collecting the semen and artificial insemination must be sterile and pre-warmed, to avoid a negative temperature effect on the semen.

Nymphomania

Bitches allow mating outside oestrus. There are often severe vaginal injuries (mating injuries, see Chapter 70).

Antipathy

A dog selected by the breeder is not accepted by the bitch in heat. On the same day she allows mating with another dog with no problems. Be careful: a mongrel from round the corner might be the chosen one.

Therapy
Change the dog, or inseminate artificially (see above).

Aggression

An aggressive bitch can discourage a dog who is ready to mate, or vice versa.

Therapy
Change the dog or inseminate artificially (see above).

Animal–Human Relationship

The bitch or dog has a much stronger relationship with the owner than with the mate.

Therapy
The owner should not be present. A person who knows the dog well, but who does not have nearly so intense a relationship with it should be present instead of the owner.

Disorders of the Oestrus Cycle

Anoestrus

Anoestrus is understood to be the absence of the oestrus cycle. The cause is a lack of ovarian activity (malfunction). According to the clinical criteria, this is subdivided into:

- Anoestrus of puberty: in animals of 14 months or late maturing bitches of 20 months; no signs of the oestrus cycle have yet occurred.
- Juvenile anoestrus: after the first or second oestrus cycle, ovarian activity is suspended.
- Anoestrus of parturition: no further oestrus cycles occur after parturition.
- Alternating anoestrus: a 6-monthly interval between periods of heat increases to 10 months and more.

The clinical picture of the bitch in anoestrus is not remarkable. Sometimes there are slight traces of dried secretions on the labia. The vaginal mucosa is smooth, not very moist, without profile and of a pinky-red, low-grade cyanotic colour. The dorsal fold can be clearly recognised. The cervix is flaccid and slightly open. The vaginal smear is difficult to produce and contains cells from the deep tissue layers (basal, parabasal and intermediary cells), mucus, mucous cells and isolated leucocytes. The whole smear is basophil stained. Findings on palpation show a bilaterally subsided uterus.

Therapy

Every other day, according to the size of the animal, 0.1 to (0.3) mg oestrogen (oestradiol benzoate) are administered s.c. or i.m. Treatment is carried out while checking the vaginal cytology so as to recognise incorrect treatment as early as possible. In the author's experience, the treatment begins to be successful from the second, or at the latest from the fourth injection. If the vaginal cytology does not show that the cycle has been induced after the fourth or fifth administration of oestrogen, treatment should be discontinued, as the therapy should not now be expected to succeed, and there is also the danger that side-effects could occur, e.g. bone marrow toxicity. If pro-oestrus occurs as a result of the oestrogen therapy, the induced oestrus cycle can be reinforced from the fourth day after the appearance of the cycle with follicle stimulating hormone (FSH, Folligon™). Every other day 25–100 IU FSH are administered s.c., i.m. or i.v. until oestrus occurs. Oestrus cycles that are established after such combination treatment usually have a pro-oestrus of 8–14 days and an oestrus of 8 days. The treatment is 84% successful (Arbeiter & Dreier 1972).

Suboestrus

Suboestrus is caused by weak ovarian function (subfunction). The beginning of the oestrus cycle can be clearly recognised, but the cycle remains static in this phase. Suboestrus is diagnosed by the following findings: slight to moderate oedema of the labia, only superficial changes to the vaginal mucosa, moderately swollen cervix and bloody mucous discharge. Abdominal palpation reveals a low-grade contracted uterus. The clinical picture of suboestrus can be confirmed by hormone analysis, as both oestrogen and progesterone levels are well below the values of the normal cycle.

Therapy

Treatment is based on substitution therapy.

- According to the size of the bitch, 25–100 IU follicle stimulating hormone (FSH, Folligon™) are administered s.c., i.m. or i.v. at 2–3-day intervals, while checking the vaginal cytology. Usually two injections are sufficient, and the bitch can be mated up to 4 days after the last FSH treatment. If this is unsuccessful, oestrogen therapy can be attempted.
- Every other day, according to the size of the patient, 0.1 mg to a maximum 0.3 mg oestrogen (oestradiol benzoate) are administered s.c. or i.m. The vaginal cytology is checked while treatment is carried out in order to recognise incorrect treatment as early as possible. In the author's experience, the treatment is successful after the second or, at the latest, after the fourth injection.
- If the vaginal mucosa does not show that the cycle has been induced after the fourth/fifth administration of oestrogen, treatment should be discontinued, as side-effects could occur. If pro-oestrus occurs as a result of oestrogen therapy, the induced oestrus cycle can be reinforced from the fourth day after the cycle has appeared with follicle stimulating hormone (FSH, Folligon™). Every other day 25–100 IU FSH are administered s.c., i.m. or i.v. until oestrus occurs. Cycles that are established after such combination treatment usually have a pro-oestrus of 8–14 days and an oestrus of 8 days.
- The success of treatment is 64% if FSH is used alone, and 29% with oestrogen treatment after unsuccessful FSH administration. A normal litter size for the breed was not achieved in all cases (Arbeiter & Dreier 1972).

Silent Heat

The oestrus cycle passes quite unremarkably, so that this condition is only recognised by very careful monitoring.

Therapy

Recognition that the bitch is in heat is made easier if her bed is covered with a white sheet so that isolated drops of blood can indicate heat. It can be helpful to leave the bitch with another bitch in heat, or with a dog. It is not advisable to use such a bitch for breeding.

Anovular Cycle

Pro-oestrus and the transition to early oestrus take place normally. The bitch is sent for mating and after either a successful mating or non-acceptance of the dog by the bitch, the P_4 level is found to be too low on examination. Alternatively a further examination takes place during oestrus, and the decrease in the P_4 level is found at examination on the third or fourth day after mating (Fig. 71.8).

Therapy
In the author's experience it is better not to attempt hormone therapy. Wait for the next cycle and again observe this very carefully.

Prolonged Pro-oestrus and Normal Oestrus

Bitches can occasionally have a prolonged pro-oestrus of up to 24 days. This is not the same as the 'prolonged oestrus cycle' (see Chapter 70, page 720). In the author's experience the duration of the subsequent oestrus is normal.

Therapy
Patience for many clinical and endocrinological tests.

Normal Oestrus Cycle with Hyperoestrogenaemia

See Chapter 70, page 720.

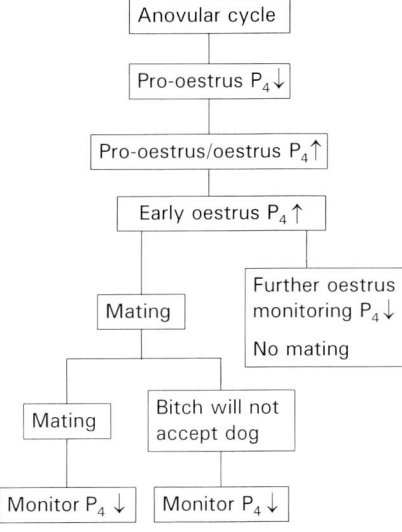

Fig. 71.8   Algorithm of an anovular cycle.

Hyperoestrogenaemia After Mating

Non-ovulating or atretic follicles continue to produce oestrogen, so that there is a negative effect on egg migration and the nidation process. The result is a reduced reproductive output.

At examination on the third day after mating, the expected clinical picture is of very early metoestrus with, usually, a red-brown discharge which should no longer be detectable on the eighth day after mating. However, here there is a brown bloody discharge as before. The vaginal speculum is very easily introduced, the vaginal mucosa still displays clear signs of oestrus, and there are predominantly mid-layer and surface cells, mucus, leucocytes and erythrocytes in the smear. Progesterone and oestrogen are both high.

Therapy
Subcutaneous progesterone or oral gestagen therapy (See Hypoluteidism, therapy, page 743).

Subclinical Infection of the Genital Organs During the Normal Oestrus Cycle (Fig. 71.9)

An on-going subclinical bacterial infection of the genitals during the oestrous phase of the cycle can be the cause of deficient fertility (Dreier 1978) or prepare the way for inflammation of the uterus during metoestrus.

Diagnosis can be made both by bacteriological investigation and by examination of the vaginal cytology. If there is a positive bacterial result, which can also be found in healthy breeding animals (Bjurstrom & Linde-Forsberg 1992), then the effective antibiotic should be determined. The most common disease organisms detected are *Pasteurella multocida*, β-haemolytic streptococci, *Escherichia coli*, *Mycoplasma* spp., *Proteus mirabilis*, staphylococci and *Pseudomonas*. The vaginal cytology shows that staining ability is affected ('washed out'; not clearly basophilic or acidophilic) and varying amounts of cell detritus can be seen (Dreier 1978) (Fig. 71.10).

Therapy

Antibiotics.

Mycoplasma and Ureaplasma Infections

According to Bjurstrom & Linde-Forsberg (1992) mycoplasmas and ureaplasmas can be cultivated from the vaginal

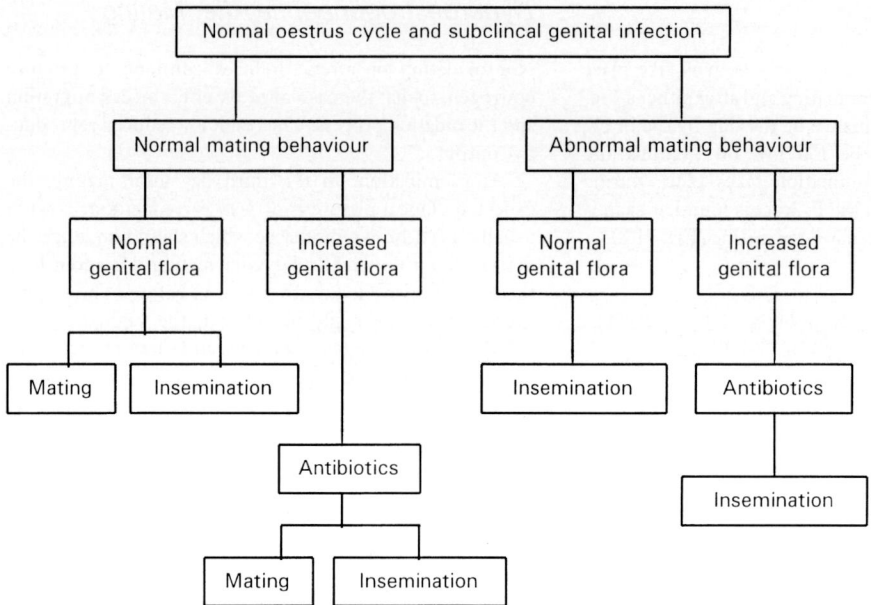

Fig. 71.9   Normal oestrus cycle in the bitch. Normal and abnormal mating behaviour, normal and pathological genital flora, mating and insemination.

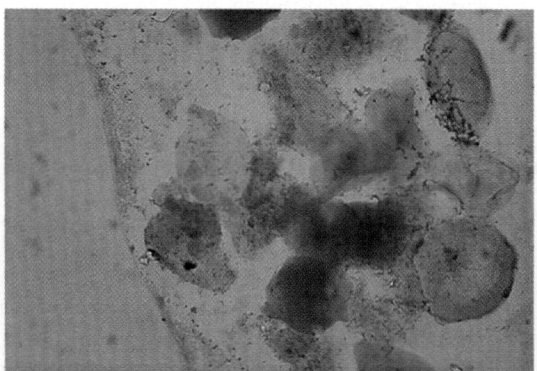

Fig. 71.10   Vaginal smear: subclinical infection of the genital organs during the normal oestrus cycle.

area of up to 59% of healthy bitches. They prevent conception, or are responsible for a reduced rate of conception. They also cause reabsorption of the fetus, abortion, premature birth, weak fetuses and neonatal death (Doig *et al.* 1981; Lein 1989).

Therapy

Tetracyclines, chloramphenicol, lincomycin, nitrofurantoin, tiamulin or aminoglycosides can be used (Rosendal 1990). Tetracyclines and chloramphenicol should not be used during pregnancy (Lein 1989).

Brucella Canis Infection

Brucella canis causes late abortion. The vaginoscopic findings are reddened vaginal mucosa and a profuse greenish-brown discharge. *Brucella canis* titre is positive.

Brucella canis can result in reabsorption of the fetuses, and according to Feldman & Nelson (1996), both dead and diseased fetuses can be delivered.

Therapy

Tetracyclines, aminoglycosides, streptomycin. A combination of tetracyclines (14 days) and aminoglycosides (7 days) gives the best results (Feldman & Nelson 1996).

PREGNANCY

Hypoluteidism

Clinically, hypoluteidism is characterised by a red-black/black-red mucous vaginal discharge varying in quantity, or, in rare cases, by high-grade bleeding from the vagina accompanied by coagula which can be as large as a hen's egg, from about the 20th day after mating. Abdominal palpation around the 25th/30th day of pregnancy reveals smaller ampullae of pregnancy which are tenser in tone, and fetal compartments which do not slip through the fingers as typically as in a normally developing pregnancy at the same stage (pathognomonic). A further consequence can even be abortion.

Therapy

With a timely diagnosis and subcutaneous administration of progesterone or oral administration of progestagens, hypoluteidism can be successfully treated. This is especially possible when breeding bitches are consistently monitored gynaecologically. However, if the vaginal discharge is still bloody after the eighth day following mating, a progesterone substitute (Luteosan™) should be started subcutaneously in a dosage of 12.5mg, 25.0mg or 50.0mg according to the size of the patient. In many cases, 2 days later a normal metoestrus can be observed. It can then be assumed that hypoluteidism was not present, and a state of delayed oestrogen decrease existed after mating, from follicles which had not ovulated and which had not become completely atretic at this time. The therapy can therefore be discontinued. The owner should be advised to carry out daily checks for any bloody vaginal discharge. If the discharge is red-brown as before, the treatment started must now be continued at 2-day intervals. The more frequently progesterone injections have to be administered to normalise a pregnancy, the sooner an oral progestagen maintenance dose (Nia 15mg™, Perlutex™) is necessary, in a dosage of 1.25–5.0mg per animal per day.

Abortion

See Chapter 70 on vaginal discharge.

CLINICAL EXAMINATION OF THE STUD DOG

In contrast to the bitch, the breeding dog is rarely subjected to an andrological–spermatological examination. This is because, in the mind of the breeder, fertility problems are mainly to be found in the bitch. Detailed explanation has only brought about limited improvements in breeders' attitudes to this issue. A breeding dog is therefore usually only presented to the vet when:

(1) a dog has mated frequently but the bitches have not conceived, or have only had small litters, and when
(2) the dogs' mating behaviour is abnormal.

The clinical andrological examination consists of:

- history,
- clinical examination,
- inspection of the prepuce and scrotum,
- palpation of the prepuce, testes and epididymes,
- inspection of the completely externalised penis,
- rectal palpation of the prostate,
- assessment of mating behaviour,
- collection of semen,
- examination of semen,
- bacteriological examination of semen,
- blood and urine tests,
- fine needle aspiration and biopsy and,
- X-ray and ultrasound examination.

History

When preparing the preliminary report, a record is made of breed, age, type of accommodation and feeding, vaccinations, general ill-health and treatments, any hormone treatment, stress, sexual behaviour, frequency of mating, results of mating and offspring.

Inspection of the Prepuce and Scrotum

Note is taken of the position, attachment to the abdomen, size (hypoplasia) and changes in the circumference of the prepuce, of any discharge (recognisable by hairs stuck together by secretions), and of changes to the opening of the prepuce (phimosis, paraphimosis). For the scrotum, changes to the surface of the skin are noted (pigmentation, inflammation, injury, tumour).

Palpation of the Prepuce, Testes, Epididymes and Spermatic Cord

During palpation of the prepuce, any oedema (allergy, infection) is noted, together with any increase in girth (tumours, injuries, haematoma) or pain (abscesses). When palpating the testicles, note should be made of the size, symmetry, consistency, temperature and any pain. With the epididymes, the head, tail and body should be differentiated. The spermatic cord (funiculus spermaticus) consists of the vas deferens, the testicular artery, the pampiniform plexus, the lymph system, nerves and cremaster muscle. These cannot be differentiated on palpation, but it should be noted whether there is any thickening and/or pain.

Inspection of the Completely Externalised Penis

When the penis is externalised, note should be taken of the size of the penis (hypoplasia), any phimosis or paraphimosis, persistent frenulum, balanoposthitis, injury, foreign body, prolapse of the urethral mucosa, neoplasm on the tip of the penis or in the region of the bulbus gland.

Digital Palpation of the Prostate Per Rectum

The gloved index finger is introduced into the rectum and the prostate is examined for size, consistency, and any pain.

Mating Behaviour

The dog shows increased interest in the bitch when she is in heat. He demonstrates his claim to ownership by marking with urine and faeces, often followed by impressive digging and scratching. When she is in oestrus, the bitch will, with few exceptions, accept the dog, allow him to mount and grasp her, and introduce the incompletely erect penis. During vigorous rubbing movements, the preliminary secretion is emitted. When the penis is fully erect, the dog changes position and ejaculates the main fraction of the semen. While still tied, which can last up to 60 min, the final secretion is discharged.

Collection of Semen

If the dog or the bitch is unwilling to mate, semen collection and artificial semen transfer are justifiable measures in the context of an investigation into breeding fitness, or to produce deep-frozen semen. Emission of the semen is effected either by manual massage of the penis (masturbation) or by allowing the dog to mount a bitch in heat. In both cases, the semen is collected either in a tulip glass or in an artificial vagina. Electroejaculation is unusual, and would require a general anaesthetic.

Semen collection is most easily carried out in tranquil surroundings in the presence of a bitch in heat. The dog is excited merely by the scent of the bitch in oestrus, so that mounting is not necessary. The prepuce is grasped with the hand and the glans penis massaged. The dog reacts by making vigorous rubbing movements. The back is arched and the penis incompletely erect (semi-erect). The preliminary secretion is now released (first fraction; duration approximately 10 s; quantity: 0.25–2 ml). The penis is externalised from the prepuce and clearly increases in circumference (full erection), and massage of the bulbus takes place. The dog changes position so that the penis is shifted caudally by 180°. The thumb and index finger encircle the bulbus in order to imitate 'tying' by gentle pulling. The main fraction of the semen (second fraction; duration: approx. 1–2 min; quantity 1–10 ml) and the prostatic secretion as the final fraction (third fraction; duration: up to 30 min; quantity: up to 20 ml) are collected in separate pre-warmed tulip glasses. The penis is held until it detumesces.

Examination of the Semen

A spermatological examination is an important addition to the clinical andrological examination process. It takes place in the context of investigations into fitness for breeding, and of artificial insemination with fresh or frozen semen. The main fraction of the ejaculate ('original sperm') is evaluated.

It should be remembered that the quality of the semen is dependent on the age of the dog, the frequency of mating, and also on the time of year. If the dog has been mated once or twice a day for several months, there can be a reduction in quantity and density. Semen quality will be normal if there are two to three ejaculations weekly (Feldman & Nelson 1996).

According to Taha *et al.* (1981), the semen is of a higher quality in spring and early summer than in late summer and autumn, possibly because of the influence of daylight and temperature.

The basic equipment for the production of a spermiogram should include a microscope with a warming plate and additional attachment for a phased optical contrast examination, a warming plate with microscope slides, cover slips, Pasteur pipettes, Bürker-Türk counting chamber, leucocyte mixer and a water-bath.

Volume

Method: Rough assessment in graduated tulip glass.

Normal value: Total ejaculate   5–25 ml

                 Main fraction   1–10 ml

Colour

Method: Subjective assessment
Normal value: Grey-white to white-grey

Consistency

Method: Subjective assessment
Normal value: Watery-milky to milky-watery

pH

Method:
- ○ Colorimetry with indicator paper.
- ○ Electronically with a pH measuring apparatus.

Normal value:
Semen   6.3 ± 0.2 (Chaffaux 1979)
Prostatic fluid 6.8 ± 0.3 (Chaffaux 1979)
Increase: Incomplete ejaculation, inflammation of testes, epididymes or prostate.

Concentration

Method:
- ○ Determination of number of sperm using Bürker-Türk counting chamber.
  10 ml Hayem's solution + 0.1 ml sperm
- ○ Determination of density with a Karras spermiodensimeter.
- ○ In a leucocyte mixing pipette, draw up semen to the 0.5 mark and 0.1 N HCl solution to the 11 mark, agitate, and assess in the Bürker-Türk counting chamber.

Normal value: 100 000–300 000/mm^2

Motility

Method: Assessment of forward, backward, localised and circular motion, and absence of movement takes place immediately after semen collection.
Using a pre-warmed pipette, one drop of sperm is placed on a pre-warmed degreased microscope slide.
Thick sperm is diluted 1 : 100, and the drop covered with a pre-warmed cover slip. Microscopic assessment at 300–500 times magnification:

Normal value: Forward movement >70%
Localised, circular and backward movement and absence of movement <30%

Differentiation of Living and Dead Spermatozoae

Method: Supravital stain: eosin stain
Using a small glass rod, carefully mix a drop of sperm with 1–2 drops yellowish eosin solution on a degreased, pre-warmed microscope slide and spread out thinly with a cover slip.
Air dry or heat.
Assessment of 200 sperms at 400–500 times magnification:
living sperms: colourless
dead sperms: red

Normal value: Up to 80% living sperm

Differentiation of Abnormal Spermatozoae

Method: (1) *Fluid fixing after Hancock*
Reagents:
NaCl parent solution:
NaCl 9 g
Dist. water to 500 ml
Buffer solution:
(a) $Na_2HPO_4 \cdot 2H_2O$ 21.68 g
Dist. water   to 500 ml
(b) KH_2PO_4 22.25 g
Dist. water   to 500 ml
200 ml (a) and (b) give 280 ml buffer parent solution
Production of formalin–salt solution (Hancock's solution)
Formalin 35%   6.25 ml
NaCl parent solution   150 ml
Buffer parent solution 150 ml
Dist. water   to 500 ml
Pipette 0.5 ml Hancock's solution + 0.1 ml sperm into a 1.5 ml Eppendorf vessel and agitate.
Phased optical contrast result at 1000 times magnification
(2) *Phased contrast examination*
Thinly spread 1 drop of sperm on a degreased pre-warmed microscope slide; air dry or fix by heating; phased optical contrast assessment at 1000 times magnification.

(3) *Karras-Kördel staining of head*

Reagents:

Metachromatic yellow parent solution:

   Metachromatic yellow   20 g

   Dist. water   to 2000 ml

Victoria blue parent solution:

   Victoria blue   15 g

   Methanol   500 ml

Oak bark solution:

   Oak bark   1 g

   Dist. water   20 ml

   Boil for 5 min, filter, let filtrate stand for
      24 h, boil again.

Production of a thin smear on a degreased,
   pre-warmed microscope slide.

Air dry for 24 h at room temperature.

Fixing: dip briefly into methanol twice.

Air dry for 30 min.

Dip into metachromatic yellow solution
   for 90 s.

Rinse with H_2O until the rinse water no
   longer stains the filter paper yellow.

Dip in oak bark solution for 60 s.

Rinse with H_2O.

Dip into Victoria blue solution for 10–15 s.

Rinse with H_2O.

Air dry.

200 sperms are assessed under the
   microscope at 1000 times magnification.

Assessment: Healthy semen has less than 30%
           pathological spermatozoa. Of these:
           Primary pathological forms: <10%
           Secondary pathological forms: <20

Cytology

In some cases, epithelial cells and red and white blood corpuscles can be found in the ejaculate.

Bacterial Culture of Semen

Examination of the main fraction of the semen (= second fraction in semen collection) for bacteria (with special reference to *Brucella canis*) and mycoplasmas should be carried out in every case. This can confirm testicular and/or epididymal inflammation. The third fraction is of significance in the diagnosis of prostatic disease. Where there is a positive bacterial result, which can also occur in healthy breeding animals (Bjurstrom & Linde-Forsberg 1992), the effective antibiotic should be elucidated. The most commonly found disease organisms in the semen are *Pasteurella multocida*, β-haemolytic

streptococci, *Escherichia coli*, *Mycoplasma* spp. and staphylococci.

Seminal Alkaline Phosphatase

This is detected in the semen. It originates from the epididymis and is a marker of epididymal secretions in the semen (Frenette *et al.* 1986). According to Johnston *et al.* (1991), it amounts to more than 5000 U/l in dogs with a normal ejaculate. The third fraction of the ejaculate which originates from the prostate has lowered alkaline phosphatase (England *et al.* 1990). It can be detected in dogs with azoospermia (Feldman & Nelson 1996).

Haematological Findings and Urinalysis

Complete blood and urine analyses are necessary to exclude or confirm systemic disease. Serological investigations for leptospirosis, salmonellosis, toxoplasmosis and brucellosis are indicated.

Fine Needle Aspiration and Biopsy of the Testis and Epididymis

These techniques are used for differentiation of normal and pathological germinative tissue, like inflammation (orchitis, epididymitis) and tumours (Sertoli cell tumour, seminoma, Leydig's interstitial cell tumour).

X-Ray and Ultrasound Examination

These are used in cryptorchidism, testicular tumours and diseases of the epididymis, vas deferens and prostate.

HORMONAL INFLUENCE ON MALE GENITAL FUNCTION AND SPERMATOGENESIS (FIG. 71.11)

Environmental stimuli influence hormonal activity via the central nervous system and the hypothalamus. Gonadotrophin releasing hormone is released by the hypothalamus and stimulates the secretion of the gonadotrophins follicle stimulating hormone and luteinising hormone in the anterior lobe of the pituitary. Luteinising

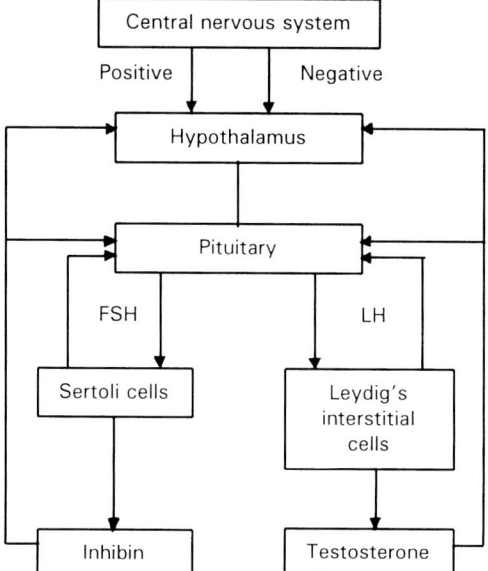

Fig. 71.11 Hormone regulation in the dog.

hormone activates Leydig's interstitial cells in the testes to secrete testosterone. Follicle stimulating hormone stimulates the Sertoli cells in the seminiferous tubules which produce inhibin. The high concentrations of testosterone are necessary for uninterrupted spermatogenesis, control of epididymal function, the action of the seminiferous tubules and the vas deferens, and for the maintenance of libido. Via a feedback mechanism, inhibin regulates follicle stimulating hormone in the blood, and testosterone regulates leutenising hormone secretion (Kumar *et al.* 1980; Falvo *et al.* 1982). Primary leutenising hormone plasma concentration is usually less than 20 ng/ml, but can fluctuate to more than 90 ng/ml (Amman 1982). Primary follicle stimulating hormone plasma concentration is less than 20 ng/ml and does not fluctuate like leuteinising hormone (Shille & Olson 1989). Follicle stimulating hormone and testosterone are necessary for sperm production. The testosterone concentration in the testes is 50–100 times higher than in the blood. In the healthy dog, the testosterone level in the blood is between 0.4 and 10.0 ng/ml (Larsen & Johnston 1980).

The germinal epithelial cycle (spermatogenesis) comprises eight stages, and takes an average of 13.6 days. The life of the primary spermatocytes is 20.9 days, and that of the secondary spermatocytes 0.5 days. Spermiohistogenesis lasts for 21.1 days (Foote *et al.* 1972).

INFERTILITY IN THE DOG
Differentiation of Infertility

Infertility in the dog is either congenital or acquired (Fig. 71.12) and is accompanied either by a normal, reduced, or completely absent libido. Congenital causes of sterility should be assumed in a dog that has accomplished several matings without a positive reproductive result. Infertile dogs with a normal libido have a defect in the testes, epididymes or prostate, and display normal activity in Leydig's interstitial cells with normal plasma testosterone levels. Where the libido is reduced or absent, Leydig's interstitial cells also seem to be defective. A reduced or absent libido is not only caused by reduced testosterone secretion, but also by psychological problems. It is difficult to obtain ejaculate from a dog with reduced libido.

Endocrine disorders (hypopituitarism, hypothyroidism, hyperadrenocorticism), hormone-producing tumours of the testes, hormones administered by the vet or an unqualified person (e.g. methyltestosterone), general disease, infections, stress and behavioural disturbances caused by trauma and/or pain on mating can all be the cause of fertility problems with or without a loss of libido (Fig. 71.13).

Stress is difficult to interpret; it can result in temporary infertility. Three or four weeks after azoospermia has been diagnosed, therefore, a dog can produce a completely normal ejaculate (Fig. 71.14).

Levels of the gonadotrophins follicle stimulating hormone (FSH) and luteinising hormone (LH), and of testosterone indicate functional disorders of the germinative tissue (functional disorders of the seminiferous tubules, Leydig's interstitial cell tumour, Sertoli cell tumour, seminoma) (Soderberg 1984; Freshman *et al.* 1988) as summarised in Fig. 71.15.

Testicular Atrophy

There is a varying degree of destruction of the seminiferous tubules (Sertoli cells, Leydig's interstitial cells, spermatogonia). The causes are general disease, orchitis, prostatitis, erosion and burning of the scrotum and testes, retrograde ejaculation, drugs such as oestrogens or anabolic agents, hypopituitarism, hypothyroidism, hyperadrenocorticism, oestrogen-producing Sertoli cell tumours, intersexuality (XXY syndrome) and *Brucella canis* infection. Idiopathic testicular hypertrophy occurs in middle-aged dogs. The cause of non-inflammatory testicular atrophy is unknown.

Therapy depends on the cause. Prognosis is doubtful to poor.

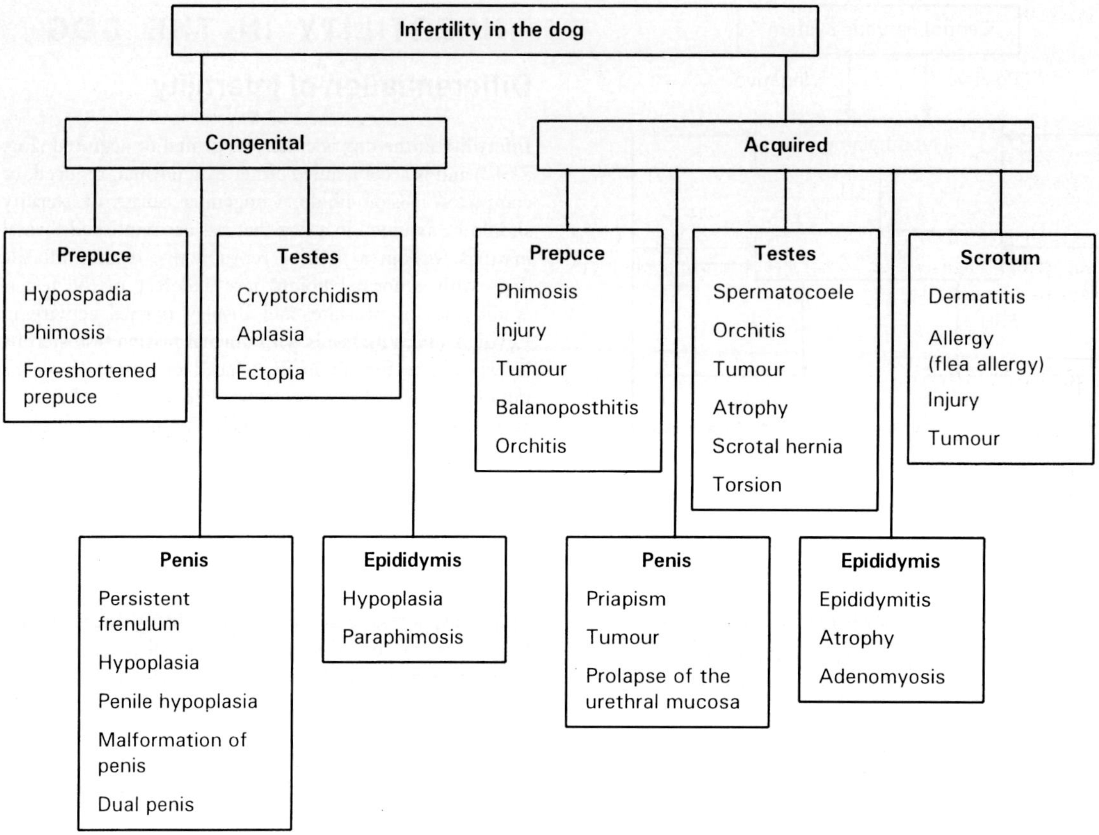

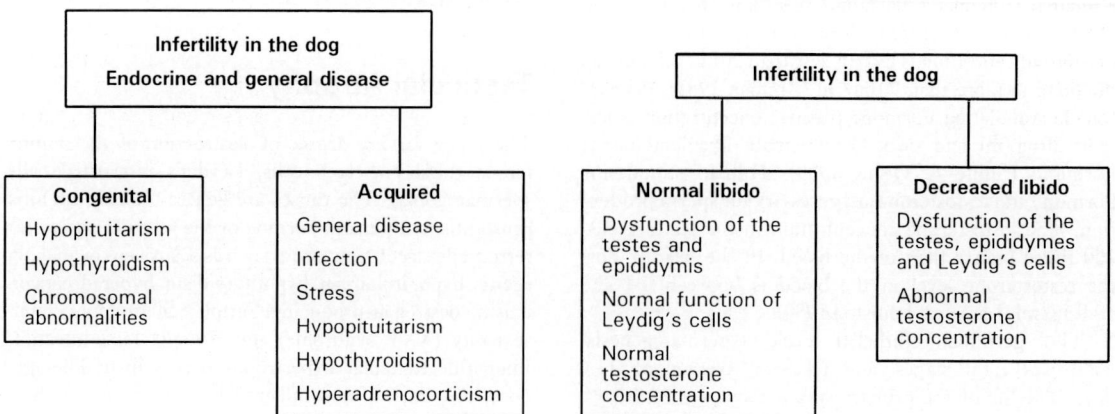

Fig. 71.12 Congenital and acquired causes of infertility in the dog.

Fig. 71.13 Congenital and acquired infertility caused by endocrine and general disorders, and stress.

Fig. 71.14 Causes of infertility with reference to normal and decreased libido.

Pathological Ejaculate

Spermatogenesis takes 55–70 days and its progress cannot be altered. Inhibitory or stimulating factors have different effects on the individual stages of spermatogenesis. The period between the operation of a factor and its effect on the ejaculate or on fertility can be relatively lengthy. If, for example, the spermatogonia are affected, this period will be at least 50 days. Changes in the semen can take the form of azoospermia, oligospermia, abnormal sperm morphology and altered motility (see Fig. 71.15).

Azoospermia

No sperm are detectable in the ejaculate. Several ejaculates collected at 6–8-week intervals are required to diagnose azoospermia. The causes of azoospermia (temporary or permanent) are general disease, orchitis, prostatitis, erosion and burning of the scrotum and testes, retrograde ejaculation, drugs such as oestrogens or anabolic agents, hypopituitarism, hypothyroidism, hyperadrenocorticism, oestrogen-producing Sertoli cell tumours, intersexuality (XXY syndrome) and *Brucella canis* infection. Some back-flow of semen into the bladder can occur during normal ejaculation (Dooley *et al.* 1990). Retrograde ejaculation is actually rare, but should be considered in azoospermia (Feldman & Nelson 1996).

Oligospermia

The number of sperm in the ejaculate is reduced. Sperm morphology can be normal or pathological. A very high rate of ejaculation (once or twice a day for several months) can cause oligospermia (Schäfer *et al.* 1996, 1997). Other causes

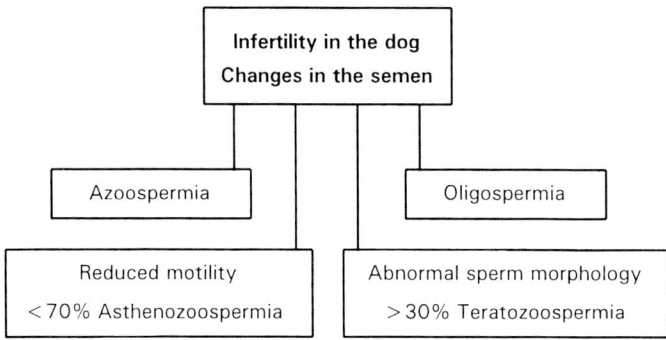

Fig. 71.15   Changes in semen that can cause infertility.

Table 71.3   Determination of testosterone and the gonadotrophins follicle stimulating hormone (FSH) and luteinising hormone (LH) in dogs with various percentages of normal seminiferous tubules, and in dogs with testicular tumours (Soderberg 1984; Freshman *et al.* 1988).

Degree of damage (number of dogs)	FSH (ng/ml ± s.e.m.)	LH (ng/ml ± s.e.m.)	Testosterone (ng/ml ± s.e.m.)
I (17)	73 ± 7	34 ± 9	3 ± 0.5
II (18)	84 ± 9	85 ± 32	3 ± 0.6
III (21)	236 ± 49	96 ± 18	3 ± 0.7
IV (14)	321 ± 58	95 ± 26	3 ± 0.6
ICT (7)	237 ± 104	70 ± 32	5 ± 1.2
SCT (2)	104 ± 23	44 ± 11	2 ± 0.6

Grade I: All seminiferous tubules have active spermiogenesis.
Grade II: Some or all of the seminiferous tubules have a lowered spermiogenesis or reduced number of spermatogonia.
Grade III: Some, but not all the seminiferous tubules have no spermiogenesis and contain only Sertoli cells.
Grade IV: None of the seminiferous tubules have spermiogenesis; they contain only Sertoli cells.
ICT Leydig's interstitial cell tumour.
SCT Sertoli cell tumor.

are the same as for azoospermia, but not so pronounced. Azoospermia can develop from oligospermia.

Abnormal Sperm Morphology (Teratozoospermia)

Present when the number of pathological sperm is more than 30%. The density and motility of the semen can be normal or pathological.

The morphologically altered spermatozoa are differentiated into those with primary damage and those with secondary damage. Primary damage is caused during spermiogenesis. The secondary morphological changes occur during passage along the epididymis and ejaculation. Sperm with primary damage include those with macrocephaly, microcephaly, bicephaly, pointed head, thickened neck, eccentrically attached neck, irregularly thickened or emaciated middle piece, duplicated middle piece, thin tail and double tail. Secondary changes are free heads, detached head plate, swollen acrosome, detached acrosome, drops of cytoplasm at the neck, middle piece (proximal, middle, distal) and tail, and tail coiled up to various degrees.

Reduced Motility (Asthenozoospermia)

The healthy ejaculate contains >70% sperm with forward movement, and <30% sperm with localised, circular and backward movement, and immobility. There is no information on what percentage causes infertility. If there are less than 50% forward moving sperm, the assessment of motility would be negative.

Therapy

The therapy would depend on the cause under consideration, such as orchitis, epididymitis, tumour, prostatitis and behavioural problems. Dogs with azoospermia and oligospermia must be monitored more frequently before this diagnosis can be pronounced definitively.

REFERENCES

Amann, R.P. (1982). Use of animal models for detecting specific alterations in reproduction. *Fundamental and Applied Toxicology*, 2, 13–26.

Arbeiter, K. & Dreier, H.-K. (1972). Pathognostik und Behandlungsmöglichkeiten der Sub-, Anöstrie und Anaphrodisie bei Zuchthündinnen. *Berliner und Münchener Tierärztliche Wochenschrift*, 18, 341–360.

Austad, R., Lunde, A. & Pearson, O.V. (1976). Peripheral plasma levels of oestradiol-17 beta and progesterone in the bitch during the oestrous cycle, in normal pregnancy and after dexamethasone treatment. *Journal of Reproduction and Fertility*, 46, 129–136.

Bjurstrom, L. & Linde-Forsberg, C. (1992). Long-term study of aerobic bacteria of the genital tract in breeding bitches. *American Journal of Veterinary Research*, 53, 665.

Chaffaux, S. (1979). Pathologie de la prostate de chien. *Recueil de Médecine Vétérinaire*, 155, 421–427.

Chakraborty, P.K. (1987). Reproductive hormone concentration during estrus, pregnancy and pseudopregnancy in the labrador bitch. *Theriogenology*, 27, 827–840.

Christie, D.W., Bell, E.T., Horth, C.E. & Palmer, R.F. (1971). Peripheral plasma progesterone levels during the canine oestrus cycle. *Acta Endocrinologica*, 68, 543–550.

Concannon, P.W. (1980). Effects of hypophysectomy and of LH administration on luteal phase plasma progesterone levels in the beagle bitch. *Journal of Reproduction and Fertility*, 58, 407–410.

Concannon, P.W. (1985). Endocrinology of canine estrous cycles, pregnancy and parturition. In: *Proceedings of the Society Theriogenology*, Denver, 1984. pp. 1–24. Society for Theriogenology, Hastings, Nebraska.

Concannon, P.W. & Castracane, V.D. (1982). Serum androstendione and testosterone concentrations during pregnancy and nonpregnant cyclesin dogs. *Biology of Reproduction*, 33, 1078–1083.

Concannon, P.W. & Hansel, W. (1975). Effects of estrogen and progesterone on plasma LH, sexual behavior and pregnancy in Beagle bitches. *59th Annual Meeting Federation of American Societies for Experimental Biology. Federation Proceedings*, 34 (3), 323.

Concannon, P.W., Hansel, W. & McEntee, K. (1977). Changes in LH, progesterone and sexual behavior associated with preovulatory luteinization in the bitch. *Biology of Reproduction*, 17, 604–613.

Concannon, P.W., Whaley, S. & Anderson, P.S. (1986). Increased LH pulse frequency associated with termination of anestrus during the ovarian cycle of the dog. *Biology of Reproduction*, 34 (Suppl.), 119 (Abstract).

Concannon, P.W., Weinstein, P., Whaley, S. & Frank, D. (1987). Suppression of luteal function in dogs by luteinizing hormone antiserum and bromocriptine. *Journal of Reproduction and Fertility*, 19, 1113–1118.

DeCoster, R., Beckers, J.F., Beerens, D. & DeMay, J. (1983). A homologous radioimmunoassay for canine prolactin: plasma levels during the reproductive cycle. *Acta Endocrinologica*, 103, 473–478.

Doig, P.A., *et al.* (1981). The genital mycoplasma and ureaplasma flora of healthy and diseased dogs. *Canadian Journal of Comparative Medicine*, **45**, 233.

Dooley, M.P., *et al.* (1990). Retrograde flow of spermatozoa into the urinary bladder of dogs during ejaculation or after sedation with xylazine. *American Journal of Veterinary Research*, **51**, 1574.

Dreier, H.K. (1978). Fruchtbarkeitsstörungen bei der Hündin. *Kleintierpraxis*, **23**, 313–356.

Dreier, H.K., Coreth, H. & Kopschitz, M.M. (1987). Progesteron- und Östrogen-bestimmung bei der Hündin im Verlauf des Normo- und Pathozyklus. *Kleintierpraxis*, **32**, 337–342.

Edquist, L.E., Johansson, E.D.B., Kasstrom, H., Olsson, S.E. & Richkind, M. (1975). Blood plasma levels of progesterone and oestradiol in the dog during the oestrus cycle and pregnancy. *Acta Endocrinologica*, **78**, 554–564.

England, G.C.W., *et al.* (1990). An investigation into the origin of the first fraction of the canine ejaculate. *Research in Veterinary Science*, **49**, 66.

Falvo, R.E., *et al.* (1982). Testosteron pretreatment and the response of pituitary LH to gonadotropin-releasing hormone (GnRH) in the male dog. *Journal of Andrology*, **3**, 193.

Feldman, E.C. & Nelson, R.W. (1996). *Canine and Feline Endocrinology and Reproduction*, 2nd edn. W.B. Saunders, Philadelphia.

Fernandez, P.A., Bowen, R.A., Kostas, A.C., Sawyer, H.R., Nett, T.M. & Olson, P.N. (1987). Luteal function in the bitch: changes during diestrus in pituitary concentration of and the number of luteal receptors of luteinizing hormone and prolactin. *Biology of Reproduction*, **37**, 804–811.

Foote, R.H., Swierstra, E.E. & Hunt, W.L. (1972). Spermatogenesis in the dog. *Anatomical Record*, **173**, 341–352.

Frenette, G., *et al.* (1986). Origin of alkaline phosphatase of canine seminal plasma. *Archives of Andrology*, **16**, 235.

Freshman, J.L., Amann, R.P., Bowen, R.A., *et al.* (1988). Clinical evaluation of infertility in the dog. *Compendium on Continuing Education for the Practicing Veterinarian*, **10**, 443.

Graf, K.J. (1978). Serum oestrogen, progesterone and prolactin concentrations in cyclic, pregnant and lactating beagle dogs. *Journal of Reproduction and Fertility*, **52**, 9–14.

Johnston, G.R. *et al.* (1991). Diagnostic imaging of the male canine reproductive organs. *Veterinary Clinics of North America*, **21**: 553.

Jones, E.G., Boyns, A.R., Cameron, E.H.D., Bell, E.T., Christie, D.W. & Parkes, M.F. (1973). Plasma oestradiol, luteinizing hormone and progesterone during the oestrus cycle in the beagle bitch. *Journal of Endocrinology*, **57**, 331–332.

Kumar, M.S.A., *et al.* (1980). Distribution of luteinizing hormone releasing hormone in the canine hypothalamus: Effect of castration and exogenous gonadal steroids. *American Journal of Veterinary Research*, **41**, 1304.

Larsen, R.E. & Johnston, S.D. (1980). Management of canine infertility. In: *Current Veterinary Therapy VII*, (ed. R.W. Kirk), pp. 1226–1231. W.B. Saunders, Philadelphia.

Lein, D.H. (1989). Mycoplasma infertility in the dog: diagnosis and treatment. *Proceedings of the Annual Meeting of the Society for Theriogenology*, 307.

McCann, J.P., Temple, M. & Concannon, P.W. (1987). Pregnancy-specific alterations in the metabolic endocrinology of domestic dogs including insulin resistance and modified regulation of growth hormone secretion. *Proceedings of the 11th International Congress on Animal Reproduction and Artificial Insemination*, **2**. p. 103. University College Dublin.

Nett, T.M., Akbar, A.M., Phemister, R.D., Holst, P.A., Reichert, L.E., Jr. & Niswender, G.D. (1975). Levels of luteinizing hormone, estradiol and progesterone in serum during the estrous cycle and pregnancy in the Beagle bitch. *Proceedings of the Society for Experimental Biology and Medicine*, **148**, 134–139.

Olson, P., Bowen, R., Behrendt, M., Olson, J.D. & Nett, T.M. (1982). Concentrations of reproductive hormones in canine serum throughout late anestrus, proestrus and estrus. *Biology of Reproduction*, **27**, 1196–1206.

Olson, P.N., Bowen, R.A., Behrendt, M.D., Olson, J.D. & Nett, T.M. (1984). Concentrations of testosterone in canine serum during late anestrous, proestrous, estrous and early diestrous. *American Journal of Veterinary Research*, **45**, 145–148.

Phemister, R.D., Holst, A.P., Spano, J.S. & Hopwood, L.M. (1972). Time of ovulation in the beagle bitch. *Biology of Reproduction*, **8**, 74–82.

Reimers, T., Phemister, R. & Niswender, G. (1978). Radioimmunological measurement of follicle stimulating hormone and prolactin in the dog. *Biology of Reproduction*, **19**, 673–679.

Rosendal, S. (1990). Mycoplasmal infections. In: *Infectious Diseases of the Dog and Cat*, (ed. C.E. Greene), pp. 446–449. W.B. Saunders, Philadelphia.

Schäfer, S., Holzmann, A. & Arbeiter, K. (1996). Beeinflussung der Qualitätsmerkmale des Ejakulates bei Beagle-Rüden durch Dauerbelastung. *Tierärztliche Praxis*, **24**, 385–390.

Schäfer, S., Holzmann, A. & Abeiter, K. (1997). The influence of frequent semen collection on the semen quality of Beagle dogs. *Deutsche tierärztliche Wochenschrift*, **104**, 26–29.

Shille, V.M. & Olson, P.N. (1989). Dynamic testing in reproductive endocrinology. In: *Current Veterinary Therapy X*, (ed. R.W. Kirk), pp. 1282–1288. W.B. Saunders, Philadelphia.

Smith, M.S. & McDonald, L.E. (1974). Serum levels of luteinizing hormone and progesterone during the estrous cycle, pseudopregnancy in the dog. *Endocrinology*, **94**, 404–412.

Soderberg, S.F. (1984). Pathophysiology of infertility and testicular atrophy in male Beagles and its relationship with endocrine disease. PhD thesis, Colorado State University.

Taha, M.B., Noakes, D.E. & Allen, W.E. (1981). The effect
of season of the year on the characteristics and composition
of dog semen. *Journal of Small Animal Practice*, **22**, 177–
184.

Wildt, D.E., Chakraborty, P.K., Panko, W.B. & Seager, S.W.J.
(1978). Relationship of reproductive behaviour, serum luteinizing hormone and time of ovulation in the bitch. *Biology of
Reproduction*, **18**, 561–570.

Wildt, D.E., Panko, W.B., Chakraborty, P. & Seager, S.W.J. (1979).
Relationship of serum estrone, estradiol-17 beta and proges-
terone to LH, sexual behavior and time of ovulation in the bitch.
Biology of Reproduction, **20**, 648–658.

Chapter 72

Conditions of the Male External Genital System

D. E. Noakes

CLINICAL EXAMINATION

A careful examination of the genital system of the male dog is important particularly in the puppy and also in the adult male where there is a history suggesting a genito-urinary disorder or infertility. The clinical examination is mainly dependent upon palpation and visual examination; supportive diagnostic procedures such as radiography, haematology, bacteriology and semen evaluation are useful in establishing a diagnosis. It is important to stress that the assay of reproductive hormones is of limited value, particularly if performed on a single sample, since there are large variations in normal values both within, and between, individual animals.

Testes and Scrotum

The scrotum of the dog is soft and thin walled. The testis is oval in shape, firm but not hard on palpation. There is considerable variation in the size of the testes in different breeds (Woodall & Johnstone 1988). The average dimensions are $3 \times 2 \times 1.5\,cm$, with an average weight of $11\,g$; the testes are normally of similar size in any individual dog.

The longitudinal axis is almost horizontal in the normally descended testis with the epididymis closely attached to the dorsolateral surface. The tail of the epididymis is palpable as a firm, but not hard, nodule on the caudal pole of each testis. Occasionally the testes appear to be positioned in tandem, especially in the Greyhound, but the normal position is readily established on palpation.

Penis and Prepuce

The penis can be readily examined by digital retraction of the prepuce. The integument is smooth, pink and moist.

The glans penis consists of two parts, the distal *pars longa glandis*, which is 5–6 cm in length, and the thicker, proximal bulbus glandis. Palpation of the *os penis* is usually possible in the non-erect penis.

The prepuce should be soft and mobile and the preputial orifice large enough to allow protrusion of the non-erect penis.

SCROTAL LESIONS

These are common in dogs kennelled on concrete floors or may be part of a generalised dermatitis. Trauma to the scrotum also occurs in hunting dogs (due to damage from thick vegetation) and as a result of dog fights.

Scrotal lesions cause great discomfort and are exacerbated by the dog licking. Affected dogs may be anorexic and reluctant to urinate.

Topical treatment (corticosteroid creams, acriflavine emulsion) may be difficult to administer due to the dog's discomfort. Systemic corticosteroids, tranquillisers or a collar to prevent self-trauma may be required.

TESTICULAR ABNORMALITIES

The testes of the dog may be the primary site of disease, as in cryptorchidism, orchitis or neoplasia, or be involved secondarily, as in Cushing's disease (see Chapter 58). The testes have a dual function, so that disease can be demonstrated in two ways – it can affect the production of testosterone by the interstitial cells, or the generation of spermatozoa.

Cryptorchidism

The testes of the dog are intra-abdominal at birth but normally descend soon afterwards (7–10 days). In some puppies it may be possible to palpate them in the scrotum or inguinal region at 2 weeks of age, but the presence of scrotal fat makes this difficult. It should be possible to palpate the testes at 6–8 weeks of age, however clinicians should exercise great care before confirming their presence. For this reason, it may be necessary to wait until the dog reaches puberty (5–12 months of age) before a definite diagnosis of cryptorchidism can be made; puberty occurs earlier in small breeds of dog.

A cryptorchid is an animal with one or both testes retained somewhere along the normal path of testicular descent. Retention is usually classified as inguinal or abdominal according to whether the testis is outside or inside the deep (internal) ring. Inguinal testes usually lie cranial to the scrotum alongside the penis, while abdominal testes lie close to the deep inguinal ring. An ectopic testis is one which has deviated from the normal pathway of descent, usually after passing through the deep inguinal ring, ectopic testes are rare in the dog.

A monorchid is an animal with only one testis. The term should not be applied to an animal with only one scrotal testis, as true monorchidism is extremely rare. An animal with only one testis must be presumed to have the second testis retained, and is thus a unilateral cryptorchid. An anorchid is an animal in which neither testis has developed.

Anorchidism is also extremely rare, and an animal with no history of castration and no scrotal testes must be presumed to have two retained testes, i.e. a bilateral cryptorchid. In cases of doubt, plasma samples can be taken before, and one hour after, an intravenous injection of human chorionic gonadotrophin (50 IU/kg). A rise in testosterone concentration indicates testicular tissue (England *et al.* 1989).

Incidence

Cryptorchidism is the commonest abnormality of sexual development. There are few surveys that describe the incidence; Cox *et al.* (1978) quote levels of 0.8–9.8%, while a surprisingly high frequency of 13% was reported in an earlier survey.

Aetiology

Normal descent of the testes is a complex process. The reasons for failure of descent are obscure but probably involve both endocrine and mechanical defects.

In certain breeds of dog, a high prevalence of the defect has been identified. These are: Toy and Miniature Poodle, Pomeranian, Yorkshire Terrier, Miniature Dachshund, Cairn Terrier, Chihuahua, Maltese, Boxer, Pekingese, English Bulldog, Miniature Schnauzer and Shetland Sheepdog. Such an observation would suggest that, as in other species, cryptorchidism is an inherited defect. Although the genetics of isolated cryptorchidism have not been completely characterised, it is likely that both males and females are carriers of the trait. This should be taken into account when reviewing the policy of breeding from either parent of affected animals, as well as the cryptorchid dog which should not be used (Burke 1986).

Clinical Significance

There are two important conditions that are associated with retained testes: an increased risk of neoplasia and a predisposition to torsion of the spermatic cord. These will be described in greater detail below.

Abdominal testes are aspermic, so that dogs with both testes retained are sterile, but will have normal libido and secondary sex characteristics. In unilateral retention, the descended testis functions normally and the dog is likely to be fertile.

Treatment

Since cryptorchidism is inherited, treatment that might induce descent should be discouraged. Testosterone and human chorionic gonadotrophin (hCG) have been used to try to induce testicular descent; apparent success probably occurs in those dogs that have inguinal testes in which descent would have occurred irrespective of treatment. The technique of orchipexy has been described, but with little proven success.

Any retained testis should be removed surgically after puberty to avoid the development of neoplasia. If it is likely that the dog will mate bitches, the descended testis should also be removed.

Testicular Neoplasia

Three types of testicular tumour have been described and have been classified according to the main cell type involved, i.e. Sertoli cell, interstitial cell and seminomas. Neoplasia of the testes is relatively frequent and is closely related to failure of normal gonadal descent. The relative risk of Sertoli cell tumours is 23 times greater, and that of seminomas is 16 times greater, in retained compared with descended testes (Pendergrass & Hayes 1976). Furthermore, neoplasia is twice as common in inguinal compared with abdominal testes (Reif *et al.* 1979).

Interstitial Cell Tumour

This is the commonest type of tumour recorded in old dogs. Frequently it causes no change in testicular size, and is rarely diagnosed; the only readily identified change is that affected testicles become hard. It rarely occurs in retained testes, is not malignant, and is generally endocrinologically inactive, although sometimes androgens are produced which result in the development of perineal tumours and prostatic hyperplasia.

Seminoma

This tumour occurs in middle-aged and old dogs. The main characteristic is marked testicular enlargement which is painless and usually unilateral. Commonly it is endocrinologically inactive, although there are reports of oestradiol production; metastases occur occasionally, especially from abdominal testes.

Sertoli Cell Tumour

This usually occurs in middle-aged and old dogs. The testis can be enlarged, firm and non-resilient, but on occasions there is no change in size. This tumour generally produces oestrogen, especially when intra-abdominal, and as a consequence there are signs of feminisation. This hormone causes gynaecomasty, pendulous sheath, penile and preputial atrophy, atrophy of the other testis if it is a unilateral lesion, prostatic enlargement (metaplasia) and bilateral symmetrical alopecia. Metastases are quite common and the dog is attractive to other males.

Treatment

In all cases of testicular neoplasia the only treatment is castration. Since the condition is frequently reported in retained testes it emphasises the need to remove these gonads before the dog reaches middle age. Frequently, and especially with Sertoli cell tumours and seminomas, both testes are involved even though there may not be obvious clinical signs.

Torsion of the Spermatic Cord (Testicular Torsion)

Torsion of the spermatic cord occurs rarely in the dog, but it is most frequently reported in retained or ectopic testes, probably due to instability of the suspension of the gonad thus allowing rotation. Torsion may also be associated with neoplastic enlargement of the testis. There does not appear to be any predisposition to side, and although the Boxer, Pekingese and Airedale Terrier have been most frequently identified with the condition, the numbers involved preclude any interpretation of a breed susceptibility (Zymet 1975).

Clinical Signs

These are dependent upon the site of the affected testis. There is usually the sudden onset of pain with a reluctance to move. The dog will be anorexic, will vomit and the gait will be stiff and abnormal. If the condition occurs in a descended testis then the scrotum will be swollen, oedematous and painful. Lethargy, dysuria and abdominal pain are sometimes seen.

Treatment

Orchidectomy should be performed as soon as possible, but fatalities may occur. The degree of torsion ranges from 360° to 720°.

Orchitis

Inflammation of one or both testes and associated epididymis is not a common condition in the dog in the UK; infection can result from trauma or haematogenous spread. The raised temperature of the testis can temporarily affect spermatogenesis, but if it is allowed to remain untreated it can result in testicular degeneration.

Clinical signs usually are a stiff gait, and scrotal and testicular enlargement which is very painful and has to be differentiated from torsion of the spermatic cord. Treatment consists of systemic antibiosis or orchidectomy.

Clinical cases of *Brucella canis* infection have not been reported in the UK, although there is serological evidence that it may exist (Taylor 1980). Onset can be insidious in dogs, causing seminal abnormalities for some time before the clinical signs of epididymitis and orchitis are evident (Barton 1977).

CONGENITAL DEFECTS

Normal mammalian sexual differentiation and development is dependent upon the successful completion of a number of sequential changes that are under genetic control. These are: (1) the establishment of chromosomal sex, (2) the development of gonadal sex, (3) the development of phenotypic sex.

An individual in which differentiation and development is abnormal and ambiguous is sometimes referred to as an intersex. However, the degree of abnormality and ambiguity can vary from slight, involving just part, to severe, in which the whole genital system is involved. Although intersexes are not common in dogs, when they do occur, they can cause dismay for breeders and disappointment for the owners of affected puppies. When an intersex occurs, there must be a failure at one of the stages of sexual development listed above.

Abnormalities of chromosomal sex can be identified by karyotyping. These can be phenotypic females (XO, XXX) or phenotypic males (XXY). In both, the genitalia is usually underdeveloped rather than ambiguous. In addition, chimaeras and mosaics can arise where individuals have at least two cell populations with different chromosomal constitutions. Some chimaeras can result in true hermaphrodites in which individuals have either an ovary and testis, or ovotestes with both ovarian and testicular tissue contained within the same organs.

When there are abnormalities of gonadal sex, there is disagreement between the chromosome constitution and the gonads; this is also referred to as sex reversal. In the dog, XX reversal has been identified in a number of different breeds. Individual animals will have a XX chromosomal constitution but with varying amounts of testicular tissue resulting in XX males which are sterile, and XX true hermaphrodites with both testicular and ovarian tissue.

Abnormalities in the development of phenotypic sex are seen in individuals where both chromosomal and gonadal sex agree, but the internal and external genital organs show varying degrees of ambiguity. These are referred to as either male or female pseudohermaphrodites. Female pseudohermaphrodites have an XX chromosome constitution, two ovaries but with varying degrees of masculinisation ranging from a slight displacement of the vulva ventrally, the presence of a rudimentary prepuce (Fig. 72.1), clitoral enlargement (Fig. 72.2), to near normal male genitalia. In some cases, where relatively slight, the condition is brought to the attention of the owner because the bitch comes into pro-oestrus with the development of a blood-stained discharge from the prepuce. Male pseudohermaphrodites have an XY chromosome constitution and testes, but with varying degrees of development of female genitalia. This can be due to defects in Müllerian duct regression resulting in the presence of parts, or the whole, female tubular genital system (Fig. 72.3). It can also be due to defects in androgen-dependent masculinisation. Examples of the latter are incomplete urethral formation in which the urethra opens at some place other than the tip of the penis; this is referred to as hypospadia. If the opening is sited near the tip of the penis it is referred to as glandular hypospadia and causes few problems. However, more severe forms have been identified with the urethra opening at the pars longa glandis (penile hypospadia), or the scrotum (scrotal hypoplasia), or sub-ischially (perineal hypospadia). Surgical repair can be difficult because frequently the urethra distal to the opening is not patent.

Aetiology

Frequently the precise cause is unknown. The possibility of it being inherited should always be considered, particularly if it occurs frequently in puppies of certain breeds and familial lines. Female pseudohermaphrodism has been

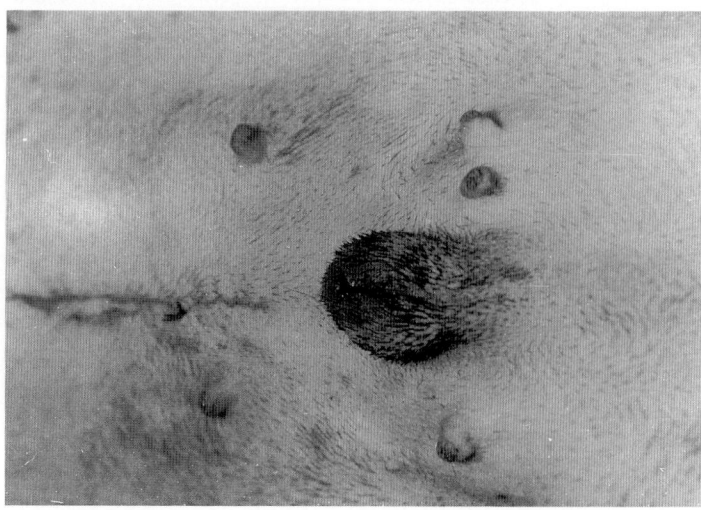

Fig. 72.1 Rudimentary prepuce which contains no penis. This female pseudohermaphrodite was first noticed to be abnormal when a haemorrhagic pro-oestrus preputial discharge began.

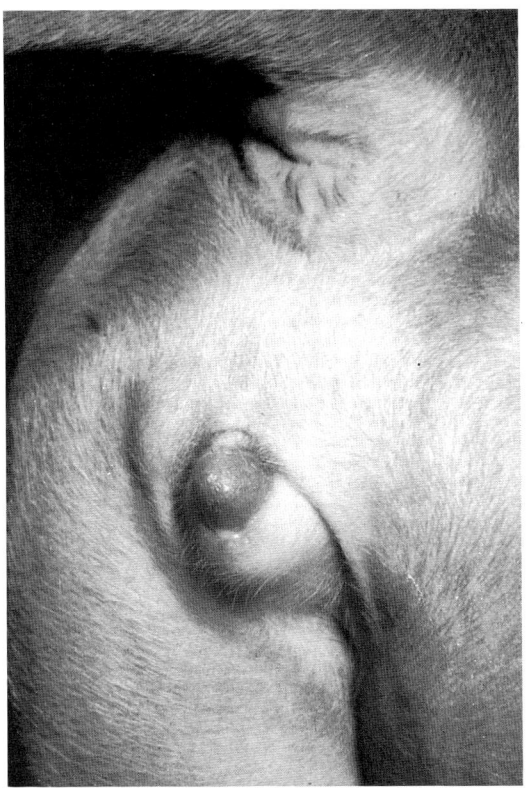

Fig. 72.2 Female pseudohermaphrodite with ventrally situated vulva and large clitoris.

reported in puppies where the dam has received androgens or progestagens during pregnancy.

Diagnosis

The ease of diagnosis of intersexuality will depend upon the severity of the developmental abnormality, in some mild forms it can be overlooked in young puppies. Karyotyping may be necessary for confirmation.

Treatment

Cosmetic surgery can make it more acceptable to the owner, as well as preventing some complications, particularly trauma to the enlarged clitoris. This will involve amputation of the phallus and reconstruction of the vulva/prepuce. Gonadectomy is indicated, especially if a testis is retained.

ABNORMALITIES OF THE PENIS AND PREPUCE

Transmissible Venereal Tumour

This tumour occurs mainly on the external genitalia of both dogs and bitches. The disease is rare in Britain and is

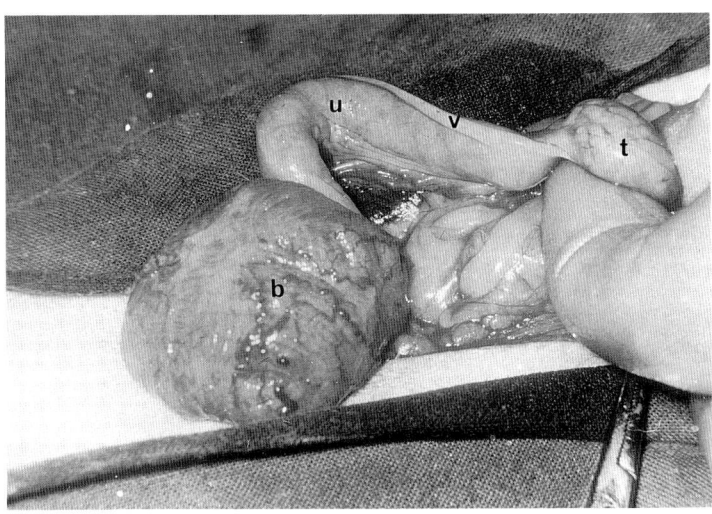

Fig. 72.3 Urogenital organs of male pseudohermaphrodite intersexual dog at laparotomy. b, urinary bladder; u, uterine horn; v, vas deferens; t, testis.

most likely to be seen in dogs in quarantine. Over the years there have been isolated reports of the disease in particular areas. It is very common world-wide, especially in tropical and subtropical climates where there are large numbers of stray and wild dogs.

The disease, which is probably of viral origin, is spread at coitus, although there are also reports of its transmission to cutaneous sites following the contamination of bites and scratches. Younger, healthier individuals tend to be more resistant to experimental transmission than older dogs.

Clinical Signs

The history of a blood-stained preputial discharge should encourage the clinician to retract the prepuce so that the surface of the penis can be examined. The lesion usually appears as a pinkish-red, nodular non-encapsulated mass, measuring up to 15 mm in diameter. Rarely metastases may involve the inguinal lymph nodes.

Cutaneous lesions have been described in dogs that are in poor health. The lesions involve the skin and subcutaneous regions and consist of raised areas up to 6 cm in diameter over the back, flank, neck and limbs.

Diagnosis

This is based on the appearance of the lesions on the glans penis. When they are small the initial sign may only be the presence of a blood-stained preputial discharge, especially after mating. In the early stages there is rarely a purulent discharge, but as the disease progresses there is necrosis and ulceration of the tumour and subsequent infection. A biopsy of the tumour mass may be taken to confirm the diagnosis.

Treatment

Since the dog will develop an immunity, the tumour will regress spontaneously in about 6 months provided that the dog is in good health. Surgical excision and cryosurgery have proved successful (Craig *et al.* 1986). In addition, a number of chemotherapeutic agents have been used: vincristine, methotrexate and cyclophosphamide (MacEwen 1989).

Balanoposthitis

This describes inflammation of the penile integument and preputial lining and is quite a common condition. Young male dogs, around the age of puberty, frequently develop a preputial discharge which, apart from the inconvenience to

the owner, has no effect on the dog. All entire male dogs have some degree of preputial discharge, which, although it contains neutrophils, is not associated with signs of inflammation. It is often difficult to decide what degree of discharge is abnormal.

Clinical Signs

There is usually a history of a preputial discharge which is purulent or slightly blood-stained. The dog will frequently lick and bite the prepuce and there may be evidence of self-inflicted trauma. He may resent palpation of the prepuce and exposure of the penis. There is rarely any systemic involvement. Exposure of the glans penis shows a red and inflamed integument with small raised nodules and in severe cases there may be ulceration.

Diagnosis

This is based on the clinical signs, especially on the appearance of the glans penis and preputial lining. Bacterial culture of the discharge or preputial swabs is of limited value. There is an extensive and varied bacterial flora on the surface of the penis and preputial lining. *Staphylococcus aureus* and mycoplasmas are most frequently isolated, although a large number of other bacterial species have also been isolated in mixed aerobic cultures. The isolation of *Proteus* spp. and *Pseudomonas* spp. in pure or nearly pure cultures may be significant.

Treatment

In many cases, especially in the young dog, treatment is unnecessary. Broad-spectrum parenteral antibiotics coupled with local application should be tried. If antiseptic washes are used care must be taken to use them at the recommended dilutions since in many cases concentrated solutions are irritant. Saline irrigation may also be tried as an alternative. Progestogens may be given in an attempt to reduce sexual self-interest, or the dog may be castrated.

Dog Pox

This is the name given to an eruptive condition of the mucous membranes of dogs and bitches, probably caused by a canine herpesvirus. The infection can occur in the colon and the recto-anal area as well as the penis of the dog and the vestibule of the bitch.

The lesions are small papules which may be present as scattered discrete eruptions or, if numerous and almost contiguous, as a moist granular mass. Individual lesions may appear haemorrhagic (although actual haemorrhage is rare) or they may glisten like vesicles. In over 90% of cases the lesions are asymptomatic, but they may, however, be associated with abnormal preputial discharge and irritation (see above). The signs may be as vague as the dog turning round suddenly to nibble in a random manner at the hindquarters, hindlegs and inside of the thighs.

Treatment

When required, treatment comprises instillation of antibiotics into the sheath and gentle massage towards the base of the penis. Cautery may render the lesions less 'active' (2–5% silver nitrate washed off with saline immediately appears effective). Although venereal transmission to bitches can take place, this appears to be a relatively uncommon method of spread.

Phimosis

This is the condition where, because of an abnormally small preputial opening, the dog is unable to protrude the partially erect penis. As a consequence erection may occur within the prepuce, causing discomfort and may ultimately result in a balanoposthitis. If severe, the dog may dribble urine that has accumulated in the prepuce. The condition is usually congenital and can be corrected by surgical enlargement of the preputial opening.

Paraphimosis

This occurs when the erect or partially erect penis has protruded from the prepuce, but the preputial orifice is restricted and acts as a tourniquet, thus preventing detumescence and return to the prepuce. It is most likely to be seen in young dogs and perhaps after coitus. It is sometimes difficult to differentiate this from persistent erection (priapism) which is probably due to some neurological or circulatory defect.

As well as causing embarrassment to owners it causes discomfort to the dog and if left untreated can result in severe trauma to the penis. Tranquillisers, cold compresses and attempted manual replacement may be successful. However, in some cases replacement under general anaesthesia, with adequate lubrication to the glans penis, may be necessary.

If the condition is persistent it may be necessary to enlarge the preputial orifice surgically.

Penile Bleeding

This may occur apparently spontaneously, or after trauma. Bleeding is usually intermittent and occurs commonly when the dog is excited, e.g. when its owner returns home. Suturing the wound with fine absorbable material may be effective if carried out when the lesion is fresh. In long-standing cases it may be necessary to excise the affected part or amputate the penis. Castration helps to prevent post-operative haemorrhage.

REFERENCES

Barton, C.L. (1977). Canine brucellosis. *Veterinary Clinics of North America*, 7(4), 705–710.

Burke, T.J. (1986). Causes of infertility. In: *Small Animal Reproduction and Infertility*, (ed. T.J. Burke), pp. 233–236. Lea & Febiger, Philadelphia.

Cox, V.S., Wallace, L.J. & Jessen, C.R. (1978). An anatomic and genetic study of canine cryptorchidism. *Teratology*, 18, 233–240.

Craig, J.A., Richardson, R.C. & Rudd, R.G. (1986). A practical guide to clinical oncology – 4: chemotherapy and immunotherapy. *Veterinary Medicine*, 81, 226–241.

England, G.C.W., Allen, W.E. & Porter, D.J. (1989). The evaluation of the testosterone response to human chorionic gonadotrophin and the identification of a presumed anorchid dog. *Journal of Small Animal Practice*, 30, 441–443.

MacEwen, E.G. (1989). Canine transmissible venereal tumour. In: *Veterinary Oncology*, (eds S.J. Withrow & E.G. MacEwen), pp. 421–424. Lippincott, Philadelphia.

Pendergrass, T.W. & Hayes, H.M. (1976). Cryptorchidism and related defects in dogs: epidemiologic comparison with man. *Teratology*, 12, 51–55.

Reif, J.S., Maguire, T.G., Kenney, R.M. & Brodey, R.S. (1979). A cohort study of canine testicular neoplasia. *Journal of the American Veterinary Medical Association*, 175, 719–723.

Taylor, D.J. (1980). Serological evidence for the presence of *Brucella canis* infection in dogs in Britain. *Veterinary Record*, 106, 102–103.

Woodall, P.F. & Johnstone, I.P. (1988). Scrotal width as an index of testicular size in dogs and its relationship to body size. *Journal of Small Animal Practice*, 29, 543–547.

Zymet, C.L. (1975). Intrascrotal testicular torsion in a sexually aggressive dog. *Veterinary Medicine and Small Animal Clinician*, 70, 1330–1331.

Chapter 73

Diagnosis and Management of Canine Prostatic Disease

N. T. Gorman

INTRODUCTION

Prostatic disease is a common clinical presentation particularly in the older dog. The purpose of this chapter is to highlight the major clinical conditions that affect the canine prostate and how these may be diagnosed accurately and treated appropriately.

The clinical signs associated with prostatic disorders include: tenesmus, constipation, haematuria, recurrent urinary tract infections, pain and/or weakness in the rear quarters. There are many other conditions that can produce these clinical signs and it is therefore important to have a clear diagnostic plan when evaluating such patients to ensure that the correct diagnosis is established.

Diagnostic Techniques

The clinical presentation will give an index of suspicion that the prostate may be involved. There are a number of simple practical techniques that can be used to help make the diagnosis and these are summarised below.

Rectal Palpation of Prostate

- This examination determines the size, conformation, symmetry, mobility, consistency of the prostate and whether or not it is movable within the pelvic canal, the abdominal cavity or firmly adhered to another structure such as the pelvic floor.
- A painful prostate generally indicates inflammatory and septic processes whereas an immovable prostate is often associated with primary neoplasia or a large prostatic cyst (especially in Doberman Pinschers).

- It is important to consider the patient's age, breed and whether it is entire or neutered. Of particular note is the Scottish Terrier, in which relatively large prostate glands are found routinely.

Radiography

Plain Lateral and Ventrodorsal Examination
The key important features on plain radiography are:

- symmetrical enlargement,
- asymmetrical enlargement,
- variation in density,
- loss of contrast detail in the caudal abdomen,
- mineralisation of the prostate and associated structures, e.g. cysts,
- sublumbar lymphadenopathy,
- bony proliferation of the pelvic brim and the base of the L6, L7 and sacrum.

Positive Contrast Urethrography

- Narrowing of the prostatic urethra and significant leakage of the contrast material into the prostate is deemed to be associated with prostatic pathological changes.
- This technique has been reported to predispose the patient to recurrent bacterial infections and bladder rupture and so should not be performed unless other imaging techniques have proved equivocal.
- A small amount of leakage into the parenchyma is not necessarily a pathological finding.

Excretory Urography

- This technique is of limited value in assessing the degree of prostatic disease but can be of value in cases when prostatic enlargement causes partial urethral obstruction.

- In such cases there is every likelihood that there will be distension of the ureters, hydroureter and hydronephrosis.

Ultrasonography

- This is a more powerful tool than radiography for imaging the prostate. Ultrasonography gives details relating to size, density, structure, consistency, prostatic urethral diameter and related structures such as cysts and abscesses.

Prostatic Massage

- This can yield important information on the cellular infiltrates in the prostate and prostatic urethra.
- Harvesting of bacteria from the prostate is sometimes possible but difficult to interpret, particularly if the urine is infected.
- The bladder is emptied and flushed a number of times with sterile saline. A male catheter is inserted into the urethra and advanced to the level of the prostate and a sample of the fluid in the prostatic urethra collected.
- The prostate is massaged per rectum and 5–10 ml of saline are instilled slowly into the catheter with the urethra occluded around the catheter to avoid leakage.
- The catheter should be advanced into the bladder and repeated samples collected. The pre-massage sample should be compared with the post-massage sample for bacterial load, cell count and cell morphology.

Semen Evaluation

- In the case of bacterial infection of the prostate, a semen sample will yield the most accurate information provided there is not a concomitant infection of any of the other male reproductive organs.
- The difficulty with collection is that the majority of dogs with prostatic disease have little or no inclination to ejaculate under normal or artificial means.
- If an ejaculate can be collected, the presence of high cell numbers and bacterial numbers are indicative of infection.

Urinalysis

- Routine urinalysis of an end of stream voided urine sample is invaluable in cases of urinary tract disease.

- In prostatic disease useful information relating to cell morphology, bacterial load, bacterial type and cell counts can be gained by this simple procedure.
- It must be appreciated that the urine sample will not always be a true indicator of the prostatic disease but it helps in establishing the degree of disease within the lower urinary tract.

Prostatic Fine Needle Aspiration

A number of techniques have been developed for obtaining an aspirate from the prostate. The principle ones are:

- transrectal aspiration,
- pararectal aspiration, and
- transabdominal aspiration.

Of these, the transabdominal route is by far the safest and easiest when there is prostatomegaly. This is particularly so when the aspiration can be undertaken with the aid of ultrasound-guided needles.

Prostatic Biopsy

- Prostatic biopsy can be undertaken as either a percutaneous or an open procedure and is indicated where a tissue sample is required for a definitive diagnosis to be made.

CLINICAL CONDITIONS

The major clinical conditions that affect the canine prostate are listed in Table 73.1.

Table 73.1 Clinical conditions affecting the canine prostate.

Benign prostatic hyperplasia
Squamous metaplasia of the prostate
Acute prostatitis
Chronic prostatitis
Prostatic abscesses
Prostatic cysts
Paraprostatic cysts
Neoplasia

Benign Prostatic Hyperplasia

This is characterised by an insidious enlargement of the prostate due to prostatic epithelial proliferation, usually in the older dog. This process is related to an imbalance between androgen and oestrogen production and androgen receptors on the surface of the epithelial cells. There is a gradual increase in size starting from early adulthood and the pathology is generally one of a uniform increase in the number and size of the prostatic epithelial cells. It is possible for there to be some cystic changes within the gland, some of which can bleed. The clinical signs are usually related to tenesmus and constipation or to obstructive lower urinary tract disease particularly urinary retention.

In nearly all these cases there is a dramatic response to castration. The prostatomegaly should begin to resolve within the first week and there should be a notable difference on rectal palpation within 2 weeks. If this is not the case then a further tissue sample should be taken.

There are times when castration is not feasible and medical treatment has to be considered. The most potent medical therapy is diethylstilboestrol (DES) which depresses gonadotrophin production by the pituitary gland thus inhibiting the circulating androgen levels. This inhibitory effect results in the reduction in the size of the prostate. There are many negative effects of using this drug the principle one being bone marrow suppression which can result in thrombocytopenia, anaemia, leukopenia or pancytopenia. DES can be effective but has the potential to induce squamous cell metaplasia, cyst formation within the prostate and infection which can complicate further the management of the case.

Squamous Metaplasia

Squamous metaplasia is associated with either the administration of exogenous oestrogens or with an oestrogen-secreting Sertoli-cell tumour. In cases of Sertoli-cell tumour, the clinical signs of the hyperoestrogenism and feminisation are also present (attractiveness to other males, monorchid or cryptorchid, an atrophied testicle, bilateral alopecia, gynecomastica, pendulous prepuce, bone marrow disorders). The treatment of a Sertoli-cell tumour is removal of both testes. In cases of administration of DES, the therapy should be discontinued.

Bacterial Prostatitis

Acute Bacterial Prostatitis

This usually arises from an ascending bacterial infection and is characterised by an acute systemic illness manifested by fever, caudal abdominal pain, haematuria and there is extreme pain upon rectal palpation of the prostate gland. There can be an asymmetry of the gland. In some cases, the infection rapidly progresses to an endotoxic shock and sepsis and death can occur if the disease is not managed quickly. The infection may be superimposed upon a pre-existing prostatic disease, such as benign prostatic hyperplasia, or affect a comparatively normal prostate. While it is believed that the majority of infections ascend from the urinary tract, there are a number of cases that will arise from systemic infection which localises within the prostate.

The therapy of a simple bacterial infection of the prostate has been dealt with in the previous section. A reasonable number of these cases will not fully recover and the animal will be left with a recurrent chronic prostatitis.

Chronic Bacterial Prostatitis

Clinically, these animals present with a history of a recurrent pyrexia of unknown origin, recurrent urinary tract infection with or without a urethral discharge. In contrast to the acute disease, the animal is not systemically ill and there may be few signs referable to the prostate. It is usual for there to be a concomitant urinary tract infection in these cases, and this needs managing as well. Diagnosis of these cases is dependent upon all the ancillary aids but a culture of prostatic fluid is particularly helpful. This may be collected via prostatic massage or, if the animal can be stimulated appropriately, by an ejaculate sample. The treatment of these cases is wholly dependent upon the sensitivity of the bacterial infection and the delivery of the antibacterial drugs to the site. A prolonged course (4–6 weeks) of antibacterial drugs such as trimethoprim–sulphadiazine or erythromycin is recommended and the animal should be castrated after 4 weeks of antibiotic therapy.

Treatment of chronic prostatitis is not easy and is focused at decreasing the bacterial load within the prostate and the urinary tract. There is a very powerful barrier that inhibits the passage of antibacterial agent from the blood into the gland. This is compounded by the variation of pH within the gland and the secretions and a number of proteins that have been shown to bind to antibiotics yielding them inactive. It has been documented for some time that the pH of the prostatic fluid in the dog is around 6.4 which is a full 1.0 pH unit difference from that of the blood. This difference can be used to therapeutic advantage by using antibiotics that concentrate in acidic conditions. Weak bases such as trimethoprim and erythromycin are ion-trapped and concentrated in the prostatic fluid. Fluoroquinolones and chloramphenicol also reach reasonable concentration within the prostate gland It is essential that therapy be continued for at least 6 weeks. Even after this time there can be pockets of infection which remain active despite the therapy. In such cases, repeated protracted therapy is required. Castration of a dog with chronic prostatitis is of benefit in that it does cause a reduction in the size and activity of the gland.

Prostatic Abscessation

This is a chronic prostatitis where the inflammatory purulent exudate accumulates in the parenchyma of the prostate. The clinical signs are variable and can be similar to acute bacterial prostatitis but less fulminating or exaggerated than signs of chronic prostatitis. There is caudal abdominal pain and the prostate gland is asymmetrical, a soft fluctuant swelling may be felt within the prostate and it is often painful upon palpation. Diagnosis of this condition is usually confirmed either by ultrasonography or by exploratory laparotomy. The abscess can either be predominantly within the body of the gland or sitting on the surface. In the latter case many adhesions can be associated with the major pathological change.

Treatment of this condition requires drainage of the prostatic abscess. This is achieved by ventral or paramedian drainage (Basinger & Rawlings 1987) or by omentalisation of the prostate (White & Williams 1991, 1995). Castration should accompany all forms of prostatic drainage to reduce the activity of the residual glandular tissue.

Whatever the method of drainage, it is essential to administer appropriate antibiotics for a period of not less than 3 weeks. The sample of purulent material taken early in the surgery should be cultured so that the most effective antibiotic can be used for the appropriate length of time. In some cases, the dogs undergo serious postoperative sepsis and attention must be given to controlling the bacteraemia and the shock that can follow.

Prostatic Cysts

There are a number of cystic conditions that affect the canine prostate. These can be divided broadly into those within the parenchyma and those outwith the main parenchyma. Within the parenchyma they can be single (retention cyst) or multiple (cystic prostatic hyperplasia). Non-parenchymal cysts can either be paraprostatic or be periprostatic

Parenchymal-Retention Cysts

These cysts develop within the parenchyma of the prostate and clinical signs only occur when the cysts become large. The clinical signs are similar to those described previously relating to an enlarged non-infected prostate. Multiple

cysts may respond to castration and surgery is only warranted if one of the cysts becomes large enough to protrude from the surface of the prostate.

Non-parenchymal

Paraprostatic cysts are the most common non-parenchymal cyst. These cysts do not originate within the prostate but are thought to arise from remnants of the Mullerian ducts. The cysts are fluid filled and can often attain such a size that they can be palpated through the abdominal wall and can be confused with the urinary bladder on a caudal abdominal radiograph. The walls of the cysts are often calcified.

The treatment of these cysts is either by drainage or resection, the latter being the most effective where it is possible. There are cases where resection is impossible and drainage through the abdominal wall is the only real alternative. This process of marsupialisation simply attaches the inner wall of the cyst to the skin and allows drainage for about 2–3 weeks. There is a tendency for the drainage stoma to heal over and daily digital examination of the wound is required to ensure that the adhesions are broken down. The walls of the cysts eventually adhere together and usually prevent formation of further cysts. Unfortunately, in some of these cases drainage is insufficient and the cyst reappears. In all cases the dog requires castration.

Prostatic Neoplasia

Benign forms of prostatic neoplasia other than benign prostatic hypertrophy are rare in the dog. Adenocarcinoma is the commonest malignant neoplasm of the prostate but is still comparatively uncommon and presents late in the disease. The clinical signs vary widely and include weight loss, rear limb weakness, tenesmus, lumbar pain, haematuria and stranguria. The majority of cases of prostatic neoplasia are diagnosed when local and distant metastases (particularly to bone) have already occurred. It is difficult to explain fully the propensity and the ability of prostatic metastases to spread to the bone but it is undoubtedly the commonest site that is seen. There have been many attempts to treat these cases surgically, with intra-operative radiotherapy or with chemotherapy and all continue to produce poor results. The most promising has been the use of radiation therapy, initially with intra-operative orthovoltage therapy and more recently with deep electron-beam therapy. Castration can in some cases cause a temporary halt to the progression of the primary disease and amelioration of the clinical signs. Most cases have a survival time without treatment of around 2 months following diagnosis and with radiation therapy of up to 9 months. The number of patients reported in clinical trials is, however, few.

Prostatectomy

It is possible to remove the prostate, either in total with a prostatectomy and anastomsis of the urethra, or partially by an intracapsular partial prostatectomy. Both procedures carry a high risk to the patient and there are very few instances where either procedure is warranted in veterinary practice. In man there have been great strides in prostatic surgery by the use of transurethral partial prostatectomy, which is a procedure that is performed from within the urethra via a cystoscope.

REFERENCES AND FURTHER READING

Barsanti, J.A. & Finco, D.R. (1989). Canine prostatic diseases. In: *Textbook of Veterinary Internal Medicine*, (ed. S.J. Ettinger), pp. 1881–1891. W.B. Saunders, Philapdelphia.

Basinger, R.R., Robinette, C.L., Hardie, E.M., *et al.* (1993). The prostate. In: *Textbook of Small Animal Surgery*, (ed. D.H. Slatter), 2nd edn. pp. 1349–1364. W.B. Saunders, Philadelphia.

Basinger, R.R. & Rawlings, C.A. (1987). Surgical management of prostatic diseases. *Compendium on Continuing Education for the Practicing Veterinarian*, 9, 993–1000.

Gourley, L.G. & Osborne, C.A. (1966). Marsupialisation. A treatment of prostatic abscess in the dog. *Journal of the American Animal Hospital Association*, 2, 100–105.

Johnston, D.E. (1985). Prostate. In: *Textbook of Small Animal Surgery*, (ed. D.H. Slatter), pp. 1635–1650. Lea & Febiger, Philalelphia.

White, R.A.S. & Williams, J.M. (1991). Prostatatic parenchymal omentalization – a new technique for management of prostatic cysts and abscesses. *Veterinary Surgery*, 20, 335.

White, R.A.S. & Williams, J.M. (1995). Intracapsular prostatic omentalization – a new technique for management of prostatic abscesses in dogs. *Veterinary Surgery*, 24, 390–395.

Zolton, G.M. & Greiner, T.P. (1978). Prostatic abscess – a surgical approach. *Journal of the American Animal Hospital Association*, 14, 698–702.

Section 10

Skeletal Disorders

Edited by Chris May

Chapter 74

Introduction to Joint Diseases

C. May

INTRODUCTION

A joint is the union of adjacent bones by fibrous, cartilaginous or elastic tissues. Joints are usually classified on the basis of the type of motion that they allow:

- diarthrosis (synovial joint, freely movable),
- amphiarthrosis (cartilaginous joint, partially movable),
- synarthrosis (fibrous joint, immobile).

Synovial joints and cartilaginous joints (intervertebral discs) are of most importance in the clinical context. The chapters in this section assume an understanding of synovial anatomy (reviewed by Bennett & May 1995) and intervertebral disc anatomy (reviewed by Wheeler & Sharp 1994).

CLASSIFICATION OF ARTHRITIS

Joint disease is most frequently classified as 'degenerative' or 'inflammatory' depending on the *predominant* pathology within the affected joint. This is ascertained most simply and reliably by synovial fluid analysis (Table 74.1).

DEGENERATIVE JOINT DISEASES

- osteoarthritis
- traumatic arthritis
- haemophilic arthritis
- neuropathic arthritis

Neuropathic arthritis and haemophilic arthritis are rare clinical entities. Traumatic arthritis may be short-lived (e.g. mild sprains and contusion) or severe enough to warrant surgical intervention (e.g. luxation or severe subluxation). Osteoarthritis is the most important degenerative joint disease from a medical viewpoint.

INFLAMMATORY JOINT DISEASES

- bacterial infective synovitis (including endocarditis and arthritis)
- discospondylitis
- Lyme disease
- tuberculosis (rare, but an important zoonosis)
- mycoplasma (rare, significance in dogs uncertain)
- fungal (rare, fungal synovitis not recorded in the UK)
- protozoan (leishmaniasis is endemic in some Mediterranean countries. Rare in UK)
- viral (significance uncertain in dogs)

Immune-Based

Erosive

- canine rheumatoid arthritis
- canine periosteal proliferative polyarthritis
- Felty's syndrome: rheumatoid arthritis complicated by splenomgaly and neutropenia. Prognosis is very poor
- polyarthritis of Greyhounds

Non-erosive

- systemic lupus erythematosus
- polyarthritis/polymyositis

Table 74.1 Synovial fluid analysis in the dog.

	Normal joint	Degenerative joint disease	Immune Mediated arthritis	Bacterial Infective arthritis
Colour	Clear/pale yellow	Yellow	Yellow (+/– blood tinged)	Yellow (+/– blood tinged)
Clarity	Transparent	Transparent	Transparent or opaque	Opaque
Viscosity	Very high	High	Low/very low	Very low
Mucin clot	Good	Good-fair	Fair-poor	Poor
Spontaneous clot	None	+/–	often	often
White cells (/mm^3)	<1000	1000–5000	>5000	>5000
Neutrophils	<5%	<10%	10–95%	>90%
Mononuclear cells	>95%	>90%	5–90%	<10%
Protein (g/dl)	2.0–2.5	2.0–3.0	2.5–5.0	>4.0

- polyarthritis/meningitis
- polyarteritis nodosa
- Sjögren's syndrome (polyarthritis with keratitis sicca, sialoadenitis)
- plasmacytic/lymphocytic gonitis (inflammatory synovitis of the stifles)
- Arthritis of Japanese Akitas
- Shar Pei fever syndrome
- Drug-induced or vaccination 'reactions'
- Idiopathic
  Type I   (no associations)
  Type II   ('reactive')
  Type III   (enteropathic)
  Type IV   (neoplastic)

Crystal Arthropathies

- gout
- pseudogout
- hydroxyapatite

All crystal arthropathies are rare in dogs.

APPROACH TO THE PATIENT

The initial steps in investigation of all joint disease are conveniently divided into an ordered series of logical steps.

History

Signalment and Background Information

Many joint diseases show predilections to a particular age or type of dog and the signalment is the first clue to this. Further background information might include the use of the animal (pet or working dog) and details of the general medical history of the dog.

Owner's Complaint

The problems identified by the owner are frequently the foundation for the remainder of the clinical examination. It is important to establish clearly and precisely the problem, or problems that the owner identifies and it may be useful to list these on the clinical record.

Specific History

The specific history should be both full and accurate. In complex or long-standing cases, obtaining an adequate history can be both painstaking and time-consuming. However, the importance of care at this stage in the examination cannot be over-emphasised. Specific points of history useful in joint disease include:

- Was the onset sudden or gradual?
- How long has the lameness been present?
- Does the severity of lameness vary with time of day, physical activity or rest?

- Does the severity of lameness vary with climatic conditions?
- Has the owner noticed any swellings, deformities or muscle wastage?
- Is there any history to suggest a systemic illness?
- What is the dog's normal exercise routine?
- During the illness has the dog been unable to perform activities previously considered normal?

> With few exceptions, a history of stiffness after rest is an indicator of joint disease.

Physical Examination

An orthopaedic examination should always be preceded by a general physical examination and may need to be supplemented by a neurological examination. The orthopaedic examination should be performed in a routine and systematic fashion. Specific aspects of the examination include:

(1) *Observation* – both standing and at one or more gaits. Particular attention should be paid to obvious limb lameness (not always the one identified by the owner!), general demeanour, conformation, posture, body contours, evidence of muscle wastage and any deformities.
(2) *Palpation* – palpation supplements observation in detecting changes in body contour (swelling or wastage). Joint swelling invisible to the eye can often be sensed by palpation. Palpation also adds information about the texture of any swellings and the presence of local heat or pain, often associated with inflammation.
(3) *Manipulation* – for both normal and abnormal movements. Each joint should be manipulated through its normal expected range of movement to assess deformity or displacement of a joint (luxation and subluxation), increases or decreases in range of movement,

pain and crepitus. The integrity of supporting structures of the joint can often be assessed by attempting manipulation for abnormal movements. The cranial draw test for investigating the integrity of the cranial cruciate ligament is a good example of this type of manipulation. It is often rewarding to repeat such manipulations with the dog sedated or anaesthetised; this is often conveniently combined with further investigations of the joint disease.

Investigation

Once a physical examination is complete, a differential diagnosis list should be drawn up and a diagnostic plan developed. Aids to the diagnosis of joint disease include:

(1) *Imaging* – most often radiology (including contrast arthrography). Other imaging techniques that have been used to evaluate joint disease include ultrasonography, linear tomography, computerised tomography, magnetic resonance imaging and scintigraphy.
(2) *Synoviocentesis and synovial fluid analysis* – this is one of the most accessible and powerful aids to the diagnosis of joint disease (Table 74.1). The information gained from simply performing total and differential white cell counts on joint fluids is often invaluable.
(3) *Inspection of joint* – achieved by either exploratory arthrotomy or by arthroscopy.
(4) *Biopsy of synovial membrane* – for histological examination, culture or immunohistochemical studies.

REFERENCES

Bennett, D. & May, C. (1995). Joint diseases of dogs and cats. In: *Textbook of Veterinary Internal Medicine*, (eds S.J. Ettinger & E.C. Feldman), pp. 2032–2077. W.B. Saunders, Philadelphia.

Wheeler, S.J. & Sharp, N.J.H. (1994). *Small Animal Spinal Disorders. Diagnosis and Surgery*. Mosby-Wolfe, London.

Chapter 75

Osteoarthritis

A. R. Coughlan

INTRODUCTION

> *Definition*
> Osteoarthritis (OA) is a condition of synovial joints characterised by chondropathy and typical associated changes in the surrounding bone and soft tissues (Fig. 75.1).

Osteoarthritis presents as a syndrome of joint pain and dysfunction. Although it is difficult to produce an aetiological framework applicable to all cases of osteoarthritis, one currently accepted model is presented in Fig. 75.2.

Traditionally, osteoarthritis has been classified as either primary (idiopathic no cause identified) or secondary (a major causative factor identified). As more is understood about the development of osteoarthritis, it is likely that an alternative classification system will emerge. Most cases of canine osteoarthritis are secondary, with common aetiologies including cranial cruciate ligament failure, hip dysplasia and articular osteochondrosis. The management of these conditions is largely surgical and is covered in detail elsewhere (see Bennett 1990), however a compact overview of articular osteochondrosis is given in Box 75.1 due to the increasing importance and ongoing controversy of this condition (see also Bennett & May 1995).

Osteoarthritis is not a passive 'falling apart' of articular cartilage; it is a dynamic process. A deeper understanding of the molecular mechanisms involved in osteoarthritis is crucial for developing therapies capable of arresting, or even reversing, progression of the disease. Reliable markers for earlier diagnosis and accurate staging of osteoarthritis are also required. Advances in these areas have been made and will be discussed in this section. Established principles of diagnosing and managing canine osteoarthritis will also be reviewed.

PATHOPHYSIOLOGY OF CHONDROPATHY IN OSTEOARTHRITIS

The remarkable physical properties of articular cartilage are dependent on a complex and specific arrangement of macromolecules in the extracellular matrix (ECM) (Fig. 75.3). It is, perhaps, surprising that chondrocytes, whose *raison d'être* is the formation and maintenance of this matrix, should be the main players in its destruction. A switch in chondrocyte metabolism to a more catabolic state is central to osteoarthritis.

Turnover of the Extracellular Matrix (ECM)

Physiological remodelling of the ECM occurs throughout life, with degraded matrix continually being replaced to maintain homeostasis. Matrix components (collagens, proteoglycans, glycoproteins) are broken down by proteinases. All four classes of mammalian proteinases (serine, cysteine, aspartate and metallo) are involved but the matrix metalloproteinases (MMPs) (stromelysins, gelatinases and collagenases) probably play the major role. The MMPs are secreted by chondrocytes as inactive proenzymes and require the removal of a short peptide for activation. Extracellular activation mechanisms for MMPs *in vivo* are poorly understood but an activation 'cascade' (cf. the coagulation cascade), involving other enzyme systems, may operate. In addition to secreting MMPs, chondrocytes also secrete local inhibitors, the tissue inhibitors of metalloproteinases (TIMPs). These are important extracellular regulators of MMP activity and hence of matrix turnover (Fig. 75.4). The reader is referred to Woessner (1991) and Birkdel-Hansen *et al.* (1993) for more detailed discussion of matrix-degrading proteinases and their inhibitors.

Box 75.1   Articular osteochondrosis in focus.

DEFINITION
The osteochondroses are a group of idiopathic conditions characterised by abnormal endochondral ossification. They can therefore affect primary and secondary centres of ossification, and the epiphyseal and metaphyseal growth cartilages. Generally there is a peristence of the cartilage template. Osteochondrosis of ossification centres and of epiphyseal growth cartilage can directly affect joints.

AETIOLOGY
- genetic factors
- overnutrition
- rapid growth
- unknown factors

MANIFESTATIONS
Osteochondrosis involving epiphyseal growth cartilage
may form cartilage flap (osteochondrosis dissecans, OCD)
- Shoulder
  - humeral head*, caudal rim of glenoid
- Elbow
  - medial humeral condyle*
- Stifle
  - femoral condyles*, patella
- Hock
  - medial and lateral ridges of the talus*
Osteochondrosis involving centres of ossification
- Shoulder
  - abnormal ossification of the proximal humeral epiphysis
- Elbow
  - delayed ossification of the proximal ulna
  - delayed ossification of the distal humeral epiphysis
- Stifle
  - delayed ossification of the tibial crest
  - abnormal ossification of the fabellae
- Hock
  - abnormal ossification of the medial malleolus
- Sacro-iliac joint
  - abnormal ossification of the cranio-dorsal sacrum
Unclassified
- Elbow
  - separated/fragmented medial coronoid process of the ulna (FMCP)*
  - ununited anconeal process (UAP)*
  - ununited medial epicondyle

* Most common manifestations

CLINICAL PRESENTATION
- persistent, mild to moderate lameness
- onset at 4–10 months of age
- affected joint painful on manipulation
- decreased range of joint motion (hock)
- synovial effusion
- often larger breeds e.g. Labrador, German Shepherd Dog, Rottweiler
- males > females (shoulder)

DIFFERENTIAL DIAGNOSES
- panosteitis
- periarticular soft tissue injury, e.g. sprain
- elbow incongruity secondary to growth disturbance
- cranial cruciate ligament pathology (juvenile cruciate disease)
- congenital dysplasia
- developmental dysplasia, e.g. hip dysplasia, patellar luxation

INVESTIGATION – Radiography:
may see radiolucent defect in subchondral bone representing persistence of cartilage e.g. OCD shoulder, hock, elbow

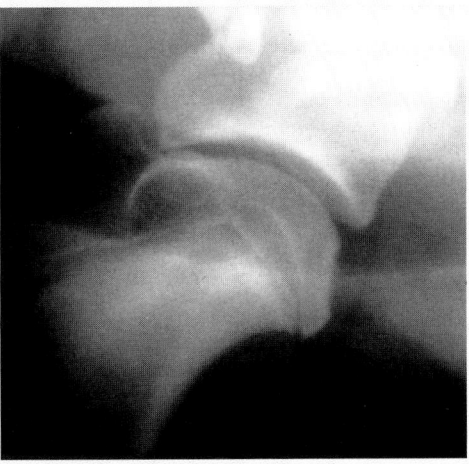

Box 75.1   *Continued*

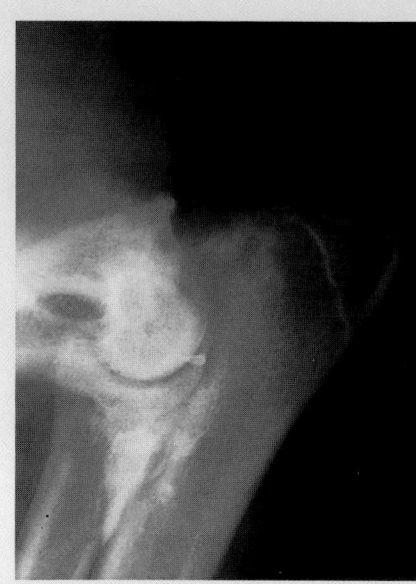

may only see evidence of secondary osteoarthritis
e.g. elbow with FMCP

MANAGEMENT GUIDELINES
Conservative – light lead exercise +/– NSAIDs

- FMCP – The general concensus is that surgery does not favourably affect outcome. Some cases with persistent or severe lameness may respond to fragment removal.
- OCD glenoid
- OCD humeral head
- OCD medial humeral condyle
- delayed/incomplete ossification

Surgery – flap/fragment removal
- OCD humeral head – may choose conservative approach initially
- OCD stifle and hock – *early* surgery probably beneficial
- OCD medial humeral condyle – may choose conservative approach initially
- FMCP if lameness persistent
- UAP

NB. Surgery is only indicated if there is a clinical problem

PROGNOSIS
The severity of secondary OA is the major determinant of long-term outcome
- shoulder   good – excellent
- stifle   fair – good
- elbow   poor – fair (guarded)
  and hock

Chondrocyte Metabolism in Osteoarthritis

In osteoarthritic cartilage, increased synthesis and secretion of proteinases, and a relative decrease in the production of local inhibitors, tips the metabolic balance in favour of inappropriate (pathological) matrix breakdown (Dean *et al.* 1989). These changes are seen initially in the superficial layers of cartilage. Some chondrocytes attempt to make up the deficit by increasing the synthesis of matrix molecules (*compensated osteoarthritis*) but eventually, catabolism becomes the dominant feature and there is a widespread net loss of matrix proteoglycans (*decompensated osteoarthritis*). This structurally weakened cartilage is more susceptible to further biomechanical damage.

The chondrocyte is responsive to a wide range of environmental factors such as mechanical stress, local pH and soluble mediators. The sum of these factors determines the metabolic profile of the cell. In health, these factors ensure homeostasis. Cytokines have a profound effect on chondrocyte metabolism. They act via cell surface receptors and

probably play a key role in the progression of osteoarthritis. The pro-inflammatory cytokines interleukin-1 (IL-1) and tumour necrosis factor a (TNFa) induce chondrocytes to increase (upregulate) MMP production and decrease (downregulate) TIMP production, causing a rapid depletion of the ECM. In cartilage, they can therefore be regarded as a *catabolic* cytokines. The growth factors, transforming growth factor β (TGFβ) and insulin-like growth factor 1 (IGF-1) downregulate MMP production and upregulate the synthesis of matrix molecules, hence exerting an *anabolic* effect.

IL-1 is considered to play an important role in the development of osteoarthritic chondropathy. Increased levels of IL-1 have been demonstrated in osteoarthritic cartilage and synovial membrane (Pelletier *et al.* 1993). Phagocytosis of matrix breakdown products provokes IL-1 synthesis by activated synovial lining cells; this could generate an important positive feedback loop in osteoarthritis (Fig. 75.5). In addition, chondrocytes in osteoarthritis appear less responsive to growth factors thus reinforcing the catabolic phenotype (Doré *et al.* 1994).

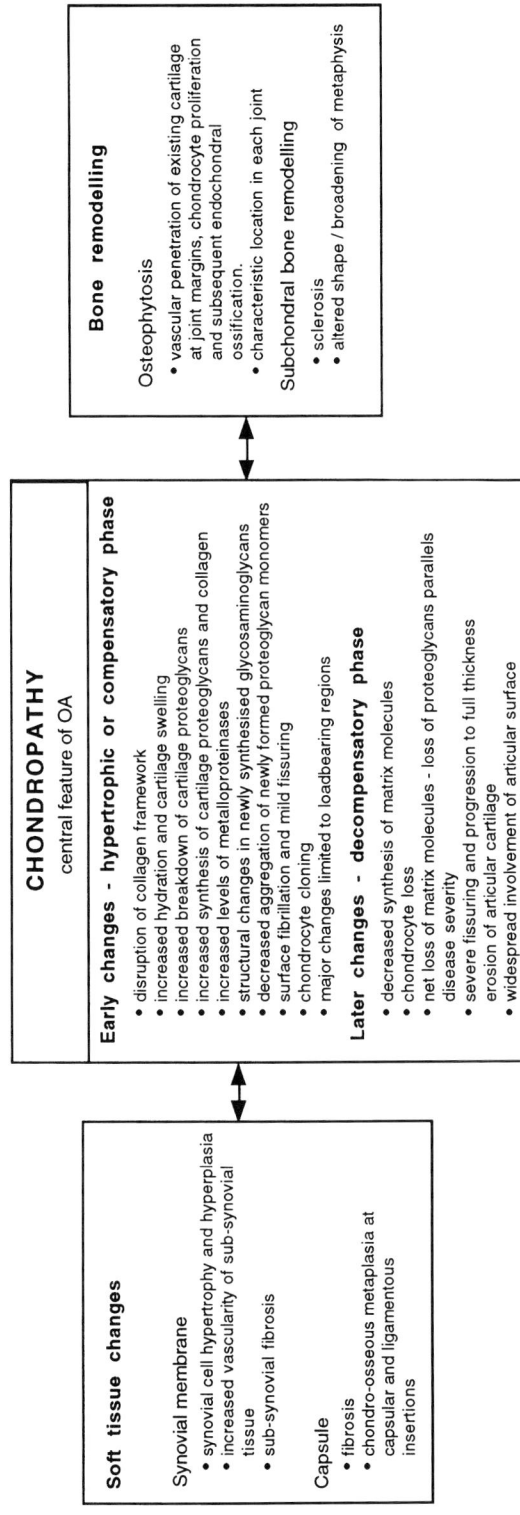

Fig. 75.1 The characteristic features of osteoarthritis.

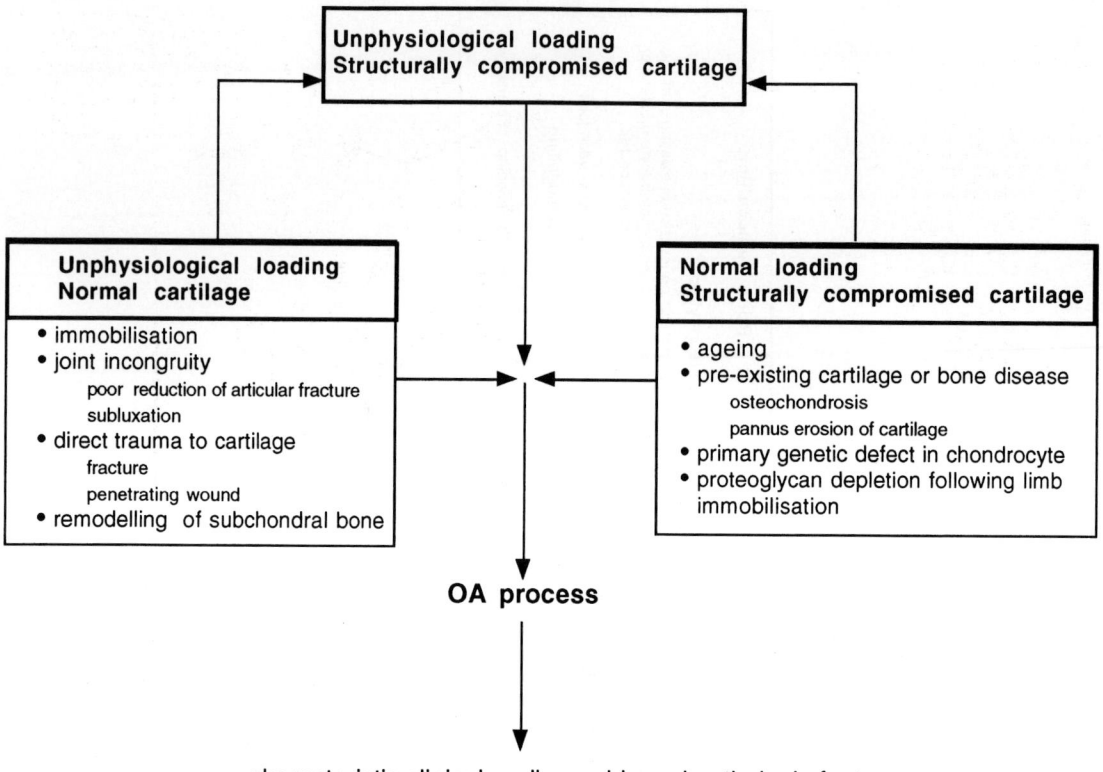

Fig. 75.2   An aetiological model for the development of osteoarthritis.

APPROACH TO THE PATIENT

The approach to the patient is as outlined in Chapter 74. Osteoarthritis is currently diagnosed on the basis of clinical presentation (Table 75.1) and typical radiographic features (Fig. 75.6). In some cases the diagnosis is difficult to confirm despite the application of clinical and radiographic criteria and in these cases synovial fluid analysis is helpful. It is rare to need synovial membrane biopsy to confirm a diagnosis of osteoarthritis.

There are shortcomings to the current methods of diagnosis in osteoarthritis:

• There is a poor correlation between radiographic changes and disease severity.
• Chondropathy is often well advanced at the time of diagnosis.

These difficulties have fuelled research to find more sensitive and accurate disease indicators in osteoarthritis. Interest has focused on biochemical markers of disease and on advanced imaging technology. Several cartilage matrix molecules have been investigated as putative biochemical markers including; proteoglycan fragments, hyaluronan and collagen cross-links. The role of these molecules in diagnosing and staging osteoarthritis is still being defined (Arican *et al.* 1994a & b; Lohmander 1994; Rorvik & Grondahl 1995). Advanced imaging techniques which may have a future role in the diagnosis of osteoarthritis include 3-D magnetic resonance imaging (MRI) and scintigraphy. MRI provides a means of non-invasive assessment of articular cartilage integrity and quantity (Pilch *et al.* 1994). Scintigraphy shows promise for predicting the eventual outcome in patients with early osteoarthritis (Innes 1995; Sharif *et al.* 1995). Cost and access to suitable facilities currently limits the widespread development of these imaging techniques in veterinary rheumatology.

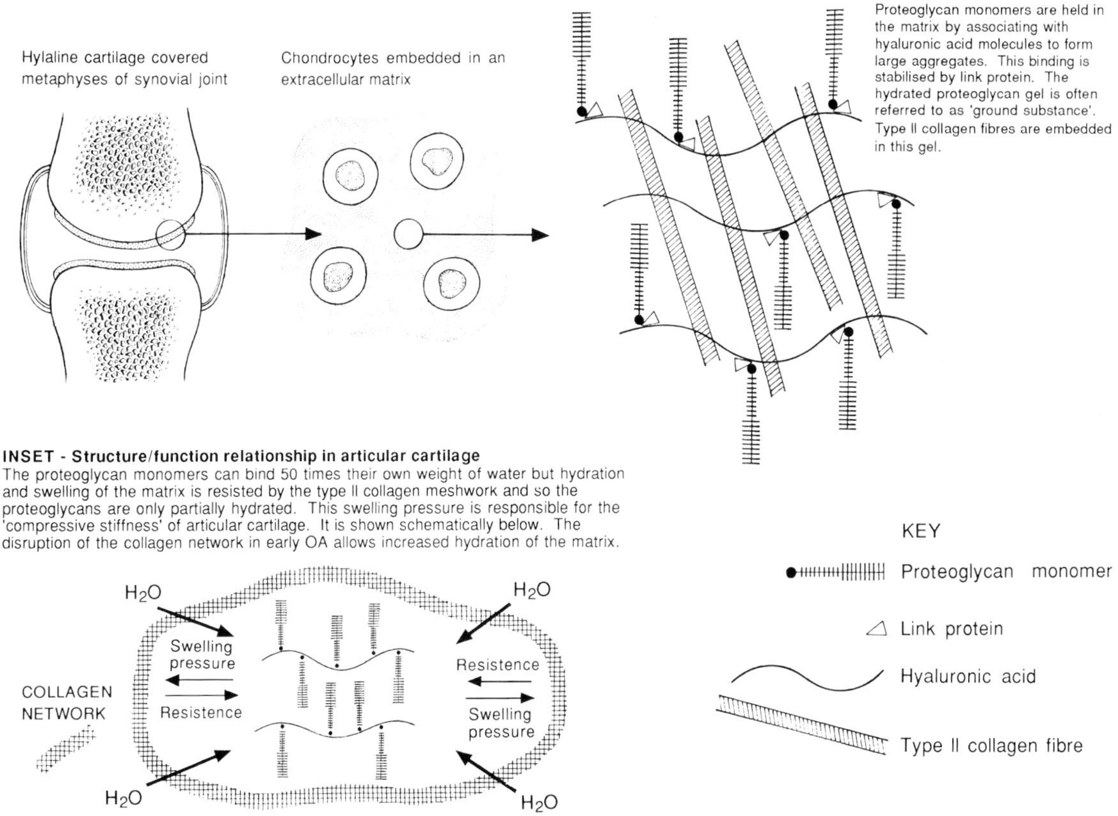

Hylaline cartilage covered metaphyses of synovial joint

Chondrocytes embedded in an extracellular matrix

Proteoglycan monomers are held in the matrix by associating with hyaluronic acid molecules to form large aggregates. This binding is stabilised by link protein. The hydrated proteoglycan gel is often referred to as 'ground substance'. Type II collagen fibres are embedded in this gel.

INSET - Structure/function relationship in articular cartilage
The proteoglycan monomers can bind 50 times their own weight of water but hydration and swelling of the matrix is resisted by the type II collagen meshwork and so the proteoglycans are only partially hydrated. This swelling pressure is responsible for the 'compressive stiffness' of articular cartilage. It is shown schematically below. The disruption of the collagen network in early OA allows increased hydration of the matrix.

H_2O

H_2O

Swelling pressure

Resistence

COLLAGEN NETWORK

Resistence

Swelling pressure

H_2O

H_2O

KEY

●━━┅┅┅╫╫╫╫ Proteoglycan monomer

△ Link protein

Hyaluronic acid

Type II collagen fibre

Fig. 75.3 The structure of articular cartilage.

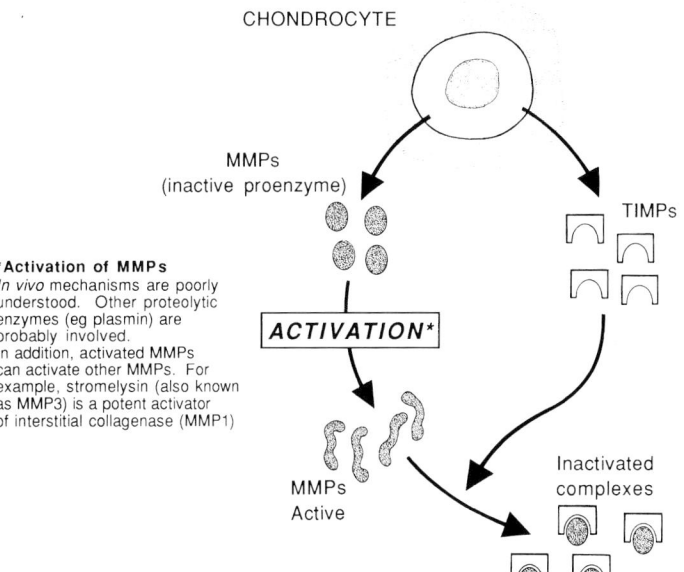

CHONDROCYTE

MMPs (inactive proenzyme)

TIMPs

*Activation of MMPs
In vivo mechanisms are poorly understood. Other proteolytic enzymes (eg plasmin) are probably involved.
In addition, activated MMPs can activate other MMPs. For example, stromelysin (also known as MMP3) is a potent activator of interstitial collagenase (MMP1)

ACTIVATION*

MMPs Active

Inactivated complexes

Fig. 75.4 The interaction of matrix metalloproteinases (MMPs) and tissue inhibitors of metalloproteinases (TIMPs).

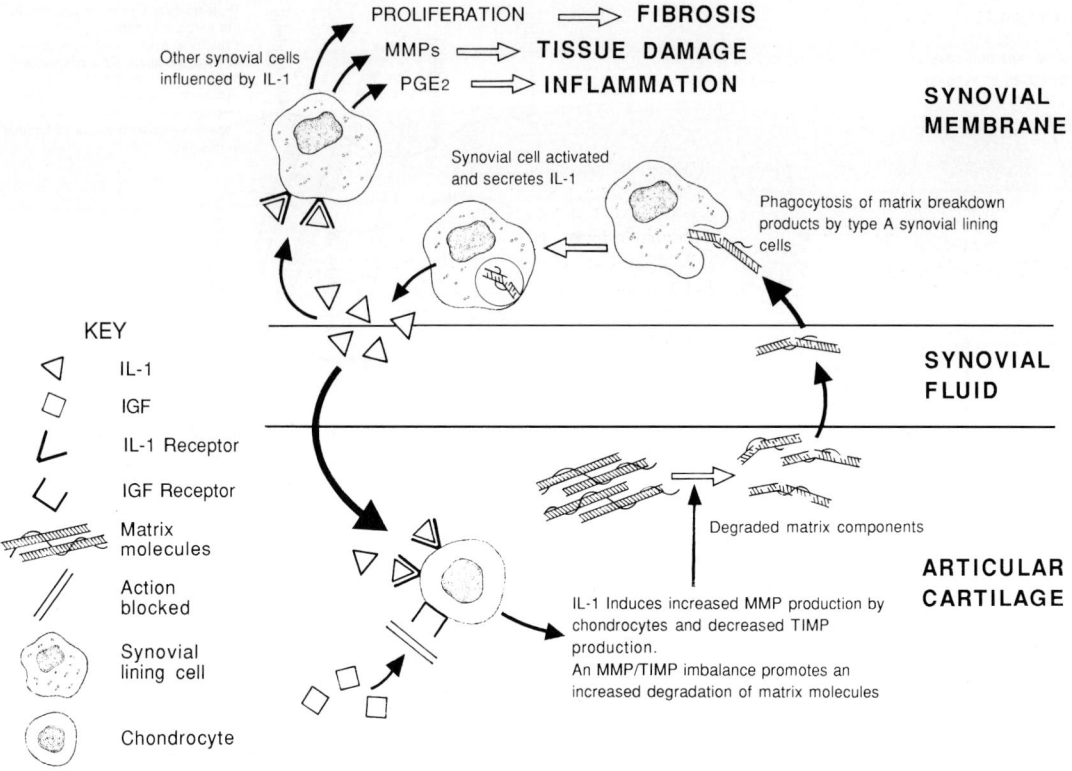

PROLIFERATION ⟹ **FIBROSIS**

MMPs ⟹ **TISSUE DAMAGE**

PGE2 ⟹ **INFLAMMATION**

Other synovial cells influenced by IL-1

SYNOVIAL MEMBRANE

Synovial cell activated and secretes IL-1

Phagocytosis of matrix breakdown products by type A synovial lining cells

SYNOVIAL FLUID

KEY

◁   IL-1

▢   IGF

∠   IL-1 Receptor

⟨   IGF Receptor

Matrix molecules

//   Action blocked

Synovial lining cell

Chondrocyte

Degraded matrix components

ARTICULAR CARTILAGE

IL-1 Induces increased MMP production by chondrocytes and decreased TIMP production.
An MMP/TIMP imbalance promotes an increased degradation of matrix molecules

Fig. 75.5   A possible positive feedback loop operating in the development and progression of osteoarthritis.

MANAGEMENT OF OSTEOARTHRITIS

Although promising new pharmacological targets have emerged, current management regimes are still primarily aimed at alleviating joint pain and avoiding factors that precipitate or worsen it. Management strategies can be classed as conservative, medical and surgical.

Conservative Management

Control of Body Weight

Excessive body weight aggravates the clinical signs of osteoarthritis and probably accelerates its progression

Table 75.1   The major clinical features of canine osteoarthritis.

History
  Stiffness after rest (usually short-lived)
  Overt lameness
  Reluctance to climb or jump
  Hesitant circling before lying down
  Restlessness at night
  Reduced exercise tolerance
  Occasionally animals become aggressive

Physical examination
  Pain on manipulation of the joint
  Crepitus (inconsistent finding)
  Joint thickening (capsular fibrosis, osteophytosis)
  Synovial effusion
  Decreased range of movement

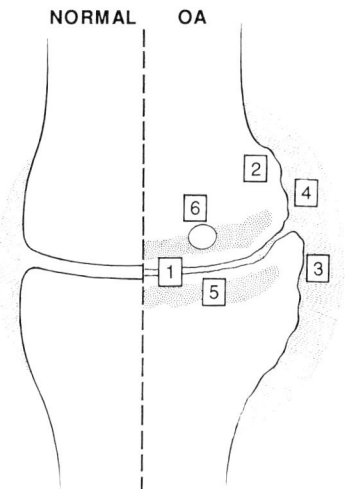

1. Joint space narrowing - often difficult to appreciate in the dog
2. Altered shape of metaphysis
3. Osteophyte formation
4. Soft tissue reaction - effusion/fibrosis
5. Sub-chondral bone sclerosis
6. Sub-chondral cyst formation - rare in the dog

Fig. 75.6 A diagramatic summary of the radiographic features of canine osteoarthritis.

(Felson 1995). Weight reduction or control is a fundamental, yet often overlooked, part of managing osteoarthritic patients.

Exercise Modification

Properly controlled exercise is important in maintaining muscle tone and reducing joint stiffness. Regular, gentle exercise should be encouraged. Excessive exercise leads to acute, and often severe, exacerbation of joint pain. An appropriate level of exercise that is acceptable to both patient and owner can usually be found, but it may need periodic adjustment.

> *Appropriate exercise*
> 'Exercise within the capability of the patient that does not induce pain, lameness or excessive stiffness, either during or following the exercise period' (Bennett & May 1994).

In mild cases, weight control and exercise modification alone are often sufficient to control clinical signs adequately. In more severe cases they will reduce the requirements for analgesic and anti-inflammatory medication.

Medical Therapy

Attention has focused on developing drugs that can halt or reverse the cartilage pathology. Agents that favourably modify the prognosis for the joint are termed *chondroprotective* or *disease modifying osteoarthritis drugs* (DMOADs).

> *Properties of DMOADs*
> Arrest or moderate the degradative processes occurring in articular cartilage.
> and/or
> Support the anabolic pathways essential for cartilage repair.
> (Burkhardt & Gosh 1987; Lequesne *et al.* 1994)

Of equal importance are drugs that can exacerbate the chondropathy, for example by decreasing proteoglycan synthesis in chondrocytes. The terms *chondrotoxic* and *chondroaggressive* have been applied to these compounds. *Chondroneutral* describes drugs with no discernible effects on chondrocyte metabolism or the cartilage matrix.

Most of our knowledge in this area has come from *in vitro* studies with cultured chondrocytes or from animal models of osteoarthritis where cartilage changes are assessed post mortem. The major challenge in assessing chondroprotection and chondrotoxicity in naturally occurring osteoarthritis has been the objective assessment of joint pathology. Patients may show symptomatic improvement but this does not equate to chondroprotection. The use of biochemical markers and advanced imaging techniques should be of great benefit in future studies.

Non-Steroidal Anti-Inflammatory Drugs

Non-steroidal anti-inflammatory drugs (NSAIDs) are the most commonly used drugs in managing canine osteoarthritis (Table 75.2). Many animals with osteoarthritis requiring pain relief are geriatric and the incidence of renal and hepatic disease is high in this group. This increases the risk of NSAID-induced toxicity and great caution is required when using NSAIDs in these animals (see Chapter 7). However, in many cases it is necessary to make a clinical judgement of the risks of NSAID therapy versus the potential benefit to the patient in terms of quality of life. NSAIDs should be regarded as an adjunct to other conservative means of management. Using NSAIDs to permit a high plane of exercise is generally poor clinical practice as the increased wear and tear to biomechanically compromised osteoarthritic cartilage will hasten disease progression (Brune 1992).

The effects of NSAIDs on chondrocyte metabolism, and hence the progression of osteoarthritis, have been extensively studied (Brandt 1987; Vignon 1994), with some, such as aspirin, being chondrotoxic. They suppress proteoglycan synthesis by chondrocytes *in vitro* and exacerbate chondropathy in experimentally-induced osteoarthritis (Brandt 1993). The importance of these observations for clinical practice has yet to be definitively established (Brune 1992; Vignon 1994). However, the chondroneutral nature of some NSAIDs licensed for use in the dog, e.g. meloxicam (Metacam™), makes them attractive choices for pain relief in canine osteoarthritis. The effects on chondrocyte metabolism of many NSAIDs commonly used in the management of canine osteoarthritis have not been investigated.

Glucocorticoids (see Chapter 6)

The use of glucocorticoids in osteoarthritis is controversial because of the potential for systemic side-effects and because there is conflicting evidence about their effects on cartilage metabolism (Johnson & Davis 1993). Glucocorticoids can reduce chondrocyte biosynthesis and hence promote the loss of cartilage matrix molecules in osteoarthritis. However, in low doses, corticosteroids have been shown to moderate the chondropathy in osteoarthritis, hence exerting a chondroprotective effect (Pelletier *et al*. 1994). Until further clarification is available, care should be exercised when using any glucocorticoids for managing osteoarthritic patients and intra-articular use cannot be routinely recommended. Bennett (1990) suggested the following guidelines for using oral glucocorticoids in canine osteoarthritis:

- to control sudden exacerbation of clinical signs, using a low dose for a few days only;
- where there is marked synovitis caused by cartilage debris or crystals;
- for advanced cases that have become refractory to other medications.

Hyaluronic Acid (HA)

Diminished viscoelasticity of synovial fluid in osteoarthritis may contribute to the mechanical damage of articular cartilage (Pelletier & Martel-Pelletier 1993). The use of hyaluronic acid and its derivatives in osteoarthritis ('viscoelastic supplementation') is attracting renewed interest.

Table 75.2 NSAIDS commonly used in the management of canine osteoarthritis.

Drug	Dose
Aspirin	20–25 mg/kg t.i.d. p.o. (anti-inflammatory dose)
	10–15 mg/kg t.i.d. p.o. (analgesic dose)
Phenylbutazone	1–5 mg/kg t.i.d. p.o. maximum 800 mg daily. Reduce to lowest effective dose for maintenance. May be given on alternate days
Cincophen/prednisolone	Cincophen 12.5 mg/kg. Prednisolone 0.125 mg/kg b.i.d. p.o.
Flunixin	1 mg/kg daily for a maximum of 3 days. i.m. or meglumine p.o.
Carprofen	2 mg/kg b.i.d. p.o. Reduce to lowest effective dose for maintenance
Ketoprofen	2 mg/kg s.c., i.m or i.v daily for a maximum of 3 days *or* 1 mg/kg p.o. daily for a maximum of 5 days
Meloxicam	0.2 mg/kg daily p.o. on the first day, reducing to 1 mg/kg for 5–7 days then the lowest effective dose for maintenance

Note: All NSAIDs carry a risk of side effects, most commonly gastrointestinal disturbance and nephrotoxicity. Always consult the drug insert before using.

HA can reduce the quantity of inflammatory enzymes in the synovial fluid, reduce synovial inflammation and alleviate pain (Balazs & Denlinger 1993). Its use in the dog requires clearer definition.

Polysulphated Polysaccharides

Polysulphated glycosaminoglycan (Adequan™) and pentosan polysulphate (Cartrophen™) are generally considered as DMOADs. Polysulphated glycosaminoglycan has been used intra-articularly in the dog but it is only licensed for use in the horse. Pentosan polysulphate is licensed for use in the dog. Polysulphated polysaccharides have shown the following *in vitro* properties:

- inhibition of proteolytic enzymes (e.g. metalloproteinases),
- increased glycosaminoglycan production by chondrocytes,
- scavenging of free radicals,
- induction of a highly polymerised hyaluronic acid by synovial cells.

In an experimental model of acute canine osteoarthritis, pentosan polysulphate had a protective effect on the severity of histological change in articular cartilage and prevented some of the early biochemical alterations associated with the disease. A greater protective effect in this model was observed when pentosan polysulphate was combined with IGF-1 (Rogachefsky *et al.* 1993).

Surgical Management

Management of Underlying Disease

It is generally accepted that early restoration of joint congruity following more severe ligament disruption, and the accurate anatomical reduction of articular fractures, will reduce the severity of secondary osteoarthritis. In some situations, such as elbow osteochondrosis and cruciate disease, osteoarthritis appears to progress regardless of surgery.

Triple pelvic osteotomy in immature dogs with hip dysplasia is a controversial area. In correctly selected dogs, it is claimed to slow the radiographic progression of osteoarthritis (Slocum & Slocum 1992). Interestingly, in human hip osteoarthritis, improved joint congruity following femoral osteotomy has also been shown to halt or even reverse the radiographic changes of osteoarthritis (Stauffer 1993). The interested reader is referred to Slocum & Slocum (1992) and Millis *et al.* (1995) for excellent reviews of this area.

Joint Lavage

Humans with knee osteoarthritis have shown symptomatic relief several months after joint lavage (Schnitzer 1993). Inflammatory mediators and wear particles are removed from the joint but a placebo effect has also been suggested. Further evaluation in the dog is necessary before recommendations can be made for its use in the management of canine osteoarthritis.

Surgical Salvage Procedures

These are reserved for end-stage joints where *correct conservative management is failing*. Included in this group are arthrodesis, excision arthroplasty and replacement arthroplasty.

Joint Resurfacing

Transplantation resurfacing of articulations is an area of active research. Tissues that have been used include perichondral and periosteal autografts, chondral and osteochondral autografts and cultured autogenous chondrocytes.

THE FUTURE OF OSTEOARTHRITIS MANAGEMENT

The crucial features that need to be addressed are:

- earlier diagnosis of the osteoarthritis process,
- the ability to stage the disease,
- the development of accurate, non-invasive methods of assessing joint pathology,
- the development of well defined chondroprotective strategies in osteoarthritis therapeutics.

The ultimate goal of medical therapy is the development of effective chondroprotective strategies. The greatest promise lies in metalloproteinase inhibitors and the modulation of chondrocyte metabolism by cytokine/anticytokine therapy. Earlier diagnosis of osteoarthritis will give chondroprotective strategies the maximum chance of modifying the course of the disease. Drug combinations targeting different points in the osteoarthritis process may be more effective than a single agent and surgical reconstruction of the articular surface may become established practice. The next few years will see major advances in the diagnosis and management of osteoarthritis.

REFERENCES

Arican, M., Carter, S.D., Bennett, D. & May, C. (1994a). Measurement of glycosaminoglycans and keratan sulphate in canine arthropathies. *Research in Veterinary Science*, **56**, 290–297.

Arican, M., Carter, S.D., May, C. & Bennett, D. (1994b). Hyaluronan in canine arthropathies. *Journal of Comparative Pathology*, **111**, 185–195.

Balazs, E.A. & Denlinger, J.L. (1993). Viscosupplementation: A new concept in the treatment of osteoarthritis. *Journal of Rheumatology*, **20** (Suppl. 39), 3–9.

Bennett, D. (1990). Joints and joint diseases. In: *Canine Orthopaedics*, (ed. W.G. Whittick), 2nd edn. pp. 761–857. Lea and Febiger, Philadelphia.

Bennett, D. & May, C.M. (1995). Joint diseases of dogs and cats. In: *Textbook of Veterinary Internal Medicine*, (eds S.J. Ettinger & E.C. Feldman), pp. 2032–2077. W.B. Saunders, Philadelphia.

Birkdel-Hansen, H., Moore, W.G.I., Bodden, M.K., *et al.* (1993). Matrix metalloproteinase: A review. *Critical Reviews in Oral Biology and Medicine*, **4**, 197–250.

Brandt, K.D. (1987). Effects of nonsteroidal anti-inflammatory drugs on chondrocyte metabolism in vivo. *American Journal of Medicine*, **83** (Suppl. 5A), 29–34.

Brandt (1993). Compensation and decompensation of articular cartilage in osteoarthritis. *Agents and Actions*, **40**, 232–233.

Brune, K. (1992). Prophylactic and therapeutic use of drugs in joint destruction. In: *Articular Cartilage and Osteoarthritis*, (eds K. Kuettner *et al.*), pp. 559–564. Raven Press, New York.

Burkhardt, D. & Gosh, P. (1987). Laboratory evaluation of antiarthritic drugs as potential chondroprotective agents. *Seminars in Arthritis and Rheumatism*, **17**, 3–34.

Dean, D.D., Martel-Pelletier, J., Pelletier, J-P., Howell, D.S. & Woessner, J.F. (1989). Evidence for metalloproteinase and metalloproteinase inhibitor imbalance in human osteoarthritic cartilage. *Journal of Clinical Investigation*, **84**, 678–685.

Doré, S., Pelletier, J-P., DiBattista, J.A., Tardif, G., Brazeau, P. & Martel-Pelletier, J. (1994). Human osteoarthritic chondrocytes possess an increased number of insulin-like growth factor 1 binding sites but are unresponsive to its stimulation. *Arthritis and Rheumatism*, **37**, 253–263.

Felson, D.T. (1995). Weight and osteoarthritis. *Journal of Rheumatology*, **22** (Suppl. 43), 7–9.

Johnson, K.A. & Davies, P.E. (1993). Drug therapy in surgical musculoskeletal disease. In: *Disease Mechanisms in Small Animal Surgery*, (ed. M.J. Bojrab), 2nd edn. pp. 1105–1111. Lea and Febiger, Philadelphia.

Innes, J. (1995). Diagnosis and treatment of osteoarthritis in dogs. *In Practice*, **17**, 102–109.

Lequesne, M., Brandt, K., Bellamy, N., Moskowitz, R., Menkes, C.J. & Pelletier, J.P. (1994). Guidelines for testing slow acting drugs in osteoarthritis. *Journal of Rheumatology*, **21**, (WHO/ILAR Suppl. 41), 65–81.

Lohmander, J. (1994). Articular cartilage and osteoarthrosis. The role of molecular markers to monitor breakdown, repair and disease. *Journal of Anatomy*, **184**, 477–492.

Millis, M.B., Murphy, S.B. & Poss, R. (1995). Osteotomies about the hip for the prevention and treatment of osteoarthrosis. *Journal of Bone and Joint Surgery*, **77A**, 626–647.

Pelletier, J-P. & Martel-Pelletier, J. (1993). The pathogenesis of osteoarthritis and the implication of the use of hyaluronan and hylan as therapeutic agents in viscosupplementation. *Journal of Rheumatology*, **20** (Suppl. 39), 19–24.

Pelletier, J-P., Faure, M-P., DiBattista, J.A., Wilhelm, S., Visco, D. & Martel-Pelletier, J. (1993). Coordinate synthesis of stromelysin, Interleukin-1, and oncogene proteins in experimental osteoarthritis. *American Journal of Pathology*, **142**, 95–105.

Pelletier, J-P., Mineau, F., Raynauld, J-P., Woessner, F.J., Gunja-Smith, Z. & Martel-Pelletier, J. (1994). Intraarticular injections with methylprednisolone acetate reduce osteoarthritic lesions in parallel with chondrocyte stromelysin synthesis in experimental osteoarthritis. *Arthritis and Rheumatism*, **37**, 414–423.

Pilch, L., Stewart, C., Gordon, D., *et al.* (1994). Assessment of cartilage volume in the femorotibial joint with magnetic resonance imaging and 3D computer reconstruction. *Journal of Rheumatology*, **21**, 2307–2319.

Rogachefsky, R.A., Dean, D.D., Howell, D.S. & Altman, R.D. (1993). Treatment of canine osteoarthritis with insulin-like growth factor-1 (IGF-1) and sodium pentosan polysulphate. *Osteoarthritis and Cartilage*, **1**, 105–114.

Rorvik, A.M. & Grondahl, A.M. (1995). Markers of osteoarthritis: A review of the literature. *Veterinary Surgery*, **24**, 255–263.

Schnitzer, T.J. (1993). Management of osteoarthritis. In: *Arthritis and Allied Conditions*, (eds D.J. McCarty & W.J. Koopman), pp. 1761–1769. Lea and Febiger, Philadelphia.

Sharif, M., George, E. & Dieppe, P. (1995). Correlation between synovial fluid markers of cartilage and bone turnover and scintigraphic scan abnormalities in osteoarthritis of the knee. *Arthritis and Rheumatism*, **38**, 78–81.

Slocum, B. & Slocum, T.D. (1992). Pelvic osteotomy for axial rotation of the acetabular segment in dogs with hip dysplasia. *Veterinary Clinics of North America, Small Animal Practice*, **22**, 645.

Stauffer, R.N. (1993). Correction of arthritic deformities of the hip. In: *Arthritis and Allied Conditions*, (eds D.J. McCarty & W.J. Koopman), pp. 969–980. Lea and Febiger, Philadelphia.

Woessner, J.F. (1991). Matrix metalloproteinases and their inhibitors in connective tissue remodelling. *FASEB Journal*, **5**, 2145–2154.

Vignon, E. (1994). Non-steroidal anti-inflammatory drugs (NSAIDs) and cartilage. *Rheumatology in Europe*, **23**, 27–28.

Chapter 76

Inflammatory Arthropathies

C. May and D. Bennett

INTRODUCTION

Inflammatory joint disease is characterised by synovitis with or without accompanying systemic illness. Most cases of canine inflammatory joint disease have either infectious or idiopathic (immune-mediated) aetiologies.

APPROACH TO THE PATIENT

The approach to patients with inflammatory joint disease is as outlined in Chapter 74. It is often necessary to obtain radiographs, perform synovial fluid analyses and obtain synovial membrane biopsies for bacterial culture or for histopathology to fully investigate dogs with infective or immune-mediated joint disease.

Specific steps to establish a definitive diagnosis and disease management are covered below under each disease heading.

INFECTIVE ARTHROPATHIES

Infective arthropathies are most commonly associated with bacteria. They may also be caused by viruses, fungi, mycoplasmas, protozoa and rickettsia, but these are rare or not documented in the UK. Bacterial infective arthritis and discospondylitis (see Chapter 81) are the most commonly presenting infective arthropathies.

Bacterial Infective Arthritis (Suppurative Arthritis)

Pathophysiology

Dogs with bacterial infective arthritis usually present with acute onset lameness in a single limb and heat, pain, swelling and disuse in a single joint. Less common presentations include a low-grade, gradual onset lameness or simultaneous infection in more than one joint. Multifocal infective arthritis is often associated with haematogenous spread of infection from a distant focus such as bacterial endocarditis, urinary tract infection or omphalophlebitis. Most dogs with bacterial infective arthritis have no signs of systemic illness (Bennett & Taylor 1988a), but cases of bacterial endocarditis may succumb to severe systemic illness which shows a poor response to therapy (Bennett & Taylor 1988b). Bacterial endocarditis has a particularly poor prognosis and is sometimes complicated by an immune-mediated arthropathy (see below).

Bacterial infective arthritis is most common in large breeds and there is a preponderance in males. It may occur in any age group. Most cases are associated with either staphylococci or β haemolytic streptococci, but many different organisms have been isolated from infected joints and mixed infections, including anaerobes, can occur. Bacteria gain access to the joint by any one of several routes (Fig. 76.1).

> Most cases of bacterial infective arthritis in dogs are the result of haematogenous localisation of infection. Penetrating wounds are a *very rare* cause.

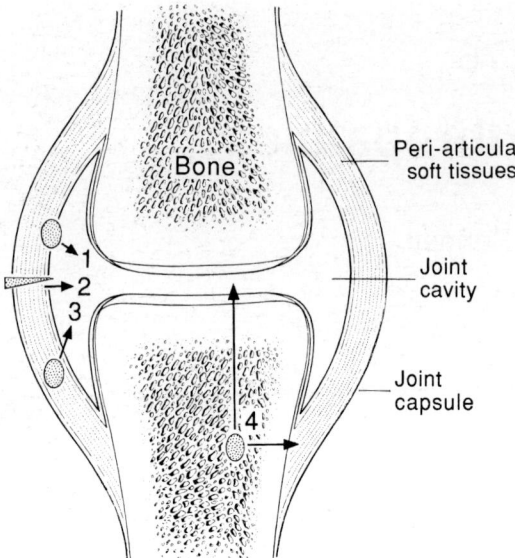

Fig. 76.1 A schematic diagram to show the potential routes of infection in infective arthritis: (1) haematogenous spread to the synovial membrane (most common route in dogs); (2) penetrating wound; (3) by extension from neighbouring soft tissues; (4) by extension from neighbouring osteomyelitis.

Table 76.1 Radiographic changes in bacterial infective arthritis.

Early changes (1–5 days)
   Intra-articular soft tissue swelling
   Periarticular soft tissue swelling
   Gas within soft tissue

Late changes (>5 days)
   Periarticular new bone formation
   Mineralisation of periarticular soft tissues
   Decreased joint space
   Subchondral bone erosion/increased joint space
   Bony sclerosis
   Regional osteopenia

Diagnosis

It is sometimes difficult to differentiate bacterial infective arthritis from traumatic joint disease especially in the early stages of disease when there may be minimal radiographic changes (Table 76.1 and Fig. 76.2). This is particularly important since infective arthritis can be preceded by an episode of traumatic arthritis.

Synovial fluid cytology is useful in differentiating traumatic joint disease from infective joint disease since the synovial fluid white-cell cytology in traumatic injuries resembles that of degenerative joint disease (see Chapter 74). However, further investigations are needed to confirm the diagnosis (Fig. 76.3). Attempts at bacterial culture can be met with false negative results. Culture is often most successful from synovial membrane (Bennett & Taylor 1988a). Biopsies should be kept moist for transport by suspension in a small volume of sterile saline. Culture of synovial fluid with pre-incubation in blood culture medium also has a high diagnostic yield (Abercromby 1994).

Management

Treatment is by prolonged (4–8 weeks) systemic antibiotic therapy. A broad-spectrum, bactericidal antibiotic should be given initially and should only be changed if specifically indicated by bacteriological culture and sensitivity results. Suitable antibiotics for initial therapy include:

- cephalosporin derivatives,
- clavulanate potentiated amoxycillin,
- quinolone carboxylic acid derivatives (e.g. enrofloxacin, ciprofloxacin).

Gentamicin impregnated polymethylmethacrylate beads may also be useful in the management of joint infections, particularly when the causative agent shows multiple antibiotic resistance (Brown & Bennett 1989). Surgical drainage and lavage may be used to supplement systemic antibiotic therapy in cases with particularly severe and rapidly progressive disease.

> *Special care of young dogs*
> Surgical drainage of infected joints is an essential emergency procedure in immature animals to prevent the increase in intra-articular pressure damaging the developing cartilage on the joint surface and in the growth plates neighbouring the joint.

Adjunctive therapies of use in bacterial infective arthritis include:

- protection and support of the joint by bandaging in the acute phase;
- analgesia;
- rest in the initial phases of treatment;

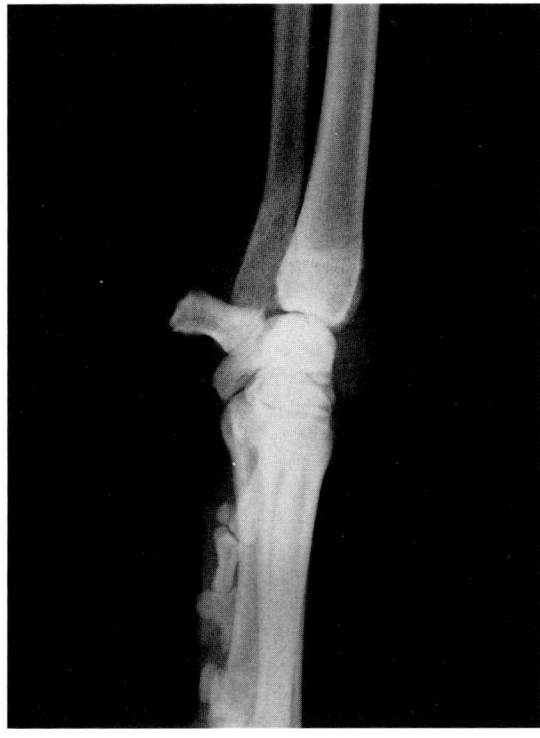

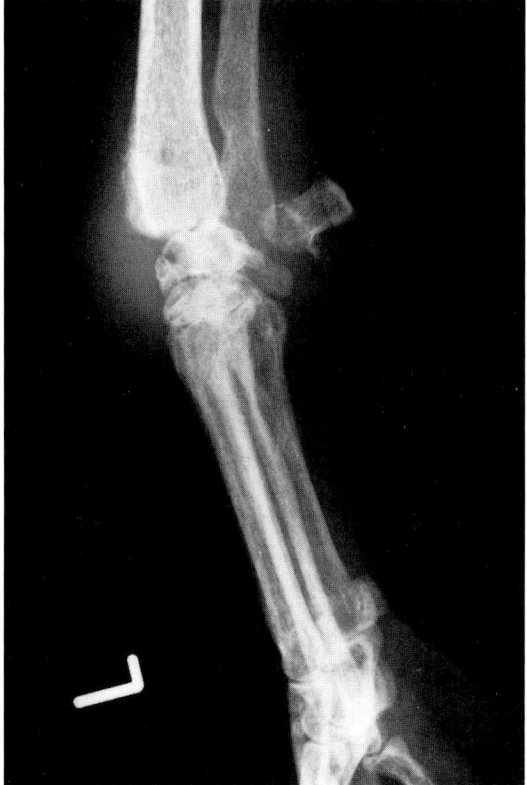

Fig. 76.2 (a) Lateral radiograph of the carpus showing soft tissue swelling on the cranial aspect with an area of calcification. There is no bony destruction or proliferation. This was a case of a low-grade bacterial infective arthritis. (b) Lateral radiograph of the carpus showing marked soft tissue swelling, bony lysis particularly within the radial carpal bone and peri-osteal new bone particularly on the distal radius. This was a case of bacterial infective arthritis which was not diagnosed and not treated correctly. The advanced joint pathology means a poor prognosis. This case necessitated a carpal arthrodesis once the infection had been cleared.

- gentle exercise and passive motion to limit adhesions in the recovery phase.

Occasionally, bacterial infective arthritis is superseded by sterile inflammation associated with persistence of bacterial antigens and/or immune complexes. Such cases respond to anti-inflammatory therapy with corticosteroids, but it is essential that the joint is sterile before these are administered (Bennett & Taylor 1988a). The prognosis for return of normal joint function in bacterial infective arthritis is guarded to poor, expecially if diagnosis and therapy has been delayed, and the long-term prognosis is limited by the progression of secondary osteoarthritis.

Lyme Arthritis

Lyme disease is a multisystemic inflammatory disorder associated with infection by the tick-borne spirochaete *Borrelia burgdorferi* (Steere 1989; Appel 1990). Many different syndromes have been associated with *B. burgdorferi* infection, including dermatological, neurological, cardiological and rheumatological diseases. However, lameness associated with inflammatory synovitis is probably the most common manifestation in dogs. Joint disease usually manifests as pauciarthritis and normally occurs weeks or months after exposure to ixodid ticks and may be associated with mild signs of systemic illness (see Chapter 21). Most cases

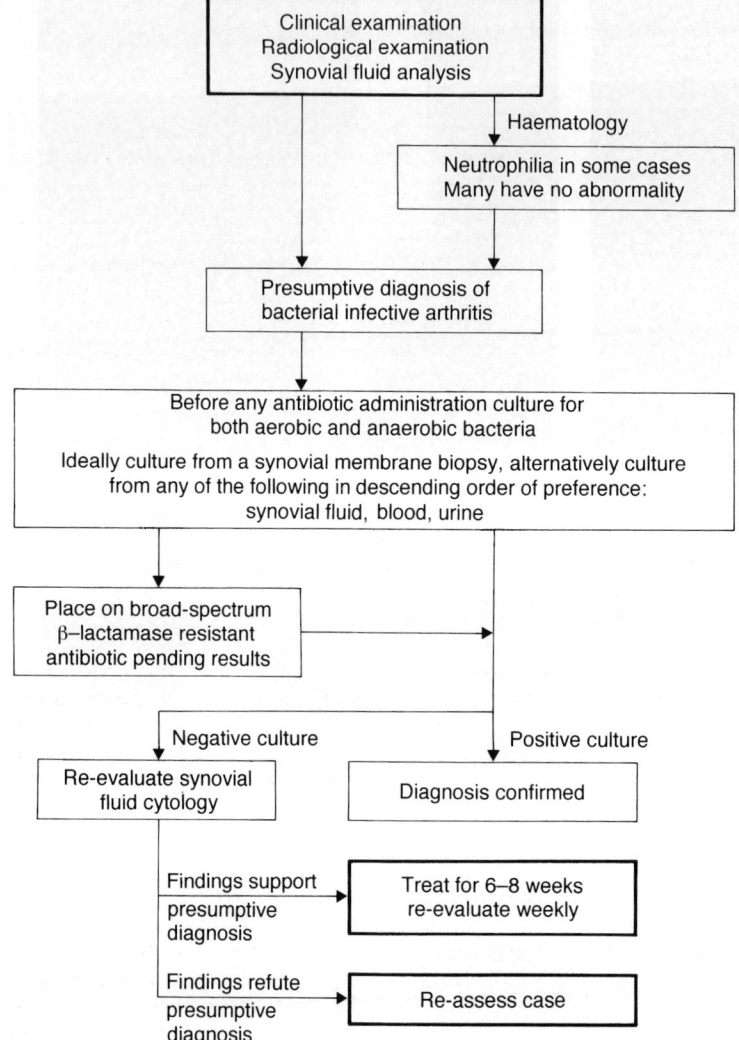

Fig. 76.3 Algorithm for the investigation of suspected bacterial infective arthritis.

of Lyme arthritis in dogs respond to antibiotic therapy. Oxytetracycline is commonly recommended, but ampicillin and its derivatives are also effective. Therapy should be continued for a minimum of 4 weeks even if complete resolution of clinical signs occurs earlier.

IMMUNE-MEDIATED ARTHROPATHIES

Classification

The classification of immune-mediated joint disease hinges on the presence or absence of erosive changes in the joints

(see Chapter 74). Specific diagnosis can be difficult and it is always useful to bear the classification in mind when considering cases of immune-mediated arthritis.

Pathophysiology

In the early stages of all types of immune-mediated arthritis there is synovitis characterised by damage to the microvascular endothelium in the synovial membrane. Such changes suggest that the factor inciting synovitis is carried to the joint by the circulation and it is widely believed that the inciting factor is an infectious agent (Schumacher 1975; Quimby *et al.* 1978; Schumacher *et al.*

1980; Bell *et al.* 1991; May *et al.* 1994). Chronic disease may result from the continued or recurrent presence of inciting antigens or from a derangement in the normal downregulation of the immune system once the inciting antigens are eliminated. The production and phagocytosis of immune complexes in response to a persistent antigenic stimulus is thought to be central to the development of chronicity in immune mediated synovitis.

In erosive forms of immune-mediated joint disease the chronic synovitis leads to the production of a proliferative granulation tissue known as pannus which invades the articular cartilage and subchondral bone. Both the inflamed synovium and the pannus are a source of enzymes which are directly responsible for destruction of the joint.

Extra-articular manifestations of disease are important features of many of these diseases, the classic example being systemic lupus erythematosus. Systemic manifestations are usually due to immune complex hypersensitivity (e.g. immune complex glomerulopathy giving rise to proteinuria) or to auto-antibody formation (e.g. anti-red-cell antibodies producing Coombs' positive anaemia).

Diagnosis

Immune-mediated joint disease should be considered in the differential diagnosis of dogs with the following signs:

- any age, breed or sex,
- generalised stiffness,
- pyrexia with, or without, signs of systemic illness.

It is helpful to subdivide investigation of suspected polyarthritis into two stages. First, establish the certain presence of immune-mediated arthritis, then go on to establish the specific diagnosis. Radiographic examination of multiple joints to give an initial classification of the disease as 'erosive' or 'non-erosive' is an important early diagnostic step.

> The classification of immune-based polyarthritis is important to help with prognosis and therapy.

Making A Diagnosis of Immune-Mediated Arthritis

The clinical presentation of dogs with polyarthritis can vary considerably from a vague stiffness or shifting lameness, an obvious limp in one or more limbs or, in severe cases, a total inability to stand and ambulate. Important clinical characteristics of most cases of immune mediated polyarthritis are:

- multiple joint involvement (polyarthritis),
- symmetrical joint involvement,
- pyrexia (see Chapter 37).

> Immune-mediated polyarthritis cases may account for 40% of dogs presenting with 'pyrexia of unknown origin' at referral centres.

Typically, there is stiffness after rest which is more severe and persistent than that seen in degenerative joint diseases. Affected joints are usually swollen and painful when palpated although this may not always be obvious on clinical examination. Assessment of synovial fluid cytology (see Chapter 74) is a more sensitive indicator of articular pathology.

> Synovial fluid arthrocentesis from several joints and its cytological examination is *the* most relevant diagnostic investigation of suspected polyarthritis.

Joint deformities, instability and crepitus may occur, particularly in the erosive forms of disease. Investigations useful in confirming the presence of immune-mediated polyarthritis are outlined in Table 76.2. Once this diagnosis is established, diagnosis of the specific syndrome can be pursued.

Making A Specific Diagnosis

Criteria have been established to help standardise the diagnosis of the immune-mediated arthropathies (Table 76.3). A specific diagnosis is made when the criteria for that disease are satisfied and all other causes of immune-mediated arthritis have been excluded. Diagnosis of specific syndromes assists in prognostication and in forming a therapeutic plan. There is a great deal of overlap between the different syndromes which probably reflects similar pathogeneses.

Erosive Joint Disease

Canine Rheumatoid Arthritis (Bennett 1987a, 1987b)

> A destructive, symmetrical, arthropathy simultaneously affecting several joints is almost invariably rheumatoid.

Table 76.2   Diagnosis of immune mediated joint disease

Diagnostic findings supporting a diagnosis of immune-mediated joint disease

Haematology
    Anaemia (auto-immune or anaemia of chronic disease)
    Leucocytosis
    Neutrophilia and left shift
    Leucopenia and/or thrombocytopenia in some cases, especially in systemic lupus erythamatosus.

Serum biochemistry
    Serum urea, creatinine, alkaline phosphatase, alanine transferase and aspartate transferase levels may be raised
    Raised creatine kinase and aldolase levels may indicate complication of myositis
    Total protein levels may vary from normal, globulins increased (immunoglobulin production), albumin decreased
        (protein losing nephropathy; immune complex glomerulopathy, amyloidosis, protein losing enteropathy)

Urinanalysis
    Proteinuria (immune complex glomerulopathy; amyloidosis)

Radiography
    Periarticular soft tissue swelling
    Joint erosions
    Periosteal new bone
    Osteophyte formation
    Symmetrical changes in multiple joints

Synoviocentesis
    Typical cytological changes (see Chapter 74)
    Several joints affected
    Symmetrical distribution
    (These findings are often diagnostic for immune-mediated joint disease)

Synovial membrane
    Histopathology typical of immune-mediated joint disease
    Biopsy (confirmatory in cases with equivocal synovial fluid cytology)
    Negative culture may help exclude bacterial synovitis

Others
    CSF protein, cell counts and creatine phosphokinase increased in cases complicated by meningitis
    Biopsy of the tissues to diagnose other complications, e.g. amyloidosis, glomerulopathy, dermatitis etc.

Although erosions are typical of canine rheumatoid arthritis (CRA) (Fig. 76.4), they may not be present in the early stages of disease and a diagnosis of CRA can be made in the absence of subchondral bone destruction. In some cases, destructive changes are only seen in one or two joints, although soft tissue swelling may be present in several joints. In chronic cases, there is collapse of the joints, excessive laxity, subluxation, luxation and deformity. There may be peri-articular bone proliferation and calcification in periarticular soft tissues.

Approximately 25% of dogs with CRA do not have significant levels of circulating rheumatoid factor (RF)

(Bennett & Kirkham 1987). Furthermore, high circulating levels of RF can be found in other chronic disease states.

> A high circulating rheumatoid factor value does not, in itself, justify a diagnosis of canine rheumatoid arthritis.
> Diagnosis should only be made on the basis of specific criteria (Table 76.3).

An antinuclear antibody (ANA) test and an anti-Borrelia antibody test should be performed to help

Table 76.3 Summary of the criteria for the diagnosis of immune-mediated arthropathies.

Erosive

Canine rheumatoid arthritis
(1) Stiffness after rest
(2) Pain or tenderness on motion of at least one joint
(3) Swelling of at least one joint
(4) Swelling of one other joint within 3 months
(5) Symmetrical joint swelling
(6) Subcutaneous nodules
(7) Erosive changes on joint radiographs
(8) Serological test positive for rheumatoid factor
(9) Abnormal synovial fluid
(10) Histopathology of synovium
(11) Histopathology of subcutaneous nodules

Seven criteria must be fulfilled, including two of criteria (7), (8) and (10). Criteria (1), (2), (3), (4) and (5) should be present for at least 6 weeks. Subcutaneous rheumatoid nodules are rare in dogs, so criteria (6) and (11) are rarely satisfied.

Canine periosteal proliferative polyarthritis
(1) At least four joints affected
(2) Periosteal articular new bone on radiographs
(3) Erosive changes on joint radiographs
(4) Enthesopathies

Criteria (1), (2) and (3) must be satisfied. More common disease in the cat, especially males.

Felty's syndrome
(1) Rheumatoid arthritis
(2) Splenomegaly
(3) Leucopenia

Polyarthritis of Greyhounds
(1) Breed specific
(2) Erosive polyarthritis (possible *Mycoplasma spumans* infection)

Non-erosive

Canine systemic lupus erythematosus (SLE)
(1) Multisystem disease. Most common manifestations include polyarthritis, skin disease, anaemia, glomerulonephritis, myositis, thrombocytopenia
(2) Antinuclear antibody present in blood
(3) Immunopathological features consistent with clinical involvement should be present, e.g. antibodies should be shown against *rbc* in haemolytic anaemia, platelets in thrombocytopenia and antibody/complement deposits shown in tissue biopsies in cases of glomerulonephritis, dermatitis, arthritis

Criteria (1) and (2) must always be satisfied. All three criteria should be satisfied to establish a definite diagnosis of SLE. However, satisfying criterion (3) is sometimes impractical and a probable diagnosis of SLE is made if only criteria (1) and (2) are satisfied.

Polyarthritis/polymyositis syndrome
(1) Non-erosive polyarthritis
(2) Clinical signs of muscle disease, e.g. myalgia, atrophy, contracture
(3) Chronic active myositis in at least two muscle biopsies
(4) Increased serum creatinine kinase and aldolase levels
(5) Negative for antinuclear antibody

Table 76.3 *Continued.*

Polyarthritis/meningitis syndrome
(1) Non-erosive polyarthritis
(2) Clinical signs of neck pain
(3) Abnormal CSF-increased protein content, increased white cell count, increased creatinine kinase levels
(4) Negative for antinuclear antibody

Heritable polyarthritis of the adolescent Akita
(1) Breed specific
(2) Young dogs – less than 1 year of age
(3) Other organ involvement, e.g. meningitis
(4) Negative for antinuclear antibody

Familial renal amyloidosis in Shar-Pei dogs
(1) Breed specific
(2) Swollen hock or carpus (or other joints)
(3) Other organ involvement (renal or liver failure due to amyloidosis)
(4) Enthesiopathies
(5) Negative for antinuclear antibody

Polyarteritis nodosa
(1) Symmetrical polyarthritis
(2) Necrosis and inflammation of blood vessels seen on biopsy of synovium, and other tissues
(3) Negative for antinuclear antibody

Canine Sjögren's syndrome
(1) Symmetrical polyarthritis (erosive or non-erosive)
(2) Keratitis sicca (dacryoadenitis)
(3) Xerostomia (sialoadenitis)

Idiopathic
Includes all cases of polyarthritis which do not satisfy criteria for the above.

Type I	No associations (uncomplicated idiopathic arthritis)
Type II	Arthritis associated with infection elsewhere in body (reactive arthritis)
Type III	Arthritis associated with gastrointestinal disease (enteropathic arthritis)
Type IV	Arthritis associated with neoplastic disease remote from the joints (arthritis of malignancy)

Some cases originally classified as idiopathic may require reclassification as the disease process progresses, e.g. some Type I cases progress to erosive rheumatoid arthritis. Idiopathic cases can show multisystemic disease. Circulating antinuclear antibodies are absent.

Miscellaneous

'Vaccination reactions'
● Arthritis develops within 5–7 days of inoculation
● Arthritis normally resolves within 1–3 days
● (Mainly associated with calicivirus vaccination in the cat)

Plasmacytic/lymphocytic synovitis of stifle joints
● Often present as cranial cruciate ligament failure
● Typical synovitis seen on biopsy
● (Not recognised in the UK)

Drug-induced
● Arthritis associated with drug administration
● Usually antibiotic
● Previous exposure to drug
● Arthritis resolves within 5–7 days of stopping drug
● Challenge studies can confirm diagnosis

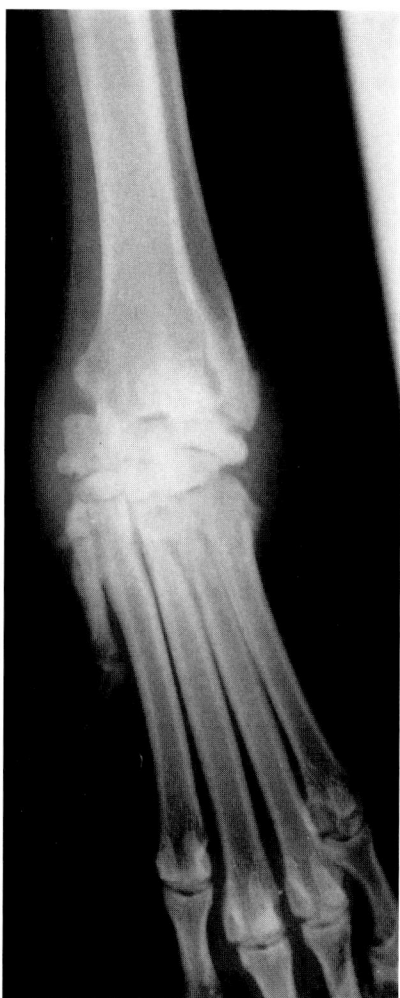

Fig. 76.4 Craniocaudal radiograph of the carpus of a dog with rheumatoid arthritis. There is obvious soft tissue swelling, subluxation of the antebrachiocarpal joint and small erosions within the carpal bones. Small areas of periosteal new bone are also evident.

differentiate CRA from systemic lupus erythematosus and Lyme disease. However, some dogs with CRA can be positive for ANA and for anti-Borrelia antibodies.

Other Erosive Joint Disease

Peri-osteal proliferative polyarthritis is very occasionally seen in the dog, although it is more common in the cat. It is characterised by an erosive polyarthritis accompanied by

extensive periosteal new bone often extending beyond the confines of the joint. Bony destruction and proliferation may be seen at ligament and tendon attachments (enthesiopathy), although these lesions can be seen in many other of the immune-based arthropathies but less consistently. Felty's syndrome is where rheumatoid arthritis is complicated by splenomegaly and leucopenia; it is very rare. Polyarthritis of Greyhounds, originally reported in Australia, is more likely to be a mycoplasma infective arthritis rather than being immune based. Greyhounds in the UK can suffer immune-based polyarthritis, but it is generally of a non-erosive nature.

Non-Erosive Joint Diseases

A number of non-erosive joint diseases have been recognised in dogs (Table 76.3). Canine idiopathic polyarthritis is the most common presentation of non-erosive polyarthritis. Systemic lupus erythematosus is characterised by the presence of circulating antinuclear antibodies, it is important because of its multisystemic nature. Other non-erosive polyarthritides include those complicated by involvement of another body system, such as polymyositis (Bennett & Kelly 1987), keratitis sicca, or sterile meningitis, those associated with certain breeds such as the Chinese Shar-Pei (DiBartola *et al.* 1990; May *et al.* 1992) or the Japanese Akita (Dougherty *et al.* 1991), and a syndrome of inflammatory synovitis of the stifles which may predispose to cranial cruciate ligament rupture. Drug induced polyarthritis is occasionally seen, especially with certain antibiotics (Table 76.5).

Systemic Lupus Erythematosus

Most dogs with systemic lupus erythematosus (SLE) present with pyrexia and a symmetric, non-erosive inflammatory polyarthritis. Other manifestations of this multi-systemic disease include auto-immune haemolytic anaemia, immune-mediated thrombocytopenia, leucopenia, immune-complex glomerulonephritis, dermatitis, polymyositis, CNS disorders including sterile meningitis, pleuritis and gastrointestinal disease.

The diversity of possible clinical presentations makes SLE easy to over-diagnose. However, it is a rare disease in dogs in the UK so care must be taken to base the diagnosis on established criteria (Bennett 1987c) (Table 76.3).

The presence of circulating ANA is an important feature of this disease, although some authorities diagnose 'seronegative SLE' in the absence of ANA (Halliwell 1982). ANA is actually a collective term for a group of antibodies to a variety of cell nuclear antigens. Immune complexes formed from the reaction of these antigens with

ANA are deposited in many tissues throughout the body and tissue damage may ensue as a result of immune complex hypersensitivity.

> Elevated serum ANA levels may occur in other chronic diseases and a positive ANA test does not, on its own, prove a diagnosis of SLE. However, a positive serum ANA titre is essential for the diagnosis of canine SLE.

Radiographs of the joints of dogs with SLE may show no obvious abnormalities and this is true of all the non-erosive polyarthropathies. Peri-osteal reaction is rare, but soft tissue swelling or synovial effusion may be seen (Fig. 76.5).

Confirmation of the diagnosis usually rests on laboratory evaluations, including:

- synovial fluid analyses typical of immune-mediated polyarthritis (see Chapter 74);
- haematology and biochemistry profiles (Table 76.2);
- urinanalysis (Table 76.2);
- a positive immunofluorescence test for serum ANA;
- antibodies to red blood cells demonstrated by either:
  - a positive Coombs' antiglobulin test, or
  - auto-agglutination (precludes the use of a Coombs' test);
- antibodies to white cells demonstrated by the anti-globulin consumption test (Bennett 1987c);
- antibodies to thrombocytes demonstrated by the platelet factor 3 test (Wilkins *et al.* 1973) or by immunofluorescence.

Tissue biopsies may be submitted for histopathological analyses in 10% formalin. However, to satisfy the third criterion, fresh tissue sections must be frozen and sectioned for immunohistopathological examination. Immune complex deposition in frozen sections may be demonstrated by a direct immunofluorescence test for the presence of immunoglobulins, fibrinogen and complement.

Polyarthritis/Polymyositis Syndrome

This syndrome is seen mainly in the Spaniel breeds and is confirmed by synovial and muscle biopsies. Increased levels of serum creatine phosphokinase and aldolase can help in establishing the diagnosis. Myositis can result in muscle fibrosis and contracture producing obvious restriction of joint motion.

Polyarthritis/Meningitis Syndrome

The meningitis is characterised by neck pain and CSF analysis generally shows an increased white cell count, increased protein levels and an increased creatine phosphokinase level. Occasionally the CSF sample may appear haemorrhagic. Certain breeds appear to be predisposed to this syndrome and include the Weimaraner, German Short-Haired Pointer, Boxer and Bernese Mountain dog. The Akita often shows meningitis and polyarthritis together.

Heritable Polyarthritis of the Adolescent Akita

The Akita is prone to polyarthritis, sometimes with meningitis. It is characterised by early onset (usually during puppyhood) and a poor prognosis.

Familial Renal Amyloidosis in Shar-Pei Dogs

These dogs present with episodes of fever and swelling of one or both hock joints and occasionally other joints. Enthesiopathies are also seen. The age of onset is variable as are the periods between the episodes of illness (generally 4–6 weeks) and each attack generally lasts 24–72 h. Amyloid deposits occur in several organs and eventually these animals show renal or liver failure, anytime between $1\frac{1}{2}$ and 6 years of age.

Polyarteritis Nodosa

This is an inflammatory disease of small arteries, often of a granulomatous nature and is only diagnosed from synovial (and other) biopsies. Meningitis and myositis can complicate the polyarthritis, and may occur in the absence of joint disease.

Canine Sjögren's Syndrome

This is a rare condition in which polyarthritis, which can be erosive or non-erosive, is accompanied by inflammation of lacrimal glands and/or salivary glands. The former can lead to clinical 'dry eye', and 'dry mouth' (xerostomia) is reported in man. This has not been reported in the dog, although swelling and inflammation of the salivary glands has.

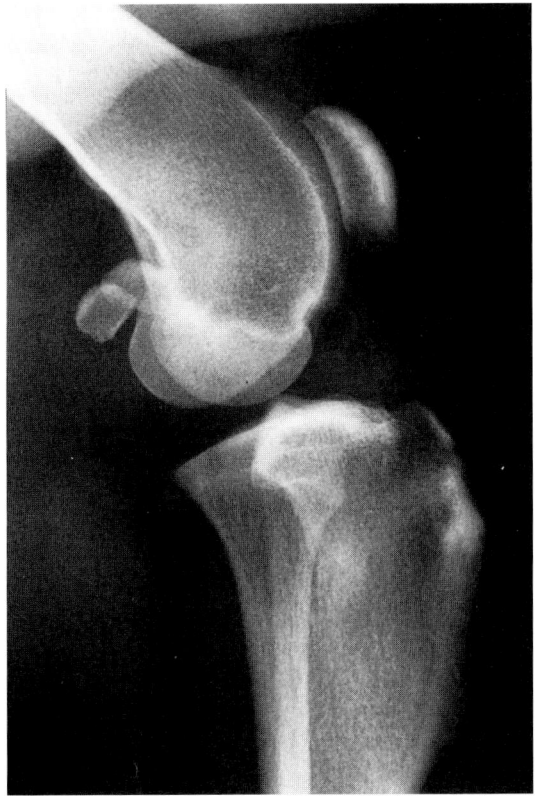

a

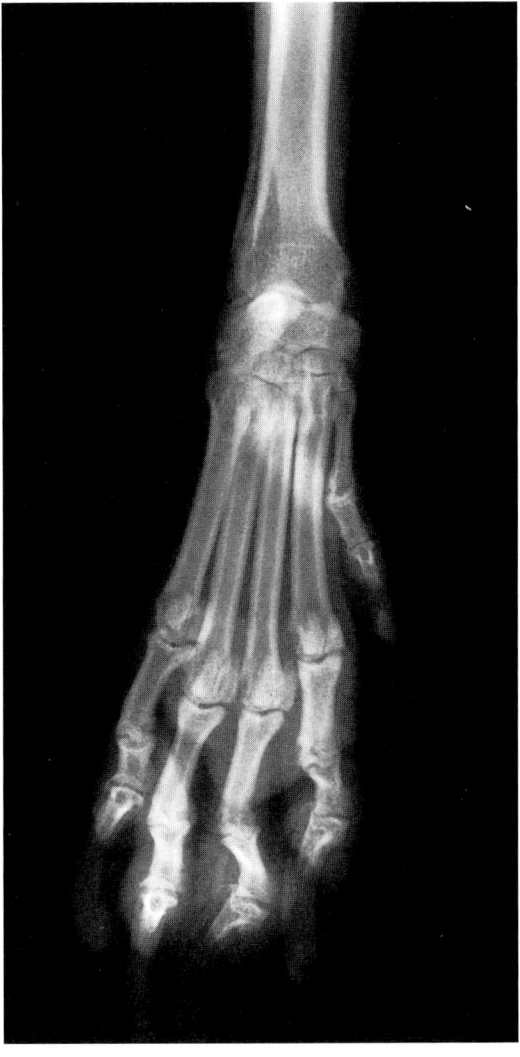

b

Fig. 76.5 (a) Lateral radiograph of the stifle joint of a dog with non-erosive immune-mediated polyarthritis. There is loss of the infra-patellar fat pad and distension of the caudal joint capule. These soft tissue changes are typical but not specific for immune-based joint disease. Other differential diagnoses include infective arthritis, traumatic arthritis and early cruciate disease. (b) Craniocaudal radiograph of the carpus and foot of a dog with immune-mediated non-erosive polyarthritis. Soft tissue thickening around the carpus is the only feature.

Canine Idiopathic Polyarthritis

Canine idiopathic polyarthritis is the most common form of immune-mediated arthropathy in dogs (Bennett 1987d). Differential diagnoses of rheumatoid arthritis, polyarthritis/polymyositis, polyarthritis/meningitis, Lyme disease, bacterial endocarditis and multiple joint infection should be excluded before establishing a diagnosis of canine idio-

pathic polyarthritis. Most cases are in young adults (1–3 years), but dogs of any age can be affected. Male dogs are apparently more commonly affected than females. Any breed of dog may be affected, but there is an apparent predilection in the following breeds:

- German Shepherd Dogs,
- Irish Setters,

- Shetland Sheepdogs,
- Spaniels,
- Collies.

Canine idiopathic polyarthritis is a collective term within which four sub-types of disease are recognised. The sub-types are classified by association with concomitant pathology. It is possible that the co-existing pathology contributes to immune complex formation and thus leads to immune complex hypersensitivity in the synovial membrane. Immune complex deposition elsewhere in the body can produce multi-system disease in some cases, but the absence of significant levels of ANA is sufficient to rule out systemic lupus erythematosus. The complicating lesions may include:

- dermatitis,
- glomerulonephritis,
- uveitis,
- retinitis.

Type I: Uncomplicated Idiopathic Arthritis

This is the most common subgroup, accounting for 50% of all cases of canine idiopathic polyarthritis. No concomitant pathology is found.

Type II: Idiopathic Arthritis Associated with Infections Remote from the Joint (Reactive Arthritis)

This group accounts for 25% of cases of canine idiopathic polyarthritis. Infections associated with polyarthritis include:

- endocarditis,
- respiratory tract infections,
- tonsillitis,
- urinary tract infections,
- pyoderma (including anal furunculosis),
- pyometra,
- abscessation.

Type III: Idiopathic Arthritis Associated with Gastrointestinal Disease (Enteropathic Arthritis)

Polyarthritis associated with some form of gastrointestinal disease accounts for approximately 15% of canine idiopathic polyarthritis cases. This is most commonly vomiting and diarrhoea.

Type IV: Idiopathic Arthritis Associated with Neoplasia Remote from the Joints

Type IV polyarthritis may occur with any malignancy since tumour cells provide a source of chronic antigenic stimulus for persistent immune complex formation.

In all types of canine idiopathic polyarthritis, the clinical signs, radiographic findings and synovial fluid analyses are typical of immune-mediated, non-erosive arthropathy. The signs are similar in all four sub-types of disease, but may be more severe in types I and II. Types III and IV may be mild with only a few joints affected, sometimes asymmetrically. Careful clinical assessment is needed to identify these other lesions which might be aetiologically important.

Vaccination Reactions

Occasionally, an immune-based arthritis can follow vaccine inoculations, most often the first injection of a primary vaccination course in a young puppy. It is usually self-limiting and clears within 2–3 days, without the need for therapy.

Drug-induced Arthritis

Immune-based polyarthritis can be associated with the administration of certain drugs, particularly antibiotics (Table 76.4). They are hypersensitivity diseases involving the deposition of drug/antibody complexes within and around blood vessels. The drug may act directly as an antigen or may combine with host proteins as haptens to form neo-antigens. Other manifestations besides polyarthritis may be seen, e.g. dermatitis, glomerulonephritis, myositis, thrombocytopenia. The dog rapidly improves (2–7 days) once the drug administration is stopped. The Doberman is apparently predisposed to polyarthritis associated with sulphonamide drugs.

Plasmacytic-lymphocytic Synovitis of the Stifle Joints

This is thought to be an immune-based disorder leading to cranial cruciate ligament failure (Pedersen *et al.* 1989), but its existence in the UK has not been demonstrated.

Table 76.4   Antibiotics associated with polyarthritis reactions.

Sulphonamides
Erythromycin
Lincomycin
Cephalosporins
Penicillin derivatives

PROGNOSIS AND THERAPEUTIC PRINCIPLES IN POLYARTHRITIS

The classification of immune-mediated arthritis into specific syndromes allows for a more accurate prognosis to be given. Prognoses are summarised in Table 76.5.

The principal aim of therapy in all idiopathic immune-mediated arthropathies is to provide symptomatic relief by suppression of the immune response and by control of inflammation. In some cases therapy can eventually be completely withdrawn without relapse of the disease. However, many animals require lifelong treatment, especially those with CRA or multisystemic diseases. Prednisolone is the mainstay of therapy for immune-mediated polyarthritis and many cases can be managed with this drug alone. However, in refractory cases, multisystemic disease or erosive disease, more aggressive drug therapy may be merited (Table 76.6). Cases of immune-mediated polyarthritis associated with infections, neoplasia and drug idiosyncrasies may resolve following removal of the inciting factor, but some of these cases also need prednisolone therapy to control the inflammatory joint disease.

Surgical treatment is rarely indicated in the management of dogs with chronic immune-mediated joint disease. Synovectomy, arthrodesis and excision arthroplasty may be considered as potential salvage procedures for relief from chronic pain. Surgical repair of subluxations and ligament injuries may also be of benefit in selected cases. However, surgical failure rates in these animals are high because of the ongoing pathology and the deleterious effects that the therapeutic agents have on wound healing.

Lifestyle management is an important adjunct to all therapies for immune-mediated arthritides. Particular attention should be paid to maintaining a low-stress existence for the dog and exercise should be moderated to the

Table 76.5 Summary of the prognoses of the immune-mediated arthropathies.

Syndrome	Prognosis
Rheumatoid arthritis	Poor. Progressive erosion and destruction of the joints. Periosteal proliferative. Therapy may preserve quality of life polyarthritis. Euthanasia may ultimately be necessary
Felty's syndrome	Poor. For canine rheumatoid arthritis and Felty's syndrome, consider chrysotherapy or cyclophosphamide or azathioprine (Table 76.6)
Systemic lupus erythematosus	Guarded, especially if there is renal involvement. In some dogs the disease can be controlled satisfactorily for prolonged periods. Consider cyclophosphamide or azathioprine therapy (Table 76.6)
Polyarthritis/polymyositis syndrome	Guarded. 30% may make a complete recovery. Most animals have permanent stiffness or relapse once therapy is withdrawn
Polyarthritis/meningitis syndrome	Most cases respond well to therapy
Polyarthritis in adolescent Akita	Poor. Euthanasia often necessary
Chinese Shar-Pei	Guarded to poor. The main prognostic factor in fever syndrome is the tendency to develop amyloidosis
Polyarteritis nodosa	Good. Generally responds well to therapy
Vaccination reactions	Good. Generally self-limiting
Drug-induced	Excellent. Complete recovery once drug is stopped
Canine idiopathic polyarthritides	
Type I	Good. Many dogs are cured with therapy. In others the disease can usually be adequately controlled. Some cases progress to an erosive rheumatoid disease
Types II, III and IV	Good, provided the primary disease can be resolved. The primary disease is often the main prognostic factor

Table 76.6 Drugs used to treat immune-mediated polyarthritis.

Drug	Recommendations for use
Prednisolone	Immunosuppressive dose (1–2 mg/kg every 8 h p.o.) for 'acute' cases. This dose continued for 2–3 weeks and then gradually reduced over 3–4 months Anti-inflammatory dose (e.g. 0.25 mg/kg every 8 h p.o.). Smallest dose that provides clinical improvement for 'chronic' cases
Cyclophosphamide	1.5 mg/kg dogs >30 kg 2.0 mg/kg dogs 15–30 kg 2.5 mg/kg dogs <15 kg and cats Given on 4 consecutive days each week for up to 16 weeks. Give in conjunction with a daily anti-inflammatory dose of prednisolone. Haematology every 7–14 days; if WBC <6000/mm², or platelets count <125 000/mm², reduce cyclophosphamide by 25%, if WBC <4000/mm² or platelets count <100 000/mm² discontinue for 2 weeks, then recommence at 50% original dose. In addition to myelosuppression can cause haemorrhagic cystitis
Azathioprine	2.0 mg/kg EOD, p.o. Used as an alternative to cyclophosphamide. Give with prednisolone (each drug given on different days). Haematology every 7–14 days (see cyclophosphamide)
Sulphasalazine	25 mg/kg every 12 h p.o. Most often indicated in cases of enteropathic polyarthritis although can be used in rheumatoid arthritis. Can cause keratitis sicca
Sodium aurothiomalate (gold salt)	0.5 mg/kg by intramuscular injection once a week for 6 weeks. Usually given with daily oral prednisolone (anti-inflammatory doses). Can be repeated after 2–3 months. Give small test dose first. Haematology every 7–14 days. Gold therapy is most often used in cases of rheumatoid arthritis. In addition to myelosuppression can cause renal impairment, pulmonary fibrosis, corneal ulceration and dermatoses
Auranofin	0.05–2.0 mg/kg b.i.d. p.o. (max. 9 mg/day). An alternative to the intramuscular use of sodium aurothiomalate. Can be given with prednisolone. Can be given as a continuous regime. Haematology every 7–14 days. Can cause osmotic diarrhoea which is often a severe problem
Colchicine	0.03 mg/kg once daily p.o. Used in cases potentially complicated by amyloidosis, e.g. 'Shar-Pei fever syndrome' to reduce the progression of amyloidosis
Dimethyl sulfoxide	Up to 250 mg/kg. Can be given orally, intravenously, subcutaneously, topically or intra-articularly. Used in cases complicated by amyloidosis, but no evidence of any obvious benefit. Produces unpleasant garlic odour
Levamisole	3–7 mg/kg EOD, p.o. Max. dose of 150 mg per day. Used for up to 4 months. Anti-inflammatory dose of prednisolone used initially. Useful for cases showing multisystemic disease. Very unpleasant taste so needs strong flavouring, e.g. orange juice

Note: This table is intended as a guide only. Administration of immunomodulatory drugs is not recommended without a thorough understanding of their use in clinical practice.
EOD, every other day.

dog's abilities, although some form of regular exercise is desirable. Routine vaccination of affected dogs should be avoided if the animal is on immunosuppressive therapy. Vaccination while receiving anti-inflammatory doses of steroid is acceptable. The possible involvement of canine distemper virus in canine immune-based polyarthritis (May *et al.* 1994) means that distemper vaccination should be avoided if possible. It is desirable to measure serum distemper antibody levels before vaccination and if the levels are high enough to be protective, vaccination with the distemper component is not justified.

REFERENCES

Abercromby, R. (1994). Infective arthritis. In: *Manual of Small Animal Arthrology*, (eds J.E.F. Houlton & R.W. Collinson), pp. 100–114. BSAVA Publications, Cheltenham.

Appel, J.G. (1990). Lyme disease in dogs and cats. *Compendium on Continuing Education for the Practicing Veterinarian*, **12**, 617.

Bell, S.C., Carter, S.D. & Bennett, D. (1991). Canine distemper viral antigens and antibodies in dogs with rheumatoid arthritis. *Research in Veterinary Science*, **50**, 64.

Bennett, D. (1987a). Immune based erosive inflammatory joint disease of the dog. Canine rheumatoid arthritis 1. Clinical radiological and laboratory investigation. *Journal of Small Animal Practice*, **28**, 779.

Bennett, D. (1987b). Immune based erosive inflammatory joint disease of the dog. Canine rheumatoid arthritis 2. Pathological investigations. *Journal of Small Animal Practice*, **28**, 799.

Bennett, D. (1987c). Immune based non-erosive inflammatory joint disease of the dog 1. Canine systemic lupus erythematosus. *Journal of Small Animal Practice*, **28**, 871.

Bennett, D. (1987d). Immune based non-erosive inflammatory joint disease of the dog 3. Canine idiopathic polyarthritis. *Journal of Small Animal Practice*, **28**, 909.

Bennett, D. & Kelly, D.F. (1987). Immune based non-erosive inflammatory joint disease of the dog 2. Polyarthritis/polymyositis syndrome. *Journal of Small Animal Practice*, **28**, 891.

Bennett, D. & Kirkham, D. (1987). The laboratory identification of serum rheumatoid factor in the dog. *Journal of Comparative Pathology*, **97**, 542.

Bennett, D. & Taylor, D.J. (1988a). Bacterial infective arthritis in the dog. *Journal of Small Animal Practice*, **29**, 207.

Bennett, D. & Taylor, D.J. (1988b). Bacterial endocarditis and inflammatory joint disease in the dog. *Journal of Small Animal Practice*, **29**, 347.

Brown, A. & Bennett, D. (1989). The use of gentamycin impregnated methylmethacrylate beads for the treatment of bacterial infective arthritis. *Veterinary Record*, **123**, 625.

DiBartola, S.P., Tarr, M.J., Webb, D.M. & Giger, U. (1990). Familial renal amyloidosis in Chinese shar pei dogs. *Journal of the American Veterinary Medical Association*, **197**, 483.

Dougherty, S.A., Center, S.A., Shaw, E.E. & Erb, H.A. (1991). Juvenile-onset polyarthritis syndrome in Akitas. *Journal of the American Veterinary Medical Association*, **198**, 849.

Halliwell, R.E.W. (1982). Autoimmune disease in domestic animals. *Journal of the American Veterinary Medical Association*, **181**, 1088.

May, C., Hammill, J. & Bennett, D. (1992). Chinese Shar-Pei fever syndrome: a preliminary report. *Veterinary Record*, **131**, 586.

May, C., Carter, S.D., Bell., S.C. & Bennett, D. (1994). Immune responses to canine distemper virus in joint diseases of dogs. *British Journal of Rheumatology*, **33**, 27.

Pedersen, N.C., Wind, A., Morgan, J.P. & Pool, R.R. (1989). Joint diseases of dogs and cats. In: *Textbook of Veterinary Internal Medicine*, (ed. S.J. Ettinger), 3rd edn. pp. 2329–2377. W.B. Saunders, Philadelphia.

Quimby, F.W., Gebert, R., Datta, S., *et al.* (1978). Characterisation of a retrovirus that cross-reacts serologically with canine and human systemic lupus erythematosus. *Clinical Immunology and Immunopathology*, **9**, 194.

Schumacher, H.R. (1975). Synovial membrane and fluid morphologic alterations in early rheumatoid arthritis. Microvascular injury and virus-like particles. *Annals of the New York Academy of Science*, **256**, 39.

Schumacher, H.R., Newton, C.D. & Halliwell, R.E.W. (1980). Synovial pathological changes in spontaneous canine rheumatoid-like arthritis. *Arthritis and Rheumatism*, **23**, 412.

Steere, A.C. (1989). Lyme disease. *New England Journal of Medicine*, **321**, 586.

Wilkins, R.J., Hurvitz, A.J. & Dodds-Laffin, W.J. (1973). Immunologically mediated thrombocytopenia in the dog. *Journal of the American Veterinary Medical Association*, **163**, 277.

Chapter 77

Bone Diseases

H. A. W. Hazewinkel

INTRODUCTION

Bone diseases are a heterogeneous group which are difficult to classify because many have unknown or multi-factorial aetiologies. Two major groups of bone disease include infectious bone diseases (see Box 77.1) and nutritional bone diseases. The remainder may be considered as inherited, endocrinological or miscellaneous conditions (Table 77.1).

NUTRITIONAL BONE DISEASES

Introduction

Nutritional bone diseases are primarily a problem in young, rapidly growing breeds of dog. Normal skeletal development is dependent on a balanced intake of protein, calories, calcium, inorganic phosphorous and vitamin D. Both excesses and deficiencies in these dietary constituents have been associated with abnormal skeletal development.

Dietary requirements for calcium, phosphorous and vitamin D in growing dogs are:

- calcium 1–2% of dry matter weight of diet,
- phosphorous 1% of dry matter weight of diet,
- calcium:phosphorous ratio 1:1 to 2:1,
- vitamin D 500 IU/kg of diet.

These dietary requirements are most easily met by feeding a commercially prepared diet without added supplementation.

Normal calcium levels in extracellular fluid are essential for a variety of vital processes (e.g. blood clotting, nerve action, muscle contraction). Calcitriol (the active form of vitamin D), parathyroid hormone (PTH) and calcitonin are the hormones maintaining calcium and phosphorous homeostasis in dogs. Briefly, calcitriol elevates serum calcium levels by encouraging calcium uptake from the gut and by enhancing resorption of calcium from bone. PTH similarly elevates serum calcium levels, primarily by an action on bone. Calcitonin depresses serum calcium levels. These hormones are controlled by a series of feedback loops which are extremely sensitive and maintain serum calcium levels within the normal range, even in the face of severe dietary derangement (Figs 77.1 and 77.2). The reader is referred to more detailed texts for further reading on calcium and phosphate physiology (Capen & Rosol 1993).

Diseases of Overnutrition

Excessive energy intake can be harmful for young growing dogs with a cartilaginous skeleton, as well as for adult dogs with arthritic joints. Increased intake of minerals also has negative effects on skeletal development, since the absorption process is less well regulated in young dogs than in adults.

Overnutrition, including high calcium intake, is important in the aetiology of several skeletal diseases in young, rapidly growing dogs (Table 77.2). Absolute calcium intake per kilogram of body weight has to be taken into account. Large amounts of calcium (with or without phosphorus) together with restricted feeding is as harmful as large amounts of a balanced diet which result in the same calcium intake. Young dogs of large breeds should be raised on a limited amount of good quality food specifically formulated for the requirements of growing dogs.

> The protein and mineral content of good quality commercial adult dog food is sufficient for raising large breed dogs.
> Overfeeding and oversupplementation must be avoided.

Box 77.1   Osteomyelitis in focus.

- Literally = inflammation of bone. Usually refers to bone infections.
- Fungal osteomyelitis rare in the UK. (For review, see Wolf & Troy 1995)
  Aspergillus spp. may cause disseminated osteomyelitis or discospondylitis, especially in German Shepherd Dogs (Day & Penhale 1988; Neer 1988)
- Viral osteomyelitis (hypertrophic osteodystrophy)
- Bacterial osteomyelitis = most common

Common organisms

Staphylococcus spp. (>50% of cases)
Streptococcus spp.
Gram negatives (e.g. *E.coli*, pseudomonads, *Proteus*)

Anaerobes and mixed infections may occur (especially in bite wounds)

Nocardia, *Brucella* and tuberculosis are rare causes of osteomyelitis

Pathophysiology

For infection to establish need:
(1)   Contamination with bacteria
  - penetrating wound
  - haematogenous spread
(2)   Diminished local host defences
  - poor local blood supply
  - foreign material implanted
  - fracture instability
  - associated soft tissue trauma
  - sequestration

Diagnosis of bacterial osteomyelitis

Acute

Signs: Systemic (pyrexia, inappetance, depression, weight loss).
               Local (heat, pain and swelling of bone, periosteum and surrounding tissues).

Radiography: Soft tissue swelling. May be no osseous changes.

Laboratory: *Usually* a neutrophilia and left shift.

Chronic

Signs: Systemic (uncommon)
               Local (abscessation, sinus tracts, lymphadenopathy, muscle atrophy, fibrosis and contracture)

Radiography: Often extensive periosteal new bone formation, bone lysis, ±involucrum and sequestrum formation.
               Cannot reliably differentiate from malignant neoplasia by radiography

Laboratory: Often haematologically *normal*

CONFIRM BY BONE BIOPSY FOR BACTERIAL CULTURES, ANTIBIOTIC SENSITIVITES AND HISTOPATHOLOGY

Treatment and prognosis

Antibiotic choice guided by culture results. Consider clavulanate potentiated amoxycillin, cephalosporins or quinolones. Clindamycin or metronidazole may be indicated when anaerobes are involved. Reserve aminoglycosides (e.g. gentamicin, lincomycin) for specific indications because of toxicity risks and consider using as antibiotic impregnated polymethylmethacrylate beads (Brown & Bennett 1988)

Acute

4–6 weeks of antibiotic therapy usually curative, provided osseous damage is minimal.

Chronic (includes those with established osseous change complicating fracture repair)

Prolonged and expensive. Recurrences can occur months or years after cessation of treatment.
Surgical debridement and removal of any implants essential in addition to antibiotic therapy. Debridement and drainage may need to be repeated. Fractures must be *rigidly* stabilised and autologous cancellous bone grafts are advisable.

Table 77.1 Classification of bone diseases of the canine appendicular skeleton.

Disease	Age	Diagnosis
Endocrinological (Jezyk 1985)		
Dwarfism	Young	C, R
Hypothyroidism	Young	C, R, B
Hyperadrenocorticism	Mature	C, B
Infectious		
Osteomyelitis (Herron 1993)	All ages	C, R, M, B
Hypertrophic osteodystrophy (Johnson *et al.* 1995)	Young	C, R
Nutritional (Capen & Rosol 1993; Hazewinkel 1994; Hazewinkel & Schoenmakers 1995)		
Nutritional hyperparathyroidism	Young	C, R, M
Rickets (hypovitaminosis D)	Young	R, B, M
Hypercalcitoninism		
Panosteitis (enostosis)	Young	C, R
Retained cartilage cores	Young	C, R
Osteochondrosis	Young	C, R
Inherited		
Dwarfism (Fletch *et al.* 1973; Jezyk 1985)	Young	C, R, M
Craniomandibular osteopathy (Riser & Newton 1985)	Young	C, R
Osteochondrosis (Olsson 1993)	Young	C, R
Fragmented coronoid process (Olsson 1993)	Young	C, R
Aseptic necrosis of femoral head (Legg–Perthes disease) (Nunamaker 1985)	Young	C, R
Miscellaneous		
Neoplasia (see Chapter 78)	Mature	C, R, M
Multiple cartilaginous exostoses (Pool 1993)	Young	C, R
Renal hyperparathyroidism (see Chapter 62)	All	C, R, B
Bone cysts	Young–mature	R, M
Hypertrophic osteopathy (Lenehan & Fetter 1985)	Mature	C, R
Disuse osteoporosis	All ages	R

C, clinical; R, radiological; B, biochemical; M, microscopical (smears, biopsies).

Table 77.2 Skeletal disorders associated with overnutrition in dogs.

Disorder	Dietary factors	Clinical significance
Osteochondrosis	Calcium, calories	Disturbed enchondral ossification disrupts normal articular and growth plate development. A major cause of morbidity in large breeds of dog
Retained cartilage cones	Calcium, calories	Small cones seen temporarily in dogs of large breeds between 15 and 21 weeks of age without clinical significance. Large (>2 cm) cones may disturb normal gain in bone length
Hip dysplasia	Calories, protein, minerals	Overloading of the cartilaginous skeleton in growing dogs. High mineral intake may hinder skeletal remodelling and adaptation of the hip joint
Cervical spondylomyelopathy ('wobbler' syndrome)	Calcium	Reduced osteoclastic resorption of the vertebral canal results in canal stenosis and spinal cord impingement
Panosteitis	Calcium	Reduced osteoclastic resorption may hinder intra-osseous blood flow and initiate oedema, fibrosis and subsequent new bone formation

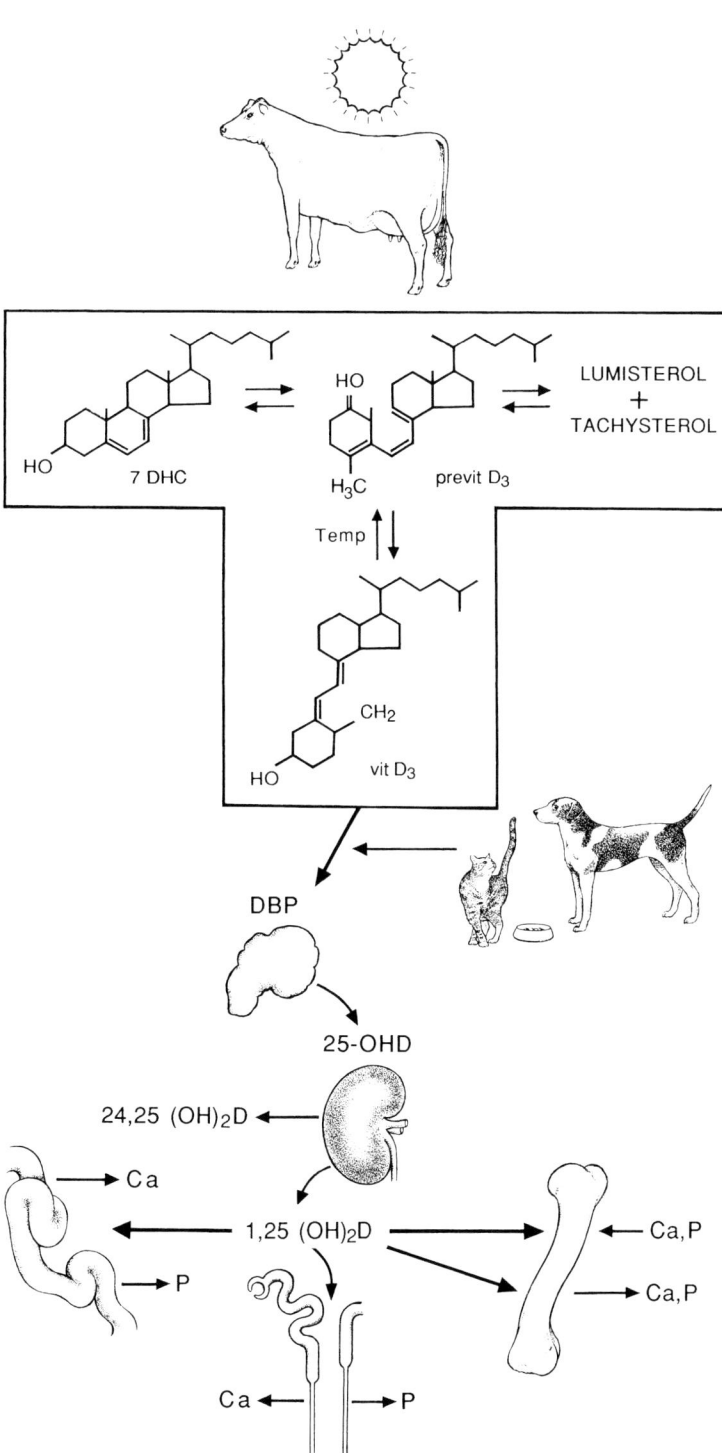

Fig. 77.1 As a result of irradiation with sunlight, vitamin D is synthesised in the skin of a variety of species but not dogs and cats, which need dietary vitamin D intake (Hazewinkel *et al.* 1994). Carried by vitamin D binding proteins (DBP), vitamin D is transported to the liver where a first hydroxylation into 25-hydroxycholecalciferol (25-OHD) occurs, followed by a second hydroxylation into 24,25-dihydroxycholecalciferol (24,25-$(OH)_2$D), or the biological more potent 1,25-dihydroxycholecalciferol (1,25-$(OH)_2$D) in the kidneys. The latter metabolite plays a significant role in intestinal absorption and renal reabsorption of calcium and phosphorus, and the mineralisation of cartilage and osteoid as well as the resorption of bone.

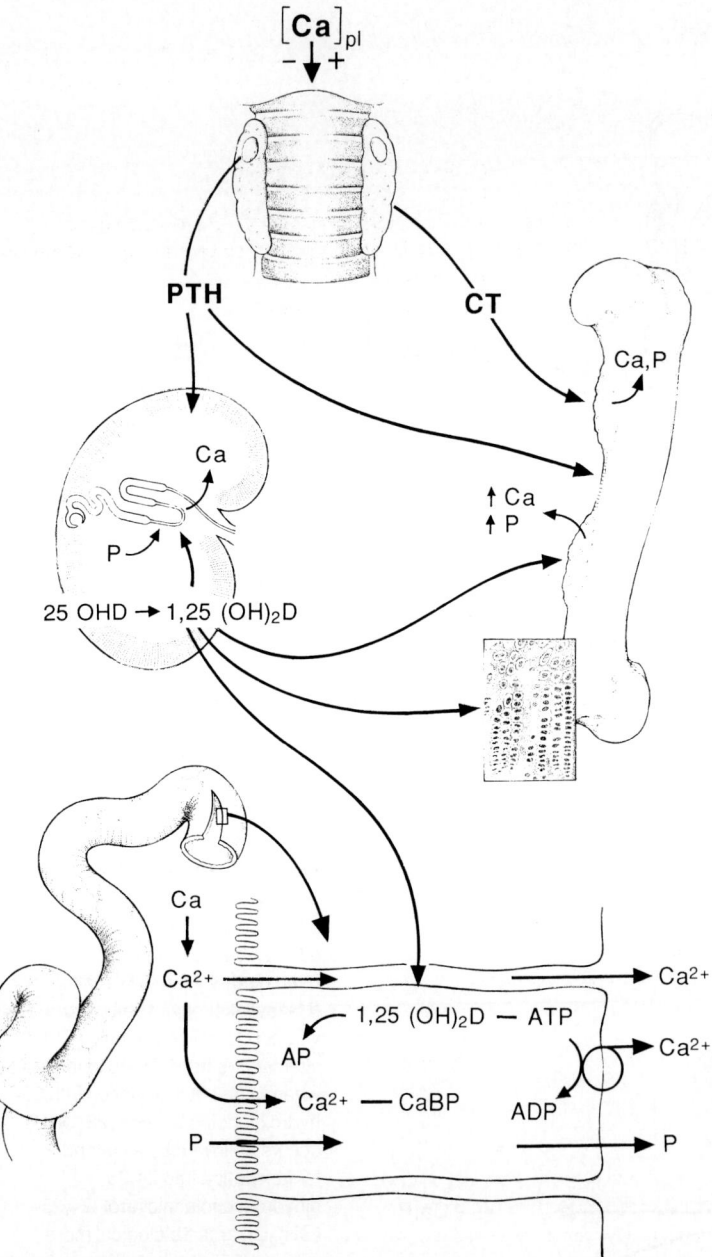

Fig. 77.2 Decreasing plasma Ca concentrations, [Ca]$_{pl}$, cause an increase in parathyroid hormone (PTH) secretion from the parathyroid glands, resulting in increased osteoclasia (thus liberating Ca and P from the skeleton), an increased Ca reabsorption from the renal tubules and an increased urinary excretion of P. In addition, PTH stimulates hydroxylation of 25-hydroxycholecalciferol (25-OHD) to 1,25-dihydroxycholecalciferol (1,25-(OH)$_2$D). 1,25-(OH)$_2$D increases the effect of PTH on bone resorption, increases active Ca and P absorption in intestinal cells and Ca and P reabsorption in the kidneys. It is also a permissive factor for osteoid and cartilage mineralisation.

Increasing [Ca]$_{pl}$ causes an increased calcitonin (CT) secretion from the thyroid glands. CT has an immediate effect on osteoclasts to retract their ruffle border enabling osteoblasts to deposit bone, thus reducing [Ca]$_{pl}$ by increasing Ca and P storage in the skeleton.

Diseases of Undernutrition or Malnutrition

Alimentary Hyperparathyroidism

> Alimentary hyperparathyroidism occurs when there is a prolonged period of insufficient dietary calcium intake or of calcium malabsorption.

Aetiopathogenesis

The factors that create calcium deficiency in alimentary hyperparathyroidism include:

- *Predominantly meat or meat by-products in the diet* (low calcium content; 'all meat syndrome', 'butcher's dog syndrome').
- *Poor quality diet with low digestibility may bind calcium to phytates.* This effectively causes calcium malabsorption, especially in young dogs of large breeds.

In these circumstances, excessive PTH is synthesised and secreted (hyperparathyroidism) to help normalise the calcium concentration in the extracellular fluid. PTH has three main actions:

- to increase osteoclastic activity;
- to increase calcitriol synthesis in the kidney from 25-hydroxy-vitamin D;
- to increase calcium and decrease phosphorous re-absorption in the renal tubules.

When the increase in absorption of calcium from the intestine is insufficient for daily requirements, the only remaining source of calcium is the skeleton. The cortex is resorbed at its endosteal surface, but cartilage mineralisation and endochondral ossification proceed undisturbed.

History and Examination

Affected dogs are young animals raised on an imbalanced diet. They are usually of large breeds and in otherwise good condition. Clinical signs include:

- reluctance to stand and walk,
- bone deformity,
- ±pathological (folding) fractures of long bones,
- ±paralysis due to spinal compression by pathological fractures of vertebrae,
- pain on skeletal palpation.

Investigation

Routine blood parameters are often normal. PTH and calcitriol levels are elevated (Table 77.3), but determination of these is sophisticated, time consuming and expensive.

Radiological findings are often diagnostic (Fig. 77.3). Bone biopsies reveal normal mineralisation but increased resorption and thus a thin cortex and thin cancellous bone spiculae.

Skeletal radiology in alimentary hyperparathyroidism (Fig. 77.3) shows:

- thin cortices,
- poor mineral opacity ('ghost bones'),
- wide medullary cavities,
- bowing of protuberances by muscle traction,
- growth plates normal width,
- wide, relatively radiopaque, metaphyses,
- folding or greenstick fractures of diaphyses,
- compression fractures of the cancellous bone of epiphyses and vertebrae.

Differential Diagnosis

Calcium deficiency can be complicated by vitamin D deficiency when solely lean meat (which is low in calcium and vitamin D) is fed. Some bone diseases due to inborn errors of metabolism may resemble alimentary hyperparathy-

Table 77.3 The range or mean (± s.e.m.) plasma concentrations of total calcium, phosphorus, parathyroid hormone (PTH), and the dihydroxy and monohydroxy vitamin D metabolites as found in research dogs with nutritional hyperparathyroidism (HyperPTH) or rickets of 3 months of age compared with normal young dogs and determined by the techniques as described in Hazewinkel *et al.* (1987).

	Calcium mmol/l	Phosphorous mmol/l	PTH pg/ml	1,25-$(OH)_2$D pg/ml	25-OHD ng/ml
Normal	3.03 ± 0.09	2.33 ± 0.16	24.7 ± 2.1	40 ± 8	20–60
HyperPTH	2.92 ± 0.06	3.12 ± 0.4	>35	260 ± 40	20–60
Rickets	2.7 ± 0.1	2.5 ± 0.2	>35	38.8 ± 7	0.1–5

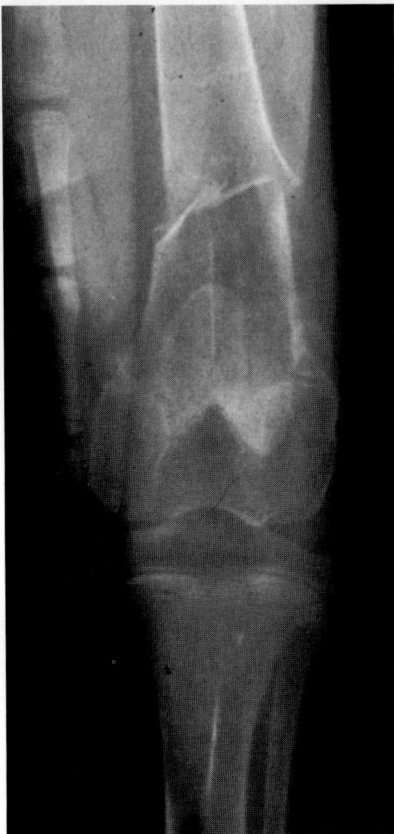

Fig. 77.3 Alimentary hyperparathyroidism. A 3-month-old German Shepherd Dog with 'ghost bones' with wide medullae, thin cortices and a greenstick fracture in the distal femur. Note the normal growth plates and relatively radiopaque metaphyses.

roidism. These include osteogenesis imperfecta, muco-polysaccharidosis and other rare diseases (for review, see Jezyk 1985).

Management
Strict cage rest is essential to prevent further pathological fractures (especially of the vertebrae). No bandages or splints can be applied, since the bone will fracture at the ends of splints where there is a stress riser effect. Similarly, analgesics are undesirable without strict confinement as they facilitate early mobility and increase the risk of pathological fracture. Definitive treatment is by normalisation of the diet:

- Provide a diet with calcium content up to 1.1% on a dry matter basis. The skeleton will mineralise within 3–4

weeks. Calcium absorption of almost 100% will take place due to the hyperparathyroid-induced high calcitriol activity.
- Extra calcium can be provided as calcium carbonate or calcium lactate. Calcium supplementation of 50 mg Ca/kg body weight may accelerate osteoid mineralisation.
- Avoid calcium supplementation with bone meal, or other forms containing phosphorous.
- Avoid vitamin D supplementation as this may further increase osteoclast activity.

If necessary, corrective osteotomies can be planned once the skeleton is normally mineralised.

Hypovitaminosis D

> In young animals, hypovitaminosis D is known as rickets.
> In adults hypovitaminosis D is known as osteomalacia.

Aetiopathogenesis
Unlike many other species (including man, but excluding cats), dogs are unable to synthesise vitamin D in their skin under the influence of sunlight. Vitamin D is absorbed from the intestine and is sequentially hydroxylated in the liver and kidney to the active metabolite 1,25-dihydroxy-vitamin D (calcitriol) or to an inactive metabolite (24,25-dihydroxy-vitamin D) (Fig. 77.1). Functions of calcitriol include:

- To stimulate active absorption of calcium (from the proximal small intestine) and phosphorus (from the distal small intestine).
- To increase reabsorption of calcium and phosphorus by the renal tubular cells.
- To facilitate osteoid and cartilage mineralisation in developing bone and to increase osteoclastic activity.

The absorption and first hydroxylation of vitamin D are loosely controlled, whereas the hydroxylation into calcitriol is directly and indirectly influenced by serum calcium and phosphorus concentration, parathyroid hormone, and increased mineral needs during growth, reproduction and lactation.

The pathogenesis of hypovitaminosis D in young puppies may occur in one of two ways:

- *Dietary deficiency of vitamin D*: When a vitamin D deficient diet is fed at an early age, puppies first metabolise the vitamin D from maternal origin (placenta and milk) and then develop hypovitaminosis D.

- *Excessive calcium supplementation*: When a diet highly supplemented with calcium is fed to young puppies, hypoparathyroidism develops resulting in a shut down of calcitriol synthesis (Fig. 77.2). Despite the high calcium and normal vitamin D content of the diet, the animal may develop clinical signs of rickets.

History and Examination

Hypovitaminosis D mostly occurs when an imbalanced diet (either low in animal fat or enriched with calcium salts) is fed from an early age onwards. It is rare as a clinical problem in adult dogs. Clinical signs are superficially similar to hyperparathyroidism and include:

- reluctance to stand and walk,
- bone deformity,
- metaphyseal flaring – most often noticeable at the distal radius and ulna or at the costochondral junctions ('rosary bead ribs'),
- ±pathological (folding) fractures of long bones,
- ±paralysis due to spinal compression by pathological fractures of vertebrae,
- pain on skeletal palpation.

Investigation

Routine blood parameters are often within the normal range. Determination of vitamin D and its metabolites may be useful (Table 77.3), but such evaluations are both specialised and expensive. Decreased levels of 25-hydroxy-vitamin D are seen with dietary deficiency, whereas normal levels of the 25-hydroxy metabolite combined with low levels of the 1,25-metabolite indicates hypoparathyroidism or renal disease.

Rapidly growing long bones, such as the radius and ulna are useful targets for radiography.

Skeletal radiology in rickets (Fig. 77.4) shows:

- thin cortices,
- bowed and/or fractured diaphyses,
- 'flaring' of the metaphyses,
- extremely wide growth plates are almost pathognomonic, but can be mimicked by some rare congenital disorders.

Clinical and radiological findings are usually diagnostic, but confirmation can be achieved by biopsy of cancellous bone and growth plate cartilage (e.g. a core biopsy of the greater trochanter). Biopsy may also be helpful to exclude rare congenital disorders, including chondrodysplasia (Fletch *et al.* 1973), metaphyseal chondrodysplasia (Jezyck 1985) and enchondrodystrophy (Breur *et al.* 1989; Bennett 1990).

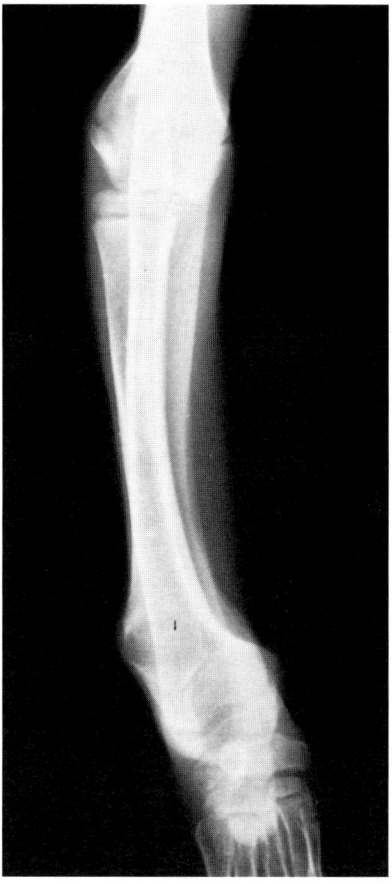

Fig. 77.4 Rickets (hypovitaminosis D). A 3-month-old mongrel dog with wide medulla, thin cortices and extremely wide, mushroom shaped, growth plates owing to poor mineralisation of cartilage and bone.

Management

Normalisation of the diet is most easily achieved by feeding a commercial prepared dog food, known to contain sufficient vitamin D to cure or prevent rickets (Hazewinkel 1994). After 3 weeks the patient should be evaluated radiographically for cortical mineralisation, callus formation at pathological fractures and mineralisation at growth plates. In cases of dietary hypovitaminosis D a dramatic improvement will be seen.

Additional supplementation of vitamin D is reserved for *confirmed* cases (by biopsy or vitamin D metabolite determination) that *do not respond* to dietary normalisation.

Inappropriate vitamin D oversupplementation may cause hypercalcemia and hyperphosphatemia with mineralisation of soft tissues, heart valves, and kidneys. This can be fatal.

MISCELLANEOUS BONE DISEASES

Hypertrophic Osteodystrophy (HOD) (Metaphyseal Osteopathy)

Aetiopathogenesis

The aetiology of HOD remains unclear and may be associated with either environmental or inherited factors. Proposed hypotheses on the aetiology of HOD have included:

- Hypovitaminosis C causes inferior collagen formation in bone and blood vessels in primates and guinea pigs and was hypothesised to be the cause of HOD in dogs. This has not proved to be the case.
- Other proposed dietary aetiologies include:
  ○ copper deficiency,
  ○ overfeeding and oversupplementation with minerals.

More recent evidence indicates a possible infective aetiology. Grøndalen (1979) demonstrated that blood taken from dogs with HOD caused clinical canine distemper virus (CDV) infection when infused into recipient dogs.

Mee *et al.* (1992) demonstrated RNA and mRNA of CDV in osteoblasts, osteocytes and bone marrow cells of CDV infected dogs and within the affected metaphyses of dogs with HOD. Metaphyseal bone lesions have also been recognised in dogs with systemic distemper (Baumgartner *et al.* 1995).

History and Examination

Often an episode of respiratory or gastrointestinal disease precedes the onset of HOD. The animal may be recently vaccinated against CDV.

Typical clinical findings in HOD (Fig. 77.5) are:

- young dogs (2–8 months old);
- predominantly larger (fast growing) breeds;
- depression;
- anorexia;
- pyrexia (rectal temperature may be >40°C);
- painful, multiple limb lameness or unable to stand;
- warm, firm, painful metaphyseal swelling;
- distal radius and ulna primarily affected;
- litter-mates may also be affected.

Investigation

The white blood cell count (especially neutrophils), globulins and alkaline phosphatase may be increased. Calcium and phosphorus are usually within normal limits. Radiological findings are diagnostic.

Radiological findings in hypertrophic osteodystrophy (Fig. 77.6) are:

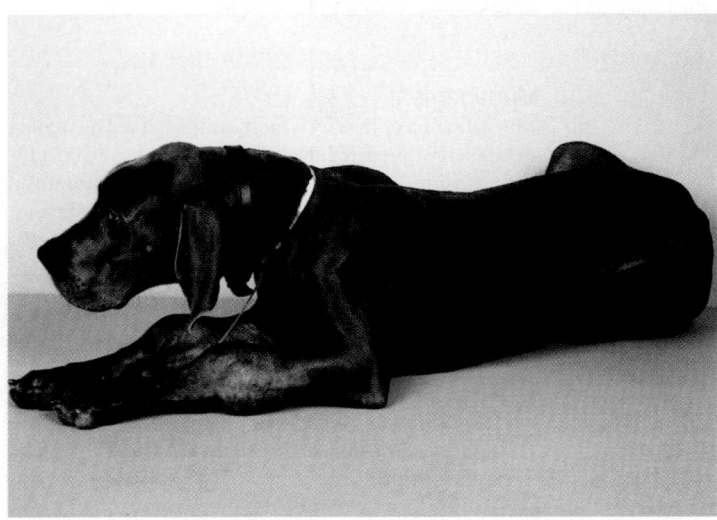

Fig. 77.5 Hypertrophic osteodystrophy. A 3-month-old Great Dane with pyrexia, inability to stand and painful firm swollen metaphyses.

- multiple, symmetrical bone involvement, especially the distal radius and ulna;
- an irregular radiolucent line in the metaphyseal area parallel to the growth plate;
- in sub-acute cases a cuff of soft tissue calcification surrounds the metaphyseal area;
- the calcified cuff eventually remodels to a near normal bone shape.

Management

Treatment of HOD centres on good nursing care which may include:

- intravenous fluid therapy,
- analgesia with NSAIDs (see Chapter 7) but not corticosteroids,
- antibiotics may be indicated.

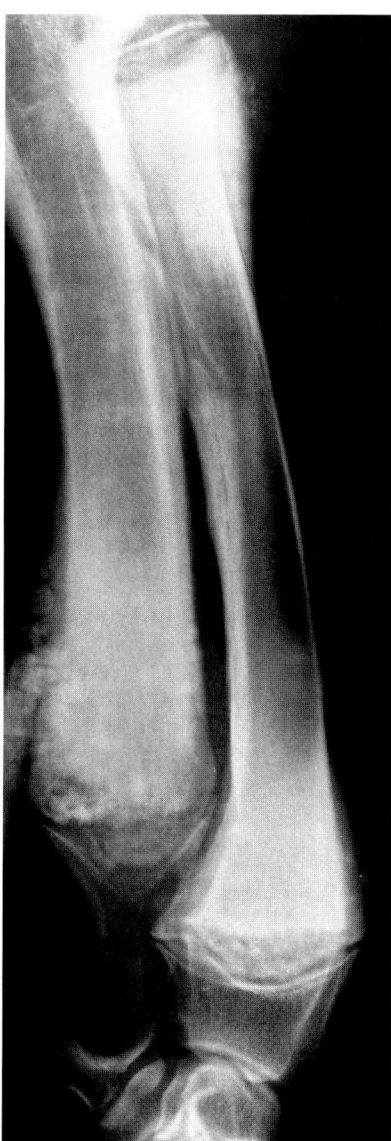

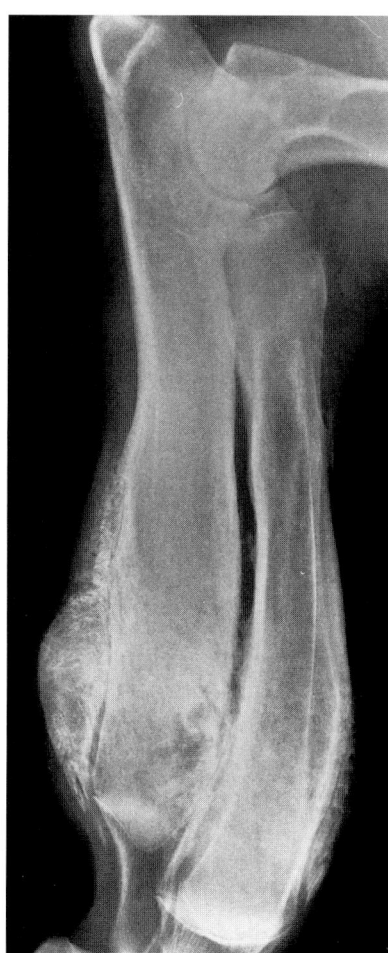

Fig. 77.6 Hypertrophic osteodystrophy. Radiographs of the same dog as Fig. 77.5: (a) radiolucent lines parallel to the growth plate, periosteal and even extra periosteal new bone formation becoming more pronounced 3 weeks later (b).

Rarely, cases may die in shock. Most survive and heal clinically, with or without remnants of diaphyseal bone deformity. Relapses may occur until the dog is fully grown.

Hypertrophic Osteopathy (HO) (Hypertrophic Pulmonary Osteoarthropathy; Morbus Marie – Bamberger; Marie's Disease)

Aetiopathogenesis

HO is characterised by symmetrical periosteal new bone formation on the long bones of the appendicular skeleton. It is associated with an increase in local blood flow to the bone. The skeletal changes are a manifestation of underlying systemic disease, including:

- Any space-occupying process in the thorax (98% of cases):
  - o primary or secondary pulmonary neoplasia (92% of thoracic cases),
  - o tuberculosis,
  - o granulomas,
  - o foreign bodies,
  - o oesophageal granulomas or sarcomas,
  - o chondrosarcoma of the rib,
  - o cardiac disease (valvular endocarditis, heartworm).
- Any space-occupying process in the abdomen (2% of cases):
  - o liver tumour,
  - o neoplasia of the urinary bladder,
  - o pyometra.

It is probable that a neurovascular reflex changes periosteal blood flow, which induces the periosteal new bone formation. The phalanges and metatarsal and metacarpal bones are initially affected followed by the more proximal bones. Vagotomy on the affected side of the space-occupying process causes remission of the periosteal reactions and regression of elevated peripheral blood flow to the extremities.

History and Examination

Depending on the underlying cause, HO may manifest in young dogs (e.g. embryonal rhabdomyosarcoma of urinary bladder), or older dogs (e.g. neoplasia, pyometra). Affected dogs may show pain, a reluctance to move and firm swellings, particularly apparent in the metacarpal and metatarsal regions (Watson 1990).

Investigation

Serum alkaline phosphatase levels may be elevated. Other haematological parameters may be affected by the primary pulmonary or abdominal pathology. Typical radiological findings are diagnostic for HO (Fig. 77.7a,b,c).

Skeletal radiological findings in hypertrophic osteopathy are:

- multiple limbs affected,
- multiple long bones affected (especially in the distal limb),
- generalised and uniform diaphyseal periosteal new bone formation,
- associated soft tissue swelling of the limbs,
- periosteal new bone may be spiculated,
- epiphyses spared of changes.

Management

The recognition of HO should lead to a search for the underlying cause (e.g. by thoracic and abdominal radiography). Removal of the primary lesion, if possible, often leads to remission of signs, but remodelling of the established periosteal new bone is a prolonged process. Vagotomy is not often a realistic therapy because of undesirable side-effects.

Panosteitis

Aetiopathogenesis

Panosteitis has had many proposed aetiologies (genetic predisposition, vascular anomaly, metabolic disease, allergy, hyperoestrogenism and parasitic migration) but a conclusive aetiopathogenesis is not yet established (Lenehan *et al.* 1985).

Panosteitis has been associated with high calcium intake in Great Danes (Hedhammar *et al.* 1974; Goedegebuure & Hazewinkel 1986). The proposed pathogenesis of panosteitis in calcium excess relates to changes in blood flow in the developing bone. Chronic calcium excess in young dogs causes an increased calcium accretion and decreased skeletal remodelling, including a decreased adaptation of vascular channels (Volkmann's canals, haversian canals) to soft tissue growth. This may result in oedema formation within the medullary cavity, degeneration of the cytoplasm of adipose bone marrow, fibrosis and new bone formation. Changes are first seen near the nutrient foramen. Oedema may also accumulate beneath the periosteum and thus make the periosteum more vulnerable to pressure and pull causing additional sub-periosteal lamellar bone deposition.

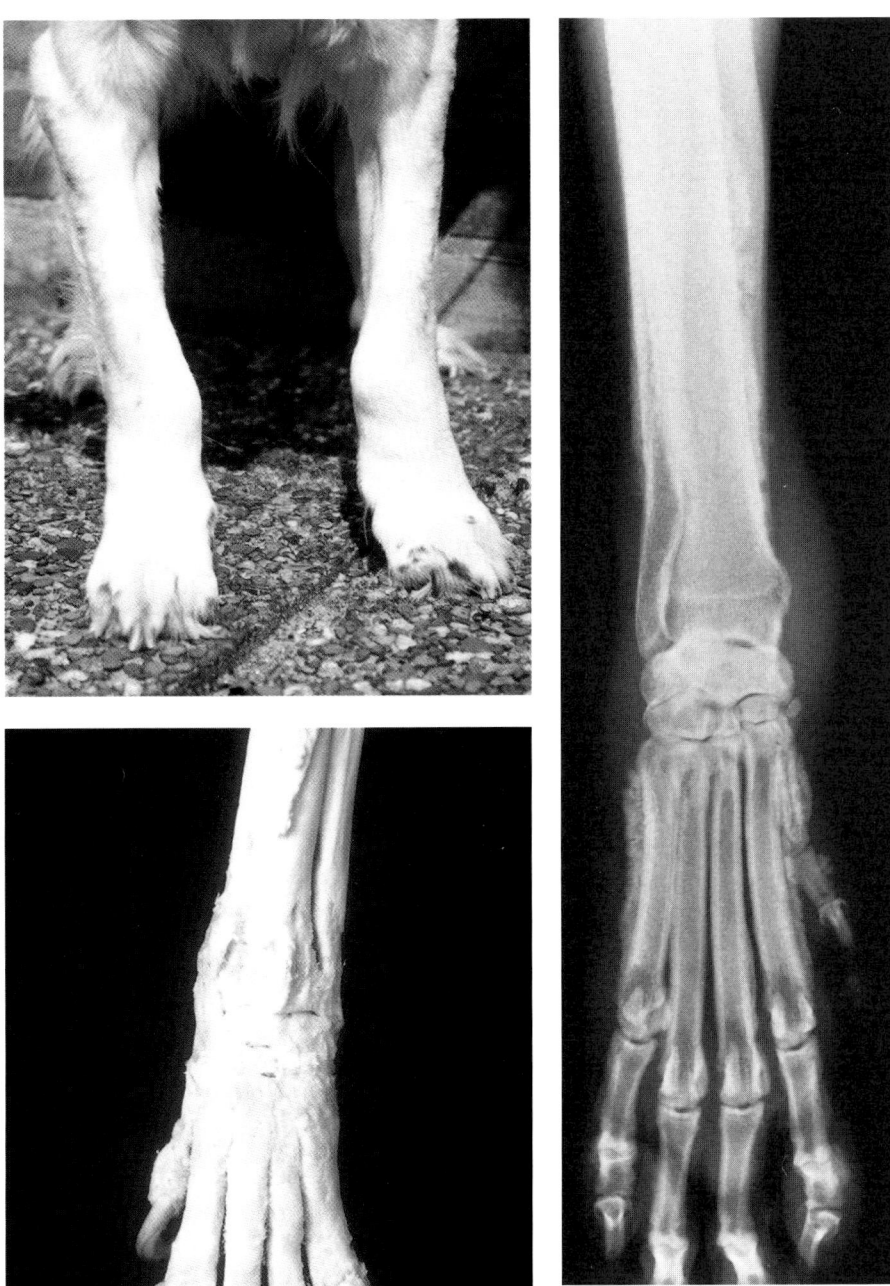

Fig. 77.7 Hypertrophic osteopathy. An 8-year-old dog with pulmonary metastasis and firmly swollen legs (a). The radiograph (b) and specimen (c) of this dog show periosteal proliferative reaction of the diaphyses of digits, metacarpals and radius and ulna but not of the epiphyses, joints or small bones of the carpus.

History and Examination

Panosteitis is mainly seen in medium-sized and large-breed dogs and is over-represented in German Shepherd Dogs. Onset is usually between 6 and 18 months of age and it is rare in older dogs. The diet may be rich in calcium.

Clinical signs of panosteitis are:

- sudden onset of shifting lameness;
- lameness increasingly severe over several days;
- intermittent lameness and remission;
- depression, inappetance and pyrexia.

A pain reaction is elicited on deep palpation of several long bones, especially the lateral-proximal ulna, distal humerus and mid-tibia. Manipulation of the elbow or shoulder joint, as part of the investigation for joint pathology, may be extremely painful in panosteitis. This is because of pressure on the long bones exerted by the clinician's grip during the manoeuvre, or because of tendon traction on the affected bone.

Investigation

Haematological parameters are often normal. Radiological changes are diagnostic, but they may be absent during acute painful episodes. When there is a high index of suspicion of panosteitis, it is often worth repeating radiographs after a 2-week delay.

Radiological features of panosteitis (Fig. 77.8) are:

- immature or young adult dogs,
- multiple bone involvement (primarily radius, ulna, humerus and tibia),
- blurring of the trabecular pattern,
- increased medullary radiopacity associated with endosteal new bone formation (especially near the nutrient foramen),
- in chronic cases smooth, well-defined sub-periosteal and endosteal cortical thickening is seen.

Management

Since the disease is self-limiting and is not often diagnosed in dogs over 22 months of age, treatment is limited to supportive therapy and nursing:

- Give analgesia in acute episodes.
- Warn the owner that other episodes will probably follow.
- In mature dogs, corticosteroids at an initial dose of 1 mg/kg body weight can be prescribed.
- Dietary correction includes reducing the calcium and vitamin content to the minimal requirements for dogs.

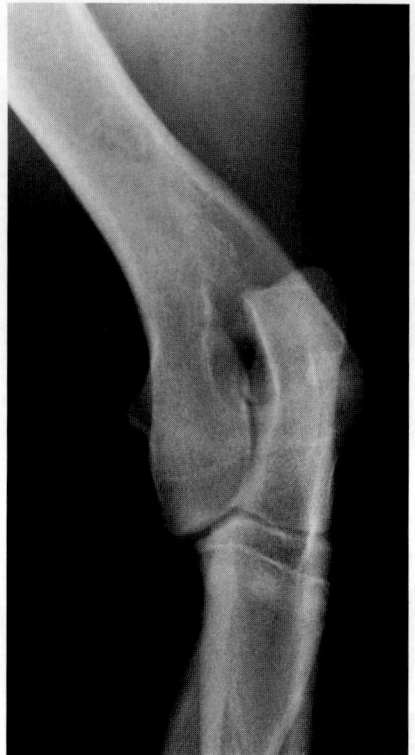

Fig. 77.8   Panosteitis. A 7-month-old Retriever with shifting lameness together with a permanent lameness of the right front leg. The dog revealed pain on deep palpation of multiple long bones and a swollen, painful elbow joint. The radiograph demonstrates medullary radiopacity of the distal humerus, especially in the area of the nutrient foramen. In addition there is an osteochondritis dissecans lesion of the medial humeral condyle which may occur coincidentally in the same patient.

Prognosis is excellent as the disease is self-limiting with few dogs displaying clinical signs beyond 2 years of age.

Craniomandibular Osteopathy (CMO) (Mandibular Periostitis, Lion- Westy- or Scotty-Jaw, Caffey–Silverman Syndrome)

Aetiopathogenesis

The precise aetiology of CMO remains unknown. In Scottish and West Highland White Terriers retrospective investigation of pedigrees implies an autosomal recessive inheritance (De Vries & Watering 1972; Padgett &

Mostosky 1986). The expression may be variable since some dogs have radiological signs of CMO in the absence of a clinical problem.

History and Examination

CMO is most frequently seen in terriers (West Highland White, Scottish, Cairn and Boston). It is occasionally seen in Great Danes, Retrievers and other dogs of larger breeds of either gender. Affected dogs are usually 3–8 months of age and present with reluctance to open the jaws or difficulty in eating. Several dogs from one litter may be affected.

Differential diagnoses of unwillingness or inability to open the mouth are:

- craniomandibular osteopathy,
- retrobulbar abscess,
- temporomandibular joint arthritis,
- intra-oral foreign body,
- masticatory myositis or fasciculitis,
- tetanus.

Clinical findings which help to differentiate CMO include:

- age and breed predisposition,
- dog may be lethargic and in poor condition,
- intermittent pyrexia (to 40.5°C),
- firm mandibular swelling,
- drooling salivation,
- pain on palpation of the mandible on one or both sides,
- pain on opening of the jaws and restricted jaw movement,
- enlarged regional lymph nodes,
- repetitive coughing (enlarged tympanic bullae displacing the trachea or retropharyngeal lymphadenopathy),
- atrophy of the muscles of mastication,
- sometimes there is rhinitis, conjunctivitis, otitis externa or stomatitis,
- there may be periods of remission between painful episodes.

Investigation

There may be increased or decreased plasma globulins, and an increased serum alkaline phosphatase. Radiological findings are diagnostic.

Radiological findings in craniomandibular osteopathy (Fig. 77.9) are:

- Enlargement and broadening of the mandibular rami are observed, ±involvement of the tympanic bullae.

- Changes are usually bilateral, but may be asymmetric or unilateral.
- Other bones of the skull (occipital, parietal, frontal and maxillary bones) may be affected.
- In exceptional cases long bones of the appendicular skeleton are affected.
- New bone does not involve the alveolar aspect of the mandible.
- Tympanic bullae may fill with new bone and can triple in size, causing tracheal displacement.

Management

In severe acute cases, affected dogs are unable to eat and drink and may need fluid therapy. Generally, NSAIDs or corticosteroids are given for symptomatic relief. According to some, corticosteroids diminish the new bone formation (De Vries & Watering 1972; Riser & Newton 1985). Surgical removal of new bone will not lead to permanent improvement, but hemimandibulectomy may be of benefit in selected cases (Riser & Newton 1985; Johnson et al. 1995).

In most cases the prognosis is good as the clinical signs disappear at the age of 11–13 months. In severe cases, with extensive changes on the tympanic bullae, the prognosis is more guarded as adhesions may permanently restrict normal mandibular function.

Bone Cysts

Bone cysts are extremely rare in dogs. They are fluid filled and are benign in nature but may increase in size. They are mostly important as a differential diagnosis for bone tumours (see Chapter 78). Small cysts may be an incidental finding during radiography for other reasons.

History and Examination

Clinically affected dogs are usually immature or young adults (1–30 months of age) of larger breeds with lameness due to mechanical hindrance or pathological fracture. Local bone thickening and abnormal alignment can be palpated.

Investigation

Clinical and radiological investigation will lead to suspicion of a bone cyst.

Radiological findings (Fig. 77.10) are:

- bone destruction with apparently little new bone production;
- expansion and thinning of the overlying bone cortex;

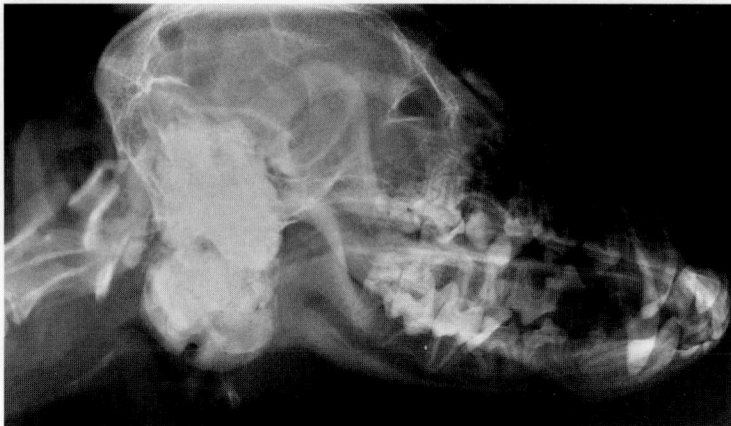

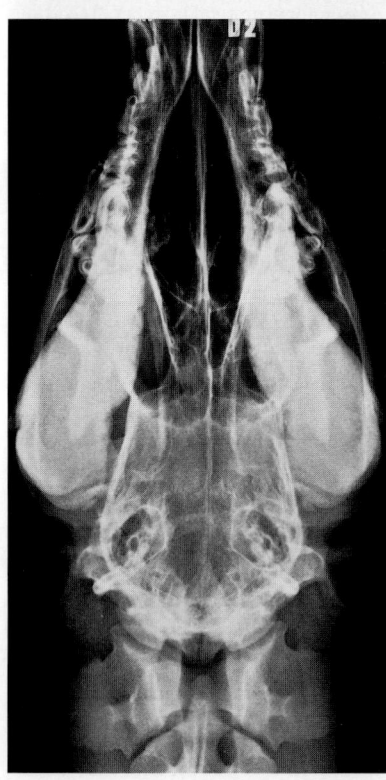

Fig. 77.9 a,b Craniomandibular osteopathy. A 6-month-old West Highland White Terrier with pyrexia and inability to open the mouth. There is bilateral new bone formation on the mandibles and tympanic bullae.

- a distinct border to the lesion and a short zone of transition between normal and abnormal tissue;
- often there are septa throughout the lesion producing a bubble-like appearance.

Further imaging may reveal more cysts in other bones (polyostotic cysts – Fig. 77.10b). If necessary, the diagnosis is confirmed by biopsy and histopathological examination.

Management

Some cysts heal spontaneously. The wall of large cysts may be curetted and the lesion packed with cancellous bone. Supportive fixation may be indicated. Uncomplicated cases generally have a good prognosis.

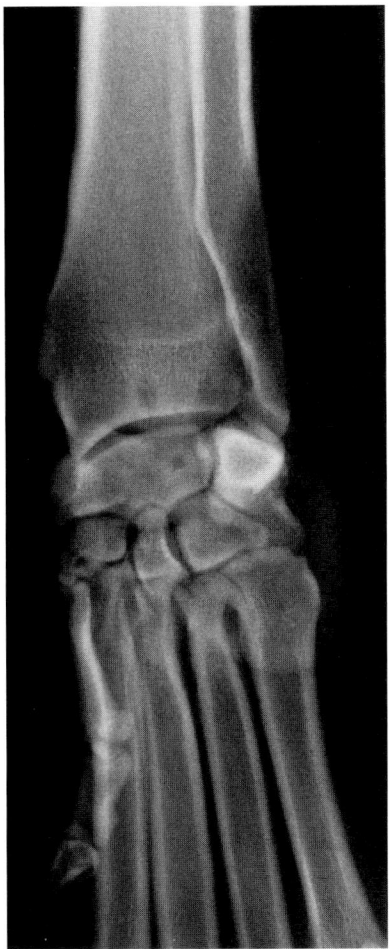

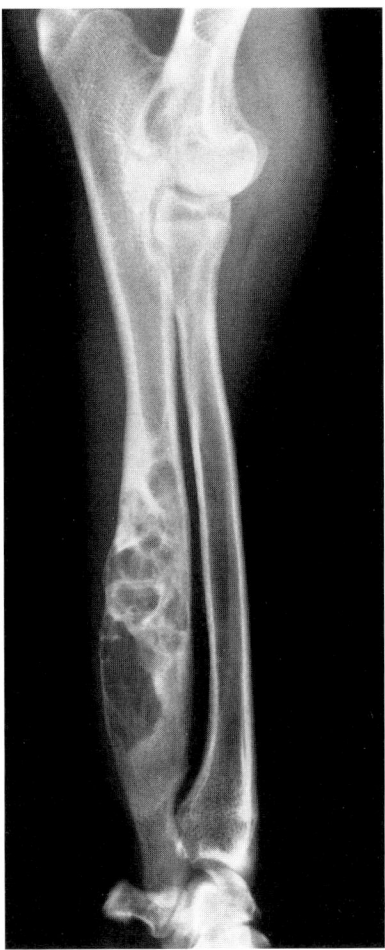

a

b

Fig. 77.10 Subchondral bone cyst (a) of the radius and radial carpal bone of a 2-year-old police dog with lameness during heavy exercise. Polyostotic bone cysts (b) in the distal ulna of a young Rottweiler.

ACKNOWLEDGEMENTS

The author wishes to thank The Department of Veterinary Radiology, University of Utrecht (headed by Professor Dr K. J. Dik) for providing radiographs and Mrs Yvonne Pollak for artwork.

REFERENCES

Baumgartner, W., Boyce, R.W., Alldinger, S., *et al.* (1995). Metaphyseal bone lesions in young dogs with systemic canine distemper virus infection. *Veterinary Microbiology*, **44**, 201–209.

Bennett, D. (1990). Joints and joint diseases. In: *Canine Orthopedics*, (ed. W.G. Whittick), 2nd edn. pp. 761–853. Lea & Febiger, Philadelphia.

Brown, A. & Bennett, D. (1988). Gentamicin-impregnated polymethyl beads for the treatment of septic arthritis. *Veterinary Record*, **123**, 625.

Breur, G.J., Zerbe, C.A., Padgett, G.A. & Braden, T.D. (1989). Clinical, radiographic, pathologic and genetic features of osteochondrodysplasia in Scottish Deerhounds. *Journal of the American Veterinary Medical Association*, **5**, 606–612.

Capen, C.C. & Rosol, T.J. (1993). Hormonal control of mineral metabolism. In: *Disease Mechanisms in Small Animal Surgery*, (eds M.J. Bojrab, D.D. Smeak & M.S. Bloomberg), 2nd edn. pp. 841–857. Lea & Febiger, Philadelphia.

Day, M.J. & Penhale, W.J. (1988). Humoral immunity in disseminated *Aspergillus terreus* infection in the dog. *Veterinary Microbiology*, **16**, 283.

De Vries, H.W. & Van de Watering, C.C. (1972). Prednisone in the treatment of craniomandibular osteopathy. *Netherlands Journal of Veterinary Science*, **5**, 123–127.

Fletch, S.M., Smart, M.E., Pennock, P.W., *et al.* (1973). Clinical and pathological features of chondrodysplasia (dwarfism-anemia) syndrome in review. *Journal of the American Veterinary Medical Association*, **162**, 257–261.

Goedegebuure, S.A. & Hazewinkel, H.A.W. (1986). Morphological findings in young dogs chronically fed a diet containing excess calcium. *Veterinary Pathology*, **23**, 594–605

Grøndalen, J. (1979). Letter to the editor. *Journal of Small Animal Practice*, **20**, 124.

Hazewinkel, H.A.W. (1994). Skeletal disease. In: *The Waltham Book of Clinical Nutrition of the Dog and Cat*, (eds J.M. Wills & K.W. Simpson), pp. 395–423. Pergamon, Oxford.

Hazewinkel, H.A.W. & Schoenmakers, I. (1995). Influence of protein, minerals and vitamin D on skeletal development of dogs. *Veterinary Clinical Nutrition*, **2**, 93–99.

Hazewinkel, H.A.W., Hackeng, W.H.L., Bosch, R., *et al.* (1987). Influences of different calcium intakes on calciotropic hormones and skeletal development in young growing dogs. *Frontiers in Hormone Research*, **17**, 221–232.

Hedhammar, A., Fu-Ming, W.U., Krook, L., *et al.* (1974). Overnutrition and skeletal disease, an experimental study in growing Great Dane dogs. *Cornell Veterinarian*, **64**, (Suppl. 5), 1–160.

Herron, M.R. (1993). Osyeomyelitis. In: *Disease Mechanisms in Small Animal Surgery*, (eds M.J. Bojrab, D.D. Smeak & M.S. Bloomberg), 2nd edn. pp. 692–696. Lea & Febiger, Philadelphia.

Jezyk, P.F. (1985). Constitutional disorders of the skeleton in dogs and cats. In: *Textbook of Small Animal Orthopaedics*, (eds C.D. Newton & D.M. Nunemaker), pp. 637–654. Lippincot, London.

Johnson, K.A., Watson, A.D.J. & Page, R.L. (1995). Skeletal diseases. In: *Textbook of Veterinary Internal Medicine, Diseases of the Dog and Cat*, (eds S.J. Ettinger & E.C. Feldman), pp. 2077–2103. WB Saunders, Philadelphia.

Lenehan, T.M. & Fetter, A.W. (1985). Hypertrophic osteopathy. In: *Textbook of Small Animal Orthopaedics*, (eds C.D. Newton & D.M. Nunemaker), pp. 603–610. Lippincott, London.

Lenehan, T.M., Van Sickle, D.C. & Biery, D.N. (1985). Canine panosteitis. In: *Textbook of Small Animal Orthopaedics*, (eds C.D. Newton & D.M. Nunemaker), pp. 591–601. Lippincott, London.

Mee, A.P., Gordon, M.T., May, C., Bennett, D., Sharpe, P.T. & Anderson, D.C. (1992). Detection of canine distemper virus in bone cells in the metaphysis of distemper dogs. *Journal of Bone and Mineral Research*, **7**, 829–834.

Neer, T.M. (1988). Disseminated aspergillosis. *Compendium on Continuing Education for the Practicing Veterinarian*, **10**, 465.

Nunamaker, D.M. (1985). Legg-Calve-Perthes disease. In: *Textbook of Small Animal Orthopaedics*, (eds C.D. Newton & D.M. Nunemaker), pp. 949–952. Lippincott, London.

Olsson, S-E. (1993). Pathophysiology, morphology and clinical signs of osteochondrosis in the dog. In: *Disease Mechanisms in Small Animal Surgery*, (eds M.J. Bojrab, D.D. Smeak & M.S. Bloomberg), 2nd edn. pp. 777–796. Lea & Febiger, Philadelphia.

Padgett, G.A. & Mostosky, U.V. (1986). Animal model: the mode of inheritance of craniomandibular osteopathy in West Highland White Terrier dogs. *American Journal of Medical Genetics*, **25**, 9–13.

Pool, R.R. (1993). Osteochondromatosis. In: *Disease Mechanisms in Small Animal Surgery*, (eds M.J. Bojrab, D.D. Smeak & M.S. Bloomberg), 2nd edn. pp. 821–833. Lea & Febiger, Philadelphia.

Riser, W.H. & Newton, C.D. (1985). Craniomandibular osteopathy. In: *Textbook of Small Animal Orthopaedics*, (eds C.D. Newton & D.M. Nunemaker), pp. 621–626. Lippincott, London.

Watson, A.D.J. (1990). Diseases of muscle and bone. In: *Canine Orthopedics*, (ed. W.G. Whittick), pp. 657–689. Lea & Febiger, Philadelphia.

Wolf, A.M. & Troy, G.C. (1995). Deep mycotic diseases. In: *Textbook of Veterinary Internal Medicine, Diseases of the Dog and Cat*, (eds S.J. Ettinger & E.C. Feldman), pp. 439–465. W.B. Saunders, Philadelphia.

Chapter 78

Skeletal Neoplasia

T. J. Anderson

INTRODUCTION TO BONE TUMOURS

Primary bone tumours are relatively rare compared with primary tumours of other organs. They are predominantly sarcomas, with rare benign tumours (Table 78.1). Osteosarcoma is the most common and represents about 80% of all primary bone tumours in dogs. Chondosarcoma represents about 10% of primary bone tumours and a further 7% are haemangiosarcomas and fibrosarcomas.

The aetiology of primary malignant bone tumours is unknown, but genetic influences are possible as osteosarcoma is over represented in certain breeds (Goldschmidt & Thrall 1985). The clinical features and approach to diagnosis are similar for all bone malignancies. Pathogenesis, management and prognosis for bone sarcomas other than osteosarcoma are summarised in Table 78.2 and osteosarcoma is covered in more detail below.

Bone may also be invaded by soft tissue tumours particularly on the extremities and in the oral cavity (e.g. malignant melanoma, squamous cell carcinoma). Multiple myeloma is a tumour of the lymphoreticular system which may present with skeletal signs (see Chapter 35). Some malignant tumours, particularly carcinomas, have a propensity to metastasise to bone.

CANINE OSTEOSARCOMA

Pathogenesis

Osteosarcoma develops in both the appendicular and axial skeleton. The most commonly affected sites are metaphyseal regions in the appendicular skeleton (Fig. 78.1).

Appendicular Osteosarcoma (Fig. 78.2)

Appendicular osteosarcoma develops almost exclusively within the medulla. Metastasis is rapid and may occur before identification of the primary tumour (Bech-Neilsen *et al.* 1976). Features of metastasis in canine osteosarcoma include:

- almost exclusively by the haematogenous route;
- primarily to the lungs;
- only 10% of cases have radiographic evidence of metastasis at the time of initial diagnosis;
- only 5% metastasise via lymphatics – local lymph node enlargement may be associated with inflammatory reaction;
- parosteal osteosarcoma (developing from the periosteum) is rare in dogs, but has a less aggressive nature (Pool 1994).

Axial Osteosarcoma

This is less common than appendicular disease (Fig. 78.1) (Goldschmidt & Thrall 1985; Heyman *et al.* 1992). The bones of the skull, particularly the mandible and maxilla are mostly affected. Whether tumours of the mandible and maxilla have a lower metastatic potential than those at other sites is controversial.

Diagnosis

The Box 78.1 provides a flow-chart of the principles of osteosarcoma diagnosis.

Table 78.1 Classification of primary bone tumours and tumour-like lesions.

Tumour classification	Distinguishing features
Malignant tumours	
Osteosarcoma	Cells produce osteoid. Not necessarily mineralised.
Chondrosarcoma	Cells produce neoplastic cartilage. There may be areas of calcification which are not areas of osteoid. Bone may develop in chondrosarcomas by endochondral ossification.
Fibrosarcoma	Cells produce varying amounts of collagenous matrix.
Haemangiosarcoma	Areas of undifferentiated sarcoma admixed with primitive vascular channels.
Liposarcoma	Fat may be demonstrated within tumour cells.
Giant cell tumour (osteoclastoma)	Large numbers of giant cells. Care must be taken as giant cells are a common feature of the pathology of many bony lesions, including osteosarcoma and some benign lesions.
Benign tumours and tumour-like lesions	
Osteoma	Slow, progressive growth over months to years. No metastasis or malignant transformation reported.
Enchondroma	Benign cartilaginous (hyaline) tumour originating within the medullary canal.
Haemangioma	Highly tortuous, large calibre blood vessels. Slow, expansive growth.
Multiple cartilaginous exostosis	A developmental condition, with cartilage capped, exostotic bone lesions developing on long bone surfaces. May be monostotic or polyostotic. Growth is in synchrony with skeletal development, ceasing with skeletal maturity. Malignant transformation has been recorded in dogs (Pool 1994).
Bone cyst	Rare in dogs. May be monostotic or polyostotic.
Fibrous dysplasia	Rare condition in which cancellous bone is replaced by fibro-osseous matrix.

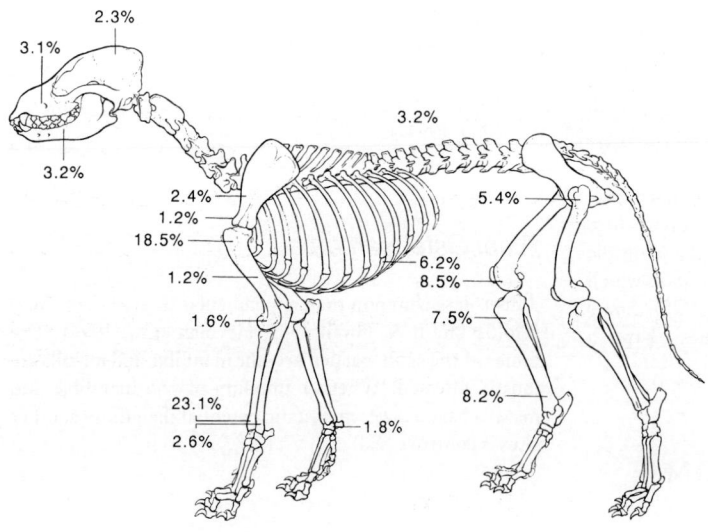

Fig. 78.1 Site of origin of 1215 primary osteosarcomas in the dog (with permission from Goldschmidt & Thrall 1985).

Box 78.1   Diagnosis of canine osteosarcoma in focus.

EXAMINATION

Lameness
   May be chronic with disuse atrophy
Firm swelling
   May not detect in well muscled areas
General examination
   To include search for metastases

MINIMUM DATA BASE

Radiography
   Affected area
   Thorax
   Any other indicated site

Haematology/biochemistry profiles

DIFFERENTIAL DIAGNOSIS

Other primary malignant bone tumour
Skeletal metastasis
Local invasion by soft tissue tumour
Bacterial osteomyelitis
Fungal osteomyelitis
Trauma
Myeloma

BIOPSY

(1)   Open biopsies may need an extensive surgical approach.
(2)   Take multiple samples if using needle technique (Fig. 78.5)
(3)   There is often a surrounding area of intense bone activity and inflammation which may confuse histological assessment. Especially if only one sample is obtained.
(4)   Risk of iatrogenic fracture with large wedge or core biopsies.
(5)   There are special considerations of the site of the biopsy if limb salvage is planned – Consult the team that will perform limb salvage.
(6)   Very bony samples need extensive decalcification before histological assessment, increasing the time to diagnosis

INTERPETATION BY AN EXPERIENCED VETERINARY PATHOLOGIST IS ADVISED

RADIOLOGICAL FEATURES (Figs 78.3 and 78.4)

(1)   Bone destruction
   • Loss of trabecular detail
   • Loss of cortical integrity
(2)   Bone production
   • Periosteal proliferation
   • Sclerosis
(3)   Soft tissue swelling
(4)   Poorly defined margin between normal and abnormal tissue
(5)   The tumour is usually confined by the physeal scar
(6)   Codman's triangle
   A smooth triangle of new bone associated with periosteal elevation

No radiographic change is tumour specific

History and Examination

The typical signalment of canine osteosarcoma patients is outlined in Box 78.2.

The clinical findings with osteosarcoma vary with the site of the lesion (Table 78.3).

Investigation

Radiography

Radiography of the primary tumour site and of thorax for detection of metastatic disease is an essential step in staging the disease. Micrometastases are almost certainly present at

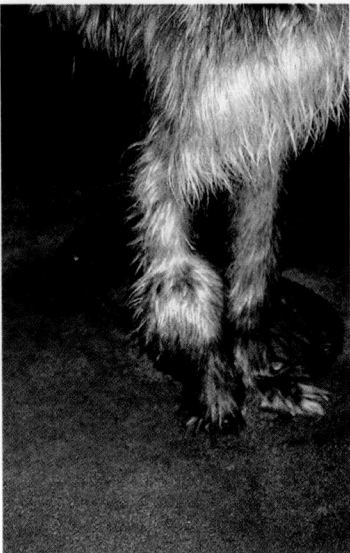

Fig. 78.2   Swelling associated with the development of
primary bone sarcoma of the distal radius.

Box 78.2   Typical signalment of canine osteosarcoma
patients.

Appendicular	Axial
Large breed (>30 kg)	Medium to large breed (Boxer may be over-represented)
Males predominate	Possibly more females (Heyman *et al.* 1992)
Median age 7.5 years	Median age 7.5 years (5.4 years for rib tumours)

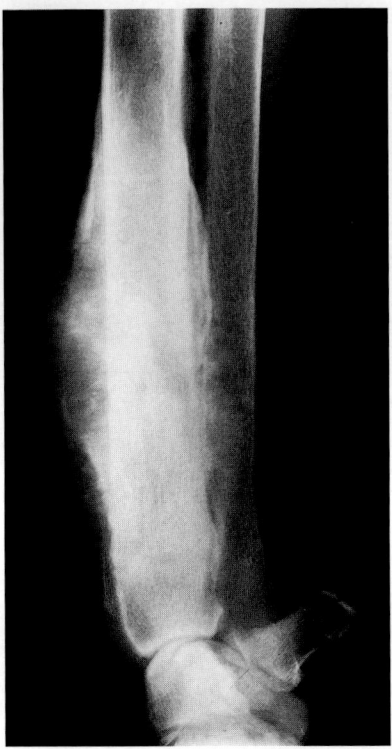

Fig. 78.3   Radiographic features of a primary bone
sarcoma (osteosarcoma) showing bone lysis, Codman's
triangle and new bone production.

the time of diagnosis (in appendicular osteosarcoma), but
they are only detectable on radiographs once they reach
approximately 0.5 cm in diameter (Dennis 1991). The right
lateral recumbent view with the lungs inflated is most
useful and if possible the radiographs should be viewed by
more than one person (Lang *et al.* 1986). Ventrodorsal
views are not essential for the detection of lesions.

Biopsy

Obtaining a diagnostic biopsy can sometimes be difficult.
Biopsies may be obtained by open (wedge biopsy, trephine
biopsy) or closed (needle biopsy) methods. The Jamshidi

needle gives accurate results (Box 78.1) (Powers *et al.* 1988).
Following ablation, the tumour should be submitted for full
pathological examination.

> *Specific diagnosis of tumour type can only be
> achieved by biopsy.*
> The nature of the tumour has a great bearing on
> management and prognosis. Current
> osteosarcoma chemotherapy protocols are not
> suitable for the management of other primary
> sarcomas of bone.

Management

Treatment Options

- palliative therapy – analgesia or amputation,
- surgery (amputation or limb salvage) and adjuvant
  chemotherapy,

Table 78.2   Clinical synopsis of none-osteosarcomatous primary bone malignancies.

Tumour	Biological behaviour	Treatment	Prognosis
Chondrosarcoma	Predominantly affects flat bones. Long clinical course compared to osteosarcoma. Some metastasise by the haematogenous route.	Amputation (limb salvage reported). Hemipelvectomy for suitable pelvic tumours (Straw *et al.* 1992). Wide excision for rib tumours.	May survive many years. Pulmonary metastasis in some cases
Fibrosarcoma	Rare tumour. Behaviour uncertain, rate of metastasis variable (Pool 1994).	Amputation	Guarded
Haemangiosarcoma	Difficult to determine if the bone lesion is primary or metastatic. The proximal humerus may be a predilection site.	Amputation	Poor
Liposarcoma	Very rare tumour. Behaviour uncertain.	Amputation	Unknown
Multilobar tumour of bone. (Chondroma rodens; Multilobar osteochondrosarcoma)	Tend to develop in bones of the skull. Locally invasive. Metastasis slow, but occurs in about 60% of cases (Straw *et al.* 1989)	Radical excision	Tumour free margins very difficult to achieve. Regrowth likely.
Giant cell tumour	Benign and malignant forms exist. Difficult to differentiate.	Amputation	Uncertain because of difficulties in histological grading.

Table 78.3   Clinical signs associated with malignant primary bone tumours.

Anatomical site	Clinical features	Remarks
Appendicular skeleton	Lameness, which is initially subtle. Onset of lameness may be associated with an observed trauma. Disuse muscle atrophy is seen with chronic lameness.	A firm local swelling develops quickly (Fig. 78.2), but can be difficult to appreciate in heavily muscled areas such as the proximal humerus.
Skull	Tumours of superficial bones have readily appreciable swelling. They tend to expand outwards initially and often do not induce neurological signs until late in the course of the disease. Can induce exophthalmus or dysphagia.	Tumours of the mandible or maxilla often expand into the oral cavity and may be quite large before they attract the attention of the owner.
Vertebrae	Spinal pain, which may be severe. Neurological deficits may develop and can have a sudden onset if there is pathological fracture of the affected vertebra.	
Ribs	Often cause no clinical problems until quite large because they initially have little effect on thoracic function.	The mass is often first noticed by the owner when stroking the dog, rather than by sight or by its effect on thoracic function.
Pelvis	May interfere with limb function, causing lameness. If within the pelvic canal, the mass may interfere with normal defecation and/or urination.	The mass may be very large before clinical signs become apparent.

- euthanasia:
  - advanced disease,
  - treatment unacceptable to the client,
  - other significant health problems in the dog.

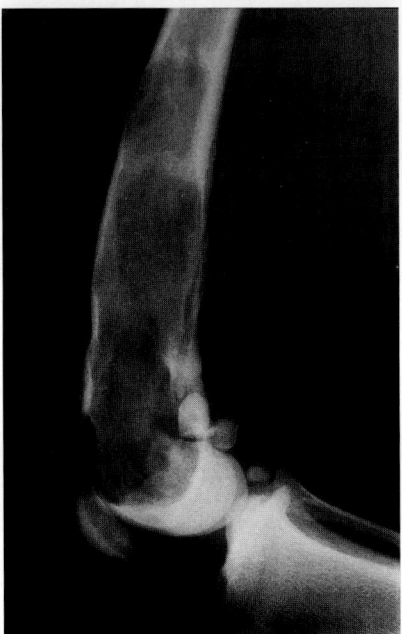

Fig. 78.4 Primary bone sarcoma (osteosarcoma) with atypical radiographic appearance.

Both *local disease* (the primary tumour site) and *distant disease* (metastatic sites) should be considered as targets for therapy. Current therapeutic goals are:

- to control local disease and alleviate the associated pain;
- to slow (or eliminate) the development of distant disease;
- elimination of distant disease is an unrealistic goal at present.

Management of Local Disease

Appendicular Osteosarcoma

Initially the discomfort may respond to palliative analgesia (e.g. with non-steroidal anti-inflammatory drugs). However, the lesion becomes progressively more painful until even opiates have little beneficial effect. Surgical ablation definitively controls the pain and eliminates tumour progression. Surgery alone is considered palliative because of the high risk of metastatic disease. Currently there are two major surgical methods for appendicular tumours (Table 78.4):

(1) Amputation – It is recommended that a full quarter amputation is undertaken.
(2) Limb salvage (Fig. 78.6) (Straw & Withrow 1993) – Limb salvage surgery involves ablating the tumour, spanning the defect with a fresh-frozen allograft of bone supported with a plate, and concurrent arthrodesis of adjacent joints. Function after limb salvage is related to the success associated with

Table 78.4 Comparison of amputation and limb salvage.

Amputation	Limb salvage
Only need general surgical experience	Need specialist surgical training/experience
No specialist equipment needed	Specialist equipment essential
Minimal morbidity and complication rate	Significant morbidity and complication rate
Prompt pain relief	
Usually excellent tumour control	Regrowth in approximately 25% of cases
Minimal infection rate with routine aseptic precautions	Up to 40% incidence of infection even with extensive aseptic precautions
Suitable for all appendicular locations	Most suited to distal radius. Other localities possible (e.g. proximal humerus)
Applicable to all breeds but some adaptation problems in giant dogs	Applicable to all breeds but often restricted to large breeds as smaller breeds cope well with amputation
Unacceptable to some owners	Often acceptable to owners rejecting amputation
Abnormal function	Potential for excellent function (e.g. distal radius site)
Cheap	Expensive

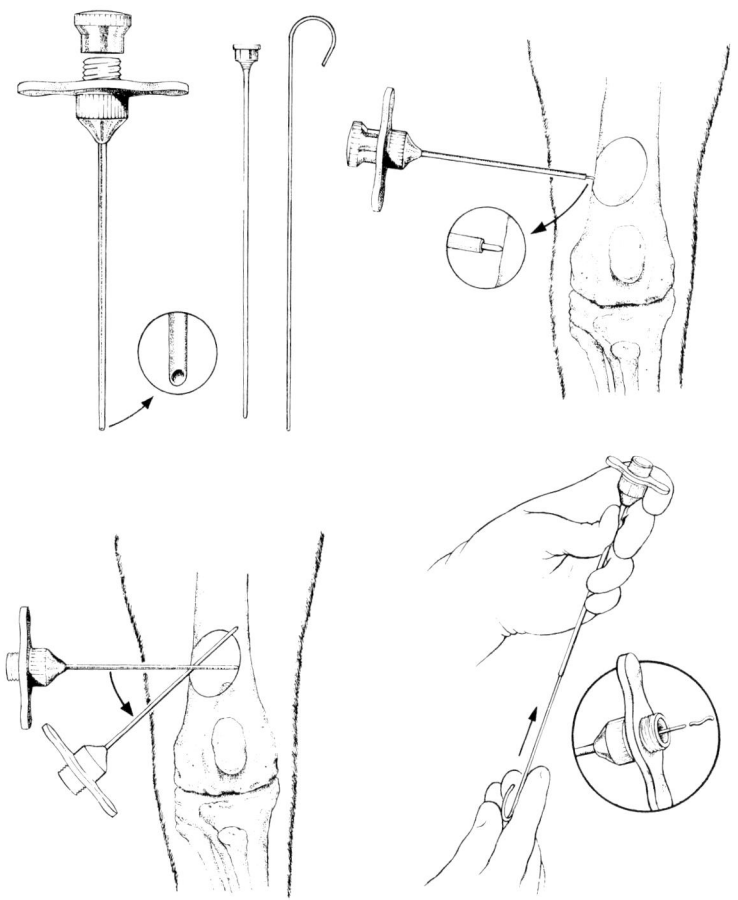

Fig. 78.5 The use of the Jamshidi needle for biopsy of bone tumours. (Reproduced from Powers *et al.* (1988) by permission of the *Journal of the American Veterinary Medical Association.*)

arthrodesis of the joints involved. Limb salvage is not recommended for tumours that would result in arthrodesis of the hock and stifle. The complication rates in limb salvage surgery are high, even in experienced hands (O'Brien *et al.* 1993a).

Axial Osteosarcoma

Treatment is by surgical ablation. The proximity of vital structures in many cases makes wide surgical margins difficult or impossible to achieve. Postoperative radiotherapy and cisplatin chemotherapy have been used as an adjunct in tumours of the maxilla and nasal sinuses (Heyman *et al.* 1992).

Management of Distant Disease

The development of chemotherapeutic techniques has had the greatest impact on the survival of appendicular osteosarcoma patients. The usefulness of similar protocols for axial osteosarcoma patients has not been established. The literature focuses on platinum based drugs (cisplatin, carboplatin). Although the ideal protocol has not been defined there is evidence that the use of three or more doses of cisplatin is important (O'Brien *et al.* 1993a). Metastases present at diagnosis, and deposits that develop subsequent to chemotherapy being instigated, do not respond to cisplatin (Ogilvie *et al.* 1993).

Cisplatin is a known teratogen and suspected carcinogen. Public health (and, in the United Kingdom, COSHH regulations) must be considered in relation to staff and clients. Direct contact of the patient with pregnant women and children should be avoided and all waste and contaminated materials should be disposed of according to local rules. Over 80% of the cisplatin is excreted in urine in the first 48h and much of the rest is excreted in faeces. Potential sources of hazard when dealing with cisplatin include:

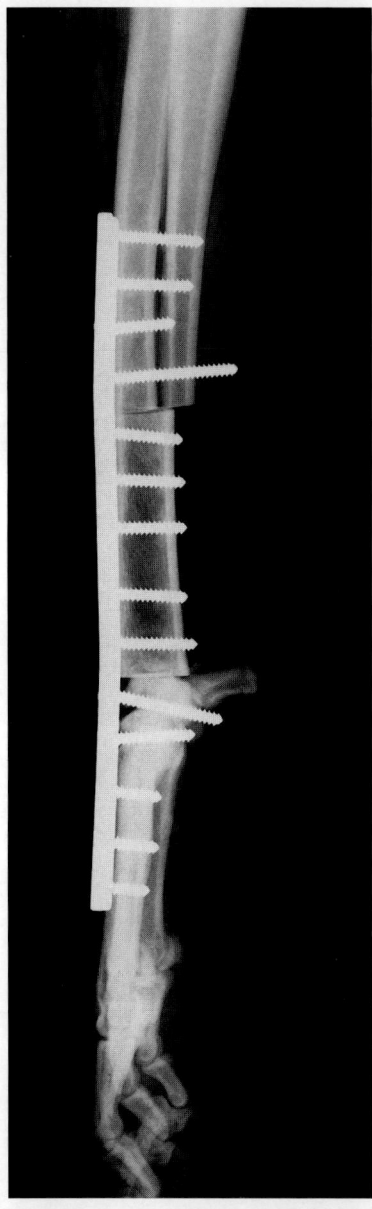

Fig. 78.6 The use of an allograft for reconstruction of the radius in a limb salvage procedure following excision of an osteosarcoma (courtesy of Mr S. Carmichael, University of Glasgow).

- aerolisation of drug during reconstitution from the powdered form,
- direct spillage of drug on to the skin,
- patient's urine,
- patient's faeces.

Cisplatin chemotherapy should not be undertaken unless the facilities and procedures exist to deal adequately with these sources of hazard.

Recently another platinum containing drug, carboplatin, has been described for the treatment of canine osteosarcoma (Bergman *et al.* 1996). This has the advantage of being less toxic than cisplatin. Doxorubicin has also been advocated in chemotherapeutic protocols for canine osteosarcoma, but its use is limited by its toxicity for cardiac muscle (Berg *et al.* 1995) (see Chapter 5).

In selected cases surgical excision of isolated metastases (metasectomy) may be of value to the patient (O'Brien *et al.* 1993b).

Prognosis

The presence of metastatic disease at the time of presentation is a poor prognostic sign. Currently there are no techniques that are of use in selection of patients for aggressive management. However, quantitative scintigraphy may be of use in identifying aggressive tumours subject to early metastasis (Forrest *et al.* 1992).

Appendicular osteosarcoma is an ultimately fatal disease. Death or euthanasia usually results from metastatic disease, but tumour ablation and the use of cisplatin adjuvant chemotherapy can increase the life span of selected patients (see Box 78.3, Table 78.5).

Survival of Dogs with Appendicular Osteosarcoma

Most dogs with axial osteosarcoma die or are euthanased owing to problems with the primary tumour rather than the

Table 78.5 Survival of dogs with osteosarcoma.

Appendicular osteosarcoma (treatment by amputation only)	
Mean survival time	19.8 weeks
Median survival time	19.2 weeks
Survival after 1 year	11.5%
Survival after 2 years	2.0%

Spodnick *et al.* (1992)

Axial osteosarcoma	
Median survival time	22 weeks
Survival after 1 year	26%

Heyman *et al.* (1992)

Box 78.3   Cisplatin chemotherapy in dogs in focus.

IMPORTANT NOTE

CISPLATIN CHEMOTHERAPY IS A SPECIALISED AREA AND THESE BRIEF NOTES ARE *NOT* INTENDED AS
THOROUGH INSTRUCTION, BUT AS AN OUTLINE OF THE PROTOCOLS

CONSULT A SPECIALIST CENTRE

PATIENT SELECTION

(1) Histologically confirmed osteosarcoma
(2) No other pathology that might be expected to
     reduce life span to less than one year
(3) No sign of disseminated neoplastic disease
     (thorax/abdomen radiographs)

(4) Suitable client and animal temperament
(5) Primary tumour amenable to surgery
(6) Renal function not significantly impaired
(7) Bone marrow not significantly impaired
     (routine heamatology)

▼

PATIENT EVALUATION

Before each chemotherapy cycle

1. Full clinical examination

2. Thoracic (±abdominal & skeletal) radiographs
    (metastasis search)

3. Haematology/biochemistry profiles

CISPLATIN TOXICITY

► Myelosuppression ◄
    May need to withhold therapy temporarily and/or
    reduce the dose
Nausea and Vomiting
► Nephrotoxicity ◄
    Manage by aggressive diuresis in the protocol
    May need to abandon therapy

▼

CISPLATIN PROTOCOLS

Reference	Dose	Diuresis	Survival
Kraegel *et al.* (1991)	50 mg/m^2 6 doses 4-week interval	0.9% saline 105 ml/m^2 per hour 12–18 h pre-cisplatin 6 h post-cisplatin. Mannitol pre-cisplatin	Median 59 weeks 62.5% alive at 1 year
Straw *et al.* (1991)	60 mg/m^2 1–6 doses 3-week interval	0.9% saline (5 ml/kg per hour) 12 h pre-cisplatin 8 h post-cisplatin. Mannitol pre-cisplatin	Median 46.4 weeks 45% alive at 1 year 21% alive at 2 years
Dobson & Blackwood (1995)	70 mg/m^2 4 doses 28-day interval	0.9% saline (25 ml/kg per hour) 3 h pre-cisplatin 3 h post-cisplatin. Then Hartmann's solution for 1–2 h	Not stated

effects of metastasis. There is a high incidence of regrowth following surgical excision which probably reflects the difficulties in attaining good surgical margins.

JOINT TUMOURS (SYNOVIAL SARCOMA)

Aetiology and Epidemiology

The aetiology of joint tumours is currently unknown. The most clinically relevant tumour of joints is the synovial sarcoma, but others include, liposarcoma, lipoma and synovial chondrosarcoma (Bennett 1990). Extra-articular tumours may occasionally invade joints.

Pathogenesis

Synovial sarcomas arise from synovioblasts rather than from the differentiated synoviocytes. In dogs they may arise

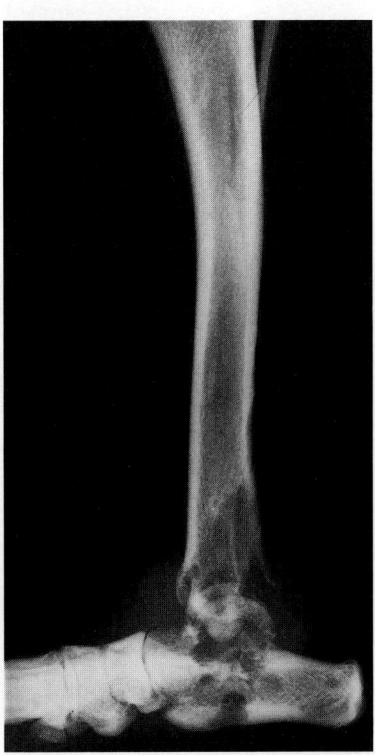

Fig. 78.7   Synovial sarcoma of the hock. Note joint swelling and lysis of multiple bones.

from the synovial membrane or from synovial sheaths associated with tendons. They are slow growing and locally invasive. Metastasis is late, to local lymph nodes and eventually to the lungs.

Clinical Features

Patients are around 7–8 years of age (McGlennon *et al.* 1988). Synovial sarcoma most commonly affects the elbow and stifle. There is firm joint swelling and pain with associated lameness. The diagnosis may be suspected on the basis of clinical and radiographic features (Fig. 78.7), but is ultimately proven by biopsy of the tumour mass.

Management

Synovial sarcoma is as an aggressive malignancy. Local excision is not recommended because of the locally invasive nature and the current recommendation is for amputation (McGlennon *et al.* 1988). There is one case report of successful chemotherapy (Tilmant *et al.* 1986).

Prognosis

Prognosis is guarded with 1-year survival following amputation being approximately 25% (McGlennon *et al.* 1988).

REFERENCES

Bech-Nielsen, S., Reif, J.S. & Brodey, R.S. (1976). The use of tumour doubling time in veterinary clinical oncology. *Journal of the American Veterinary Radiological Society*, **17**, 113–116.

Bennett, D. (1990). Joints and joint diseases. In: *Canine Orthopaedics*, (ed. W.G. Whittick), 2nd edn. pp. 761–853. Lea and Febiger, Malvern.

Berg, J., Weinstein, M.J., Springfield, D.S. & Rand, W.M. (1995). Results of surgery and doxorubicin chemotherapy in dogs with osteosarcoma. *Journal of the American Veterinary Medical Association*, **206**, 1555–1559.

Bergman, P.J., Macewan, E.G., Kurzman, I.D., *et al.* (1996). Amputation and carboplatin for treatment of dogs with osteosarcoma: 48 cases (1991–1993). *Journal of Veterinary Internal Medicine*, **10**, 76–81.

Dennis, R. (1991). Diagnostic imaging of the tumour patient. In: *Manual of Small Animal Oncology*, (ed. R.A.S. White). BSAVA Publications, Cheltenham.

Dobson, J. & Blackwood, L. (1995). *Notes on the Use of Cisplatin.* The University Press, Cambridge.

Forrest, L.J., Dodge, R.K., Page, R.L., *et al.* (1992). Relationship between quantitative tumour scintigraphy and time to metastasis in dogs with osteosarcoma. *The Journal of Nuclear Medicine*, **33**, 1542–1547.

Goldschmidt, M.H. & Thrall, D.E. (1985). Malignant bone tumors in the dog. In: *Textbook of Small Animal Orthopaedics*, (eds C.D. Newton & D.M. Nunamaker), pp. 887–898. J.B. Lippincott, Philadelphia.

Heyman, S.J., Diefenderfer, D.L., Goldschmidt, M.H. & Newton, C.D. (1992). Canine axial skeletal osteosarcoma: A retrospective study of 116 cases. *Veterinary Surgery*, **21**, 304–310.

Kraegel, S.A., Madewell, B.R., Simonson, E. & Gregory, C.R. (1991). Osteogenic sarcoma and cisplatin chemotherapy in dogs: 16 cases (1986–1989). *Journal of the American Veterinary Medical Association*, **199**, 1057–1059.

Lang, J., Wortman, J.A., Glickman, L.T., Biery, D.N. & Rhodes, H. (1986). Sensitivity of radiographic detection of lung metastases in the dog. *Veterinary Radiology*, **27**, 74–78.

McGlennon, N.J., Houlton, J.E.F. & Gorman, N.T. (1988). Synovial sarcoma in the dog – a review. *Journal of Small Animal Practice*, **29**, 139–152.

Ogilvie, G.K., Straw, R.C., Jameson, V.J., *et al.* (1993). Evaluation of single agent chemotherapy for treatment of clinically evident osteosarcoma metastases in dogs: 45 cases (1987–1991). *Journal of the American Veterinary Medical Association*, **202**, 304–306.

O'Brien, M.G., Straw, R.C. & Withrow, S.J. (1993a). Recent advances in the treatment of canine appendicular osteosarcoma. *Compendium on Continuing Education for the Practicing Veterinarian*, **15**, 939–946.

O'Brien, M.G., Straw, R.C., Withrow, S.J., *et al.* (1993b). Resection of pulmonary metastases in canine osteosarcoma: 36 cases (1983–1992). *Veterinary Surgery*, **22**, 105–109.

Pool, R.R. (1994). Tumours of bone and cartilage. In: *Tumours in Domestic Animals*, (ed. J.E. Moulton), 4th edn. pp. 157–220. University of California Press, California.

Powers, B.E., Larue, S.M., Withrow, S.J., Straw, R.C. & Richter, S. (1988). Jamshidi needle biopsy for diagnosis of bone lesions in small animals. *Journal of the American Veterinary Medical Association*, **193**, 205–210.

Spodnick, G.J., Berg, J., Rand, W.M. *et al.* (1992). Prognosis for dogs with appendicular osteosarcoma treated by amputation alone. 162 cases (1978–1988). *Journal of the American Veterinary Medical Association*, **200**, 995–999.

Straw, R.C. & Withrow, S.J. (1993). Limb-sparing surgery for dogs with bone neoplasia. In: *Textbook of Small Animal Surgery*, (ed. D. Slatter), 2nd edn. pp. 2020–2026. W.B. Saunders, Philadelphia.

Straw, R.C., Lecouteur, R.A., Powers, B.E. & Withrow, S.J. (1989). Multilobular osteochondrosarcoma of the canine skull: 16 cases (1978–1988). *Journal of the American Veterinary Medical Association*, **195**, 1764–1769.

Straw, R.C., Withrow, S.J., Richter, S. *et al.* (1991). Amputation and cisplatin chemotherapy for the treatment of canine osteosarcoma. *Journal of Veterinary Internal Medicine*, **5**, 205–210.

Straw, R.C., Withrow, S.J. & Powers, B.E. (1992). Partial or total hemipelvectomy in the management of sarcomas in nine dogs and two cats. *Veterinary Surgery*, **21**, 183–188.

Tilmant, L.L., Gorman, N.T., Ackerman, N., *et al.* (1986). Chemotherapy of synovial sarcoma in the dog. *Journal of the American Animal Hospitals Association*, **188**, 530–532.

Section 11

Neurology and Neuromuscular Disorders

Edited by Chris May

INTRODUCTORY COMMENTS

The aim of this Section is to provide the reader with insight into neurological problems as they appear in the clinical setting. Disease processes affecting the nervous system are therefore grouped and discussed according to their typical clinical presentation. Some disease processes manifest themselves as different neurological problems depending on the location of the nervous system affected (e.g. intervertebral disc disease may produce paraplegia or quadriplegia depending on whether the lumbar or cervical spinal cord is affected). Pertinent features of the neurological examination will be discussed· at the beginning of each problem section although a degree of awareness of neuroanatomy is assumed (for reviews, see Chrisman 1991; De Lahunta 1983; Oliver *et al.* 1987). In evaluating any patient with neurological disease it is helpful to adopt a consistent approach. The recommended sequence of patient evaluation is history, general physical and then neurological examination. When evaluating animals with neurological problems it is useful to keep five questions in mind:

(1) Does the animal have neurological disease?
(2) Where is the lesion?
(3) What is the lesion?
(4) How bad is the lesion?
(5) What can be done about it?

Attention to these questions allows a logical, diagnostic, prognostic and therapeutic approach to a case. The first question is intended to remind clinicians that non-neurological conditions may masquerade as neurological disorders. For example, orthopaedic disorders such as hip dysplasia, bilateral cruciate ligament rupture and polyarthritis are well known for luring unwary clinicians down the wrong diagnostic path.

The precise, consistent layout of the nervous system lends it to easy graphic representation and it is helpful to generate a mental image of the location of the neurological lesion to help in consideration of differential diagnoses and diagnostic procedures. Recognition of several different lesion locations within one patient, sometimes referred to as multifocal disease, is very suggestive of inflammatory or disseminated neoplastic disease.

REFERENCES

De Lahunta, A. (1983). *Veterinary Neuroanatomy and Clinical Neurology*. W.B. Saunders, Philadelphia.

Chrisman, C.L. (1991). *Problems in Small Animal Neurology*. Lea and Febiger, Philadelphia.

Oliver, J.E., Hoerlein, B.F. & Mayhew, I.G. (1987). *Veterinary Neurology*. W.B. Saunders, Philadelphia.

Chapter 79
Seizures and Behavioural Change

A. Hopkins

INTRODUCTION

- Seizure is the clinical manifestation of excessive, disorderly, paroxysmal cerebral neuronal discharge. Synonyms include ictus, fit and convulsion.
- Behavioural changes include increased timidity or aggression, circling, head pressing, aimless or compulsive wandering.
- Epilepsy is a state of recurrent seizures regardless of aetiology. Only after a thorough diagnostic evaluation has been completed, can one ascribe a cause or classification to the type of epilepsy.

Seizures are typically classified as generalised or partial (focal) (Table 79.1). Generalised seizures result from involvement of both cerebral hemispheres and typically manifest as loss of consciousness, recumbency, tetany, paddling, salivation, urination and defaecation. This is the most common type of seizure seen in dogs and is also sometimes referred to as a 'tonic-clonic' seizure. Use of the terms grand mal and petit mal are probably best avoided as they are human terms frequently used incorrectly by veterinarians.

Partial seizures occur when the seizure activity is restricted to a discrete area of one hemisphere. The clinical manifestation depends on the function of the part of the brain involved. A focal seizure can spread to involve the whole cortex and become a generalised seizure. Although generalised seizures must have a focal origin, rapid spread of seizure activity throughout the hemispheres results in bilateral dysfunction.

Status epilepticus refers to generalised seizures continuing for more than 15 min or repeated seizures with no return to consciousness in between.

STRUCTURE AND FUNCTION

Seizures and behavioural changes indicate disease of the forebrain (cerebral hemispheres and thalamus, Fig. 79.1).

Recognition of a partial seizure can be useful in localising the lesion to a particular part of the brain (e.g. twitching of one leg may suggest a lesion in the motor cortex on the opposite side to the abnormal limb). It has been suggested that fly biting in dogs is a form of partial seizure whose focus is in the visual cortex.

APPROACH TO THE PATIENT

The causes of seizures can be conveniently divided into being of intracranial or extracranial origin. Extracranial causes should be investigated first as this can be done with attention to a good history and serum biochemical evaluation. If the results of this evaluation are normal, the clinician may proceed with the evaluation of intracranial causes which requires computed tomography (CT) or magnetic resonance imaging (MRI) of the brain and cerebrospinal fluid analysis.

When a cause is identified the term symptomatic seizures or epilepsy is sometimes used. If, despite thorough investigation, no abnormalities are found, the term idiopathic seizures or epilepsy is used. Dogs falling into this category are frequently pure-bred animals, 1–5 years old at the time of their first seizure, and otherwise healthy (Table 79.2).

Table 79.1   Classification of seizures.

Generalised seizures
   Tonic-clonic seizures (grand mal)
   Absence seizures (petit mal, humans only?)
Partial (focal) seizures
   Simple partial seizures
      Motor
      Sensory
   Complex partial seizures
      Temporal lobe (psychomotor) seizures
      'Running fits'

Table 79.2   Differential diagnosis of seizures.

Idiopathic
Symptomatic
Extracranial causes
   Hypoglycaemia
   Hepatic encephalopathy
   Hypo/hypernatraemia
   Hypocalcaemia
   Toxins
   Hypoxia
Intracranial causes
   Lysosomal storage disorders
   Hydrocephalus
   Neoplasia
   Meningoencephalitis
   Granulomatous meningoencephalitis (GME)
   Distemper
   Toxoplasma gondii (*Neospora caninum*)
   Rickettsial diseases
   Miscellaneous bacterial and fungal infections
   Vascular disease, thromboemboli
   Trauma

History

Verification that the owner is indeed reporting a seizure is vital. With generalised seizures this is rarely a problem. Focal muscle spasms due to pain may be mistaken for partial seizures. Thorough examination is indicated to avoid misdiagnosis.

- Seizure type – partial seizures are very suggestive of a focal, structural, intracranial lesion.
- Age is very important (Table 79.3).
- Sex – oestrous appears to lower the seizure threshold.
- Tumour – previous or concurrent malignancy may be associated with brain metastasis.
- Drugs – acepromazine lowers seizure threshold.
- Episodic behavioural abnormalities are suggestive of extracranial metabolic disorders.
- Toxins – any age group may be affected. Careful questioning may reveal potential exposure.

Table 79.3   Relationship of age to common seizure aetiologies.

0–1 year	Hypoglycemia, portosystemic shunt, encephalitis, hydrocephalus
1–5 years	Idiopathic epilepsy
5 years +	Neoplasia, hypoglycemia (inslinoma)

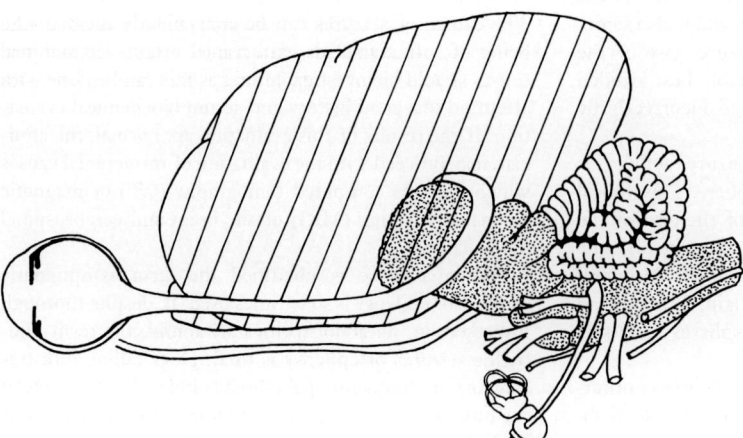

Fig. 79.1 Diagrammatic representation of the areas of the brain responsible for seizures (hatched area), behavioural changes (hatched area), and altered mentation (hatched and dotted area).

Examination

- Persistent interictal neurological abnormalities (e.g. circling, proprioceptive deficits, blindness) are very suggestive of a structural intracranial lesion. Note: obvious, but usually temporary, neurological deficits may result from the seizure itself (and also any anticonvulsant drugs that may have been administered). These deficits often last several hours, sometimes 1–3 days and rarely up to a week. Serial neurological evaluations are required to establish the presence of persistent deficits.
- Active ocular lesions may be seen in infectious diseases (e.g. distemper).
- Cardiac abnormalities (e.g. arrythmia) may result in hypoxic seizures.
- Neoplasia detected on physical examination raises the possibility of metastatic disease.

Investigation

Haematology

- Leukocyte abnormalities may suggest an inflammatory process.
- Distemper virus inclusions are occasionally seen in neutrophils.

Biochemistry

- Glucose levels are important in all seizure patients.
- Cholesterol, urea, bilirubin and albumin levels are indicators of hepatic function.
- Serum bile acid levels (preprandial and 2 hours postprandial) are the best liver function test.
- Electrolyte levels should be assessed.

Immunology

- Serology for distemper, toxoplasma, rickettsial diseases.
- Immunofluorescence of conjunctival scrapings for distemper antigens.

Physical Procedures

- ECG if an arrhythmia is suspected. Thorough cardiac evaluation may be indicated.
- Cerebrospinal fluid (CSF) analysis if index of suspicion of meningoencephalitis is high or following CT or MRI scan.

Diagnostic Imaging

- CT or MRI is indicated if no extracranial causes can be identified.
- Ultrasound – persistent fontanelle allows visualisation of brain in hydrocephalus. Abdominal ultrasound may be used for detection of portosystemic shunts.
- Nuclear scintigraphy in portosystemic shunts helps confirm shunt presence and quantify its magnitude (Daniel *et al.* 1991)
- Radiographs of thorax and abdomen should be considered to evaluate for neoplasia. Plain radiography of the head is of little value.
- Portal venography clearly demonstrates portosystemic shunt anatomy.

Management

The primary goal in the management of patients with seizures is the recognition and treatment of underlying disease. Attention should also be directed at dealing with precipitating factors (e.g. drugs, oestrous cycle). If this is not possible or successful, then symptomatic therapy is indicated. The seizure frequency should be established before beginning therapy so treatment efficacy can be assessed (two to four seizures are usually sufficient). The decision of when to commence therapy is somewhat dependent on the client and seizure severity. One treatment guideline is to medicate if the seizure frequency is greater than one every 2 months. Severe clusters of seizures, even if infrequent, generally warrant daily medication and often an increase in anticonvulsant drug dose during anticipated cluster episodes. Client communication is essential and it is important that you both have the same goals in therapy (Table 79.4). Realistically this is the best reduction in seizure frequency or severity for the least drug-induced side-effects. Monitoring drug levels is important for optimal management of the seizure patient. Levels should be assessed after a steady state has been achieved and just before a dose being administered so that a trough level can be ascertained.

SPECIFIC DISEASES

Idiopathic Epilepsy

This is the most common type of epilepsy in the dog. It is also referred to as true, inherited or primary epilepsy. Affected dogs are typically 1–5 years old and a pure breed. The seizures are generalised from the onset, frequently when the animal is resting, of short duration (30 s to 3 min)

Table 79.4   Treatment of seizures.

Maintenance therapy

Drug	Dose	Serum level
Phenobarbitone	2–3 mg/kg p.o. b.i.d.	15–40 μg/ml
Primidone	5–10 mg/kg p.o. t.i.d.	15–40 μg/ml (phenobarbitone)
Potassium bromide	22 mg/kg p.o. s.i.d.	1500–2000 μg/ml

Phenobarbitone is the first choice drug (Lane & Bunch 1990). Although widely used, primidone is more hepatotoxic and largely metabolised to phenobarbitone. If acceptable seizure control has not been achieved with serum phenobarbitone levels of 35 μg/ml, little is usually gained at higher serum levels, while increasing the risk of hepatotoxicity. Addition of potassium bromide is then recommended (Podell & Fenner 1993). This may result in excessive drowsiness and require a decrease of the phenobarbitone dose by 10–25%.

Status epilepticus – first priority stop the seizure!

(1)   Diazepam 0.25–0.5 mg/kg i.v., i.m., or per rectum (Podell 1995). Repeat twice if necessary.
       If ineffective,
(2)   Pentobarbitone 3–15 mg/kg i.v.

Phenobarbitone (2–4 mg/kg i.v.) has been used in place of or before pentobarbitone. The author prefers the diazepam, pentobarbitone combination for speed and efficacy and begins intravenous phenobarbitone at a maintenance dose after termination of the immediate crisis. Care should be taken to avoid/minimise the respiratory depression seen with barbiturates.

NB. Take diagnostic blood samples before further therapeutics

---

and followed by a rapid recovery. Urination and defaecation frequently accompany the event. While dramatic, these seizures are not usually life threatening because of their short duration. Prolonged seizures (>5 min) rapidly result in hyperthermia, hypoxia, hypercapnia and acidosis which can rapidly achieve life threatening status. Results of previously discussed diagnostic procedures are normal.

Neoplasia

Advanced diagnostic and therapeutic techniques have led to increased recognition and demand for therapy of brain tumours. Usually seen in older dogs, seizures may be the only presenting sign (Fig. 79.2). A wide range of tumours has been reported with meningiomas, oligodendrogliomas and astrocytomas being the most common. Pituitary tumours may be associated with signs of endocrinological dysfunction (e.g. hyperadrenocorticism, diabetes insipidus, diabetes mellitus). Analysis of CSF does not often help with definitive diagnosis of brain tumours, although abnormal results may serve to confirm the presence of intracranial pathology. Owing to the risk of brain herniation it is safer to reserve judgement as to the necessity of CSF sampling until a CT or MRI scan has been performed. It is often possible to identify the tumour type from the brain scan although confirmation usually requires biopsy.

Long-term survival times in excess of 2 years are becoming more common especially with pituitary tumours and meningiomas and owners should be aware of the increasing treatment possibilities (Table 79.5) (Heidner *et al.* 1991; Evans *et al.* 1993).

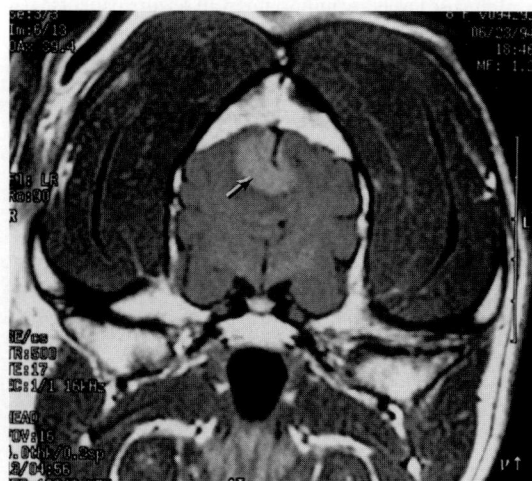

Fig. 79.2   Magnetic resonance image of the brain (transverse section, contrast-enhanced) of an 8-year-old female Rottweiler. A large meningioma originates from the falx cerebrum. Seizures were the only clinical sign.

Table 79.5   Brain tumour therapy.

(1) *Corticosteroids.* Palliative therapy. Alleviation of peritumoural oedema may produce temporary improvement for up to 4–6 months.
(2) *Radiation therapy.* Alone or after surgery. Studies have indicated its effectiveness in treatment of meningiomas and pituitary tumours.
(3) *Surgery.* Offers advantages of gross total or subtotal resection, tissue diagnosis and alleviation of intracranial pressure. Usually followed by radiation therapy or chemotherapy.
(4) *Chemotherapy.* Although used in treatment of human gliomas and CNS lymphoma, veterinary experience is largely empirical and based on use of lomustine or carmustine

Hypoglycaemia

A continual supply of glucose is necessary for normal brain activity. Hypoglycaemia results in neuronal energy depletion, tissue acidosis and altered neurotransmitter function. Causes of hypoglycaemia include:

- hypothermia, endoparasites, anorexia and stress in puppies;
- insulinomas (β-cell pancreatic tumours) may be associated with a paraneoplastic peripheral neuropathy causing generalised weakness, muscle atrophy and decreased spinal reflexes;
- other tumours, e.g. hepatoma, which are thought to secrete insulin-like factors;
- insulin overdose in diabetic dogs;
- septicaemia.

Hepatic Encephalopathy (HE)

Deficient liver function leads to the accumulation of neurotoxins and abnormal neurotransmitters. Hepatic encephalopathy is most commonly associated with a single portosystemic (portal-azygous or portal-caval) shunt. Extrahepatic shunts are more common in small dogs while intrahepatic shunts are more common in large dogs (Bostwick & Twedt 1995). Affected animals are young and typically exhibit episodic disturbances in mentation and behaviour. Single shunts are usually surgically managed, although intrahepatic shunts with more difficulty. Diffuse hepatic disease or multiple shunts are usually managed medically. The goal of medical therapy is to reduce the level of circulating toxins which accumulate as a result of the hepatic insufficiency.

Medical Management of Hepatic Encephalopathy

Bacterial degradation of proteins in the colon is thought to be the main source of neurotoxins in HE. Therapeutic strategies largely aimed at reducing this process include:

- vegetable- or dairy-protein based diet;
- lactulose 0.5 ml/kg p.o. t.i.d. (may be administered as an enema in an encephalopathic crisis) and;
- neomycin 20 mg/kg p.o. t.i.d. *or* metronidazole 7.5 mg/kg p.o. b.i.d.

Encephalitis

The most common causes of encephalitis are canine distemper virus and granulomatous meningoencephalitis (GME). Sporadic cases of protozoal (*Toxoplasma gondii* and *Neospora caninum*), bacterial and fungal encephalitis are also seen. Young dogs are more commonly affected. Seizures may be associated with other signs (e.g. head tilt, nystagmus, chorioretinitis) suggesting a multifocal disease process. Fever may be present. Multifocal, contrast-enhancing lesions may be seen on CT or MRI. This, in conjunction with abnormal CSF (increased protein level and leukocyte count) is strong evidence for the presence of meningoencephalitis. Culture of CSF should be considered if >50 neutrophils per µl or infectious agents are seen on CSF microscopy. Serology for infectious agents in CSF and serum may aid in the diagnosis. Although eradicated from Britain, the increasing incidence of rabies on the continent indicates the necessity for a continuous level of awareness. Rabies infection may present in a number of ways including behavioural changes (typically towards aggression), salivation, dysphagia, ataxia and quadriparesis. Although incubation periods vary from 3 weeks to 6 months once neurological signs are apparent, death usually occurs in 2–7 days.

REFERENCES

Bostwick, D.R. & Twedt, D.C. (1995). Intrahepatic and extrahepatic portal venous anomalies in dogs: 52 cases (1982–1992). *Journal of the American Veterinary Medical Association*, **206**, 1181–1185.

Daniel, G.B., Bright, R. & Shull, R. (1991). Per rectal portal scintigraphy using 99 m technetium pertechnetate to diagnose portosystemic shunts in dogs and cats. *Journal of Veterinary Internal Medicine*, **5**, 23–27.

Evans, S.M., Dayrell-Hart, B., Powlis, W., Christy, G. & Van

Winkle, T. (1993). Radiation therapy of canine brain masses. *Journal of Veterinary Internal Medicine*, 7, 216–219.

Heidner, G.L., Kornegay, J.N., Page, R.L., Dodge, R.K. & Thrall, D.E. (1991). Analysis of survival in a retrospective study of 86 dogs with brain tumours. *Journal of Veterinary Internal Medicine*, 5, 219–226.

Lane, S.B. & Bunch, S.E. (1990). Medical management of recurrent seizures in dogs and cats. *Journal of Veterinary Internal Medicine*, 4, 26–39.

Podell, M. (1995). The use of diazepam per rectum at home for the acute management of cluster seizures in dogs. *Journal of Veterinary Internal Medicine*, 8, 68–74.

Podell, M. & Fenner, W.R. (1993). Bromide therapy in refractory canine idiopathic epilepsy. *Journal of Veterinary Internal Medicine*, 7, 318–327.

Chapter 80

Altered Consciousness (Stupor and Coma)

A. Hopkins

INTRODUCTION

Altered levels of consciousness are classified as:

- *Depression* – Note that animals with systemic illness may be depressed in the absence of neurological disease.
- *Delirium* – A state of excessive, inappropriate response to the environment or stimulation. Usually represents forebrain disease.
- *Stupor* – A state of unconsciousness from which the animals can be aroused with painful stimuli (although not to a state of normal consciousness).
- *Coma* – A state of unconsciousness from which the animal cannot be aroused.

Also included in this section is the sleep disorder narcolepsy.

STRUCTURE AND FUNCTION

Altered levels of mentation result from disease of either both cerebral hemispheres or the brainstem. The brainstem contains the ascending reticular activating system (ARAS) which acts as a central conduit for sensory information from the body and head to activate the cerebral cortex. Interruption of the ARAS depresses cortical activity. Assessment of animals with abnormal mentation requires determination of whether disease of the cerebral hemispheres or brainstem is the cause. This is usually achieved by the recognition of cranial nerve abnormalities in the latter location.

APPROACH TO THE PATIENT

The differential diagnoses and diagnostic approach discussed in Chapter 79 can be applied here as all the conditions causing seizures can also cause altered mentation (Table 80.1). Extracranial disorders exert their effects diffusely on the forebrain while most of the previously discussed intracranial disorders can affect either the brainstem or the forebrain.

Diagnostic Imaging

- skull radiography in head trauma and bite wounds
- CT or MRI
- thoracic and abdominal radiographic evaluation for neoplasia

SPECIFIC DISEASES

Head Trauma

The sequelae to head injury may be divided into primary and secondary components (Dewey *et al.* 1992, 1993). Primary components are the immediate effects of haemorrhage and axonal injury. Secondary events are related to the release of inflammatory mediators from extravasated blood and severed axons. Neurovascular damage is accompanied by the release of enzymes, iron and vasoactive agents into the surrounding neuropil. Arachidonic acid metabolites and free radical generation contribute to the development of vasogenic and cytotoxic oedema in the surrounding area (Brown & Hall 1992). Small insults may be contained.

Table 80.1 Examination of the patient with altered consciousness.

Mentation. Classify as normal, depressed, delirious, stuporous, comatose.

Gait and posture. The more normal patient mobility is, the better the prognosis. Patient monitoring is essential however as any patient with head trauma can deteriorate.

Cranial nerves. These project to and from the brainstem and thus reflect its functional status. The most useful reflexes for assessing brainstem function are:

- pupil size and reactivity,
- palpebral reflex,
- oculovestibular reflex.

In the absence of drugs and ocular disease, if the pupils are not of normal size or reactivity then significant brain disease exists, often with a poor to guarded prognosis. Any trend away from normal size and reactivity indicates progressive brain disease.

- A classic sign associated with herniation and brainstem compression is progressive dilatation and loss of reactivity of one or both pupils.

Cardiorespiratory system. Brainstem damage may result in abnormalities of breathing patterns, heart rate and blood pressure.

Table 80.2 Management of head trauma.

Baseline examination & regular monitoring essential whatever the initial severity.
Ensure good oxygenation
Ensure adequate blood pressure
Head level or slightly elevated (10–20°)

Fluid therapy
  Care to avoid over hydration and raised intracranial pressure
  Use isotonic fluids for maintenance
  Hypertonic (7%) saline 2–4 ml/kg at 0.5–1.0 ml/kg per hour best choice for treatment of systemic shock as lowers intracranial pressure

Corticosteroids
  Controversial. Not advocated in humans.
  Prednisolone 0.5–1.0 mg/kg p.o. b.i.d.
  Methylprednisolone sodium succinate (30 mg/kg i.v., Braughler & Hall 1985)

Hypersomotic therapy
  Indications: Coma (due to intracranial disease) on initial presentation. Deteriorating neurological status in face of other therapy. Not indicated in the responsive stable patient.
  Mannitol 0.25–1.0 g/kg i.v. over 3–5 min
  Frusemide 0.7 mg/kg i.v./i.m. 15 min after mannitol (Roberts *et al.* 1987)

Antibiotics
  Indicated in penetrating injuries of the cranial vault
  Potentiated sulphonamides 15 mg/kg b.i.d. i.m., i.v.
  Metronidazole 20 mg/kg i.v., p.o. t.i.d.
  Chloramphenicol 50 mg/kg p.o., i.v. t.i.d.

Anticonvulsants
  Diazepam, phenobarbitone, pentobarbitone (see seizure management)

Surgery
  Decision to operate difficult and ideally based on CT or MRI. Benefits include, decompression, evacuation of haematoma, removal of bone fragments, lavage of penetrating wound. Indications: bite wound with calvarial penetration, depression fracture, deterioration of unilateral forebrain injury in face of medical therapy. Disadvantages include; risk of anesthesia, not finding anything, infection.

Larger lesions can produce a self-reinforcing process of oedema and ischaemia with further expansion of the lesion and a rise in intracranial pressure. In the confines of the rigid cranial vault this may have the disastrous consequences of compromising intracranial blood flow and producing physical brain tissue displacement (herniation). Such an event is usually manifest clinically as decreasing consciousness and dilation of the pupils and is often terminal. Successful management of head trauma can be difficult, requiring aggressive diagnostic, monitoring and therapeutic techniques. In veterinary medicine these are limited in terms of availability and cost. As a result, management of head trauma is still largely empirical.

The brainstem contains many vital centres and pathways compacted into a small area. Relatively small lesions can have dramatic, sometimes rapidly fatal consequences. Brainstem involvement may be primary or secondary (compression by an expanding forebrain lesion, e.g. oedema or haematoma) and is indicated by abnormal cranial nerve function. Serial neurological evaluation is indicated for detecting secondary development of brainstem signs. The relative redundancy of the dog forebrain means that larger lesions can be sustained with less severe consequences.

Open skull fractures and penetrating bite wounds carry a high risk of infection and haemorrhage. Antibiotic therapy is essential in such cases. Bite wounds should be thoroughly inspected and cleaned, even if this means making a hole in the calvarium larger to inspect the lesion.

Management of head trauma is summarised in Table 80.2.

Narcolepsy

A sleep disorder characterised by sudden daytime sleep attacks associated with abnormal brainstem function. Sleep attacks are usually associated with muscle paralysis and loss of tendon reflexes referred to as cataplexy. Rarely, cataplexy may occur by itself in which case the recumbent animal is alert and follows objects with its eyes. Attacks are usually brought on by excitement, e.g. eating, exercise, sexual arousal. Diagnosis is often quite easy and the attacks can be reproduced intentionally, e.g. by feeding. Yohimbine ($25-50\,\mu g/kg$ i.v. bolus) and imipramine ($0.5\,mg/kg$ i.v. bolus) challenges may be used to decrease the attacks. The inherited disease is not curable and animals usually remain symptomatic, although the prognosis is good and the disease not fatal. Some animals with the inherited form improve with advancing age. Treatment involves the administration of imipramine ($0.5-1.0\,mg/kg$ p.o. t.i.d.).

REFERENCES

Braughler, J.M. & Hall, E.D. (1985). Current application of high dose steroid therapy for CNS injury. *Journal of Neurosurgery*, **62**, 806–810.

Brown, S.A. & Hall, E.D. (1992). Role of oxygen-derived free radicals in the pathogenesis of shock and trauma, with focus on central nervous system injuries. *Journal of the American Veterinary Medical Association*, **200**, 1849–1859.

Dewey, C.W., Budsberg, S.C. & Oliver, J.E. (1992). Principles of head trauma management in dogs and cats – Part I. *Compendium on Continuing Education for the Practicing Veterinarian*, **14**, 199–207.

Dewey, C.W., Budsberg, S.C. & Oliver, J.E. (1993). Principles of head trauma management in dogs and cats – Part II. *Compendium on Continuing Education for the Practicing Veterinarian*, **15**, 177–193.

Roberts, P.A., Pollay, M., Engles, C., Pendleton, B., Reynolds, E. & Stevens, F.A. (1987). Effect on intracranial pressure of furosemide with varying doses and administration rates of mannitol. *Journal of Neurosurgery*, **60**, 440–446.

Chapter 81

Ataxia, Weakness and Paralysis of the Pelvic Limbs

A. Hopkins

INTRODUCTION

Ataxia is inco-ordination of the pelvic limbs manifest as swaying and altered step length (dysmetria) when walking. This may be the earliest sign of spinal cord disease. Ataxia often coexists with paraparesis.

Paraparesis is weakness of the pelvic limbs, usually manifest as difficulty rising, a low gait when walking, and difficulty standing. To help in staging severity of spinal cord disease a distinction is made between ambulatory and non-ambulatory paraparesis. In the former the animal can stand but has a tendency to drag its legs, and fall. In the latter the animal is too weak to rise by itself but when supported and encouraged to move, will show weak movements in the limbs.

Paraplegia represents complete absence of voluntary movement in the pelvic limbs (paralysis). This is determined by supporting the animal in a standing position and dragging it forward.

STRUCTURE AND FUNCTION

Weakness (paraparesis) or absence (paraplegia) of pelvic limb movement may result from lesions affecting:

- the spinal cord caudal to T2,
- the peripheral nerves supplying the pelvic limbs,
- the vascular supply to the pelvic limbs (Fig. 81.1)

If spinal cord segments T3 to L3 are affected then the pelvic limb spinal reflexes (patellar and withdrawal) and anal reflex will be normal, or, in the case of the patellar reflex, even increased. If the spinal cord segments L4 to S3,

or the peripheral nerves arising from these segments are affected the spinal reflexes will be depressed or even absent. Deep pain sensation should always be evaluated in paraplegic animals and is assessed by pinching the nail bed with haemostats and observing a *behavioural response* (turning, crying, biting, snarling). The presence of a withdrawal reflex does *not* evaluate deep pain. The absence of a withdrawal reflex does *not* indicate loss of deep pain. In animals with only paresis, evaluation of deep pain sensation is unnecessary (see Table 81.1).

> The presence or absence of deep pain is the single most important prognostic factor in the evaluation of animals with spinal cord (or peripheral nerve) disease.

Animals with mild compression of the cervical spinal cord can appear significantly worse in the pelvic limbs. Unless critical attention is paid to the thoracic limbs, an error in localisation and subsequent diagnostic evaluation may be made. Likewise animals with neuromuscular disease may appear worse in the pelvic limbs early in the course of the disease.

APPROACH TO THE PATIENT

History

- Breed – intervertebral disc disease (IVDD) is very common in chondrodystrophic dogs. Discospondylitis is seen in larger breed dogs. Degenerative myelopathy (DM) is seen more commonly in German Shepherd Dogs.
- Pain is an important localising sign in intervertebral disc disease, discospondylitis, fractures and some

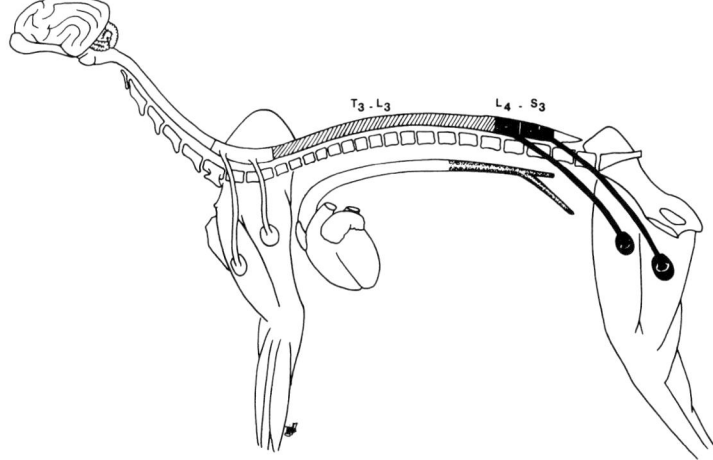

Fig. 81.1 Diagrammatic representation of lesion locations causing pelvic limb dysfunction.

spinal tumours. Pain is notably absent in dogs with fibrocartilaginous embolism and degenerative myelopathy.
- Speed of onset of clinical signs is important. Fibrocartilaginous emboli are typically peracute in onset. Spinal tumours and intervertebral disc prolapse may be acute or chronic.
- Age – degenerative myelopathy occurs in older dogs.

Examination

A valuable step in assessing animals with pelvic limb dysfunction is to grade the severity of the problem (Table 81.1). This aids in decision making, especially with respect to the management of intervertebral disc disease and fractures. It also allows objective monitoring of an animal's progress.

- Neoplasia detected elsewhere on physical examination raises concerns of metastatic disease.
- Trauma often involves multiple body regions.
- Retinal lesions may be seen with distemper and protozoal infections.

Table 81.1 Grades of pelvic limb dysfunction.

Grade	
1	Pain only, no neurologic deficits
2	Paraparesis, ambulatory
3	Paraparesis, non-ambulatory
4	Paraplegia, deep pain sensation present
5	Paraplegia, deep pain sensation absent

- Cold, pulseless limbs may be seen with aortic thromboembolism.

Investigation

Differential diagnosis is outlined in Table 81.2.

Haematology

- Leukocytosis may be observed in discospondylitis, but is an inconsistent feature.

Immunology

- Serology for *Brucella canis* in cases of discospondylitis.
- Serology for infectious agents causing myelitis.

Microbiology

- Infectious organisms may be cultured from blood, urine or the disc space itself.

Physical Procedures

- CSF analysis typically reveals mild to moderate non-specific elevations in protein levels and leukocyte count. Myelitis is usually associated with mononuclear pleocytosis. CSF analysis is of most value if evaluated in conjunction with myelography.
- Electrodiagnostic evaluation may be used to investigate lesions of the lumbosacral intumescence and

Table 81.2   Differential diagnosis of pelvic limb ataxia and weakness.

Degenerative
  Degenerative myelopathy
  Afghan myelopathy
  Hound ataxia
Anomalous
  Spinal dysraphism
  Arachnoid cysts
  Osteochondromatosis
  Hemivertebrae
  Spina bifida (myelomeningocoele)
Neoplasia
  Vertebral neoplasia
  Meningioma, astrocytoma, neurofibroma
Inflammatory
  Discospondylitis
  Myelitis (distemper, toxoplasmosis, neosporosis,
    granulomatous meningoencephalomyelitis (GME))
Trauma
  Intervertebral disc disease (IVDD)
  • Thoracolumbar
  • Lumbosacral
  Road traffic accident
Vascular
  Fibrocartilaginous embolism
  Aortic thromboembolism

peripheral nerves as these may be accompanied by denervation.

Diagnostic Imaging

- Plain radiography and myelography form the mainstay for the evaluation of spinal disorders. Thoracic and abdominal radiographs should be considered when evaluating for neoplasia.
- Fluoroscopy may permit biopsy of some spinal tumours.
- CT or MRI may be used to obtain images of greater detail.

MANAGEMENT

General guidelines are presented in Table 81.3. Many complications arise in dealing with paraparetic/paraplegic animals, resulting from the recumbent state itself or the drugs frequently administered.

SPECIFIC DISEASES

Degenerative Myelopathy (DM)

Demyelination of the thoracic spinal cord results in progressive, non-painful paraparesis. Most often seen in older German Shepherd Dogs, other large breeds are affected sporadically. The cause is unknown. Typical early clinical signs include pelvic limb ataxia, scuffing of the toes and wearing of the nails. Signs may be asymmetric initially. Most affected animals have normal or exaggerated pelvic limb spinal reflexes. In about 25% of cases one or both patellar reflexes are decreased or absent due to dorsal (sensory) root involvement. Such cases are responsible for the term chronic degenerative radiculomyelopathy (CDRM). Signs often progress from mild ataxia to paraplegia or non-ambulatory paraparesis within 6 months. Faecal and urinary continence are maintained. Diagnosis is based on history and exclusion of other spinal cord diseases via plain radiography, myelography and CSF analysis. The prognosis is guarded. There is anecdotal evidence about the benefit of corticosteroids or a combination of vitamin E, aminocaproic acid and vitamin B (Clemmons 1989). Exercise is encouraged.

Neoplasia

A wide variety of tumours may affect the spinal cord with the commonest being primary or metastatic vertebral body tumours (e.g. osteosarcoma, haemangiosarcoma and carcinomas). Most vertebral body tumours are painful. Vertebral body lysis may be seen radiographically although loss of 25% of the bone density is required before lytic change is apparent. Clinical signs vary from acute to slowly progressive. Although most affected dogs are middle aged to older, any age can be affected. Diagnosis is based on plain radiography, myelography and surgical biopsy. While the overall prognosis for dogs with spinal cord neoplasia is poor, some benefits may be gained in treatment of tumours such as meningiomas, ependymomas and lymphoma.

Discospondylitis

Discospondylitis results from bacterial or, rarely, fungal infection of the intervertebral disc and adjacent vertebral bodies. The most commonly isolated organisms are *Staphylococcus intermedius*, although many Gram-negative and Gram-positive organisms have been identified. Less common, but well recognised, are fungal infections (e.g. *Aspergillus*). Any disc may be involved although mid-thoracic, lumbosacral and caudal cervical sites are the most common. Spinal cord compression may result from soft

Table 81.3 Medical management of paraplegic dogs.

Cage rest. Advocated for some cases of IVDD and some spinal fractures. Clean, soft bedding to avoid decubitus ulcers

Physiotherapy. Massage and manipulate limbs 5–10 min twice a day. Sling walking for animals not at risk from deterioration. Whirlpool baths. Exercise encouraged in dogs with degenerative myelopathy.

Pain relief

Diazepam	0.5 mg/kg p.o. t.i.d. or,
Methocarbamol	22–44 mg/kg p.o. t.i.d. or,
Prednisolone	0.25–0.5 mg/kg p.o. b.i.d. or,
Aspirin	10–25 mg/kg p.o. b.i.d. (*not* if anticipating surgery)

Immediate postoperative period:

Butorphanol	0.2–0.8 mg/kg i.v./s.c. every 2–6 h
Morphine sulphate	0.2–0.6 mg/kg s.c. as required
Fentanyl patches (Hardie 1995)	

Dogs with IVDD managed medically MUST BE CAGE CONFINED as pain relief leads to increased mobility and risk of further prolapse of disc material.

Management of micturition is of PARAMOUNT importance in animals with spinal disease. Bladder dysfunction is common in paraplegic animals. Overflow dribbling often misinterpreted as evidence of urination. If unattended, extreme distension may damage the bladder wall and result in permanent atony.

- Manual expression t.i.d., or
- Catheterisation t.i.d. (sterile technique).
- In-dwelling catheter with sterile collection bag if repeated catheterisation is too traumatic.
- Pharmacological assistance:
    For the turgid (upper motor neurone) bladder:
    ○ Diazepam 0.5 mg/kg p.o. t.i.d.
    ○ Phenoxybenzamine 0.25–0.5 mg/kg p.o. t.i.d.
    For the flaccid (lower motor neurone) bladder:
    ○ Bethanechol 5–15 mg/kg p.o. t.i.d.

Urinary tract infections and urine scalding are comon. Antibiotic therapy is best guided by the results of urine culture and sensitivity.

---

tissue inflammation or collapse of the intervertebral disc space. Clinical signs are typically seen in adult, large breed dogs, are progressive and include:

- focal spinal pain,
- fever,
- paraparesis or quadriparesis,
- loss of condition/weight loss.

The characteristic radiographic lesion is loss of intervertebral disc space, lysis of adjacent vertebral end plates and bony proliferation of the vertebral bodies (Fig. 81.2). Early lesions may be characterised by collapse of the disc space and lysis of the end plates. Occasionally clinical signs appear before development of a radiographic lesion. Radionucleotide imaging may identify such cases although an alternative is to repeat the radiographs in 2–4 weeks. Treatment is ideally guided by results of culture (from blood, urine or disc itself) and sensitivity. Empirical se-

lection may be based on relative frequency of bacterial isolates, with *Staphylococcus intermedius* being the most common.

- For Gram-positive infections:
    ○ cloxacillin (20–40 mg/kg p.o. t.i.d.) or
    ○ cephalexin (22 mg/kg p.o. t.i.d.)
- For Gram-negative infections:
    ○ enrofloxacin (5 mg/kg p.o. b.i.d.)
- Broad-spectrum treatment:
    ○ trimethoprim–sulphadiazine (30 mg/kg p.o. b.i.d.)

Treatment should be continued for 8 weeks. The best indication for efficacy of treatment is clinical response with a positive effect usually being noted in 3–4 days. Resolution of radiographic abnormalities may take several months. Surgery may need to be considered in dogs with evidence of spinal cord compression that show a poor response to antibiotic therapy, loss of deep pain sensation due to severe

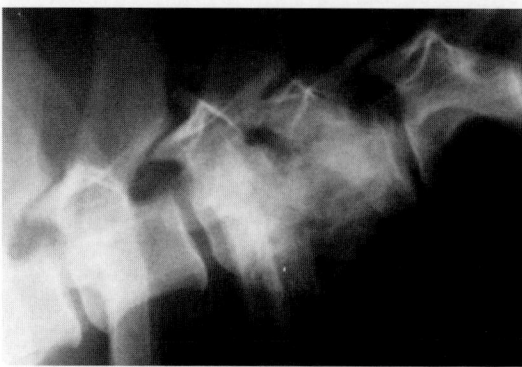

Fig. 81.2 Typical radiographic features of discospondylitis; disc space collapse, end plate lysis and proliferative osteomyelitis of adjacent vertebral bodies.

spinal cord compression and deterioration in the face of antibiotic therapy.

Myelitis

Inflammation of the spinal cord may result from infectious and non-infectious (e.g. granulomatous meningoencephalomyelitis (GME)) causes. Canine distemper virus can cause an acute transverse myelitis in young dogs resulting in signs of focal spinal cord disease. Affected dogs may have other clinical signs (e.g. seizures or active retinal lesions) to suggest the multifocal inflammatory nature of the disease. Infections with the protozoal parasites *Toxoplasma gondii* and *Neospora caninum* result in widespread involvement of many organ systems, liver, lungs, peripheral and central nervous system and muscles. However a clinical presentation common to both infections appears to be progressive paraparesis and rigid, extended pelvic limbs associated with muscle contracture, myositis, neuritis and myelitis. Therapy with clindamycin or potentiated sulphonamides may be considered, but the neurological deficits are often too far advanced for significant recovery.

Intervertebral Disc Disease (IVDD)
(see Box 81.1)

This is the most common cause of spinal disease in all breeds of dog. Clinical signs can be acute or chronic. Diagnosis requires radiography. Plain radiographic features include narrow intervertebral disc space, narrow interarticular joint space, intervertebral foramen opacification and calcified material in the vertebral canal (Fig.

81.3a). These findings may be subtle and sometimes misleading (Fig. 81.3b). Myelography is essential for accurate localisation of the lesion when considering surgery (Olby *et al.* 1994). Calcification of intervertebral discs is common in chondrodystrophoid dogs and does *not* necessarily indicate the site of the lesion. In animals without deep pain sensation, lack of improvement after 2 weeks indicates a guarded prognosis and lack of improvement after 1 month indicates a grave prognosis for functional recovery. Many paraplegic animals can be successfully cared for although the situation seems easier if the dog is small.

Lumbosacral degenerative disc disease is characterised by a dorsal, bulging disc that protrudes into the vertebral canal, compressing the cauda equina (Ness 1994). These structural changes are thought to be a reaction and compensation to chronic instability of the lumbosacral articulation. It is most commonly seen in large breed dogs, especially the German Shepherd Dog. Clinical signs are often restricted to pain, usually manifest on climbing up or down steps. More severe compression is associated with paraparesis, conscious proprioceptive deficits, urinary and faecal incontinence. If ignored the damage sustained may be permanent. Diagnosis requires demonstration of the protruded disc. This may be achieved by a variety of different techniques including:

- myelography,
- epidurography,
- discography,
- CT or MRI.

Denervation of tail muscles associated with nerve compression may be demonstrated by electromyography. Decompression via dorsal laminectomy affords a good prognosis if performed before incontinence develops. While some recovery is possible in the latter situation more caution should be exercised regarding the prognosis.

Spinal Trauma

This category includes injuries sustained in road traffic accidents, falls, fights and malicious wounding. Similar evaluation and treatment guidelines to those used in IVDD are used here. The wide variety of possible spinal traumas make it difficult to make fixed recommendations. Many fractures and luxations can be managed conservatively. However if there is concern for spinal instability then surgical stabilisation should be considered to minimise continued spinal cord trauma. Myelography can provide important information as to the integrity of the cord and presence and severity of any compression. This is important in animals without deep pain sensation with regards to prognosis and treatment.

Box 81.1 Intervertebral disc disease (IVDD) in focus.

Epidemiology. Any breed of dog may be affected. IVDD is typically seen in chondrodystrophic dogs aged 1–5 years and non-chondrodystrophic dogs aged >5 years.

Aetiology and pathogenesis. Degeneration of the disc impairs its flexibility. Altered stress distribution in the disc leads to tearing of the annulus fibrosus, prolapse of the nucleus pulposus and fibrous proliferation. Spinal injury results from combinations of compression and contusion. IVD prolapse is seen in the thoracolumbar, lumbar and cervical spine. In chondrodystrophoid dogs, 70% of disc prolapses occur between and including T11–12 and L1–2.

Clinical signs
- Paraparesis/paraplegia (acute or chronic)
- Focal pain

Surgical therapy		*Medical therapy*
Hemilaminectomy		Cage rest
& fenestration		Analgesics

Recovery rate	Grade of severity	*Recovery rate*
95%	1 (Pain only)	75–85%
95%	2 (Ambulatory paraparesis)	75–85%
95%	3 (Non-ambulatory paraparesis)	55–85%
95%	4 (Paraplegia)	55–85%
50% (if surgery in 24 h)	5 (Deep pain absent)	5–10%

(Kornegay 1992)

Corticosteroids in IVDD
Grades 1–4: Prednisolone (see medical management). Use is personal choice. Can be very effective but tend to be overused.

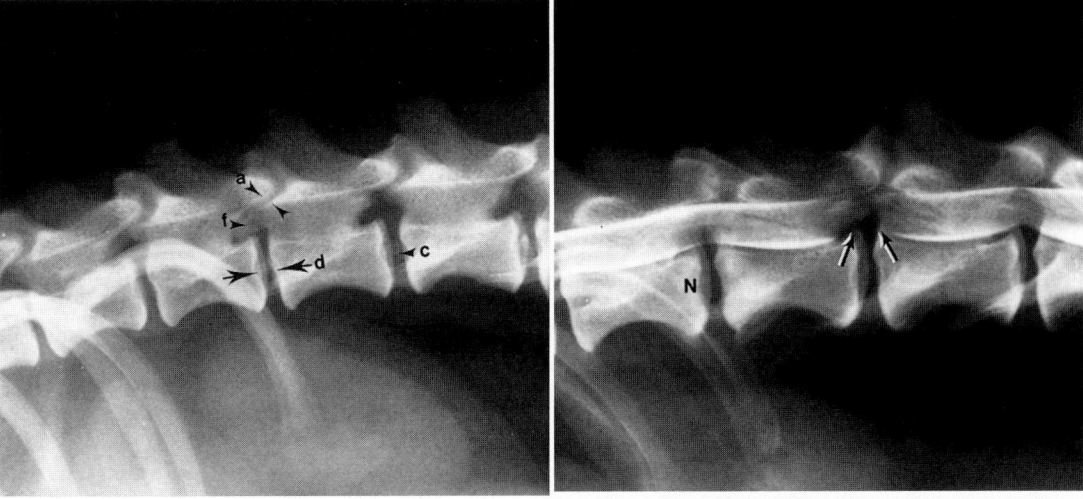

a   b

Fig. 81.3   (a) Typical radiographic features of intervertebral disc disease; narrow intervertebral disc space and articular joint space, opacification of the intervertebral foramen and calcification of intervertebral disc material. (b) Myelogram of a dog with intervertebral disc prolapse. The narrow disc is not associated with spinal cord compression demonstrating the value of myelography in confirming lesion location.

Box 81.1 *Continued.*

Grade 5: High dose therapy with methylprednisolone sodium succinate (Solu-Medrone™):
   30 mg/kg i.v. within 8 h of spinal cord injury
   15 mg/kg i.v. 2 and 6 h after initial dose
   2.5 mg/kg per hour i.v. for next 18–42 h

   This drug regime is extrapolated from experimental studies in cats (Braughler *et al.* 1987) and clinical trials in humans (Bracken *et al.* 1992). Its benefit is not proven in dogs and several variations on the regime exist (Coughlan 1993).
   High doses of corticosteroids (especially dexamethasone) can be associated with severe gastrointestinal complications (Toombs *et al.* 1980).

Avoid combinations of steroids and NSAIDs

Fibrocartilaginous Embolism (FCE)

Peracute, sometimes catastrophic spinal cord dysfunction results from a shower of thromboemboli to the microvasculature of the spinal cord. The embolic material is thought to originate from the intervertebral discs although the path of entry into the spinal cord vasculature is not understood. Any part of the spinal cord may be affected. Typical clinical features include:

- larger breed dogs,
- peracute onset associated with some form of exercise,
- lack of pain (brief discomfort sometimes reported at the onset),
- asymmetric neurological deficits. Severe lesions however may result in an extensive, bilaterally symmetrical lesion.

Prognosis depends on the location and severity. Lesions affecting the spinal cord intumescences at C6–T2 and L4–S3 carry a poorer prognosis than lesions elsewhere. Again the presence or absence of deep pain is the best guide to the prognosis. There is no treatment of proven value although most clinicians use corticosteroids in a similar way to the treatment of IVDD.

Aortic Thromboembolism

This is a rare condition in dogs associated with hyperadrenocorticism and the nephrotic syndrome (caused by renal loss of antithrombin III). The clinical signs are similar to the feline counterpart and the prognosis equally poor.

REFERENCES

Bracken, M.B., Shepard, M.J., Collins, W.F., *et al.* (1992). A randomized, controlled trial of methylprednisolone or naloxone in the treatment of acute spinal-cord injury. Results of the second national acute spinal cord injury study. *New England Journal of Medicine*, **322**, 1405–1411.

Braughler, J.M., Hall, E.D., Means, E.D., Waters, T.R. & Anderson, D.K. (1987). Evaluation of an intensive methylprednisolone sodium succinate dosing regimen in experimental spinal cord injury. *Journal of Neurosurgery*, **67**, 102–105.

Clemmons, R.M. (1989). Degenerative myelopathy. In: *Current Veterinary Therapy X: Small Animal Practice*, (ed. R.W. Kirk), pp. 830–833. W.B. Saunders, Philadelphia.

Coughlan, A.R. (1993). Secondary injury mechanisms in acute spinal cord trauma. *Journal of Small Animal Practice*, **34**, 117–122.

Hardie, E.M. (1995). New horizons in pain management: Transdermal fentanyl patches. *Perspectives*, **Jan/Feb**, 35–37.

Kornegay, J.N. (1992). Intervertebral disk disease: treatment guidelines. In: *Current Veterinary Therapy XI. Small Animal Practice*, (eds R.W. Kirk & J.D. Bonagura), pp. 1013–1018. W.B. Saunders, Philadelphia.

Ness, M.G. (1994). Degenerative lumbosacral stenosis in the dog: A review of 30 cases. *Journal of Small Animal Practice*, **35**, 185–190.

Olby, N.J., Dyce, J. & Houlton, J.E.F. (1994). Correlation of plain radiographic and lumbar myelographic findings with surgical findings in thoracolumbar disc disease. *Journal of Small Animal Practice*, **35**, 345–350.

Toombs, J.B., Caywood, D.D., Lipowitz, A.J. & Stevens, J.B. (1980). Colonic perforation following neurosurgical procedures and corticosteroid therapy in four dogs. *Journal of the American Veterinary Medical Association*, **177**, 68.

Chapter 82

Ataxia, Weakness and Paralysis of all Four Limbs

A. Hopkins

INTRODUCTION

Weakness and paralysis of all four limbs are referred to as quadriparesis (or tetraparesis) and quadriplegia (or tetraplegia) respectively.

Structure and Function

Quadriparesis may result from lesions affecting:

- the brain,
- the cervical spinal cord or
- the neuromuscular system (Fig. 82.1).

A careful neurological examination, with particular attention to the spinal reflexes, is very important in separating these different locations.

Brain Disorders

Brain disorders causing tetraparesis are usually associated with other signs of intracranial disease (e.g. seizures, altered mentation and behaviour). These diseases have been covered previously and will not be discussed here. (See Chapters 79 and 80.)

Spinal Cord Disorders

Spinal cord disorders causing quadriparesis can be divided into two locations:

- C1–C5: conscious proprioceptive deficits in all four limbs. Spinal reflexes are intact and even increased in all four limbs. Extensor rigidity of all four limbs may be seen (Table 82.1).

- C6–T2: conscious proprioceptive deficits in all four limbs. Thoracic limb spinal reflexes are depressed to absent, while pelvic limb reflexes are normal to increased. Pelvic limbs may demonstrate rigidity while the thoracic limbs are flaccid.

Occasionally spinal cord lesions may lateralise significantly and produce weakness that is worse on one side (hemiparesis, hemiplegia). Close evaluation often reveals involvement of all four limbs but the asymmetry may be dramatic. In most cases of cervical cord compression the pelvic limbs are clinically more affected. In some cases however weakness may be worse in the thoracic limbs.

A similar scale to that used for the assessment of paraparetic dogs can be used here. Lesions of the cervical spinal cord severe enough to cause loss of deep pain sensation in the limbs however, are rarely compatible with life because of interruption of respiratory neural pathways.

Neuromuscular Disorders

Neuromuscular disorders can be divided into those affecting the lower motor neurone (neuropathy), neuromuscular junction (junctionopathy) and muscle cell (myopathy) (Table 82.2).

Clinical signs of neuromuscular disease affect all four limbs and are typically progressive but may be episodic and related to exercise. Weakness may initially or consistently be more apparent in the pelvic limbs and so critical evaluation of the thoracic limbs is important to confirm the diffuse nature of the disease.

- *Neuropathy*: Characteristic features of neuropathy include varying degrees of weakness, conscious proprioceptive deficits, decreased muscle tone, muscle atrophy and decreased spinal reflexes.
- *Junctionopathy*: Typically presents as exercise induced weakness that improves with rest. Spinal reflexes and

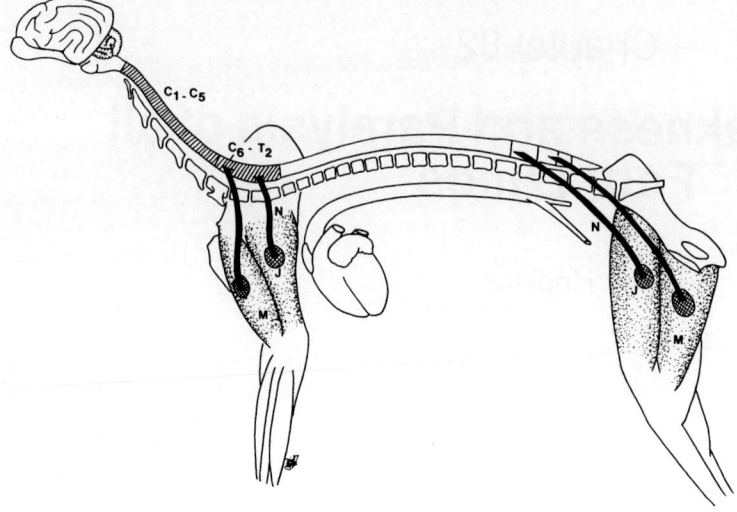

Fig. 82.1　Diagrammatic representation of lesion locations causing quadriparesis/plegia. The neuromuscular system is divided into the lower motor neuron (N), neuromuscular junction (J) and muscles (M). Spinal cord lesions are represented by the hatched area.

Table 82.1　Focal spinal causes of quadriparesis/plegia.

Degenerative
　　Leukoencephalomyelopathy and neuroaxonal dystrophy
　　　of Rottweilers (Chrisman 1993)
　　Hereditary ataxias of Smooth Haired Fox Terriers and
　　　Jack Russell Terriers
Anomalous
　　Congenital vertebral anomalies
　　Arachnoid cysts
Neoplasia Inflammatory
　　Discospondylitis
　　Meningomyelitis
Traumatic
　　Intervertebral disc disease
　　Fracture/luxation (e.g. road traffic accident)
　　Cervical stenotic myelopathy
　　Atlanto axial subluxation
Vascular
　　Fibrocartilaginous embolism

Table 82.2　Differential diagnosis of neuromuscular disease.

Neuropathy
　　Polyradiculoneuritis
　　　Protozoal (neosporosis, toxoplasmosis)
　　　Immune-mediated
　　Hypothyroidism
　　Diabetes mellitus
　　Paraneoplastic (e.g. insulinoma)
　　Lead, chronic organophosphate intoxication
　　Spinal muscular atrophy (e.g. Rottweiler, Brittany
Spaniel)
Junctionopathy
　　Myasthenia gravis
　　Tick paralysis
　　Coral snake envenomation
　　Acute/subacute organophosphate intoxication
　　Botulism
Myopathy
　　Polymyositis:　　　(toxoplasmosis, neosporosis,
immune-mediated)
Hyperadrenocorticism
Hypothyroidism
Hypo-/Hyper-kalaemia
Hypo-/Hyper-calcaemia
Mitochondrial myopathies (Clumber & Sussex Spaniel, Old
English Sheepdog (Breitschwerdt *et al.* 1992)
Muscular dystrophy (Golden Retriever, Labrador Retriever,
Irish Terrier)

conscious proprioception are normal. However, complete blockade of the neuromuscular junctions (e.g. botulism) will produce flaccid paralysis and areflexia of all four limbs.
- *Myopathy*: Typical findings are weakness (may be exercise related), muscle atrophy and possibly muscle pain. Conscious proprioception and spinal reflexes are normal.

APPROACH TO THE PATIENT

History

- Breed related problems include; atlanto-axial subluxation in Yorkshire Terriers and Toy Poodles; cervical stenotic myelopathy (CSM) in Doberman Pinschers and Great Danes; fibrocartilaginous embolism in large breed dogs; muscular dystrophy in Labrador and Golden Retrievers.
- Acute onset of clinical signs in fibrocartilaginous embolism, intervertebral disc disease and trauma.
- Exercise related weakness suggests neuromuscular disease (e.g. myasthenia gravis).

Examination

- Pain is a predominant feature of many spinal disorders (e.g. intervertebral disc disease, neoplasia, discospondylitis, atlanto-axial subluxation and meningomyelitis).
- Fever may be seen in inflammatory disorders (e.g. meningomyelitis, discospondylitis).
- General physical abnormalities may be seen in endocrine disorders.

Investigation

Haematology

- Anaemia may be found in hypothyroidism.
- Leukocytosis may occur in inflammatory disorders.

Biochemistry

- Hyperglycaemia occurs in diabetes mellitus.
- Hypercholesterolaemia may occur in hypothyroidism.
- Creatine kinase (CK) elevations are often seen in myopathies. Normal recumbent animals may have mild to moderate CK elevations.
- Thyroid levels and stimulation testing may be abnormal in neuromuscular disease.
- Post-exercise blood gas analysis may be abnormal in certain myopathies (e.g. acidosis in mitochondrial myopathies).
- Pre- and post-exercise lactate levels may be abnormal in certain metabolic myopathies.
- Potassium and calcium abnormalities may be associated with muscular weakness.

Immunology

- Serum acetylcholine receptor antibody titre is the definitive test for acquired myasthenia gravis.
- An elevated anti-nuclear antibody (ANA) titre may be seen in polymyositis associated with systemic lupus erythematosus.
- Serology for infectious diseases (e.g. *Toxoplasma*, *Neospora*).

Physical Procedures

- CSF protein and leukocytes are often increased in meningomyelitis and polyradiculoneuritis. Spinal cord compression may also be associated with mild to moderate elevations in protein and cytology values.
- Electrodiagnostic evaluation is essential in the investigation of neuromuscular diseases.
- Muscle biopsy is important in the investigation of neuromuscular disease.
- Exercise challenge with biochemical evaluation (blood gases, pyruvate and lactate levels).
- Edrophonium (Camsilon™) response test for myasthenia gravis (see Table 82.3).

Diagnostic Imaging

- Plain radiography and myelography are very important in the investigation of cervical spinal cord disease. Thoracic radiography may reveal megaoesophagus in some neuromuscular diseases.

Management

For focal spinal cord diseases most of the general recommendations discussed in Chapter 81 apply here. Specific recommendations concerned with the treatment of the underlying disease processes are discussed below.

SPECIFIC DISEASES

Intervertebral Disc Disease

This is probably the most common cervical spinal disorder. All breeds of dog are affected. Clinical signs include pain (sometimes intense), quadriparesis and quadriplegia. Plain radiography and myelography are essential for diagnosis and accurate localisation. Medical therapy (see Chapter 81) may be employed for the first episode of pain. Severe pain, chronic (>2 weeks) or relapsing pain and animals demonstrating neurological deficits are best managed surgically. Ventral slot decompression affords an excellent prognosis.

Atlanto-axial Subluxation

Increased laxity of the atlanto-axial joint associated with malformation or absence of the dens leads to spinal cord compression. Young, toy breeds are typically affected. Clinical signs include varying combinations of neck pain, quadriparesis or quadriplegia. Diagnosis is made with plain radiography by demonstrating opening of the space between the cranial aspect of the dorsal spine of C2 and the dorsal lamina of C1 during *gentle* neck flexion (Fig. 82.2a,b). Care should be taken not to over-flex the neck when performing this procedure as traction on the brainstem can have serious, sometimes fatal cardiorespiratory sequelae. Surgical fusion of C1–2 from a ventral approach and employing transarticular stabilisation carries a very good prognosis (Wheeler & Sharp 1994).

Cervical Stenotic Myelopathy (CSM) (Cervical Spondylomyelopathy, 'Wobbler' Syndrome)

A combination of vertebral malformation, increased intervertebral laxity and hypertrophy of intervertebral ligaments and articular facets causes stenosis of the vertebral canal and compression of the caudal cervical spinal cord. Most commonly seen in adult Doberman Pinschers and young Great Danes where it is referred to as the 'wobbler syndrome' CSM is occasionally recognised in other large breeds of dog. Pelvic limb ataxia is the initial clinical sign, although careful evaluation of the thoracic limbs often reveals a stiff, choppy gait. More severely affected animals demonstrate obvious neurological deficits in all four limbs and sometimes quadriplegia. Radiographic findings (Fig. 82.3) include malalignment of the caudal cervical vertebrae C5, 6, 7, associated with dorsal (ligamentum flavum) and ventral (hypertrophied dorsal annulus) compression of the spinal cord. Lateral compression associated with large articular facets may be apparent on ventrodorsal views. Prednisolone therapy may result in significant improvements sometimes for long periods of time. However progressively increasing doses are often needed. A number of different surgical techniques have been described including ventral slot, ventral slot with distraction, distraction alone and dorsal laminectomy. Ventral slot procedures are often combined with attempts to encourage fusion. Good and bad results have been reported with all the techniques and

the outcome of surgery may be affected as much by patient selection as by the procedure itself.

Meningomyelitis

The term refers to a group of diseases whose common feature is meningitis, usually manifest as neck pain and fever. Spinal cord parenchymal involvement (myelitis) produces neurological deficits ranging from ataxia to quadri-

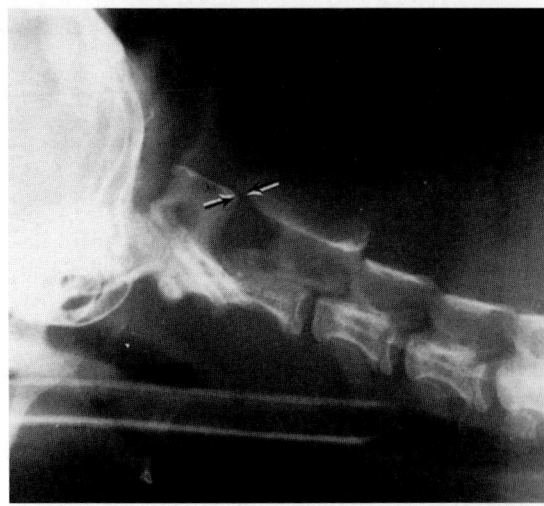

a

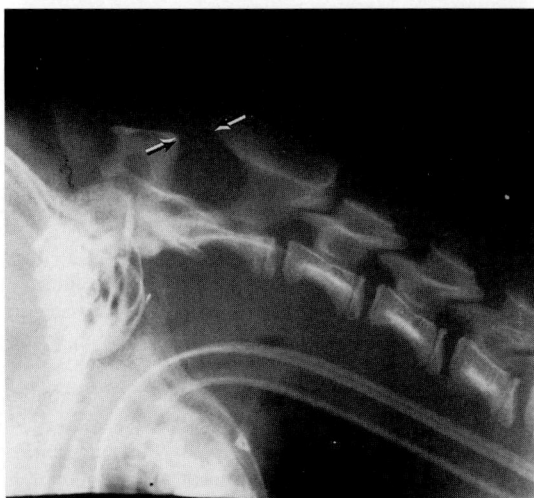

b

Fig. 82.2   (a) Radiographs of a 1-year-old Poodle with neck pain. (b) Same dog with mild neck flexion demonstrating opening of the dorsal space between C1 and C2. This space should not change in a normal dog.

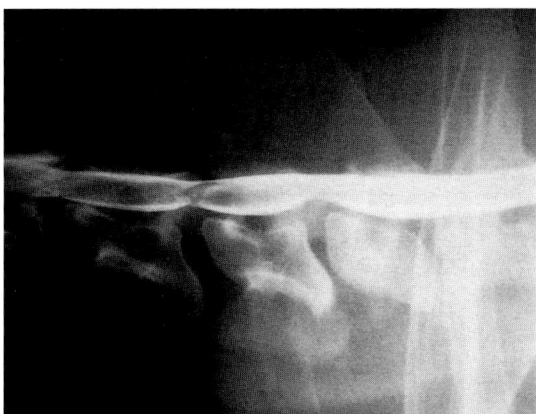

Fig. 82.3 Typical radiographic findings of cervical stenotic myelopathy in a 7-year-old Doberman Pinscher with quadriparesis. Note the abnormally shaped vertebrae, abnormal alignment and compression of the spinal cord.

plegia. This category of diseases is poorly understood and includes both infectious (e.g. distemper, toxoplasmosis) and purportedly non-infectious causes (e.g. granulomatous meningo encephalomyelitis (GME), aseptic meningitis of young large breed dogs). Some breeds (e.g. Beagle, Bernese Mountain Dogs) appear to be affected by unique forms of inflammatory disease of possible immune-mediated origin (Meric 1992). Diagnosis is based on demonstration of inflammatory CSF in the face of normal plain radiographs and myelogram. Myelography is usually not performed if the index of suspicion for meningomyelitis is high (neck pain, no neurological deficits, fever, normal plain radiographs and inflammatory CSF). Leukocyte elevations in CSF may be moderate (<50 WBCs/μl) and predominantly lymphocytic (e.g. GME) or dramatic (>200 WBCs/μl) and predominantly neutrophilic (e.g. aseptic meningitis, Beagle pain syndrome). Treatment with corticosteroids produces responses varying from temporary improvement to dramatic resolution. The latter response has led to clinical use of the term steroid-responsive meningitis although this is potentially misleading. Before administering corticosteroids the clinician should be confident that infectious agents are not involved. Culture of CSF is indicated if the neutrophil count is $>50/\mu$l.

Diabetes Mellitus

The best known peripheral neuropathy is that caused by diabetes mellitus. Affected animals may have a characteristic plantigrade stance in the pelvic limbs due to sciatic neuropathy. Varying degrees of postural deficits, muscle atrophy, weak reflexes and decreased muscle tone are found. Critical evaluation of the thoracic limbs reveals similar but sometimes less obvious findings. The clinical signs often improve with management of the diabetic state.

Hypothyroidism

A number of neurological disorders including, vestibular disease, facial paralysis, peripheral neuropathy, myasthenia gravis and laryngeal paralysis have been associated with hypothyroidism (Jaggy *et al.* 1994). The link between low thyroid function and these disorders is not understood. In many cases it is not known if the hypothyroidism is the cause of the neurological deficits or a result of the same disease process. Thyroid replacement, while indicated, may not result in resolution of the signs. Some conditions associated with hypothyroidism resolve spontaneously, without thyroid supplementation.

Myasthenia Gravis

Myasthenia gravis is an exercise-induced weakness resulting from a deficiency of acetylcholine receptor in the postsynaptic membrane. In most instances this is due to immune-mediated attack of the acetylcholine receptor, but congenital deficiency has been reported. Two clinical forms are recognised in the dog; a generalised form manifest as progressive stiffness of the gait and collapse on exercise, and a focal form resulting in mega-oesophagus and sometimes pharyngeal and laryngeal weakness. Strength improves with rest in the generalised form. Mega-oesophagus may result in aspiration pneumonia and respiratory distress. Thymomas have been associated with this condition. Diagnosis is made on the basis of a cholinesterase inhibitor response test (see Table 82.3), electrodiagnostic testing and detection of antibody to the acetylcholine receptor (Hopkins 1993).

Treatment with pyridostigmine (2 mg/kg p.o. b.i.d.) and corticosteroids often effects clinical improvement although management of mega-oesophagus can prove difficult.

Immune-mediated Polyradiculoneuritis

This is probably the most common inflammatory peripheral nerve disease. Weakness beginning in the pelvic limbs, evolves into a flaccid, areflexic, quadriplegia over 2–7 days. Pain sensation is intact. Cranial nerve and respiratory function is usually maintained. Muscle atrophy is dramatic after 2 weeks. Electrodiagnostic evaluation reveals evidence of demyelination and axonal damage. Recovery usually occurs

Table 82.3   Cholinesterase inhibitor (edrophonium/neostigmine) response testing.

- Atropine (0.04 mg/kg i.m.) is administered 10 min before testing. This reduces muscarinic overactivity which may result in bradycardia, salivation, bronchosecretion and bronchoconstriction.

Then

- Edrophonium (Camsilon™, 0.1 mg/kg i.v.) is administered at the height of weakness (induced by exercise if needed).

Or

- Neostigmine (Prostigmin™, 0.05 mg/kg i.m.) is administered before exercise. The dog's exercise tolerance is established beforehand by exercising it over a known distance. The dog is then exercised at 5-min intervals, starting 10 min after neostigmine injection.

Dramatic positive responses to cholinesterase inhibitors are strongly suggestive of myasthenia gravis. However, mild improvements (false positives) can sometimes be seen in dogs with polymyopathy or polyneuropathy.

spontaneously but may take 4–8 weeks. Good supportive care is essential to nurse the animals through the prolonged recumbency. Relapses and chronic variations of this disease have been reported. Although the condition is thought to be an auto-immune disease, corticosteroids have not been shown to be beneficial. The condition of distal denervating disease, only reported in the UK, has a similar clinical presentation.

REFERENCES

Breitschwerdt, E.B., Kornegay, J.N., Wheeler, S.J., Stevens, J.B. & Baty, C.J. (1992). Episodic weakness associated with exertional lactic acidosis and myopathy in Old English Sheepdog litter-mates. *Journal of the American Veterinary Medical Association*, **201**, 731–736.

Chrisman, C.L. (1993). Neurological disease of Rottweilers: Neuroaxonal dystrophy and leukoencephalomalacia. *Journal of Small Animal Practice*, **33**, 500–504.

Hopkins, A.L. (1993). Canine myasthenia gravis. *Journal of Small Animal Practice*, **33**, 477–484.

Jaggy, A., Oliver, J.E., Ferguson, D.C., Mahaffey, E.A. & Glaus Jun, T. (1994). Neurological manifestations of hypothyroidism: A retrospective study of 29 dogs. *Journal of Veterinary Internal Medicine*, **8**, 328–336.

Meric, S.M. (1992). Breed-specific meningitis in dogs. In: *Current Veterinary Therapy XI. Small Animal Practice*, (eds R.W. Kirk & J.D. Bonagura), pp. 1007–1009. W.B. Saunders, Philadelphia.

Wheeler, S.J. & Sharp, N.J.H. (1994). Atlanto-axial subluxation. *Small Animal Spinal Disorders: Diagnosis and Surgery*, pp. 109–121. Mosby-Wolfe, London.

Chapter 83

Monoparesis and Monoplegia

A. Hopkins

Definition
Weakness or paralysis of one limb.

STRUCTURE AND FUNCTION

Monoparesis most commonly results from damage to a peripheral nerve or plexus supplying a limb. However, spinal cord lesions behind T2 can be so focal as to cause signs restricted to one pelvic limb (Fig. 83.1). Evaluation of the spinal reflexes aids in precise localisation of the lesion.

APPROACH TO THE PATIENT

Examination

In evaluating animals with limb fractures consideration should always be given to the possibility of nerve damage. The simplest assessment of nerve integrity is determination of the presence or absence of deep pain sensation in the limb (several areas should be tested). Evaluation of the sensory fields of the affected limb allows determination of the nerves involved.

Investigation

Physical Procedures

- Electromyography confirms the presence of peripheral nerve disease and delineates the nerves involved.

Diagnostic Imaging

- Plain radiography – nerve sheath tumours may extend through and distend the intervertebral foramen.
- Myelography may reveal spinal cord compression from encroaching peripheral nerve tumours or unilateral disc protrusion.
- CT or MRI can provide detailed information regarding tumour location and anatomy.

SPECIFIC DISEASES

The differential diagnosis of specific diseases is outlined in Table 83.1.

Brachial Plexus Avulsion

Varying degrees of thoracic limb dysfunction result from traction injury of the brachial plexus. Ipsilateral Horner's syndrome (see Table 85.1) and loss of panniculus reflex are common associated findings. Most brachial plexus injuries are associated with some degree of nerve root avulsion from the spinal cord. Avulsion carries a hopeless prognosis for the nerve involved. Traction injury without avulsion, while appearing clinically similar, has some potential for regeneration although 2–6 months may be required for recovery. Prognosis for the limb depends on the extent of avulsion. There are no specific therapies. Management involves physiotherapy to keep the joints mobile while waiting to see what regeneration takes place. Complications include self-mutilation due to dysaesthesias, trauma to a dragging limb

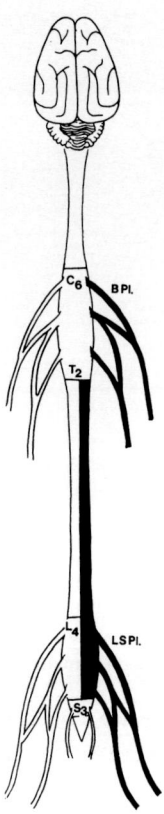

Fig. 83.1   Diagrammatic representation of lesion locations causing monoparesis/plegia. BPl, brachial plexus intumescence; LSPl, lumbar-sacral plexus intumescence.

and limb contracture. Limb salvage procedures including muscle transposition and carpal arthrodesis have not generally found favour among surgeons. Severe complications may necessitate limb amputation.

Table 83.1   Differential diagnosis of monoparesis/monoplegia.

Peripheral nerve
    Brachial plexus trauma/avulsion
    Neoplasia (schwannoma/neurofibroma/lymphoma)
Spinal cord
    Intervertebral disc disease (see Chapter 81)
    Fibrocartilaginous embolism (see Chapter 81)
    Neoplasia
    Trauma

Neoplasia

Typically seen in older dogs, nerve sheath tumours (e.g. neurofibrosarcoma) cause progressive painful limb dysfunction over several weeks to months (Targett *et al.* 1993). The problem is often initially misdiagnosed as musculoskeletal. When muscle atrophy becomes severe, the diagnosis becomes more evident. Denervation may be confirmed by electrodiagnostic evaluation. Deep palpation of the axilla may reveal a mass or marked pain response. Radiography and myelography may reveal evidence of extension into the vertebral canal. CT and MRI can be employed to delineate the tumour accurately. Good results have been reported with amputation if the tumour is confined to the limb. Spinal cord involvement confers a very poor prognosis.

REFERENCES

Targett, M.P., Dyce, J. & Houlton, J.E.F. (1993). Tumours involving the nerve sheaths of the forelimb in dogs. *Journal of Small Animal Practice*, **34**, 221–225.

Chapter 84

Ataxia of the Head and Limbs (Cerebellar Disease)

A. Hopkins

INTRODUCTION

Cerebellar diseases are uncommon (Table 84.1); however, they usually present with a characteristic group of neurological signs.

STRUCTURE AND FUNCTION

The cerebellum is largely responsible for regulation and co-ordination of motor activity. Loss of function results in overactive, poorly controlled muscular activity manifest clinically as dysmetria of all four limbs. Hypermetria is the most obvious form of dysmetria. Swaying of the trunk and head are often apparent while standing. Head tremor is often observed when the animal is trying to perform co-ordinated head movements (e.g. eating). The menace response is typically absent although affected animals are not blind. Signs may start subtly and progress over a number of weeks to months. Mentation, conscious proprioception and spinal reflexes are normal. Severe disease may result in decerebellate rigidity characterised by recumbency, extension of the head, neck and thoracic limbs and flexion of the pelvic limbs.

APPROACH TO THE PATIENT

History

- Most cerebellar diseases are insidious. More acute signs may be seen with trauma, encephalitis (e.g. distemper, granulomatous meningoencephalitis) or neoplasia.

Examination

- Fundic examination should be performed for evidence of infectious disease.

Investigation

Haematology

- Lymphocyte vacuolation may be seen in certain lysosomal storage disorders.
- Distemper virus inclusions are occasionally seen in blood leukocytes.

Immunology

- Immunofluorescence of conjunctival smears for distemper antigens.
- CSF titres for distemper antibodies.

Physical Procedures

- CSF analysis.

Table 84.1   Differential diagnosis of cerebellar disease.

Lysosomal storage disorders
Abiotrophy
Cerebellar hypoplasia
Neoplasia
Encephalitis (distemper)
Trauma

Diagnostic Imaging

* CT or MRI.

MANAGEMENT

Most diseases causing cerebellar dysfunction have a poor prognosis. Animals eventually become incapacitated by their extreme inco-ordination although this may take several months to years. Although its use is debatable in treatment of infectious encephalitis, prednisolone therapy may produce some alleviation of signs associated with distemper infection.

Chapter 85

Cranial Nerve Abnormalities

A. Hopkins

STRUCTURE AND FUNCTION

Cranial nerves carry sensory information (e.g. touch, pain) to the brainstem and motor impulses from the brainstem. Cranial nerve dysfunction may result from disease of the peripheral receptor or effector, cranial nerve trunk or brainstem nucleus (Table 85.1). Brainstem lesions are often associated with additional findings of postural deficits (e.g. knuckling) and mentation changes due to involvement of sensory and motor pathways and the reticular activating system.

Although strictly not a cranial nerve, sympathetic dysfunction is mentioned here because of its integration with the cranial nerve examination.

APPROACH TO THE PATIENT

Examination

- Otic examination
- Ocular examination
- Check for systemic evidence of hypothyroidism

Investigation

Biochemistry

- Hypercholesterolaemia may be seen in hypothyroidism.
- Thyroxine and TSH evaluation should be performed.
- Creatine kinase elevations may be seen in cases of masticatory muscle myositis.

Immunology

- Serum antibody to 2 M muscle fibres may be demonstrated in masticatory muscle myositis (Shelton & Cardinet 1989).

Physical Procedures

- CSF analysis may reveal increased cellularity and protein suggesting neuritis, encephalitis or neoplasia. Rarely, neoplastic cells (e.g. lymphoma) may be found in CSF.
- Brainstem auditory evoked response testing (BAER) is useful in assessing deafness.

Diagnostic Imaging

- CT or MRI.
- Radiographs of tympanic bullae for evaluation of vestibular disease, facial paralysis and Horner's syndrome.

Management

Therapies are presented under the discussion of specific disorders.

SPECIFIC DISEASES

Masticatory Muscle Atrophy

Mastciatory muscle atrophy may be associated with:

- polymyositis,
- masticatory muscle myositis (MMM),

Table 85.1 Aetiology of selected cranial nerve abnormalities.

Cranial nerve	Clinical sign	Aetiology
Optic (II)	Blindness	Optic neuritis
		Neoplasia
Oculomotor (III)	Strabismus	Hydrocephalus
	Mydriasis	Neoplasia
		Encephalitis
		Trauma
Trigeminal (V)	Masticatory muscle atrophy	Neuritis
	Dropped jaw	Trauma
		Neoplasia
Facial (VII)	Facial paralysis	Idiopathic
		Hypothyroidism
		Otitis media
		Neoplasia
Vestibular (VIII)	Head tilt	
	Nystagmus	(see Box 85.1)
	Strabismus	
Cochlear (VIII)	Deafness	Geriatric
		Hereditary
		Otitis externa/media
Glossopharyngeal (IX)	Dysphagia	Neoplasia
		Encephalitis
Vagus (X)	Dysphagia	Idiopathic
	Dysphonia	Neoplasia
	Laryngeal paralysis	Encephalitis polyneuropathy (e.g. T4)
	Megaoesophagus	
Sympathetic	Horner's syndrome	Otitis media
		C1–T2 cord lesion
		Brachial plexus lesion
		Neck trauma

- hyperadrenocorticism,
- neoplasia of the trigeminal nerve,
- trauma to the trigeminal nerve,
- trigeminal neuritis.

Polymyositis and MMM typically cause chronic, progressive, atrophy of the temporal and masseter muscles. Atrophy may be associated with reduced ability to open the jaw (trismus). Less commonly, acute forms of MMM are associated with pain and swelling. Muscle biopsy reveals characteristic inflammatory changes. MMM is due to immune-mediated attack of the type 2M muscle fibres found only in masticatory muscles. These antibodies may be detected and quantified to confirm the diagnosis. Treatment requires immunosuppressive doses of prednisolone for several weeks. Refractory cases may require addition of other immunosuppressive drugs (e.g. azathioprine).

Unilateral atrophy of masticatory muscles is usually associated with trauma or neoplasia of the trigeminal nerve (Fig. 85.1).

Dropped Jaw

Dropped jaw results from acute neuritis of both trigeminal nerves. The dog is unable to close its mouth but can swallow and lap if its mouth is held closed. Differentiation from physical causes (e.g. foreign body, dislocated jaw, fractured jaw) is important. The condition appears to resolve spontaneously in 2–3 weeks. Persistent or progressive cases warrant diagnostic evaluation for neoplastic cranial nerve

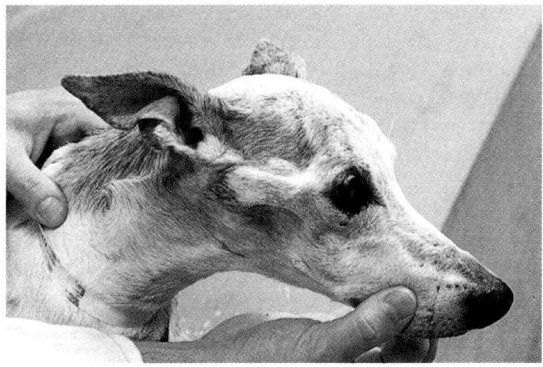

Fig. 85.1 Unilateral masticatory muscle atrophy in a 10-year-old Whippet associated with trigeminal neoplasia.

disease. Affected animals can be managed by applying a soft, elastic strap around the muzzle to substitute for masticatory muscle tone. Neurogenic atrophy becomes apparent after 10–14 days.

Vestibular Disease

Clinical signs result from lesions of either the peripheral (inner ear and vestibular nerve) or central (brainstem and ventral cerebellum) vestibular systems (Fig. 85.2). The head tilt is typically towards the same side as the lesion ('tilt to the trouble' Fig. 85.3). Distinguishing between central and peripheral vestibular disease aids in selection of differential diagnoses, prognosis and diagnostic procedures (Box

85.1). Recognition of central vestibular disease raises the suspicion of encephalitis or neoplastic disease.

Idiopathic (Geriatric) Vestibular Disease

This is the most common form of canine vestibular disease. Old dogs (>10 years) present with a peracute onset of head tilt, nystagmus and disequilibrium, severe enough to result in inability to stand, incessant rolling, and vomiting. Although peripheral in clinical appearance, the location and aetiology of the lesion are unknown. Improvement is often noted in 24–48 h but resolution of clinical signs occurs over a period of 1–4 weeks. Neither antibiotic nor corticosteroid therapy appear to influence the recovery rate. Sedation with acepromazine (0.05–0.1 mg/kg i.m./s.c.) or chlorpromazine (0.5 mg/kg i.m./s.c.) may help settle the animal and alleviate the nausea seen initially. Diagnosis is often based on history and clinical signs. The prognosis is good despite the dramatic initial clinical signs. Occasionally animals may suffer repeat episodes. Persistence or progression of clinical signs should raise concerns of progressive disease (e.g. labyrinthitis, neoplasia).

Otitis Interna (Labyrinthitis)

Otitis interna may be associated with otitis media and otitis externa. Diagnosis requires otic examination and radiography of the tympanic bullae. In difficult cases CT or MRI may provide a more detailed evaluation (Fig. 85.4a,b). Facial paralysis and Horner's syndrome (Table 85.2) may accompany the head tilt.

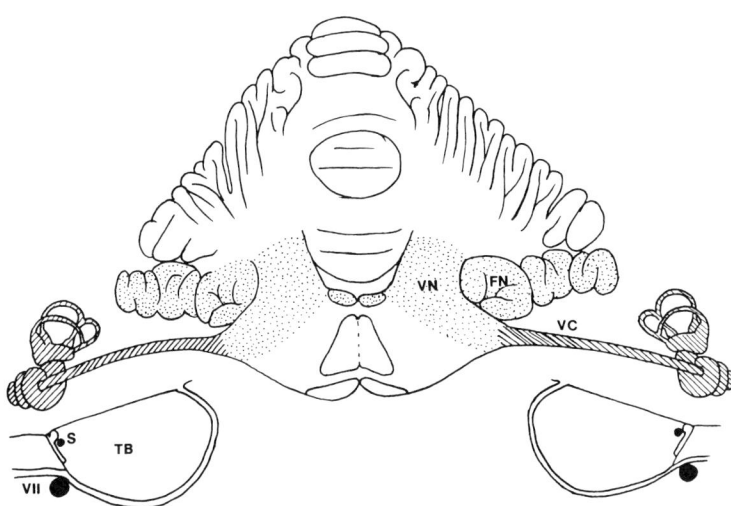

Fig. 85.2 Diagramatic representation of the central and peripheral vestibular systems. VN, vestibular nuclei; TB, tympanic bulla; VII, facial nerve; S, sympathetic nerves; VC, vestibulocochlear nerve (VIII); FN, flocculonodular lobe.

Box 85.1 Vestibular disease in focus.

Central versus peripheral vestibular disease

Nystagmus   Hallmarks of vestibular disease
& head tilt

Peripheral

Nystagmus	Horizontal or rotary
Postural deficits	None
Mentation	Alert, although distressed
Other signs	Possible involvement of cranial nerve VII

Central

Nystagmus	Horizontal, rotary or vertical
Postural deficits	Yes – ipsilateral to the lesion
Mentation	Depressed to stuporous
Other signs	Possible involvement of cranial nerves V, VII, IX, X, XII

NB Damage to the ventral cerebellum (encephalitis, neoplasia) may cause paradoxic vestibular syndrome, where the head tilts away from the side of the lesion. Unilateral hypermetria and/or conscious proprioceptive deficits indicate the side of the lesion

Differential diagnosis of vestibular disease
(1) Otic examination
(2) Radiographs of tympanic bullae
(3) CSF analysis if suspect encephalitis or neoplasia
   NB. Risk of herniation in animals with neoplasia and raised intracranial pressure.
(4) CT or MRI is the best way to evaluate the intracranial cavity as well as tympanic bullae
(5) Myringotomy (& culture) if otitis media
(6) Thyroid evaluation if no structural abnormalities detected

Peripheral vestibular disease
- Idiopathic/geriatric
- Toxic (aminoglycosides)
- Neoplastic
- Inflammatory (otitis media/interna)
- Congenital (Doberman, English Cocker Spaniel)
- Hypothyroidism

Central vestibular disease
- Encephalitis (e.g. distemper, rickettsia, granulomatous meningoencephalitis)
- Neoplasia
- Toxic (metronidazole)
- Hypothyroidism

A variety of Gram-positive and Gram-negative organisms have been isolated from infected ears, sometimes in association with neoplasia or a foreign body. Antibiotic therapy may effect temporary resolution but problem cases often require a combination of surgery (bulla ostectomy to remove inspissated purulent debris) and long-term antibiotic therapy. Even then, some infections persist. Antibiotic therapy is optimally directed by culture and sensitivity. Empirical considerations include enrofloxacin, cephalexin, chloramphenicol and potentiated sulphonamides.

Granulomatous Meningoencephalitis (GME)

GME is an inflammatory disease of the central nervous system characterised by diffuse perivascular accumulations of lymphocytes and macrophages. Young adult, small breed dogs seem to be most commonly affected. Although any part of the CNS can be involved, the cerebellum, vestibular nuclei and cerebral cortex are most commonly affected. Clinical signs reflect multifocal inflammatory disease. A common presentation is seizures and central vestibular disease. Neck pain may reflect meningitis. The overall prognosis for the disease is poor but temporary improvement of clinical signs may result from corticosteroid therapy. Radiation therapy has been used to treat some focal lesions.

Deafness

Deafness results from disease of the receptor organ of Corti (sensorineural deafness) or the mechanical conduc-

Table 85.2 Horner's syndrome.

Signs
   Enophthalmus
   Protrusion of the third eyelid
   Slight narrowing of the palpebral fissure
   Miosis
Horner's syndrome may be associated with lesions at any of the following sites:
   Cervical spinal cord
   T1–T3 spinal cord
   T1–T3 ventral nerve roots and proximal spinal nerves
   Cranial thoracic sympathetic trunk
   Cervical sympathetic trunk
   Middle ear cavity
   Retrobulbar

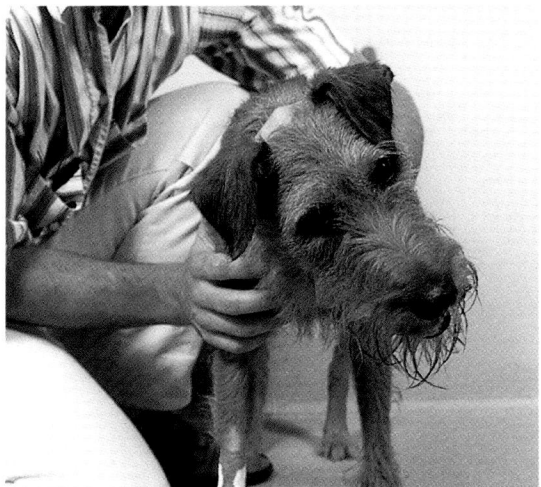

Fig. 85.3 Head tilt in a dog with otitis media and otitis interna of the right ear.

tion system (conduction deafness) which includes the ear canals, tympanic membrane and ear ossicles. Unilateral deafness may be difficult to detect clinically. Electrophysiological assessment is then required. Sensorineural deafness is usually hereditary although it may be toxic. Conduction deafness is acquired as a result of otitis externa/media. Occasionally deafness is encountered in older dogs with no otoscopic evidence of ear disease. Such cases may be the result of age-related degenerative changes in the ear ossicles and sensory apparatus.

Congenital (sensorineural) deafness is recognised in several breeds with the Dalmatian being the best recognised. Spontaneous, postnatal degeneration of the receptor takes place in the first few weeks of life. Bilaterally deaf puppies, easily detected by their lack of response to sounds, can sometimes be trained to hand signals but tend to be aggressive and difficult to manage. Affected puppies are typically euthanased. Studies have suggested up to 7% of Dalmatians exhibit bilateral deafness and up to 21% unilateral deafness.

Laryngeal Paralysis

This is a common cause of upper airway obstruction, especially in older dogs. Clinical signs include an inspiratory rattle on exertion in mild cases or inspiratory dyspnoea at rest in severe cases. Laryngeal dysfunction may result from disease of the brainstem vagal motor nucleus, vagal nerve or the laryngeal muscles themselves. Although respiratory signs may be the sole clinical complaint, laryngeal paralysis may be one manifestation of a generalised neuropathy or myopathy. Several different aetiologies have been recognised (see Table 85.3).

Diagnosis involves demonstrating failure of abduction of the vocal fold under a light plane of anesthesia. Denervation or degeneration of the dorsal cricoarytenoid muscle may be confirmed by detection of abnormal electrical potentials on electromyographic examination. Complete electrodiagnostic evaluation is required to demonstrate generalised neuropathy. Thyroid status should be evaluated. While treatment of any underlying disease is important, surgical treatment involving either

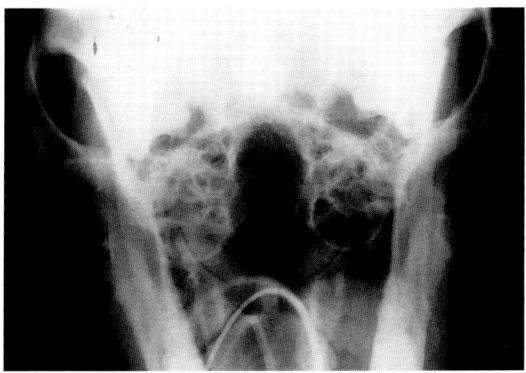

a

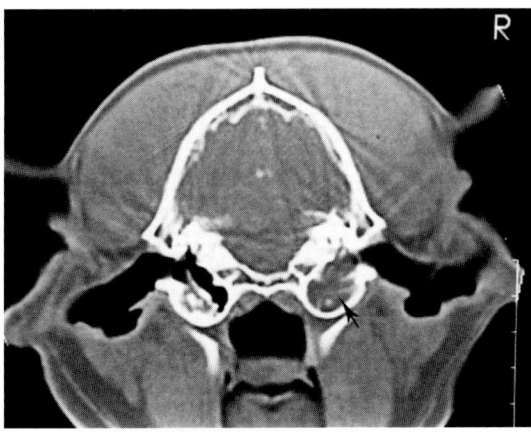

b

Fig. 85.4 (a) Bulla radiographs demonstrating opacification of the right tympanic bulla caused by otitis. (b) CT scan of the same dog illustrating accumulation of a soft tissue density (fluid and debris) in the right tympanic bulla. A lesser accumulation, not seen on the plain radiographs, is also seen in the left bulla.

Spinal muscular atrophy	Hereditary laryngeal paralysis of Bouvier des Flandres, Siberian Husky
Diabetes mellitus	
Hypothyroidism	
Neoplasia	
Polyradiculoneuritis	
Idiopathic	Older, large breed dogs.
Chronic lead intoxication	
Polymyositis	
Myasthenia gravis	

Table 85.3 Differential diagnosis of laryngeal paralysis.

vocal cordectomy or laryngeal 'tie back' may be necessary to alleviate respiratory difficulty.

Cranial Polyneuropathy

This refers to simultaneous disease of multiple cranial nerves. Recognition raises strong suspicion of neoplasia of the floor of the skull where the cranial nerves are in close proximity as they leave the brainstem. Tumours that demonstrate this propensity include lymphoma, meningioma, pituitary carcinoma and metastatic tumours. Diagnosis requires CSF analysis and CT or MRI evaluation. Acute vestibular disease is sometimes seen in association with facial paralysis and hypothyroidism in Cocker Spaniels although a causal relationship has not been proved.

REFERENCE

Shelton, G.D. & Cardinet III, G.H. (1989). Canine masticatory muscle disorders. In: *Current Veterinary Therapy X: Small Animal Practice*, (ed. R.W. Kirk), pp. 816–819. W.B. Saunders, Philadelphia.

Section 12

Dermatology

Edited by Richard Harvey

Chapter 86

Superficial Bacterial Infections

I. S. Mason

AETIOLOGY

Although superficial bacterial infections, or pyodermas, are common, they form some of the most difficult problems encountered in canine practice. They are usually associated with coagulase-positive staphylococci although occasionally other bacteria, including coagulase-negative staphylococci, have been isolated from clinical cases.

> *Staphylococcus intermedius* is isolated from around 90% of affected dogs, while *Staphylococcus aureus* and *Staphylococcus hyicus* have been isolated from 8% and 5% of cases respectively. In some instances, more than one species is found on affected animals.

It has been shown that *S. intermedius* can be readily isolated from the mucosae of most normal dogs and it is likely that these bacteria form a resident population on oral, nasal and anal mucous membranes. Self-grooming is likely to lead to spread of *S. intermedius* from these sites on to the skin and hair. Although *S. intermedius* has been isolated from normal skin and hair, it is likely that this represents contamination from the mucosae rather than true residency status. Hair has been shown to carry large numbers of bacteria. These may originate from the mucous membranes but hairs may also trap bacteria from the environment. The significance of this is unknown as the distal portion of the hair provides a nutrient-poor and arid environment and these bacteria may not be viable. The proximal portion of canine hair may support viable bacteria due to the high relative humidity and temperature along with sweat and sebum which may form a source of nutrients.

PATHOGENESIS

While it is generally accepted that pyoderma is a secondary disorder, there is little scientific information regarding the mechanisms by which normal mucosal commensal micro-organisms become cutaneous pathogens in some individuals. A wide spectrum of underlying diseases may predispose dog skin to infection (Table 86.1).

It is interesting that many of these diseases are common in other mammals such as horses, cats and man. Despite this pyodermas are uncommon in these species. This apparent anomaly may be explained by recent evidence which suggests that canine skin may be inherently more susceptible to infection than that of other species. Canine skin has the thinnest stratum corneum of any mammal yet studied. However, it has many more cell layers than that of other species. It has been postulated that a cell dense, compact, thin stratum corneum is likely to contain scant amounts of intercellular lipid and aqueous material; this has been supported by results of scanning electron microscopical studies. It is probable that the intercellular material of the stratum corneum is important in cutaneous defence. Hence, the dog may be more susceptible to bacterial skin disease than other species as a result of these ultrastructural differences. Moreover, the hair follicle infundibula of canine skin are not sealed with lipid as in other species. Again, this may contribute to the high prevalence of canine pyoderma, particularly folliculitis.

> The pathogenesis of pyoderma is complex but it is likely that the role of the underlying disease is to undermine epidermal defences so facilitating penetration by staphylococcal products.

If the underlying disease is associated with inflammation, then changes in the cutaneous microclimate (increased temperature and humidity) may promote bacterial proliferation. Investigations have shown that intradermal injection of staphylococcal extracts and purified products elicits lesions similar to those seen in clinical cases of pyoderma. Thus, increased numbers of bacteria on the skin surface provide greater amounts of staphylococcal products and the potential for the development of more numerous and more severe lesions. Pruritic primary diseases lead to licking and chewing; in this way the animal inoculates the skin with bacteria from the oral mucosa. The self-trauma and excoriation associated with pruritic disorders will degrade skin barriers. Serum and blood may ooze on to the skin surface and provide a source of nutrient for staphylococci.

The mechanisms by which non-pruritic primary diseases predispose dogs to pyoderma are less well understood and it has been assumed that systemic and endocrine disorders have a deleterious effect on cutaneous immunity and barrier function. Metabolic disease is often associated with immunosuppression and may have an effect on physical barriers within the skin (e.g. defective lipid metabolism may affect epidermal permeability barriers). Alternatively, there may be a more general effect on humoral and cellular immunity. In common with primary causes of pyoderma, metabolic diseases may also lead to changes in the surface micro-environment via effects on epidermal keratinisation and lipogenesis; such changes may promote proliferation of potentially pathogenic bacteria.

Irrespective of the cause, it is likely that once staphylococcal products enter the dermis, they induce inflammation by toxic and immune-mediated mechanisms thereby leading to further changes in the cutaneous microclimate, pruritus and further self-inoculation of bacteria into the lesions.

The term 'primary pyoderma' is used to describe cases where no underlying disease is identified. However, it is preferable to use the term 'idiopathic pyoderma' to refer to such cases. It is probable that primary pyoderma does not exist. *Staphylococcus intermedius* is usually not sufficiently virulent to cause skin disease in a normal host. Some (primary) host factor must be present which allows proliferation and penetration of this bacterium and the development of (secondary) pyoderma; failure to identify this primary factor does not mean that it is absent.

Table 86.1 Examples of underlying diseases which have been implicated in the pathogenesis of pyoderma.

Hypersensitivity	flea bite hypersensitivity
	atopy
	food intolerance
Ectoparasites	demodicosis
	sarcoptic mange (scabies)
	cheyletiellosis
	pediculosis (lice)
Endocrine/systemic diseases	
	hypothyroidism
	hyperadrenocorticism
Anatomical	skin folds
Immunodeficiency	T-lymphocyte defects
	immunoglobulin deficiency

CLINICAL FEATURES

Superficial pyoderma associated with *S. intermedius* may involve infection and inflammation of the superficial portion of the hair follicles (folliculitis) or the epidermis between the hair follicles (impetigo).

- Pustules are one of the hallmarks of pyoderma. However, pustules are quite rare in the dog despite the high incidence of pyoderma. This apparent discrepancy is explained by the fact that pustules are only present in canine skin for a short while before they rupture.
- A range of primary and secondary lesions ranging from papules and vesicles to crust formation, scaling, epidermal collarettes, hyperpigmentation and ulceration also may be present, depending on the aetiology and other factors (see Fig. 86.1). These lesions represent a chronological sequence of lesion development. The absence of pustules does not rule out a diagnosis of pyoderma.

Impetigo

Impetigo or juvenile pustular dermatitis is generally regarded as a minor disorder of young pups which either resolves spontaneously or following simple topical (and occasionally systemic) antimicrobial therapy. While it is generally accepted that pyoderma is a secondary phenomenon, there have been no published studies concerning the primary causes or pathogenesis of impetigo. It is has been stated that it occurs in poorly managed litters and may be

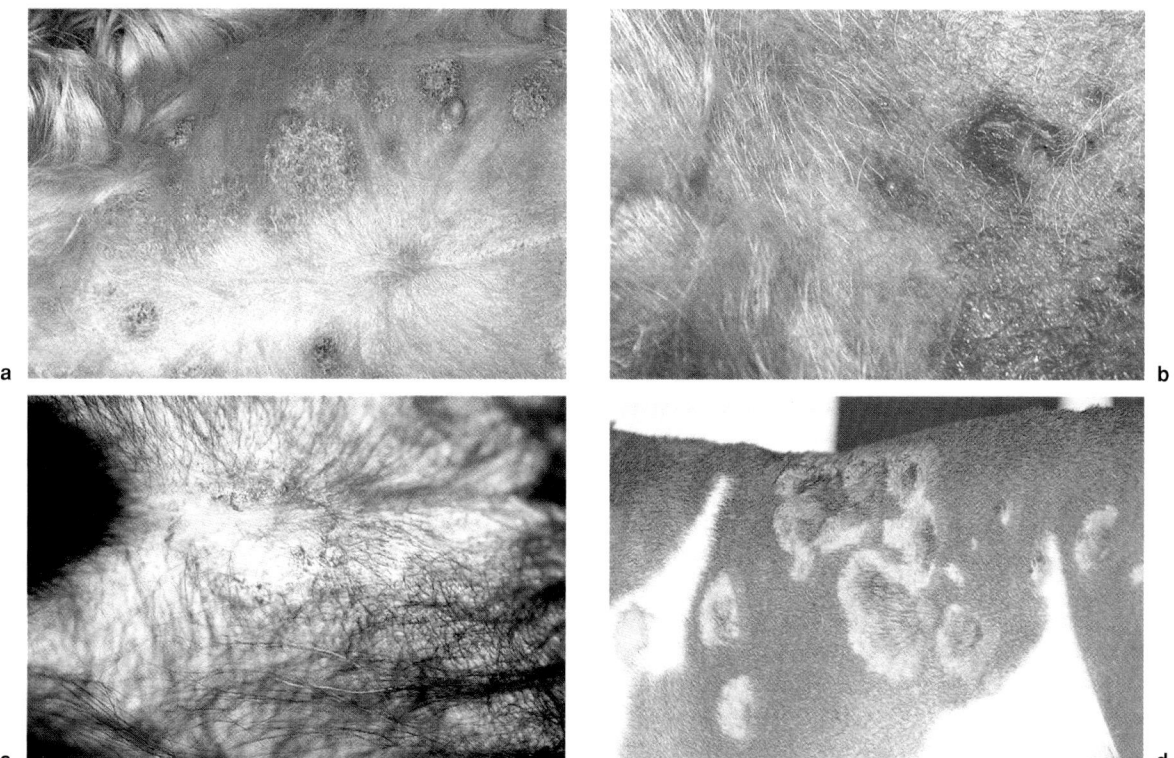

Fig. 86.1 Lesions of superficial pyoderma. Crusted patches (a), polycyclic, erythematous wheals and crusting (b), pustules and epidermal collarettes (c) and multiple patches of alopecia (d). Figures courtesy M. Vroom.

associated with endoparasitism or ectoparasitism, viral infections, poor nutrition and a dirty environment. However, this has not been subject to scientific scrutiny and impetigo is known to occur under conditions of good husbandry.

Impetigo affects the inguinal and axillary regions of sexually immature dogs, usually pups 3–9 months of age. It is not contagious and is characterised by sub-corneal pustules (i.e. pustules not involving the hair follicle) affecting the relatively glabrous areas (principally the groin and axillae). Occasionally mild pruritus may be present. The pustules rupture easily and a dried, yellowish exudate may be present. The pathogenesis is poorly understood. However, the prognosis is good and the disease usually responds to topical antimicrobial therapy. Occasionally, however, systemic treatment is needed.

Superficial Folliculitis

Superficial follicultitis is a more serious disorder and often necessitates life-long therapy. It is extremely common.

Adult dogs are more usually affected. Primary causes include hypersensitivity, ectoparasitism, endocrinopathy (especially hypothyroidism), other systemic disorders and anatomical factors. The primary lesions are papules and pustules affecting the superficial portion of the hair follicle. More typically, scale, crusts, epidermal collarettes and focal areas of hyperpigmentation are present. Superficial follicultitis is often pruritic. Pruritus may be present because the primary cause is inherently pruritic (e.g. atopic dermatitis) or due to the inflammatory effects of staphylococcal metabolites. Virtually any breed, sex or age of dog can be affected.

The clinical history may provide clues as to which primary disorder is present. For example, a pruritic superficial dermatitis in a young adult Terrier with foot chewing and facial lesions is suggestive of atopy. However, a nonpruritic pyoderma in a lethargic Golden Retriever would indicate that thyroid function should be evaluated.

Lesions usually affect the ventral relatively glabrous areas such as the axillae, abdomen and groin, although in some instances the dorsal trunk is affected; this leads to a 'moth-eaten' appearance to the coat of short-coated breeds.

DIAGNOSIS

Clinical history and physical examination are usually sufficient to indicate that impetigo is present. In some instances, biopsy and histopathology, along with culture of pustule contents, may be necessary. Clinical investigations are outlined in Box 86.1.

In the diagnosis of superficial folliculitis the history and physical examination are of paramount importance, enabling the clinician to narrow the differential diagnosis, rank the likely causes and plan the approach to the investigation of the problem.

TREATMENT

Most cases of impetigo recover spontaneously once the underlying management problem has been resolved or at sexual maturity. Topical antimicrobial therapy with an antimicrobial shampoo may be of value. Occasionally short-term systemic antimicrobial therapy is required. Glucocorticoids are contraindicated as they encourage deepening and worsening of the infection.

Management of superficial folliculitis is based on identification and treatment of the underlying cause in association with systemic and topical antimicrobial therapy.

Box 86.1   Superficial bacterial infections: clinical investigations.

Cytology

- examination of the stained contents of pustules may help to rule out other pustular disorders such as pemphigus foliaceus (absence of acantholytic cells) and sterile eosinophilic pustular dermatitis (absence of eosinophils). Neutrophils and bacteria indicate that pyoderma is present.
- examination of stained skin surface smears or adhesive tape specimens may provide positive information that pyoderma is present (bacteria, neutrophils) and help rule our *Malassezia* involvement (absence of yeasts).

Skin scrapings, coat brushings, hair plucks

- to rule out ectoparasites.

Flea control, hypoallergenic diet, intradermal testing, other allergy tests

- to rule out hypersensitivity.

Blood samples, including thyroid testing

- to screen for systemic/endocrine disease.

Bacterial culture and antimicrobial sensitivity testing

- to confirm the presence of staphylococci and aid in selection of antimicrobial agents for therapy.

Histopathology

- often of limited value in pyoderma as non-specific secondary lesions tend to predominate. May be of value in ruling out other pustular diseases such as pemphigus. May suggest or identify underlying cause of pyoderma, e.g. demodicosis or hypothyroidism.

The investigations undertaken and the order in which they are performed depend on the severity of the disorder, the clinician's assessment (based on history and physical examination) of the likely underlying causes and the commitment of the dog's owner. However, the microscopical examination of skin scrapings and other samples to rule out ectoparasites; flea eradication; cytology and dietary trials are probably the *minimum* investigation.

Antimicrobial Treatment of Superficial Pyoderma

This discussion presupposes that the primary cause of the pyoderma has been diligently searched for and, where possible, appropriately treated. The role of antimicrobial treatment is to augment specific therapy directed at the actual cause of the problem, or to manage idiopathic pyoderma. Only the general principles of antimicrobial therapy will be discussed here as the management of pyoderma is covered in detail later in Chapter 89.

Topical Therapy

Topical treatment may be usefully employed as an adjunct to systemic antimicrobial therapy in moderately severe forms of pyoderma or used alone in milder cases.

Creams and Gels

Such treatments are limited to localised lesions. They are difficult to use where hair is present. It is expensive and time consuming to treat large areas of skin. The use of creams and gels is probably confined to acute moist dermatitis or intertrigo (fold pyoderma). Suitable antimicrobial agents include neomycin, mupirocin, fusidic acid and benzoyl peroxide. (Only licensed veterinary products should be used.) These agents may be combined with glucocorticoids. The net effect of use of such antibiotic–steroid combinations is a balance between the immunosuppressive effects of the glucocorticoid and its beneficial role in reducing inflammation and self-trauma.

Shampoos

Where pyoderma is more generalised and affects haired skin, shampoos are the topical treatment of choice. Active principals of antibacterial shampoos include benzoyl peroxide, ethyl lactate, triclosan and chlorhexidine.

> It is important that the entire skin surface of the affected dog is treated and clients should be carefully instructed in the use of these products.

Systemic Therapy

Canine pyoderma should be treated with the correct drug, at the correct dose for the correct duration (guidelines are given in Box 86.2). Suitable drugs and their doses are discussed in Chapter 89. Duration of therapy depends on the depth and severity of infection with deep and severe pyodermas requiring at least 2–3 weeks more therapy than cases of superficial folliculitis. It is seldom necessary to treat cases of impetigo systemically. In general, pyoderma should be treated until 2–3 weeks beyond clinical resolution. Clinicians should be aware that the problem will inevitably recur if the primary problem has not been identified and treated. Strategies for the long-term management of idiopathic pyoderma are covered elsewhere in the section.

PROGNOSIS

In cases of impetigo, the prognosis is excellent, with spontaneous recovery being observed in the majority of cases.

In cases of superficial folliculitis, the prognosis depends on the underlying cause. For example, pyoderma secondary to flea allergic dermatitis may never recur provided that rigorous flea control is enforced. Similarly, pyoderma secondary to hypothyroidism may be 'cured' as long as adequate thyroxine supplementation is administered. Alternatively, pyoderma secondary to an incurable systemic disease, neoplasm or atopic dermatitis may be difficult to

Box 86.2 Guidelines for the antimicrobial treatment of superficial pyoderma.

> - Investigate possible primary causes thoroughly.
> - Treat primary cause specifically.
> - Evaluate severity of case. In mild cases, topical medication alone may suffice. In more severe cases, topical and systemic treatment may be necessary initially.
> - Regularly monitor response.
> - Discontinue systemic therapy 2–3 weeks after lesions resolve.
> - Evaluate effect of systemic therapy alone.
> - Gradually decrease frequency of topical agents (shampoos etc.).
> - Avoid using glucocorticoids.

control. Such cases may require long-term antimicrobial therapy.

Superficial folliculitis will usually recur unless the underlying cause is identified and treated. Before con-demning an animal to life-long symptomatic antimicrobial therapy, the clinician must ensure that all appropriate steps have been taken to identify the primary problem.

Chapter 87

Superficial Fungal Infections

R. Bond

INTRODUCTION

Mammalian skin is constantly exposed to many species of fungi but relatively few are able to induce cutaneous disease. Pathogens such as dermatophytes may be acquired from environmental or animal reservoirs. Alternatively, the resident microflora may include potential pathogens such as *Malassezia pachydermatis* which putatively induce disease subsequent to failure of the host's cutaneous defence mechanisms. This chapter will be limited to discussions of the most common superficial fungal diseases in the dog, namely dermatophytosis and *Malassezia* dermatitis.

DERMATOPHYTOSIS

Aetiology

Dermatophytosis is the infection of the hair, nail or stratum corneum by a fungus of the genera *Microsporum*, *Trichophyton* or *Epidermophyton*. Dermatophytes have adapted to digest keratin and are widely distributed in the environment. The species most often isolated from dogs in the UK are *M. canis* and *T. mentagrophytes* (Table 87.1) while *T. erinacei* and *M. persicolor* are less often seen. However, there is geographic variability in the relative incidence of the dermatophytes species; for example, *M. gypseum* occurs frequently in the southern US (Lewis *et al.* 1991) whereas it is rarely isolated from dogs in the UK (Sparkes *et al.* 1993). Occasionally, more than one species may be isolated from the same host.

Epidemiology

Dermatophytes may be classified according to their natural habitat and host preferences:

- Geophilic. Species which primarily exist in soil (e.g. *M. gypseum*)
- Zoophilic. Species adapted to animals (e.g. *M. canis*, *T. mentagrophytes*)
- Anthropophilic. Species adapted to humans (e.g. *T. rubrum*)

The zoophilic and anthropophilic species are believed to have evolved from soil organisms. The anthropophilic species tend to have a narrow host range whereas many zoophilic dermatophytes such as *M. canis* and *T. mentagrophytes* have retained affinity for keratin of both animal and humans and frequently infect other species. The zoonotic capacity of dermatophytes, especially *M. canis*, is of considerable public health importance. Exposure to the infective propagules may result from contact with an infected animal, fomite or from environmental contamination.

- Infected hairs, scales and crusts may harbour viable arthrospores for long periods; Sparkes *et al.* (1994a) demonstrated that *M. canis* arthroconidia on cat hairs may remain viable for over 12 months.
- Cats are an important source of *M. canis* infections and this dermatophyte is highly contagious (Wright 1989; Sparkes *et al.* 1993).
- Dogs with an outdoor lifestyle may be exposed to geophilic dermatophytes by digging and rooting, and dogs which hunt may acquire zoophilic species from wild rodents (Wright 1989; Foil 1990).

Dermatophyte	Bristol (n = 475)*		London (n = 49)†		Louisiana (n = 70)‡	
	Number	%	Number	%	Number	%
Microsporum canis	309	65	12	24	30	43
M. gypseum	3	<1	2	4	31	44
M. persicolor	12	<1	4	8	NR	–
Trichophyton erinacei	15	<1	5	10	§	§
T. mentagrophytes	114	24	23	47	8§	11§

Table 87.1 Frequency of isolation of various dermatophyte species from dogs at three centres in the United Kingdom and North America.

*, Sparkes *et al.* (1993); †, Royal Veterinary College Dermatology Unit unpublished data 1988–1994; ‡, Lewis *et al.* (1991),§ reported only as *Trichophyton* species; NR, not reported.

- Young dogs appear to be predisposed to dermatophytosis (Lewis *et al.* 1991; Sparkes *et al.* 1993), presumably reflecting differences in non-specific defence or lack of acquired immunity.
- In the UK, Jack Russell Terriers seem predisposed to dermatophytosis acquired from wild animals and Yorkshire Terriers appear to be at increased risk from *M. canis* infections (Wright 1989; Sparkes *et al.* 1993).

Pathogenesis

The initial event in the colonisation of the stratum corneum is the adherence of arthroconidia to corneocytes (Hay 1992). Germination results in the formation of hyphae which penetrate the layers of the stratum corneum. Invasion of corneocytes is aided by the production of keratinases. Adherent arthroconidia which fail to germinate will be shed by the normal process of epidermal desquamation. Most dermatophyte species isolated from dogs also invade hair in the anagen phase; however, *M. persicolor* and *E. floccosum* cannot and are confined to the stratum corneum (Bond *et al.* 1992). Non-specific defences such as complement and unsaturated transferrin generally restrict dermatophytes to keratinised tissues (Hay 1992).

Both humoral and cellular immune responses are induced by dermatophyte antigens; however, serum antibody is largely ineffective in protecting the host, presumably because the site of infection is isolated from the vascular system (Jones 1993). Humans who mount decisive delayed-type hypersensitivity responses are able to eliminate the infection, whereas patients with defective cellular immunity develop chronic or recurrent dermatophytosis. It is probable that a similar range of immune responses occur in dogs, accounting for the spectrum of acute, self-limiting and more chronic infections also seen in this species.

Clinical Signs

Clinical signs of dermatophytosis vary markedly in type, extent, severity and duration depending on fungal species and strain virulence factors and the response of the host.

- Skin lesions in dogs tend to be localised but there is marked individual variability in the degree of inflammation and alopecia.
- The classic 'ringworm' lesion consists of a variably erythematous, circular patch of alopecia and scaling which spreads peripherally and heals centrally and is usually associated with *M. canis* in the dog (Fig. 87.1).
- Variable degrees of 'cigarette-ash'-like crust may form.
- *Trichophyton* infections frequently cause severe inflammatory lesions of the face or limbs which slowly

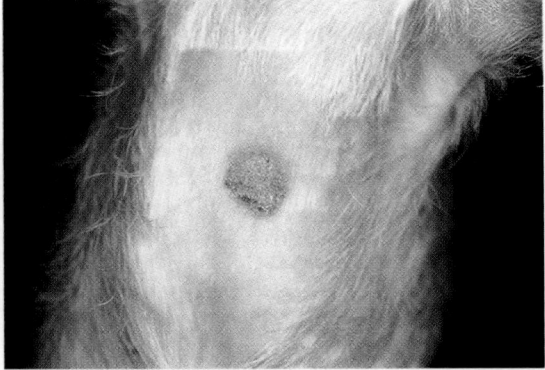

Fig. 87.1 Classical lesions of dermatophytosis. A well demarcated, circular patch of erythema and scaling caused, in this case, by *Trichophyton mentagrophytes*. The area has been clipped. Figure courtesy R. Bond.

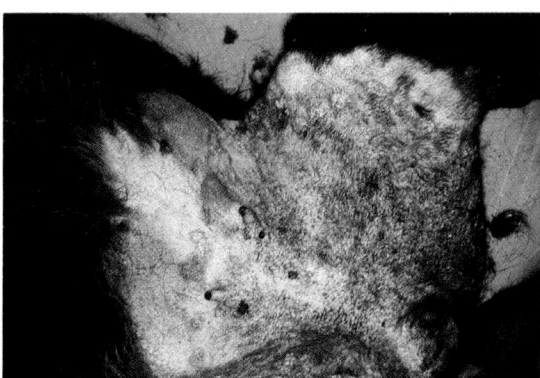

Fig. 87.2   Severe lesions of dermatophytosis. In this case infection with *Trichophyton erinacei* has resulted in extensive alopecia, hyperpigmentation and crusting. Figure courtesy R. Bond.

advance and tend to persist for long periods (Fig. 87.2). Such lesions on the face may be misdiagnosed as autoimmune diseases.

* *Microsporum canis* lesions in young dogs and *M. persicolor* infections may present as localised or generalised scaling with minimal alopecia and erythema (Wright 1989; Bond *et al.* 1992).
* A kerion is a form of dermatophytosis with deep, suppurant inflammatory lesions which present as single or multiple nodules, often caused by *M. gypseum* (Foil 1990).
* Secondary staphylococcal infection may complicate any lesion type. Onychomycosis (infection of the claw) is uncommon and may occur either alone or in association with infection of pedal skin.

Diagnosis

Dermatophytosis should be considered in the differential diagnosis of localised or generalised skin lesions characterised by alopecia, scaling, folliculitis/furunculosis or nodules. The epidermal collarette lesion of staphylococcal pyoderma in the dog is often mistaken for dermatophytosis. Diagnosis is based upon demonstration of fungal elements in skin or hair using direct light or fluorescence microscopy, Wood's light examination, culture or by histopathological examination of skin biopsy specimens. Although culture is probably the most sensitive method, demonstration of tissue *invasion* is an important consideration when dermatophytes are cultured because coat contamination may occur without infection.

Wood's Lamp Examination

Hairs infected with some strains of *M. canis* fluoresce with an apple-green colour when illuminated with ultraviolet light, possibly due to the presence of the tryptophan metabolite, pteridin. However, over 50% of *M. canis* isolates of canine origin and the *Trichophyton* species usually recovered from dogs do not fluoresce (Sparkes *et al.* 1993).

> Fluorescent hairs strongly suggests dermatophytosis caused by *M. canis* whereas absence of fluorescence has little diagnostic value.

Skin scales and fungal cultures do not fluoresce. Examinations should be performed in a darkened room and the lamp should be allowed to warm up for 5–10 min. Hairs that fluoresce are ideal material for microscopy and culture.

Direct Microscopy

Fungal spores and hyphae may be visualised in hair and scale samples microscopically. Arthrospores on hair shafts provide convincing evidence of dermatophytosis. Care must be taken not to confuse saprophytic fungal hyphae and conidia with dermatophytes; dermatophytes never produce macroconidia in tissue.

> Fungal elements can be difficult to visualise and may not be found even when samples are examined by experienced mycologists.

The use of fluorescent stains such as calcafluor white improves the sensitivity of direct microscopy (Sparkes *et al.* 1994b); however, application of this excellent technique is limited by the requirement for a microscope with an ultraviolet source.

Fungal Culture

Skin scales and hairs obtained by plucking, scraping or brushing can be incubated on a variety of media. Most mycology laboratories routinely use Sabouraud's dextrose (glucose–peptone) agar supplemented with cycloheximide and chloramphenicol to inhibit saprophytic moulds and bacteria.

Plates should be incubated at around 26°C for up to 4 weeks. Identification is based on gross colonial and microscopic morphology, especially the structure of macroconidia. Dermatophytes usually form flat white colonies within 10–14 days.

> On dermatophyte test medium, the development of white colonies coincident with a red colour change in the agar within 10–14 days suggests that a dermatophyte may have been isolated.

However, it is not possible to observe the reverse pigmentation of the colony and some strains produce few macroconidia on this medium, making identification without sub-culture more difficult. False-negative cultures may result from overgrowth of contaminants or insufficient sample material. Contamination of the hair coat by a dermatophyte without tissue invasion may result in false-positive diagnoses.

Biopsy

Histopathological examination of skin biopsy specimens may provide rapid and conclusive proof of tissue invasion, although special stains are occasionally required for identification of hyphae and spores. Inflammatory patterns recognised include perifolliculitis, folliculitis and furunculosis, or a hyperplastic superficial perivascular to superficial diffuse dermatitis with mononuclear cells predominating (Yager & Wilcock 1994a).

Treatment

Dermatophyte infections often resolve within 1–3 months. However, some infections, especially those caused by *Trichophyton* sp. and *M. persicolor*, and onychomycoses, are often very persistent.

- Trial therapy is not appropriate in dermatophytosis because the therapeutic agents are expensive and potentially toxic and long-term treatment is often needed.
- A combination of clipping, systemic and topical therapy is most appropriate.
- Localised lesions in dogs should be clipped to a margin of 5 cm to remove infected hairs, and whole body clips should be considered if lesions are generalised.

Treatment options and doses are given in Table 87.2.

Topical Therapy

Topical therapeutics reduce contamination of the environment and may aid resolution of the disease. Localised lesions may be treated with miconazole or clotrimazole-containing creams or lotions applied daily. Generalised infections are more readily treated using enilconazole (Imaverol™) applied as a dip at 3-day intervals. Chlorhexidine is widely recommended but there are doubts over its efficacy as a sole treatment; DeBoer and Moriello (1995) showed that a 2% chlorhexidine shampoo used twice weekly did not influence the course of experimental feline dermatophytosis due to *M. canis*.

Griseofulvin

Griseofulvin, a fungistatic antibiotic which inhibits cell division by disruption of spindle and cytoplasmic microtubule function (Elewski 1993), is probably the systemic treatment of first choice. The drug is poorly water-soluble and fatty meals enhance its absorption. The manufacturer's recommended dose of 15–20 mg/kg daily is substantially less than that suggested in most textbooks; Foil (1990) suggests 25–60 mg/kg twice daily. Harris and Riegelman (1969) reported that dogs metabolise griseofulvin more rapidly than most other species tested and proposed a dose of 90 mg/kg. Griseofulvin is teratogenic and is contraindicated during pregnancy. Most dogs tolerate this drug well although side-effects including haematological and gastrointestinal signs are occasionally seen. Therapy should be continued for 2 weeks after resolution of infection (clinical remission plus negative culture), and weeks or months of treatment may be required in some cases.

Ketoconazole

Ketoconazole has been used as an alternative to griseofulvin; however, this drug is not currently licensed for use in dogs in the UK. Ketoconazole inhibits the synthesis of ergosterol which is required for the integrity of the cell membrane (Elewski 1993). Suggested doses range from 10 to 30 mg/kg daily (Greene 1990). Side-effects include anorexia, vomiting, hepatotoxicity and inhibition of adrenal and gonadal hormone synthesis (Greene 1990). Ketoconazole is contra-indicated in pregnancy. This drug should only be considered when griseofulvin is either not tolerated or not effective.

Other Systemic Therapeutic Agents

Itraconazole and terbinafine have proved very useful for the treatment of dermatophytosis in humans (Elewski 1993) and studies are required to evaluate their potential in dogs.

Table 87.2 Treatment options and doses for superficial fungal infections in the dog.

Drug	Route	Dermatophytosis	Malassezia dermatitis	Comments
Griseofulvin	Oral	25–60 mg/kg b.i.d.*	Not indicated	Fatty meal aids absorption. Contraindicated in pregnancy.
Ketoconazole	Oral	10–30 mg/kg†	5–10 mg/kg b.i.d.‡	Excellent in Malassezia dermatitis. (Not licensed in UK) Expensive. Contraindicated in pregnancy.
Miconazole/ chlorhexidine (2%/2%)	Topical (shampoo)	Not reported	Every 2–3 days, initially	Excellent in Malassezia dermatitis. Not reported but probably useful in dermatophytosis
Chlorhexidine (0.5–2%)	Topical (shampoo)	Every 1–3 days	Every 1–3 days	Doubtful efficacy in dermatophytosis. Variable response in Malassezia dermatitis; highest concentrations best.
Selenium sulphide	Topical (shampoo)	Not reported	Every 2–3 days initially	Variable response in Malassezia dermatitis. More effective if followed by enilconazole rinse.
Enilconazole (0.2% emulsion)	Topical (rinse)	Every 3 days	Every 3 days	In Malassezia cases, use after shampoo if marked scaling or greasy exudate. Not licensed for Malassezia dermatitis.
Miconazole (2% cream/ supension)	Topical	Twice daily	Twice daily	Focal lesions only.
Clotrimazole (1% cream)	Topical	Twice daily	Twice daily	Focal lesions only. Not licensed for dogs in UK.

*, Foil (1990); †, Greene (1990); ‡, Mason (1993).

MALASSEZIA DERMATITIS

Aetiology

The monopolar-budding yeast, *Malassezia pachydermatis* (formerly *Pityrosporum canis*), has long been implicated as a pathogen within the canine external ear canal but it is only in recent years that it has been associated with skin disease of other regions (Dufait 1983; Mason & Evans 1991). There is now a large body of evidence, albeit circumstantial, to suggest that this yeast is an important cause of pruritic dermatitis in certain dogs.

Epidemiology

The high frequency of isolation of *M. pachydermatis* from the anus, ear canal, lip and interdigital skin of healthy dogs suggests that it normally inhabits the skin and mucosae (Dufait 1985; Bond *et al.* 1995c). Under normal circumstances, physical, chemical and immunological defence mechanisms restrict skin colonisation and infection by yeasts and other microbes (Jenkinson 1992). Although the factors which allow the transition of a cutaneous commensal to parasite are poorly understood, dogs colonised by *M. pachydermatis* are at risk of infection should the yeast acquire greater virulence or if host defence is compromised. *M. pachydermatis* should be considered to be an opportunistic rather than a primary pathogen.

The breed incidence *Malassezia* dermatitis varies with geographical location; in one US study, Basset Hounds and Dachshunds were over-represented (Plant *et al.* 1992) whereas others have recognised Poodles to be commonly affected (Dufait 1983). In a series of 40 cases seen at the Royal Veterinary College, West Highland White Terriers, Cocker Spaniels and Basset Hounds were significantly over-represented when compared with the hospital population.

Concurrent diseases such as atopic disease and other hypersensitivities, endocrinopathies and keratinisation disorders are frequently recognised in dogs with *Malassezia* dermatitis. It is not clear whether these diseases favour the development of abnormal yeast populations or merely occur coincidentally; however, these disorders are also believed to favour the development of staphylococcal pyoderma in the dog. In some cases, no other diseases are apparent. One report suggested that prior antibacterial therapy may favour the yeast (Plant *et al.* 1992) but this requires further study as high bacterial counts often co-exist with elevated yeast populations (Bond *et al.* 1995b).

Pathogenesis

Pathogenic mechanisms proposed for *M. pachydermatis* in the dog are currently speculative and have largely been extrapolated from studies of other cutaneous microbes in a variety of host species. Microscopic studies have shown that the yeast is located in the stratum corneum in close association with corneocytes and the ability to adhere to squames may be an important factor in initial colonisation. *In vitro* studies have shown that *M. pachydermatis* produces a variety of enzymes including esterases and lipases (Bond & Anthony 1995); these proteins and other products of yeast metabolism could cause skin damage directly or indirectly. Hypersensitivity to *M. furfur* is believed to be important in the pathogenesis of the 'head–neck form' of human atopic dermatitis (Kieffer *et al.* 1990) and it is tempting to speculate that some atopic dogs may become sensitised to allergens from *M. pachydermatis*.

Clinical Signs

- Affected skin is usually erythematous with varying degrees of alopecia and scaling (Fig. 87.3a&b).
- Hyperpigmentation and lichenification are frequently observed in animals with chronic disease and seem particularly common in West Highland White Terriers.
- A greasy exudate which tends to mat the lower portion of the hair is often a feature of lesions in intertriginous areas.
- Interdigital lesions are common and in more severe cases, erythema and alopecia may extend to affect the accessory carpal areas and medial aspects of the limbs. Some dogs with severe limb lesions develop marked skin thickening, resulting in the formation of erythematous, scaling, alopecic ridges.

Abdominal lesions often initially consist of symmetrical, well-demarcated, circular or elliptical areas of ery-

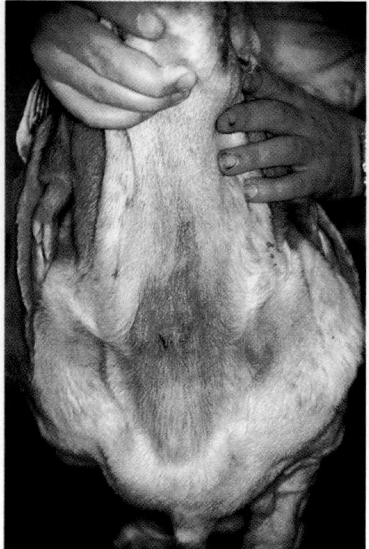

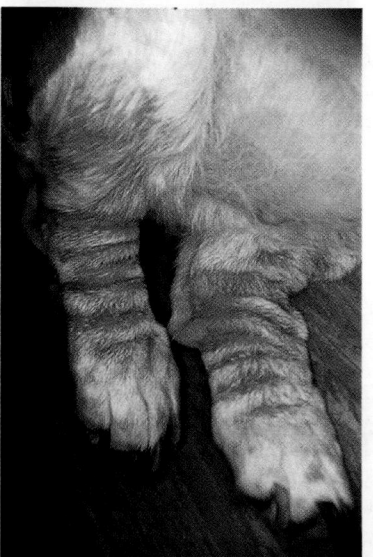

Fig. 87.3 Erythema, alopecia and greasy exudation on the ventral neck (a) and limbs (b) of a Basset Hound with *Malassezia pachydermatis* dermatitis. Figures courtesy R. Bond.

thema which develop into scaly plaques. Alternatively, more diffuse erythema with scattered papules are seen. Patches of erythema, alopecia and exudation may be found in the ventral neck, especially in Basset Hounds (Bond *et al.* 1995b) and Cocker Spaniels. Concurrent erythematous otitis externa with variable ceruminous discharge is common and pinnal lichenification and scaling may develop in some dogs. Frenzied facial pruritus is an uncommon manifestation of *Malassezia* dermatitis; some dogs will collapse when the face is stroked and these animals are often incorrectly diagnosed as having neurological disease. Peripheral lymphadenopathy is common in severe cases.

Diagnosis

Malassezia dermatitis should be considered in the differential diagnosis of pruritic dermatitis in the dog, especially if lesions affect the face, feet, ventrum or intertriginous areas.

> The clinical signs of *Malassezia* dermatitis may closely resemble, or coexist with allergic diseases, pyoderma and primary and secondary disorders of keratinisation.

Based on current knowledge, a diagnosis of *Malassezia* dermatitis is appropriate when a dog with elevated *M. pachydermatis* populations on lesional skin shows a good clinical and mycological response to appropriate antifungal therapy. A variety of methods can be used to estimate populations of the yeast.

Cytological Techniques

Cytology allows *M. pachydermatis* populations to be rapidly assessed. The author prefers a tape-strip technique; clear adhesive tape (Scotch tape is easiest to handle) is applied to lesional skin, removed, stained with Diff-Quik and examined using the high-power objective. The yeast has a characteristic 'peanut'-shaped morphology (Fig. 87.4). It is difficult to locate more than just an occasional *M. pachydermatis* cell on healthy truncal skin using this technique and populations should be considered elevated if the yeast is readily identified (Bond *et al.* 1994). Dry scrapes and impression smears are alternative cytological techniques.

Cultural Techniques

Standard swabbing techniques may enable isolation of the yeast but provide no data on population sizes. The contact plate method allows quantitative cultural assessments to be obtained simply in clinical cases; small agar plates are directly applied to lesional skin for 10s and incubated at 32–37°C for 3–7 days (Bond *et al.* 1994). Contact plates counts should be interpreted based on the anatomical site sampled; in healthy dogs, axillae and groin populations are

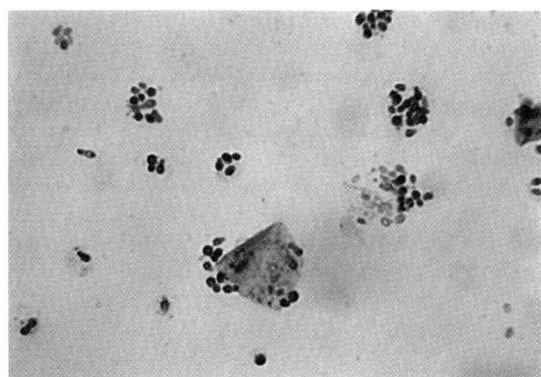

Fig. 87.4 Photomicrograph of *Malassezia pachydermatis* associated with squames. Diff Quik stain, high dry (×40) power. Figure courtesy P. Hill.

typically less than 1 colony-forming unit (cfu)/cm² but large populations can be found on lip folds and interdigital skin (Bond *et al.* 1995c). Profuse growth on plates from affected truncal skin should prompt trial therapy. The detergent scrub technique is useful for research purposes but the need for rapid sample processing (Bond *et al.* 1995a) makes it unsuitable for general use. Sabouraud's dextrose agar is widely used but occasional more lipid-dependent strains grow poorly on this medium, and the author prefers modified Dixon's agar (Bond *et al.* 1994; Bond & Anthony 1995).

Histopathology

The yeast may also be visualised in the epidermal stratum corneum by the histopathological examinations of skin biopsy specimens (Yager & Wilcock 1994b). Other features include epidermal hyperplasia and spongiosis, and a mixed superficial perivascular infiltrate of mononuclear cells. Neutrophils, eosinophils and mast cells may also be present in increased numbers. In some cases seen by the author, yeasts were not evident in histological sections, possibly due to loss of the superficial stratum corneum layers during processing. Thus, identification of the yeast should prompt trial therapy but failure to visualise the yeast histopathologically does not exclude its presence and possible pathogenic role.

Trial Therapy

Although trial therapy is required to confirm the diagnosis, a limitation of the trial therapy approach is that some antifungal agents have other actions. For example, ketoconazole is known to have immunomodulatory effects (Mason & Stewart 1993) and miconazole/chlorhexidine shampoo has substantial antibacterial activity (Bond *et al.* 1995b). It is also possible that elevated populations are not a prerequisite for a beneficial effect of anti-*Malassezia* therapy; for example, populations of *M. furfur* in humans with seborrhoeic dermatitis are usually comparable to those of normal skin but the condition responds well to anti-*Malassezia* therapy (Ingham & Cunningham 1993). It is not clear whether this reflects other effects of antifungal agents or an abnormal host response to the yeast.

Therapy

Topical Therapy

Topical therapy can be used alone or in association with systemic treatment (Table 87.2). The superficial location of the yeast renders it susceptible to topical therapy and shampoos are particularly indicated in dogs with marked exudation and malodour. A recent study showed that a 2% miconazole and 2% chlorhexidine shampoo (Sebolyse™) is an effective treatment for *Malassezia* dermatitis in Basset Hounds (Bond *et al.* 1995b). Good results have also been obtained in other breeds and the author currently considers this product (where available) to be the treatment of choice. The dual activity of this product against both the yeast and coagulase-positive staphylococci is important because many dogs also have elevated cutaneous bacterial populations.

Selenium sulphide shampoos are useful in some cases (Mason 1993; Bond *et al.* 1995b), especially if the dog is subsequently rinsed in a 0.2% emulsion of enilconazole (Imaverol™). Ketoconazole shampoos are also helpful but are not licensed for veterinary use. Attention to the frequency and duration of application of shampoos is essential if optimal results are to be obtained; as a general rule, 10 min application periods at 2- or 3-day intervals are required until the disease is controlled. Treatments suitable for focal lesions include enilconazole dips, and miconazole or clotrimazole creams and lotions. Chlorhexidine shampoos are often disappointing when used alone but the 4% surgical scrub formulation is useful in some cases.

Systemic Therapy

Ketoconazole (see section on dermatophytosis) is usually very effective when given orally at 5–10 mg/kg twice daily with food for 14–28 days. This drug is particularly helpful in severe cases, where the response to treatment is often dramatic. Disadvantages of oral ketoconazole include the potential for side-effects and the high cost in large dogs.

Preliminary reports suggest that oral itraconazole is an effective alternative but this is also expensive (Mason & Stewart 1993).

In dogs with concurrent diseases, dermatological signs may persist despite successful antimicrobial therapy, and clinical remission may not be achieved until such conditions are also treated. Many cases of *Malassezia* dermatitis are recurrent and require regular maintenance therapy, especially when any predisposing factors cannot be identified or corrected. Topical therapy is preferable to oral ketoconazole for long-term management and the treatment regimens should be tailored for the individual.

REFERENCES

Bond, R. & Anthony, R.M. (1995). Characterisation of markedly lipid-dependant *Malassezia pachydermatis* isolates from healthy dogs. *Journal of Applied Bacteriology*, **78**, 537–542.

Bond, R., Middleton, D., Scarff, D.H. & Lamport, A.I. (1992). Chronic dermatophytosis due to *Microsporum persicolor* infection in three dogs. *Journal of Small Animal Practice*, **33**, 571–576.

Bond, R., Collin, N.S. & Lloyd, D.H. (1994). Use of contact plates for the quantitative culture of *M. pachydermatis* from canine skin. *Journal of Small Animal Practice*, **35**, 68–72.

Bond, R., Lloyd, D.H. & Plummer, J.M. (1995a). Evaluation of a detergent scrub technique for the quantitation of *M. pachydermatis* on canine skin. *Research in Veterinary Science*, **58**, 133–137.

Bond, R., Rose, J.F., Ellis, J.W. & Lloyd, D.H. (1995b). Comparison of two shampoos for treatment of *M. pachydermatis*-associated seborrhoeic dermatitis in basset hounds. *Journal of Small Animal Practice*, **36**, 99–104.

Bond, R., Saijonmaa-Koulumies, L.E.M. & Lloyd, D.H. (1995c). Population sizes and frequency of *M. pachydermatis* at skin and mucosal sites on healthy dogs. *Journal of Small Animal Practice*, **36**, 147–150.

DeBoer, D. & Moriello, K.A. (1995). Inability of topical treatment to influence the course of experimental feline dermatophytosis. *Journal of the American Veterinary Medical Association*, **207**, 52–57.

Dufait, R. (1983). *Pityrosporon canis* as the cause of canine chronic dermatitis. *Veterinary Medicine/Small Animal Clinician*, **78**, 1055–1057.

Dufait, R. (1985). Presence de *M. pachydermatis* (syn. *Pityrosporum canis*) sur les poils et les plumes d'animaux domestiques. *Bulletin de la Sociéte Francaise de Mycologie Medicale*, **14**, 19–22.

Elewski, B.M. (1993). Mechanisms of action of systemic antifungal agents. *Journal of the American Academy of Dermatology*, **31**, S28–34.

Foil, C.S. (1990). Dermatophytosis. In: *Infectious Diseases of the Dog and Cat*, (ed. C.E. Greene), pp. 659–669. WB Saunders, Philadelphia.

Greene, C.E. (1990). Antifungal chemotherapy. In: *Infectious Diseases of the Dog and Cat*, (ed. C.E. Greene), pp. 649–658. WB Saunders, Philadelphia.

Harris, P.A. & Riegelman, S. (1969). Metabolism of griseofulvin in dogs. *Journal of Pharmaceutical Sciences*, **58**, 93–96.

Hay, R. (1992). Fungi and fungal infections of the skin. In: *The Skin Microflora and Microbial Skin Disease*, (ed. W.C. Noble), pp. 232–263. Cambridge University Press, Cambridge.

Ingham, E. & Cunningham, A.C. (1993). *Malassezia furfur. Journal of Medical and Veterinary Mycology*, **31**, 265–288.

Jenkinson, D.McE. (1992). The basis of the skin surface ecosystem. In: *The Skin Microflora and Microbial Skin Disease*, (ed. W.C. Noble), pp. 1–32. Cambridge University Press, Cambridge.

Jones, H.E. (1993). Immune response and host resistance of humans to dermatophyte infection. *Journal of the American Academy of Dermatology*, **28**, S12–18.

Kieffer, M., Bergbrant, I., Faergemann, J., *et al.* (1990). Immune reactions to *Pityrosporum ovale* in adult patients with atopic and seborrhoeic dermatitis. *Journal of the American Academy of Dermatology*, **22**, 739–742.

Lewis, D.T., Foil, C.S. & Hosgood, G. (1991). Epidemiology and clinical features of dermatophytosis in dogs and cats at Louisiana State University: 1981–1990. *Veterinary Dermatology*, **2**, 53–58.

Mason, K.V. (1993). Cutaneous *Malassezia*. In: *Current Veterinary Dermatology*, (eds C.E. Griffin, K.W. Kwochka & J.M. MacDonald), pp. 44–48. Mosby Year Book, St. Louis.

Mason, K.V. & Evans, A.G. (1991). Dermatitis associated with *Malassezia pachydermatis* in 11 dogs. *Journal of the American Animal Hospital Association*, **27**, 13–20.

Mason, K.V. & Stewart, J.J. (1993). *Malassezia* and canine dermatitis. In: *Advances in Veterinary Dermatology*, Vol. 2, (eds P.J. Ihrke, I.S. Mason & S.D. White), pp. 399–402. Pergamon Press, Oxford.

Plant, J.D., Rosenkrantz, W.S. & Griffin, C.E. (1992). Factors associated with and prevalence of high *Malassezia pachydermatis* numbers on dog skin. *Journal of the American Veterinary Medical Association*, **201**, 879–882.

Sparkes, A.H., Gruffydd-Jones, T.J., Shaw, S.E., Wright, A.I. & Stokes, C.R. (1993). Epidemiological and diagnostic features of canine and feline dermatophytosis in the United Kingdom from 1956 to 1991. *Veterinary Record*, **133**, 57–61.

Sparkes, A.H., Werret, G., Stokes, C.R. & Gruffydd-Jones, T.J. (1994a). *Microsporum canis*: inapparent carriage by cats and the viability of arthrospores. *Journal of Small Animal Practice*, **35**, 397–401.

Sparkes, A.H., Werret, G., Stokes, C.R. & Gruffydd-Jones, T.J. (1994b). Improved sensitivity in the diagnosis of dermatophytosis by fluorescence microscopy with calcafluor white. *Veterinary Record*, **134**, 307–308.

Wright, A.I. (1989). Ringworm in dogs and cats. *Journal of Small Animal Practice*, **30**, 242–249.

Yager, J.A. & Wilcock, B.P. (1994a). Folliculitis, furunculosis, and sebaceous adenitis. In: *Colour Atlas and Text of Surgical Pathology of the Dog and Cat. Volume 1: Dermatopathology and Skin Tumours.* pp. 179–198. Mosby Year Book, London.

Yager, J.A. & Wilcock, B.P. (1994b). Perivascular dermatitis. In: *Colour Atlas and Text of Surgical Pathology of the Dog and Cat. Volume 1: Dermatopathology and Skin Tumours.* pp. 74–76. Mosby Year Book, London.

Chapter 88

Deep Pyoderma

M. J. Day and D. H. Shearer

AETIOPATHOGENESIS

- Canine deep pyoderma is characterised by bacterial infection of the hair follicles with extension to surrounding tissue.
- Disruption of the hair follicle (furunculosis) is associated with intense local inflammation which is pyogranulomatous in nature but may also involve infiltration of eosinophils, lymphocytes and plasma cells (Day 1994).
- The inflammatory response is enhanced by the presence of released hair shaft and keratin, and follows tissue planes to extend to the deep dermis–subcutis and to the surface, resulting in the formation of draining sinus tracts.
- The causative agent in almost all cases is *Staphylococcus intermedius*, a coagulase-positive staphylococcus which may elaborate a range of toxins and enzymes (Berg *et al.* 1984; Cox *et al.* 1984; Allaker *et al.* 1991).

There is debate as to whether the organism expresses (Lachica *et al.* 1979; Cox *et al.* 1986; Fehrer *et al.* 1988) or does not express (Shearer & Day, unpublished observations) staphylococcal protein A. This discrepancy may reflect the geographical origin of the isolates examined or differences in laboratory methodology utilised. *Staphylococcus intermedius* is part of the normal transient microflora of the canine hair coat and resides in high concentration in the perianal and nasal regions (Devriese & De Pelsmeker 1987; Allaker *et al.* 1992).

> In the majority of cases of canine deep pyoderma, deep colonisation by *S. intermedius* is thought to follow an alteration of the cutaneous microclimate which occurs subsequent to an underlying systemic or cutaneous disease.

Deep pyoderma is frequently secondary to a range of disorders, including hypersensitivity dermatitis, demodicosis or endocrinopathy and may occur as a sequel to superficial pyoderma. In a percentage of cases, no such underlying condition is identified, and the skin disease is referred to as primary, idiopathic pyoderma. Particular breeds of dog appear predisposed to this form of pyoderma (e.g. German Shepherd Dog, English Bull Terrier) and it has been suggested that this susceptibility reflects an underlying immunodeficiency state (Wisselink *et al.* 1985). Although various immunological dysfunctions have been identified in dogs with pyoderma, the observed changes in many cases are likely to be an effect of, rather than a cause of, the clinical disease (Barta & Turnwald 1983; Wisselink *et al.* 1988; DeBoer *et al.* 1990a; Miller 1991). A recent study of peripheral blood lymphocytes in German Shepherd Dogs with pyoderma has identified an imbalance in the relative proportion of CD4+ and CD8+ T cells and a reduction in the number of CD21+ B cells (Chabanne *et al.* 1993).

Studies of the specific immune response to *Staphylococcus* in canine deep pyoderma have been limited. In most cases, a strong humoral immunity is induced by the infection. Specific anti-staphylococcal antibodies of the IgG, IgA and IgE classes have been identified (Morales *et al.* 1994; Shearer & Day, unpublished observations), the latter suggesting a role for Type I hypersensitivity in the pathogenesis of this disease. The IgG antibodies are predominantly of the IgG1 and IgG4 subclasses (Shearer, Corato & Day, unpublished observations) and react with a group of nine immunodominant *S. intermedius* antigens of molecular weight range 25 kD to 120 kD (Shearer & Day, unpublished observations). The serum of dogs with deep pyoderma acts as an efficient opsonin of *S. intermedius* for *in vitro* phagocytosis and killing by normal canine neutrophils (Shearer & Day 1993).

The lesions of deep pyoderma are infiltrated by plasma cells expressing IgG (IgG2 and IgG4), IgA and IgM, suggesting active local humoral immunity (Day 1994; Day &

Mazza 1995). Numerous CD3+ T lymphocytes also infiltrate affected dermis, however it is of note that German Shepherd Dogs with deep pyoderma have a paucity of infiltrating T cells when compared with affected dogs of other breeds (Day 1994). This is supportive of the hypothesis that a failure of T cell homing to inflamed skin may be an important factor in the progression of lesions in this breed.

EPIDEMIOLOGY

An epidemiological study of 313 dogs presenting to a university referral dermatology clinic with staphylococcal pyoderma has been undertaken (Shearer & Day, unpublished observations). Of these 95 were diagnosed as having idiopathic pyoderma and the major features of this group of dogs were:

- A breed predisposition for idiopathic pyoderma among dogs of the German Shepherd, West Highland White Terrier, English Bull Terrier and Cocker Spaniel breeds was noted.
- Affected dogs had a mean age of 5.6 years.
- No gender predisposition was recorded.
- There was no seasonal incidence of presentation with disease.
- The causative agent was *S. intermedius* alone in all cases.

CLINICAL FEATURES

Canine deep pyoderma has a range of clinical presentations (Table 88.1), although it is likely that the underlying pathogenesis is the same in each case.

In most cases the presenting complaint is pruritus, although in some cases this may not be present. In non-pruritic deep pyoderma, underlying diseases such as endocrinopathy (hypothyroidism, hyperadrenocorticism) or metabolic disorders (hepatocutaneous syndrome) should be considered.

The lesions of deep pyoderma are pustules or erythematous, elevated, ulcerated nodules with surface ulceration and crusting. Sinus tracts draining the subcutaneous tissues may develop which discharge a red, purulent exudate. Affected dogs often have regional lymphadenopathy. In chronic lesions the development of scar tissue may leave the skin permanently thickened, even after successful treatment of the infection. The distribution of lesions may be generalised, largely over the abdomen or trunk, or localised to specific areas such as the muzzle (Fig. 88.1), chin and lips, carpal or tarsal region (Fig. 88.2), or feet. Dogs of the German Shepherd breed appear particularly susceptible to the generalised form of disease (Fig. 88.3) (Wisselink *et al.* 1985, 1988). It has been proposed that anal furunculosis, to which German Shepherd Dogs are also predisposed, is a further local manifestation of deep pyoderma in the dog (Day & Weaver 1992).

> Deep pyoderma characteristically has a chronic, recurrent course with relapse often occurring after withdrawal of antibiotic treatment.

Table 88.1 Classification of canine deep pyoderma.

Localised	Generalised
Muzzle	Generalised pyoderma
Chin	German Shepherd Dog pyoderma
Carpal/tarsal	
Interdigital	
Callus/pressure point	
Anal and perianal	

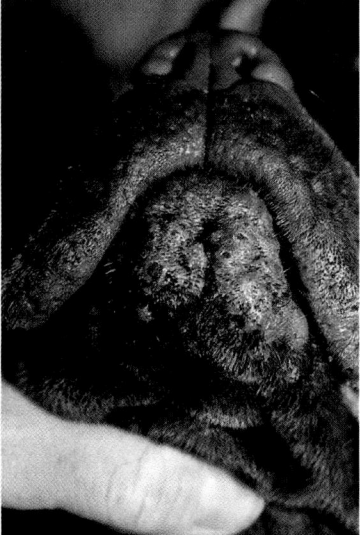

Fig. 88.1 Localised deep furunculosis (canine acne) on the rostral muzzle of a Labrador Retriever. Figure courtesy R. Harvey.

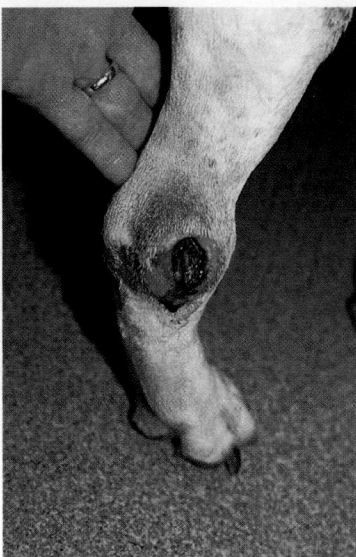

Fig. 88.2 Localised deep furunculosis and sinus formation over the lateral aspect of the hock. Figure courtesy R. Harvey.

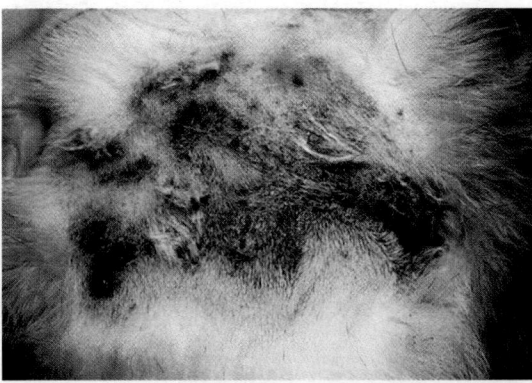

Fig. 88.3 A poorly defined area of ulceration, sinus formation and crust – German Shepherd pyoderma. Figure courtesy R. Harvey.

DIAGNOSTIC INVESTIGATION

The diagnostic assessment of deep pyoderma should include investigations that would enable detection of any underlying disease state, such as ectoparasite infestation,

Table 88.2 Diagnostic investigation of canine deep pyoderma.

Cytological examination of pustule contents
Skin scraping/hair plucking to rule out
    ectoparasites/dermatophytes
Culture and sensitivity of pustule content or biopsy of lesion
Dermatohistopathology
Investigate possible underlying causes by
●   Blood samples/specific tests for internal diseases (endocrinopathy)
●   Intradermal skin testing (atopy and flea allergy)
●   Food elimination trial

hypersensitivity or endocrinopathy. For example skin scraping, endocrine function testing, food elimination trials or intradermal skin testing may be deemed appropriate (Table 88.2). Diagnostic tests specific for deep pyoderma include:

● Cytological examination of an aspirate of pustule contents – on a stained smear, the presence of large numbers of degenerate neutrophils with colonies of coccoid bacteria is supportive of a diagnosis of pyoderma.
● Skin scraping/hair pluckings – these should be examined for ectoparasites (*Demodex canis* and *Sarcoptes scabiei*) and dermatophytes by microscopy and fungal culture.
● Bacterial culture of biopsied tissue or swabs of the contents of intact pustules.
● Skin biopsy to confirm characteristic histopathological changes and assist in the identification of any underlying disease. Biopsies are better taken from early pustular lesions than chronic ulcerated areas.
● Serological testing for the concentration and specificity of serum anti-staphylococcal antibodies is not readily available but in future may provide an adjunct to diagnosis.

MANAGEMENT

Systemic Antibacterial Therapy

An important consideration in the therapeutic approach to deep pyoderma is alleviation of any underlying disease state and removal of the causative agent, *S. intermedius*. The first line of therapy involves administration of systemic antibiotics usually based on the results of bacterial culture and sensitivity and continued until 2 weeks after clinical cure.

Topical Therapeutics

Whole body clipping or removal of hair from around lesions followed by topical therapy using antibacterial shampoos (ethyl lactate, benzoyl peroxide or chlorhexidine) is an essential adjunct to systemic antibiotics. Shampoos should be used twice weekly until the lesions resolve and can be used less frequently for control in recurrent cases. A humectant rinse should be used after each shampoo to rehydrate the coat. Localised pyodermas can be managed by clipping (if necessary) and topical antibacterial shampoos (ethyl lactate, benzoyl peroxide or chlorhexidine) or gels (mupirocin, benzoyl peroxide). These can be applied daily until resolution. In recurrent localised pyoderma the owners should be advised to apply a topical antibacterial agent as soon as signs reappear.

Modification of Immune Response

In refractory cases, modifying the immune response may be considered as an adjunct to systemic antibiotic treatment. Commercially prepared *S. aureus* bacterin (*Staphylococcus* phage lysate) in conjunction with antibiotic has been of use in cases of superficial recurrent pyoderma (DeBoer *et al.* 1990a) but does not appear to increase serum levels of anti-staphylococcal IgG (DeBoer *et al.* 1990b). A preparation derived from *Propionibacterium acnes* (Immunoregulin) together with antibiotic therapy, has also been successful in some dogs (Kern 1985; Becker *et al.* 1989). Finally, the use of autogenous vaccination may be considered. This approach involves culture of the causative organism from the skin of the affected animal and the production of a crude killed extract. The extract is administered by subcutaneous injection, usually every 1–2 weeks for up to 12 weeks. The effectiveness of this form of therapy remains a point of debate and there is no clear direction and definitive proof.

REFERENCES

Allaker, R.P., Lamport, A.I., Lloyd, D.H. & Noble, W.C. (1991). Production of 'virulence factors' by *Staphylococcus intermedius* isolates from cases of canine pyoderma and healthy carriers. *Microbial Ecology in Health and Disease*, **4**, 169–173.

Allaker, R.P., Lloyd, D.H. & Bailey, R.M. (1992). Population sizes and frequency of staphylococci at mucocutaneous sites on healthy dogs. *Veterinary Record*, **130**, 303–304.

Barta, O. & Turnwald, G.H. (1983). Demodicosis, pyoderma, and other skin diseases of young dogs, and their associations with immunologic dysfunctions. *Compendium on Continuing Education for the Practicing Veterinarian*, **5**, 995–1002.

Becker, A.M., Janik, T.A., Smith, E.K., Sousa, C.A. & Peters, B.A. (1989). *Proprionibacterium acnes* immunotherapy in chronic recurrent pyoderma. *Journal of Veterinary Internal Medicine*, **3**, 26–30.

Berg, J.N., Wendell, D.E., Vogelweid, C. & Fales, W.H. (1984). Identification of the major coagulase-positive *Staphylococcus* sp. of dogs as *Staphylococcus intermedius*. *American Journal of Veterinary Research*, **45**, 1307–1309.

Chabanne, I., Marchal, T., Denerolle, P., *et al.* (1993). Lymphocyte subset abnormalities in German Shepherd dog pyoderma (GSP). *Veterinary Immunology and Immunopathology*, **49**, 189–198.

Cox, H.U., Newman, S.S., Roy, A.F. & Hoskins, J.D. (1984). Species of Staphylococcus isolated from animal infections. *Cornell Veterinarian*, **74**, 124–135.

Cox, H.U., Schmeer, N. & Newman, S.S. (1986). Protein A in *Staphylococcus intermedius* isolates from dogs and cats. *American Journal of Veterinary Research*, **47**, 1881–1884.

Day, M.J. (1994). An immunopathological study of deep pyoderma in the dog. *Research in Veterinary Science*, **56**, 18–23.

Day, M.J. & Mazza, G. (1995). Tissue immunoglobulin G subclasses observed in immune-mediated dermatopathy, deep pyoderma and hypersensitivity dermatitis in dogs. *Research in Veterinary Science*, **58**, 82–89.

Day, M.J. & Weaver, B.M.Q. (1992). Pathology of surgically resected tissue from 305 cases of anal furunculosis in the dog. *Journal of Small Animal Practice*, **33**, 583–589.

DeBoer, D.J., Moriello, K.A., Thomas, C.B. & Schultz, K.T. (1990a). Evaluation of a commercial staphylococcal bacterin for management of idiopathic recurrent superficial pyoderma in dogs. *American Journal of Veterinary Research*, **51**, 636–639.

DeBoer, D.J., Schultz, K.T., Thomas, C.B. & Moriello, K.A. (1990b). Clinical and immunological responses of dogs with recurrent pyoderma to injections of Staphylococcus phage lysate. In: *Advances in Veterinary Dermatology*, Vol. 1, (eds C. Von Tscharner & R.E.W. Halliwell), pp. 335–346. Balliere Tindall, London.

Devriese, L.A. & De Pelsmaecker, K. (1987). The anal region as a main carrier site of *Staphylococcus intermedius* and *Streptococcus canis* in dogs. *Veterinary Record*, **121**, 302–303.

Fehrer, S.L., Boyle, M.D.P. & Halliwell, R.E.W. (1988). Identification of protein A from *Staphylococcus intermedius* isolated from canine skin. *American Journal of Veterinary Research*, **49**, 697–701.

Kern, J.F. (1985). Immunotherapy for canine dermatoses. *Canine Practice*, **12**, 30–32.

Lachica, R.V.F., Genigeorgis, C.A. & Hoeprich, P.D. (1979). Occurrence of protein A in *Staphylococcus aureus* and closely related *Staphylococcus* species. *Journal of Clinical Microbiology*, **10**, 752–753.

Miller, W.H. (1991). Deep pyoderma in two German shepherd dogs associated with a cell-mediated immunodeficiency.

Journal of the American Animal Hospital Association, **27**, 513–517.

Morales, C.A., Shultz, K.T. & DeBoer, D.J. (1994). Antistaphylococcal antibodies in dogs with recurrent staphylococcal pyoderma. *Veterinary Immunology and Immunopathology*, **42**, 137–147.

Shearer, D.H. & Day, M.J. (1993). An *in vitro* assay for the measurement of phagocytosis and killing of *Staphylococcus intermedius* by canine neutrophils. *Proceedings of the European*

Society of Veterinary Dermatology Annual Congress, Aalborg, Denmark, pp. 262.

Wisselink, M.A., Willemse, A. & Koeman, J.P. (1985). Deep pyoderma in the German shepherd dog. *Journal of the American Animal Hospital Association*, **21**, 773–776.

Wisselink, M.A., Bernadina, W.E., Willemse, A. & Noordzij, A. (1988). Immunologic aspects of German shepherd dog pyoderma. *Veterinary Immunology and Immunopathology*, **19**, 67–77.

Chapter 89

Treatment of Pyoderma

M. W. Vroom

INTRODUCTION

Bacterial skin infections are one of the most common dermatoses of the dog. *Staphylococcus intermedius* is the most important organism isolated from cases of canine pyoderma, although other organisms, such as *Staphylococcus aureus*, coagulase-negative staphylococci, *Streptococci* spp., *Proteus mirabilis*, *Escherichia coli* and *Pseudomonas* spp., may occasionally be associated with infection. This chapter discusses the clinical approach to, and the management of, canine pyoderma. The pitfalls in treatment and the problem of recurrent pyoderma will also be discussed.

APPROACH TO THE PATIENT

History

A complete history is important, as it may help to identify the cause of the pyoderma. In particular it is very important to ask the owner if there is any pruritus, and whether or not it is present in the absence of lesions since this may give clues to the existence of underlying diseases. The detailed approach of superficial and deep pyoderma is discussed elsewere but hypersensitivities, ectoparasite infestations and endocrine disturbancies should all be considered as possible underlying disorders.

Examination and Clinical Investigations

When considering the possibility of pyoderma in a clinical case it is important to consider a number of points:

- Pustules, or a purulent exudate, are not always associated with pyoderma.
- The lesions of pyoderma may mimic those of other dermatoses.
- Pruritus can be an important feature of the pyoderma but may not always be apparent.
- Pyoderma may be localised or generalised and may occur anywhere on the body.

Clinical examination of the dog and a detailed examination of the skin should allow the clinician to differentiate superficial pyoderma from deep pyoderma (Table 89.1).

Aspiration or Impression Cytology

This is a helpful procedure which is very easy to perform. It is cheap, quick and gives immediate information. Some practice may be necessary to obtain readable smears but the effort is worth while. Cytological examination of the contents of a pustule, or a smear of the exudate from a sinus may allow identification of the type of organism associated with the lesion. In particular it may allow identification of cocci, presumed to be *Staphylococcus intermedius*, and other bacterial forms such as bacilli.

The pustule is opened with a sterile 25 G needle and a clean glass slide gently pressed against the opened pustule. This procedure is repeated several times at different places on the slide. The exudate is allowed to air dry (the process may be accelarated by directing a hairdrier on to the slide), stained with a rapidly acting stain such as Diff-Quik and covered with a cover slip. The preparation is initially examined under the lowest magnification and then under high dry (×40). This degree of magnification is sufficient to recognise cocci, bacilli, neutrophils, and other cells, which may be present, and examination under oil immersion is not usually necessary.

Table 89.1   The distinguishing features of superficial and deep pyoderma.

The clinical signs of superficial pyoderma:

- papules, pustules, erythema and crusts
- polycyclic lesions with central hyperpigmentation and an erythematous, slightly raised margin
- a patchy alopecia giving a 'moth eaten' appearance to the coat
- small groups of raised hairs, which can easily be plucked out, or will fall out spontaneously. The base of the hairs are attached to a small crust. No purulent exudate is visible

The clinical signs of deep pyoderma:

- dark red, raised nodules containing haemorrhagic exudate
- fistulous draining tracts, necrotic and ulcerated skin beneath crust
- a very thin, often oedematous skin around the lesions
- enlarged lymph nodes and an elevated body temperature
- depression, lethargy and anorexia

A number of diagnostic investigations may be performed in order to characterise the disease and obtain information on the organisms which may be involved:

- aspiration or impression cytology of the contents of a pustule
- adhesive tape stripping of the intact skin
- microbiological culture and sensitivity testing
- punch biopsy, for both histopathology and microbiological culture and sensitivity testing

---

Adhesive Tape Stripping

Adhesive tape strips are taken from the surface of the skin. The area is clipped and then a short length of clear, adhesive tape is pressed firmly into contact with the skin. It is then removed, stained (Diff-Quik is suitable) covered with a cover slip and laid across a microscope slide, adhesive side down. Microscopic examination will reveal squames and micro-organisms.

Bacteriological Culture and Sensitivity Testing

The result of a culture and susceptibilty will not only provide information about the antibacterial susceptibility of the organisms isolated but also the identification of the organisms. This information is important as it may provide clues about the nature of the disease process. Thus, the most frequently isolated pathogen is *Staphylococcus intermedius*. Recovery of a pure growth of *Staphylococcus epidermidis* (a non-pathogenic inhabitant of the skin) might suggest immuno-incompetence. It is therefore important not to accept an antibacteriological susceptibility panel only: it is very important to know if one is dealing with pathogenic bacteria. Occasional discrepancies arise between *in vitro* susceptibility and the perceived response *in vivo*. This may relate to testing procedures, incorrect dosage, poor compliance or the development of bacterial resistance. Bacteriological culture and sensitivity testing are indicated in four clinical situations:

- deep pyoderma,
- recurrent superficial pyoderma,
- pyoderma which is not responding as one would expect,
- doubt whether the lesions represent is a pyoderma.

Bacteriological Sampling in Cases of Superficial Pyoderma
Do not disinfect the pustule as the alcohol may penetrate and kill the bacteria. Lift the top of the pustule (or gently elevate a crust) with a sterile 25 G needle. Gently press the swab on to the exposed surface and allow time for the contents to be absorbed. Place the swab into appropriate transport medium and send it to a laboratory with experience in dealing with veterinary samples.

Bacteriological Sampling in Cases of Deep Pyoderma
The surface of the affected area should be clipped and disinfected with alcohol which is allowed to dry. The area is then gently squeezed to express exudate and this is then sampled with the swab.

Bacteriological Sampling Using Skin Biopsy Punches
In the absence of pustules or sinuses, in situations where surface contamination is thought to be great, or where

unusual pathogens (such as mycobacteria or actinomycetes) are suspected samples may be obtained by biopsy. In contrast to the normal biopsy procedure the skin has to be clipped and aseptically prepared. Biopsy samples are taken with a punch (or occasionally by excision) and sent to the laboratory in a sterile transport medium. No formaldehyde should be used.

MANAGEMENT

A number of factors are taken into account when selecting an appropriate antibacterial agent such as selecting an agent that reaches the skin in sufficiently high concentration and using an antibacterial agent that is likely to be effective against *S. intermedius*. The potential for side-effects, the likely duration of treatment and the costs of the medication are also factors that should be considered before prescribing medication. Important considerations are listed in Table 89.2 and an outline of the management regime for a case of pyoderma are given in Tables 89.3 and 89.4.

Good empirical choices for superficial pyoderma include lincomycin, trimethoprim–sulfadiazine with clavulanic acid-potentiated amoxycillin and cephalosporins reserved for difficult cases. For deep pyoderma a good first choice might be trimethoprim–sulfadiazine with cephalosporines or enrofloxacin reserved for difficult cases. Suggested doses are given in Table 89.5.

Table 89.2 The do's and don'ts of successful medication for canine pyoderma.

Do's:
- weigh the dog
- supply a minimum of 3 weeks of treatment for a superficial pyoderma
- supply a minimum of 6 weeks of treatment for a deep pyoderma
- ensure that the dog is re-examined during the last week of therapy
- combine systemic treatment with supportive topical therapy
- ensure that the owner understands the dose and rationale
- keep a proper clinical record

Don'ts:
- guess the dose
- provide topical glucocorticoid-containing ointments
- combine glucocorticoids with systemic antibacterial agents
- attempt too many treatments (antibacterial, antiparasitic, restricted diet, contact screen) at the same time.

Table 89.3 Treatment schedule for a case of superficial pyoderma.

First visit	• Inspect the whole dog, including otoscopy
	• Look for ectoparasites such as fleas and lice
	• Perform two or more skin scrapings and look for *Demodex canis*, *Sarcoptes scabiei* and *Cheyletiella* spp.
	• Provide systemic antibacterial treatment on an empirical basis and anticipate treatment for 3 weeks (i.e. 2–3 weeks plus 1 week after lesions have healed)
	• Provide antibacterial shampoo for weekly application
Second visit	Has the owner performed the right treatment schedule?
	• good response, no further treatment
	• good response but pyoderma relapsed within weeks and still pruritic. If no ectoparasites can be detected then consider food allergy or atopy
	• partial response: continue therapy for another 3 weeks and submit a sample for bacterial culture and sensitivity.
	• no response and no pruritus: sample for culture and sensitivity and repeat skin scrapings. Perform a skin biopsy. Consider endocrinopathies such hypothyroidism and hyperadrenocorticism
Third visit	It is important to check a good response, do not rely on the owner's impression.

Table 89.4 Treatment schedule of a deep pyoderma.

First visit	• Consider the location of pyoderma:
	   ○ flea related
	   ○ generalised
	   ○ pressure point
	   ○ acne
	• Perform skin scrapings
	• Bacterial culture and sensitivity testing is mandatory
	• Start with 3–4 weeks antibiotic treatment (anticipate 4–6 weeks therapy) and provide supportive shampoo. Clip the affected areas

Second visit	Has the owner performed the right treatment scedule?
	• partial response: continue therapy.
	• no response:
	   ○ flea related: make sure there are no fleas or flea faeces
	   ○ generalised: perform minimal three skin biopsies
	   ○ acne (or other localised form): check for other skin problems such as allergy, hypothyroidism, contact allergy, demodicosis

Third visit	Has the owner performed the right treatment schedule? • Good response: discharge • Partial response: repeat the clipping if necessary, change to a more potent antibiotic and shampoo. Perform further investigations such as haematology and biochemistry

Table 89.5 Suggested dose rates for systemic antibacterial agents.

Agent	Suggested dosage
Lincomycin	20 mg/kg b.i.d. empty stomach
Clindamycin	5–10 mg/kg b.i.d. or 11 mg/kg once daily
Trimethoprim-sulfa	5–25 mg/kg b.i.d.
Amoxycillin with clavulanic acid	12.5–20 mg/kg b.i.d.
Cephalexin	15–20 mg/kg b.i.d.
Enrofloxacin	5–10 mg/kg b.i.d.

Systemic Antibacterial Therapy

Lincomycin Group

Lincomycin is a macrolide agent which acts by interfering with bacterial protein synthesis. It is a narrow spectrum, bacteriostatic antibacterial agent. Lincomycin achieves good penetration into the skin and it is excreted by the bile and urine. Resistance to lincomycin can occur rapidly (especially in staphylococci) and there is cross-resistance with other antibiotics in the macrolide-group, such as erythromycin. Side-effects are seldom, loose stools have been observed. It is preferable to give the drug on an empty stomach, i.e. 2h before or after feeding.

Clindamycin is a more recently developed agent which also is effective against Gram-negative bacteria. The oral absorption of the drug is more efficient than that of lincomycin and feeding has no influence on the absorption. Clindamycin appears to enhance the opsonisation of *S. aureus* and the drug accumulates in the polymorphonuclar granulocytes. The development of resistance is rather rapid.

Trimethoprim-Potentiated Sulphonamides

The combination of these two agents results in a double blockade in the bacterial synthesis of dihydrofolic acid. Thus, the sulphonamide fraction inhibits the synthesis of dihydrofolic acid from para-aminobenzoic acid (PABA) and trimethoprim inhibits the subsequent step from dihydrofolic acid to tetrahydrofolic acid. *In vitro* this combination is bacteriocidal but in the action may only be bacteriostatic *in vivo*. Trimethoprim-potentiated sulphonamides are very well absorbed from the gut and penetrate into the skin in high concentrations. They are excreted by the kidney into the urine. Recently a new combination has been made available in which trimethoprim has been replaced with orthoprim. The orthoprim–sulphonamide combination requires only once daily dosage and is reported to have fewer side-effects than trimethoprim-potentiated sulphonamides. Only time will tell.

Idiosyncratic drug eruptions have been reported with trimethoprim-potentiated sulphonamides. These include polyarthritis and pyrexia, cutaneous drug eruptions, keratoconjunctivitis sicca, blood dyscrasia (anaemia, lymphadenopathy and thrombocytopenia) and hepatitis. Doberman Pinschers, in particular, seem to be prone to polyarthritis (Crabb 1989). Sulphonamides also suppress the serum concentration of thyroxine.

Clavulanic Acid-Potentiated Amoxycillin

This broad-spectrum, bactericidal combination is absorbed very well by the stomach with excretion taking place via the kidney. Clavulanic acid is a non-competitive inhibitor of many β-lactamase enzymes and, in combination with β-lactamase containing agents, such as amoxycillin, it renders them resistant against β-lactamase, commonly produced by *S. intermedius*. Side-effects are rare, although animals that are allergic to penicillins and/or cephalosporins should not receive this antibiotic. There is clinical data which suggests that the dermatological dosage of clavulanic acid-potentiated amoxycillin should be higher than usually recommended and a dose of 22 mg/kg twice daily has been suggested as more appropriate. The drug is inactivated by moisture and the tablets should be stored dry.

Cephalosporins

Cephalosporins are a group of broad-spectrum, bactericidal agents which can be classified into three groups, based on spectrum of antibacterial activity. In veterinary medicine only the first-generation drugs are used, such as cephalexin. Cephalosporins act in an identical manner to penicillin: the β-lactam ring binds the transpeptidase enzyme, which is necessary for synthesis of the peptidoglycan bacterial cell wall. Cephalosporins are β-lactamase resistant and therefore effective against penicillin resistant strains of *Staphylococcus intermedius*. Cephalosporins are eliminated predominantly by the kidneys and side-effects (lethargy, anorexia, vomiting and diarrhoea) are rare.

Quinolones

The modern quinolone antibacterial agents are broad-spectrum and bactericidal. They are excreted by the kidney. The absorption of quinolones is not influenced by food in the stomach and they may be administered with or without food. These drugs inhibit bacterial gyrase, an enzyme essential for DNA replication. Quinolones are effective against most strains of *S. intermedius* and bacterial resistance is rare. Caution should be used when medicating immature dogs as the agents induce damage to articular cartilages. They should not be used in dogs less than 12 months of age, or less than 18 months of age in giant breeds where maturity is slower.

Topical Therapy

Antibacterial shampoos play a very useful supportive role in the management of pyoderma. In addition to their potential antibacterial effects they help to remove scale and crust. Appropriate use of topical therapeutics, as adjuncts to systemic antibacterial agents, may reduce the length of therapy and long-term use may help to prevent relapse. There are many different shampoos, with various combinations of ingredients (Table 89.6) and clinicians should ensure that they understand fully the properties and indications of the products that they use. It may be better to concentrate on a few, regularly used, products rather than attempting to stock, and failing to understand the indications of, a larger range.

Iodine 1%	Antibacterial. May be irritant, because it is drying. It may stain light coloured hair coats
Chlorhexidine 0.5%	Effective antibacterial agent.
Ethyl lactate 10%	Lowers skin pH, inhibits bacterial growth, keratoplastic
Benzyl peroxide 3%	Antibacterial, follicular flushing, lowers skin pH, good degreasing agent, keratolytic, may be irritant

Table 89.6 Properties of ingredients which are commonly used in topical products.

Superficial pyoderma	Deep pyoderma
Demodicosis	Demodicosis
Dermatophytosis	Panniculitis
Scabies	Neoplasia
Subcorneal pustular dermatosis	Drug eruption
Drug eruption	Immune-mediated diseases
Pemphigus foliaceus	Foreign bodies
Pemphigus erythematosis	Sterile granuloma
Leishmaniasis	Leishmaniasis
Hepatocutaneous syndrome	

Table 89.7 The differential diagnoses of superficial and deep pyoderma.

The frequency of shampooing in a case of superficial pyoderma may start from two, or even three, times a week at first. If response is noted, the frequency of shampoo may be reduced to once a week, or less. Cases of extensive, deep pyoderma may, ideally, benefit from daily shampooing, or even whirlpools which remove the surface debris. However, focal forms of deep pyoderma will also benefit from the application of regular, topical therapeutics.

The regular application of topical medications, particularly to areas of skin which are alopecic, may be adversely drying and almost all cases will benefit from post-shampoo application of humectants or moisturisers such as propylene glycol, lactic acid, urea and glycerine. These products help to maintain epidermal hydration, and integrity, in the face of regular degreasing shampoos.

RECURRENT PYODERMA

Recurrent superficial pyoderma can be a frustrating experience. The clinician should consider dose, compliance, the potential for bacterial resistance, the duration of treatment and the possibility of underlying disease. In addition, the diagnosis of superficial, or deep, pyoderma, should be reconsidered (Table 89.7).

Sometimes no primary cause can be found and empirical therapy is necessary. Good communication is necessary in these cases as they are frustrating for the clinician and expensive for the owner. Occasionally, regular application of topical antibacterial shampoos may be effective. In more severe cases, systemic antibacterial agents are necessary. Pulse therapy is one solution: systemic antibacterial agents (at full therapeutic doses) are administered on a 1 week on and 1 week off basis, or 3 days on and 3 days off. Another possibility is once daily administration, again at the full therapeutic dosage. These regimes have the added advantage of considerable cost savings for the owner, if long-term treatment is necessary. However, these extended, low dose regimes should be reserved for cases which defy definitive diagnosis.

Immunostimulants may be helpful in some cases. The efficacy of immunotherapy with various regimes has been reported. The use of *Propionibacterium acnes* was discussed by Becker *et al.* (1989) while DeBoer *et al.* (1990) reported the efficacy of a staphylococcal-derived antigen. It is difficult to obtain conclusions from these studies because of the limited numbers of dogs used in the trials.

COMBINATION OF GLUCOCORTICOIDS AND ANTIBACTERIAL AGENTS

The combination of glucocorticoids and antibacterial agents should be avoided. While the use of glucocorticoids results in a rapid reduction of erythema the anti-inflammatory effect is only temporary and, as soon as the steroids are tapered, the pyoderma will relapse. The use of systemic glucocorticoids also hampers interpretation of the response, if any, to the treatment. Topical treatment with corticosteroid containing ointments will also suppress the erythema and may give a false impression of efficacy.

REFERENCES

Becker, A.M., Janik, T.A., Smith, E.K., Sousa, C.A. & Peters, B.A. (1989). *Propionibacterium acnes* immunotherpay in recurrent canine pyoderma. *Journal of Veterinary Internal Medicine*, **3**, 26–30.

Crabb, A.E. (1989). Idiosyncratic reactions to sulfonamides in dogs. *Journal of the American Veterinary Medical Association*, **195**, 1612–1614.

DeBoer, D.J., Moriello, K.A., Thomas, C.B. & Schultz, K.T. (1990). Evaluation of a commercial staphylococcal bacterin for management of isiopathic recurrent superficial pyoderma in dogs. *American Journal of Veterinary Research*, **51**, 636–639.

Chapter 90

Clinical Approach to Pruritus in the Dog

P. B. Hill

INTRODUCTION

Pruritus, or itch, is a sensation in the skin that leads to a desire to scratch. It is one of the most common reasons for dogs to be presented to veterinary surgeons in general practice, and is the most frequent clinical sign associated with canine skin disease. In addition to scratching, pruritus can lead to chewing, licking, rubbing, rolling or head shaking. It can result in considerable discomfort to the dog, and much anxiety for the owner. Pruritus is a multifactorial problem that can be caused by a number of different diseases. However, in general, most pruritic diseases encountered in general practice are caused by ectoparasites (Fig. 90.1), infectious agents or allergies (Fig. 90.2). Table 90.1 lists the common skin diseases that should be considered in all cases when pruritus is the chief complaint on initial presentation.

> It is essential to remember that more than one disease may be present in the same patient (Fig. 90.4).

For example, veterinary dermatologists commonly see cases of atopy, flea bite hypersensitivity, superficial pyoderma, and *Malassezia* dermatitis all in the same dog. In such cases, each dermatosis contributes to the overall level of pruritus (a process known as summation), and failure to recognise one component can result in failure to manage the pruritus successfully. It is crucial when approaching the problem of pruritus to diagnose every disease that is present and treat each one specifically with appropriate therapy.

In order to make a specific diagnosis, or diagnoses, the various diseases that cause pruritus must be differentiated.

This requires a logical and systematic approach which includes:

- obtaining a relevant history;
- a complete physical examination;
- establishment of differential diagnoses;
- diagnostic tests to rule in or out the differential diagnoses;
- specific treatment for each disease diagnosed.

OBTAINING A HISTORY

Many veterinary dermatologists use a questionnaire to obtain a complete history. This can be filled out by the client while in the waiting room reducing the need for exhaustive questioning in the consulting room. If a questionnaire is not used, certain questions should be committed to memory so that the history provides the following information.

(1) Age, breed and sex – many pruritic skin diseases have age and breed distributions (Table 90.2) although it should be remembered that this list is only a guide as these diseases can occur in any breed.
(2) Description of complaint
 - Does the dog scratch, chew, bite or lick itself?
 - What areas are affected?
 - How long has it been present?
 - Was it sudden or gradual onset?
 - Is there loss of hair?
(3) Severity
 - How often does the dog scratch?
 - Does it stop the dog from sleeping?
(4) Seasonality
 - Is the problem continual or intermittent?
 - Is it worse at certain times of year?

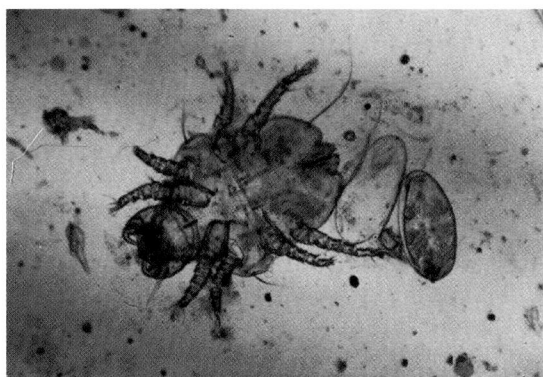

Fig. 90.1   Cheyletiellid mite, and egg, found on microscopic examination of skin scrapings. Figure courtesy P. Hill.

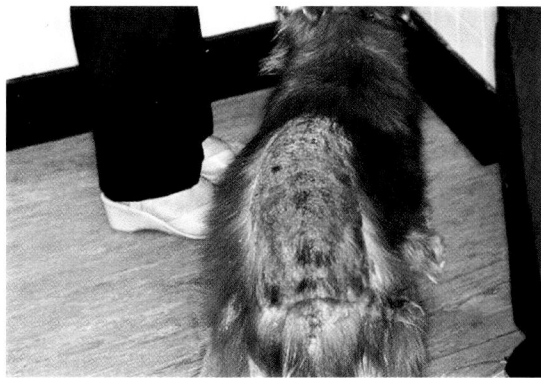

Fig. 90.3   Flea bite hypersensitivity. Alopecia, lichenification and hyperpigmentation over the dorsal lumbosacral region of a dog with a severe flea bite hypersensitivity. Figure courtesy P. Hill.

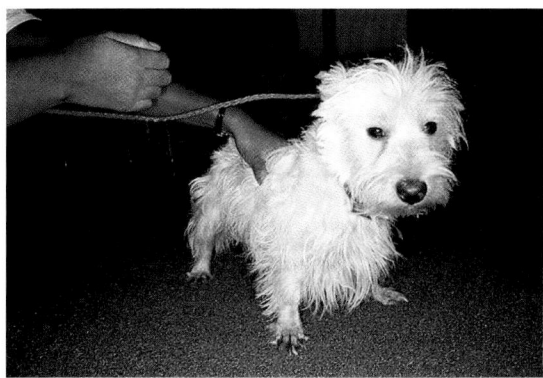

Fig. 90.2   Pedal erythema and alopecia in a dog with atopy. Figure courtesy P. Hill.

Table 90.1   Pruritic skin diseases of dogs commonly encountered in practice.

Ectoparasitic
   Scabies
   Cheyletiella dermatitis
   Demodicosis

Infectious agents
   Superficial pyoderma (*Staphylococcus intermedius*)
   Malassezia dermatitis

Allergies
   Flea bite hypersensitivity (Fig. 90.3)
   Atopy
   Food
   Contact

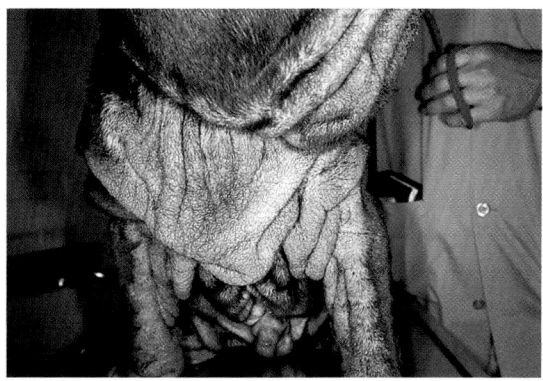

Fig. 90.4   *Malassezia pachydermatis* and pyoderma on the ventral neck and thorax of a dog. The increase in humidity and local maceration which occurred with the depths of the skin folds was a contributing factor in the aetiology of this case. Figure courtesy P. Hill.

(5)   Possible contagion
   • Where was the dog acquired from?
   • Has the dog been to the kennels or groomers recently?
   • Do any other pets in the household have skin problems?
   • Do any members of the family have skin problems?
(6)   Diet
   • Describe the dog's diet.
(7)   Possible contact materials
   • What does the dog lie and sleep on?

Table 90.2   Age and breed distribution for common pruritic skin diseases.

Disease	Typical age when starts	Breed commonly affected
Flea bite hypersensitivity	Any age	Any breed
Scabies	Any age	Any breed
Cheyletiella dermatitis	More common in puppies	Any breed
Pyoderma	Any age	Any breed
Demodicosis	3–12 months	Afghan Hound, Beagle, Bull Terrier, Bulldog, Boxer, Boston Terrier, Chinese Shar-Pei, Chihuahua, Collie, Dachshund, Dalmation, Dobermann Pinscher, German Shepherd, Great Dane, Old English Sheepdog, Pointer, Pug
Malassezia dermatitis	Young to middle age	Basset Hound, Chihuahua, Dachshund, German Shepherd Dog, Poodle, Spaniel, Shetland Sheepdog, West Highland White Terriers
Atopy	1–3 years	Beagle, Bulldog, Chinese Shar-Pei, Dalmation, English Setter, Golden Retriever, Labrador Retriever, German Shepherd Dog, Terriers,
Food allergy	Any age	Any breed
Contact allergy	Any age	Any breed

- What does the dog contact indoors (rugs, bedding etc.) and outdoors (grass, trees etc.)?
(8) Previous diseases and treatments
    - Has the dog ever had fleas?
    - What treatments have been given in the past, and did they work?
    - What treatment is the dog on now?
    - How often is the dog bathed or groomed and when was the last time?
    - Does your dog have any other medical problems or abnormal signs?

A thorough history provides clues that allow prioritisation of the differential diagnoses (Box 90.1). For example, the owner's description of the initial complaint and the areas affected may describe a typical pattern of lesions that characterise certain diseases, before generalisation and chronic changes occur. If a skin disease has been present for a number of months, or years, it is likely that secondary changes will have altered the appearance of the condition making the physical examination less rewarding.

Details of the dog's diet can help to formulate a hypoallergenic diet if food allergy is suspected and details of contact materials can help to establish a diagnosis of contact dermatitis (irritant or allergic).

The response, or lack of response, to previous treatments can help to assess the likelihood of particular dis-

Box 90.1   Clues to differential diagnoses

- Extremely severe pruritus is commonly associated with scabies (Figs 90.5a, b&c).
- Seasonal pruritus, especially in the summer and autumn, is usually due to atopy or flea bite hypersensitivity.
- Lesions occurring in other pets or members of the family suggest ectoparasitic diseases.
- Flea infestations may cause a papular rash on the legs of the owners.
- The bites of sarcoptic and cheyletiellid mites often affect the arms or abdomen of in-contact people.
- Recent visits to kennels or groomers may reveal a potential source of contagion for these ectoparasites.

eases. However, recent treatment may have altered the appearance of the disease and if the dog has been bathed the likelihood of finding ectoparasites is reduced. Finally, most dogs with pruritic skin diseases do not have systemic signs, but diarrhoea or increased frequency of bowel motions can be associated with food allergy.

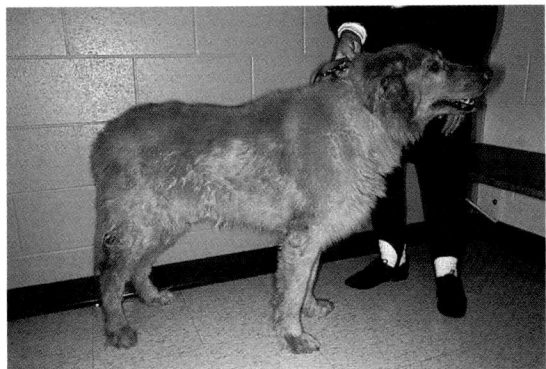

a

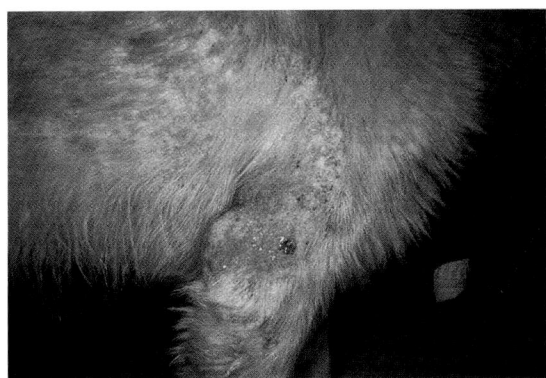

b

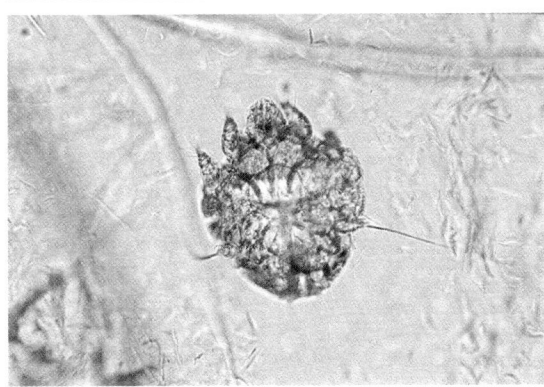

c

Fig. 90.5 (a) Labrador retriever with scabies. Note the signs of self-trauma on the flank and lateral thigh. The erythematous papular dermatitis on the elbow (b) is highly suggestive of scabies. Finding the mite on microscopic examination of skin scrapings (c) is diagnostic. Figures courtesy P. Hill.

PHYSICAL EXAMINATION

A general physical examination with a complete dermatological examination is essential when assessing pruritus.

> The aim of the dermatological examination is to determine the nature of the skin lesions and their distribution.

It is important to establish a routine when examining the skin so that the whole body area is covered. Usually, the examination starts at the head and proceeds caudally. The ears, ear margins, periocular region, ventral neck, axillae, ventral abdomen, interdigital areas and perineum should receive as much attention as the trunk. The skin and hair coat should be carefully examined by running the fingers against the lie of the hair. At this stage it may be possible to see grossly visible ectoparasites such as fleas or lice, or clues to their presence such as flea dirt or lice eggs. If necessary, the hair coat may need to be clipped in order to visualise the lesions. Visible evidence for the pruritic nature of the disease includes salivary staining of the feet (a reddish brown discoloration indicating licking), hair trapped under the gumline of the incisors (indicating chewing) and linear excoriations (indicating scratching).

The lesions that are present must be characterised and recorded. The clinician must be familiar with the various types of lesion that occur on the skin, and what they represent. It is also important to be able to distinguish primary lesions (which occur as a direct result of the disease process) from secondary lesions such as hyperpigmentation and lichenification which occur as a result of progression of the disease or self-trauma. Secondary changes can be associated with any untreated pruritic skin diseases and should not be regarded as specific for any condition. The distribution of the lesions is also extremely helpful in prioritising differential diagnoses, as many pruritic diseases have characteristic distribution patterns (Table 90.3).

FORMATION OF A DIFFERENTIAL DIAGNOSIS

The differential diagnosis is formulated by correlating the information obtained from the history and physical examination. A common mistake is failure to include potential diagnoses because of an inadequate history or incomplete

Table 90.3 Typical lesions and distribution seen in common pruritic skin diseases.

Disease	Associated lesions	Distribution
Flea bite hypersensitivity	Papules Alopecia Pyotraumatic dermatitis (hot spots)	Dorsal lumbo-sacral
Scabies	Papules Scaling Erythema	Ear margins Pinnae Legs Ventrum
Cheyletiella dermatitis	Scaling (dandruff)	Dorsal
Demodicosis	Alopecia Follicular casts and comedones	Head, legs
Superficial pyoderma	Papules Pustules Epidermal collarettes	Trunk Ventrum
Malassezia dermatitis	Papules Greasy scale Erythema	Ventral neck Interdigital areas Ears Perineum Axillae Otitis externa
Atopy and food allergy	None Erythema	Face Periocular Otitis externa Axillae Feet Ventrum
Allergic/irritant contact allergy	Papulo pustular eruption	Hairless areas Ventrum Feet Axillae

physical examination. For example, failure to ascertain that the owner had developed a rash may allow a diagnosis of scabies to be overlooked. Such cases can be misdiagnosed as allergic and managed inappropriately for many months. Also, failure to recognise the significance of some of the lesions listed in Table 90.3 can lead to misdiagnosis. This most commonly occurs when epidermal collarettes are not identified as the lesions of a superficial pyoderma. Inappropriate therapy may then be instituted which results in a protracted course of relapsing skin disease. The clinician must also be aware that some diseases are quite similar (scabies and atopy), whereas others may not appear as classically described (atopy may mimic the distribution of flea bite hypersensitivity). For these reasons, even with a com-

plete history and a thorough physical examination, it is usually not possible to make a specific diagnosis without the aid of diagnostic tests.

DIAGNOSTIC TESTS

Diagnostic tests are used to determine the presence, or absence, of diseases considered in the differential diagnosis so that a specific diagnosis (or diagnoses) can be established. Most of the tests required for dermatological diagnosis are simple, economical and easy to perform in general practice, but it is essential to be aware of the meaning of a positive or negative result. Interpretation of positive results is usually straightforward, but negative results can be misleading because they only occasionally rule out the disease for which the test is being used. For example, finding *Sarcoptes scabiei* mites on a skin scraping is diagnostic for scabies. However, failure to find mites in no way rules out the diagnosis, and the dog should still be treated for the disease if it

Table 90.4 Appropriate diagnostic tests for common pruritic skin diseases, and the significance of positive and negative results.

Disease	Appropriate tests	Positive result (diagnostic finding)	Interpretation of negative result
Flea bite hypersensitivity	Flea combing	Fleas or flea dirt	May still be flea bite hypersensitivity
	Intradermal flea antigen test	Wheal at injection site immediate or delayed	(1) Not FAD (2) Antigen lost potency
Scabies	Skin scraping	Mites or eggs	Could still be scabies – treat if suspect
Cheyletiella dermatitis	Flea combing Skin scraping	Mites or eggs attached to hairs	Could still be *Cheyletiella* – treat if suspect
Demodicosis	Deep skin scraping	Adult mites, eggs, larvae, nymphs	Very unlikely to be *Demodex*, as mites are easy to find
Superficial pyoderma	Cytology of pustule contents	Neutrophilic inflammation with phagocytosed cocci	(1) Poor sample (2) Poor staining (3) May be sterile pustular disease
Malassezia dermatitis	Impression smears Sellotape imprints	Peanut shaped budding yeast organisms	(1) Not *Malassezia* dermatitis (2) Poor sample (3) Poor staining
Atopy	Intradermal skin test	Positive reactions (wheals)	(1) Not atopic (2) Tested out of season (3) Dog been on recent glucocorticoids or antihistamines (4) Antigens lost potency
	ELISA	Positive scores – may be atopic or may be false positive reactions	(1) Not atopic (2) Appropriate antigens not tested (3) Test insensitive (mixtures of antigens used)
Food allergy	3–10 week hypoallergenic diet trial	Cessation or reduction in pruritus	(1) Not food allergy (2) Wrong diet chosen
Contact allergy	Remove dog from usual environment	Cessation or reduction in pruritus	(1) Not contact allergy (2) Offending material still present
	Patch testing	Positive (delayed) reactions	(1) Not contact allergy (2) Appropriate antigens not tested

FAD, flea allergic dermatitis.

is suspected. Table 90.4 lists the appropriate tests for particular diseases, and the significance of a positive or negative result.

TREATMENT OF PRURITUS

Treatment for pruritus can be specific (which can lead to resolution of the disease), and symptomatic (which alleviates the discomfort associated with pruritus).

- Specific treatments include antiparasitic agents, antibacterial drugs, antifungal agents, hyposensitisation therapy and 'hypoallergenic' diets.
- Symptomatic treatments include glucocorticoids, antihistamines, essential fatty acid supplements and moisturising baths.

Whenever possible, specific treatments should be prescribed based on specific diagnoses. However, because of the difficulties associated with negative test results (Table 90.4), it is sometimes necessary to treat pruritic diseases without making a specific diagnosis. In these cases it is essential to choose a treatment that will also act as a diagnostic test. For example, it is not unusual to fail to find mites in cases of scabies. These patients should be treated with specific therapy for scabies so that if the dog makes a complete recovery, the diagnosis can be made retrospectively.

In addition to specific therapy, symptomatic therapy is a very useful adjunct in the treatment of pruritus and when used judiciously can hasten the recovery of the patient. However, symptomatic therapy should be used for the minimal period of time and should *never* be used as a substitute for an accurate diagnosis. In some cases (such as canine atopy), symptomatic therapy may be required for extended periods of time, but it is essential that the diagnosis is correct before embarking on such a course of treat-

Table 90.5 Specific and symptomatic treatments for common pruritic skin diseases.

Disease	Specific treatment	Symptomatic treatment
Flea bite hypersensitivity	Topical insecticides Household treatment	Glucocorticoids
Scabies	Topical miticide Ivermectin	Glucocorticoids
Cheyletiella dermatitis	Topical miticide	Anti-seborrheic shampoo
Demodicosis	Amitraz/benzoyl peroxide	None required. DO NOT USE GLUCOCORTICOIDS
Pyoderma	Systemic antibiotics/topical antibacterials	None required. DO NOT USE GLUCOCORTICOIDS
Malassezia dermatitis	Topical antifungal shampoo (miconazole/chlorhexidine) Ketoconazole (systemic or topical)	Anti-seborrheic shampoo
Atopy	Hyposensitisation	Glucocorticoids Antihistamines Essential fatty acids Antipruritic baths (colloidal oatmeal)
Food allergy	Hypoallergenic diet	Glucocorticoids Antihistamines Essential fatty acids Antipruritic baths
Contact allergy	Avoidance	Glucocorticoids Antihistamines Essential fatty acids Antipruritic baths

Table 90.6 A summary of the options to consider when faced with a case that defies early diagnosis.

Consider less common diseases
- dermatophytosis – perform a fungal culture
- intestinal parasite hypersensitivity – perform a faecal examination
- autoimmune diseases – skin biopsy
- keratinisation defects – skin biopsy
- neoplastic diseases (mycosis fungoides and mast cell tumours) – skin biopsy

Consider treatment resistance
- resistance to antibiotics – perform a culture and sensitivity
- resistance to antiparasitic agents – choose an alternative

Consider poor client compliance
- treatment not been given

Consider referral to a specialist

ment. Specific and symptomatic treatments for the common pruritic skin diseases are shown in Table 90.5.

SPECIFIC APPROACH FOR CASES PRESENTING WITH PYODERMA AND PRURITUS

In cases presenting with a clinically obvious superficial pyoderma with associated pruritus, the most appropriate course of action (after ruling out underlying parasitic causes), is to treat the infection with systemic antibiotics and topical antibacterials for 3 weeks. At this stage, the patient should be re-evaluated. If the pyoderma has resolved but the pruritus is still present, the clinician should investigate for other underlying pruritic diseases. If the pyoderma and pruritus has completely resolved the antibiotics can be stopped and the dog may require no further treatment. If the pyoderma subsequently relapses, the dog should be investigated for underlying causes of pyoderma which are not themselves pruritic.

APPROACH FOR CASES THAT REMAIN UNDIAGNOSED

The most common reason for pruritus to remain undiagnosed is that one of the common diseases discussed above has been missed. The first step is therefore to re-evaluate the case to ensure that the necessary approach has been adopted to completely rule out all the possibilities. If the patient is still undiagnosed, the clinician should consider less common diseases, treatment resistance, lack of owner compliance and the possibility of referral (Table 90.6).

FURTHER READING

Griffin, C.E. (1993). Pruritus in the dog. In: *Manual of Small Animal Dermatology*, (eds P.H. Locke, R.G. Harvey & I.S. Mason), pp. 45–51. British Small Animal Veterinary Association, Cheltenham.

Griffin, C.E., Kwochka, K.W. & MacDonald, J.M. (1993). *Current Veterinary Dermatology – The Science and Art of Therapy*, pp. 3–137. Mosby Year Book, St Louis.

Muller, G.H., Kirk, R.W. & Scott, D.W. (1989). *Small Animal Dermatology*, 4th edn. pp. 92–149. WB Saunders, Philadelphia.

Reinke, S.I. (1988). The clinical approach to the pruritic dog. *Veterinary Clinics of North America*, 18, 983–998.

Scarff, D.H. (1993). Approach to dermatological diagnosis. In: *Manual of Small Animal Dermatology*, (eds P.H. Locke, R.G. Harvey & I.S. Mason), pp. 23–32. British Small Animal Veterinary Association, Cheltenham.

Chapter 91

The Diagnosis and Management of Allergic Skin Disease

J. I. Henfrey

INTRODUCTION

Allergic skin disease is the commonest cause of pruritus in dogs in the UK. The most common allergic reaction is to parasites, in particular the flea, and this is covered in Chapter 92. Of the non-parasitic allergies, atopic disease is the commonest followed by food intolerance (commonly, but sometimes inappropriately, known as food allergy), contact irritant/allergic reactions and, more rarely, allergies to drugs, bacteria and hormones. Pruritus is the hallmark of allergic skin disease in dogs. As veterinary surgeons and owners have become more aware of the adverse effects of long-term glucocorticoid use, successful control of pruritus requires accurate identification of significant allergens if possible, with a logical approach to management.

PATHOGENESIS

Allergic reactions can be divided into atopic and non-atopic allergic reactions.

- Atopic disease can be defined as an inherited predisposition to develop IgE antibodies to environmental allergens resulting in allergic disease (Halliwell & Gorman 1989).
- Atopic disease is mediated by the interaction of allergen and IgE on the mast cell surface, and is a classic example of a type 1 hypersensitivity reaction.

Traditionally the route of access of allergen to the skin of atopic dogs has always been assumed to be via the respiratory tract, but there is increasing evidence that percutaneous penetration of allergens through the thin canine epidermis may be important in the pathogenesis of atopic disease.

- Non-atopic allergic skin diseases are those in which there is no inherited predisposition to develop an IgE response to an allergen.
- Non-atopic allergic skin diseases are thought to be associated with type 3 and 4 allergic reactions (but may include a type 1 reaction) and include food allergy, contact allergy, parasite allergy and reactions to drugs, endoparasites, hormones and bacteria.

An important concept in the pathogenesis of clinical disease associated with allergic skin disease is that of the 'threshold' of allergy. It is common in clinical practice to see dogs with two or more subclinical allergies, for example atopic disease and flea allergy dermatitis. It is the summation of the two allergies which causes pruritus and clinical disease, hence control of one alone may render the animal asymptomatic.

CLINICAL FEATURES

Atopic Disease

The hallmark of atopic disease is pruritus (Figs 91.1–91.4):

- Pruritus may initially be seasonal, but often becomes perennial.
- Pruritus is usually evident on the face, ears, feet and ventrum.
- Pruritus may be generalised pruritus or localised.
- Otitis externa may be the sole presenting sign of atopic disease.

Atopic disease is the commonest non-parasitic allergy seen in the UK. Clinical signs usually commence between 1 and 3 years of age. Occasionally it develops between 6 and 12 months of age, and only rarely after 6 years of age.

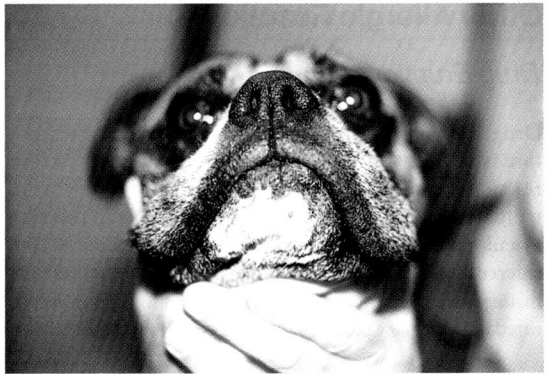

Fig. 91.1   Erythematous muzzle of a Boxer with atopy. Figure courtesy J. Henfrey.

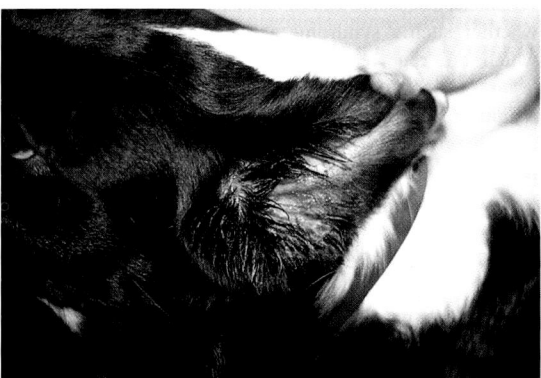

Fig. 91.2   Erythematous otitis externa in a dog with atopy. Figure courtesy J. Henfrey.

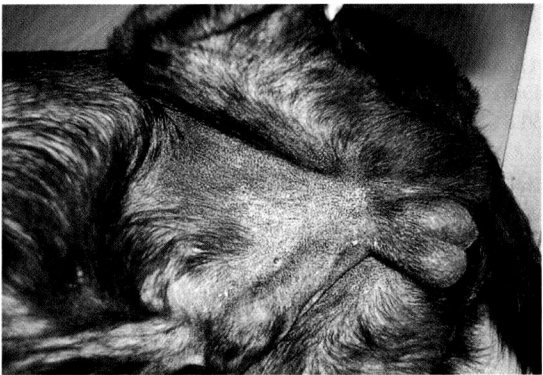

Fig. 91.3   Patchy alopecia, erythema. Patchy hyperpigmentation and surface scale in the groins and ventral abdomen of a dog with atopy. Figure courtesy J. Henfrey.

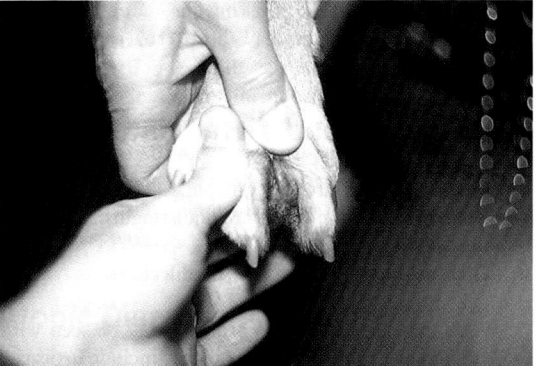

a

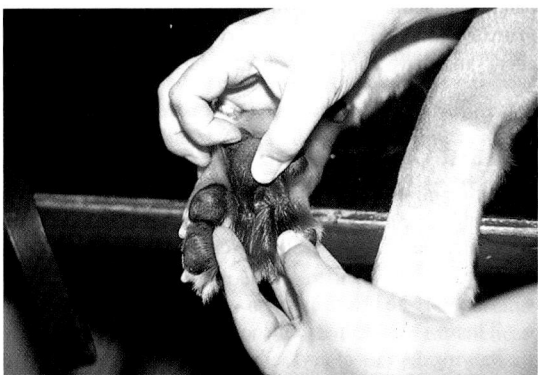

b

Fig. 91.4   Dorsal (a) and plantar (b) interdigital erythema in dogs with atopy. Figures courtesy J. Henfrey.

Certain breeds are predisposed, and in the UK English Setters, Boxers, West Highland White Terriers, Labrador Retrievers, Staffordshire Bull Terriers and Golden Retrievers are frequently affected.

While a primary eruption may be evident in some cases the majority of clinical signs are caused by self-trauma. Clinical signs include pedal erythema of both surfaces of all four feet, often with saliva staining of the fur. Dogs with atopic disease commonly chew and lick at the palmar metacarpus, between the accessory carpal and stop pads. Ventral erythema, alopecia and hyperpigmentation (especially in West Highland White Terriers) is common, and many dogs exhibit varying degrees of seborrhoea and secondary pyoderma. Most cases of pyoderma are superficial and most prominent in the glabrous regions, but some dogs develop deep pyoderma particularly of the face and feet and this may be associated with prolonged glucocorticoid therapy. *Malassezia pachydermatis* infection is common, particularly in the West Highland White Terrier. Some cases have conjunctivitis and sneezing similar to hay fever in man. Otitis externa initially may be episodic and confined to the vertical portions of the external ear canals

91.5), and it is worthwhile trying two or three examples before discarding them from the therapeutic armoury (Paterson 1994). They are at their most useful for dogs with housedust mite allergy and if used in combination with essential fatty acids, topical therapy and a programme of allergen avoidance, control of pruritus may be achieved in around one-third of cases.

Immunotherapy

The object of immunotherapy is to hyposensitise the animal to its allergens by repeated low doses of allergen. Several preparations are available commercially. Allergens in an aqueous suspension require frequent injections, and adverse anaphylactic reactions are possible. Alum-precipitated allergens require fewer injections, the risk of anaphylaxis is less but they are slightly more expensive than aqueous solutions. Allergens for inclusion should be selected on the basis of an intradermal test; by convention, only 10 allergens are included in each preparation, therefore selection should be made based on the strength of the skin test reaction and the animal's exposure to the allergens. Adverse reactions are uncommon. Anaphylaxis is extremely rare, but it is prudent to insist the dog remains in the surgery for half an hour after the first few injections.

Table 91.5 Antihistamines which may be useful in the management of atopy.

Drug	Group	Dosage
Chlorpheniramine	Alkylamine	0.4 mg/kg t.i.d.
Clemastine	Ethanolamine	0.05 mg/kg b.i.d.
Cyproheptadine	Piperadine	0.1 mg/kg b.i.d.
Hydroxyzine	Ataraxics	2 mg/kg t.i.d.
Trimeprazine	Phenothiazine	0.5 mg/kg b.i.d.

More commonly, some dogs exhibit an increase in pruritus around the time of each injection. This can usually be controlled with a short course of antihistamines or glucocorticoids. Therapy should be continued for 9 months before the full effect is seen. Quoted success rates vary, but in this author's referral practice approximately one-third of dogs will stop scratching completely, one-third will improve and the rest will exhibit little change. Some dogs will initially improve and then relapse; some of these animals have added further allergens to their repertoire and benefit from repeated intradermal testing and hyposensitisation. During the hyposensitisation period it is imperative that any pyoderma or *Malassezia* infection is controlled, and a programme of allergen avoidance is followed if possible. Intermittent courses of low dose, alternate day prednisolone or antihistamines with concurrent essential fatty acid therapy will often reduce pruritus to an acceptable level during hyposensitisation, and do not appear to affect the efficacy of hyposensitisation.

REFERENCES

Bond, R., Thorogood, S.C. & Lloyd, D.H. (1994). Evaluation of two enzyme-linked immunosorbent assays for the diagnosis of canine atopy. *Veterinary Record*, **135**, 130–133.

Halliwell, R.E.W. & Gorman, N.T. (1989). Atopic diseases. In: *Veterinary Clinical Immunology*, pp. 232–233. W.B. Saunders, Philadelphia.

Lewis, L., Morris, M. & Hand, M. (1987). *Small Animal Clinical Nutrition*. Mark Morris Associates, Kansas.

Paterson, S. (1994). Use of antihistamines to control pruritus in atopic dogs. *Journal of Small Animal Practice*, **35**, 415–419.

Willemse, T. (1986). Atopic disease: a review and reconsideration of diagnostic criteria. *Journal of Small Animal Practice*, **27**, 771–777.

Chapter 92

Fleas, Flea Bite Hypersensitivity and Flea Control: An Update

M. A. Fisher

INTRODUCTION

Fleas are the most ubiquitous ectoparasites of dogs in the UK and are responsible for causing a number of diseases in dogs, cats and humans. Each year, while a great deal of money and effort is spent on controlling them, the perception is that the annual 'flea problem' is certainly not being contained and, if anything, is increasing. There are a number of factors that tend to assist the continued success of the flea population, not least the increased numbers of dogs and cats. The dog population increased by 22% and the cat population by 33% in the decade 1981–1991 (PFMA 1992). Many of these dogs and cats are pets, living alongside us in the house. Alterations made to the interior of houses such as wall-to-wall carpeting, upholstered furniture and increased draught proofing have been cited as factors that may assist flea proliferation (Kristensen *et al.* 1978). Mild, humid winters are a further factor that may increase survival of immature fleas in the home environment.

A large number of dogs (and cats) develop hypersensitivity to components of flea saliva and exhibit symptoms of flea bite hypersensitivity (FBH), also known as flea allergic dermatitis. Fleas from pets are also responsible for causing papular urticaria in man (Maunder 1984).

The aim of this chapter is to outline understanding of the epidemiology and biology of the flea and flea-related skin disease in the light of developments in the past 15 years and to examine how innovations in flea control can be integrated into a rational flea control programme. An overall target is to ensure that pet owners understand the basis of flea control so that the money spent on flea control can be used judiciously and to good effect, particularly in households where one or more members suffer from flea-bite hypersensitivity, where the aim must be to eliminate or strictly control the flea population. Apologies are due for the frequent reference in the text to cats rather than dogs,

however the bulk of the research into *Ctenocephalides felis felis* has been carried out on cats and not dogs.

THE FLEA POPULATION ON DOGS IN GREAT BRITAIN AND IRELAND

It is common for owners to blame the cat or hedgehogs for the fleas on their dog. Limited survey evidence from Great Britain and Ireland, summarised in Table 92.1, suggests that, more often than not, it is the 'cat' flea *Ctenocephalides felis felis* (*C. felis*) that is present on the majority of dogs.

The *C. felis* is known to be a polyxenous parasite, that is it is capable of maintaining its lifecycle on a large number of hosts, including dogs. Therefore, while cats may have been the original source of the flea and may act as a reservoir, equally the dog can maintain its own supply of fleas, with the animal's environment as the main reservoir. The next most common species is the 'dog' flea, *Ctenocephalides canis*, which tends to be the predominant flea in certain circumstances, for example in the kennel situation (Fisher *et al.* 1989) and in some areas such as Dublin (Baker & Hatch 1972; Baker & Mulcahy 1986). This flea is less tolerant of other hosts (Baker & Elharam 1992), so other mammals acting as reservoirs are less likely. There is circumstantial evidence and a perception that *C. canis* is displaced from dogs by *C. felis* in urban areas (Kristensen *et al.* 1978; Amin 1966), though the mechanism for this remains unclear. Only a small proportion of fleas found on dogs are hedgehog (*Archaeopsylla erinacei erinacei*), human (*Pulex irritans*) or other fleas (Table 92.1). Moreover, a mixed population of flea species on the same dog is a relatively infrequent finding.

Table 92.1 Prevalence of flea species on dogs in the UK and Ireland.

Reference	Area	No. dogs	C. felis	C. canis	Others
Edwards (1969)	GB	–	22 (16)	113 (84)	–
Baker & Hatch (1972)	Dublin	50*	2 (1.3)	120 (81)	26Pi
Beresford-Jones (1981)	London	65†	10‡ (71)	4‡ (2.9)	–
Geary (1977)	UK	173†	81 (81)	18 (18)	1Sc, 1B, 5A
Else et al. (1977)	E. Anglia	272†			60‡F (11)
Beresford-Jones (1981)	London	193†	33‡ (87)	5‡ (13)	1‡Oh
Baker & Mulcahy (1986)	Dublin	97*	4 (1.0)	381 (99)	1Pmm
Hatch & Dooge (1986)	Dublin	5*	–	–	6A
Coward (1991)	S. England	66*	54	7	2Sc, 5A
Chesney (1995)	S.W. England	60*	85 (74)	30 (26)	2A

Values in parentheses are percentage of total.
*, Total number infected.
†, Total number examined.
‡, Number of dogs with this flea present.
Pi, *Pulex irritans*; A, *Archaeopsylla erinacei erinacei*; Sc, *Spilopsylla cuniculi*; B, bird flea; Pmm, *Paraceras melis melis*; Oh, *Orchopeas howardi*; F, fleas.

THE BIOLOGY OF *CTENOCEPHALIDES FELIS FELIS*

The adult flea remains on the host, though fleas may move from host to host, particularly when they lie in close contact. Up to 15% of fleas were observed to move from one host to another when infected cats were allowed to contact one another (Rust 1994), with fleas often showing a marked preference for some individuals. The female flea may begin to lay eggs 24–48 h after her first blood meal and she can continue to produce up to 50 eggs per day during peak production (Dryden 1989). Fleas can live on cats for at least 113 days, but the majority of fleas survive for only a few days when cats are allowed to groom normally (Dryden 1989).

The eggs are like small, oval pearls and are just visible to the naked eye. They are smooth so they quickly fall off the coat into the environment (Rust 1992). Studies have shown that there is a diurnal rise and fall in egg production, with peak egg-laying timed to coincide with the time when the host is most likely to be in the 'nest' (Kern *et al.* 1992; Rust 1992). Development from the egg, through the larval and pupal stages, to the adult occurs in the environment, with temperature and humidity exerting profound effects on the duration and survival of each immature stage (Table 92.2). It should be remembered that the conditions in the parasite's immediate environment or microclimate will not nec-essarily be identical to those of the macroenvironment of the room or garden.

The flea larvae look like small, white maggots and measure between 2 and 5 mm. They feed off organic debris in the environment and, to a large extent, the flea faeces. Larvae that have fed on flea faeces acquire a discoloured gut, visible as a brown line running through them. Though flea faeces are not essential for larval development (Silverman & Appel 1994) survival rates are markedly better when larvae have access to flea faeces. It has been suggested that, since the composition of the faeces differs very little from the blood ingested by the flea, that the adult flea has evolved faeces specifically to feed its young (Silverman & Appel 1994). The larvae are negatively phototactic and positively geotactic and move down into the base of carpets (Byron 1987). This ensures that some larvae, and the pupae in particular, will be well protected from the effects of vacuum cleaning and/or sprays applied to the surface of the carpet. Larvae are the stage most susceptible to adverse environmental conditions, particularly desiccation (Table 92.2).

After two moults the mature larva spins a sticky, silken cocoon and pupates. In normal circumstances the pupa becomes coated in environmental debris so is difficult to identify. Pupae are often the most troublesome stage of the flea life-cycle to control, partly due to their protected location and to the duration of pupation in some environmental conditions (Table 92.2).

Even when pupation is completed, the adult flea may emerge immediately or may remain in the cocoon for a

Table 92.2 Effects of temperature and humidity on development and survival of the immature stages of *C. felis*.

Egg

  3°C for 5 days lethal
  13°C 75% r.h.: 50% of eggs hatch within 6 days
  16°C 2% r.h.: only 15% of eggs hatched
  27°C 75% r.h.: 50% of eggs hatch within 2 days

Larvae

  10°C: First instar larvae die
  13°C 75% r.h.: 50% fully developed in 26 days
  21°C 75% r.h.: 50% fully developed in 11 days
  27°C 75% r.h.: 50% fully developed in 5 days
  Less than 33% r.h.: 100% larval mortality
  10% soil moisture: good survival
  <or> 10% soil moisture: decreased survival

Pupae

  3°C for 5 days killed 100% pupae
  13°C 75% r.h.: 99 days for 50% of pupae to develop
  21°C 75% r.h.: 26 days for 50% of pupae to develop
  27°C 75% r.h.: 11.5 days for 50% of pupae to develop
  35°C: pupae developed but adults failed to hatch

r.h., relative humidity.
Silverman *et al.* (1981), Silverman & Rust (1983).

considerable time (Silverman & Rust 1985). *Ctenocephalides felis* are stimulated to leave the cocoon by pressure and increased temperature in the environment (Silverman & Rust 1985). Emergence may occur rapidly after appropriate stimulation, accounting for the stories of people entering an empty house and being bitten by fleas shortly afterwards.

> The difficulty of controlling the pupal stage and the pre-emergent adult flea has been recognised as providing the flea with a window of opportunity, the 'pupal window', by which the flea can evade the control measures exerted against it.

Once emerged, the small unfed adult fleas actively seek a host, exhibiting positive phototaxis (Dryden & Broce 1993). They jump towards heat, CO_2 and light, particularly intermittent light (Dryden & Broce 1993). Unfed fleas that are not immediately successful in locating a host may survive for up to 62 days in ideal environmental conditions (Silverman & Rust 1983).

THE BIOLOGY OF *CTENOCEPHALIDES CANIS*

There is less detailed information available about the biology of *C. canis*, and while the parasite is similar in many ways to *C. felis*, it cannot be assumed to be identical. For example, it appears to be markedly less tolerant of low humidity and temperature than *C. felis*. Baker & Elharam (1992) found that no larvae survived at 22°C and 50% r.h., while 36.5% developed to adults when the relative humidity was increased to 75%. Similarly <1% of larvae developed to adults at 25°C and 50% r.h., while 48.6% developed when the relative humidity was increased to 75%.

An understanding of the conditions necessary for flea development helps to explain the success or failure of particular locations to act as reservoirs of infection, and why successful locations provide a continuous or an intermittent source of reinfection. For instance, marked fluctuations in the flea populations of dogs kept in unheated kennels have been observed (Fisher unpublished 1992). In contrast, in many heated houses, where an appropriate environment is maintained almost continually, such fluctuations are likely to be less marked. There has been no work conducted to examine the importance of the garden as a source of infection in the UK, but, given the requirements (Table 92.2) for development of the immature stages, certain areas within the garden may be suitable for flea development, at least in the summer months.

FLEA BITE HYPERSENSITIVITY / FLEA ALLERGY DERMATITIS

Repeated exposure to flea bites from *C. felis* and *C. canis* can initiate FBH. *Archaeopsylla erinacei erinacei* and *Spilopsylla cuniculi* can also provoke the hypersensitive state (Baker & Mulcahy 1986; Coward 1991 and personal communication). It is unusual to find FBH in an animal under 6 months of age, with clinical signs usually first observed in animals between 1 and 6 years of age, though later onset is not unusual (Baker & O'Flanagan 1975; Halliwell & Gorman 1989). There is consensus that there is no sex predisposition but, while most authors have reported no breed predisposition (Baker & O'Flanagan 1975; Muller *et al.* 1989), Sischo & Ihrke (1990) have reported increased incidence in some breeds of dog.

It appears that intermittent exposure to fleas is important for the development of FBH. For example, 28 dogs exposed to fleas once a week for 10 weeks all developed hypersensitivity reactions (Gross & Halliwell 1985). The immunological reactions involved in hypersensitivity to fleas in the dog appear complex and our understanding is, as yet, incomplete. For example, there does not appear to be one clearly defined antigen, indeed sera from different dogs showing flea hypersensitivity vary in their recognition of flea antigens (McKeon & Opdebeeck 1994). The response to flea bites may consist of immediate, later and delayed hypersensitivity reactions. The immediate and delayed hypersensitivities are the classic Gell and Coombs Type I and Type IV reactions. The intermediate stage, characterised by local infiltration with large numbers of basophils is termed cutaneous basophil hypersensitivity (Halliwell & Schemmer 1987). Moreover, some dogs will show each of these stages in turn, while others will show one or two of the three (Gross & Halliwell 1985). Once sensitised, it requires only a relatively small number of bites to re-establish the itch–scratch–lick syndrome that results in severe skin lesions. The clinical signs associated with FBH are summarised in Table 92.3 (Fig. 92.1).

It remains unclear what happens to the hypersensitive animal that remains exposed to fleas. There are reports of the animals becoming less pruritic and erythematous as hyperkeratinisation occurs (Baker & O'Flanagan 1975) but Muller *et al.* (1989) state that FBH animals become more sensitive with time. The poor and variable results achieved when hyposensitisation of FBH dogs is attempted (Halliwell 1981) would suggest that desensitisation does not occur in a set pattern in the dog.

Some dogs that are continually exposed to fleas show signs of immunotolerance, particularly when exposure

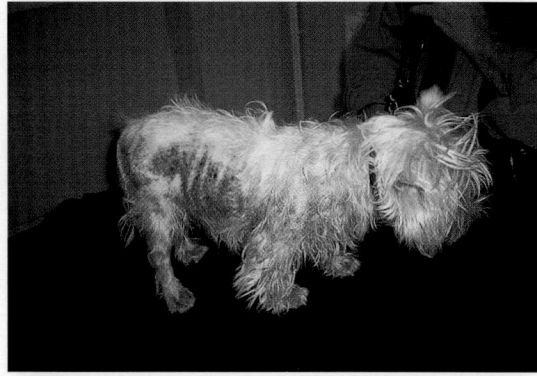
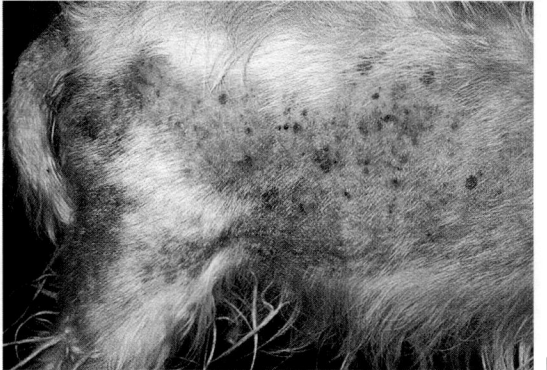

Fig. 92.1a,b   Severe erythema and alopecia in a West Highland White Terrier consistent with flea bite hypersensitivity. Figures courtesy M. Craig.

began at an early age (Halliwell & Longino 1985). Levels of anti-flea IgG and IgE are low in these animals (Halliwell & Longino 1985), while both anti-flea IgG and IgE levels are raised in the hypersensitive animal.

Diagnosis of Flea Bite Hypersensitivity

Diagnosis of FBH is summarised in Table 92.4.

There is a seasonal pattern in the number of cases that parallels the increase in the flea population through the latter part of the summer and into the winter. Therefore, there is a greater probability that dermatitis is associated with FBH when presented in September than in February, though the *C. felis* 'flea season' seems to be becoming a year-round event. There may be collaborative evidence for indicating the presence of fleas, for example, *Dipylidium caninum* infection of the affected animal or humans in the household that have been bitten by fleas. A thorough clinical examination is essential in order to eliminate differential

Table 92.3   Dermatological signs associated with flea bite hypersensitivity (FBH).

Initial signs that may be associated with FBH
  Erythematous papule
  Pruritus

Secondary changes associated with FBH
  Papulocrustous dermatitis
  Self-excoriation with broken, truncated hairs
  Local alopecia (especially over caudal dorsum and
    caudal ventrum, (particularly the medial aspect of the
    thighs))
  Pyotraumatic dermatitis (wet eczema, hot spot)
  Secondary superficial pyoderma
  Lichenification
  Hyperpigmentation

Table 92.4   Diagnosis of flea bite hypersensitivity.

History, e.g. season late summer/autumn or early winter
Clinical examination, including coat combing (perhaps
    including other members of the household)
Response to treatment
• control of symptoms (as necessary)
• vigorous flea control
Intradermal skin test or other test for the presence of
    hypersensitivity

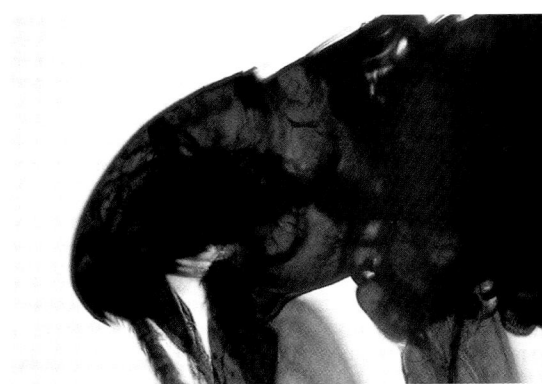

a

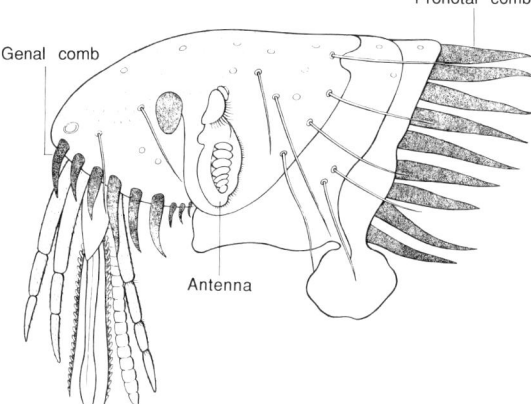

b

Pronotal comb

Genal comb

Antenna

Fig. 92.2   (a) Photomicrograph and (b) line drawing, of
the anterior part of a flea, *Ctenocephalides felis*. This is the
view that the clinician would see if a flea was examined
under low power of a microscope and is adequate for
identifying most of the common fleas to species level.
Clarity may be improved by placing the flea in a suitable
clearing fluid (10% KOH for example) for 12–24 hours.
Photomicrograph courtesy of M. Craig. Illustration
reproduced from *Veterinary Parasitology*, 2nd edn
(ed. G. M. Urquhart *et al.*), Blackwell Science, Oxford.

diagnoses and to support the diagnosis of FBH. Lesions
(Table 92.3) are typically confined to the caudal back and
caudal ventrum (Fig. 92.1a&b). Diagnosis is supported
by demonstration of fleas on the animal (Fig. 92.2a&b),
though finding these may be confounded by the effectiveness of flea and flea dirt removal during the excess grooming and scratching carried out by these animals. It is
essential that a very fine-tooth comb (approximately 15
teeth to the centimetre e.g. Dust/Flea Comb, Hindes,
Birmingham, UK) is used, together with a systematic
approach to grooming to maximise the chance of demonstrating fleas and/or flea faeces ('flea dirt'). Suspect black
material removed from the coat may be confirmed to be flea
dirt by placing on wet cotton wool: a red ring will be seen
around the edge of flea dirt (Fig. 92.3). It may be necessary
to groom other members of the household in order to prove
that fleas are present in the animal's environment. In many
cases the animal's improvement following the removal of
fleas serves to confirm the diagnosis.

Occasionally it will be necessary to carry out a wider
examination in order to confirm a diagnosis of FBH.
Intradermal skin tests can be a useful diagnostic tool. It is
important to obtain a reliable source of antigen and the
person performing the test should be familiar with the
technique. The animal should not have received any systemic glucocorticoids or antihistamines in the recent past.
The test site should be checked 15 min after injection, then
again at 24 h so that dogs showing only delayed reactions
are not missed (Halliwell & Gorman 1989). The presence of
a rise in circulating eosinophils may provide supportive
evidence, but skin biopsy is usually inconclusive.

Even when the test is carried out well, some dogs with
FBH will fail to respond. This observation has led to the
suggestion that 'provocative testing', by applying a vial
containing unfed adult fleas to a shaved area of skin for

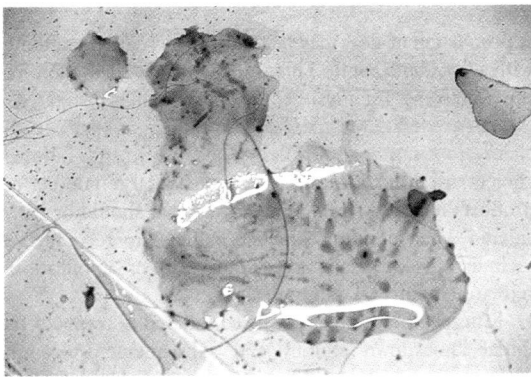

Fig. 92.3   Flea faeces on damp paper. The red
discoloration of the paper confirms the presence of flea
faeces since they contain blood. Figure courtesy M. Craig.

Aerosol products for application to the environment may appear to be ineffective after a shorter period than that claimed by the manufacturer due to incomplete application or the inability of the spray to penetrate down to the base of the carpet. By the time that the young adult emerges from the cocoon the insecticidal cover may have passed, particularly in the case of the combined insecticide/IGR containing methoprene and pyrethrins, where insecticidal control may be extended by repeating the treatment after 1–3 weeks. Control in this case may be improved by reapplying the product after 1–3 weeks to obtain an extended duration of activity (Lloyd personal communication 1993). Borax (sodium polyborate) containing products, e.g. Fleeban™, have been introduced into the UK. The substance is applied to the carpet and has been used extensively in the US to control flea larvae (Dryden & Rust 1994). One study (Hinkle 1992) found 100% mortality of flea larvae after treatment of carpet with boric acid at $200\,g/cm^2$.

Lufenuron (Program™) is a novel approach to control of the early environmental stages. A tablet containing lufenuron is administered to the dog once monthly. All female fleas receive treatment with the active ingredient that prevents chitin synthesis as they feed. Subsequently, eggs that are laid fail to hatch or the larvae fail to develop (Hink *et al.* 1994). More than 99% of flea eggs failed to develop to adulthood from day 7 to day 32 after treatment with a single dose of lufenuron given to dogs at a mean dose rate of $12.8\,mg/kg$ bodyweight (Hink *et al.* 1994). However, there is likely to be a marked lag period before fleas are controlled, especially as the product has no effect against pupae or adult fleas, either in the environment or on the animal. The length of the lag period will be variable (Blagburn *et al.* 1994) but is likely to be longest when the generation time is prolonged for example in cooler weather. It is therefore recommended that both the animal and the environment are treated with insecticide in the face of an existing problem. Obviously, it is essential to treat all cats and dogs in the household, not just the pet with FBH.

There are some basic 'flea traps' on the UK market; these act by luring the unfed flea, using the light and heat of an electric light bulb, to jump on to an attractively smelling sticky pad. These are capable of catching a small proportion of fleas but an improved design, capable of catching >86% of fleas within 20 h in a carpeted room $3.1 \times 3.3\,m$, has been described by Dryden & Broce (1993). This trap utilises the attraction of changes in light intensity by having an intermittently illuminated green-yellow light. Unfortunately, this trap is not commercially available in the UK at the present time.

Designing a Control Programme

The dog owner wishing to instigate a flea control strategy may possess anything from a flea-free environment to a flea-ridden, multi-animal household with one or more animals already showing FBH. It is inappropriate to give the same advice to all owners so each of these extreme situations will be considered separately.

First, there is the owner who intends to put a newly purchased puppy into a dog- and cat-free environment and wants to instigate a prophylactic strategy to prevent fleas becoming a problem. It is possible to carry out such prophylaxis using either an on-animal or an environmental product, beginning in the spring and terminating treatments in mid- to late-autumn. This should be coupled with owner observation, preferably by using regular combing to monitor evidence of the control measures failing. Where owners are concerned about unnecessary use of chemical control, regular combing may be used in the first instance before stepping in with a treatment strategy at the first sign of fleas or flea dirt.

At the other end of the spectrum is the dog owner who has a dog showing signs of severe FBH or whose dog is covered in fleas and flea dirt. Alternatively, the owners may be getting severely bitten themselves by newly-emerged fleas from the environment. In this situation a quick resolution may be brought with a two-part approach, using both environmental and adulticide control, for the following reasons:

(1) In any of these situations there will be eggs, larvae and cocoons, containing either developing pupae or preemergent adults, all at various stages of development in the animal's environment. The numbers of these will normally far outweigh the number of adult fleas present on the animal.

(2) It is essential to reduce the risk of subsequent flea bite challenge to any dog with FBH otherwise control of the condition will not be achieved or there will be a subsequent breakdown of control.

(3) The owner is more likely to be satisfied if they observe an immediate improvement in the situation.

A combined approach (Table 92.7) using fenthion (Tiguvon™) and lufenuron (Program™) was found to control flea burdens on cats living in a flea-infested environment more effectively than either product given alone (Jacobs personal communication 1995). Staggering on-animal and environmental treatments may assist in reducing the opportunity for fleas to reproduce successfully during the final days before retreatment when the efficacy of some treatments may be in decline.

Once the initial problem has been brought under control, it may be possible to maintain control using either an adulticide or by controlling the immature stages, particularly where the animal is kept in a closed environment and/or the newer products such as imidacloprid spot-on or fipronil spot-on or spray are used. In other situations,

Table 92.7 A combined approach to flea control.

Control on the animal
  Comb
  Treat with insecticide
  Treat in-contact animals

Control of immature stages in the environment
  Vacuum cleaner
  Wash animal's bedding regularly
  Apply environmental insecticide/larval growth inhibitor or
     treat animal with chitin synthesis inhibitor (lufenuron)

however, a long-term dual approach to control may be necessary, either because there is unlikely to be 100% control with an on-animal or an environmental treatment or because there is occasional re-infection occurring from outside.

Owner understanding and compliance is essential if flea control is to be effective. The advice given to owners may be reinforced with an information sheet outlining the flea lifecycle and the basis for control, together with details of the treatments recommended and the retreatment interval. The practitioner should bear in mind that it is, from the dermatological viewpoint, perhaps better not to introduce a flea control strategy into a household where the dog is covered in fleas but shows no hypersensitivity (Muller *et al.* 1989) if there is a chance that the control measures and/or owner compliance could lead to the animal receiving intermittant exposure to fleas, which might induce development of FBH.

Apparent Failure of Flea Control

It is worth while, in the event of apparent breakdown of the instigated flea control, to carry out an investigation of *exactly* what the owners have done to control the flea problem. It is also appropriate to check the species of flea present and that there are no other underlying causes of skin disease. Having eliminated the possibility of an unusual source of fleas and other causes of skin disease, a flea-control programme may be tailored to particular circumstances. For example, if it is suspected that there may be outdoor reservoirs of immature fleas then lufenuron (Program™) might form part of the treatment as this will 'go where the animal goes'. Methoprene is degraded by sunlight so is not suitable for outdoor application and there are no environmental outdoor products in the UK equivalent to the 'yard' treatments in the US. Resistance to flea control products is a recognised problem in the US but has not been identified in the UK.

SAFETY CONSIDERATIONS

The practitioner should consider the potential toxicity of the chemicals recommended for flea control and, in particular, take care to ensure that different chemical groups, with different modes of action, are used on the animal and in the environment. An exception occurs in the case of Nuvan Top™ and Nuvan Staykil™, where both the adulticide and environmental treatments contain organophosphate compounds but there is a data sheet recommendation to use the two together. The potential toxicity of the chemicals used for flea control has been reviewed by Kwochka (1987) and in *Clinical Veterinary Toxicology* (Lorgue *et al.* 1996).

FUTURE DEVELOPMENTS FOR THE CONTROL OF FLEAS

Research in the United States, examining natural pathogens of the flea, has resulted in the introduction of the first 'biological control' for fleas. 'Interrupt' consists of a canister of nematodes that attack flea larvae. The product is for application to outdoor areas where flea development may be occurring. These products may be introduced into Europe. To date, research to create a 'flea vaccine' has produced variable results (Opdebeeck & Slacek 1993; Heath *et al.* 1994).

REFERENCES

Amin, O.M. (1966). The fleas (Siphonaptera) of Egypt: distribution and seasonal dynamics of fleas infesting dogs in the Nile Valley and Delta. *Journal of Medical Entomology*, **3**, 293–298.

Baker, K.P. & Elharam, S. (1992). The biology of *C. canis* in Ireland. *Veterinary Parasitology*, **45**, 141–146.

Baker, K.P. & Hatch, C. (1972). The species of fleas found on Dublin dogs. *Veterinary Record*, **91**, 151–152.

Baker, K.P. & Mulcahy, R. (1986). Fleas on hedgehogs and dogs in the Dublin area. *Veterinary Record*, **119**, 16–17.

Baker, K.P. & O'Flanagan, J. (1975). Hypersensitivity of dog skin to fleas – a clinical report. *Journal of Small Animal Practice*, **16**, 317–327.

Baker, N.F. & Farver, T.B. (1983). Failure of Brewer's yeast as a flea repellent on dogs. *Journal of the American Veterinary Medical Association*, **183**, 212–218.

Beresford-Jones, W.P. (1981). Prevalence of fleas on dogs and cats in an area of central London. *Journal of Small Animal Practice*, **22**, 27–29.

Blagburn, B.L., Vaughan, J.L., Lindsay, D.S. & Tebbitt, G.L. (1994). Efficacy dosage titration of lufenuron against developmental stages of fleas (*C. f. felis*). *American Journal of Veterinary Research*, **55**, 98–101.

Byron, D.W. (1987). Aspects of the biology, behaviour, bionomics and control of immature stages of the cat flea *Ctenocephalides felis felis* (Bouche) in the domicillary environment. PhD thesis. Cited by Dryden, M.W. & Rust, M.K. (1994). The cat flea: biology, ecology and control. *Veterinary Parasitology*, **52**, 1–19.

Chesney, C.J. (1995). Flea species found on cats and dogs in Southwest England: further evidence of the polyxenous state, with implications for flea control. *Veterinary Record*, **136**, 356–358.

Coward, P.S. (1991). Fleas in southern England. *Veterinary Record*, **124**, 272.

Dryden, M.W. (1989). Host association, on-host longevity and egg production of *C. f. felis*. *Veterinary Parasitology*, **34**, 117–122.

Dryden, M.W. & Broce, A.B. (1993). Development of a trap for collecting newly emerged *Ctenocephalides felis* (Siphonaptera: Pulicidae). *Journal of Medical Entomology*, **30**, 901–906.

Dryden, M.W. & Rust, M.K. (1994). The cat flea: biology, ecology and control. *Veterinary Parasitology*, **52**, 1–19.

Dryden, M.W., Long, G.R. & Gaafar, S.M. (1989). Effects of ultrasonic flea collars on *Ctenocephalides felis* on cats. *Journal of the American Veterinary Medical Association*, **195**, 1717–1718.

Edwards, F.B. (1969). Correspondence. *Veterinary Record*, **85**, 665.

Else, R.W., Bagnall, B.G., Phaffs, J.J.G. & Potter, C. (1977). Endo- and ecto-parasites of dogs and cats: a survey from practices in the East Anglian Region, BSAVA. *Journal of Small Animal Practice*, **18**, 731–737.

Fisher, M.A., Pilkington, J.G. & Jacobs, D.E. (1989). Efficacy of cythioate against fleas on dogs and cats. *Veterinary Dermatology*, **1**, 46–48.

Fisher, M.A., Hutchinson, M.J., Jacobs, D.E. & Dick, I.G.C. (1993). Efficacy of fenthion against the flea, *C. felis*, on the cat. *Journal of Small Animal Practice*, **34**, 434–435.

Fisher, M.A., Hutchinson, M.J., Jacobs, D.E. & Dick, I.G.C. (1994). Comparative efficacy of fenthion, dichlorvos/fenitrothion and permethrin against the flea, *Ctenocephalides felis*, on the dog. *Journal of Small Animal Practice*, **35**, 244–246.

Geary, M.R. (1977). Ectoparasite survey. *Veterinary Dermatology Newsletter*, **2**, 2–3.

Gross, T.L. & Halliwell, R.E.W. (1985). Lesions of experimental flea bite hypersensitivity in the dog. *Veterinary Pathology*, **22**, 78–81.

Halliwell, R.E.W. (1981). Hyposensitisation in the treatment of flea bite hypersensitivity: results of a double-blind study. *Journal of the American Animal Hospital Association*, **17**, 249–253.

Halliwell, R.E.W. (1982). Ineffectiveness of thiamine (vitamin B1) as a flea repellent in dogs. *Journal of the American Animal Hospital Association*, **18**, 423–426.

Halliwell, R.E.W. & Gorman, N.T. (1989). Nonatopic allergic skin diseases. In: *Veterinary Clinical Immunology*. pp. 262–266. W.B. Saunders, Philadelphia.

Halliwell, R.E.W. & Longino, S.J. (1985). IgE and IgG antibodies to flea antigen in differing dog populations. *Veterinary Immunology and Immunopathology*, **8**, 215–223.

Halliwell, R.E.W. & Schemmer, K.R. (1987). The role of basophils in the immunopathogenesis of hypersensitivity to fleas (*Ctenocephalides felis*) in dogs. *Veterinary Immunology and Immunopathology*, **15**, 203–213.

Hatch, C. & Dooge, D.J. (1986). Fleas on hedgehogs and dogs. *Veterinary Record*, **119**, 162.

Heath, A.W., Arfsten, A., Schriefer, M.E., *et al.* (1994). Vaccination against the cat flea *C. f. felis*. *Parasite Immunology*, **16**, 187–191.

Hink, W.K., Zakson, M. & Barnett, M.S. (1994). Evaluation of a single oral dose of lufenuron to control flea infestations in dogs. *American Journal of Veterinary Research*, **55**, 822–824.

Hinkle, N.C. (1992). Biological factors and larval management strategies affecting the cat flea (*Ctenocephalides felis felis* Bouche) populations. PhD thesis. Cited by Dryden, M.W. & Rust, M.K. (1994). The cat flea: biology, ecology and control. *Veterinary Parasitology*, **52**, 1–19.

Kern, W.H., Koehler, P.G. & Patterson, A. (1992). Daily patterns of cat flea (Siphonaptera: Pulicidae) egg and faecal deposition. *Journal of Medical Entomology*, **29**, 203–206.

Kristensen, S., Haarlov, N. & Mourier, H. (1978). A study of skin diseases in dogs and cats IV: Patterns of flea infestation in dogs and cats in Denmark. *Nordisk Veterinær Medicin*, **30**, 401–413.

Kwochka, K.W. (1987). Fleas and related disease. *Veterinary Clinics of North America: Small Animal Practice*, **17**, 1235–1261.

Lorgue, G., Lechenet, J. & Rivière, C. (1996). *Clinical Veterinary Toxicology*, (ed. M.J. Chapman). Blackwell Science, Oxford.

McKeon, S.E. & Opdebeeck, J.P. (1994). IgG and IgE antibodies against antigens of the cat flea, *Ctenocephalides felis felis*, in sera of allergic and non-allergic dogs. *International Journal for Parasitology*, **24**, 259–263.

Maunder, J.H. (1984). Entomological components to urticaria. *Practitioner*, **228**, 1051–1055.

Muller, G.H., Kirk, R.W. & Scott, D.W. (1989). *Small Animal Dermatology*, 4th edn. pp. 482–489. W.B. Saunders Philadelphia.

Opdebeeck, J.P. & Slacek, B. (1993). An attempt to protect cats against infestation with *C. felis* using gut embrane antigens as a vaccine. *International Journal for Parasitology*, **23**, 1063–1067.

Osbrink, W.L.A., Rust, M.W. & Reierson, D.A. (1986). Distribution and control of cat fleas in homes in Southern California (Siphonaptera: Pulicidae). *Journal of Economic Entomology*, **79**, 135–140.

PFMA (Pet Food Manufacturers Association) (1992). *Profile*. PFMA, London.

Rust, M.K. (1992). Influence of photoperiod on egg production of cat fleas (Siphonaptera: Pulicidae) infesting cats. *Journal of Medical Entomology*, **29**, 242–245.

Rust, M.K. (1994). Interhost movement of adult cat fleas (Siphonaptera: Pulicidae). *Journal of Medical Entomology*, **31**, 486–489.

Silverman, J. & Appel, A.G. (1994). Adult cat flea (Siphonaptera, Pulicidae) excretion of host blood proteins in relation to larval nutrition. *Journal of Medical Entomology*, **31**, 265–271.

Silverman, J. & Rust, M.K. (1983). Some abiotic factors affecting the survival of the cat flea *C. f. felis* (Siphonaptea: Pulicidae). *Environmental Entomology*, **12**, 490–495.

Silverman, J. & Rust, M.K. (1985). Extended longevity of the pre-emerged cat flea (Siphonaptera; Pulicidae) and factors stimulating emergence from the pupal cocoon. *Annals of the Entomological Society of America*, **78**, 763–768.

Silverman, J., Rust, M.K. & Reierson, D.A. (1981). Influence of temperature and humidity on survival and development of the cat flea, *C. felis* (Siponaptera: Pulicidae). *Journal of Medical Entomology*, **18**, 78–83.

Sischo, W.M. & Ihrke, P.J. (1990), Unpublished data. Cited in: *Veterinary Dermatopathology.*, (eds T.L. Cross, P.J. Ihrke & E.J. Walder), pp. 119–122. Mosby Year Book, St Louis.

Slacek, B. & Opdebeeck, J.P. (1993). Reactivity of dogs and cats to feeding fleas and to flea antigens injected intradermally. *Australian Veterinary Journal*, **70**, 313–314.

Chapter 93

Current Methods of Mite and Tick Control in the Dog

C. F. Curtis

INTRODUCTION

Mites and ticks belong to the class Arachnida and are members of the order Acari. The mite species commonly causing skin infestations in dogs in Britain and Europe are *Sarcoptes scabiei* var. *canis*, *Otodectes cynotis*, *Neotrombicula autumnalis*, *Demodex canis* and *Cheyletiella* spp. Environmental pyroglyphid mite species such as *Dermatophagoides farinae* and *D. pteronyssinus* ('house dust mites') are believed to be important in the aetiology of canine atopy and a recent survey of 418 intradermal allergen test results revealed that 82% and 63% of atopic dogs in the UK developed a positive skin test reaction to these allergens respectively (Ferguson 1991).

Sarcoptes scabiei and *Cheyletiella* spp. and, to a lesser extent, *Otodectes cynotis* may be transmitted to humans (Thoday 1979; Scott & Horn 1987). Infestation in man causes a pruritic rash but this usually resolves once the source of parasites is removed, despite the fact that *Sarcoptes scabiei* var. *canis* has been known to produce ova in human hosts (Kummel 1981).

> The accepted method for the diagnosis of mange is the identification of mature or immature mites or their eggs in skin scrapings suspended in mineral oil or potassium hydroxide (Muller *et al.* 1989a).

Some mites, particularly *Sarcoptes scabiei*, can be difficult to find as they may only be present in low numbers so it is advisable to subject any animal presenting with historical and clinical features suggestive of sarcoptic mange to a therapeutic trial, even if the mite cannot be detected in skin scrapings. Recent studies of canine antibody responses to *Sarcoptes scabiei* infestations have led to the development of a diagnostic enzyme-linked immunosorbent assay (ELISA) for sarcoptic mange (Bornstein & Zakrisson 1990) but this is not yet commercially available in the UK.

Approximately 800 species of ticks are recognised world-wide, the majority of which act as obligate parasites. The two families of veterinary importance are the Ixodidae (hard ticks), and the more primitive Argasidae (soft ticks). In northern Europe, the hard ticks *Ixodes ricinus* (castor bean or sheep tick), *Ixodes hexagonus* (hedgehog tick), *Ixodes canisuga* (kennel tick), *Haemaphysalis punctata* and *Dermacentor reticulatus* are known to parasitise domestic animals. Isolated reports of the tropical tick *Rhipicephalus sanguineus* have appeared in the literature (Fox & Sykes 1985). *Ixodes ricinus* is the species most frequently isolated from dogs in Britain, particularly those which have been exercising in fields or on moors where sheep and cattle, the ticks' principal hosts, have been grazing. Tick bites are a source of irritation to animals and man and large numbers may result in anaemia. They pose a more serious threat to human health as vectors and reservoirs of viral, rickettsial, protozoal and bacterial organisms responsible for zoonotic diseases such as the spirochete *Borrelia burgdorferi*, the cause of Lyme disease (Cupp 1991). Currently, tick vaccines based on 'concealed' gut antigens are being developed (Willadsen & Kemp 1988). These have shown promising results with high killing rates and reduced egg production but are not yet commercially available.

The first part of this chapter will describe the products currently available in Britain for the control of mite and tick infestations in dogs. In the second part, methods of environmental control of house dust mites will be discussed.

PRODUCTS USED IN THE CONTROL OF MITE AND TICK INFESTATIONS IN THE DOG

Organophosphates

Phosmet

There are two licensed canine scabicides in the UK: phosmet (Vet-Kem Sponge-On for Dogs™) and amitraz (Aludex™). Phosmet is also approved for the control of ticks and, although not specifically licensed for the treatment of cheyletiellid, trombiculid and psoroptid mites, it is effective against these species. Like all organophosphates, it is a potent anti-cholinesterase and should not be used in sick or debilitated animals, puppies under 12 weeks of age, pregnant or nursing bitches. Phosmet treatment failures have been reported (Moriello 1992) but may reflect geographical variation in organophosphate efficacy, misuse of the product or re-infestation. When treating canine scabies, the manufacturers recommend that if no improvement is seen within 14 days, retreatment may be necessary (Table 93.1). For tick control, a single application is recommended, unless the dog is repeatedly re-infested.

When controlling scabies or tick infestations, in-contact dogs should always be treated concurrently. The risk of transmission of *Sarcoptes scabiei* var. *canis* to cats is low (Hawkins *et al.* 1987) but *Cheyletiella yasguri* and *Otodectes cynotis* are less host specific so in-contact cats should also be treated when dealing with these mite species. An acaricidal spray such as iodofenphos with dichlorvos (Nuvan Staykil) should be applied around the dog's environment and on to grooming equipment as mange mites (with the possible exception of *Demodex canis*) and ticks can survive off the

host and the eggs of *Cheyletiella* spp. may be attached to dropped dog hairs.

Diazinon

Diazinon is an organophosphate approved for tick control in Europe and is available as a topically applied 'spot-on' liquid or as the active component of a number of insecticidal collars. The 'spot-on' product (20% w/v diazinon; Droplix) is absorbed through the skin following application to the dorsal neck and enters the circulation. Feeding ticks ingest the product during a blood meal and are paralysed and killed as a result of its anti-cholinesterase action. This preparation can be used at monthly intervals on puppies from 3 months of age. It is claimed to be effective against ticks for 2 weeks following application.

The major disadvantage of this type of product is that the tick has to bite before it is killed and is therefore still able to spread disease and cause discomfort. One alternative is to use surface-active preparations with immediate knock-down and repellent properties. Insecticidal collars incorporating 15% diazinon are claimed to act in this way (Preventef insecticidal collars for dogs, Derasect insecticidal collar for dogs). The drug is gradually released from the surface of the collar on to the coat over a 4-month period and is reputed to kill ticks within days and prevent re-infestation for up to 120 days. The collars can be used on puppies from 2 and 3 months of age respectively.

Cythioate

Cythioate (Cyflee™), marketed as a systemic insecticide and acaricide, is approved for use as an aid in the control of demodectic mange in dogs over 12 weeks of age. The manufacturer's recommended dosage is 3.0 mg/kg twice a week for at least 6 weeks. This product is easy to use but is not generally considered effective in the treatment of canine demodecosis (Kwochka 1993).

Sulphur Compounds

Selenium Sulphide

For many years, sulphur has been employed topically as an anti-parasitic agent (Humphreys 1958). Although not specifically licensed for ectoparasite control in the dog, 1% selenium sulphide shampoo (Seleen™) is safe and effective against *Cheyletiella* spp. mites. Grant (1991) recommends its use at weekly intervals for at least 3 weeks, with concurrent treatment of in-contacts and the environment.

Table 93.1 The use of 11.74% phosmet for canine scabies.

1. Consider clipping medium and long-haired breeds before application to ensure maximal skin contact.
2. Dilute phosmet with tepid water, according to manufacturer's instructions.
3. Wearing gloves and an apron, apply to entire body surface with a sponge.
4. Do not rinse.
5. Allow dog to dry in a well ventilated area (ideally outdoors).
6. Repeat steps 2–5 after 14 days.

Formamidines

Amitraz

The formamidine pesticide amitraz is approved for the treatment of demodectic mange caused by *Demodex canis*, or the short bodied unnamed demodex species (Mason 1993), at a variety of concentrations and frequencies of application in different countries of the world. A recent study in which 0.125% amitraz solution (Taktic™) was applied to half the body of 50 dogs with generalised demodecosis on alternate days, reported a cure rate of 61% with a median duration of treatment of 6.5 weeks (range 3 weeks to 9 months) (Medleau & Willemse 1995). Dogs that were considered cured remained free of disease for a follow-up period of 2 to 4.5 years (median 3 years). 'Taktic' is only licensed for the control of mange, lice and ticks in cattle, sheep and pigs.

In the United States, solutions of 0.025% amitraz (Mitaban™) can be applied at 2-week intervals but this regime has been associated with treatment failure rates of 47–100% (White & Stannard 1983; Kwochka *et al.* 1985; Scott & Walton 1985). Studies investigating the use of 0.05% amitraz solution, applied weekly, claimed much higher cure rates of 65–80% (Kwochka *et al.* 1985; Bussieras & Chermette 1986) but the subjects were not monitored for long follow-up periods, making their interpretation difficult.

In Britain, 0.05% amitraz solution (Aludex™) is approved for use at weekly intervals in the dog (Table 93.2). It is contraindicated in Chihuahuas, pregnant or nursing bitches and puppies less than 3 months of age. Demodecosis is frequently complicated by pyoderma and a bactericidal antibacterial drug should be used concurrently for a minimum of 3 weeks.

Table 93.2   The use of 0.05% amitraz solution for the control of canine demodecosis.

---

1. Clip medium and long-haired breeds.
2. Pre-wash with a de-greasing, keratolytic shampoo such as 2.5% benzoyl peroxide.
3. Allow to dry.
4. Dilute amitraz with tepid water, according to manufacturers' instructions.
5. Wearing gloves and an apron, apply to the entire body surface using a sponge (persons receiving monoamine oxidase inhibiting drugs should not handle amitraz).
6. Do not rinse. Allow dog to dry in a well-ventilated area (ideally outdoors).
7. Repeat steps 2–6 weekly until successive skin scrapings are free of mites (see below).

Perhaps the most important part of any demodecosis treatment regime is the monitoring and regular reassessment of affected animals. Multiple skin scrapings should be taken every 4 weeks and the ratios of dead:live and mature:immature mites noted to assess progress. If repeated scrapings do not contain mites, treatment should be continued for a further 2–4 weeks and only withdrawn if repeated scrapings fail to demonstrate the mite. Persistent, focal infestations, for example otodemodecosis and podo-demodecosis, may respond to localised therapy with 5.0% amitraz (Aludex™) diluted 1 in 60 with mineral oil, applied daily (Chester 1988). Owners should be warned that there is high incidence of relapse with this disease and that re-institution of therapy may be necessary if clinical signs recur. Demodectic mange is unique in that the treatment of in-contact animals, premises and grooming equipment is not considered necessary as transmission of *Demodex canis* between adult dogs is only believed to be possible under experimental conditions (Folz *et al.* 1978; Folz 1983).

Amitraz is also licensed for the treatment of sarcoptic mange. Three applications of a 0.025% solution at fortnightly intervals, has been shown to have effective scabicidal activity (Folz 1984).

Avermectins

Ivermectin

Ivermectin, a fermentation product of *Streptomyces avermitilis*, has been used for several years as an anthelmintic, insecticide and acaricide. It stimulates the pre-synaptic release of γ-aminobutyric acid (GABA) and potentiates its binding to receptors, resulting in paralysis and death of parasites in which GABA is a peripheral neurotransmitter (Bennett 1986).

The drug is currently licensed in many counties of the world as an ivermectin preparation used as a heartworm preventative (Heartgard™), given orally once a month at a dosage of 5–7 µg/kg. The 1% injectable bovine ivermectin product (Ivomec™) is known to be effective against *Sarcoptes scabiei*, *Otodectes cynotis* and *Cheyletiella yasguri* infestations in the dog when given by two subcutaneous injections, 2 weeks apart, at 200–300 g/kg (Yazwinski *et al.* 1981; Paradis & Villeneuve 1988).

A number of workers have investigated its efficacy against *Demodex canis* in chronic cases of amitraz-resistant, generalised demodecosis. Scott & Walton (1985) and Paradis (1989) concluded that weekly subcutaneous injection of the 1% bovine product at 400 g/kg for 2 months was without benefit but a single case which was treated orally with 600 g/kg per day had mite-free skin scrapings after 7 months (Paradis & Laperriere 1992). It is unlikely that these doses of ivermectin will obtain approval for use in dogs because of the risk of neurotoxicity in this species, particularly in collies, sheepdogs and their crosses (Pulliam *et al.* 1985; Pulliam & Preston 1989).

Milbemycin Oxime

Milbemycin oxime is a fermentation product of *Streptomyces hygroscopicus aureolacrimosus*. This compound is currently licensed for use in dogs in North America and in some European countries as an anthelmintic which is given orally once a month for the prevention of heartworm and control of hookworms (Interceptor™). It has the advantage of being less toxic to collies than ivermectin and doses of up to 20 times the recommended 0.5 mg/kg dosage for heartworm prevention have been used in this breed without adverse effects (Talbot 1990). Two studies investigating the use of milbemycin oxime in the treatment of 76 chronic generalised demodecosis cases, the majority of which had not responded to therapy with amitraz, reported cure rates of 42% and 53% using dosages ranging from 0.5 to 4.6 mg/kg administered over 60–210 days (Garfield & Reedy 1992; Miller *et al.* 1993). Dogs were considered cured if they remained free of clinical signs and mites were absent from skin scrapings for a follow-up period of at least 12 months after medication was withdrawn. However 60 of the 76 dogs described had 'juvenile-onset' demodecosis, a form of the disease which may resolve spontaneously in 30–50% of cases (Muller *et al.* 1989b), so the cure rates quoted may be exaggerated.

Pyrethroids

Permethrin (Table 93.3)

Pyrethroids are more frequently used as insecticides than acaricides but two products containing permethrin are currently approved for tick control in Britain. Permethrin is toxic to ticks on contact and if a sufficiently high concentration is present on the skin and coat, it has a repellent effect and prevents re-infestation. One product is available as a liquid containing 65% w/w permethrin (Exspot™ insecticide for dogs) which is applied to the skin of the dorsal neck (also the lumbar area if dog is >15 kg) once a month. The drug spreads over the skin in epidermal lipids but is not absorbed systemically. It is approved for use in puppies from 2 weeks of age. Treated animals should not be handled for 6 hours following application and should be prevented from swimming for 12 hours. The second product incorporates 8% w/w permethrin into an insecticidal collar (Natura™ insecticidal collar for dogs) and is approved for tick control in dogs over 3 months of age. Permethrin is continually released from the collar for 4 months.

Chemically impregnated collars have been reported to induce contact irritant or allergic reactions and owners should be advised to check their animals regularly for signs of dermatitis.

Phenylpyrazoles

Fipronil (Table 93.3)

Fipronil is a novel molecule which acts as an insecticide and acaricide by inhibiting the γ-aminobutyric acid (GABA)-mediated chloride ion flux into arthropod peripheral nerve cells through binding at a site within the chloride channels of GABA receptors. This results in muscular paralysis and death of the arthropod (Colliott *et al.* 1992). It is licensed in the UK as a 0.25% solution in an isopropanol base for the control of fleas and ticks in dogs from 2 days of age and for the treatment of fleas in cats from 7 weeks of age (Frontline™ spray). The fipronil is thought to bind to hair and skin and form a 'reservoir' within pilosebaceous units although the exact mechanism of its persistence has not yet been fully determined. Absorption through the epidermis into the dermis is negligable (Penaliggon, personal communication). Anecdotal reports of its use against *Neotrombicula autumnalis* infestations (Famose 1995) suggest it may also be an effective miticidal agent with a residual action of approximately 1 month. The author has used it successfully to treat an outbreak of scabies in a litter of 5-week-old puppies but to her knowledge, no studies investigating the product's action against *Sarcoptes scabiei* have been reported in the literature.

METHODS FOR THE CONTROL OF HOUSE DUST MITES IN THE ENVIRONMENT

Human atopic patients sensitised to house dust mites are routinely given advice on measures designed to limit allergen exposure. Recently, the British Society for Allergy and Clinical Immunology (Anon. 1991) has described the relative efficacy of various control methods. Environmental control of house dust mites is often neglected during the treatment of canine atopy and should be considered.

The most important factors influencing house dust mite population levels are relative humidity and temperature. Reductions in both parameters can significantly retard the growth and egg production rates of these mites and accelerate their mortality rate (Colloff 1987). Therefore animal bedding, which often supports elevated populations of

Table 93.3 Products currently recommended for the control of canine mite and tick infestations.

Parasite species	Product	Active principle	Directions*	Method of application	Comments
Sarcoptes scabiei	Aludex™	2.5% mitraz	Apply solution to skin and allow to dry	Once weekly	Do not use on Chihauhaus
	Vet-Kem Sponge-On™ for dogs	11.74% phosmet	As above	Two treatments at 2-week intervals	Treat in contact dogs. Wash bedding and grooming equipment. Spray house with acaricidal spray (e.g. Nuvan Staykil™)
Cheyletiella yasguri	Vet-Kem Sponge-On™ for dogs	11.74% phosmet	As above	As above	As above.
	Seleen	1% selenium sulphide	Lather into coat	Three treatments at weekly intervals	Neither product holds UK licence for the treatment of *C heyletiella* sp.
Demodex canis	Aludex™	5% amitraz	Apply solution to skin and allow to dry	Once weekly until obtain 2 mite-free skin scrapes, 4 weeks apart	Not necessary to treat in-contacts or environment
Otodectes cynotis	Auroto™ GAC™ Oterna™ Canaural™	4% thiabendazole 1% permethrin 5% monosulfiram Unknown	After cleansing, apply two to three drops to each ear, massage after use	Use twice daily for 3 weeks	Treat the ears of in-contact dogs and cats. In generalised cases, treat entire dog with Vet-Kem Sponge-On™ for dogs. Treat house with acaricidal spray (e.g. Nuvan Staykil)
Ixodes sp.	Vet-Kem Sponge-On™ for dogs	11.74% phosmet		One dip or spot-on treatment alone may be necessary	Avoid exercising dogs in tick-infested areas.
	Natura™ and Preventef™ insecticidal collars for dogs	8% permethrin and 15% diazinon respectively	Follow manufacturers' instructions	Collars may help to prevent re-infestation	Treat house with acaricidal spray (e.g. Nuvan Staykil™)
	Derasect™ insecticidal collar for dogs	15% diazinon			
	Droplix™ Exspot™	20% diazinon 65% permethrin			

* Summarised – always read and follow manufacturers' directions for use.

these mites, should not be subjected to wet cleaning methods.

Routine vacuuming has been shown to significantly increase airborne levels of Der p1, the principal house dust mite allergen believed to trigger human atopic disease. This can be prevented by using an approved 'Medivac' cleaner with a superior filter which minimises the amount of allergen recirculated by the vacuuming process (Kalra *et al.* 1990). However, these machines are expensive and financial constraints may prohibit their use.

Environmental miticidal sprays and liquid nitrogen freezing techniques have been suggested as additional methods of decreasing house dust mite populations. Clinical trials with such products have been disappointing. One possible explanation is that despite a reduction in mite numbers, levels of airborne Der p1 allergen in the form of mite faeces remain unaffected by these treatments (Taylor 1992). Perhaps the most useful, affordable method of house dust mite avoidance for dogs is the use of bedding covers which are non-permeable to house dust mites and their faeces. A number of these products are available for pillows and mattresses of various sizes and they are reported to be efficacious in reducing allergenic challenge in atopic people (Taylor 1992).

REFERENCES

Anon (1991). The control of dust mites and other domestic allergens. A position paper from the workshop meetings of the British Society for Allergy and Clinical Immunology, Southampton, 21 June and 29 July.

Bennett, D.G. (1986). Clinical pharmacology of ivermectin. *Journal of the American Veterinary Medical Association*, **189**, 100–104.

Bornstein, S. & Zakrisson, G. (1990). Ny diagnostik av hundens rævskabb (*Sarcoptes scabiei*). *Svensk Veterinærtidning*, **42**, 180–181.

Bussieras, J. & Chermette, P. (1986). Amitraz and canine demodicosis. *Journal of the American Animal Hospital Association*, **22**, 779–782.

Chester, D.K. (1988). Medical management of otitis externa. *Veterinary Clinics of North America, Small Animal Practice*, **18**, 799–812.

Colliott, F., Kukorowski, K.A., Hawkins, D.W. & Roberts, D.A. (1992). Pests and diseases. *Proceedings of the Brighton Crop Protection Conference*, Brighton 1992, pp. 29–34.

Colloff, M.J. (1987). Effects of temperature and relative humidity on development times and mortality of eggs from laboratory and wild populations of the European house dust mite: *Dermatophagoides pteronyssinus* (Acari: *Pyroglyphidae*). *Experimental and Applied Acarology*, **3**, 279–289.

Cupp, E.W. (1991). Biology of ticks. *Veterinary Clinics of North America: Small Animal Practice*, **21**, 1–26.

Famose, F. (1995). Ectoparasites and their control. *Proceedings of the Royal Veterinary College Occasional Seminar in Dermatology, Autumn 1995*, pp. 28–30. The Royal Veterinary College, London.

Ferguson, E.A. (1991). A review of intradermal skin testing in the United Kingdom. *Veterinary Dermatology Newsletter*, **14**, 13–18.

Folz, S.D. (1983). Demodicosis (*Demodex canis*). *Compendium on Continuing Education for the Practicing Veterinarian*, **5**, 116–121.

Folz, S.D. (1984). Canine scabies (*Sarcoptes scabiei* infestation). *Compendium on Continuing Education for the Practicing Veterinarian*, **6**, 176–180.

Folz, S.D., Geng, S., Nowakowski, L.H. & Conklin, R.D. (1978). Evaluation of a new treatment for canine scabies and demodecosis (amitraz). *Journal of Veterinary Pharmacology and Therapeutics*, **1**, 199–204.

Fox, M.T. & Sykes, T.J. (1985). Establishment of the tropical dog tick, *Rhipicephalus sanguineus*, in a house in London. *Veterinary Record*, **116**, 661–662.

Garfield, R.A. & Reedy, L.M. (1992). The use of oral milbemycin oxime (Interceptor) in the treatment of chronic generalised canine demodicosis. *Veterinary Dermatology*, **3**, 231–235.

Grant, D.I. (1991). Parasitic skin diseases. In: *Skin Diseases in the Dog and Cat*. pp. 28–52. Blackwell Science, Oxford.

Hawkins, J.A., McDonald, R.K. & Woody, B.J. (1987). *Sarcoptes scabiei* infestation in a cat. *Journal of the American Academy of Veterinary Medicine*, **190**, 1572–1573.

Humphreys, M. (1958). *Cheyletiella parasitovorax* infestation of the dog. *Veterinary Record*, **70**, 442.

Kalra, S., Owen, S.J., Hepworth, J. & Woodcack, A.A. (1990). Airborne house dust mite antigen after vacuum cleaning. *Lancet*, **336**, 449.

Kummel, B. (1981). Case presentation. *Proceedings of American Academy of Veterinary Dermatology*, Atlanta, April 1981.

Kwochka, K.W. (1993). Demodicosis. In: *Current Veterinary Dermatology*, (eds C.E. Griffin, K.W. Kwochka & J.M. McDonald), pp. 72–84. Mosby Year Book, Philadelphia.

Kwochka, K.W., Kunkle, G.A. & Foil, C.S. (1985). The efficacy of amitraz for generalised demodicosis in dogs : a study of two concentrations and frequencies of application. *Compendium on Continuing Education for the Practicing Veterinarian*, **7**, 8–17.

Mason, K.V. (1993). A new species of Demodex mite with *Demodex canis* causing canine demodecosis: a case report. *Proceedings, American Academy of Veterinary Dermatology Annual Meeting*, San Diego, p. 92.

Medleau, L. & Willemse, T. (1995). Efficacy of daily amitraz on generalised demodicosis in dogs. *Journal of Small Animal Practice*, **36**, 3–6.

Miller, W.H., Scott, D.W., Wellington, J.R. & Panic, R. (1993). Clinical efficacy of milbemycin oxime in the treatment of generalised demodicosis in adult dogs. *Journal of the American Veterinary Medical Association*, **203**, 1426–1429.

Moriello, K.A. (1992). Treatment of Sarcoptes and Cheyletiella infestations. In: *Current Veterinary Therapy XI*, (ed. R.W. Kirk), pp. 558–560. W.B. Saunders, Philadelphia.

Muller, G.H., Kirk, R.W. & Scott, D.W. (1989a). Diagnostic methods. In: *Small Animal Dermatology*, 4th edn. pp. 92–149. W.B. Saunders, Philadelphia.

Muller, G.H., Kirk, R.W. & Scott, D.W. (1989b). Cutaneous parasitology. In: *Small Animal Dermatology*, 4th edn. pp. 347–426. W.B. Saunders, Philadelphia.

Paradis, M. (1989). Ivermectin in small animal dermatology. In: *Current Veterinary Therapy X*, (ed. R.W. Kirk), pp. 560–563. W.B. Saunders, Philadelphia.

Paradis, M. & Villeneuve, A. (1988). Efficacy of ivermectin against *Cheyletiella yasguri* infestation in dogs. *Canadian Veterinary Journal*, **29**, 633–635.

Paradis, M. & Laperriere, E. (1992). Efficacy of daily ivermectin treatment in a dog with amitraz-resistant, generalised demodicosis. *Veterinary Dermatology*, **3**, 85–88.

Pulliam, J.D. & Preston, J.M. (1989). Safety of ivermectin in target animals. In: *Ivermectin and Abamectin*, (ed. W.C. Campbell), pp. 157–161. Springer-Verlag, New York.

Pulliam, J.D., Seward, R.L., Henry, R.T. & Steinberg, S.A. (1985). Investigating ivermectin toxicity in collies. *Veterinary Medicine Small Animal Clinics*, **80**: 33–40.

Scott, D.W. & Horn, R.T. (1987). Zoonotic dermatoses of dogs and cats. *Veterinary Clinics of North America: Small Animal Practice*, **17**, 117–144.

Scott, D.W. & Walton, D.K. (1985). Experiences with the use of amitraz and ivermectin for the treatment of generalised demod-icosis in dogs. *Journal of the American Animal Hospital Association*, **21**, 535–541.

Talbot, R.B. (1990). In: *Veterinary Pharmaceuticals and Biologicals*, 7th edn. pp. 441–442. Veterinary Medicine Publishing Company, Lenexa.

Taylor, C. (1992). House dust mite allergen avoidance measures. In: *Fighting the Mite – a Practical Guide to House Dust Mite Allergy*. pp. 13–28. The Wheatsheaf Press, Cheshire.

Thoday, K.L. (1979). Skin diseases of dogs and cats transmissable to man. *In Practice*, **1**, 5–15.

White, S.D. & Stannard, A.A. (1983), Canine demodicosis. In: *Current Veterinary Therapy VIII*, (ed. R.W. Kirk), pp. 484–487. W.B. Saunders, Philadelphia.

Willadsen, P. & Kemp, D. (1988). Vaccination with 'concealed' antigens for tick control. *Parasitology Today*, **4**, 196–199.

Yazwinski, T.A., Pote, L., Tilley, W., Rodriguez, C. & Greenway, T. (1981). Efficacy of ivermectin against *Sarcoptes scabiei* and *Otodectes cynotis* infestations in dogs. *Veterinary Medicine Small Animal Clinics*, **76**, 1749–1751.

Chapter 94

Advances in the Diagnosis of Canine Endocrine Dermatoses

D. Heripret

INTRODUCTION

Canine endocrinopathies are relatively common. Endocrinopathies with cutaneous manifestations include hyperadrenocorticism, hypothyroidism, sex hormone imbalances, growth-hormone responsive dermatosis, diabetes mellitus and perhaps seasonal flank alopecia.

The typical, but not exclusive, clinical appearance is of a non-pruritic, symmetrical alopecia of the trunk of an adult dog. However, other important dermatoses can mimic this pattern and must be ruled out before assessing the endocrine status of the dog. A careful history, complete physical and dermatological examinations and a good differential diagnosis should progress to the application of non-specific and specific diagnostic tests, in order to provide a definitive diagnosis and allow for appropriate treatment.

The aims of this chapter are to present the differential diagnosis of non-pruritic symmetrical alopecia in the dog. The reader is referred to Chapters 54–59 in the endocrine section for cross reference, in particular Chapter 54 which covers the basic test methodology for assessing endocrine function.

DIFFERENTIAL DIAGNOSIS

The course of an endocrine dermatosis is usually slowly progressive. Few of the presenting signs are pathognomonic and a detailed history and clinical examination are mandatory to establish a thorough differential diagnosis. There are no short cuts to attaining a definitive diagnosis. For example, several sections from a number of biopsy samples may need to be examined if the typical histopathological features of endocrine dermatoses are to be found,

and these are rarely pathognomonic (Gross & Ihrke 1990; Gross *et al.* 1992). The most common presenting syndrome is uncomplicated symmetrical alopecia (i.e alopecia in the absence of systemic disease) (Table 94.1).

Dogs with Typical Signs of Non-pruritic, Symmetrical Alopecia Exhibiting No Primary or Secondary Lesions

The essential diagnosis to rule out is colour dilution alopecia. This condition is a genodermatosis based on a recessive gene transmission. It can be seen in blue, red, fawn, black coated dogs from many breeds. Colour dilution alopecia can look very similar to endocrine alopecia. Current recommendations are to rule out this dermatosis, by histopathological examination of biopsy samples, before assessing the various endocrine functions in a dog of a predisposed breed.

Dogs with Symmetrical Alopecia and Pruritus with or without Primary and Secondary Lesions

Infective or parasitic diseases should first be ruled out. Demodicosis, superficial pyoderma, dermatophytosis and *Malassezia pachydermatis* dermatitis may complicate an endocrine dermatosis or mimic it. Thus hyperadrenocorticism may present as a pruritic dermatosis in 25% of cases (White *et al.* 1989) because of calcinosis cutis or bacterial, fungal or parasitic complications. Skin scrapings, tape strips, direct smears, bacteriological or mycological cultures are mandatory before assessing endocrine status. If the alopecia persists after the pruritus and lesions have resolved with treatment then an endocrine dermatosis should be

Dermatosis	Prominence in the differential	Main diagnostic keys
Genodermatoses		
Colour dilution alopecia (& black hair follicular dysplasia)	++++	Biopsy
Hypotrichosis	+	History, breed
Pattern baldness	+	History, breed
Follicular dysplasia	++	Biopsy
Short hair syndrome of silky breed	+	Aspect, breed
Infectious causes		
Demodicosis	+++	Skin scraping
Superficial pyoderma	++	Smear, culture
Dermatophytosis	++	Wood's light, culture
Malassezia dermatitis	+++	Tape strip, smear, culture
Miscellaneous causes		
Telogen and anagen defluxation	+	History
Post-clipping alopecia	+	History, breed
Sebaceous adenitis	+	Biopsy
Alopecia areata	+	Aspect, biopsy
Superficial pemphigus	+	Aspect, biopsy
Epidermotropic lymphoma	+	Aspect, biopsy

Table 94.1   Principal causes of non-pruritic, symmetrical alopecia in the dog.

considered. If pruritus, or lesions, remain then other conditions must be considered, such as hypersensitivities.

Atypical Presentations

- Facial dermatosis in hyperadrenocorticism (White *et al.* 1989)
- Patchy alopecia in seasonal flank alopecia
- Xanthomatosis in diabetes mellitus
- Pituitary dwarfism (mainly in German Shepherd Dogs)

HYPERADRENOCORTICISM
(SEE CHAPTER 59 PAGE 611)

History and Clinical Signs

Canine hyperadrenocorticism is a systemic disease: the cutaneous changes observed are only a small proportion of the signs potentially encountered. The cutaneous signs of hyperadrenocorticism are observed in only 65% of the cases although skin lesions are often the first obvious signs noticed by the owner. Hyperadrenocorticism is typically a disease of middle-aged dogs (mean 11 years old) but it may be seen in dogs as young as 12 months or less (White *et al.* 1989).

General Signs

- Polyuria/polydipsia (85%)
- Polyphagia
- Pendulous abdomen (potbellied appearance)
- Hepatomegaly
- Anoestrous
- Polypnoea
- Muscle wasting (Fig. 94.1)
- Pseudomyotonia
- Thromboembolism
- Behavioural changes

Dermatological Signs

- Truncal symmetrical
- Non-pruritic alopecia (60%)

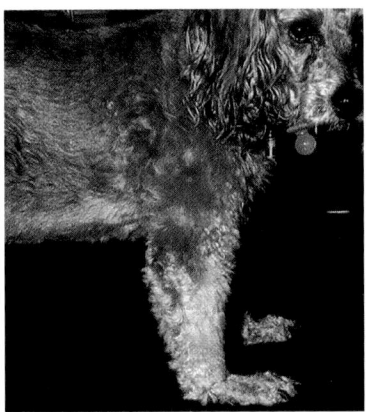

Fig. 94.1 Carpal hyperextension associated with pituitary dependent hyperadrenocorticism. Figure courtesy D. Heripret.

- Thin and hypotonic skin
- Seborrhoea
- Comedones (5–35%)
- Pigmentary disturbances
- Telangiectasia
- Phlebectasia
- Non-truncal alopecia
- Calcinosis cutis (2–40%)
- Secondary fungal or bacterial infections
- Demodicosis (Figs 94.2a&b)

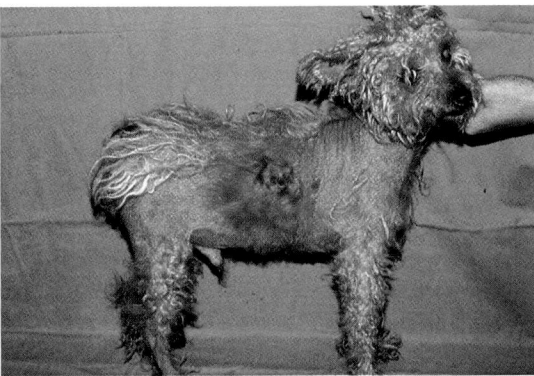

Fig. 94.2 Alopecia associated with pituitary dependent hyperadrenocorticism showing minimal cutaneous signs (a) and with erythema and crusting (b). Figures courtesy D. Heripret.

Non-specific Tests

Haematology

Stress leucogram: neutrophilia (capillar demargination, medullary stimulation), lymphopenia (destruction) and eosinopenia (medullary retention).

Elevated Alkaline Phosphatase (ALP)

Affected dogs produce a unique isoenzyme of ALP induced either by endogenous or exogenous glucocorticoids and most dogs with hyperadrenocorticism have total ALP above the normal range. Although this specific ALP isoenzyme can be measured (by heat inhibition or by levamisole inhibition) the test lacks specificity and should therefore not be used as a screening test (Jensen & Poulsen 1992).

Miscellaneous

Elevation of ALT (glycogenic hepatic storage), hypercholesterolaemia (stimulation of lipolysis), low urinary specific density, low total T_4 in 40% to 60% of the cases – euthyroid sick syndrome (Feldman & Nelson 1987; Ferguson & Peterson 1992; Jensen & Poulsen 1992; Hansen *et al.* 1994).

Specific Diagnostic Tests

Normal values depend on the laboratory (the author recommends that clinicians use a veterinary laboratory that will measure enough samples to establish adequate normal values and thus validate their measurements).

ACTH Stimulation Test

See Chapter 54 page 583.

Interpretation
In normal animals the post-ACTH cortisol should be >100 < 500 nmol/l. Exaggerated response (>500 nmol/l) is consistent with spontaneous hyperadrenocorticism. Poor or no response is consistent with iatrogenic hyperglucocorticoidism (<100 nmol/l) or adrenocortical insufficiency.

Comment
The ACTH test is a good screening test for pituitary dependent disease but if hyperadrenocorticism is supected, the diagnosis should not be excluded on the basis of a normal response to ACTH stimulation.

Urine Cortisol/Creatinine Ratio (UCCR)

This test is very sensitive (near 100%) (Rijnberk *et al.* 1988), but its specificity is very low (25%) (Smiley & Peterson 1993; Heripret 1995). Hyperadrenocorticism can be ruled out on the basis of a negative UCCR but cannot be diagnosed if UCCR is high since many other conditions (all the causes of polyuria/polydipsia in particular) may also cause a high value. The UCCR does not allow diagnosis of iatrogenic hyperglucocorticoidism.

Method
Measurement of urine creatinine (mmol/l) and urine cortisol (nmol/l) in a morning urine sample.

Interpretation
UCCR < 10×10^{-6} rules out hyperadrenocorticism.

Comment
This test must only be used to rule out hyperadrenocorticism. It can be very useful when interpreted along with ACTH stimulation test.

Low-Dose Dexamethasone Suppression Test (LDDST)

See Chapter 54 and page 583.

Interpretation
Suppression at 8 h and cortisol value < decision point (dependent on the laboratory value, 40 nmol/l) is consistent with a normal response (Heripret 1995).

Comment
This is the best diagnostic test but it is technically difficult to perform and to interpret.

Aetiological Diagnostic Tests

Low-Dose Dexamethasone Suppression Test (LDDST)

This test must only be used to diagnose hyperadrenocorticism, but a good suppression at 3 h with rebound over the decision point at 8 h is diagnostic of a pituitary dependent hyperadrenocorticism (PDH). However, PDH cannot be ruled out when suppression and rebound do not occur.

High-Dose Dexamethasone Suppression Test (HDDST)

This test is used to distinguish between pituitary and adrenal disease in those cases in which the LDDST is not pathognomonic.

Interpretation
Suppression to less than 50% of basal concentration with cortisol at the 8 h sample < decision point (depend on the laboratory value) is consistent with a diagnosis of PDH.

Comment
Some 15–20% of PDH cases respond similarly to an adrenal tumour (i.e. no suppression). A clear cut suppression is diagnostic of PDH but an unsuppressed test does not rule out PDH.

ACTH Measurement

See Chapter 54 and page 584.

This test is the best one to differentiate PDH and adrenal tumour (AT) but is very difficult to perform owing to technical problems. The ACTH concentration is high in PDH (ACTH hyperproduction by the pituitary gland) and low in AT (negative feed-back on the pituitary gland by the large amount of cortisol produced by the tumour).

Imaging Techniques

Radiography

The normal or hypertrophied glands can usually not be seen; however 30% of the adrenal tumours become calcified.

Ultrasonography

The left adrenal gland can be seen in 96% of the cases and the right one in 72% of the cases (Grooters *et al.* 1994). The ultrasonographer must visualise both adrenal glands (same size – PDH; very different size – adrenal tumour). If he cannot see both of them, no conclusion can be drawn. Ultrasonography is also useful to detect hepatic metastases of an adrenal adenocarcinoma.

Tomodensitometry

This technique allows visualisation of the pituitary gland and adrenal glands. It is a very useful technique but is still quite expensive to perform.

Proposed Diagnostic Pathway

The most accurate way to diagnose hyperadrenocorticism involves performing all of the three tests simultaneously (UCCR in the morning then LDDST and ACTH stimulation test over a $9^1/_4$-h period). However, this is not very practical and is economically questionable.

The author currently recommends an initial ACTH stimulation test simultaneously with a UCCR and if there is no clear-cut answer (i.e. ACTH normal and UCCR positive) an LDDST is performed. To obtain the aetiological diagnosis, the HDDST is still rewarding but ultrasonography is becoming more and more important in this regard.

HYPOTHYROIDISM (SEE ALSO CHAPTER 56 PAGE 590)

Canine hypothyroidism is, like hyperadrenocorticism, a systemic disease. The cutaneous changes are generally more obvious to the owner.

History and Clinical Signs

(Figs 94.3 & 94.4)

Breed Predisposition

Doberman Pinscher, Boxer, Great Dane, Irish Setter, Schnauzer and many other breeds are predisposed to hypothyroidism. The age of onset varies: the more a breed is predisposed, the earlier the disease begins: 2–3 years 22%, 4–6 years 32%, 7–9 years 22% (Milne & Hayes 1991). There is no sex predisposition (neutered females are at higher risk than intact dogs).

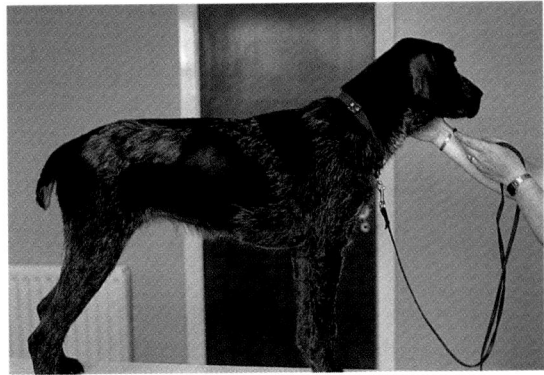

Fig. 94.3 Hypothyroidism in a Pointer. Note the good condition and alert disposition in this case. Bilateral alopecia was the only clinical sign. Figure courtesy R. Harvey.

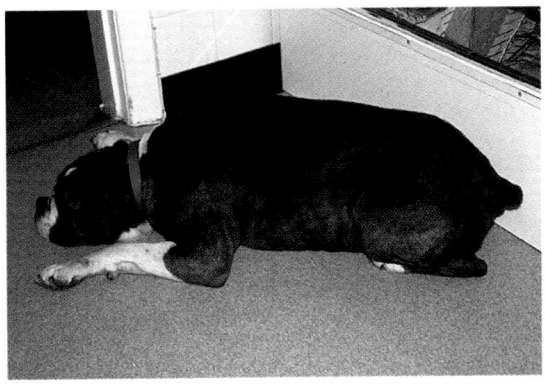

Fig. 94.4 Hypothyroidism. Note the obesity and lethargy in this (unsedated) Boxer with hypothyroidism. Figure courtesy R. Harvey.

General Signs

- Skeletal abnormalities (almost only in congenital forms)
- Neuromuscular abnormalities (facial palsy, laryngeal paralysis, polyneuropathy, myopathy, megaoesophagus)
- Bradycardia and hypocontractility (diminished number of β-receptors)
- Hyperlipaemia
- Immunosuppression
- Mild normocytic non-regenerative anaemia
- Anoestrus or testicular atrophy
- Abnormality in the secretion of prolactin (inappropriate galactorrhoea)

Dermatological Signs

- Haircoat alteration (dull, dry)
- Symmetrical non-pruritic alopecia occuring first in frictional areas
- Involvement of the ventral neck, the tail
- Hypermelanosis
- Seborrhoea (altered lipid profile)
- Secondary infections (*Staphylococcus* spp., *Malassezia* sp.)

Non-specific Tests

- Mild normocytic non-regenerative anaemia (23%) (Panciera 1994)
- Mild elevation of serum creatinine kinase activity (18%) (Panciera 1994)
- Hypercholesterolaemia (73%) (Panciera 1994)
- Histopathology: (Gross & Ihrke 1990; Gross *et al.* 1992) generally non-diagnostic changes although some changes suggestive of hypothyroidism may be seen, such as increased dermal mucin (except in Shar-Pei breed), vacuolated and hypertrophied erector pili muscles.

Specific Tests

Proposed tests: measurement of total thyroxine (T_4) (TT_4), free T_4 (FT_4), total triiodothyronine (T_3) (TT_3), thyroid-stimulating hormone (TSH) stimulation test, thyrotrophin-releasing hormone (TRH) stimulation test, K value, serum antithyroglobulin.

Many non-thyroidal factors can affect circulating thyroid hormone concentrations (decreased serum TT_4 and TT_3, increased rT_3), resulting in misdiagnosis of hypothyroidism in a euthyroid dog (Ferguson 1988). Some drugs can produce the same effect (Tables 94.2 and 94.3).

Table 94.2 Main causes of euthyroid sick-syndrome.

Chronic weight loss
Cancer cachexia
Hyperadrenocorticism (low resting T_4 and suppressed response to TSH)
Diabetes mellitus
Renal insufficiency
Hepatic insufficiency
Chronic infection
Deep pyoderma
Generalised demodicosis

Table 94.3 Principle drugs which may lower serum T_4.

Glucocorticoids
Androgens
Heparin
Phenobarbitone
Diazepam
Phenothiazines
Trimethoprim–sulfamethoxazole
Phenylbutazone
Penicillin
Propylthiouracil
Salicylates
Dopamine

Basal Total T_4 (TT_4)

A TT_4 value well in the normal range (>20 nmol/l) makes hypothyroidism unlikely. A very low T_4 concentration (particularly if associated with hypercholesterolaemia) with compatible clinical signs is strongly indicative of hypothyroidism. Values in the borderline low normal range are not as diagnostically definitive and other testing procedures (TSH stimulation test, FT_4, repeating T_4 measurement) are required.

Interpretation

Normal values are in the range 12–55 nmol/l; hypothyroidism is unlikely in a dog that has TT_4 >20 nmol/l, but likely when TT_4 <7 nmol/l.

Comment

Measurement of TT_4 concentration is an easy, inexpensive and useful screening procedure. Normal TT_4 value rules out hypothyroidism but borderline or low TT_4 is not diagnostically definitive of hypothyroidism.

Free T_4 Measurement (FT_4)

Only few laboratories assay FT_4 by equilibrium dialysis (the standard reference method). Other assays, more widely used, reveal great variations when compared with equilibrium dialysis (variation range 13–115% over 12 laboratories) (Ferguson 1990). Moreover, measurement of serum FT_4 concentration using the single-stage radioimmunoassay, does not provide additional information about thyroid gland function to that gained by measurement of serum TT_4.

Interpretation
Normal values are within the range 8–40 pmol/l.

Comment
This test is not recommended except as an occasional second procedure in case of equivocal TT_4 value.

K Value

The K value is derived from the serum-free T_4 and serum cholesterol concentrations according to the formula

$$K = 0.7 \times FT_4 (pmol/l) - cholesterol \, (mmol/l)$$

Although the derived K value has a reasonable degree of diagnostic accuracy there is a large grey zone.

Interpretation
$K < -4$: hypothyroidism; $K > +1$: euthyroid; $-4 < K < +1$: TSH stimulation test is mandatory.

Comment

(1) Free T_4 (FT_4) is determined by radio-immuno assay and not by equilibrium dialysis.
(2) The FT_4 values may vary from one laboratory to another.
(3) No dogs with euthyroid sick syndrome were included in the study.
(4) Sampling for cholesterol must be made in fasted patients in order to avoid abnormally high values due to diet. Furthermore, cholesterol concentration may vary from dog to dog in accordance with other parameters such as renal or hepatic disease, or even bodyweight.
(5) Cholesterol concentrations are normal in some 30% of hypothyroid dogs.
(6) In practice there is always a large indecisive range and the Larsson K value test is not recommended (Rosychuck & Vroom 1993).

Basal Total T_3 Measurement (TT_3)

TT_3 can be profoundly affected by non-thyroidal diseases. Furthermore, a lowering of serum T_3 usually occurs later than a fall in TT_4 because of the autoregulatory mechanisms of the body.

Interpretation
Normal values are within the range 0.5–2.5 nmol/l.

Comment
This test is of limited usefulness and has no advantage over T_4 measurement.

Reverse T_3 (rT_3)

In human euthyroid sick syndrome, rT_3 (an inactive de-iodination product of T_4), is usually increased. However, there is no evidence that this assay helps to distinguish dogs with hypothyroidism from those with non-thyroidal suppression of T_4.

TSH Stimulation Test

This test is a direct test of thyroidal reserve and often provides good distinction of hypothyroid from euthyroid dogs following borderline TT_4 measurement. Dogs with non-thyroidal illness will often respond to TSH, but not always.

Intrepretation

- post-TSH <12 nmol/l: hypothyroidism
- post-TSH >30 nmol/l: euthyroidism
- post-TSH 12–30 nmol/l: indecisive range. If the difference between pre-TSH and post-TSH TT_4 value is <10 nmol/l, hypothyroidism is likely; if the difference is >10 nmol/l, the diagnosis is uncertain.

Comment
TSH is expensive and the results of the TSH stimulation test are not always clear, that is why the author recommends it as a second-stage diagnostic test after TT_4 measurement.

TRH Stimulation Test

In healthy dogs, TRH stimulation test results in only a small increase in the serum concentration of T_4 (mean 6 nmol/l) and is less useful than TSH stimulation test (Kaufman *et al.* 1985). An abnormal response is not specific for hypothyroidism.

Interpretation
In normal animals the TT_4 post-TRH should reach 1.5 × basal and a minimum level of 30 nmol/l.

Comment
The author does not recommend the TRR stimulation test.

Thyroid Biopsy

This is the most definitive test to identify thyroid pathology. Unfortunately, lymphocytic thyroiditis and thyroidal atrophy result in progressive loss of the thyroid parenchyma, making an aspiration biopsy a poorly reliable procedure. A surgical biopsy is required (Feldman & Nelson 1987).

Comment

Most owners are not willing to consider general anesthesia for thyroid biopsy.

Antithyroglobulin Antibodies (ATAc)

In dogs, ATAc are demonstrable in more than 50% of cases of naturally occurring hypothyroidism by means of ELISA or indirect immunofluorescence techniques.

Therapeutic Trial with Levothyroxine

When hypothyroidism is suspected and the dog shows low or borderline basal concentrations of TT_4, or a TSH stimulation test result which is not in the decisive range, a therapeutic trial (T_4 supplementation $10g/kg$ b.i.d.) can be proposed (Nachreiner 1990). The serum T_4 concentrations should be monitored (before and 5h after oral administration of T_4) to confirm that adequate therapeutic concentrations are achieved. Those that do not respond after 6–8 weeks can be assumed to be euthyroid (Nachreiner 1990). However, it should be remembered that hair regrowth may be due to non-specific actions of thyroid hormone.

Comment

This test can only be done after a correct diagnostic work-up, an attempt to rule out non-thyroidal illness and must be based upon a high suspicion of hypothyroidism without direct biological proof.

SEX HORMONE IMBALANCES (TABLE 94.5)

While there is no doubt that the sex hormones have a role in the maintenance of cutaneous homeostasis, the relationships between sex hormones and the skin, the interaction between other steroids and hormones, the importance of the skin receptors and the importance of adrenal secretion are not currently fully understood in dogs. Furthermore, the sex hormones measurement is usually limited (testosterone, progesterone and oestradiol); the values vary greatly with the method used; we lack information regarding reference values of these hormones in animals with non-endocrine or other endocrine illness; and the values may vary between breeds, individuals and with the sexual status of an individual (Schmeitzel & Lothrop 1990a,b).

These facts make the definitive diagnosis of sex hormone imbalance very difficult and best made on clinical

Table 94.5   Sex hormone imbalances.

- Dermatoses related to hyposexualism with absence of puberty: hypothalamic, pituitary or gonadal origin
- Dermatoses related to hyposexualism with normal puberty (adults): hypothalamo-pituitary hyposexualism (tumours, hyperadrenocorticism); gonadal hyposexualism (oestrogen secreting testicular tumours, idiopathic male feminisation syndrome, ovarian imbalance type II, testosterone responsive dermatosis of the castrated dog, idiopathic testosterone responsive dermatosis)
- Dermatoses related to hypersexualism: hyperandrogenism (Leydig cell neoplasia, hyperprogesteronaemia–hyperandrogenism of the Miniature Spitz), hyperoestrogenism (ovarian imbalance type I, dermatoses related to oestrogen administration), hyperprogesteronism
- Castration responsive dermatosis in male dogs.
- Post-partum telogen defluxion

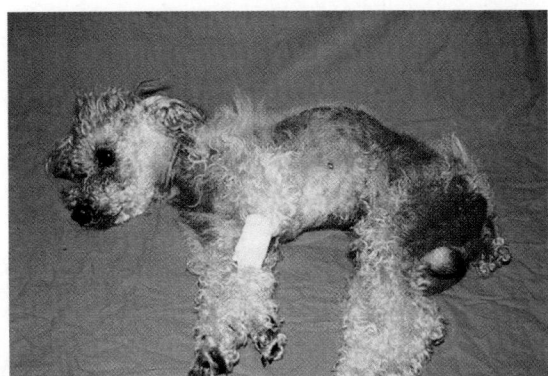

Fig. 94.5   Alopecia associated with severe anaemia in a Miniature Poodle with Sertoli cell tumour. Figure courtesy D. Heripret.

and historical grounds (Fig. 94.5) together with the elimination of differential diagnoses (Ferguson 1993).

History

The goal of the questions is to try to classify the disease.

- How old was the dog at the beginning of the disease?
- Is the dog neutered?
- Has the dog a normal puberty with secondary sexual manifestations?

- Did the sexual behaviour change?
- If the dog is a female: are the sexual cycles appearing on a regular basis?
- Are the symptoms permanent or cyclic?
- What were the treatments (systemic and topic)?
- Are there any non-dermatological problems?

Evaluation of Endocrine Sexual Function in the Male (Table 94.6)

Testosterone Measurement

Luteinising hormone (LH) is secreted in pulses in the male with a peak approximately every 60–90 min, inducing a peak in testoseterone levels. A single measurement of testosterone is unreliable to evaluate the endocrine function of the testis (Miller & Dunstan 1993). Stimulation is required with an analogue of LH (human chorionic gonadotrophin (HCG) stimulation test).

Method

- Take an initial sample (serum pot) for measurement of basal testosterone.

Table 94.6 Interpretation of sex hormone assay in the male dog.

HCG stimulation test:
Failure to stimulate (<20 nmol/l after 24 h) suggests
 hypogonadism (hyperadrenocorticism must be ruled out
 in adult dog)
Hyperoestradiolaemia:
Functional testicular tumour (Sertoli-cell tumour,
 seminoma)
Hyperprogesteronaemia:
May be suggestive of adrenal sex hormone abnormality.
 Perform an ACTH stimulation test with measurement of
 other sex hormones if possible
*Xylazine or clonidine stimulation test with glucose and/or
 GH measurements*:
Castration is indicated in male dogs when there is no
 response to the stimulation

HCG, human chorionic gonadotrophin.
Note. Normal sex hormone measurement does not rule out sex
hormone imbalance (some cases of testicular neoplasia, idiopathic
feminising syndrome, castration responsive dermatitis). In some
castrated dogs, oestradiol concentration may be higher than in
intact dogs (adrenal production).
Gonadal function is controlled by pituitary hormones, Luteinising
hormone (LH) and follicle stimulating hormone (FSH) which are in
turn controlled by an hypothalamic hormone, gonadotrophin-
realising hormone (GnRH).

- Inject (i.m.) 50 IU/kg of HCG.
- Take a second sample collected after 24 h.

Intrepretation

Basal samples will usually fall between 1 and 15 nmol/l and stimulated samples should exceed 25 nmol/l.

Comment

Castrated dogs will show minimal or no response; dogs with cryptorchid testes will have similar results to normal dogs. This test mainly explores hyposexualism without puberty; in the adult (which has undergone normal puberty), hyper-adrenocorticism can be responsible for the lack of stimulation and should be ruled out before diagnosing a true hyposexualism (i.e. testosterone responsive dermatosis).

Other Sex-hormone Measurements

Oestradiol is usually but not invariably elevated in Sertoli-cell tumours and some seminomas. A normal oestradiol measurement does not rule out a secreting testicular neoplasia. In idiopathic feminisation syndrome, there is no change in oetradiol value.

Progesterone, dehydroepiandrosterone sulphate (DHEAS), androstenedione or 17-hydroxyprogesterone may be elevated after an ACTH stimulation test when adrenal sex hormone abnormality is present (Schmeitzal & Lothrop 1990a,b).

Evaluation of Endocrine Function in the Female Dog (Table 94.7)

Blood concentrations of female sex hormones vary during the sexual cycle. Thus hormone concentrations must be interpreted in the light of repeated cytologic examination of vaginal smears. Moreover, other endocrine disease may interact:

- Alopecia and anoestrus of the mature female may be due to hypothyroidism, hyperadrenocorticism or iatrogenic hyperglucocorticism.
- Telogen defluxion: may result from raised progesterone concentrations at parturition (Hubert & Olivry 1990) or after rapid fall in oestrogen concentrations (Schmeitzel & Lothrop 1990a,b).

Unless there are very high concentrations of serum oestradiol or progesterone, it is unlikely that basal sex hormone assay will be helpful. History, clinical aspect, elimination of differential diagnoses and response to treatment (hormone supplementation or neutering) are still the only way to confirm a sexual aetiology.

Table 94.7   Interpretation of sex hormone assay in the bitch.

There is a physiological peak of oetradiol during oestrus, and of progesterone during dioestrus.

Hyperoestradiolaemia:

Ovarian imbalance (Type 1) may result from excessive ovarian function (i.e. ovarian cyst or neoplasia). Most functional ovarian neoplasms are granulosa cell tumours. Nymphomania may be present.

Hyperprogesteronaemia:

Hyperprogesteronaemia may be seen in intact female Boxers and be responsible for cyclic alopecia during dioestrus.

Note. In neutered females, the measurement of sex hormones is mandatory when adrenal sex hormone imbalance is suspected. (Test ACTH with measurement of progesterone and other sex hormones if possible.)

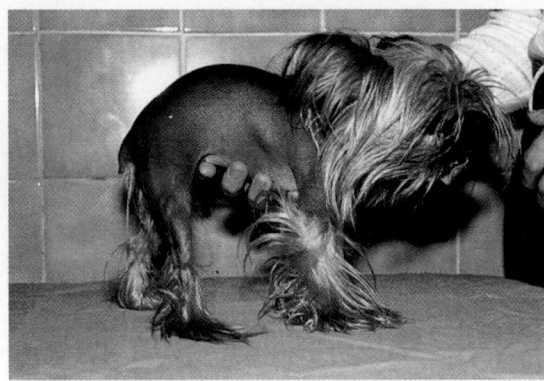

Fig. 94.6   Suspected adult-onset growth hormone responsive dermatosis in a 2-year-old Yorkshire Terrier bitch. Figure courtesy D. Heripret.

SEASONAL FLANK ALOPECIA

Canine recurrent flank alopecia is a skin disorder of unknown origin characterised by episodes of truncal hair loss often encountered on a seasonal basis. The condition is mostly recognised in Airedale Terriers, Boxers (Miller & Dunstan 1993), English Bulldogs, Doberman Pinschers, Korthals, Miniature Schnauzers and Miniature Poodles. It has been recognised in dogs of either sex and of any reproductive status. Alopecia frequently starts in the autumn and resolves in spring or summer.

The diagnosis is based on the history, the appearance (patchy or annular to polycyclic, well-circumscribed alopecia confined to the flanks), and the elimination of other endocrine dermatoses and histopathology.

Histopathological examination of biopsy samples may show features suggestive of this dermatosis such as follicular atrophy and infundibular hyperkeratosis which extends into openings of secondary follicles and sebaceous ducts (Gross *et al.* 1992).

Some of these cases may respond to melatonin injection (Paradis 1995).

GROWTH HORMONE RESPONSIVE DERMATOSIS

Pituitary dwarfism can easily be diagnosed, based on the clinical appearance of the dog and after the elimination of

congenital hypothyroidism (Fig. 94.6). The existence of an entity called 'growth hormone responsive dermatosis of the adult dog' is controversial for several reasons. The xylazine or clonidine stimulation tests show individual and breed variations, in Pomeranians the response to the stimulation tests can be the same in normal or in alopecic individuals, the regrowth of the hair coat after treatment with GH may be non-specific (Rosser 1990; Schmeitzel & Lothrop 1990a,b). Furthermore, some alopecic dogs with abnormal GH-stimulation tests have an impaired secretion of adrenal sexual hormones (Schmeitzal & Lothrop 1990a,b). A good response was obtained with mitotane (o,p'-DDD) treatment. These facts cast doubt on the true role of GH in these dogs, despite a demonstration of poor GH response to stimulation in some cases.

GH Stimulation Tests

Only a few laboratories are able to measure GH. To avoid this problem, the elevation of blood glucose during xylazine or clonidine induced GH secretion may be helpful in evaluating somatotroph function (GH-insulin antagonism). In the normal dog, the peak increase in plasma glucose concentration occurs between 45 and 90 min after xylazine or clonidine administration (Feldman & Nelson 1987). If this peak occurs, an abnormality of GH secretion can be ruled out without measuring GH.

Method

- Take a basal blood sample (serum pot) for growth hormone measurement.
- Inject xylazine (0.2 mg/kg) or clonidine (0.01 mg/kg) i.v.

Summary
The clinical similarity of endocrine dermatoses, the numerous and unknown interactions between the different endocrine systems, the impact of other illness on these systems make the diagnosis of these dermatoses quite difficult. A systematic diagnostic process must be followed in every case.

A proposed diagnostic pathway:

- Rule out hypothyroidism, hyperadrenocorticism, iatrogenic hyperglucocorticism.
- Rule out evident sexua, imbalances and measure sex hormones.
- Rule out colour dilution alopecia.
- GH-glucose stimulation test
  - □ if there is a peak in glucose concentration, GH responsive dermatosis can be ruled out and sexual imbalance must be considered;
  - □ if there is no increase in glucose level after the stimulation test, measurement of GH concentration during the stimulation test is mandatory;
  - □ if there is no increase in GH concentration and the dog is a male, castration must be considered (Rosser 1990). If the dog is a female, a tentative diagnosis of GH responsive dermatosis can be made.

- Further samples are collected at 15, 30, 45, 60, 90 min.

Interpretation

A strong response to stimulation rules out GH responsive dermatosis. However, a lack of elevation in GH concentration may be seen in normal dogs.

REFERENCES

Feldman, E.C. & Nelson, R.W. (1987). *Canine and Feline Endocrinology and Reproduction*. W.B. Saunders, Philadelphia.

Ferguson, D.C. (1988). The effect of non-thyroidal factors on thyroid function tests in dogs. *Compendium on Continuing Education and the Practicing Veterinarian*, **10**, 1365–1377.

Ferguson, D.C. (1990). The value of free hormone measurements in clinical diagnosis: fact or fiction? In: *Proceedings of the 8th Annual Meeting of the American College of Veterinary Internal Medicine Forum*, pp. 769–772.

Ferguson, D.C. & Peterson, M.E. (1992). Serum free and total iodothyronine concentrations in dogs with hyperadrenocorticism. *American Journal of Veterinary Research*, **53**, 1636–1640.

Ferguson, E.A. (1993). Symmetrical alopecia in the dog. In: *A Manual of Small Animal Dermatology*, (eds P.H. Locke, R.G. Harey & I.S. Mason), pp. 101–103. BSAVA Cheltenham.

Grooters, A.M., Rooters, A.M., Biller, D.S., Miyabayashi, T. & Leveille, K. (1994). Evaluation of routine abdominal ultrasonography as a technique for imaging the canine adrenal gland. *Journal of the American Animal Hospital Association*, **30**, 457–462.

Gross, T.L. & Ihrke, P.J. (1990). The histologic analysis of endocrine-related alopecia in the dog. In: *Advances in Veterinary Dermatology*, Vol. 1, (eds C. Von Tscharner & R.E.W. Halliwell), pp. 77–88. Baillière Tindall, London.

Gross, T.L., Ihrke, P.J. & Walder, E.J. (1992). Atrophic diseases of the hair follicle In: *Veterinary Dermatopathology*. pp. 273–297. Mosby Year Book, St Louis.

Hansen, B.L., Kemppainen, R.J. & McDonald, J.M. (1994). Synthetic ACTH (Costyntropin) stimulation tests in normal dogs: comparison of intravenous and intramuscular administration. *Journal of the American Animal Hospital Association*, **30**, 38–41.

Heripret, D. (1995). Etude des différents tests diagnostiques de l'hypercorticisme spontané du chien. *Pratique Médical et Chirurgicale Animale Compagne*, **30**, 309–317.

Hubert, B. & Olivry, T. (1990). Dermatologie et hormones sexuelles chez les carnivores domestiques. 1° partie: physiopathologie. *Pratique Médicale et Chirurgicale Animale Compagne*, **25**, 477–482.

Jensen, A.L. & Poulsen, J.S.D. (1992). Preliminary experience with the diagnostic value of the canine corticosteroid-induced alkaline phosphatase isoenzyme in hypercorticism and diabetes mellitus. *Journal of the American Veterinary Medical Association*, **39**, 342–348.

Kaufman, J., Olson, P.N., Reimers, T.J., *et al.* (1985). Serum concentrations of thyroxine, 3,5,3′-triiodothyronine, thyrotropin, and prolactin in dogs before and after thyrotropin-releasing hormone administration. *American Journal of Veterinary Research*, **46**, 486–492.

Miller, M.A. & Dunstan, R.W. (1993). Seasonal flank alopecia in Boxers and Airedale Terriers: 24 cases (1985–1992). *Journal of the American Veterinary Medical Association*, **203**, 1567–1572

Milne, K.L. & Hayes, H.M. (1991). Epidemiologic features of canine hypothyroidism. *Cornell Veterinarian*, **71**, 3–14.

Nachreiner, R.F. (1990). Controversies in the diagnosis of hypothyroidism. *Proceedings of the 8th Annual Meeting of the American College of Veterinary Internal Medicine Forum*, pp. 349–350.

Panciera, D.L. (1994). Hypothyroidism in dogs: 66 cases (1987–1992). *Journal of the American Veterinary Medical Association*, **204**, 761–767.

Paradis, M. (1995). Canine recurrent flank alopecia: treatment with melatonin *Proceedings of the 11th Annual Meeting of the American Association of Veterinary Dermatology and the American College of Veterinary Dermatology*, p. 49.

Rijnberk, A., Van Wees, A. & Mol, J.A. (1988). Assessment of two tests for the diagnosis of canine hyperadrenocorticism. *Veterinary Record*, **122**, 178–180.

Rosser, E.J. (1990). Castration responsive dermatosis in the dog. In: *Advances in Veterinary Dermatology*, Vol. 1, (eds C. Von Tscharner & R.E.W. Halliwell), pp. 34–42. Baillière Tindall, London.

Rosychuck, R.A.W. & Vroom, M.W. (1993). Workshop Report 2: Hypothyroidism In: *Advances in Veterinary Dermatology*, Vol. 2, (eds P.J. Ihrke, I.S. Mason & S.D. White), pp. 403–408. Pergamon Press, Oxford.

Schmeitzel, L.P. & Lothrop, C.D. (1990a). Hormonal abnormalities in Pomeranians with normal coat and Pomeranians with growth hormone-responsive dermatosis. *Journal of the American Veterinary Medical Association*, **197**, 1333–1341.

Schmeitzl, L.P. & Lothrop, C.D. (1990b). Sex hormones and skin disease. *Veterinary Medicine Report*, **2**, 28–41.

Smiley, L.E. & Peterson, M.E. (1993). Evaluation of a urine cortisol:creatine ratio as a screening test for hyperadrenocorticism in dogs. *Journal of Veterinary Internal Medicine*, **7**, 163–168.

White, S.D., Ceragioli, K.L., Bullock, L.P., Mason, G.B. & Stewart, C.J. (1989). Cutaneous markers of canine hyperadrenocorticism. *Compendium on Continuing Education for the Practicing Veterinarian*, **11**, 446–465.

Chapter 95

Treatment of Defects in Cornification of Canine Skin

A. H. Werner

INTRODUCTION

Seborrhoea, dandruff and scaley skin are common complaints from clients when presenting dogs to the veterinary practitioner. Excessive scale production or retention is indicative of a primary or secondary cornification disorder. One study indicated that scaley skin represents the fourth most common disease of the skin in North American dogs (Sischo 1989).

The term keratinisation refers to one aspect of epidermopoiesis, although it is frequently used interchangeably with cornification to summarise the complex cascade of biochemical events that transforms the epidermis from viable, dividing stem cells into the dead and selectively permeable stratum corneum. Like many tissues, the epidermis is continuously self-renewing, proliferating and differentiating. Significant steps in our understanding of the pathways followed during the cornification process have been recently made through studies of epidermal cell cultures.

PATHOPHYSIOLOGY

The viable epidermis contains a cycling stem cell compartment consisting of both resting and actively dividing cells. Dividing cells proliferate in response to tissue demands.

- The normal process of epidermopoiesis in dogs, also known as the cell renewal time, is approximately 22 days (Kwochka 1993a).
- Injury or inflammation produces a greatly increased activity, with cell renewal time decreasing to as much as half of normal (Scott *et al.* 1995).
- Certain disease states, such as primary seborrhoea, are defined by epidermal renewal times of as little as 7 days (Kwochka 1993a).

Epidermopoiesis involves four distinct biochemical events, which are listed in Table 95.1.

In simplistic terms, the epidermis consists of a natural armour made up of individual cell links, each link created by the cell envelope, held together by keratin fibres, with the entire structure coated with lipids and other molecules. Eventually, each link is disconnected from the group and is shed individually into the environment as replacements are created at the epidermal base (Kwochka (1993a) contains an excellent overview).

The production and dissolution of the epidermis requires the normal progression of each of the four epidermopoietic events. Alteration in the formation of the constituents of the epidermis, including sebaceous and apocrine gland secretions, results in cornification defects. Studies of skin scales from human beings with seborrhoeic dermatitis, atopic dermatitis, and psoriasis reveal an absence of the highest molecular-weight keratins (Soter & Baden 1991). Defects in hydrolytic enzymes, leading to abnormalities in the intercellular substances, result in abnormal shedding of keratinocytes (Kwochka 1993a). Abnormalities in the levels of fatty acids within the epidermis of seborrhoeic dogs have been demonstrated, perhaps leading to alterations in transepidermal water loss as well as changes in keratinocyte shedding (Kwochka 1993a).

> The epidermis is continuously turning over, with new cells being created and dead cells being shed imperceptibly. Any disruption of this cycle may lead to thickening of the epidermis (acanthosis) and thickening or thinning of the stratum corneum (hyperkeratosis or hypokeratosis, respectively). Severe abnormalities may lead to premature cell death (dyskeratosis).

934   Dermatology

Table 95.1 The four major processes in keratinisation.

(1) Keratinisation – the formation of the fibrous protein keratin molecules. Keratin is the major intermediate filament present in all epithelial cells.
(2) Keratohyaline granule synthesis – keratohyaline is an amorphous, histidine-rich material that causes the aggregation of keratin subunits into filaments.
(3) Cell envelope development – the cell envelope is a highly cross-linked, extremely insoluble layer located deep to the plasma membrane of epidermal cells and serves as a structural scaffold for the insertion of keratin filaments, as well as potentially regulating the hydration of the epidermis.
(4) Deposition of intercellular lipid bilayer – lamellar bodies synthesise and secrete their contents into the intercellular spaces which, after modification, become neutral lipids rich in sterol esters, free cholesterol, cholesterol esters, and diester waxes; there are lesser quantities of triglycerides and free fatty acids. Intercellular lipids are major components of the epidermal barrier function.

CLINICAL ASPECTS

Table 94.2 lists the common canine cornification defects.

Differentiation between congenital and acquired (primary and secondary) cornification disorders is most often based upon the breed of animal and the age of onset; development before the age of 2 years is usual for congenital disorders. Differentiation is important from both a treatment and a prognostic aspect:

- Secondary cornification disorders have an excellent prognosis for resolution or control, assuming that the underlying aetiology can be identified and treated.
- Primary cornification defects have a more guarded prognosis, as control is more difficult and requires management over the lifetime of the patient.

Interestingly, although cornification defects in the various breeds may appear clinically similar, they are different pathophysiologically, as response to a specific treatment in one breed does not predict response in another (Figs 95.1–95.3). For example, the cornification defect of West Highland White Terriers and the idiopathic seborrhea of Bassett Hounds are apparently not identical to the cornification disorder of the Cocker Spaniel, as positive response to treatment with retinoids has been noted in the Cocker Spaniel but has not been noted in these other breeds (Werner & Power 1994).

Table 95.2 Common canine cornification defects.

Congenital defects	Acquired defects
Primary seborrhoea	Secondary seborrhoea
Ichthyosis	Vitamin A-responsive
Schnauzer comedo syndrome	dermatosis
Epidermal dysplasia of West	Acne
Highland White Terriers	Ear margin dermatosis
Psoriasiform–lichenoid	Tail gland hyperplasia
dermatitis of	
Springer Spaniels	
Footpad hyperkeratosis	

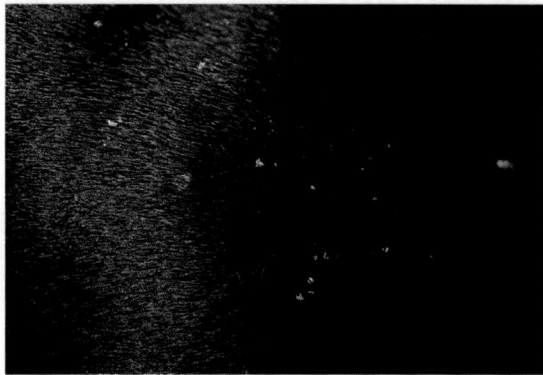

Fig. 95.1 Large, pale, rather dry scale on the dorsum of a Doberman Pinscher. This breed suffers from primary defects in keratinisation as well as being prone to the more common secondary causes such as hypothyroidism. Figure courtesy of Richard Harvey.

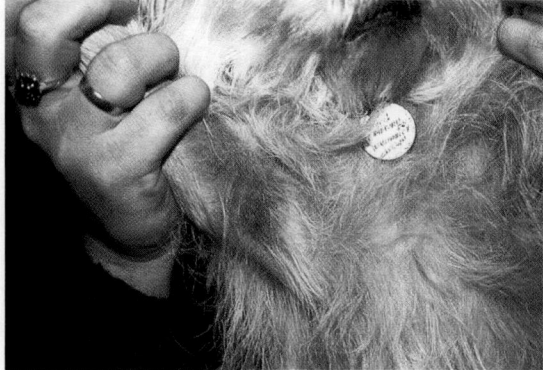

Fig. 95.2 Greasy scale and hyperpigmentation in the axilla of a West Highland White Terrier. This case was due to *Malassezia pachydermatis* secondary to atopy. Figure courtesy of Richard Harvey.

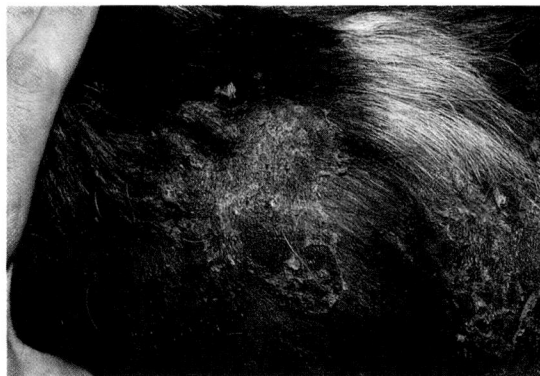

Fig. 95.3 Crusted papules, scale and alopecia on the flank of a Cocker Spaniel with a primary defect in keratinisation. Figure courtesy of Richard Harvey.

Specific treatment of cornification disorders is based on three principles:

- diagnosis and control of contributory disease,
- removal of excessive epidermal debris,
- restoration of normal epidermopoiesis.

Regardless of the cause of the cornification defect, resolution of clinical signs requires similar therapies. Specific treatments, as they relate to individual diseases, will be mentioned in the following text when applicable. The reader is referred to more complete publications for the diagnosis and treatment of specific disorders.

DIAGNOSIS OF CONTRIBUTORY DISEASES

Cornification defects are frequently caused, or exacerbated by, contributory diseases that must be controlled. Table 95.3 summarises the most common contributory diseases, however, any disease affecting the skin is likely to result in excessive scale formation and exfoliation.

TOPICAL THERAPY

Treatment to remove the scales and crusts is paramount to restoring a normal appearance and symptomatic topical therapy is the major form of treatment for cornification disorders. The purpose of topical agents is to loosen intercellular adhesion, separate keratinocytes and hydrate the cells to permit easy removal.

Water is an excellent solvent and also hydrates the stratum corneum although excessive hydration (leading to maceration) must be avoided in order to maintain the protective barrier function of the epidermis. However, shampoos must have an adequate contact time with the skin in order for the active ingredients to be maximally effective. To prevent maceration, baths should be limited to less than 15 min, with a contact time of at least 5 min for each topical agent. Encouraging the client to use a clock to time the bath can help standardise the patient's care. In general, this author recommends the use of an appropriate shampoo and conditioner once to twice per week initially, with maintenance baths at least biweekly once the condition has stabilised. Individual case variation may necessitate more frequent bathing for maintenance. Table 95.4 lists the most common active ingredients used in veterinary formulations for control of excessive scale.

Many excellent topical products are available to the veterinary practitioner. Unfortunately, it is not uncommon for the practitioner to carry multiple products with similar ingredients, and to lack an adequate understanding of the indications for each active ingredient. A detailed description of topical therapy is found in Kwochka (1993b). In the author's opinion, sulphur/salicylic acid combination shampoos are the mainstay of antiseborrhoeic therapy, while tar-based shampoos are perhaps used excessively. One recent study stabilised seborrhoeic Cocker Spaniels with frequent baths using a sulphur/salicylic acid shampoo during a double-blind placebo-based study of the effects of retinoids on cornification disorders. While treated dogs improved, on a histological grading, more than untreated dogs, both groups of dogs responded dramatically to topical therapy (Werner *et al.* 1990). It must be remembered that all patients are different, therefore the client may need to try several shampoos before finding the most effective and accepted topical therapy.

There are other, less utilised, active ingredients found in veterinary shampoo formulations. Most of these ingredients address other symptoms, such as pruritus or coat dryness. During the past 3 years, the use of after-shampoo moisturisers and conditioners has gained attention. Conditioners, emollients, emollient–emulsifier combinations, and humectants attempt to restore epidermal hydration by trapping water within, or attracting water to, the epidermis. Epidermal hydrators are best applied immediately after a bath, while the epidermis and hair coat are still wet. Maintaining a hydrated epidermis enhances the keratolytic effect of subsequent shampoos, leading to a faster clinical response.

Table 95.3 Contributing diseases with cornification defects.

Disease	Cutaneous signs	Diagnosis	Treatment
Pyoderma	Epidermal collarettes Pustules, crusted papules 'Rancid fat odour'	Tzanck preparation Biopsy	Three weeks or longer of appropriate antibiotic Antiseptic shampoo
Malassezia dermatitis	Erythroderma Greasy exudation or fine scale	Epidermal prepration Biopsy	Ketoconazole 10 mg/kg daily for 6 weeks. Antifungal shampoo
Hypothyroidism	Lack of hair regrowth Excessive scale Recurrent pyoderma	Routine blood work TSH testing	Thyroxine supplementation
Hyperadrenocorticism	Lack of hair regrowth Recurrent pyoderma Calcinosis cutis	Routine blood work ACTH stimulation Dexamethasone suppression	Mitotane (*o,p'*-DDD) therapy Adrenalectomy Ketoconazole
Ectoparasitism	Pruritus Hair loss Recurrent pyoderma	Skin scrapings Biopsy	Appropriate parasiticide therapy
Hypersensitivity	Pruritus Erythroderma Recurrent pyoderma	Intradermal skin test Food elimination trial RAST/ELISA	Hyposensitization Allergen avoidance
Dermatophytosis	Hair loss Erythroderma Fine scale	Fungal culture Biopsy Positive Wood's lamp for 6 weeks	Griseofulvin 25–50 mg/kg daily Itraconazole 5 mg/kg b.i.d. for 6 weeks. Antifungal rinse or shampoo
Pemphigus foliaceus immunosuppression	Vesicles/pustules Scale and crusts	Tzanck preparation Biopsy	Selective

RAST, radioallergosorbent test; ELISA, enzyme-linked immunosorbent assay.

Table 95.4 Shampoo therapy: Common ingredients and mode of action.

Active Ingredient	Antiseptic action?	Keratolytic action?	Keratoplastic action?	Antipruritic effect?
Glycerin, Urea, lactic acid	Mild	No	No	No
Solubilised sulphur	Yes	Yes	Mild	Yes
Salicylic acid	Yes	Yes	Mild	Mild
Benzoyl peroxide	Yes	No	No	Yes
Coal tar extract	Yes	Yes	Yes	Mild

SYSTEMIC THERAPEUTICS

Systemic Therapy with Retinoids

The retinoids are a class of pharmacological compounds, some of which occur naturally (vitamin A, β-carotene), others which have been synthesised (13-cis-retinoic acid, etretinate, the arotinoids) and all of which have profound affects on epithelial tissues. Naturally occurring vitamin A (retinol) and its metabolites, retinoic acid and retinal, are essential requirements for reproduction and vision, as well as normal growth, differentiation and maintenance of epithelial tissues. Medical use of vitamin A began in the

1920s based on the recognition of clinical and histological similarities between vitamin A deficient animals and certain dyskeratotic skin conditions (Werner & Power 1994).

Synthetic retinoid drugs are formed by modifications of the retinol molecule. Synthetic retinoids have direct effects on cell nuclei and their delivery to the target tissues differs from that of vitamin A, thus they do not interfere with normal vitamin A metabolism. Although more than 1500 analogues of vitamin A have been synthesised, only four have been developed into useful drugs. At appropriate dosages, the retinoids are essential regulators of epithelial growth and differentiation. The therapeutic benefits and the side-effects of synthetic retinoids are based on their vitamin-like A activity, but the mechanisms of action of the synthetic retinoids are not entirely understood. Multiple nuclear receptors that are modulated by the retinoids have been identified (Werner & Power 1994). Clinically, these drugs promote desquamation and help normalise the hyperproliferative epidermis.

Currently available synthetic retinoid drugs are tretinoin, isotretinoin, etretinate and acitretin. Clinical experience over the last 20 years has shown that, although these drugs are chemically related, they are not interchangeable. In human medicine, the primary indications for tretinoin are acne and photo-aging; isotretinoin for severe cystic acne and etretinate for psoriasis and disorders of cornification (Heller & Schiffman 1985; Ellis & Voorhees 1987; Peck & DiGiovanna 1987). Acitretin is the active metabolite of etretinate (etretin) and has the same indications.

Veterinary dermatologists began evaluating synthetic retinoid therapy for diseases of companion animals in the early 1980s. Initial reports found that isotretinoin was ineffective for the treatment of the primary cornification disorder of Cocker Spaniels or for the treatment of solar-induced squamous cell carcinoma of cats (Power & Ihrke 1990). Recent successes with etretinate therapy have encouraged investigations using retinoids for the treatment of a variety of veterinary dermatoses. Most information on retinoids is based on demonstrated efficacy in clinical trials or on successful use in clinical settings with limited numbers of animal patients.

> The primary cornification disorder of Cocker Spaniels has been treated with etretinate at dosages of 1 mg/kg once daily or divided twice daily (Werner & Power 1994). Response is usually noted within 60 days, with decreases in scaling, softening of plaques and relief of pruritus.

Severely affected dogs may gradually improve over 6 months and continued therapy is required to maintain the improvement. Alternate dosing during maintenance, such as one week on medication followed by one week off, has not generally been successful. The dosage of isotretinoin, although not considered effective for most seborrhoeic Cocker Spaniels, is the same as for etretinate. The proposed disorders of cornification seen in other breeds may selectively respond to retinoid therapy. Because the exact pathomechanism of each disorder is not currently known, it is difficult to predict which patients are likely to respond to these drugs. Therefore, a 90-day trial of each drug is recommended.

Side-effects of the synthetic retinoids are related to their vitamin A activity. The most common side-effects seen in dogs include inappetance, vomiting, diarrhoea, pruritus, increased thirst, conjunctivitis, cheilitis and joint stiffness (Werner & Power 1994). Overall, the incidence of side-effects in dogs has been extremely low, and signs resolve when therapy is discontinued or when the dosage is lowered. One side-effect that occurs slightly more frequently is keratoconjunctivitis sicca (Werner & Power 1994). Elevations in serum liver enzymes and triglycerides are also uncommon in dogs, but values should be monitored. Isotretinoin is more likely to cause side-effects, thus etretinate is preferred when extended treatment is anticipated. The most serious side-effect of synthetic retinoids is teratogenicity. Etretinate is stored in body fat resulting in lengthy withdrawal times (up to 2 years after discontinuation of therapy). Intact females and breeding males *must not* be treated and clients must be carefully instructed on the potential human hazard if accidentally ingested.

Recommendations for proper monitoring of retinoid therapy include pre-treatment and day 30 serum chemistry and triglycerides, with subsequent retesting if indicated. Tear production should be measured pre-treatment and monthly for several months. Routine monitoring every 3–6 months thereafter is prudent. Significant elevations in liver enzymes can be lowered by dose reduction; elevations in cholesterol and triglycerides may respond to dietary fat restriction; and lowered tear production often responds to topical cyclosporin.

Systemic Therapy with Vitamin A

Perhaps lost in all of the excitement of the potential of the synthetic retinoids, vitamin A itself has been overlooked. Vitamin A-responsive dermatosis is a seborrhoeic skin disease of adult-onset primarily in Cocker Spaniels characterised histologically by striking follicular plugging. Treatment with 600–800 IU/kg of vitamin A (retinol) daily resolves lesions within 10 weeks while response to synthetic retinoids is poor (Scott *et al.* 1995). Although primary cornification defects, as mentioned above, rarely respond to this therapy, it would not be inappropriate to begin a limited trial with vitamin A before initiating treatment with a synthetic retinoid, especially when economic concerns prohibit retinoid use.

Systemic Use of Vitamin D and its Derivatives

The skin has long been known to be a source of vitamin D when exposed to ultraviolet light. However, the skin has more recently been identified as one of the target organs of the hormone form of this vitamin, $1,25(OH)_2D_3$ (Blumenberg *et al.* 1992; Kragballe 1992). Specific nuclear receptors for $1,25(OH)_2D_3$ have been identified in keratinocytes and have been shown to regulate growth, enhancing differentiation and suppressing proliferation of these cells in cultures. Side-effects of excessive $1,25(OH)_2D_3$ in humans include hypercalcaemia, hypercalciuria, soft tissue calcification, renolith formation and bone resorption. Similar to development of synthetic retinoids, synthetic vitamin D analogues (including calcipotriol) have been developed and are currently being studied. It is likely that during the next few years, more information on their uses and potential side-effects in veterinary medicine will be forthcoming.

LOCAL APPLICATION OF RETINOIDS AND VITAMIN D DERIVATIVES

The use of medicinal lotions is limited in veterinary medicine because of practicality. Applying creams and ointments through a thick hair coat is difficult and messy, leading to poor efficacy and compliance. However, for select patients in whom cornification abnormalities are localised or large patches of alopecia afford easy access to the skin, medicinal lotions can be applied. Both vitamin A and vitamin D classes of drugs have topical formulations. Although they are used topically, their mode of activity is not similar to shampoos. These topical drugs alter the formation of epidermis rather than simply removing excessive accumulations of debris, and therefore they are more appropriately described as systemic medications. The vitamin A derivative for topical use is tretinoin. Severe cases of canine (and feline) acne have responded to tretinoin application (Power & Ihrke 1995). Tretinoin is applied as either a lotion or cream daily to every other day until results are noted, then discontinued or reduced to once weekly for maintenance. The epidermis of dogs and cats is thinner than that of human beings (0.1–0.5 mm vs. 0.04–1.5 mm) and irritant side-effects of tretinoin can be

Summary
Treatment of cornification disorders requires an understanding of the normal formation of the epidermis and the abnormalities that produce disease. Cornification disorders occur from the increases in the proliferation, decreases in the differentiation and reduction in the desquamation of the keratinocyte. Sebaceous and apocrine gland secretions also play a role in the normal functioning of the epidermis. The hallmarks of the cornification disorder are excessive scaling and accumulation of keratinaceous debris. Specific treatment is based on controlling contributory disease, removing the excessive epidermal debris, and restoring normal epidermopoiesis. In all patients with cornification disorders, the majority of therapeutic response results from topical cleansing, while systemic control remains adjunctive.

more severe. A retinoid 'rash' or 'burn' is a characteristic side-effect of application. The use of tretinoin should be reserved for those cases of acne that do not respond to topical or systemic antimicrobial therapy, or to topical follicular flushing and cleansing with benzoyl peroxide shampoos.

In human beings, a topical vitamin D derivative $(1,24(OH)_2D_3$-tacalcitol ointment) produces dramatic reduction in the severity of psoriatic lesions, with a significant change towards normalisation of proliferation and reduction in inflammation. The adhesion of keratinocytes to each other is also affected, producing more normal desquamation. Specific uses of this compound in veterinary medicine have not been elucidated, most likely due to its potentially severe side-effects. However, its use for acne and localised skin lesions, such as seborrhoeic plaques or acanthosis nigracans, merits future study.

REFERENCES

Blumenberg, M., Connoly, D.M. & Freedberg, I.M. (1992). Regulation of keratin gene expression: The role of the nuclear receptors for retinoic acid, thyroid hormone, and vitamin D_3. *Journal of Investigative Dermatology*, **98**, S42–S49.

Ellis, C.N. & Voorhees, J.J. (1987). Etretinate therapy. *Journal of the American Academy of Dermatology*, **16**, 267–291.

Heller, E.H. & Shiffman, N.J. (1985). Synthetic retinoids in dermatology. *Canadian Medical Association Journal*, **132**, 1129–1136.

Kragballe, K. (1992) Vitamin D_3 and skin diseases. *Archives of Dermatological Research*, **284**, S30–S36.

Kwochka, K.W. (1993a). Overview of normal keratinization and cutaneous scaling disorders of dogs. In: *Current Veterinary Dermatology: The Science and Art of Therapy*, (eds C.E. Griffin, K.W. Kwochka, & J.M. MacDonald), pp. 169–175. Mosby Year Book, St. Louis.

Kwochka, K.W. (1993b). Symptomatic topical therapy of scaling disorders. In: *Current Veterinary Dermatology: The Science and Art of Therapy*, (eds C.E. Griffin, K.W. Kwochka & J.M. MacDonald), pp. 191–202. Mosby Year Book, St. Louis.

Peck, G.L. & DiGiovanna, J.J. (1987). Retinoids. In: *Dermatology in General Medicine*, (eds T.B. Fitzpatrick *et al.*), pp. 2582–2608. McGraw Hill, New York.

Power, H.T. & Ihrke, P.J. (1990). Synthetic retinoids in veterinary dermatology. *Veterinary Clinics of North America Small Animal Practice*, **20**, 1525–1539.

Power, H.T. & Ihrke, P.J. (1995). The use of synthetic retinoids in veterinary medicine. In: *Kirk's Current Veterinary Therapy XII*, (ed. J. Bonagura), pp. 585–590. W.B. Saunders, Philadelphia.

Scott, D.W., Miller, W.H. & Griffin, C.E. (1995). *Muller & Kirk's Small Animal Dermatology*, 5th edn. pp. 26 and 830–831. W.B. Saunders, Philadelphia.

Sischo, W.M. (1989). Regional distribution of ten common skin diseases in dogs. *Journal of the American Veterinary Medical Association*, **195**, 752.

Soter, N.A. & Baden, H.P. (1991). *Pathophysiology of Dermatologic Diseases*, 2nd edn. McGraw-Hill, New York.

Werner, A.H. & Power, H.T. (1994). Retinoids in veterinary medicine. *Clinics in Dermatology*, **12**, 579–586.

Werner, A.H., Power, H.T., Ihrke, P.J., *et al.* (1990). Double-blinded study of the efficacy of etretinate (Tegison®) in the treatment of Cocker Spaniels with a keratinization disorder. In: *Proceedings, Annual Members' Meeting AAVD & ACVD*, San Francisco, p. 41.

Chapter 96

Neoplasia of the Skin and Associated Tissues

N. T. Gorman and J. M. Dobson

INTRODUCTION

The skin and subcutis is the largest and most accessible organ of the body. Cutaneous neoplasms are diagnosed more frequently than tumours of other organs and skin tumours represent approximately 30% of all canine neoplastic disease (Theilen & Madewell 1987; Dobson & Gorman 1988; Pully & Stannard 1990; Goldschmidt & Schofer 1992).

DEFINITION

The skin and subcutis are composed of many different types of tissue which may be affected by a vast array of different tumours. These may be divided broadly into the following categories:

(1) *Primary tumours which arise within the dermis or subcutis.*
    Primary tumours arise within the dermis, subcutis and adjacent connective tissues. Primary tumours can either be malignant or benign and can occur as solitary or multiple lesions.
(2) *Secondary tumours which arise at a distant site and metastasise to the skin.*
    These are tumours that are part of a systemic malignant neoplastic condition. These may present as solitary or multiple lesions.

Thus tumours of the skin may be benign or malignant, primary or secondary and may present as solitary or multiple lesions. The classification of primary tumours of the skin is shown in Table 96.1. Skin tumours must also be differentiated from a diverse array of non-neoplastic,

tumour-like conditions including hyperplastic lesions, granulomatous lesions, inflammatory lesions and developmental lesions. It is not possible to illustrate all the skin tumour types in this text but a few examples are included in Table 96.1.

CLINICAL APPROACH TO CUTANEOUS NEOPLASMS

A prerequisite to the successful management of any neoplastic condition is an accurate definition of the nature and extent of the disease. Diagnosis of a skin tumour requires a detailed history and an appropriate clinical examination. The tissue type of the mass must be defined. This can be achieved in two complementary ways: cytology and histology.

Cytology

It is easy to obtain samples from lesions of the skin and subcutis for cytological examination. Exfoliative cytology may be performed by fine-needle aspirate, tissue imprint or exudate smear. Cytological examination provides information regarding the appearance of neoplastic cells and can show whether they are epithelial, round cell or spindle cell in type. In some cases, for example the mast cell tumour, this information may give a definitive diagnosis. It cannot be over-emphasised what an important diagnostic tool cytology is in the early diagnosis of cutaneous tumours.

Histology

Definitive diagnosis of a neoplasm invariably depends on microscopic examination of tumour architecture, cell type,

Table 96.1 Classification of primary cutaneous neoplasms in domestic animals.

Epithelial tumours
  Papilloma
  Basal cell tumour
  Squamous cell carcinoma (Fig. 96.1)
  Sebaceous gland tumours
    Sebaceous adenoma
    Sebaceous epithelioma
    Sebaceous adenocarcinoma
  Tumours of perianal glands
    Hepatoid gland adenoma/Adenocarcinoma
  Sweat gland tumours
    Adenoma/adenocarcinoma (Fig. 96.2)
  Tumours of hair follicles
    Pilomatricoma
    Trichoepithelioma
  Intracutaneous cornifying epithelioma
Melanocytic tumours
  Benign melanoma
  Malignant melanoma
Mesenchymal tumours
  Fibrous tissue
    Fibroma
    Fibrosarcoma
    Canine haemangiopericytoma
    Malignant fibrous histiocytoma
  Adipose tissue
    Lipoma
    Liposarcoma
  Vascular tissue
    Haemangioma
    Haemangiosarcoma (Fig. 96.3)
    (Also myxoma, myxosarcoma,
    leiomyoma, leiomyosarcoma
    rhabdomyosarcoma)
Mast cell tumour (Figs 96.4 and 96.5)
Lymphohistiocytic
  Lymphoma
    Primary lymphoma (Fig. 96.6)
    Mycosis fungoides (Figs 96.7–96.10)
    Histiocytic lymphoma
    Plasmacytoma
  Histiocytic disease
    Histiocytoma
    Histiocytosis (Fig. 96.11)
    Systemic histiocytosis (Fig. 96.12)

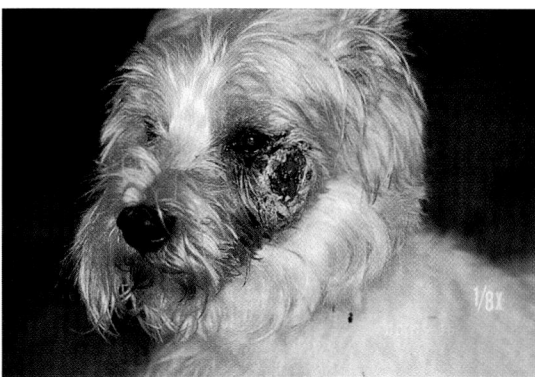

Fig. 96.1 Infiltrating squamous cell carcinoma.

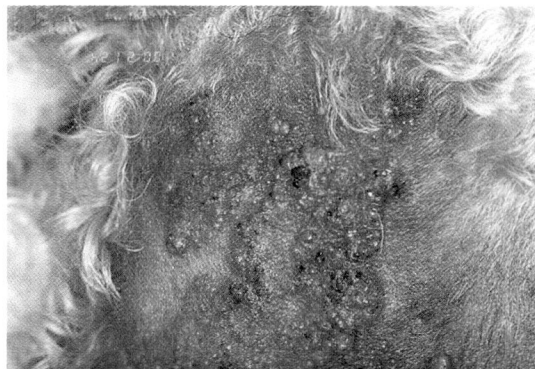

Fig. 96.2 Infiltrating nodules of a sweat gland adenocarcinoma.

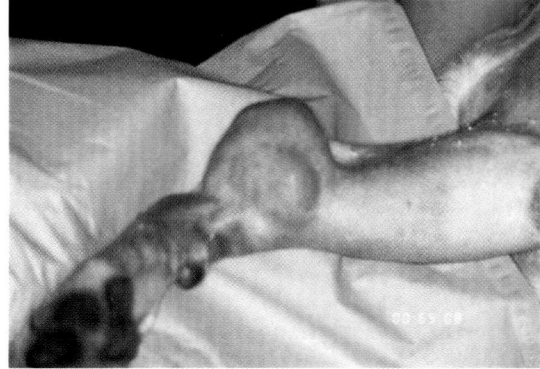

Fig. 96.3 Soft tissue sarcoma – haemangiosarcoma.

mitotic rate and relationship of the neoplastic cells with adjacent normal tissues. This can only be achieved by histological examination of representative tissue from the lesion. Histological diagnosis, clinical staging of a tumour and a

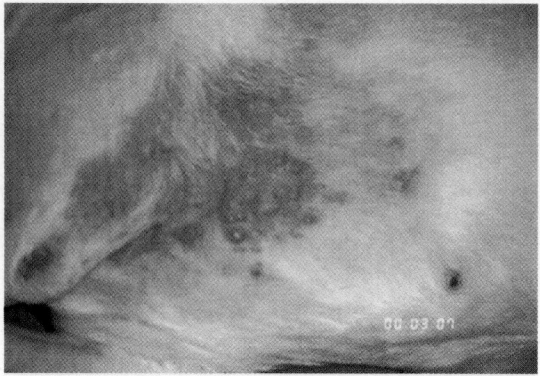

Fig. 96.4   Infiltrating mast cell tumour in the axilla.

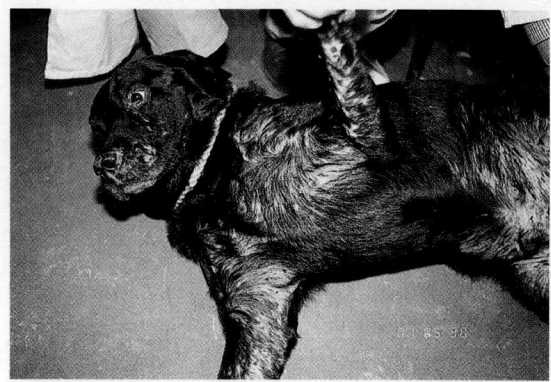

Fig. 96.7   Mycosis fungoides.

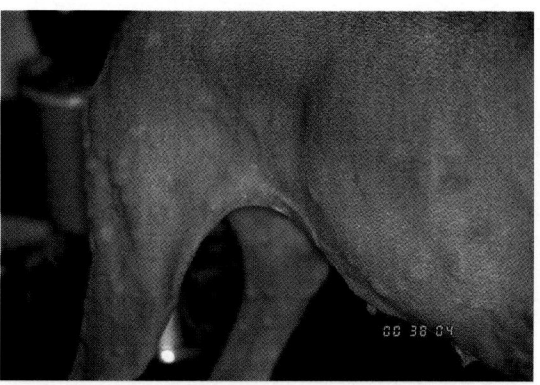

Fig. 96.5   Disseminated mast cutaneous mast cell tumours.

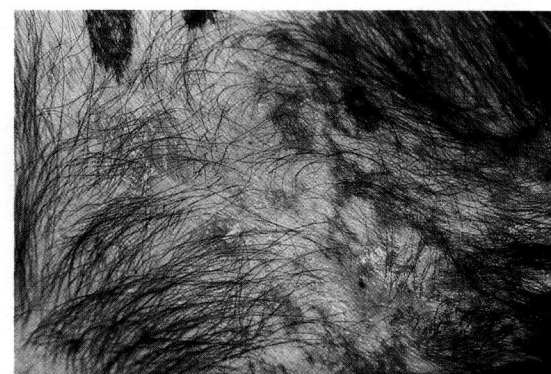

Fig. 96.8   Mycosis fungoides.

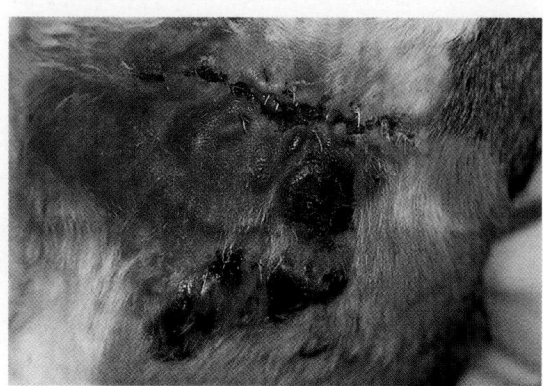

Fig. 96.6   Primary cutaneous lymphoma.

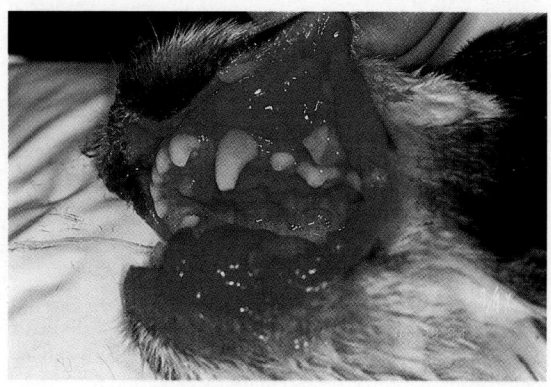

Fig. 96.9   Mycosis fungoides.

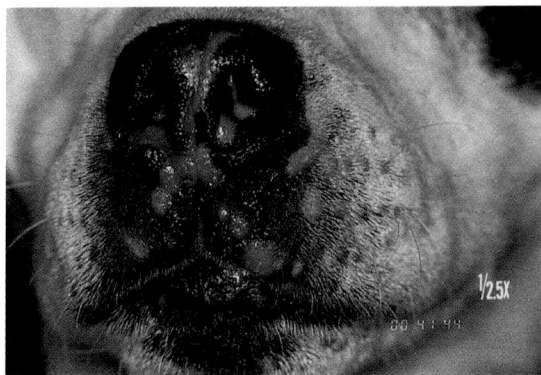

Fig. 96.10   Mycosis fungoides.

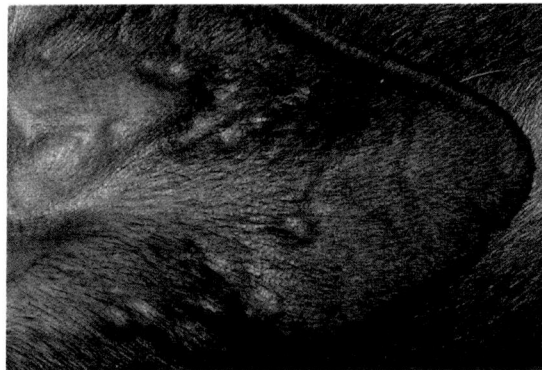

Fig. 96.11   Cutaneous histiocytosis.

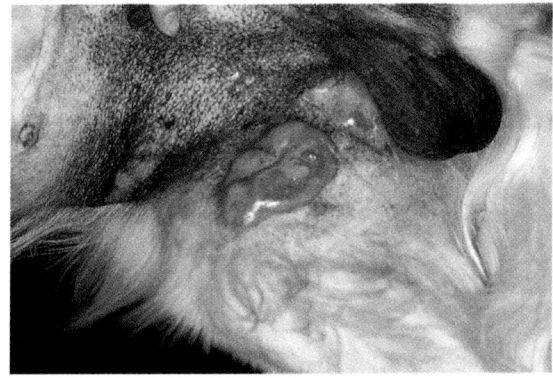

Fig. 96.12   Systemic histiocytosis.

knowledge of the likely biological behaviour of the tumour provide the information upon which to base prognosis and select treatment.

SPECIFIC TUMOUR TYPES

Neoplasms that usually present as solitary cutaneous lesions include the epithelial tumours (basal cell and squamous cell tumours), adnexal tumours, melanocytic tumours and tumours of mesenchymal origin (fibroma, lipoma, fibrosarcoma etc. (see Table 96.1). Approximately 25–35% of canine skin tumours are malignant. The general principles of diagnosis and management previously described apply to all such tumours.

Squamous Cell Carcinoma

Squamous cell carcinoma (SCC) is one of the most common malignant cutaneous tumours in the dog representing between 4 and 18% of all canine cutaneous tumours. Sites of occurrence include the limbs, particularly the digits, and the head (lips and nose). In the majority of cases the aetiology is unknown. However, long-term exposure of non- or lightly-pigmented skin to ultraviolet light can result in development of SCC, as seen in the pinna, eyelids, rhinarium and occasionally on the trunk.

Squamous cell carcinomas arise from the squamous epithelial cells of the epidermis and infiltrate into the underlying dermal and subcutaneous tissues. The tumour may be 'productive' forming a papillary growth with a cauliflower like appearance, or 'erosive' forming a shallow ulcer with raised edges. In both instances the lesion is frequently ulcerated, infected and associated with a chronic inflammatory infiltrate. *It is not uncommon for these tumours to be dismissed as infective/inflammatory lesions on initial presentation.* The majority of SCCs arising in the skin are well differentiated and if adequate surgical resection can be achieved, the prognosis is good.

The most malignant cutaneous SCC in the dog is that which arises in the nail bed region of the digit (Susaneck & Withrow 1989). This is an aggressive tumour, invasion and destruction of the distal phalanx is frequent. Amputation of the affected digit(s) is the treatment of choice but these tumours frequently metastasise to regional lymph nodes and therefore the prognosis is extremely guarded. Anaplastic squamous cell tumours at other sites may also metastasise via the lymphatic route, and disseminated metastases have been observed.

Squamous cell carcinomas arising on the nasal rhinarium, present a particular problem. These tumours have a tendency to infiltrate the alar cartilage and are often more extensive than may be appreciated. Radical surgical resection of some SCCs affecting the rhinarium and the alar cartilage can be performed with appropriate reconstruction of the area using skin flaps to close the defect. Squamous cell carcinomas are considered to be radiosensitive and SCC of the nose or at sites where surgery is not feasible may respond favourably to radiation therapy. One year control rates of 34–46% have been reported for radiation therapy of all SCCs but there is considerable variation depending on tumour site and on the fractionation schedule employed.

Mast Cell Tumours

Mast cell tumours are important cutaneous tumours, representing 9–21% of all canine skin tumours (Macy & Withrow 1989; Gorman & Dobson 1991). The terms mast cell tumour, mastocytoma, mastocytosis and mast cell sarcoma are often used interchangeably although the two latter terms tend to be reserved for cases with systemic involvement. Mast cell tumours present a considerable challenge to the clinician and a knowledge of their unique biological aspects is essential in the management of these tumours.

Mast cells are found throughout the body in loose connective tissues and are involved in a wide variety of physiological reactions. They are widely known for their importance in Type I hypersensitivity reactions but their primary function is related to the induction of acute inflammatory reactions in response to injury. The cytoplasm of mast cells contains granules containing numerous biologically active vasoactive peptides which include histamine, heparin, proteolytic enzymes and many other amines. It is these granules that stain metachromically to give the mast cell its characteristic appearance under light microscopy.

Mast cell tumours have many presentations and probably should be included in the list of differentials for any cutaneous mass no matter what its appearance. Mast cell tumours may arise in the dermis or in subcutaneous tissues, they may be solitary or multiple and internal organs (particularly the spleen and liver) may be involved. MCTs have been reported in all age groups, the mean age for dogs is 8.5 years. The brachiocephalic breeds notably the Boxer, are reported to have the highest incidence of MCT, but all breeds and cross-bred dogs may be affected. In the United Kingdom Labradors and Golden Retrievers seem to be over represented in the affected population.

There is no typical appearance of a MCT but some features are characteristic. Cutaneous tumours range from well circumscribed, firm raised plaques within the dermis, the surface of which is often erythematous or ulcerated, to poorly circumscribed, subcutaneous lesions. The tumour may be associated with inflammatory swelling and fluctuating oedema may be a presenting feature.

Many attempts have been made to categorise the clinical behaviour of MCT and to correlate this with histological criteria. There are three grades of mast cell tumour: anaplastic poorly differentiated or undifferentiated; intermediate or moderately differentiated and well differentiated/mature. These grades do bear some correlation to patient survival but they are by no means absolute and in this respect the classification of MCT remains a grey area (see Table 96.2).

There have been attempts to correlate the argyrophilic nucleolar organiser regions in mast cells to the histological grade and prognosis with variable results (Bostock *et al.* 1989; Kravis *et al.* 1996). Clinically, one can recognise two basic types of MCT: solitary slowly growing tumours and rapidly growing tumours which invariably metastasise to regional lymph nodes. However, it is not unknown for a slowly growing, apparently benign tumour to suddenly change into the aggressive variety, therefore the distinction is not definitive.

A proportion of mast cell tumours' release of histamine, heparin, other vasoactive amines and enzymes from the cytoplasmic granules may have local and systemic effects which are important in both the diagnosis and management of the tumour. Locally, release of histamine may result in acute inflammation, erythema, oedema, ulceration and irritation. In some circumstances these reactions may confuse the diagnosis but a history of fluctuating swelling and ery-

Table 96.2 The prognosis following surgical removal of mast cell tumours.

Histological grade	% disease-free survival at 12 months
Well differentiated mast cell tumour	90%
Intermediate/moderately differentiated mast cell tumour	75%
Poorly differentiated mast cell tumour	<25%

Bostock *et al.* (1989).

thema should alert the clinician to the possibility of a MCT. Increased bleeding times may result from heparin release by tumour cells, this may occur spontaneously in ulcerated lesions or may be noted subsequent to surgical interference. Delayed wound healing may result from release of proteolytic enzymes at the time of surgery. It is because of this activity that the authors consider mast cell tumours in two categories: those that are physiologically active and those that are not.

Any interference with a mast cell tumour, particularly where there has been a history that suggests that the mass has been releasing the vasoactive amines, be it physical manipulation, surgical incision or cryosurgery may precipitate histamine release from the tumour. Rare cases of anaphylaxis have been reported and premedication with antihistamine (H_1) agents is a wise precaution where the mast cell tumour is clearly physiologically active. More frequent systemic effects include gastrointestinal ulceration, owing to chronic stimulation of H_2 histamine receptors on gastric parietal cells which results in an increased acid secretion and gastric hypermotility. Gastrointestinal ulceration must not be overlooked, it is debilitating and distressing to the patient and in severe cases duodenal perforation will occur and the associated peritonitis can be fatal. Other paraneoplastic syndromes associated with MCT include hypergammaglobinaemia and inflammatory glomerular disease.

The management of MCT depends on the stage of the disease at presentation, the histological grade of the tumour and whether or not there are systemic effects associated with the release of heparin and the other vasoactive amines. Surgical excision is the treatment of choice for solitary lesions without local lymph node involvement. Excision margins of at least 2–3 cm should be achieved since neoplastic cells may extend into peripheral and deep tissues much further than expected. Where the grade of the tumour is known then the margin of excision should be adjusted accordingly. Surgical removal of a well differentiated mast cell tumour is often curative.

Where lymph nodes are involved and/or the primary lesion is too extensive to allow adequate surgical excision, radiotherapy or chemotherapy (or both), may be appropriate but the prognosis is guarded to poor. Any treatment that damages the tumour cells *in situ* may provoke a marked inflammatory response which will result in swelling and erythema, giving the impression that the lesion is progressing. Considerable effort has been afforded by oncologists to evaluating chemotherapeutic agents in the management of mast cell tumours. Despite this effort little progress has been made and it still appears that prednisolone is probably the most useful agent for systemic therapy and significant tumour regression may be achieved and maintained using which regimen based on this drug (see Tables 96.3 and 96.4).

Table 96.3   Treatment recommendations for the management of mast cell tumours.

Well differentiated tumours	Wide local excision – if incomplete resection further surgery. Irradiate tumour bed – least favoured option
Intermediate or moderately differentiated tumours with no nodal involvement	Radical surgical excision – if not feasible cytoreductive surgery with postoperative irradiation
Intermediate tumours with nodal involvement and poorly differentiated mast cell tumours	Surgery and/or radiation of the primary mass/nodes plus chemotherapy
Any tumour with distant metastases	Treat with chemotherapy

Table 96.4   Cytotoxic drug protocols for mast cell tumours.

Prednisolone	40 mg per m^2 daily for 2 weeks (or until a tumour response is seen) then 40 mg per m^2 alternate day treatment aiming to reduce in 10 mg increments to a maintenance dose of 20 mg per m^2
Prednisolone and cyclophosphamide	Prednisolone 40 mg per m^2 daily for 2 weeks (or until a tumour response is seen) then 40 mg per m^2 alternate day treatment aiming to reduce in 10 mg increments to a maintenance dose of 20 mg per m^2
Cyclophosphamide	50 mg per m^2 every 48 h
Cimetidene	5 mg/kg every 6 h should be used in any cases where there is evidence of histamine release

An important systemic effect of mast cell tumours is duodenal ulceration. This is seen in those patients who have mast cell tumours that release significant amounts of the vasoactive amines alluded to previously. The use of anti-H_2 agents such as cimetidene, ranitidene and omeprazole to block the H_2 receptor has proved to be invaluable in the long-term management of these cases and prevents the development of duodenal ulceration.

CUTANEOUS LYMPHOPROLIFERATIVE DISEASE

Lymphoproliferative disease is well characterised in the dog where there is a wealth of information on the various common types as detailed in Chapter 35. It has long been recognised that the skin can be involved but the true incidence of cutaneous lymphomas in the dog remains unknown (Goldschmidt & Bevier 1981). This is largely because the definition of the various forms of lymphoid infiltrate into the skin is still unclear and needs careful examination.

There are two major forms of cutaneous lymphoma in the dog that will be dealt with separately below:

(1) *Primary cutaneous T-cell lymphoma*: In this case the lymphocyte that becomes malignant is one that normally recirculates through the skin and is a T cell. There are two forms of primary cutaneous T-cell lymphoma:
   ● primary cutaneous lymphoma,
   ● mycosis fungoides.
(2) *Secondary cutaneous lymphoma*: In this case the skin becomes involved because of dissemination from a lymphoma at another site be it multicentric, alimentary or thymic. The lymphocytes in this case are not all T-cell lymphomas but reflect the phenotype of the original tumour.

Primary Cutaneous T-cell Lymphoma

Primary Cutaneous Lymphoma

The clinical presentation of cutaneous lymphoma is varied. In the majority of cases multiple lesions including nodules, plaques, erythroderma and exfoliative dermatitis are present. There is a rapid progression of the neoplasm following the initial appearance of the lesion. In the early stages dogs do not appear systemically ill but once the disease has progressed the systemic signs associated with lymphomas, particularly hypercalcaemia, are a characteristic feature. The aggressive nature of this form of the disease is remarkable and the response to treatment is poor in comparison to other forms of canine lymphoma.

The clinical diagnosis of primary canine lymphoma can sometimes be difficult but is readily confirmed on cytological and histological examination of tissue samples. There is a diffuse infiltrate of the dermis with lymphoblasts which can extend into the epidermis. The treatment of this form of lymphoma is similar to the treatment of other systemic lymphomas. It is folly to think that as the tumour is 'simply in the skin' that the treatment needs to be less aggressive. There are a number of regimens available for the treatment of lymphoma and each clinician has their own particular one with which they are comfortable.

Mycosis Fungoides

This is the epitheliotropic form of cutaneous lymphoma that is characterised by a lymphoid infiltrate into the epidermis rather than the dermis. There is a long clinical course to this disease and it is fair to say that there is no classical presentation of the disease. There are three stages to the disease: premycotic, mycotic or plaque, and the tumour stage. The first two stages can be present for many months or years before there is progression to tumour stage. In the premycotic stage there is generally a history of either an erythroderma or a generalised exfoliative, pruritic dermatitis. In this particular stage the clinical presentation can be very similar to exfoliative seborrheic condition. The premycotic lesions may have had a very protracted course before some of them progress to the plaque stage, which is characterised by firm elevated plaques. In an individual animal the premycotic and mycotic stages can occur concurrently and present a very confusing clinical presentation. The final progression is to the tumour stage which is characterised by the development of multiple raised plaques in the skin. Once the disease has progressed to this stage there is usually a rapid clinical course with dissemination to the regional lymph nodes and then systemic spread of the lymphoma. At this stage the clinical signs are those associated with a disseminated lymphoma.

Diagnosis of mycosis fungoides can only be achieved by a biopsy of the affected site(s). There is a characteristic lymphocytic infiltrate into the epidermis and the associated Pautrier's microabscesses. The epidermal changes also include hyperkeratosis and acnathosis but there is great variation in the severity of these changes.

Secondary Cutaneous Lymphoma

In these cases the skin becomes infiltrated with lymphoma cells secondary to an underlying lymphoma. As a consequence of this the clinical presentation is usually one of lymphoma rather than skin disease. Where present these are usually multiple lesions and are often ulcerated.

Canine Histiocytic Lymphoma

It is well recognised by histopathologists that there can be a diffuse infiltrate of mononuclear cells that have a histiocytic appearance, into the dermis. These histiocytic-like cells have the morphological characteristics that one would expect of a malignant cell population. However it is clear that there is considerable variation in the characteristics of this histiocytic infiltration and it is more than likely that there are a number of neoplastic diseases that hide under the guise of histiocytic lymphoma. This point will only be clarified once the exact phenotype and lineage of the cells is defined. (In human histopathology histiocytic lymphoma is clearly of lymphoid lineage.)

The variation that is noted on histopathology is echoed by the clinical course of the histiocytic lymphoma. There is a predilection for young to middle-aged dogs to be affected with Spaniels and Collies over-represented in this hospital population. The course of the disease is generally not as aggressive as primary cutaneous lymphoma and this group appears to be more sensitive to combination chemotherapy than other forms of cutaneous lymphoma although this finding needs to be substantiated.

CANINE HISTIOCYTIC DISEASES

There is a lack of clarity about the true spectrum of histiocytic diseases in the dog. The original classification of histiocytic disease is being challenged as there is an increase in the ability to classify the various phenotypes and genotypes of both histiocytic and lymphoid cell phenotypes in the dog (see Table 96.5, data from Moore *et al.* 1996). The following is an overview of the current position but this may well change over the next year or two.

Canine Cutaneous Histiocytoma

The canine cutaneous histiocytoma is a tumour that is unique to the skin of the dog. It is a relatively common

Table 96.5 Cell surface antigens in canine histiocytic disorders.

Antigenic marker	CD1	Thy1	CD4
Cutaneous histiocytoma	+	–	–
Cutaneous histiocytosis	+	+	+
Systemic histiocytosis	+	+	+
Malignant histiocytosis	+	–	–
Histiocytic sarcoma	+	–	–

All these conditions are Langerhans cell histiocytoses.
Cutaneous histiocytoma shows epidermal Langerhans cell phenotype: upregulates CD44, CD49d, CD54.
Cutaneous and systemic histiocytosis are reactive histiocytoses of dermal Langerhans cells, arising in the context of disordered immune regulation.

tumour, representing up to 10% of all canine cutaneous neoplasms. There are several characteristic features: cutaneous histiocytoma is more often seen in young dogs than older animals, 50% of tumours occur in dogs under 2 years of age. The tumours are most commonly found on the head, especially the pinna, the hind limbs, feet and trunk. The Boxer and Dachshund appear to be predisposed to development of cutaneous histiocytoma.

Cutaneous histiocytoma presents as a rapidly growing, circular, intradermal lesion. The surface may be alopecic and is often ulcerated but rarely does the lesion cause any discomfort to the animal. Histological sections show infiltration of the epidermis and dermis by histiocytic tumour cells with round to oval nuclei. Numerous mitotic figures give the lesion the appearance of a highly malignant neoplasm. This appearance may be misdiagnosed by non-veterinary pathologists who are unfamiliar with the condition, since the tumour resembles the human malignant cutaneous histiocytoma, a tumour which carries a poor prognosis. Despite the histological appearance and the rapid growth rate, cutaneous histiocytoma is a benign tumour which may even regress spontaneously; local surgical excision is usually curative. A clear lymphocytic infiltrate of the histiocytoma can be seen in many cases, which is often interpreted as an anti-tumour cellular response.

Cutaneous Histiocytosis

This is characterised by multifocal cutaneous histiocytic lesions and in all cases there are dermal infiltrates of large histiocytic cells (Calderwood-Mays & Bergeron 1986). Although there appears to be a higher incidence in Collies there is no age predisposition. Clinically these present as one or more erythematous cutaneous plaques or nodules around the head, nose and ears. This can extend into the nasal mucosa and as a result may lead to respiratory stridor. Histologically cutaneous histiocytosis is characterised by dermal infiltrates of large histiocytic cells. There is some question as to whether or not these nodules are true neoplastic disease or an extension of or related to idiopathic sterile granulomatous, pyogranulomatous dermatoses, periadnexal multinodular granulomatous dermatitis. Moore *et al.* (1996) considers this to be a reactive condition with an underlying disorder of immune regulation. The response to immunosuppressive treatment usually good.

Malignant Histiocytosis

Malignant histiocytosis is a rare disease characterised by widespread neoplastic proliferation of malignant histiocytes. Although this is rare in the dog population as a whole the Bernese Mountain Dog is disproportionately affected (Ramsey *et al.* 1996). Affected dogs are usually 6–8 years of age with a male predisposition. It has also been seen in other breeds especially in Golden Retrievers and Rottweilers. This a very aggressive disease with a short course and is rapidly fatal. It is characterised by multiple tumours affecting especially spleen, liver, lymph nodes and lungs with or without bone marrow involvement. Signs are relatively non-specific depending upon which organs are affected but include weight loss, dyspnoea, severe non-regenerative anaemia. Unlike systemic histiocytosis the skin and eyes are rarely affected (see below). The histopathological appearance is one of sheets of pleiomorphic cells with foamy cytoplasm, often with erythrophagocytosis and multinucleate giant cells. There is a high mitotic index with abnormal mitoses and appearance invariably appears as that of a very anaplastic tumour. There is clearly a strong genetic component to this condition and a polygenic mode of inheritance has been reported in the Bernese Mountain Dog (Padgett *et al.* 1995).

Systemic Histiocytosis

A rare histiocytic disorder characterised by a prolonged and fluctuating course in which a variety of tissues are infiltrated by atypical histiocytes. The incidence is rare but there is familial occurrence in the Bernese Mountain Dog. Clinically the skin and eyes are consistently affected (Moore 1984; Paterson *et al.* 1995). Skin lesions include nodules and plaques on the flanks, muzzle, nasal planum, eyelids and scrotum. Ocular involvement may manifest as conjunctival and episcleral nodules, exophthalmos, uveitis and glaucoma. In time lymph nodes and other internal organs may become involved. The disease waxes and wanes with periods of exacerbation and remission. Unlike malignant histiocytosis systemic histiocytosis is rarely fatal, but

chronic and debilitating in nature. Histopathologically the histiocytic infiltrates do not demostrate any features of malignancy. It is unresponsive to antibiotic and immunosuppressive therapy. Two modes of inheritance have been proposed: autosomal recessive Moore (1984) and polygenic Padgett *et al.* (1995).

SOFT TISSUE SARCOMAS

The term soft tissue sarcoma describes malignant neoplasms that arise from mesenchymal tissues, including dermal and subcutaneous connective tissues. Tumours of fibrous, adipose, muscular and vascular tissues and tumours arising from peripheral nervous tissue are included in this definition. In total these tumours represent 9–14% of all canine skin soft tissue neoplasms. Irrespective of tissue type, soft tissue sarcomas may be considered as a group since they are characterised by common morphological and behavioural features. However these tumours do vary in their degree of malignancy and a definitive diagnosis including histological garde is necessary for prognosis.

The most common soft tissue sarcomas are the tumours of fibrous tissue, traditionally classified as fibrosarcoma and canine haemangiopericytoma (see Table 96.1). Some soft tissue sarcomas lack sufficient differentiation for definitive classification and may be described as spindle cell sarcoma or anaplastic sarcoma. A group of tumours containing mixtures of spindle (fibroblast-like) cells, rounded (histiocyte-like) cells and pleomorphic giant cells is also recognised; some of these tumours resemble the fibrohistiocytic tumours of man, e.g. the malignant fibrous histiocytoma. Malignant fibrous histiocytomas are thought to arise from a pluripotent mesenchymal cell that differentiates into histiocyte-like cells and fibroblast-like cells and cells with intermediate morphology. The soft tissue sarcomas that are seen in the flat coated sarcoma may be of this type. As a group soft tissue sarcomas display a spectrum of biologic behaviour and therapeutic response.

Soft tissue sarcomas usually develop in older animals with a mean age of 9 years in dogs and cats. Fibrosarcomas have occasionally been found in dogs as young as 6 months of age. The distribution of soft tissue sarcomas is widespread and sites include the head, limbs and trunk. The rate of growth is variable, haemangiopericytoma and solitary fibrosarcoma may be slow growing while the anaplastic tumours often grow at an alarming rate. As a group, these tumours are characterised by an infiltrative pattern of growth. The tumours may appear to be encapsulated due to the formation of a pseudocapsule from compressed normal tissues. The tumour invariably extends into and beyond this structure. The treatment of choice is radical surgical excision; in most cases it is necessary to resect the entire anatomic compartment if all neoplastic cells are to be eradicated. Failure to achieve this aim accounts for the high rate of local recurrence. It is therefore essential to identify the tumour and to carefully plan the surgical procedure before attempting therapy. Although sarcomas are often considered to be radioresistant tumours, radiation therapy may play a role in their management, especially as an adjunct to surgical excision. Doxorubicin is the most effective agent for the treatment of soft tissue sarcoma although the use of other agents, e.g. cyclophosphamide and vincristine, in mulit-drug regimes has been described. The role of chemotherapy in the management of soft tissue sarcoma is palliative and the prognosis for the more maligant tumours is generally poor.

The potential for metastatic spread from soft tissue sarcomas is variable. Haemangiopericytoma is notorious for local recurrence but rarely metastasises. Approximately 25% of fibrosarcomas metastasise and although metastasis is frequently stated as being via haematogenous dissemination to the lung, in the authors' experience lymph node involvement is quite common. The incidence of metastasis is higher in the anaplastic tumours where haematogenous spread is more common.

Other soft tissue sarcomas such as liposarcoma, haemangiosarcoma etc. display similar behaviour to the tumours already described. Haemangiosarcoma is a particularly malignant tumour that may arise at any site and metastatic rates as high as 90% are documented (see Table 96.6).

MELANOCYTIC TUMOURS

Melanomas arise from melanocytes situated in the basal layer of the epidermis or the epithelium of the gingiva.

Table 96.6 Soft tissue sarcomas.

Tumour	Metastatic potential
Canine haemangiopericytoma	Low grade tumour metastasis-rare
Fibrosarcoma (well differentiated)	Low grade tumours approximately 25% metastasise
Neurofibrosarcoma	
Synovial cell sarcoma Rhabomyosarcoma	Intermediate-high grade 50 > 75% metastasise
Haemangiosarcoma	High grade tumour >90% metastasise

Cutaneous melanomas are less common than oral melanomas but the majority that arise on the distal extremities or mucocutaneous junctions (e.g. the lip and eyelid) are highly malignant. Those arising in the skin are usually benign.

Benign melanomas of the dermis are classically small, pigmented nodules. Instances of spontaneous regression of such lesions are documented. Malignant melanomas may be pigmented but amelanotic forms are recognised. Ulceration and secondary infection are common features. Regional lymph node metastasis and widespread distant metastases frequently occur early in the course of the disease. It is essential that clinical staging includes a thorough physical evaluation of drainage lymph nodes and radiographic evaluation of thoracic and abdominal cavities.

Therapy for primary malignant tumours requires radical surgical excision, surgical margins of up to 3 cm are necessary to ensure complete resection. Melanoma of an extremity requires at least amputation of the affected digit – limb amputation may be necessary to achieve an adequate margin.

Canine melanomas are radiosensitive but require large individual fractions to achieve response. Prophylactic irradiation of lymph nodes is indicated if this form of therapy is undertaken. Various chemotherapeutic regimes have been advocated for treatment of malignant, disseminated melanoma but efficacy is unproven.

REFERENCES

Bostock, D.E. (1973). The prognosis following surgical removal of mastocytomas in dogs. *Journal of Small Animal Practice*, **14**, 27–40.

Bostock, D.E., Crocker, J., Harris, K., *et al.* (1989). Nucleolar organising regions as indicators of post-surgical prognosis in canine spontaneous mast cell tumours. *British Journal of Cancer*, **59**, 915–918.

Calderwood-Mays, M.B. & Bergeron, J.A. (1986). Cutaneous histiocytosis in dogs. *Journal of the American Veterinary Medical Association*, **188**, 377–381.

Dobson, J.M. & Gorman, N.T. (1988). A clinical approach to the management of skin tumours in the dog and cat. *In Practice*, **10**, 55–68.

Goldschmidt, M.H. & Shofer, F.S. (1992). *Skin Tumours of the Dog and Cat*. Pergamon Press, Oxford.

Goldschmidt, M.H. & Bevier, D.E. (1981). Skin tumours in the dog. Part III Lympho-histiocytic and melanocytic tumours. *Compendium of Continuing Education for the Practicing Veterinarian*, **3**, 588–594.

Gorman, N.T. & Dobson, J.M. (1991). The skin and associated tissues. In: *Manual of Small Animal Oncology*, pp. 187–200. The British Small Animal Veterinary Association, Cheltenham, UK.

Kravis, L.D., Vail, D.M., Kisseberth, W.C., *et al.* (1996). Frequency of arygyrophilic nucleolar organiser regions in fine-needle aspirates and biopsy specimens from mast cell tumours in dogs. *Journal of the American Veterinary Medical Association*, **209**, 1418–1420.

Macy, D.W. & Withrow, S.J. (1989). Mast cell tumors. In: *Clinical Veterinary Oncology*, (ed. E.G. MacEwen), pp. 156–167. J.B. Lippincott, Philadelphia.

Moore, P.F. (1984). Systemic histiocytosis of Bernese Mountain dogs. *Veterinary Pathology*, **21**, 554–563.

Moore, P.F., Schrenezel, M.D., Affolter, V.K., *et al.* (1996). Canine spontaneous histiocytoma is an epidermotropic Langerhans cell histiocytosis which expresses CD1 and specific β2 integrin molecules. *American Journal of Pathology*, **148**, 1699–1708.

Padgett, G.A., Madewell, B.R., Keller, E.T., Jodar, L. & Packard, M. (1995). Inheritance of histicytosis in Bernese mountain dogs. *Journal of Small Animal Practice*, **36**, 93–98.

Paterson, S., Boydell, P. & Pike, R. (1995). Systemic histiocytosis in the Bernese mountain dog. *Journal of Small Animal Practice*, **36**, 233–236.

Pulley, L.T. & Stannard, A.A. (1990). Tumours of the skin and soft tissues. In: *Tumours in Domestic Animals*, (ed. J.E. Moulton), 3rd edn. pp. 23–82. University of California Press, Berkley.

Ramsey, I.K., McKay, J.S., Rudorf, H. & Dobson, J.M. (1996). Malignant histiocytosis in three Bernese mountain dogs. *Veterinary Record*, **138**, 440–444.

Susaneck, S.J. & Withrow, S.J. (1989). Tumors of the skin and subcutaneous tissues. In: *Clinical Veterinary Oncology*, (ed. E.G. MacEwen), pp. 139–155. J.B. Lippincott, Philadelphia.

Theilen, G.H. & Madewell, B.R. (1987). Tumours of the skin and subcutaneous tissues. In: *Veterinary Cancer Medicine*, (ed. G.H. Theilen & B.R. Madewell), 2nd edn. p. 233. Lea & Febiger, Philadelphia.

Section 13

Ophthalmology

Edited by Simon Petersen-Jones

Chapter 97

Introduction to the Ocular System

S. Petersen-Jones

ANATOMY AND PHYSIOLOGY

The important aspects of ocular anatomy and physiology are discussed under the relevant parts of this section.

EXAMINATION

The transparent nature of many of the ocular structures often allows direct visualisation of ocular disease processes, allowing diagnosis and close monitoring of progression or resolution of lesions. An ophthalmic examination should form part of every clinical examination because the eye may be involved as part of a systemic disease and the retina is the only part of the central nervous system that can be directly visualised. Neglecting to perform an ophthalmic examination may mean that important clues to the aetiology of disease are missed.

A careful, thorough and systematic examination of the eye is the key to ophthalmological diagnosis. Careful recording of findings is also essential. A certain amount of basic equipment is required to perform an ophthalmic examination (Table 97.1).

A suitable protocol for examination is shown in Table 97.2.

Signalment

The breed age and sex of the animal can be of importance. Inherited or breed related ocular problems are common in certain breeds of dog.

History

A full history should be taken and include the points listed in Table 97.3.

Hands-off, Lights on Examination

While the history is being taken the unrestrained dog can be observed (initial distant 'Hands-off, lights on' part of the examination). This is followed by a closer examination of the unrestrained animal, which is useful for the assessment of eyelid conformation (restraining the animal can pull on the skin of the head, altering the position of the eyelids).

Hands-on, Lights on Examination

Vision Testing

Owners' assessment of vision can be unreliable, for example, many owners do not notice if their dog has a unilateral visual deficit or they may not realise the extent of loss of vision if it has been slowly progressive giving the dog a chance to adapt.

The vision of dogs can be tested in a number of different ways (Table 97.4). Attempts should be made to test vision from both medial and lateral visual fields of each eye and to also test vision under both bright and dim lighting conditions. The latter is particularly useful for investigating early retinal disease.

A set routine is advised for the examination of the adnexa and eye and a suggested routine for the adnexa, lids and anterior portion of the eye is shown in Table 97.5. The Schirmer tear test should be performed early in the examination.

Table 97.1   Equipment.

- *Examination room that can be darkened*
- *Focal illuminator* (e.g. pen torch/Finhoff transilluminator)
- *Magnifying device* (e.g. loupe, direct ophthalmoscope, slit-lamp biomicroscope)
- *Direct ophthalmoscope*
- *Indirect ophthalmoscope* (pen torch and condensing lens provides a cheap alternative)
- *Schirmer tear test strips* (to measure tear production)
- *Fluorescein dye* (to stain ulcers)
- *Nasolacrimal cannulae* (to flush nasolacrimal ducts)
- *Swabs* (to collect material for culture from infected eyes)
- *Spatulae* to collect material from the ocular surface for cytology

More specialist equipment includes:
- *Tonometer* – to measure intraocular pressure
- *Gonioscopy lens* – to view the iridocorneal drainage angle through which aqueous drains out of the anterior chamber of the eye
- *Electroretinography* – to investigate retinal function
- *Ocular ultrasound*

Table 97.2   Examination protocol.

History (see Table 97.3)
Hands-off, lights on examination
- From a distance – look for pain/discomfort; discharge; asymmetry
- Closer – assess eyelid conformation

Hands-on, lights on examination
- Vision testing (see Table 97.4)
- Use a systematic approach to lids and adnexa, ocular surface and anterior segment (see Table 97.5)
- Do Schirmer tear tests before manipulating eye too much (see page 979)

Hands-on, lights off examination
- Pen torch/transilluminator (repeat examination of all structures – Table 97.5)
- Pupillary light reflexes
- Other neurological tests
- Use of magnification to examine lesions (loupe, direct ophthalmoscope, slit-lamp biomicroscope)
- Stain cornea with fluorescein if indicated
- Dilate pupil (apply tropicamide and wait 20 min) to fully examine structures posterior to the iris (perform tonometry/gonioscopy, if required, before pupillary dilation)
- Ophthalmoscopy (see below)

Further tests

Table 97.3   History.

- Previous problems?
- Problems in related or in-contact dogs?
- General health, presence of other signs?
- Rate of onset?
- Known aetiology?
- Initial signs?
- Pain/discomfort?
- Vision – night and day?
- Duration?
- Previous treatment?

Hands-on, Lights-off Examination

The adnexa, lids, ocular surface and anterior segment are examined again. The lens is also examined as is the anterior part of the vitreous. Look along the beam of light to see the reflection from the tapetum, also shine the light across the eye looking both along the beam and across the beam. Full examination of the structures posterior to the iris usually requires that the pupil is dilated by application of a mydriatic such as tropicamide. The Schirmer tear test and assessment of pupillary light reflexes must be performed before the mydriatic is applied.

Table 97.4 Techniques for vision testing.

- *The menace reflex* is useful and enables assessment of both medial and lateral visual fields. Care should be taken not to create air currents that are felt on the cornea, or to touch facial hair, both of which will induce blinking regardless of the visual status of the dog.
- *Cotton wool ball test*. This involves dropping cotton wool balls across the animal's visual field and observing the reaction. Be aware that even cotton wool can make a noise when it lands causing the dog to turn towards the noise.
- *Obstacle courses*. The owner is positioned one side of the obstacles and the dog on the other side. The owner calls the dog who then negotiates the obstacles. This can be repeated under different lighting conditions and with each eye blindfolded in turn.
- *Visual placing reaction*. The animal is lifted towards a table edge (without actually touching it) and if visual it should stretch out its front legs towards the table.

Table 97.5 Systematic examination routine.

- Entire head – lesions, discharge, symmetry
- Eyelid skin
- (Conformation of eyelids – performed before restraint)
- Eyelid margin – see openings of meibomian glands and nasolacrimal puncta
- Evert eyelids and examine conjunctival lining
- Press on globe through upper eyelid to protrude third eyelid (also digital tonometry)
- Examine conjunctiva in fornix and over globe
- Assess tear film – look at lustre of cornea; see tear meniscus against lower lid
- Sclera
- Cornea – transparency and smooth surface (can check corneal blink reflex)
- Anterior chamber
- Iris
- Pupillary apertures
- Front of lens

Table 97.6 Dioptre settings for direct ophthalmoscopy.

Cornea/conjunctiva	+20 to +30 dioptres
Anterior surface of lens	+12 dioptres
Posterior surface of lens	+8 dioptres
Vitreous	0 to +8 dioptres
Fundus	0 dioptres

Assessment of Pupillary Light Reflexes

The briskness and completeness of the direct and consensual reflexes should be noted. In theory both the medial and lateral portions of the retina can be assessed, but in practice this is difficult.

Pupillary reflexes are discussed further in Chapter 106.

Magnified Examination of the Adnexa and Anterior Segment of the Eye

This can be achieved by a number of devices; a slit-lamp biomicroscope is the most useful and most expensive, alternatively a magnifying loupe or direct ophthalmoscope can be used. When using a direct ophthalmoscope set the instrument as shown in Table 97.6.

Distant Direct Ophthalmoscopy

This is a very useful technique (Table 97.7). It relies on obtaining a good reflection from the tapetum against which any opacity in the normally transparent structures of the eye are silhouetted.

Table 97.7 Distant direct ophthalmoscopy.

- Use the direct ophthalmoscope
- Start at arm's length from the animal with the ophthalmoscope set on zero and the widest beam of light selected
- Look along the visual axis of the animal until the bright tapetal reflex is seen
- Any opacities in or on the cornea, in the anterior chamber, lens or vitreous will appear as dark shadows against the reflected light

Table 97.8 Tips for direct ophthalmoscopy.

- Rest the ophthalmoscope against your eyebrow so that your eye is as close to the viewing hole as possible
- Get the ophthalmoscope close to the dog's eye
- Use the widest beam of light
- Dilate the pupil for the best view (tropicamide drops applied 20 min before examination – NB check pupillary light reflex first)
- Move your head around to see as much as possible
- Try to look through your left eye for the animal's left eye and vice versa (to prevent noses clashing)

Direct ophthalmoscopy	Indirect ophthalmoscopy
Most commonly used method in general practice	Method most commonly used by veterinary ophthalmologists
Relatively inexpensive equipment	Equipment more expensive, although indirect ophthalmoscopy is possible using a pen torch and plastic magnifying lens – (this is the cheapest method of examining the fundus)
Image is upright	Image is inverted and reversed (can be confusing for beginners)
Magnified image but narrow field of view (scanning around is required to build up a mental picture of the entire fundus)	Less magnification, but much greater field of view. This allows for rapid and easy examination of large areas of the fundus. Magnification and field of view can be altered by selection of lenses of different strength – typically between 14 dioptres (higher magnification, narrower field of view) and 30 dioptres (lower magnification and wider field of view)
Can be difficult to see through opacities (e.g. corneal or lens)	Superior view through opacities of the ocular media

Table 97.9 Comparison between direct and indirect ophthalmoscopy.

- Dilate the pupil
- Hold the examining light by your temple so that it is possible to look along the beam of light.
- Position yourself at arm's length from the patient so that the light is shining along the dog's visual axis. A good tapetal reflection should be seen.
- Interpose the lens at right angles to the examining beam of light about 5 cm from the cornea. An aerial image of the fundus should now be seen. Move the lens closer or further from the cornea until the best image is achieved. The author finds it easiest to hold the edge of the lens between finger and thumb and rest a little finger on the animal's head. The hand holding the lens then moves with any head movements.
- To view other parts of the fundus the examiner must be prepared to either move him or herself or to alter the position of the animal's head. To view the dorsal fundus, for example, the examiner needs to look up into the eye or lift the animal's nose upwards, and to view the medial fundus the examiner needs to view from the lateral side of the eye. Therefore quite a lot of moving about may be required to view the entire fundus. When changing the direction of viewing it is important to alter the lens so that it remains at 90° to the beam of the examining light.

Table 97.10 Indirect ophthalmoscopy using a pen torch and magnifying lens.

This technique is very useful for distinguishing between cataract (a true opacity of the lens) and nuclear sclerosis. A cataract will appear as a dark shadow against the fundus reflection while the denser nucleus in dogs with nuclear sclerosis has the appearance of a transparent sphere within the lens itself.

Close Direct Ophthalmoscopy

This can be a continuation of distant direct ophthalmoscopy. Once the tapetal reflection is in view the examiner moves closer until within a few centimetres of the eye. The fundus should now be in focus. This technique gives a magnified view of a small area of the fundus, the examiner needs to move around to build up a mental montage of as much of the fundus as possible (Table 97.8).

Indirect Ophthalmoscopy

This technique has some major advantages over direct ophthalmoscopy (see Table 97.9).

Simple indirect ophthalmoscopy may be performed using a pen torch and condensing lens (between 15 and 30 dioptres) (Table 97.10).

Details of further investigations are found in the relevant sections.

FURTHER READING

Cottrell, B.D. & Petersen-Jones, S.M. (1993). Special examination techniques. In: *Manual of Small Animal Ophthalmology*, (eds S.M. Petersen-Jones & S.M. Crispin), pp. 27–35. BSAVA Publications, Cheltenham.

Hopper, C.D. & Crispin, S.M. (1993). Laboratory examination. In: *Manual of Small Animal Ophthalmology*, (eds S.M. Petersen-Jones & S.M. Crispin), pp. 37–43. BSAVA Publications, Cheltenham.

Mould, J. (1993). The right ophthalmoscope for you? *In Practice*, **15**, 73–76.

Mould, J. (1993). Approach to an ophthalmic examination. In: *Manual of Small Animal Ophthalmology*, (eds S.M. Petersen-Jones & S.M. Crispin), pp. 11–25. BSAVA Publications, Cheltenham.

Chapter 98

Conditions of the Globe and Orbit

K. Abrams and C. Goodwin

ORBITAL ANATOMY

The canine orbit is conically shaped with the apex facing posteriorly and the globe filling the majority of the expanded anterior portion of the orbit. All retrobulbar tissue, including the extraocular muscles, blood vessels, nerves, lacrimal gland and fat occupy the tightly packed posterior portion of the orbit and therefore, any change in orbital volume directly affects the position of the globe.

Osseous Structure

Only the medial and dorsal portions of the canine orbit are completely protected by bone. The ventral and lateral surfaces consist mostly of soft tissue. Laterally, the orbital rim is completed by the orbital ligament which connects the frontal and zygomatic bones. Ventrally, the orbital border consists primarily of the pterygoid muscle, fat, and zygomatic salivary gland; this soft tissue orbital floor allows orbital access to oral cavity infections or migrating foreign bodies. The depth of the orbit varies between breeds, with brachycephalic dogs such as Shih Tzus and Lhasa Apsos having shallow orbits while dolichocephalic breeds such as Collies have relatively deep orbits. This variation is clinically relevant when considering normal breed-related eye position, as well as pathological conditions.

Extraocular Muscles

Seven extraocular muscles control movement of the canine globe within the orbit (Table 98.1, Fig. 98.1). Four rectus muscles originate from the orbital apex and insert at 90° apart from each other on the dorsal, ventral, lateral and medial portions of the globe behind the limbus. They move the eye in vertical and horizontal directions. Two oblique muscles, the dorsal and ventral, help to apply torsion, or rotation, to the globe. The dorsal oblique muscle passes through the trochlea on the medial orbital wall and changes direction to insert on the dorsolateral portion of the globe; it results in rotation of the dorsal globe in a ventromedial direction. The ventral oblique, after inserting on the ventrolateral portion of the globe, rotates the dorsal portion of the globe in a ventrolateral direction. Dogs also have a retractor oculi muscle, which allows the globe to be retracted into the orbit, especially during ocular pain, although this ability is limited in brachycephalics. The innervations of the extraocular muscles are shown in Table 98.1.

Orbital Fascia

Three continuous layers of fascia surround the globe and line the orbit:

- The periorbita is the outermost layer and after arising posteriorly from the optic nerve dural sheath lines the orbit until it splits into two portions at the orbital rim to become the periosteum and the orbital septum. The orbital septum becomes the tarsal plate of the eyelids, which is a poorly developed structure in dogs.
- Tenon's capsule (fascia bulbi) is the second fascial layer; it inserts at the limbus and lies between the thin conjunctiva and the thick sclera.
- The extraocular muscle fascial sheaths comprise the third type of orbital fascia.

Table 98.1 Extraocular muscles.

Muscle	Primary action	Cranial nerve innervation
Dorsal rectus	Upward rotation (elevation)	III (Oculomotor nerve)
Ventral rectus	Downward rotation (depression)	III
Lateral rectus	Lateral rotation (abduction)	VI (Abducens nerve)
Medial rectus	Medial rotation (adduction)	III
Dorsal oblique	Intorsion rotation	IV (Trochlear nerve)
Ventral oblique	Extorsion rotation	III
Retractor bulbi	Globe retraction	VI

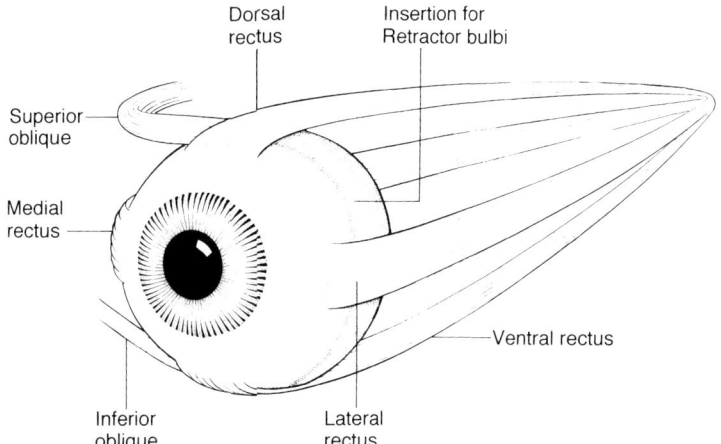

Fig. 98.1 A diagram showing the extraocular muscles.

EXAMINATION OF THE ORBIT

Clinical History

Specific items in the history can aid in investigation of orbital disease:

- Acute versus chronic disease can help differentiate inflammatory from neoplastic processes.
- General illness signs such as anorexia, lethargy, and pain upon chewing or opening the mouth tend to indicate inflammatory diseases of the orbit.
- History of travel to areas with endemic fungal infections is important to consider.

Clinical Techniques

Examination of the globe, adnexa, oral cavity and overall health of the patient can help in the general classification of orbital disease. Basic clinical examination techniques include:

- Globe position. Symmetry of globes – is each globe directed forward equally or is one globe deviated (strabismus)? Painful to patient?

> Clinical tip – examine eyes from above to help recognise exophthalmos and enophthalmos.

- Differentiate between an enlarged eye (buphthalmos) and a rostrally displaced eye (exophthalmos). Remember that a buphthalmic globe will show intraocular changes not expected in an eye which is simply displaced by an orbital space-occupying lesion.

> Clinical tip – if in doubt whether eye is enlarged or anteriorly displaced measure corneal diameter of each globe.

Chapter 99

Conditions of the Eyelids

K. Abrams and C. Goodwin

Although canine eyelids vary in shape and size, they serve the same basic functions of protecting the cornea from exposure and injury, supplying the outer portion of the tear film, and distributing the tear film across the cornea.

ANATOMY OF THE EYELIDS (FIG. 99.1)

The basic histological structure of the eyelids from superficial to deep includes (Fig. 99.2):

- skin,
- orbicularis oculi muscle,
- stroma, which contains the poorly developed tarsal plate and meibomian glands,
- conjunctiva.

Upper and lower eyelids meet at an angle medially and laterally forming the canthi. Along the upper eyelid, adjacent to the lid margin, two to four rows of cilia (eyelashes) are positioned; the lower eyelid is devoid of cilia. Surrounding the follicles of the cilia are modified sweat glands (glands of Moll) and sebaceous glands (glands of Zeis). Meibomian glands lie deep in the eyelid and can be seen through the mucous membrane surface, the conjunctiva. They secrete the outer, oily component of the tear film via their openings along the eyelid margins. The palpebral conjunctiva extends from the upper eyelid margin to line the eyelids and is reflected at the upper and lower fornices (cul-de-sac) to form the bulbar conjunctiva.

The third eyelid occupies the ventromedial portion of the conjunctival sac (Fig. 99.3). It contains a T-shaped hyaline cartilage skeleton which is positioned with the top of the T running parallel with the free edge of the lid.

Conjunctiva is reflected over the third eyelid and flaps of conjunctiva continuous with the free edge of the third eyelid extend into dorsal and ventral fornices, partly encircling the globe.

The gland of the third eyelid envelops the base of the T-shaped cartilage and produces almost half of the aqueous portion of the tear film (Helper *et al.* 1974). Ductules from the gland open on the bulbar (inner) surface of the third eyelid among lymphoid follicles.

EXAMINATION OF THE EYELIDS

Careful examination of the eyelids with good illumination and magnification is crucial for detecting subtle but significant eyelid disease. Systematic evaluation with a magnifying head loupe or by slit-lamp biomicroscopy is accomplished best by sweeping across each eyelid individually in a lateral to medial motion. The contour of the margin is evaluated first for irregularities such as swellings, depressions, or adventitious cilia. Next, the edge of the eyelid margin can be examined by pressing a finger above the margin to cause slight eversion. The meibomian gland openings can be easily seen with this technique. Finally, the eyelids should be fully everted to examine the conjunctival surface, the underlying meibomian structures, the lacrimal puncta which are positioned close to the medial canthus, and to detect the presence of any masses or abnormal cilia. Flipping (or everting) the eyelid can be accomplished either by grasping the lid near the margin and simply pulling the lid away from the cornea or by using a straight instrument such as a cotton tip applicator or tongue depressor placed on the eyelid skin to flip the lid over the instrument.

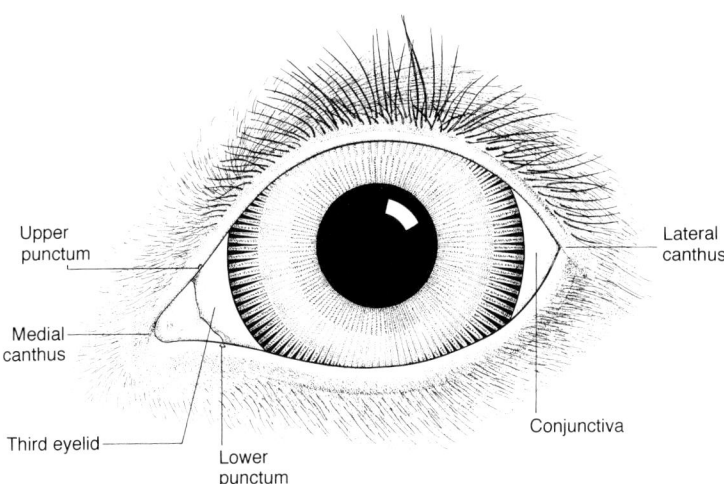

Upper punctum

Medial canthus

Third eyelid

Lower punctum

Lateral canthus

Conjunctiva

Fig. 99.1   Diagram showing the external features of the eyelids.

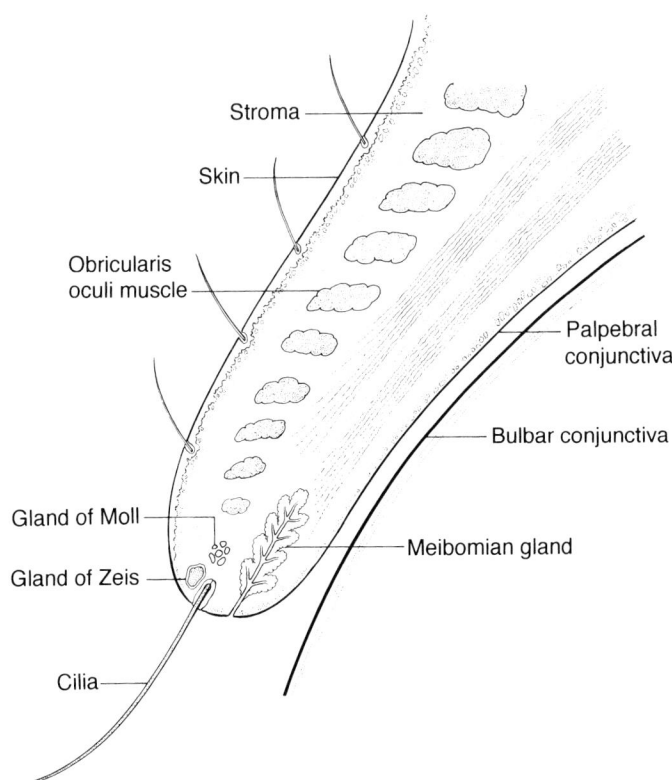

Stroma

Skin

Obricularis oculi muscle

Gland of Moll

Gland of Zeis

Cilia

Palpebral conjunctiva

Bulbar conjunctiva

Meibomian gland

Fig. 99.2   Diagram of a cross section through the upper eyelid.

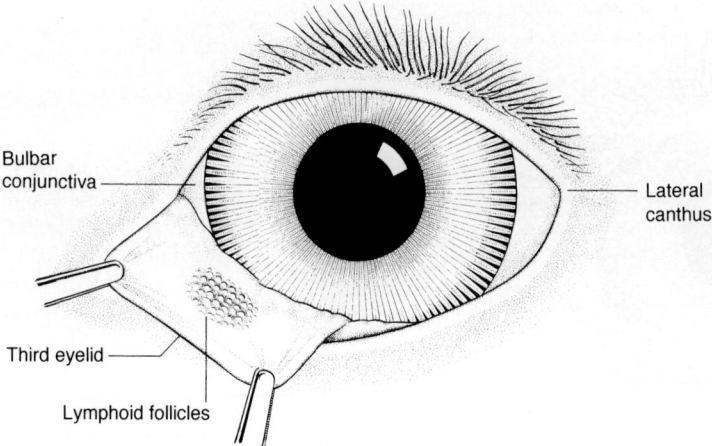

Bulbar
conjunctiva

Lateral
canthus

Third eyelid

Lymphoid follicles

Fig. 99.3 Diagram of the anatomy of
the third eyelid.

CONGENITAL DISORDERS

Some congenital disorders occur sporadically while other
anomalies tend to be breed-specific as summarised below:

- *Coloboma / agenesis* – eyelid colobomas are defects in the
  formation of a portion of the eyelid and are rare in
  dogs. The extent varies from complete agenesis of the
  lid, agenesis of a portion of the lid, or simply defective
  lid margins. Depending on the severity they can result
  in inadequate lid closure and an exposure keratitis.
  Selection of surgical technique for repair depends on
  the specific nature of the coloboma. Reported in: Jack
  Russell Terriers (Bedford 1988).
- *Dermoids* (Fig. 99.4) – a congenital mass composed of
  skin structures positioned on the eyelid, conjunctiva
  and/or cornea. Hairs arising from the dermoid can
  cause corneal irritation. Surgical removal must be complete to prevent re-growth of hairs.
  Breeds most commonly affected include: Golden
  Retriever, Rottweiler, German Shepherd, Saint
  Bernard, Dalmatian.
- *Ankyloblepharon* (fusion of the upper and lower eyelids
  along the margin length) is normal in new-born
  puppies up to about 10–14 days of life. Prolonged
  fusion occasionally occurs and in such cases the eyelids
  can be separated with blunt scissors, being sure that the
  eyelid margins are preserved.
  Occurrence: any breed.
- *Ophthalmia neonatorum* (Fig. 99.5) – This describes the
  development of a purulent ocular discharge beneath

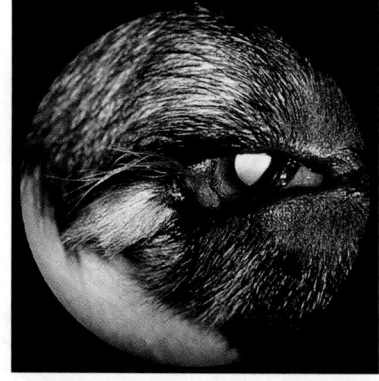

Fig. 99.4 A dermoid affecting eyelid and conjunctiva of a
young German Shepherd Dog. (Photograph courtesy of
Dr S.M. Petersen-Jones.)

the fused lids of a neonate. There is resulting swelling
of the lids and if untreated damage to the cornea. It is
treated by carefully opening the lids and thoroughly
irrigating the conjunctival sacs with saline. Purulent
material is collected for culture and until results are
available a broad-spectrum antibiotic ointment applied
to control infection and keep the ocular surface protected. Treatment should be continued until normal
tear production is established.
Occurrence: any breed.

- *Lagophthalmos* – Brachycephalic breeds tend to have
  large, prominent globes which coupled with large

palpebral fissures means that the eyelids may not completely close during the dog's natural blink. Exposure keratitis occurs during prolonged exposure such as during sleep. Surgery to shorten the palpebral fissure is beneficial in such cases.

Commonly affected breeds: Lhasa Apso, Shih Tzu, Pekingese, Cocker Spaniels.

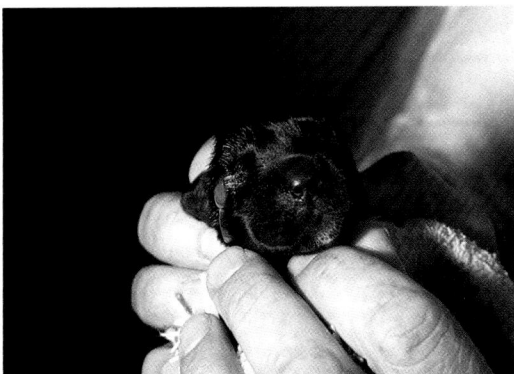

Fig. 99.5 Ophthalmia neonatorum. An ocular surface infection has developed in this puppy before the eyelids opening. The eyelids have been manually opened to release the purulent material. (Photograph courtesy of Dr S.M. Petersen-Jones.)

CONFORMATIONAL DISORDERS

Various combinations of inward rolling (entropion) and outward rolling (ectropion) of the eyelids occur in certain breeds. Entropion can result in corneal ulceration due to abrasion from eyelid hair. Ectropion usually results in less severe ocular surface disease although chronic infections or exposure conjunctivitis can occur. Characteristic features of each breed's eyelid conformational problems are listed in Table 99.1.

Entropion (Fig. 99.6)

Clinical signs of entropion can include: blepharospasm, epiphora, corneal ulceration and rubbing at the eye. Developmental, spastic and cicatricial entropion should be differentiated when deciding on the best course of action. Spastic entropion is that which arises from blepharospasm and globe retraction due to painful ocular lesions. In such cases the primary disease must be treated and the spastic entropion may resolve once the pain has diminished. In some cases temporary eversion of the eyelid may be required to allow healing of the lesion. Spastic entropion can easily be differentiated from other forms of entropion

Table 99.1 Eyelid conformational problems.

Type of anomaly	Lids usually involved	Breeds
Simple entropion	Single lower lid	Rottweilers, Retrievers, Irish Setters
	Both lower lids	Shar Pei, Chow Chow, Bulldog
	Both upper lids	Chow Chow, Bulldog, Bullmastiff
	All four lids	Shar Pei, Chow Chow, Bulldog, Bullmastiff
Lateral entropion with central ectropion (diamond eye)	Lower/upper lids	Great Dane, Newfoundland, Saint Bernard
Ectropion	Lower lids	Bloodhound, Saint Bernard, Cocker Spaniel, Bulldog
Senile upper eyelid trichiasis/ entropion and lower lid ectropion	Lower/upper lids	English Cocker Spaniel

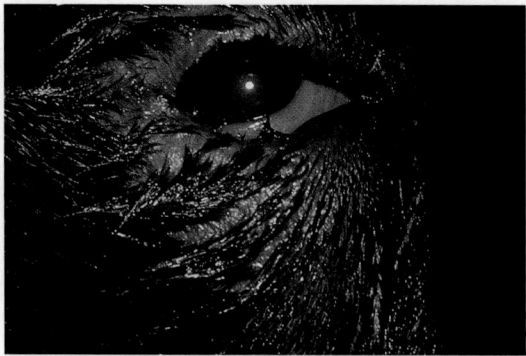

Fig. 99.6 Lower eyelid entropion in an Akita.

by anaesthetising the cornea with a topical ophthalmic anaesthetic. Anatomical entropion will persist, whereas the spastic form of the disease will be corrected.

Correction of Entropion

Temporary Repair
Some young puppies (weeks old) with entropion may grow out of the tendency towards entropion as they get larger. While waiting to see if this will happen a 'tacking' procedure should be used temporarily to correct the problem, relieve discomfort and prevent corneal damage. This procedure involves placing vertical mattress sutures along the affected eyelids temporarily to evert the eyelid margin from the corneal surface. Absorbable and non-absorbable suture materials, as well as skin staples, have been used for this technique. As the puppy grows, the procedure may have to be repeated and the client must be informed that this technique is to provide temporary relief until the dog is 4–6 months old, at which time permanent correction can be performed if necessary.

Permanent Blepharoplasty
Assorted techniques have been described to correct entropion (Miller & Albert 1988). Most methods, such as the Hotz–Celsus method, involve removal of skin and orbicularis oculi muscle near the eyelid margin followed by suturing of the incision to correct the deformity. The incision should be only a few millimetres from the eyelid margin and the amount of tissue removed is dependent on the severity of the entropion. The surgeon must evaluate the required degree of correction before sedation or general anaesthesia. It is far better to err towards under-correction and possibly have to repeat the procedure at a later date than to create ectropion with a poor cosmetic outcome.

Upper Eyelid Trichiasis/Entropion
(Fig. 99.7)

This condition occurs commonly in middle-aged and older English Cocker Spaniels. A loss of elasticity in the skin of the head leads to drooping of the facial mask and misdirection of the cilia of the upper eyelid onto the cornea. A lower eyelid ectropion is often present. The resulting keratitis and conjunctivitis are often exacerbated by reduced tear production and secondary bacterial conjunctivitis. Surgical correction (Stades 1987) will usually lead to relief of the discomfort and irritation, resolution of the inflammation and an improvement in tear production.

Ectropion (Fig. 99.8)

Compared with entropion, ectropion does not require immediate attention. Eversion of the eyelids, usually the lower lid, is more often a cosmetic concern. The degree of ectropion may vary in individuals usually worsening towards the end of the day, or following exercise. Some patients do develop chronic or intermittent conjunctivitis as a result of exposure of the conjunctival fornix and inability to clear accumulated debris and mucus from the fornix.

Repair of Ectropion

Various eyelid shortening or tensing procedures have been described such as the Kuhnt–Szymanowski method or

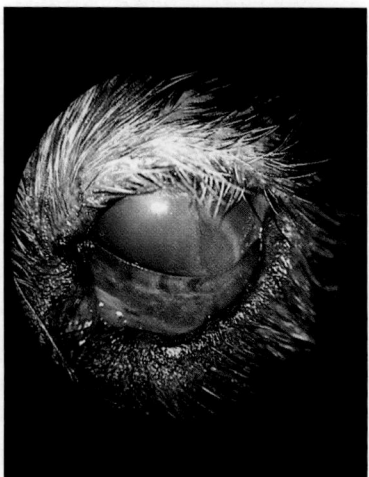

Fig. 99.7 Upper eyelid trichiasis/entropion in this English Cocker Spaniel has resulted in corneal abrasion and a superficial corneal ulcer. Surgical correction of the lid deformity is required. (Photograph courtesy of Dr S.M. Petersen-Jones.)

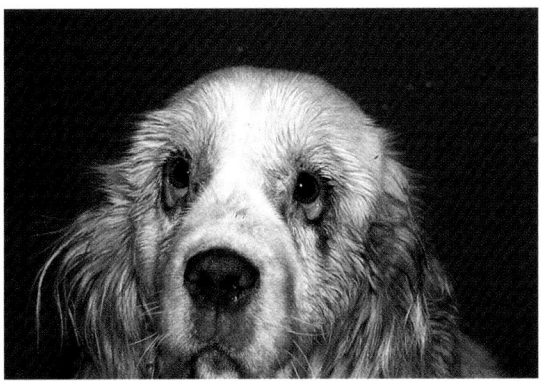

Fig. 99.8   Marked bilateral lower eyelid ectropion causing exposure of the lower conjunctival sacs. (Photograph courtesy of Dr S.M. Petersen-Jones).

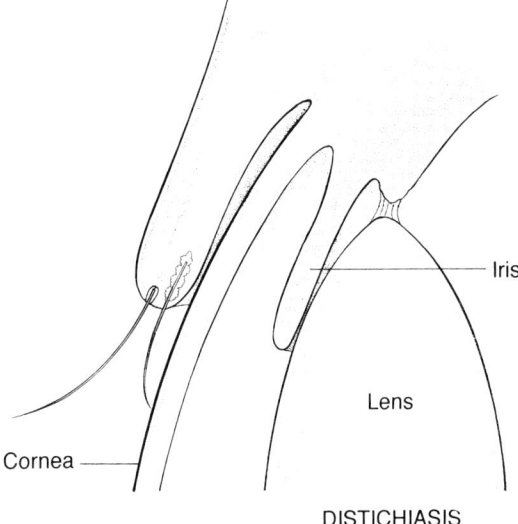

DISTICHIASIS

Fig. 99.9   Diagram of cross section of an eyelid showing position of distichia.

modifications on this technique (Munger & Carter 1984). These methods involve removal of partial or full thickness eyelid sections to reduce the eyelid laxity.

CILIA DISORDERS

Confusion often surrounds terminology associated with cilia disorders in the dog. As described above, normal cilia arise from hair follicles external to the meibomian glands. Problems occur when cilia arising from either the normal hair follicle or from the meibomian glands are misdirected towards the cornea. These disorders are described below.

Distichiasis (Figs 99.9 and 99.10)

In this disorder cilia arise from, or adjacent to the meibomian gland openings along the eyelid margin. It is a very common condition in some breeds, e.g. it has been estimated that 90% of American Cocker Spaniels have distichiasis (Gelatt 1991), other breeds commonly affected include Bulldog, Pekingese and Shetland Sheepdog. The clinician must carefully determine if the abnormal cilia are clinically significant, as many patients with distichiasis are free of clinical disease. Common clinical signs include: epiphora, 'blinking', conjunctival hyperaemia, and corneal ulcers. Often, distichiasis is blamed as the cause of ocular problems when in fact, the patient has a completely separate eye problem. One simple method to determine the significance of the distichia is to epilate the abnormal cilia; the removal of cilia should provide immediate but temporary

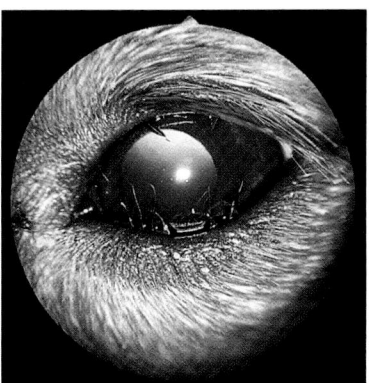

Fig. 99.10   Distichiasis in a Shetland Sheepdog. (Photograph courtesy of Dr S.M. Petersen-Jones.)

relief to the patient. If there is no improvement immediately following removal of the cilia, the clinician should look for other causes of the patient's problem.

Permanent correction of distichiasis is best accomplished by destruction of the abnormal hair follicle either by electrolysis, or trans-conjunctival cryosurgery (Chambers & Slatter 1984; Wheeler & Severin 1984). Cryosurgery is safe and although it may cause temporary depigmentation of the skin it is without any permanent cosmetic problems.

Ectopic Cilia (Fig. 99.11)

These cilia arise from meibomian glands and protrude straight through the conjunctiva. Although occurring much less frequently than distichiasis these typically short and often stout cilia almost invariably cause clinical disease such as severe blepharospasm, epiphora and corneal ulceration. Ectopic cilia can be difficult to visualise but careful evaluation of the conjunctival surface, often in the centre of the upper lid, will typically reveal a single location with one or more cilia protruding through the conjunctiva. As opposed to distichia, which do not always cause clinical disease, ectopic cilia should be strongly suspected as the cause of irritation and surgically removed as soon as possible.

Surgical destruction of ectopic cilia can be accomplished by surgical removal of a block of conjunctiva and stroma surrounding the cilia. If cryosurgery is available, the tissue remaining at the site of excision can be frozen to destroy any residual follicles.

Trichiasis

The presence of misdirected hairs from normal hair follicles is termed trichiasis and commonly occurs in brachycephalic breeds and older English Cocker Spaniels as previously described. The brachycephalic breeds may have prominent nasal skin folds that irritate the cornea or nasal

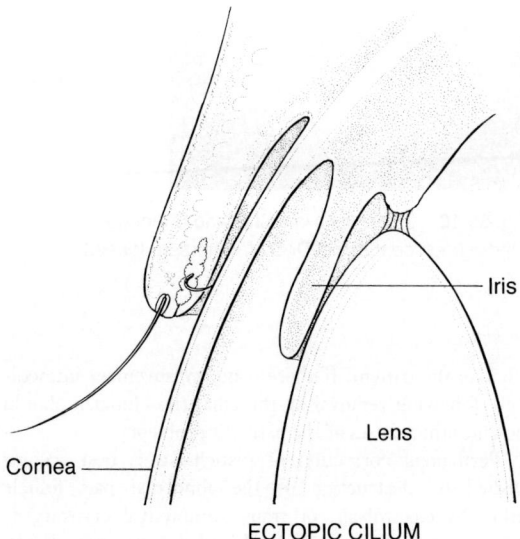

Fig. 99.11 Diagram of a cross section of an eyelid showing position of ectopic cilia.

canthal trichiasis where long hairs sweep horizontally across the cornea from the nasal canthus. Breeds such as the Pekingese are at risk of developing corneal damage from nasal fold trichiasis and in such cases the offending skin folds should be surgically removed. When medial canthal trichiasis (e.g. in breeds such as the Lhasa Apso or Shih Tzu) causes keratitis, excision or cryosurgical destruction of the nasal caruncular tissue may be indicated.

EYELID DERMATOSES

Numerous types of inflammatory and neoplastic eyelid disorders occur in the dog. Identification of the aetiology of canine blepharitis can be challenging since many of the disorders present similarly with erythematous and alopecic lesions. Table 99.2 lists the differential diagnoses of eyelid dermatoses and indicates appropriate investigative techniques.

HORDEOLUM AND CHALAZION

Much confusion exists surrounding the terms hordeolum and chalazion with the veterinary literature often contradicting itself with definitions. Hordeolum simply represents an inflammatory papule or pustule of the eyelid, often associated with staphylococcal infection (Yanoff & Fine 1989). An external hordeolum (stye) involves the hair follicle and associated glands; an internal hordeolum is inflammation of the meibomian glands. A hard and painless nodule of the eyelid resulting from chronic glandular inflammation is termed a chalazion. Whereas a hordeolum may be managed medically, chalazia require surgical intervention with curettage or excision.

EYELID NEOPLASIA (FIG. 99.12)

Tumours of the eyelids are quite common. Table 99.3 lists the most commonly reported eyelid tumours and their frequency in two studies. About 73–88% of these tumours are benign, but they may cause ocular disease or cosmetic concerns (Krehbiel & Langham 1975; Roberts *et al.* 1986). The size, shape, and location of the mass determines whether clinical signs occur; some masses appear to be solely cosmetic, whereas, others cause ocular discharge, ble-

Table 99.2 Eyelid dermatoses.

Type of disorder	Aetiologies	Diagnostic aids
Infectious blepharitis		
Bacterial	*Staphylococcus* spp. *Streptococcus* spp.	Bacterial cultures
Viral	Canine distemper virus	Systemic disease (respiratory, gastrointestinal, neurological) Cytology Fluorescent antibody test
Mycotic	*Microsporum* spp. *Trichophyton* spp.	Fungal culture KOH preparation Fluorescence
Parasitic	*Demodex canis* *Sarcoptes scabei*	Skin scraping
Immune-mediated		
Atopy	Systemic allergens	Concurrent atopy signs (chewing at paws/axillary) Skin testing
Auto-immune skin diseases	Pemphigus Bullous pemphigoid Systemic lupus erythematosus Discoid lupus erythematosus	Skin biopsy

Oculodermatological
     disease
	Vogt–Koyanagi–
	     Harada syndrome
		Associated panuveitis
		Skin biopsy

Miscellaneous disorders		
Keratoconjunctivitis sicca	Breed predilection Thyroid disease Sulpha drugs	Schirmer tear test Peri-ocular crusts/mucus
Meibomianitis	*Staphylococcus* spp. Immune-mediated	Bacterial culture Dramatic response to corticosteroids

Table 99.3 Classification of eyelid tumours.

Tumour type	Krehbiel & Langham 1975 % ($n = 202$)	Roberts *et al.* 1986 % ($n = 200$)
Sebaceous adenoma	28.7	60.0
Squamous papilloma	17.3	10.6
Sebaceous adenocarcinoma	15.3	2.0
Benign melanoma	12.9	17.6
Malignant melanoma	7.9	2.8
Histiocytoma	3.5	1.6
Mastocytoma	2.5	1.0
Basal cell carcinoma	2.5	1.2
Squamous cell carcinoma	2.0	1.0
Fibroma	2.1	
Fibropapilloma	1.0	
Lipoma	1.0	
Miscellaneous	3.5	2.2

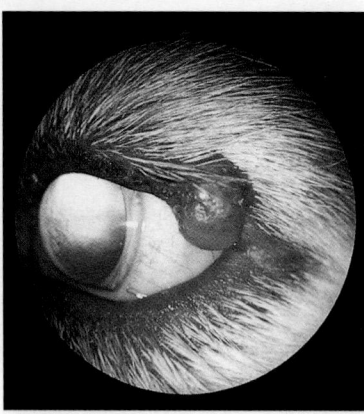

Fig. 99.12 Tumour involving the eyelid of a dog. This particular tumour was a histiocytoma.

pharospasm, conjunctival hyperaemia and corneal ulceration. Certain masses have an erosive surface and will intermittently bleed creating client anxiety for household furniture staining!

Criteria for removal of an eyelid tumour are:

- causing ocular disease or irritation;
- resulting in functional eyelid abnormalities – e.g. unable to properly close leading to an exposure keratitis;
- tumour has an erosive surface;
- consider the dog's general health – age, systemic disease, presence of other tumours?, etc.

Removal of eyelid tumours often requires full thickness wedge resection of the eyelid tissue since many masses arise from internal eyelid structures such as glandular tissue. Simple removal at the skin or eyelid margin level generally results in re-growth of the tumour within a short period of time. Full thickness resection can be V-shaped or shaped like a 'house'. After resection, the subcutaneous tissue is closed with absorbable suture and the eyelid margin is perfectly aligned with a figure of eight suture pattern. The surgeon then closes the remainder of the skin incision with simple interrupted sutures. Tumours involving up to 30% of the eyelid margin length are candidates for the simple wedge resection, but more extensive masses may require sliding skin grafts.

CONDITIONS OF THE THIRD EYELID

The third eyelid is essential for protection of the cornea, production of a portion of the aqueous tear film, and distribution of the tear film. Any disorder of structure or function can have significant consequences such as exposure keratitis, keratoconjunctivitis sicca and corneal ulceration.

Protrusion of the Third Eyelid

Protrusion of the third eyelid is a common finding with a number of possible causes (Table 99.4). Third eyelids with a lack of pigment show up well against the background of the iris and many owners wrongly think that they are abnormally prominent, particularly if the border of other third eyelid is pigmented.

Table 99.4 Causes of protrusion of the third eyelid.

Pain	Painful ocular lesions cause retraction of the globe and protrusion of the third eyelid
Abnormalities of the globe	Microphthalmos
	Phthisis bulbi
Orbital disease	Orbital space-occupying lesions (including neoplasia of the third eyelid)
	Orbital fibrosis
	Loss of orbital fat
Conjunctival adhesions	Severe conjunctival inflammation may cause adhesions between in contact conjunctival surfaces
Systemic disease	Tetanus
	Dehydration
	Cachexia

Scrolled Cartilage (Fig. 99.13)

Certain breeds including the German Shepherd, Irish Setter, Newfoundland, Weimaraner, Saint Bernard, Great Dane and German Shorthaired Pointer can develop a scrolled third eyelid cartilage as puppies or young adults. Usually the problem is primarily cosmetic. Surgical repair of scrolled cartilage is aimed at removing the abnormal portion of cartilage. Although in some cases this does not result in a satisfactory result.

Prolapsed Gland of the Third Eyelid
(Fig. 99.14)

This condition is commonly referred to as 'cherry eye' and is common in the American Cocker Spaniel, Lhasa Apso, Shar Pei, Beagle and Bulldog. In this disorder the gland dis-

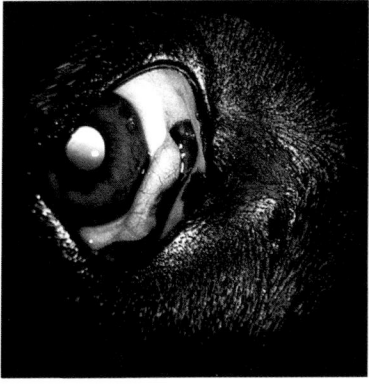

Fig. 99.13 Scrolling of the third eyelid. (Photograph courtesy of Dr S.M. Petersen-Jones.)

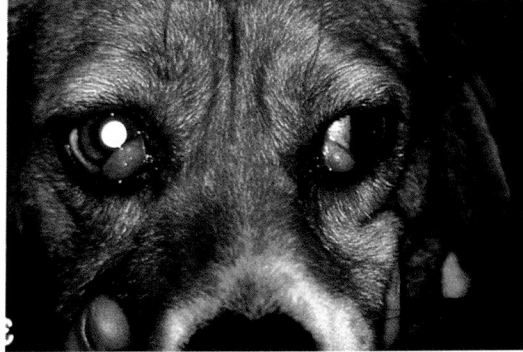

Fig. 99.14 Bilateral prolaspe of the nictitans glands.

locates from its normal position to protrude from the bulbar side of the third eyelid to appear as a pink smooth surfaced mass at the medial canthus. Often the gland becomes hyperaemic and some patients will scratch at the eye. The gland should be surgically replaced since excision predisposes to keratoconjunctivitis sicca.

Three basic methods of gland replacement include: replacement of the gland into a pocket created in the third eyelid, attachment of the gland to the ventromedial sclera (taking care not to penetrate the globe), and attachment of the gland to the periosteum of the orbit (Morgan *et al.* 1993; Stanley & Kaswan 1994). Each technique has potential for complications or failure.

Follicular Conjunctivitis

Enlargement of the follicles on the bulbar surface of the third eyelid is quite common in young dogs, especially Labrador Retrievers. Although infectious causes have been investigated, this disorder probably represents an irritant or allergic type of conjunctivitis. Clinical signs include epiphora and conjunctival hyperaemia. This may be part of a more generalised follicular conjunctivitis, as discussed on page 984.

Plasmoma (Plasma Cell Infiltration of the Third Eyelid) (see Fig. 100.20)

This condition is related to chronic superficial keratitis (pannus) which may or may not also be present. It results in third eyelid depigmentation, thickening and the development of an irregular contour to the free border. Plasmoma is seen most frequently in German Shepherds, Dachshunds and Greyhounds.

Treatment is similar to the management of chronic superficial keratitis, consisting of topical corticosteroids or cyclosporin ointment. The patient should be treated until signs resolve and then the therapy can be gradually reduced to the least possible frequency required to maintain the normal appearance of the third eyelid.

Neoplasia of the Third Eyelid

A number of different tumours may affect the third eyelid. These include those involving the conjunctival surface (such as papillomas, haemangiomas, squamous cell carcinomas etc.) and those of deeper structures such as the tear secreting gland (adenomas and adenocarcinomas).

REFERENCES

Bedford, P.G.C. (1988). Conditions of the eyelids in the dog. *Journal of Small Animal Practice*, **29**, 416–428.

Chambers, E.D. & Slatter, D.H. (1984). Cryotherapy (N_2O) of canine distichiasis and trichiasis: an experimental and clinical report. *Journal of Small Animal Practice*, **25**, 647–659.

Gelatt, K.N. (1991). The canine eyelids. In: *Veterinary Ophthalmology*, (ed. K.N. Gelatt), 2nd edn. pp. 256–275. Lea & Febiger, Philadelphia.

Helper, L.C., Magrane, W.G., Koehm, J. & Johnson, R. (1974). Surgical induction of keratoconjunctivitis sicca in the dog. *Journal of the American Veterinary Medical Association*, **165**, 172–174.

Krehbiel, J.D. & Langham, R.F. (1975). Eyelid neoplasms of dogs. *American Journal of Veterinary Research*, **36**, 115–119.

Miller, W.W. & Albert, R.A. (1988). Canine entropion. *Compendium of Continuing Education for the Practicing Veterinarian*, **10**, 431–438.

Morgan, R.V., Duddy, J.M. & McClurg, K. (1993). Prolapse of the gland of the third eyelid in dogs: a retrospective study of 89 cases (1980–1990). *Journal of the American Animal Hospital Association*. **29**, 56–60.

Munger, R.J. & Carter, J.D. (1984). A further modification of the Kuhnt–Szymanowski procedure for correction of atonic ectropion in dogs. *Journal of the American Animal Hospital Association*, **20**, 651–656.

Roberts, S.M., Severin, G.A. & Lavach, J.D. (1986). Prevalence and treatment of palpebral neoplasms in the dog: 200 cases (1975–1983). *Journal of the American Veterinary Medical Association*, **189**, 1355–1359.

Stades, F.C. (1987). A new method for surgical correction of upper eyelid trichiasis-entropion: Operation method. *Journal of the American Animal Hospital Association*, **23**, 603–610.

Stanley, R.G. & Kaswan, R.L. (1994). Modification of the orbital rim anchorage method for surgical replacement of the gland of the third eyelid in dogs. *Journal of the American Veterinary Medical Association*, **205**, 1412–1414.

Wheeler, C.A. & Severin, G.A. (1984). Cryosurgical epilation for the treatment of distichiasis in the dog and cat. *Journal of the American Animal Hospital Association*, **20**, 877–884.

Yanoff, M. & Fine, B.S. (1989). Skin and lacrimal drainage system. In: *Ocular Pathology. A Text and Atlas*, (eds M. Yanoff & B.S. Fine), 3rd edn. pp. 172–174. J.B. Lippincott, Philadelphia.

Chapter 100

Conditions of the Ocular Surface

P. Renwick

THE TEAR FILM

The tear film covers the cornea and conjunctiva and is vital for the healthy function of the ocular surface. It is a trilaminar structure comprising a superficial lipid layer, a middle aqueous layer, and an inner mucus layer (Fig. 100.1). The sites of production and the functions of each layer are shown in Table 100.1.

Tear Film Abnormalities

Lipid Layer Insufficiency

Lipid insufficiency is rarely diagnosed, but may result from damage to the eyelid margins, for example due to trauma, blepharitis or iatrogenic injury. It may result in loss of aqueous tears by evaporation and epiphora (overflow) (Fig. 100.2). Treatment comprises attention to the underlying cause (see Chapter 99) and the use of lipid substitutes (e.g. Lacri-Lube™) applied several times daily.

Mucus Layer Abnormality

A reduction in goblet cell numbers can occur as a result of chronic conjunctivitis or in association with keratoconjunctivitis sicca. A reduction in the population of goblet cells may also occur as a rarely identified separate entity, leading to conjunctival and corneal changes not dissimilar to those of keratoconjunctivitis sicca, but with a normal tear production and an absence of discharge (Moore 1990). Treatment comprises the frequent application of mucus substitutes (e.g. hypromellose or dextran) and the use of topical cyclosporin twice daily if an immune-mediated component is suspected.

Aqueous Insufficiency (Keratoconjunctivitis Sicca)

Keratoconjunctivitis sicca or 'dry eye' is a common cause of ocular surface inflammatory disease in dogs. It should be suspected in any dog presenting with signs of conjunctivitis or keratitis without obvious tear overflow. Early recognition and treatment of the disease helps to avoid its potentially blinding sequelae.

Clinical Signs

Keratoconjunctivitis sicca is generally an insidious condition although occasionally it may be of acute onset (especially in neurogenic cases and those associated with drug toxicity or canine distemper virus). The signs listed may initially be subtle, but usually advance with time:

- conjunctivitis – thickening of the conjunctiva may develop with chronicity;
- ocular discharge – usually tenacious and mucopurulent (Fig. 100.3);
- uneven corneal surface – leading to a lack-lustre appearance and an irregular corneal reflection;
- corneal vascularisation/pigmentation – often commencing dorsally;
- corneal thickening (Fig. 100.4);
- ulceration – ulcers are often small and rapidly deepening, especially in acute cases (Fig. 100.5);
- pain – more often in acute cases, less apparent in chronic disease;
- dry ipsilateral nostril in some cases.

Aetiology

The causes of keratoconjunctivitis sicca include:

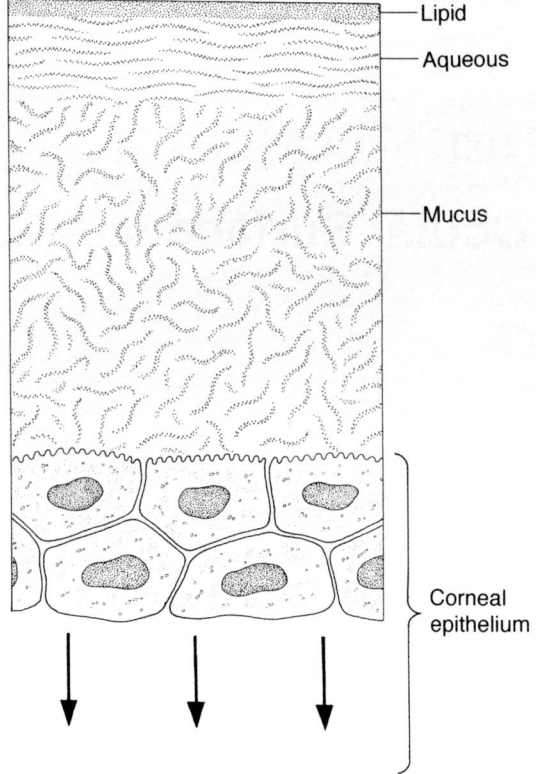

Fig. 100.1 The tear film (diagrammatic). The current understanding of the tear film is that long chains of mucins extends across what was previously thought to be predominantly the aqueous portion of the tear film.

Lipid

Aqueous

Mucus

Corneal epithelium

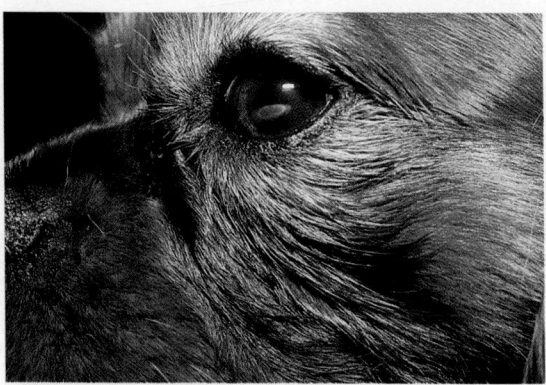

Fig. 100.2 A Cavalier King Charles Spaniel with marked epiphora due to lipid insufficiency. Meibomian gland tissue had been destroyed by juvenile cellulitis at 3 months of age.

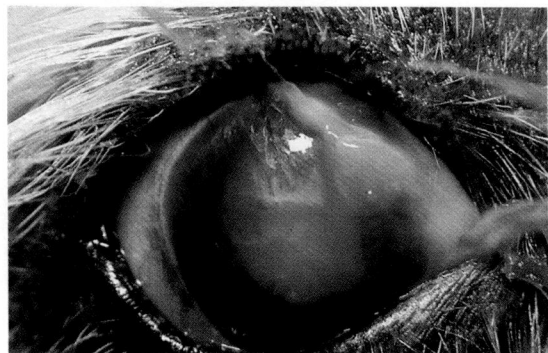

Fig. 100.3 Keratoconjunctivitis sicca causing tenacious mucopurulent discharge in a West Highland White Terrier. A cataract is also present.

Table 100.1 The tear film.

Layer	Source	Function
Mucus	Conjunctival goblet cells	Adhesion of aqueous phase to the hydrophobic corneal epithelium Lubrication
Aqueous	Lacrimal gland Nictitans gland (Accessory glands – minor) contribution	Lubrication Supply of O_2/nutrients and removal of debris/waste products Medium for transport of inflammatory cells/antibodies Create a smooth optical surface
Lipid	Meibomian glands (Accessory glands – minor contribution)	Reduce evaporation of aqueous tears Prevent spillage of tears over lid margin due to surface tension effect

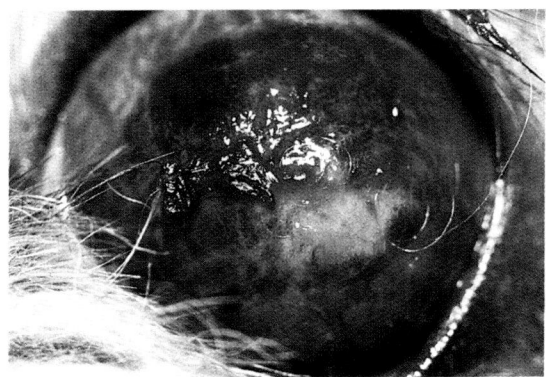

Fig. 100.4 Marked corneal pigmentation, thickening and surface irregularity in a West Highland White Terrier with advanced keratoconjunctivitis sicca.

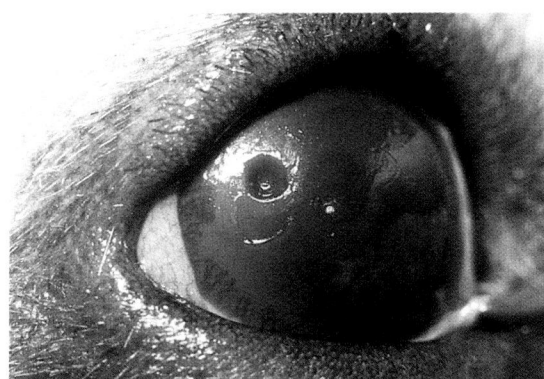

Fig. 100.5 Deep corneal ulceration associated with keratoconjunctivitis sicca in a Cavalier King Charles Spaniel. A marked vascular response and corneal oedema are present.

- congenital – uncommon;
- drug-induced, e.g. sulpha drugs – sulphasalazine/sulphadiazine and phenazopyridine (a urinary analgesic);
- canine distemper virus;
- neurogenic – damage to the parasympathetic supply to the lacrimal and third eyelid glands, e.g. following facial trauma;
- immune-mediated dacryoadenitis – the commonest cause in dogs;
- 'idiopathic' – probably immune-mediated in most cases.

Of those causes listed, immune-mediated disease is the most commonly encountered in dogs. Progressive destruc-

tion of the lacrimal and nictitans glands occurs due to immune-mediated dacryoadenitis (Kaswan & Salisbury 1990). Breeds commonly affected include the West Highland White Terrier, English and American Cocker Spaniels, English Bulldog, Shih Tzu and Lhasa Apso. Affected animals are typically middle-aged and although these cases are essentially bilateral, they may initially present with clinical disease in one eye.

Diagnosis

Diagnosis is based upon signalment, history, clinical signs and the Schirmer tear test readings (Box 100.1).

Box 100.1 Schirmer tear test (Fig. 100.6).

- Perform before the application of any drops or topical anaesthetic.
- Bend the test strip at the notch near its end and place in the ventral conjunctival sac.
- Leave in position for 1 min with the eyelids held closed if necessary.
- Normal results range from 10–25 mm/min.
- <10 mm/min is suspicious of keratoconjunctivitis sicca.
- <5 mm/min is diagnostic of keratoconjunctivitis sicca.

Treatment

The management of keratoconjunctivitis sicca is summarised in Table 100.2. The primary aim is to restore the continual production of normal endogenous tears, as these are far superior to tear substitutes, however frequently instilled. The recent introduction of cyclosporin therapy has greatly improved the prognosis for most canine patients with keratoconjunctivitis sicca. Cyclosporin has a lacrimogenic effect and also acts to reduce immune-mediated dacryoadenitis, the fundamental lesion in the majority of affected dogs. Despite the presence of secondary bacterial conjunctivitis in many cases of keratoconjunctivitis sicca, it is rarely necessary to treat this specifically; correction of the primary problem will usually rectify the opportunist bacterial infection.

Cases with advanced disease may fail to respond to medical management, and under these circumstances a parotid duct transposition is indicated (see Wyman 1979 for a description of the technique). Complications of the technique include salivary epiphora, crystalline deposition on the cornea and eyelids, and failure of the procedure due to iatrogenic parotid duct damage.

Table 100.2   Management of keratoconjunctivitis sicca.

Aim	Method
Remove cause if possible	E.g. stop sulphonamide therapy
Nursing care	Cleaning with sterile saline/water
Aqueous phase replacement	Artificial tears, e.g. hypromellose, polyvinyl alcohol, applied topically every 1–6 h
	Stimulate endogenous production:
	• topical cyclosporin twice daily
	• oral 1% pilocarpine drops (1–4 drops twice to three times daily on food)
	Parotid duct transposition (if medical management fails)
Immunosuppression (control of dacryoadenitis)	Cyclosporin topically twice daily
	Corticosteroids topically as indicated
Control of corneal pigmentation and vascularisation	Cyclosporin topically twice daily
	Corticosteroids topically (only if there is no corneal ulceration)
Treat ulceration	Therapy depends upon nature and depth of ulcer (see later section)

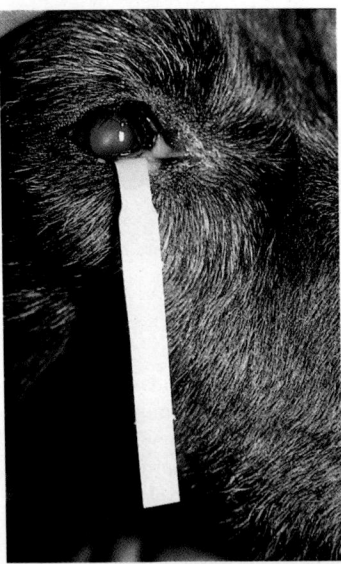

Fig. 100.6   The Schirmer tear test strip in position.

Keratoconjunctivitis sicca is generally a lifelong condition which is essentially bilateral in most cases. Monitoring over a period of months or years and considerable client education are required.

Tear Drainage

Tear drainage occurs from the tear lake within the ventral conjunctival sac. If tear drainage is inadequate or tear pro-duction is excessive (e.g. in response to painful stimuli) then epiphora (tear overflow) will result.

The nasolacrimal system in dogs (Fig. 100.7) comprises:

- two lacrimal puncta – upper and lower,
- two canaliculi – upper and lower,
- nasolacrimal sac,
- nasolacrimal duct,
- nasal ostium.

Accessory openings of the nasolacrimal duct may occur within the nasal cavity – especially in brachycephalic dogs. The nasal ostium lies several millimetres caudal to the opening of the external nares at the junction of the lateral wall and floor of the nostril.

Investigation of the Drainage System

All cases in which nasolacrimal duct disease is suspected warrant further investigation (see Habin 1993 for a review of the subject). The first test to perform in order to assess tear duct function is the fluorescein drainage test (Box 100.2).

Further investigation of the system may include:

- Nasolacrimal duct irrigation using a 23–30 G blunt-ended cannula placed in the upper punctum – the lower punctum may be temporarily occluded to facilitate flushing;
- Nasolacrimal duct cannulation using 2/0 or 3/0 monofilament nylon;
- Contrast radiography – contrast agent is injected into the nasolacrimal duct.

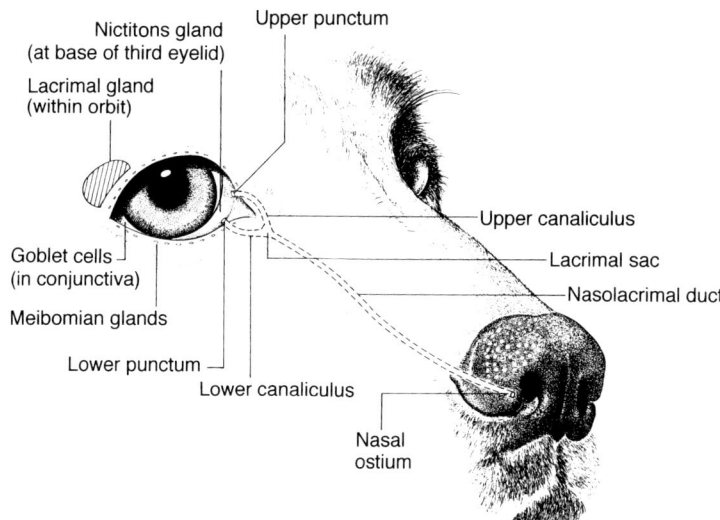

Fig. 100.7 The major structures associated with tear production and drainage.

- Used to give an indication of functional duct patency.
- Fluorescein is placed in the conjunctival sac.
- Stain normally takes less than 5 min to appear at the nostrils.
- Detection is enhanced with cobalt blue or UV light.
- A negative result does not confirm obstruction of the nasolacrimal duct, it is merely consistent with it – if a negative result is obtained, further investigation is required.

Conditions of the Drainage System

Congenital Anomalies

These generally involve absence or reduced development of one or more portions of the system:

- Imperforate lower punctum is the most frequently recognised problem.
- Micropunctum is a less extreme variant of the condition.

English and American Cocker Spaniels and the Golden Retriever are most commonly affected. The presenting sign is early onset epiphora without other ocular signs. Diagnosis is confirmed by irrigation of the duct. Treatment involves the surgical creation or enlargement of the punctum (Barnett 1979).

Dacryocystitis

Dacryocystitis is inflammation of the lacrimal sac or naso-lacrimal duct. It may be acute or chronic and may be a sequel to, or an inciting cause of conjunctivitis. It may be associated with foreign bodies, e.g. awned grass seeds (Figs 100.8 & 100.9). The accumulation of inflammatory debris and swelling of the mucosa may occlude the lumen of the duct.

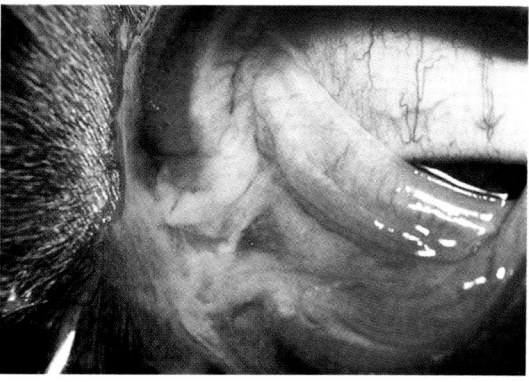

Fig. 100.8 Mucopurulent discharge from the nasolacrimal duct in an English Springer Spaniel. The discharge is mixed with normal tears and was the result of dacryocystitis caused by a grass seed lodged within the nasolacrimal duct.

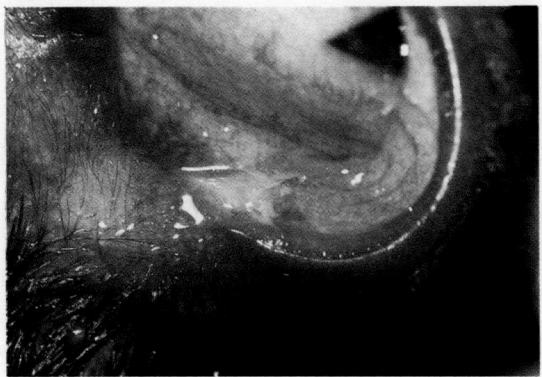

Fig. 100.9 The grass seed irrigated from the nasolacrimal duct of the dog in Fig. 100.8.

Miscellaneous Conditions of the Nasolacrimal Drainage System

In addition to dacryocystitis, acquired obstruction of the drainage system may occur due to trauma, dental disease, rhinitis, cyst formation and neoplasia.

Epiphora

Epiphora is overflow of tears. It is a common problem in some breeds, e.g. Toy Poodle and Bichon Frisé, and leads to discoloration of the hair ventral to the medial canthus (tear staining) (Box 100.3). In the toy breeds it is caused by anatomical features resulting in insufficient tear drainage with tears running on to the face at blinking.

Clinical Signs

- Epiphora
- Associated mucoid or mucopurulent conjunctivitis
- Mucopurulent material at the medial canthus – may be mixed with normal tears
- Ability to express mucopurulent material from lacrimal puncta with digital pressure
- Swelling/abscess formation in the lacrimal sac – this may rupture leading to fistula formation (differential diagnoses include malar abscess)
- Pain at the medial canthus
- Chronic cases may present as recurrent conjunctivitis, partially responsive to antimicrobials

Investigation

- Nasolacrimal duct irrigation – samples may be obtained for Gram stain, culture/sensitivity and cytology
- Radiography – obstruction/areas of bone destruction may be seen

Treatment

- Topical and systemic antibacterial therapy (broad-spectrum or based on sensitivity test results)
- Judicious use of steroids to reduce swelling/scarring
- Irrigation of the duct to dislodge foreign bodies/debris – awned grass seeds may be best dislodged by flushing from the nasal ostium (only feasible in larger dolicho-cephalic breeds)
- Catheterisation in severe cases – fine polyethylene tube is left in-situ for 2–3 weeks
- An abscess may require lancing and/or frequent irrigation

Box 100.3 Causes of epiphora.

(1) Decreased drainage of tears:
- Nasolacrimal duct dysfunction (see above)
  - congenital obstruction, e.g. duct atresia, imperforate punctum
  - acquired disease, e.g. dacryocystitis, neoplasia
- Decreased access of tears to the lower punctum
  - poor lid–globe apposition in ectropion, diamond eye and phthisis bulbi
  - shallow tear lake – the lower lid is tightly apposed to globe
  - medial lower lid entropion – not uncommon – correct surgically
- Hair from the medial canthus contacts the globe and acts as a wick

(2) Increased tear production overwhelming normal drainage capacity:
- Trichiasis (e.g. from nasal folds), distichiasis, ectopic cilia
- Conjunctival foreign body
- Conjunctivitis (allergic, irritant-induced)
- Blepharitis or other lid problems, e.g. scarring, coloboma, neoplasia, entropion
- Corneal ulceration, dermoid, foreign body, keratitis
- Episcleritis, scleritis
- Uveitis, panophthalmitis
- Glaucoma
- Retrobulbar cellulitis, abscess

CONJUNCTIVA

The conjunctiva is a thin mucous membrane which covers the posterior surfaces of the upper and lower eyelids (palpebral conjunctiva), both surfaces of the third eyelid and the anterior surface of the sclera and episclera (bulbar conjunctiva). In conjunction with the tear film it acts to protect the globe from insult. It is highly vascular and immunosensitive.

Conjunctivitis

The conjunctiva is susceptible to inflammation, and this may be of an acute or chronic nature. In acute cases hyperaemia and oedema (chemosis, Fig. 100.10) may occur along with signs of discomfort and a variable degree of discharge which may be serous, mucoid or mucopurulent.

The aetiology of conjunctivitis includes:

- irritants – dust, wind, chemicals,
- allergy,
- foreign bodies – e.g. awned grass seeds,
- mechanical irritation due to adnexal disease – e.g. entropion, ectopic cilia,
- extension of inflammation from adjacent structures
  - eyelids,
  - nasolacrimal duct,
  - episclera,
- infection
  - viral – canine distemper virus,
  - bacterial – commonly *Staphylococcus* spp. and *Streptococcus* spp. (Fig. 100.11),

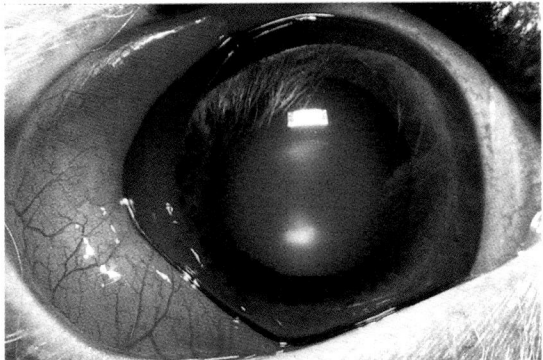

Fig. 100.10 Chemosis in an Old English Sheepdog with concurrent vomiting and diarrhoea. The signs resolved, but the cause remained undetermined.

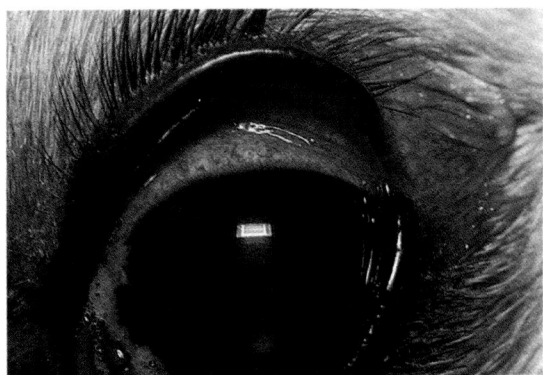

Fig. 100.11 Bacterial conjunctivitis in a crossbred dog. The signs resolved with topical antimicrobial therapy.

- keratoconjunctivitis sicca,
- immune-mediated – e.g. plasma cell infiltration of the third eyelid (part of the chronic superficial keratoconjunctivitis complex of German Shepherd Dogs) see page 975.

It is of utmost importance that conjunctivitis be differentiated from other conditions which can result in reddening of the ocular coats (see Box 100.4 for differential diagnoses).

Treatment

The treatment of conjunctivitis depends upon its aetiology. An underlying cause should always be sought before

Box 100.4 Conditions causing redness of the ocular coats.

- Conjunctivitis
- Subconjunctival haemorrhage – Fig. 100.12 (trauma, bleeding diathesis)
- Horner's syndrome – may cause conjunctival vascular engorgement
- Keratitis, e.g. keratoconjunctivitis sicca (dry eye), chronic superficial keratoconjunctivitis in the German Shepherd Dog
- Episcleritis
- Scleritis (uncommon)
- Uveitis
- Glaucoma
- Retrobulbar disease (abscess, cellulitis, neoplasia)

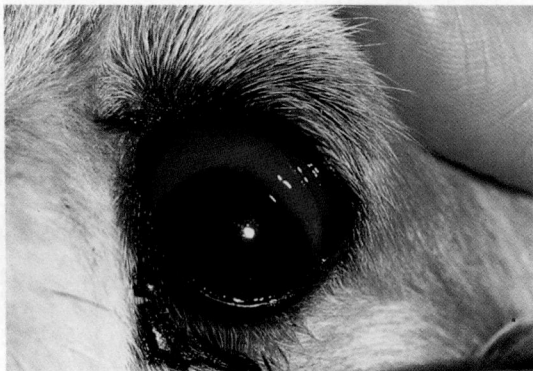

Fig. 100.12 Subconjunctival haemorrhage in a Chihuahua after a road traffic accident.

Table 100.3 Antibacterials for ocular surface infections.

Spectrum of activity	Agent
Broad-spectrum	Chloramphenicol (Neomycin) (Framycetin)
Staphylococcus spp.	Fusidic acid
Pseudomonas aeruginosa	Tobramycin Ciprofloxacin (Gentamicin)

labelling conjunctivitis as a primary bacterial problem. Where conjunctivitis is secondary to a primary problem, such as mechanical irritation, this should be dealt with accordingly. Primary (and sometimes secondary) bacterial conjunctivitis requires topical antimicrobial therapy. The agents most commonly used are listed in Table 100.3. Where necessary therapy should be adjusted according to the result of bacteriological culture and antibiotic sensitivity testing. The use of corticosteroids and systemic antimicrobial agents is rarely indicated in bacterial conjunctivitis cases. The treatment of chronic superficial keratoconjunctivitis and keratoconjunctivitis sicca are dealt with on pages 977 and 989 respectively.

Follicular Conjunctivitis

Follicular conjunctivitis describes the development of multiple, raised pink lymphoid follicles across the conjunctival surface (Box 100.5). This is a non-specific response to conjunctival insult and occurs most commonly in young dogs.

Box 100.5 Follicular conjunctivitis.

Features:
- Multiple, raised pink lymphoid follicles across the conjunctival surface
- Commoner in young dogs
- Non-specific response to conjunctival insult
- Presence of follicles may cause mild irritation

Treatment:
- Initially topical corticosteroids
- If does not resolve mechanical debridement may be required – gently scrape follicles with a No. 15 blade

Conjunctival Neoplasia

Neoplasia of the conjunctiva is infrequently encountered in dogs, but conditions such as adenoma, fibroma, fibrosarcoma, haemangioma, haemangiosarcoma, mastocytoma and lymphosarcoma may all occur.

CORNEA

Congenital Disorders

Corneal Dermoid

Corneal dermoids are the commonest congenital problem encountered. They comprise superficial masses (choristomas) which are usually located at the lateral limbus, contain elements of skin and are often hairy (Fig. 100.13). They may extend to involve the conjunctiva and, occasion-

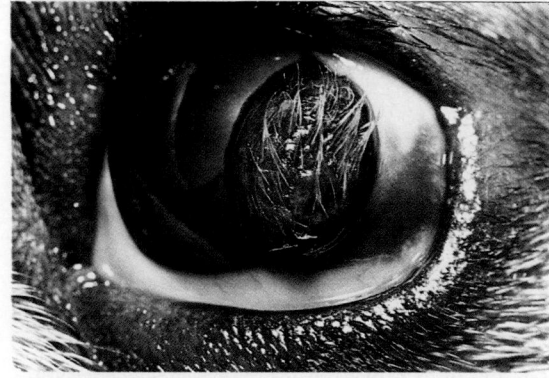

Fig. 100.13 Corneal dermoid in the left eye of a 6-week-old Bulldog.

ally, the eyelids. Surgical removal is required in the form of a superficial keratectomy.

Microcornea

Microcornea is seen most commonly in association with microphthalmos, although occasionally it may occur in an otherwise normally sized eye.

Corneal Opacities

Corneal opacity of a mild, diffuse, temporary nature is seen in normal puppies up to a few weeks of age. Permanent focal opacities may be seen as a result of persistent pupillary membranes contacting the corneal endothelium. No treatment is required.

Corneal Injuries

Chemical Injury

Chemical injury may be caused by acid or alkali burns. Acid burns tend to be self-limiting whereas alkali can penetrate straight through the cornea and continue to cause damage for several hours after the initial insult. Immediate treatment in either case comprises lavage with copious volumes of fluid. Subsequent therapy depends upon the extent of the injury, but usually involves intensive treatment as for a deep, melting corneal ulcer (see page 987).

Mechanical Injury

Mechanical injury may vary in extent from superficial abrasion to severe full-thickness laceration. A careful assessment of the intraocular structures is mandatory to detect associated injuries, for example to the iris or lens, and also the presence of any foreign material either in the cornea or within the eye (Fig. 100.14). Blunt trauma may be associated with damage to deeper structures such as the ciliary body or retina, resulting in intraocular haemorrhage. Radiography is indicated if the animal may have been shot. Treatment is outlined in Box 100.6.

Inflammatory Corneal Conditions (Keratitis)

Aetiology

Inflammation of the cornea is commonly encountered in dogs and has numerous causes including:

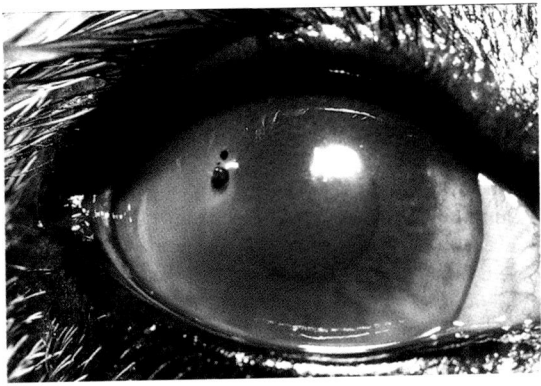

Fig. 100.14 A thorn corneal foreign body in a dog. The signs present included blepharospasm, epiphora, corneal oedema and those of a moderate anterior uveitis.

Box 100.6 Treatment of corneal injuries.

Superficial injuries:
- Topical antimicrobial therapy
- Treat any associated uveitis (see Chapter 101).

Deep lacerations (see Crispin 1993 for surgical details)
- Careful suturing
- Reform the anterior chamber in the event of a full thickness injury
- Intensive therapy to control uveitis and prevent intraocular infection – use aqueous chloramphenicol drops if there is a risk of direct installation into the anterior chamber – avoid ointments and viscous drops initially

- trauma,
- adnexal disease causing mechanical insult,
- infection
  - superficial, e.g. bacterial, fungal,
  - systemic, e.g. canine viral hepatitis, leishmaniasis,
- abnormalities of the pre-ocular tear film, e.g. keratoconjunctivitis sicca,
- immune-mediated disease,
- extension of inflammation from associated structures, e.g. episclera, uveal tract,
- idiopathic – a proportion of these may be immune-mediated.

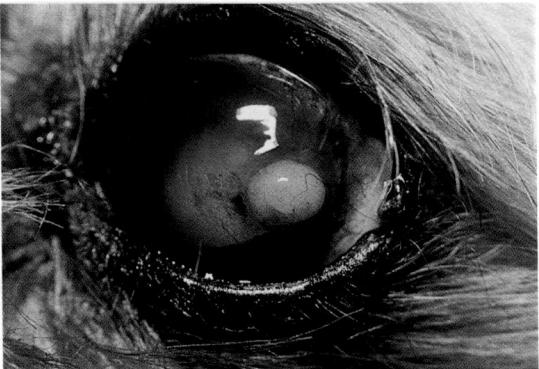

Fig. 100.21 An epithelial inclusion cyst in a Yorkshire Terrier. The lesion had developed as a sequel to a cat scratch a year previously.

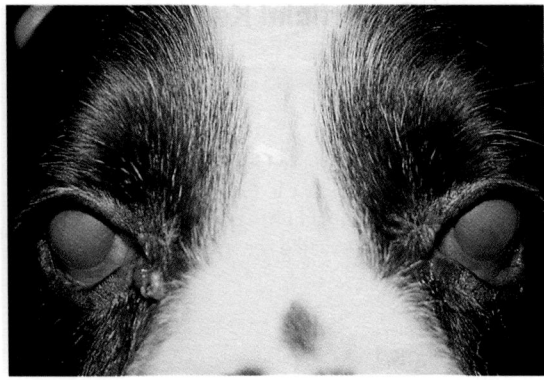

Fig. 100.22 A 9-year-old English Springer Spaniel with bilateral corneal oedema due to corneal endothelial dystrophy.

although heredity and the mode of inheritance is unproven in many instances of so-called corneal dystrophies in dogs (Cooley & Dice 1990).

Epithelial Basement Membrane Dystrophy (Recurrent Epithelial Erosion)

This condition was discussed earlier (see above).

Corneal Endothelial Dystrophy

Dysfunction of the corneal endothelium, for whatever reason, results in disturbance of the endothelial pump mechanism which is responsible for maintaining the cornea in a relatively dehydrated state. Failure of this mechanism results in the accumulation of fluid within the corneal stroma. Oedema in the cornea disrupts optical transparency and can result in the formation of fluid-filled bullae (bullous keratopathy). The bullae may rupture on the corneal surface, causing ulceration that can be very difficult to resolve.

Clinical Findings

Corneal endothelial dystrophy is a condition of middle-aged and older dogs which develop progressive corneal oedema and as a consequence visual impairment (Fig. 100.22). The condition is painless unless ulceration due to bullous keratopathy develops. Vascularisation can occur in advanced cases.

In the UK the breeds over-represented with the condition are:

- English Springer Spaniel,
- Boxer,
- Chihuahua,
- Boston Terrier.

Heredity in these breeds is, as yet, unproved. Findings similar to those of endothelial dystrophy can be seen in any elderly dog, indicative of a similar, non-hereditary, degenerative condition of the corneal endothelium in these cases.

Diagnosis

Diagnosis is based upon signalment and history and the finding of bilateral corneal oedema with no other apparent ocular disease. Corneal oedema can develop in a number of conditions and these must be differentiated from corneal endothelial dystrophy (Table 100.5).

Treatment

Treatment is generally unsuccessful. Topical hyperosmotic agents such as 5% sodium chloride ointment may be of some temporary benefit. Penetrating keratoplasty ('corneal grafting') is of limited value in dogs as the graft often becomes oedematous after surgery.

Corneal Stromal Lipid Dystrophy (Crystalline Stromal Dystrophy)

Clinical Findings

Lipid deposits, predominantly of cholesterol, occur in the anterior corneal stroma in a number of breeds of dog including the Cavalier King Charles Spaniel, Shetland Sheepdog, Rough Collie, Siberian Husky, Beagle, Afghan

Condition	Differentiating signs
Corneal endothelial dystrophy	Predisposed breeds (see text) Bilateral Diffuse, progressive oedema IOP normal Painless unless ulceration develops Little or no vascularisation
Corneal ulceration	Any breed Oedema concentrated around ulcer Painful Frequently vascularised
Corneal wounds/trauma	Evidence of injury
Persistent pupillary membranes	Membranes visible Focal, non-progressive opacity
Anterior lens luxation	Terrier breeds and Border collie Sub-central, non-progressive oedema Lens usually present in anterior chamber Iridodonesis (trembling, unsupported iris)
Anterior uveitis	Painful Often unilateral Episcleral congestion Miotic pupil Aqueous flare Keratic precipitates Low IOP Possible systemic illness
Glaucoma	Painful Often unilateral Elevated IOP Episcleral congestion Mid-dilated pupil Probable blindness
Keratitis/neovascularisation	Marked vascular reaction Often other ocular disease, e.g. • episcleritis • keratoconjunctivitis sicca • history of ulceration etc.
Drug toxicity	History of receiving corneal endothelial toxic drug • (e.g. tocainide, Gratzek *et al.* 1993)

Table 100.5 Differential diagnosis of corneal oedema and corneal endothelial dystrophy.

IOP, intra-ocular pressure

Hound, German Shepherd Dog and the Boxer. The condition presents as white crystalline opacities in the axial cornea, often as an oval or ring shape (Fig. 100.23). The overlying epithelium is intact. The deposits usually form by 4 years of age, are generally non-progressive and do not normally interfere with vision (Crispin 1993).

Diagnosis

Diagnosis is based upon the signalment and characteristic clinical appearance. Lipid deposition within the cornea can occur for other reasons (see below), but these cases are often unilateral and associated with corneal vascularisation or signs of other ocular disease.

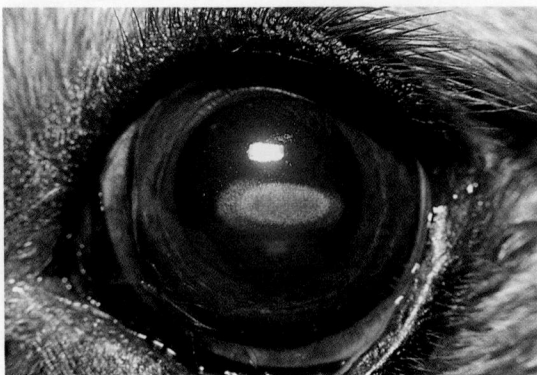

Fig. 100.23 Crystalline stromal dystrophy in an 18-month-old Cavalier King Charles Spaniel.

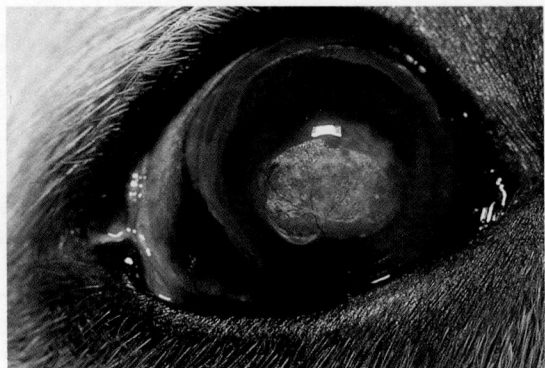

Fig. 100.24 Lipid keratopathy in a Labrador Retriever associated with previous anterior uveitis which had developed as a sequel to extracapsular cataract extraction.

Treatment

Treatment is rarely required. In severe or progressive cases, investigation of circulating lipid levels may be warranted.

Corneal Lipid Deposition

Lipid may be deposited in the cornea as a result of:

- crystalline stromal dystrophy (see above),
- previous corneal disease,
- systemic dyslipoproteinaemia.

Lipid Keratopathy

Lipid keratopathy involves both lipid deposition and vascularisation of one or both corneas (Crispin 1989). In most cases the lipid deposits are found predominantly in the anterior stroma. The vascularisation may precede or follow the deposition of lipid. The condition is not a specific entity, but rather the common end-point of a number of conditions. Not infrequently corneal lipid deposition results from previous ocular inflammation such as episcleritis (see below), keratitis or anterior uveitis (Fig. 100.24). Some cases exhibit concurrent plasma hyperlipoproteinaemia and investigation of the lipid profile and other biochemical parameters is indicated in those cases with marked corneal lipid deposition (see DeBowes 1987 for a review of canine hyperlipoproteinaemia).

Treatment

- Identify and treat any underlying cause of hyperlipoproteinaemia (Box 100.9).

Box 100.9 Causes of hyperlipoproteinaemia.

- Spontaneous (Miniature Schnauzer)
- Dietary
- Secondary (the commonest form in dogs)
  - hypothyroidism
  - hyperadrenocorticism
  - diabetes mellitus
  - nephrotic syndrome
  - pancreatitis (hyperlipoproteinaemia may also *cause* pancreatitis)
  - hepatic disease

- Control any associated ocular disease.
- Superficial keratectomy if the lesion is substantial or associated with corneal ulceration.

Corneal Calcium Deposition

Calcium deposition (sometimes accompanied by lipid) is occasionally seen in the canine cornea. It has been reported as a spontaneous problem in the Golden Retriever (Crispin & Barnett 1983), but may also be seen in association with systemic disorders such as hypercalcaemia, hypervitaminosis D and renal secondary hyperparathyroidism. In the clinical setting corneal calcification is most commonly encountered in elderly dogs (Fig. 100.25), and investigation of serum biochemical and haematological parameters is recommended in these cases.

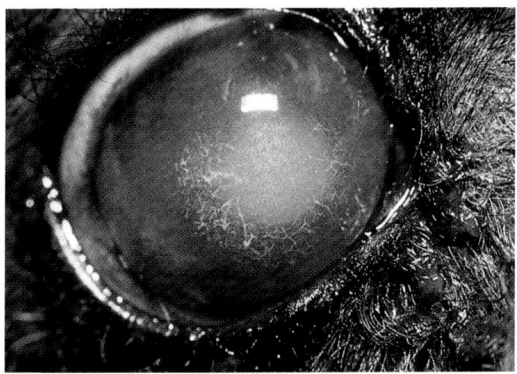

Fig. 100.25 Calcareous degeneration of the cornea in a 15-year-old Miniature Poodle with chronic renal failure.

SCLERA, EPISCLERA AND LIMBUS

Episcleral Inflammatory Disorders

Inflammation of the episclera is not infrequently encountered in dogs. The close anatomical relationship between episclera, overlying conjunctiva and underlying sclera results in a tendency for more than one layer to become involved in any inflammatory process. The nomenclature of the clinical types of episcleritis is rather confused.

Episcleritis

The commonest type encountered is either localised or diffuse. The lesions tend to be raised, erythematous and often have a yellowish tinge due to cellular infiltration (Fig. 100.26). A slightly nodular appearance may be seen. Secondary corneal involvement is common, comprising local corneal vascularisation and, not uncommonly, lipid deposition. Discomfort is generally mild. The cause of the condition is uncertain, but it may be immune-mediated.

Nodular Episcleritis

In this instance obvious nodules are present in the perilimbal episclera. This type of episcleritis is probably a variant of that described above.

Nodular Episclerokeratitis

Nodular episclerokeratitis is primarily seen in dogs in the United States and most commonly affects Collie Breeds (Paulsen *et al.* 1987). A fleshy mass or masses comprising granulomatous inflammatory tissue arise at the limbus and spread to involve the cornea. Occasionally the third eyelid and (rarely) the iris, may be involved. Control is much more difficult than in episcleritis and nodular episcleritis (see Table 100.6).

Table 100.6 Treatment of episcleral inflammatory conditions.

Type of inflammation	Therapy
Episcleritis	Topical steroids, e.g. prednisolone acetate 6 times daily initially Topical cyclosporin twice daily Systemic steroids in recalcitrant cases, e.g. prednisolone 1 mg/kg per day
Nodular episcleritis	As for episcleritis May require resection first
Nodular episclerokeratitis	Systemic immunosuppressants • azathioprine 2 mg/kg every other day • corticosteroids, e.g. prednisolone 2–4 mg/kg per day Cryotherapy Irradiation

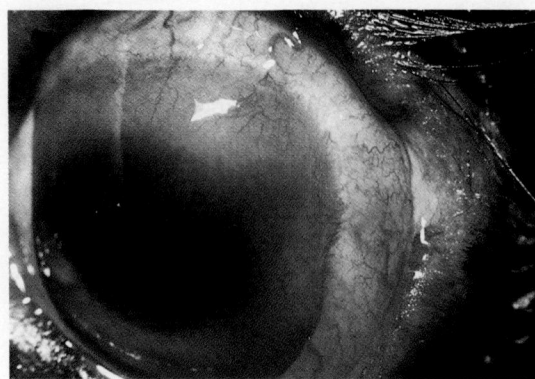

Fig. 100.26 Diffuse episcleritis in an English Springer Spaniel. Corneal involvement has developed in this case.

Scleritis

Primary scleritis is less common than episcleritis in dogs. It is usually a more painful and aggressive condition than episcleritis. The scleral vessels tend to assume a purple coloration and associated cellular infiltrates may impart a yellowish tinge to the lesion. There is a tendency for both anterior and posterior uveitis to develop in association with the disease.

Treatment

Control of scleritis can be difficult and therapy should be adjusted according to the severity and chronicity of the problem:

* topical steroid, e.g. prednisolone acetate – six times daily initially;
* systemic steroids, if necessary at immunosuppressive doses, e.g. prednisolone or methylprednisolone – 2–4 mg/kg per day;
* other systemic immunosuppressive agents, e.g. azathioprine – 2 mg/kg every other day.

Limbus

Limbal Keratomalacia

This is a rare condition in the dog involving destruction of the limbal cornea by a collagenolytic process. Toxins, *Pseudomonas aeruginosa* and possibly an immune-mediated component may be involved in its pathogenesis.

Limbal Neoplasia

Various neoplasms, such as haemangiomas, haemangiosarcomas and fibrosarcomas have been reported to affect the limbal region. However, these are rarely seen and the commonest tumour found at this site is limbal epibulbar melanoma.

Limbal Epibulbar Melanoma

Limbal epibulbar melanomas may occur in any breed, although the German Shepherd Dog is over-represented. These tumours arise from melanocytes at the corneoscleral junction, most frequently in the dorsolateral quadrant of the globe. They are usually pigmented and are first seen as a dark swelling in the perilimbal sclera (Fig. 100.27). Spread into the cornea is not uncommon and may be associated with corneal lipid deposition at the leading edge of the mass. Intraocular extension of the mass may occur, and investigation should include gonioscopy (see page 1004) to assess the extent of the lesion before treatment. An epibulbar melanoma must be distinguished from an intraocular melanoma that has subsequently invaded the sclera.

Treatment

Epibulbar melanomas are generally slow to metastasise and carry a favourable prognosis. Local resection may be possible if intraocular extension has not occurred. The defect created may be closed in a number of ways, including the use of a free graft of third eyelid cartilage and its associated conjunctiva (Blogg *et al.* 1989). Should the mass be invading the intraocular structures, cryotherapy may be attempted, although enucleation is probably the safest option in these circumstances.

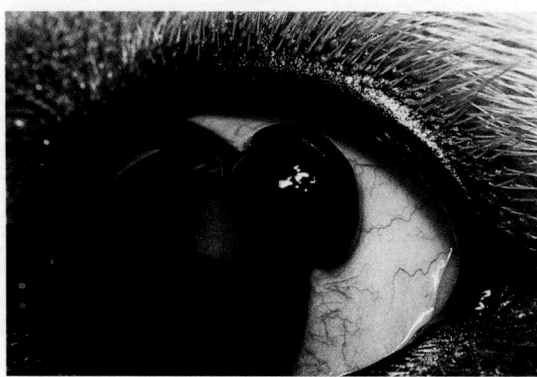

Fig. 100.27 Limbal epibulbar melanoma in a Labrador Retriever. The mass was successfully resected.

REFERENCES

Barnett, K.C. (1979). Imperforate and micro-lachrymal puncta in the dog. *Journal of Small Animal Practice*, **20**, 481–490.

Bedford, P.G.C., Grierson, I. & McKechnie, N.M. (1990). Corneal epithelial inclusion cyst in the dog. *Journal of Small Animal Practice*, **31**, 64–68.

Blogg, J.R., Dutton, A.G. & Stanley, R.G. (1989). Use of third eyelid grafts to repair full-thickness defects in the cornea and sclera. *Journal of the American Animal Hospital Association*, **25**, 505–512.

Cooley, P.L. & Dice, P.F. (1990). Corneal dystrophy in the dog and cat. *Veterinary Clinics of North America: Small Animal Practice*, **20**, 681–692.

Crispin, S.M. (1989). Lipid deposition at the limbus. *Eye* 3, 240–250.

Crispin, S.M. (1993). The pre-ocular tear film and conditions of the conjunctiva and cornea. In: *Manual of Small Animal Ophthalmology*, (eds S.M. Petersen-Jones & S.M. Crispin), pp. 137–171. BSAVA Publications, Cheltenham.

Crispin, S.M. & Barnett, K.C. (1983). Dystrophy, degeneration and infiltration of the canine cornea. *Journal of Small Animal Practice*, **24**, 63–83.

DeBowes, L.J. (1987). Lipid metabolism and hyperlipoproteinemia in dogs. *Compendium on Continuing Education for the Practicing Veterinarian*, **9**, 727–734.

Gratzek, A.T., Calvert, C.A., Martin, C.L. & Kaswan, R.L. (1993). Corneal edema in dogs treated with tocainide. *Progress in Veterinary and Comparative Ophthalmology*, **3**, 47–51.

Habin, D. (1993). The nasolacrimal system. In: *Manual of Small Animal Ophthalmology*, (eds S.M. Petersen-Jones & S.M. Crispin), pp. 91–102. BSAVA, Cheltenham.

Jackson, P.A., Kaswan, R.L., Meredith, R.E. & Barrett, P.M. (1991). Chronic superficial keratitis in dogs: A placebo controlled trial of topical cyclosporine treatment. *Progress in Veterinary and Comparative Ophthalmology*, **1**, 269–275.

Kaswan, R.L. & Salisbury, M.A. (1990). A new perspective on canine keratoconjunctivitis sicca. Treatment with cyclosporine. *Veterinary Clinics of North America: Small Animal Practice*, **20**, 583–613.

Kaswan, R.L., Martin, C.L. & Doran, C.C. (1988). Blepharoplasty techniques for canthus closure. *Companion Animal Practice*, **2**, 6–8.

Kern, T.J. (1990). Ulcerative keratitis. *Veterinary Clinics of North America: Small Animal Practice*, **20**, 643–666.

Kirschner, S.E. (1990). Persistent corneal ulcers: What to do when ulcers won't heal. *Veterinary Clinics of North America: Small Animal Practice*, **20**, 627–642.

Moore, C.P. (1990). Qualitative tear film disease. *Veterinary Clinics of North America: Small Animal Practice*, **20**, 565–581.

Morgan, R.V. & Abrams, K.L. (1994). A comparison of six different therapies for persistent corneal erosions in dogs and cats. *Veterinary and Comparative Ophthalmology*, **4**, 38–43.

Paulsen, M.E., Lavach, J.D., Snyder, S.P., Severin, G.A. & Eichenbaum, J.D. (1987). Nodular granulomatous episclerokeratitis in dogs: 19 cases (1973–1985). *Journal of the American Veterinary Medical Association*, **190**, 1581–1587.

Whitley, R.D. (1991). Canine cornea. In: *Veterinary Ophthalmology*, (ed. K.N. Gelatt), 2nd edn. pp. 307–356. Lea & Febiger, Philadelphia.

Wyman, M. (1979). Ophthalmic surgery for the practitioner. *Veterinary Clinics of North America: Small Animal Practice*, **9**, 311–348.

Chapter 101

Conditions of the Anterior Uvea

N. J. Millichamp

The uvea is made up of the vascular coats of the eye, anteriorly it comprises the iris and ciliary body, and is continuous with the posterior uvea or choroid. The iris consists of a fibrovascular structure, the stroma, bounded anteriorly by a fibroblastic anterior border region and posteriorly by a double layer of epithelium, the posterior layer of which is pigmented. Normal variations in pigmentation of the iris stroma result in differences in iris colour and in some dogs result in heterochromia iridis – areas of different coloration within an individual iris or between irises (Fig. 101.1). Two muscles, the iris sphincter muscle adjacent to the pupil margin and the dilator muscle in the posterior stroma, receive parasympathetic and sympathetic innervation respectively.

The anterior pars plicata of the ciliary body bears the ciliary processes consisting of a highly vascular stroma covered by a double layer of epithelium. The suspensory ligament, or zonule, of the lens arises from the pars plicata and attaches to the equatorial region of the lens. The posterior portion of the ciliary body, the pars plana, is less vascular and extends to the junction with the retina at the ora ciliaris retinae.

CONGENITAL UVEAL ABNORMALITIES

Persistent pupillary membranes are remnants of fetal tissue in the anterior chamber. They arise from the anterior face of the iris and either attach to other areas of iris, the anterior lens capsule or the posterior surface of the cornea. In severe cases they cause focal areas of oedema of the cornea or focal anterior capsular cataracts in the lens at points of attachment. In young dogs they may undergo further regression. No treatment is necessary. Persistent pupillary membranes are inherited in the Basenji and probably in other breeds.

Coloboma of the iris is an area where normal mesenchymal tissue of the iris failed to develop. It may appear as an irregular or notched pupil or hole in the iris stroma and epithelium. It may be associated with merling and is commonly seen in the Australian Shepherd.

ANTERIOR UVEITIS

Uveitis may affect the choroid or anterior segment structures. Inflammation localised to the iris is referred to as iritis, that of the ciliary body is cyclitis. Localised inflammation of the pars plana of the ciliary body is intermediate uveitis or pars planitis. In many cases the inflammation may involve more than one region and the terms iridocyclitis or anterior uveitis is appropriate in most cases. Acute injury to the eye including corneal abrasions or lacerations results in a breakdown of the blood aqueous barrier and formation of plasmoid or secondary aqueous due to an influx of proteins and fibrinogen. This initial acute response of the eye may be self-limiting in many cases. Persistence of an inflammatory stimulus (corneal ulceration, infection, immunological response) will be seen clinically as a persistent uveitis. Choroiditis or chorioretinitis may accompany anterior uveitis.

The highly vascular nature of the uvea is important in the development of uveitis. Immune responses and infectious organisms which cause vasculitis may localise their effects in the uvea, or the uvea may be targeted as part of multisystem vascular disease. Although the eye lacks lymphatics the uvea acts as a repository for sensitised lymphocytes. Subsequently these cells may be reactivated resulting in recurrent or persistent uveitis.

Prostaglandins play an important role as chemical mediators in uveitis in the dog. Other mediators including various cytokines are involved, although at present there is a paucity of data for the dog.

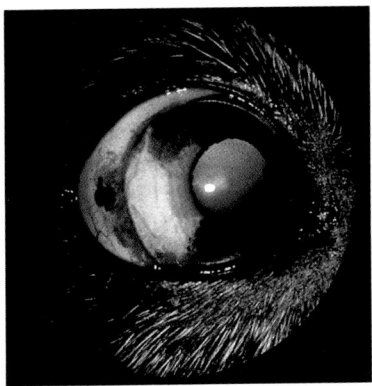

Fig. 101.1   Heterochromia iridis.

History and Examination

Most cases of uveitis are presented because the owner observes ocular pain or a change in the appearance of one or both eyes rather than because there is a loss of vision. In chronic cases with other ocular sequelae or in cases with severe chorioretinitis or optic neuritis visual impairment is likely to occur. The history should include the vaccination status of the dog, details of trauma to the head or eye and the presence of any concurrent systemic illness. The duration of the problem may be acute, chronic or recurrent.

Clinical findings in acute anterior uveitis include:

- *Ocular pain* – notably blepharospasm and increased lacrimation.
- *Enophthalmos* of the globe with *nictitans protrusion* in dolichocephalic breeds.
- '*Red-eye*' – injection of conjunctival and ciliary blood vessels.
- *Corneal oedema* because of endothelial damage.
- *Aqueous flare* due to light scattering by protein in the anterior chamber.
- *Keratic precipitates* or *hypopyon* due to inflammatory cells deposited on the posterior surface of the cornea or settling ventrally in the anterior chamber respectively.
- *Hyphaema* (haemorrhage) in the anterior chamber with vasculitis, trauma, coagulopathy or neoplasia.
- *Swollen iris* with dilated superficial blood vessels (Fig. 101.2).
- *Miosis* (pupillary constriction) and *anisocoria* (difference in size between the pupils) due to the action of chemical mediators.
- *Low intraocular pressure* (unless secondary glaucoma develops) because of reduced aqueous production and increased uveoscleral outflow.

- *Chorioretinitis and optic neuritis* (if accompanied by posterior uveal involvement).

In chronic cases of uveitis all of the above signs are often present. Additionally other sequelae develop including:

- *Posterior synechia* – adhesions between the iris and lens limiting pupil movement and distorting the pupil margin (Fig. 101.3).
- *Pigment* on the anterior lens capsule.
- *Deep neovascularisation* of the cornea.
- *Increased pigmentation* of the iris (decreased pigmentation in uveodermatological syndrome – see below).
- *Cataract* and less commonly *lens luxation*.
- *Glaucoma* – because of inflammatory cells, protein and swelling in the trabecular meshwork blocking aqueous drainage from the eye. Additionally posterior synechia

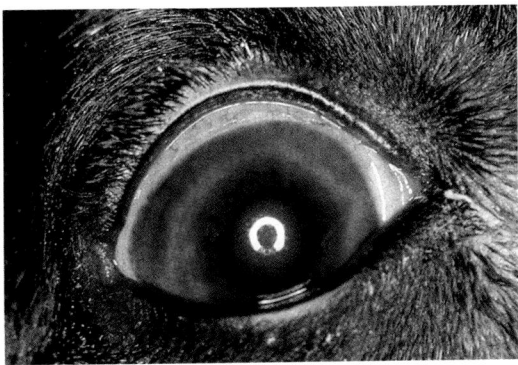

Fig. 101.2   Acute uveitis with a red eye, corneal oedema, aqueous flare and dilated iris stromal blood vessels.

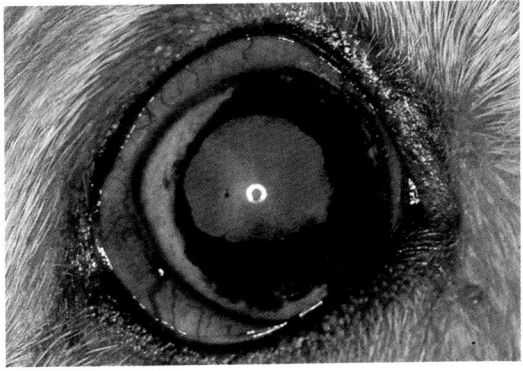

Fig. 101.3   Chronic uveitis with posterior synechia, pigment on the anterior lens capsule, iris colour change and cataract.

Table 101.3 Anterior uveitis – specific therapeutic agents.

Topical corticosteroids (do not use in cases associated with corneal ulceration)
Prednisolone acetate 1% suspension – good ocular penetration, dexamethasone 0.1% suspension; betamethasone sodium phosphate 0.1% every 4–6 h used with or without antibiotics

Systemic corticosteroids
Prednisone/prednisolone 1.2–2.2 mg/kg p.o. divided every 12 h for 1–2 weeks then dose halved for 1 week, then every 48 h for 5 treatments. Contraindicated if cornea ulcerated or with systemic infectious diseases

Non-steroidal anti-inflammatory drugs (NSAIDs)
Topical NSAIDs every 6 h
Flurbiprofen 0.03% solution
Suprofen 1.0% solution
Diclofenac Na 0.1% solution
Can use with topical corticosteroids or in cases where steroids are contraindicated (corneal epithelial abrasions, diabetes mellitus, systemic infectious disease). *Should be used with caution if IOP is elevated since these drugs may reduce aqueous drainage from the eye.*

Systemic NSAIDs
Flunixin meglumine 0.11–0.22 mg/kg i.v. every 24 h not to exceed two doses in 48 h
Aspirin 10–25 mg/kg every 12 h p.o.
Phenylbutazone 15–22 mg/kg every 12 h p.o.
Ketoprofen 1 mg/kg every 24 h p.o. (for up to 5 days)
2 mg/kg every 24 h s.c., i.m. or i.v. (for up to 3 days)

Systemic cytotoxic drugs
Azathioprine 2.2 mg/kg every 24 h p.o. reducing to 0.5–1.0 mg/kg every 24–48 h. Monitor CBC/platelet count weekly to determine if myelosuppression/leukopenia occurs.

Mydriatics/cycloplegic drugs (topical)
Atropine 1% solution/ointment every 6 h or less to effect, to maintain mydriasis and reduce ciliary muscle spasm. (Contraindicated if IOP elevated)
Phenylephrine 10% solution up to every 6 h to achieve maximal mydriasis

IOP, intra-ocular pressure; CBC, complete blood count.

pathic or secondary to iritis. They present as lightly pigmented spherical single or multiple objects in the anterior chamber, attached to the iris or free-floating (Fig. 101.4). Light reflected from the tapetum will pass through cysts, unlike solid neoplasms. No treatment is necessary.

Neoplasms of the uvea may be primary or secondary. Melanoma and ciliary body adenocarcinoma are the most commonly reported primary tumours. The most commonly described metastatic tumour in the dog is lymphosarcoma although metastasis of tumours from any other organ system is possible. The presenting signs include distortion and swelling of the iris, often by a pigmented mass, erosion of tumour through the adjacent sclera, uveitis, hyphaema, glaucoma and occasionally retinal detachment. The diagnosis of uveal neoplasia relies upon the clinical appearance and ultimately histopathology. Small uveal melanomas may be successfully removed surgically. Large

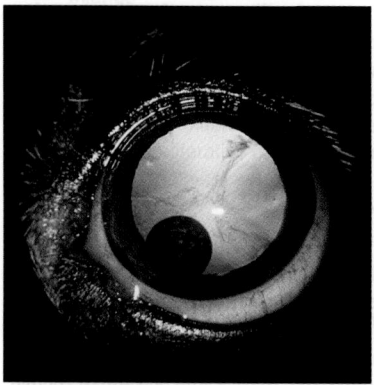

Fig. 101.4 Iris cyst and incipient posterior suture line cataract in a Boston Terrier.

intraocular tumours should be treated by enucleation and submission of the eye for histopathology.

FURTHER READING

Crispin, S.M. (1988). Uveitis in the dog and cat. *Journal of Small Animal Practice*, **29**, 429–447.

Gwin, R.M. (1988). Anterior uveitis: diagnosis and treatment. *Seminars in Veterinary Medicine and Surgery (Small Animal)*, **3**, 33–39.

Håkanson, N. & Forrester, S.D. (1990). Uveitis in the dog and cat. *Veterinary Clinics of North America: Small Animal Practice*, **20**, 715–735.

Collins, K.B. & Moore, C.P. (1991). Canine anterior uvea. In: *Veterinary Ophthalmology*, (ed K.N. Gelatt), 2nd edn. pp. 357–395. Lea & Febiger, Philadelphia.

Chapter 102

Glaucoma

N. J. Millichamp

Glaucoma encompasses a group of diseases characterised by a pathological increase in the intra-ocular pressure (IOP), resulting in damage to the optic nerve and retina and thus visual loss. If untreated permanent blindness is an inevitable outcome.

Glaucoma is a challenge for the general practitioner and specialist alike since by the time most cases are presented significant pathology has occurred resulting in varying degrees of visual loss. Owners may fail to notice early signs of elevated intra-ocular pressure which if occurring in a human patient would be readily perceived. A delay in diagnosis and treatment may have drastic consequences for the visual outcome. Unfortunately glaucoma is often misdiagnosed as some other cause of a red eye – especially uveitis or conjunctivitis. The most appropriate therapy for these conditions may be contraindicated in cases of glaucoma.

AQUEOUS PRODUCTION AND DRAINAGE

Aqueous humour, produced by the ciliary processes primarily by active secretion into the posterior chamber, passes through the pupil to the anterior chamber. Aqueous serves to nourish tissues of the anterior segment and carry away waste materials. It drains from the eye through the iridocorneal angle and trabecular meshwork gaining access to the scleral venous plexus and venous circulation. A small amount of aqueous diffuses through the iris and ciliary body to be absorbed in the suprachoroidal space (uveoscleral outflow). The iridocorneal angle, or opening into the ciliary cleft is at the iris root and is spanned by the pectinate fibres. This structure is hidden from direct visualisation by the scleral shelf which is formed by the oblique junction between the cornea and sclera at the limbus. Examination of the iridocorneal angle (gonioscopy) is important in the investigation of glaucoma and is achieved by placing a special lens (goniolens) on the cornea.

CLASSIFICATION OF CANINE GLAUCOMA

Glaucoma is classified as either primary (with no other ocular disease preceding glaucoma development) or secondary (where glaucoma develops because of other ocular disease) (Table 102.1).

Primary Glaucoma

- Most cases are inherited.
- Both eyes are affected although clinical signs of the disease usually develop in each eye at different times.

Primary glaucoma is further divided according to the morphological appearance of the iridocorneal angle:

- narrow angle,
- goniodysgenesis,
- open angle.

Narrow Angle

Dogs in which the opening into the ciliary cleft develops abnormally so that it is narrower than normal (referred to as a narrow drainage angle) are predisposed to closure of the angle later in life. Closure of the angle may be due to age-related changes in the depth of the peripheral anterior chamber. A narrow iridocorneal angle is also predisposed to blockage by inflammatory exudate or cells. Typically dogs with narrow-angle glaucoma present with acute and high elevation of IOP which commonly may reach 50–60 mmHg. Rapid therapy is needed if there is to be any hope of avoiding or postponing visual loss. Many breeds of dog are predisposed to narrow-angle glaucoma including the American and English Cocker Spaniels, Samoyed and Miniature Poodle.

Goniodysgenesis

Mesodermal goniodysgenesis is a form of primary glaucoma in which the angle does not differentiate normally and is left covered with sheets of mesodermal tissue broken by periodic holes or slits in place of the normal pectinate ligaments. How this mesodermal tissue limits aqueous outflow is uncertain. The breed in which this type of glaucoma is most often encountered is the Basset Hound in which the onset of glaucoma often appears to be associated with iridocyclitis.

Open Angle

Open-angle glaucoma develops in several canine breeds in which the width of the angle appears to be normal. In the Beagle open-angle glaucoma had been shown to be recessively inherited. The underlying abnormality is unknown although ultrastructural and biochemical abnormalities occur in the trabecular meshwork within the ciliary cleft of affected Beagles. The onset of glaucoma is usually more insidious than in the narrow-angle forms of glaucoma with a gradual increase of intra-ocular pressure into the range of 30–40 mmHg occurring over several months.

Secondary Glaucoma

Secondary glaucoma, due to either iridocorneal angle blockage or impedance of aqueous drainage through the pupil, occurs as a result of other ocular disease including:

- lens luxation where the lens interferes with normal aqueous circulation;
- uveitis resulting in swelling of the trabecular meshwork and blockage of the angle by inflammatory exudate;
- neoplasia either involving the angle or neoplastic cells deposited in the angle from the aqueous;
- intraocular haemorrhage;
- vitreous loss into the anterior chamber and angle during cataract surgery or associated with lens luxation or lens removal;

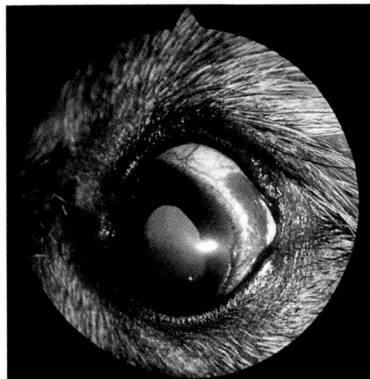

Fig. 102.1   Pigmentary glaucoma in a Cairn Terrier. Note the scleral pigmentation.

- the Cairn Terrier may develop a form of pigmentary glaucoma in which the iridocorneal angle becomes blocked by pigment (Fig. 102.1).

CLINICAL SIGNS

Although the diagnosis of glaucoma is based on measurement of the intra-ocular pressure, certain clinical features may be suggestive of the disease. The strong breed predisposition is important. In acute narrow-angle or secondary glaucoma the major clinical signs include:

- *blindness* in the affected eye,
- *ocular pain* (blepharospasm and increased lacrimation),
- *'red-eye'* due to passive engorgement of the conjunctival and scleral vessels (Fig. 102.2),
- *corneal oedema*,
- *dilated and non-responsive pupil* (due to paralysis of the iris sphincter muscle at high pressures).

In chronic glaucoma all of the above signs may be seen with the addition of:

- *buphthalmos* – an increase in the size of the eye,
- *tears in Descemet's membrane* – deep linear streaks seen in the cornea (Fig. 102.3),
- *deep perilimbal corneal neovascularisation*,
- *iris atrophy* – holes or thinned areas of iris stroma,
- *lens luxation*,
- *cupping and atrophy of the optic nerve*, retinal vessel attenuation and retinal atrophy (Fig. 102.4).

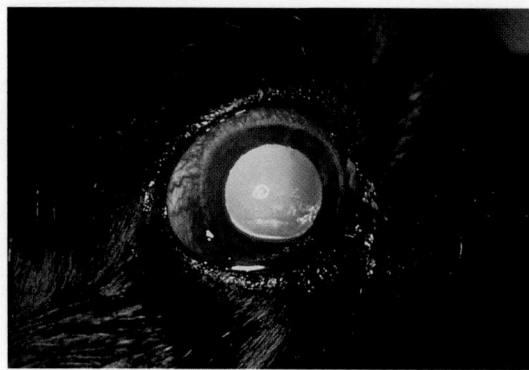

Fig. 102.2 Acute closed angle glaucoma in an American Cocker Spaniel. Conjunctival and scleral blood vessels are injected, the cornea is oedematous, the pupil dilated.

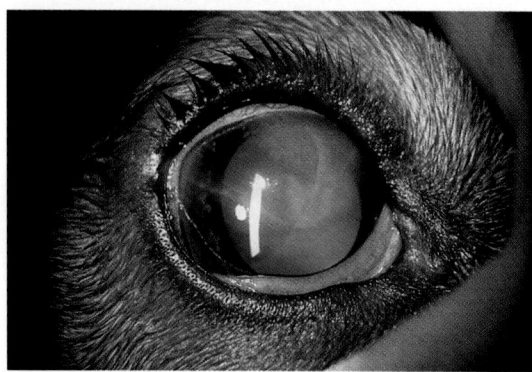

Fig. 102.3 Chronic glaucoma with buphthalmos, corneal oedema, tears in Descemet's membrane and mydriasis.

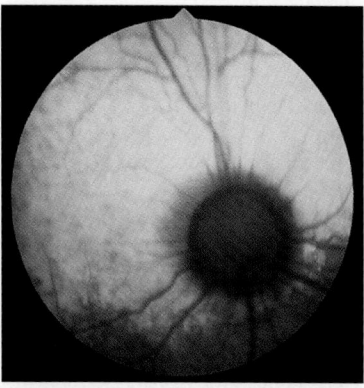

Fig. 102.4 Optic atrophy and cupping in dog with chronic glaucoma.

It is often difficult to make a definite diagnosis of uveitis in cases where this is the underlying cause of glaucoma. If there is doubt whether a dog has uveitis or glaucoma – treat for glaucoma since this is more likely to threaten sight if treated inappropriately.

INVESTIGATION (TABLE 102.1)

Tonometry

The diagnosis and management of glaucoma relies upon the ability of the veterinarian to measure the intra-ocular pressure. In the absence of a tonometer potential glaucoma cases should be expeditiously referred to a practice with a tonometer or a specialist. The normal intra-ocular pressure in the dog ranges from 15 to 25 mmHg.

- *Digital tonometry*, where the eye is palpated through the eyelids, is unreliable at best.
- *Indentation tonometry – Schiötz tonometer*. This is the most practical affordable method for general practitioners. This tonometer applies a weight to the eye resulting in corneal indentation which is measured on a scale. The scale reading may be converted to actual intra-ocular pressure by the use of canine calibration tables.
- *Applanation tonometry*. More accurate readings of intra-ocular pressure are obtained with an applanation tonometer, but the relatively high cost of these instruments limits them to specialists.

Gonioscopy

Gonioscopy is the use of a lens which is applied to the cornea to view the width and appearance of the irido-corneal angle. In unilateral cases of glaucoma gonioscopy should be used in the fellow normal eye to determine whether the glaucoma is due to developmental iridocorneal angle abnormalities (these conditions are generally bilateral).

MANAGEMENT

The therapy for glaucoma and prognosis for successful management depends upon the type of glaucoma, the extent of damage to the visual system at the time of diagnosis and the severity of the increase of IOP. The extent of damage to the optic nerve and loss of vision depends both

Table 102.1 Glaucoma – aetiology/pathogenesis.

Primary glaucoma
Bilateral with lag (usually months) between eyes

Narrow/closed angle
- American, English & Welsh Cocker Spaniel, Samoyed, Siberian Husky, Miniature & Toy Poodles and various other breeds
- Acute onset with high IOP (>40 mmHg)
- Blindness, pain, red eye, corneal oedema, dilated often fixed pupil

Mesodermal goniodysgenesis
- Basset Hound
- Iridocyclitis may be present

Open angle
- Beagle, Miniature Poodle, Norwegian Elkhound
- Gradual increase of IOP (initially 30–40 mmHg)
- Progressive buphthalmos, red eye, mild mydriasis, cupping of optic nerve, gradual visual loss and pain

Secondary glaucoma
- Lens luxation (Terrier breeds)
- Uveitis
- Neoplasia
- Hyphaema
- Pigmentary (Cairn Terrier)
- Vitreous prolapse
- Intra-ocular surgery

Glaucoma – investigation
- History – duration of problem will affect potential to restore vision
- Thorough ophthalmic examination of anterior and posterior segment (uveitis, lens luxation, neoplasia). Appearance of optic nerve and retina in chronic cases may predict visual outcome
- Tonometry (IOP > 25 mmHg) Schiötz or applanation methods
- Gonioscopy (both eyes if possible, 'normal' eye if too much corneal oedema in glaucomatous eye)

on the severity of the IOP increase and its duration. Of the primary glaucomas, open-angle glaucoma is more readily controlled than narrow-angle glaucoma. If a dog presents with very high pressures of short duration it is important quickly to restore a normal IOP in order to evaluate whether the dog still has useful vision. A dog that presents with high pressures and chronic changes (particularly optic nerve changes) is less likely to regain vision when the IOP is lowered.

Acute, primary glaucoma with severe elevations of IOP should be vigorously treated, initially with medical therapy to reduce fluid volume in the eye and return the IOP to the normal range and determine if useful vision remains. If medical therapy fails to rapidly reduce the IOP to the normal range, or vision is irretrievably lost, surgical options should be considered. Current medical treatment reduces the production and increases the drainage of aqueous from the eye. If IOPs are over 50 mmHg intensive

therapy with all of the following agents should be tried (see Table 102.2).

- *Hyperosmotics*: Agents such as mannitol and glycerol reduce intra-ocular pressure by drawing fluid from the vitreous and aqueous humour into the surrounding vasculature. Mannitol is the agent of choice since it can be given at a reliable dose intravenously. Glycerol may induce vomiting. Dogs should not have access to water for 1–2 h after administering hyperosmotics.
- *Carbonic anhydrase inhibitors (CAI)*: Agents such as dichlorphenamide or methazolamide given orally reduce aqueous production by blocking carbonic anhydrase mediated buffering involved in aqueous secretion. They cause a considerable reduction in aqueous production. Acetazolamide, which can be used orally or intravenously, may cause more systemic side effects. Long-term use of systemic CAI may result in

Ophthalmology

Table 102.2 Glaucoma – management.

Acute glaucoma (IOP > 45 mmHg) Emergency treatment:
  Mannitol i.v. (1–2 g/kg in 20 min; remove water 1–2 h)
  Methazolamide (5–10 mg/kg divided twice daily) *or* dichlorphenamide (10–15 mg/kg divided twice daily) *or* topical
    dorzolamide (one drop every 8 h)
  Pilocarpine (1–2% one drop every 6–8 h) *or* demecarium bromide (0.125–0.25% one drop every 12–24 h)
  Timolol maleate (0.5%) – one drop every 12 h
  Adrenaline (1–2%) or dipivefrine (0.1%) – one drop every 6–12 h
  Secondary glaucoma: Treat underlying disease (uveitis (see Table 101.3) lens extraction for lens luxation etc.)

Chronic glaucoma (IOP < 45 mmHg) (open-angle glaucoma)
  Use carbonic anhydrase inhibitor, parasympathomimetic and β-adrenergic blocker at dosage above. Mannitol not usually
  required

Maintenance treatment
  Continue therapy with methazolamide or dichlorphenamide orally (or topical dorzolamide), and topical pilocarpine or
  demecarium and timolol. Sympathomimetics may also be used. Intra-ocular pressure should be maintained at less than
  25 mmHg and if vision is restored by these medications medical therapy may be continued alone. If the IOP cannot be
  maintained within the normal range with medications alone but the eye remains visual the dog should be referred for
  surgical implantation of a *Drainage device or cyclophotocoagulation or cyclocryotherapy*

  If the pressures cannot be controlled by a combination of medical and surgical therapy and vision is lost in the affected eye
  the eye should undergo *enucleation or evisceration with implantation of a prosthesis or intravitreal gentamicin injection*

Glaucoma prophylaxis (primary glaucoma):
  Timolol maleate every 12 hours ± a topical parasympathomimetic and carbonic anhydrase inhibitor may prolong the
  interval until fellow eye develops disease.

---

hypokalaemia and require potassium supplementation in the diet. A topical CAI, dorzolamide hydrochloride, is now available but awaits full evaluation in dogs. Topical use of the CAI should avoid the side-effects associated with systemic treatment.

- *Parasympathomimetics*: Pilocarpine is the most commonly used drug in this class. Parasympathomimetics are believed to increase aqueous drainage by contracting the ciliary muscle and opening the trabecular meshwork. In dogs with narrow angles the miotic action of these drugs may also be beneficial in moving the iris base from the ciliary cleft. Indirect acting (cholinesterase inhibitors) parasympathomimetics such as demecarium bromide may have a stronger action than pilocarpine, but also are likely to cause more ocular and systemic side-effects. Parasympathomimetics may cause breakdown of the blood-aqueous barrier (uveitis) or cause extreme miosis and limit aqueous flow from the posterior to anterior chamber. Aqueous build-up in the posterior chamber results in forward displacement of the iris (iris bombé) which further compromises the iridocorneal angle. Formation of adhesions between the anterior iris and peripheral cornea (anterior synechiae) result in complete obstruction of the angle.

- *Sympatholytics*: Beta-blockers such as timolol maleate act by unknown mechanisms. These drugs are not potent enough to significantly reduce a grossly elevated IOP (particularly in closed angle glaucoma) when used alone, although they may be used in cases of mild elevation of IOP (particularly open-angle glaucoma).

- *Sympathomimetics*: Agents such as adrenaline or dipivefrine reduce IOP in dogs with glaucoma. They may reduce aqueous production and increase outflow. They can be used with miotic agents to limit the degree of miosis by stimulating the iris dilator muscle.

If medical therapy alone is insufficient to maintain normal IOP in a potentially visual eye surgical procedures are indicated:

- *Cyclocryoablation, cyclophotoablation*: The ciliary body may be locally destroyed using either cryotherapy or laser therapy. Destruction of the ciliary processes results in reduced aqueous production. Both procedures result in uveitis and may initially further elevate IOP. For either procedure referral to a specialist is recommended.

- *Surgical procedures to increase aqueous outflow*: Various surgical procedures have been described to increase the drainage of aqueous. All involve creating a drainage pathway from the peripheral anterior chamber into the subconjunctival space or retrobulbar space. Various drainage implants or valves have been devised to improve the flow of aqueous. All of these techniques are prone to fail after a period of time due to fibrosis at the drainage site. Use of anti-mitotic agents may, in the future, prolong the drainage potential of these surgical procedures in combination with maintenance of anti-glaucoma medical therapy. Surgical therapy is likely to be most effective in cases of primary glaucoma and especially in dogs with open-angle disease. Such cases should be referred to a specialist for specific surgery.

- *Ocular evisceration with prosthetic implants or enucleation*: In *blind eyes* with glaucoma from any cause other than neoplasia or infection the treatment of choice is evisceration and implantation of a silicone prostheses. This eliminates the need to apply expensive medications to a blind and painful eye, and maintains a cosmetic eye. If owners prefer enucleation can be performed. These surgeries may be used in blind eyes *regardless of IOP* since even eyes that have started to undergo phthisis bulbi after chronic glaucoma would appear to remain painful to some degree.

- *Pharmacological cycloablation*: Injection of 25 mg gentamicin sulphate with 1 mg dexamethasone in a volume not to exceed 0.5 ml into the vitreous will destroy ciliary processes and reduce aqueous production. A 20 g needle is directed into the vitreous space 5 mm behind the limbus and an equal volume of vitreous is removed before injecting the drugs. This technique should be reserved for *blind eyes* since the retina will also be destroyed. It is most appropriate for geriatric dogs which would represent anaesthetic risk for more appropriate therapy such as evisceration and silicone implantation. The procedure can be performed under heavy sedation and topical anaesthesia.

FURTHER READING

Bedford, P.G.C. (1980). The clinical and pathological features of canine glaucoma. *Veterinary Record*, **107**, 53–58.

Bedford, P.G.C. (1980). The aetiology of canine glaucoma. *Veterinary Record*, **107**, 76–82.

Bedford, P.G.C. (1980). The treatment of canine glaucoma. *Veterinary Record*, **107**, 101–104.

Brooks, D.E. (1990). Glaucoma in the dog and cat. *Veterinary Clinics of North America: Small Animal Practice*, **20**, 775–797.

Gelatt, K.N. (1991). The canine glaucomas. In: *Veterinary Ophthalmology*, (ed. K.N. Gelatt), 2nd edn. pp. 396–428. Lea & Febiger, Philadelphia.

Chapter 103

Conditions of the Lens

N. J. Millichamp

The lens is a transparent biconvex structure located behind and in contact with the iris. It is suspended by the zonule or suspensory ligament from the ciliary body. The lens is divided into an outer cortical and inner nuclear region enclosed by a thin capsule. An anterior epithelium lines the anterior capsule. The lens equator is the peripheral area adjacent to the zonule. Division of epithelial cells at the equator results in the formation of concentric layers of fibres which are gradually displaced inwards causing continued growth of the structure throughout life. The lens fibres form the lens sutures where their ends are opposed in the anterior and posterior cortex. The vitreous humour has a circular ring of attachment to the posterior lens capsule half way between the posterior pole of the lens and the equator.

CATARACT

A cataract is any opacity within the lens. Cataract should be differentiated from nuclear sclerosis – a normal ageing change in the nucleus which appears as a spherical grey hazy area in diffuse light. It is possible to see the fundus clearly through nuclear sclerosis and the dog's vision is not impaired.

Classification of Cataracts

Cataracts may be classified according to the aetiology, location in the lens, stage of development or progression and age of onset. The most common cause of cataract in the dog is genetic, although secondary cataracts may occur associated with various systemic and ocular conditions (Table 103.1). The majority of cataracts in the dog are recessively inherited, although in a few breeds (notably Golden and Labrador Retrievers) dominant inheritance has been sug-

gested. All inherited cataracts are bilateral and often quite symmetrical although in some breeds asymmetrical progression is usual (for instance the American Cocker Spaniel and Miniature Poodle). In many breeds the natural history of the cataract is often quite characteristic regarding the age of onset, location and progression of the opacities. This is especially true in the Boston Terrier, Golden and Labrador Retrievers, Miniature Schnauzer, Standard Poodle and Welsh Springer Spaniel. For details of inherited cataracts occurring in any particular country see the literature of the hereditary eye screening scheme of that country.

Lens opacities may involve focal areas of the lens. Early or incipient cataract involves areas of the nucleus, cortex or capsule with anterior, posterior, equatorial and polar locations in these structures (Figs 103.1 & 103.2). The cataract may progress to involve the entire lens. A cataract involving the entire lens which still allows the examiner to detect a tapetal reflection is described as immature (Fig. 103.3). A total dense cataract preventing any view of the fundus or tapetal reflection is mature (Fig. 103.4) or may be hypermature. Both immature and mature cataracts may significantly limit the dog's vision. With further progression the cataract may become hypermature and in some cases may eventually undergo resorption resulting in changes in the shape of the lens (Figs 103.5 & 103.6). Protein leaking from a progressing cataract (especially at the hypermature stage) into the eye incites uveitis (phacolytic uveitis) and in some dogs, glaucoma. Changes in lens shape due to resorption of a hypermature cataract may result in vitreous tension on the peripheral retina in some cases leading to retinal tears and detachment.

Many inherited cataracts develop during the first few years of life, although some may be congenital (present at birth and detected when the eyelids open at two weeks of age) and others (for instance in the American Cocker Spaniel and Miniature Poodle) develop in middle to old age. Designation as juvenile or senile cataracts are of little value in classification.

Table 103.1 Cataract.

Aetiology
    Inheritance (often recessive, occasionally dominant)
    Diabetes mellitus
    Other metabolic disorders, e.g. hypocalcaemia
    Uveitis/trauma
    Retinal degeneration
    Retinal dysplasia and detachment
    Glaucoma
    Associated with persistent hyperplastic primary vitreous/ persistent hyperplastic tunica vasculosa lentis
    Nutritional (arginine deficiency)
    Toxic (radiation, electric shock, drugs)

Classification
    Location in lens (capsule, cortex, nucleus)
    Age of onset (present at birth or acquired)
    Stage of progression
      Incipient/early
      Immature
      Mature (intumescent)
      Hypermature (Morgagnian)

Investigation

Rule out other primary/secondary ocular disease – perform complete ophthalmic examination:

- Uveitis – primary or secondary to the cataracts, trauma or ocular neoplasia Treat underlying cause of the uveitis. In cases of mild phacolytic (cataract induced) uveitis treat the eye for 2 weeks with topical corticosteroid/NSAID and re-examine to determine whether adequate response to allow surgery

- Diabetes mellitus – blood and urine glucose and urine ketone measurement. If dog is a poorly regulated diabetic, insulin regulation should be re-evaluated and fine tuned before referral for cataract surgery

Several ocular conditions are likely to limit the successful outcome of cataract surgery significantly, and therefore should be viewed as contraindications to surgical therapy in most cases. These include:

- Retinal degeneration (progressive retinal atrophy) – funduscopic examination of both eyes if possible around the cataracts. Electroretinography to determine state of retinal function if fundus cannot be seen

- Retinal detachment – associated with later progression of cataracts. Evidence of intra-ocular haemorrhage, reduced electroretinogram amplitudes from affected eye. Ocular ultrasound to rule out

- Glaucoma – measure intra-ocular pressure with Schiötz/applanation tonometry

- Lens luxation – examination of eye for signs of iridodonesis, vitreous in the anterior chamber, aphakic crescent

Treatment of Cataracts

Cataracts are diagnosed and classified according to their location as determined by ophthalmoscopic examination through a dilated pupil. The stage of the cataract is important when deciding when the dog should be referred to a specialist for surgery. With current surgical techniques it is preferable to operate on cataracts at an early stage to avoid the later complications of lens induced uveitis and retinal detachment. Before referring the dog for surgery any signs of lens induced uveitis should be treated with a topical corticosteroid for 10–14 days.

Currently there is no medical therapy for cataract. The only effective treatment is surgical removal. Cataract surgery requires equipment beyond the scope of most general practices thus cases should always be referred to a specialist.

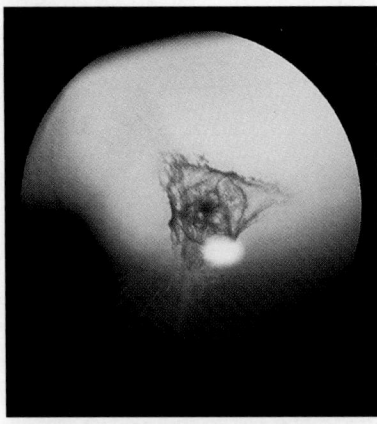

Fig. 103.1 Posterior polar suture line cataract typical of inherited cataract seen in several breeds including Golden and Labrador Retrievers.

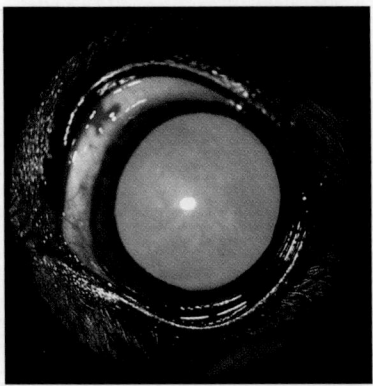

Fig. 103.4 A total mature cataract.

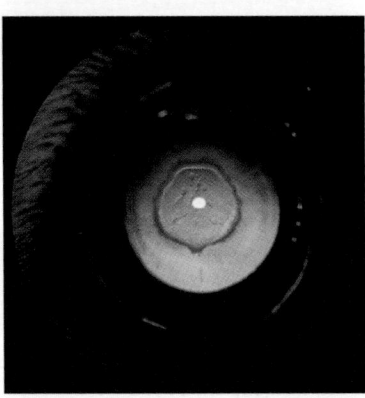

Fig. 103.2 An incipient perinuclear cataract in a puppy fed a milk replacement compound.

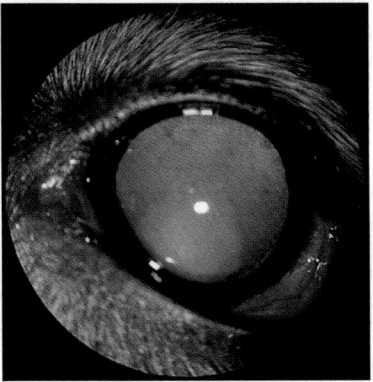

Fig. 103.5 A hypermature liquefying cataract (Morgagnian cataract). The dense lens nucleus is sinking ventrally in liquefied cortex.

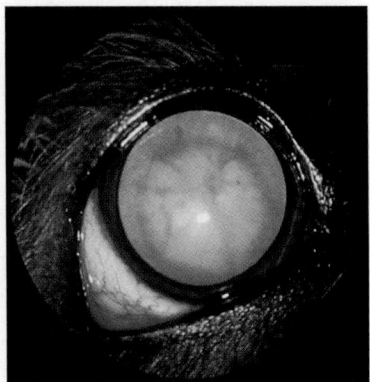

Fig. 103.3 An immature complete cataract. Although the cataract involves the whole lens the tapetal reflection is still visible.

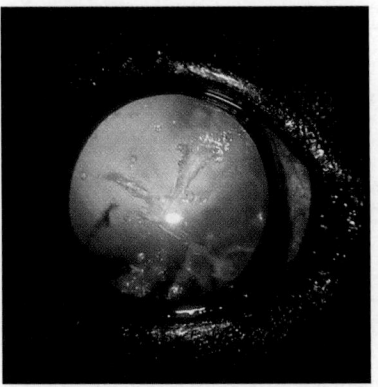

Fig. 103.6 A hypermature resorbing cataract with wrinkles in the lens capsule.

- Young dogs with progressive cataracts should be considered candidates for bilateral cataract extraction and intra-ocular lens implantation without waiting until the cataracts progress sufficiently to cause blindness, by which time they may have already caused secondary ocular disease
- Elderly dogs with bilateral cataract causing visual impairment are suitable for cataract extraction. If a cataract is incomplete and the other eye normal the progression should be monitored before electing to remove the cataract.
- Dogs with bilateral cataracts can have both removed at the same time, even if there is asymmetry in the stage of progression. This avoids the need for more than one anaesthetic procedure and reduces the cost to the client.

Upon referral to a specialist the dog should undergo evaluation for uveitis or any predisposition to glaucoma (tonometry and gonioscopy). The retinal function should be evaluated with an electroretinogram and in cases where the response is poor the eyes should undergo ultrasound to rule out retinal detachment.

Cataracts can be removed by extracapsular extraction using an 'open-sky' approach with a 160° limbal incision, anterior capsulotomy and delivery of the lens nucleus followed by irrigation/aspiration to remove the remaining lens cortex. However, removal of the lens through a small incision by ultrasonic phacoemulsification and aspiration is the method preferred by many veterinary ophthalmologists. After removal of the lens a prosthetic intra-ocular lens may be placed in the remaining lens capsule.

LENS LUXATION

Displacement of the lens from its normal location behind the iris in the patellar fossa of the vitreous occurs when breaks develop in the suspensory zonule. The lens may be partially dislocated (subluxated) if part of the zonule is broken, or totally luxated if the circumferential zonule is disrupted. The lens may remain behind the pupil, luxate into the vitreous or anterior chamber, or straddle the pupil.

Lens luxation may be primary or secondary to other ocular disease.

Primary Lens Luxation (Fig. 103.7)

The characteristics of primary lens luxation are:

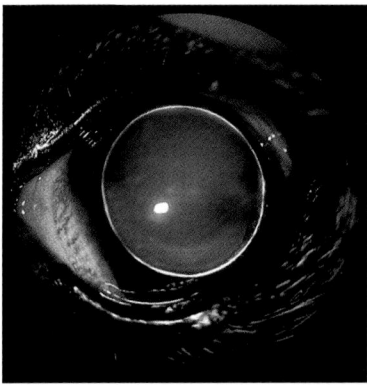

Fig. 103.7 A primary anterior lens luxation.

- affects several Terrier breeds, the Border Collie and possibly other breeds,
- autosomal recessive inheritance,
- usually develops between 3 and 6 years of age,
- bilateral,
- usually a lag between the two eyes in development of clinical signs.

Secondary Lens Luxation

Secondary lens luxation may occur due to:

- chronic glaucoma due to stretching of the zonule in a buphthalmic eye,
- severe ocular trauma,
- uveitis,
- uveal neoplasia.

Diagnosis

The most severe sequel to lens luxation is glaucoma due to impaired aqueous flow into the anterior chamber causing anterior displacement of the iris and angle closure, or obstruction of the angle by the vitreous. Posterior lens luxation may be associated with liquefaction (syneresis) of the vitreous and retinal detachment.

The diagnosis of lens luxation is based on the clinical signs. Signs of lens subluxation include:

- iridodonesis (trembling of the iris) seen when the eye or head moves due to a loss of support of the iris by the lens;
- asymmetric and variable depth to the anterior chamber in different quadrants;

- an aphakic crescent seen through the pupil in the quadrants where the zonule is broken (Fig. 103.8);
- strands of vitreous (like wispy cotton wool) in the anterior chamber.

If the lens becomes completely luxated:

- it may be seen ventrally in the vitreous;
- it may be seen sitting in the pupil;
- it may be seen in the anterior chamber (Fig. 103.7);
- contact with the corneal endothelium causes a focal area of corneal oedema;
- if the IOP is elevated there will be diffuse corneal oedema and other signs of glaucoma;
- there may be signs of anterior uveitis and discomfort (with or without glaucoma).

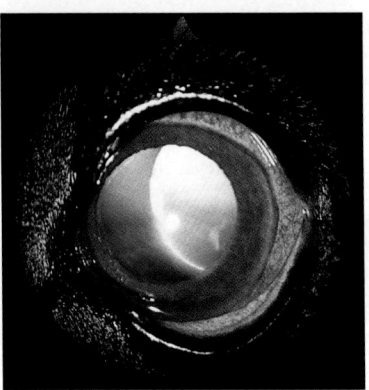

Fig. 103.8   A posteriorly subluxated lens.

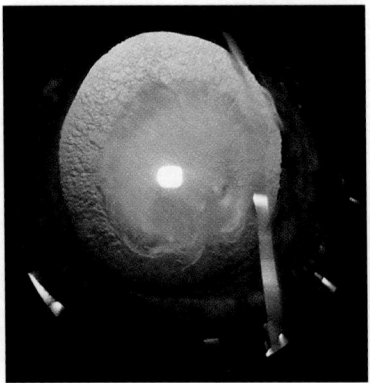

Fig. 103.9   Persistent hyperplastic primary vitreous/persistent tonica vasculosa lentis. (PHPV/PHTVL) in an English mastiff. Note the presence of a fibrovascular plaque on the posterior surface of the lens. This is partially obscured by a progressive secondary cataract.

The fellow eye should always be examined for signs of impending subluxation. If the lens is subluxated the intraocular pressure (IOP) should be measured and glaucoma treated if present. Many ophthalmologists will wait until the subluxated lens luxates fully before operating in which case the owners should be appraised of the clinical signs which would indicate total luxation and glaucoma. Complete lens luxation should be viewed as an ocular emergency regardless of the IOP and the dog referred to a specialist immediately for intracapsular lens removal, to try to avert development of sequelae. Dogs should be treated for glaucoma if present, or given topical corticosteroids until examined by an ophthalmologist.

PERSISTENT HYPERPLASTIC PRIMARY VITREOUS/PERSISTENT TUNICA VASCULOSA LENTIS (PHPV/PHTVL)

PHPV/PHTVL is a developmental disease of the vitreous which usually involves the lens. The disease may be inherited in the Doberman Pincher and the Staffordshire Bull Terrier. In some dogs multiple ocular anomalies comprising microphthalmos and developmental defects of the lens, vitreous and retinas may be present. In mildly affected animals pigment deposits are present on the posterior lens capsule. In the more severely affected dogs pigmented vascular remnants (plaques) of the embryonic vasculature, which surrounded the lens, may be seen on the back of the lens (hyperplastic primary vitreous) or equatorial lens capsule (hyperplastic tunica vascular lentis) (Fig. 103.9). Cortical cataracts, posterior lenticonus, lens colobomas, microphakia or intralenticular haemorrhage may occur. Mydriasis maintained with atropine may allow vision past small opacities. In severe cases lens removal may be considered, although there is a considerable risk of haemorrhage from vitreous blood vessels.

FURTHER READING

Barnett, K.C. (1985). The diagnosis and differential diagnosis of cataract in the dog. *Journal of Small Animal Practice*, **26**, 305–316.

Curtis, R. (1990). Lens luxation in the dog and cat. *Veterinary Clinics of North America: Small Animal Practice*, **20**, 755–773.

Davidson, M.G., Nasisse, M.P., Jamieson, V.E., English, R.V. & Olivero, D.O. (1991). Phacoemulsification and intra-ocular lens implantation: a study of surgical results in 182 dogs. *Progress in Veterinary and Comparative Ophthalmology*, **1**, 233–238.

Leon, A. (1988). Diseases of the vitreous in the dog and cat. *Journal of Small Animal Practice*, **29**, 448–461.

Nasisse, M.P., Davidson, M.G., Jamieson, V.E., English, R.V. & Olivero, D.K. (1991). Phacoemulsification and intra-ocular lens implantation: a study of technique in 182 dogs. *Progress in Veterinary and Comparative Ophthalmology*, **1**, 225–232.

Petersen-Jones, S.M. (1993). Conditions of the lens. In: *Manual of Small Animal Ophthalmology*, (eds S.M. Petersen-Jones & S.M. Crispin), pp. 213–228. BSAVA Publications, Cheltenham.

Chapter 104

Conditions of the Vitreous

S. Petersen-Jones

ANATOMY OF THE VITREOUS

The vitreous is a clear semi-gel structure filling the posterior cavity of the globe. It has a matrix of collagen fibres with some condensations which appear as faint membranes within the more amorphous gel. Cloquet's canal spans the vitreous from the posterior surface of the lens and its anterior portion can usually be visualised with good illumination and magnification.

The main function of the vitreous is to provide mechanical support for the retina and the walls of the globe, and to allow diffusion of nutrients while being optically transparent. There are firm attachments of the vitreous to the pars plana ciliaris, the ora ciliaris retinae, the posterior lens capsule and around the optic disc.

Examination of the Vitreous

Complete examination of the posterior segment of the eye is facilitated by use of a mydriatic (e.g. tropicamide). The following techniques are used:

- focal illumination (pen torch or transilluminator) – useful for anterior vitreous;
- ophthalmoscopy (direct or indirect) – used to examine the posterior portion of the vitreous;
- magnification (e.g. slit-lamp biomicroscope) – gives detailed view of anterior vitreous;
- ultrasonography – useful when opaque optical media preclude direct visualisation – retinal detachments and even detachment of the vitreous face from the retinal surface can be identified by a skilled ultrasonographer.

CONDITIONS OF THE VITREOUS

Opacities

There are a number of possible reasons for the presence of congenital or acquired opacities within the vitreous. They are summarised in Table 104.1. Persistent hyperplastic vitreous/persistent tunica vasculosa lentis, a congenital abnormality involving the vasculature which in embryonic life supplied nutrition to the developing lens is discussed under the conditions of the lens (Chapter 103).

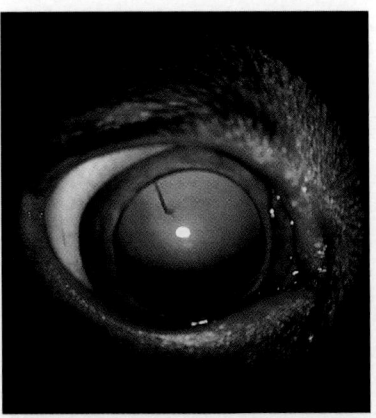

Fig. 104.1 A persistent hyaloid artery in a German Shorthaired Pointer. The hyaloid remnant can be seen inserting on the posterior surface of the lens. Ophthalmoscopically it could be followed to the optic disc.

Table 104.1 Vitreal opacities.

Appearance of vitreal opacity	Possible aetiologies
Greyish strand attached to posterior of lens snaking into vitreous, in some instances it may reach as far as the optic disc and will occasionally be blood filled	Remnant of hyaloid artery (not usually of clinical significance) (Fig. 104.1). A tiny hyaloid tag attached to the posterior lens at Mittendorf's dot can be seen in normal dogs (magnification is required)
Spherical thin-walled, semitransparent structure suspended in vitreous	These are cysts and are uncommon: Pigmented cysts probably arise from the ciliary body Grey coloured cysts probably represent hyaloid remnants
Appearance of blood in vitreous	Haemorrhage from retinal or anomalous vessels: Trauma Retinal detachment Systemic hypertension Neoplasia Coagulopathies Leakage from anomalous vessels
Grey membrane with surface blood vessels	A detached retina
Whitish membrane without surface vessels	Cyclitic membrane (may follow inflammation involving pars plana)
White, reflective, 'spots' suspended in vitreous	Asteroid hyalosis – commonly seen as an ageing change
Glittering whitish vitreal deposits combined with liquefaction of the vitreous – allowing the deposits to gravitate ventrally	Synchisis scintillans. An uncommon degenerative condition of vitreous. May follow vitreal inflammation or haemorrhage
Inflammatory material within vitreous – varies from a hazy appearing vitreous to accumulation of white purulent material	Endophthalmitis (bacterial or fungal) Penetrating wounds Intraocular foreign bodies Neoplasia such as lymphoma may result in accumulation of neoplastic cells in the vitreous

Vitreal Degeneration and Detachment

Liquefaction (syneresis) of the vitreous is a common degenerative process. Detachment of the vitreous face from the retinal surface (detectable by ultrasonography) can lead to retinal traction and detachment. Liquefied vitreous can pass through any retinal tears and holes to reach the sub-retinal space and will prevent any possibility of spontaneous reattachment.

FURTHER READING

Curtis, R., Barnett, K.C. & Leon, A. (1991). Diseases of the canine posterior segment. In: *Veterinary Ophthalmology*, (ed. K.N. Gelatt), 2nd edn. pp. 461–525. Lea and Febiger, Philapdelphia.

Leon, A. (1993). Conditions of the vitreous. In: *Manual of Small Animal Ophthalmology*, (eds S.M. Petersen-Jones & S.M. Crispin), pp. 229–235. BSAVA Publications, Cheltenham.

Chapter 105

Conditions of the Fundus

S. Petersen-Jones

ANATOMY AND PHYSIOLOGY OF THE FUNDUS

The function of the rest of the anterior part of the eye is to deliver a focused image on to the photoreceptor cells where the message is converted to an electrical signal by photo-transduction. The electrical information generated is conveyed to bipolar cells and hence on to ganglion cells, the axons of which form the optic nerve and transmit visual information to higher centres. Considerable integration of information occurs within the inner retina, with various types of cell being involved. Fig. 105.1 shows the anatomical structures of the posterior segment. It should be noted that photoreceptors point outwards with the tips of their outer segments enveloped by processes of the retinal pigment epithelial cells which phagocytose spent outer segment material. This interaction is important for the function and continued health of the photoreceptor cells. The two main classes of photoreceptor play different roles, rods are sensitive and responsible for vision in poor lighting conditions while cones function under brighter lighting conditions and provide some degree of colour vision to the dog (Miller & Murphy 1995).

The choroid lies outside the retina and has a high blood flow and is usually darkly pigmented (although pigmentation may be lacking in some individuals) and is important for the supply of nutrients and oxygen. Tight junctions in the vascular endothelium and the retinal pigment epithelium (RPE) limits the size of molecule that can reach the retina (the blood:retinal barrier) conferring immuno-privilege to the retina. Breakdown of this barrier occurs in inflammatory conditions. Within the tapetal area of the fundus (typically a triangular area in the dorsal portion of the fundus) a tapetal layer is present within the inner choroid, a lack of pigment in the RPE cells allows ophthal-moscopic visualisation of the reflective coloured tapetum. The tapetum is very useful clinically because its reflective nature aids detection of thinning or thickening of the overlying layers (i.e. the retina). Thinning results in increased reflection of light while thickening diminishes the reflection.

The term fundus describes the structures that can be seen ophthalmoscopically at the posterior of the eye and includes:

- optic nerve head,
- retina (including retinal pigment epithelium),
- superficial retinal vasculature,
- choroid underlying the retina – including in the tapetal area the tapetum,
- in some instances the underlying sclera may be visible.

Examination of the fundus is described on pages 956–957.

FUNCTIONAL INVESTIGATIONS

The overall visual abilities of an animal may be assessed by vision testing as described in Chapter 97. Electroretino-graphy allows detailed investigation of retinal function and can detect retinal dysfunction before any noticeable effect on vision or development of ophthalmoscopic changes. The technique involves stimulating the retinal photo-receptors with a flash, or flashes, of light and measuring the resulting electrical activity usually via a corneal contact lens with an in-built electrode. By using different lighting intensities, differing wavelengths of light or repeated flashes of light of selected frequencies it is possible to individually assess rod and cone function (Acland 1988; Narfström et al. 1995).

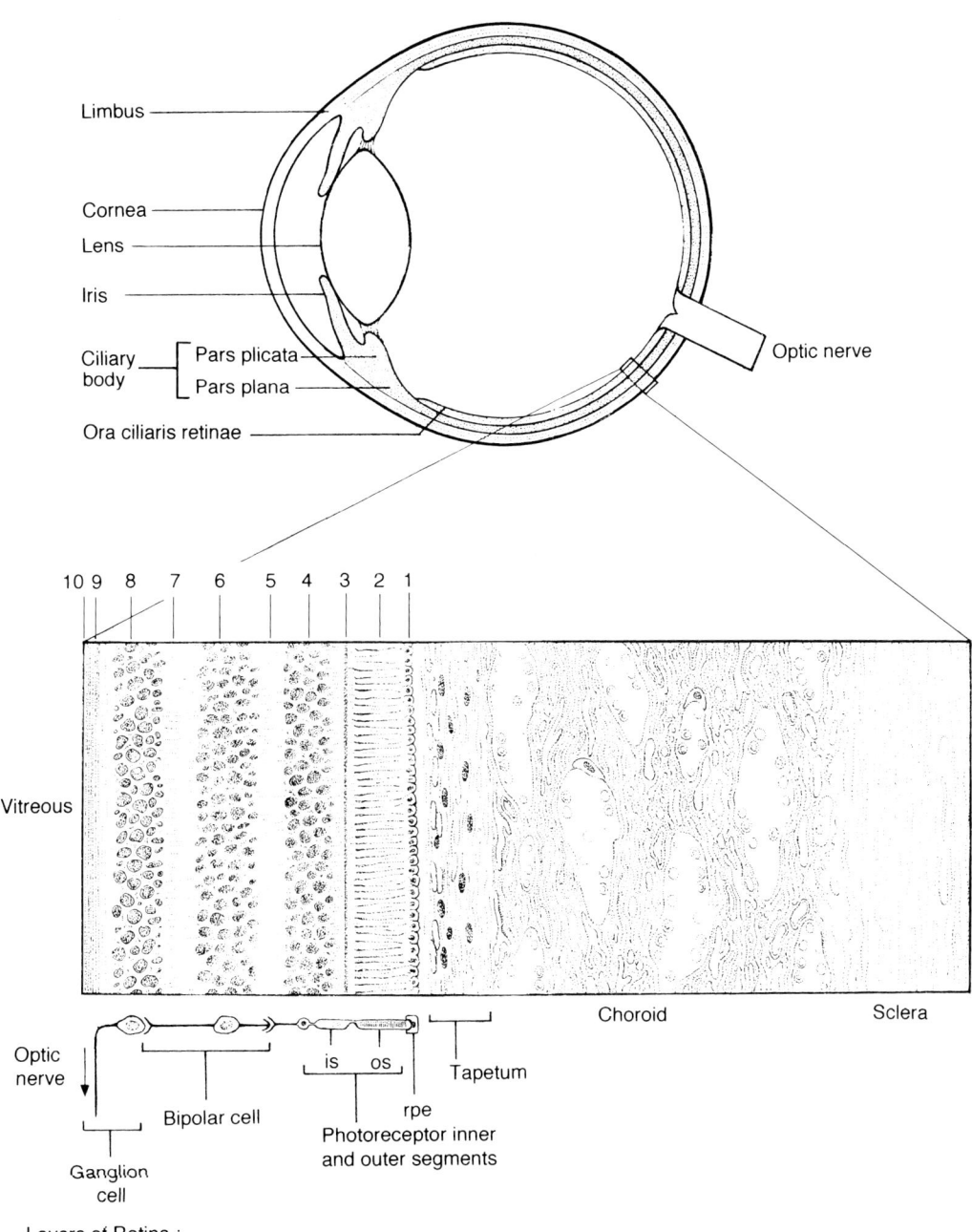

Fig. 105.1   Diagram of a cross section through an eye with detail of the posterior segment structures.

NORMAL APPEARANCE OF THE FUNDUS

The appearance of the normal fundus varies considerably between individual dogs. This wide range of normality must be appreciated before abnormality can be detected (Table 105.1, Figs 105.2–105.6).

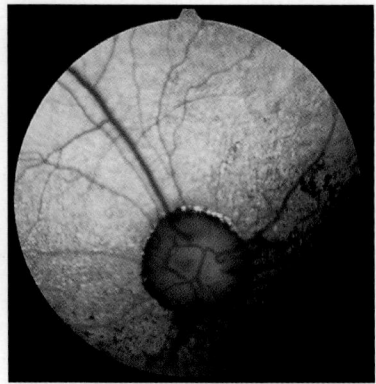

Fig. 105.4 Normal canine fundus. Note the round optic disc with a narrow zone of increased tapetal reflection partly around the disc (this is known as conus and is normal). The tapetum is orange/yellow in this dog.

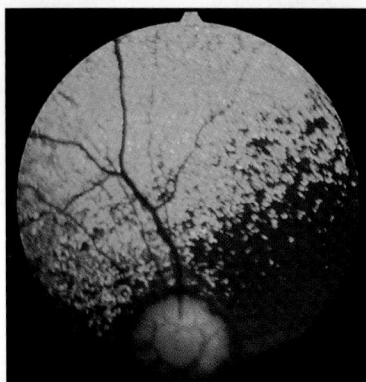

Fig. 105.2 Normal canine fundus. Note the roughly circular shape of the optic disc and the blue/green tapetal colour with a gradual transition to non-tapetal fundus.

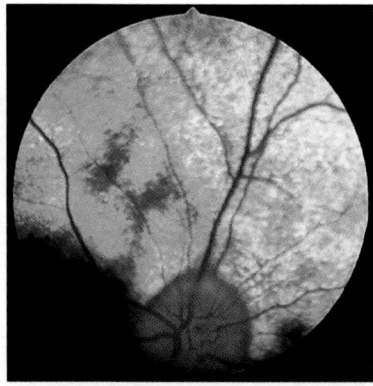

Fig. 105.5 Normal canine fundus. Note the irregular coloration of the tapetum (due to variations in the thickness of the tapetal layer).

CONDITIONS OF THE FUNDUS

There is a wide spectrum of diseases which may affect the fundus of the eye but in dogs inherited disease is common. Conditions may be congenital or acquired, may reflect primary disease or be associated with systemic disorders. The commonest external sign of retinal disease is a loss of vision.

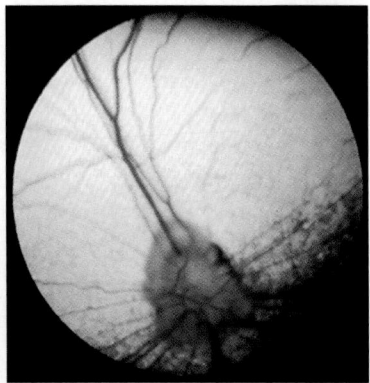

Fig. 105.3 Normal canine fundus. Note the triangular shape to the optic disc (due to myelination of nerve fibres extending further than in Fig. 105.2) and yellow tapetal colour.

Table 105.1   Normal appearance of the canine fundus.

Feature	Range of appearances (Figs 105.2–105.6)
Optic nerve head (disc)	• *Position* – just ventromedial to posterior pole, tapetal/non-tapetal junction usually close to to disc • *Shape* – circular to triangular, may be irregular, surface slightly raised, often with a central dip (physiological pit) • *Colour* – pinkish white. White colour due to myelination and pink due to blood vessels • *Surface vasculature*. Pattern varies, may be a partial or complete vascular ring visible on the surface. Retinal vasculature travels over part of the disc and radiates out from disc periphery
Tapetal fundus	Tapetal area may be reduced (particularly in miniature breeds) or even absent (e.g. often in colour-dilute individuals). Not present at birth but develops in the first 3 months of life. • *Position*. The tapetum occupies the area of the fundus just dorsal to the disc, but does not extend to the ora ciliaris retinae • *Shape*. Roughly triangular, may vary in extent. The junction with the non-tapetal area may be sharply demarcated or irregular with islands of tapetal tissue being seen in the non-tapetal area • *Colour*. Varies between grey, blue, reddish, green and yellow. Developing tapetum first appears blue in colour and then slowly develops adult coloration
Non-tapetal fundus	This describes the entire retinal area which does not have an underlying tapetum. • *Colour*. Typically dark greyish brown to black in colour. A slight mottling in pigmentation is common and should be distinguished from depigmentation resulting from pathological processes. Some animals (often those with a light coloured iris) have reduced or even absent pigmentation in the choroid and retinal pigment epithelium. This results in a reddish non-tapetal fundus or even a 'tigroid' appearance due to choroidal blood vessels superimposed on a background of sclera
Superficial retinal vasculature	Consist of arterioles and venules. • Arterioles numbering up to 20 are smaller and radiate from the edge of the disc • The major venules (approximately three to six) come together to form a venous circle on or within the substance of the optic disc The pattern of the vessels varies as does their tortuosity

Tables 105.2 and 105.3 display disorders that cause vision loss in young dogs and middle-aged or older dogs respectively.

Collie Eye Anomaly (CEA)

• Congenital
• Inherited – ? autosomal recessive (Yakely *et al.* 1968)
• Collie breeds affected (similar lesions reported in other breeds) – high incidence in Rough and Smooth Collies and Shetland Sheepdogs, low incidence in Border Collies

The condition is manifest as characteristic bilateral, but not necessarily symmetrical ophthalmoscopic lesions (Bedford 1982):

• *Choroidal hypoplasia* (CH) – this is considered to be the diagnostic lesion. It is a variable sized area of abnormal choroid adjacent and lateral to optic disc (Figs 105.7–105.9). The affected area has reduced pigmentation allowing visualisation of abnormal choroidal blood vessels and often underlying sclera. CH is clearly seen in young puppies 6–8 weeks of age. Pigment deposition after this age may partially or completely mask the lesion resulting in the so called 'go normal' dog which is

Table 105.2   Posterior segment disease capable of causing visual loss in young dogs.

Condition	Features

Collie eye anomaly	Collie breeds (see below for details)
	Vision loss due to:
	    Large optic disc coloboma
	    Retinal detachment
	    Intraocular haemorrhage (often associated with retinal
	      detachment)

Total vitreoretinal dysplasia	Inherited forms are breed specific Retinal detachment/non-attachment
Multifocal retinal dysplasia	Some affected dogs develop retinal detachment, others have large areas of retinal abnormality. Most cases show little or no visual disturbance
Optic nerve hypoplasia	Abnormally small optic disc
Early-onset generalised progressive retinal atrophy	Uncommon in the general pet population. Includes rod–cone dysplasia type 1 in Irish Setters
Posterior uveitis or retinitis	See page 1026 for a description

Table 105.3   Posterior segment disease capable of causing vision loss in middle-aged or older dogs.

Condition	Features
Progressive retinal atrophy (PRA) (generalised)	An inherited primary photoreceptor disease Reported in a large number of breeds world-wide Several different forms recognised Age of onset and rate of progression varies between and within forms of PRA Ophthalmoscopic signs between different forms are similar – see below
Sudden acquired retinal degeneration	Cause of a rapid bilateral loss of vision associated with dilated, non-responsive pupils and initially little or no ophthalmoscopically detectable retinal pathology

Retinal pigment epithelial dystrophy (central progressive retinal atrophy)	Probably due to an inherited predisposition combined with environmental factors
	    Recognised in a number of breeds, predominantly occurs in the UK
	    Incidence reduced recently
	    Characteristic fundus lesions
	    May not result in total vision loss

Retinal detachment	Inflammatory Neoplastic Vascular hypertension Idiopathic
Posterior uveitis or retinitis	See page 1026 for a description

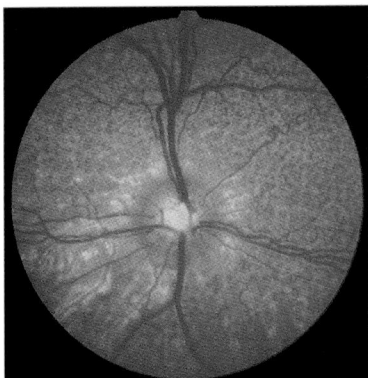

Fig. 105.6 Normal canine fundus. Note the lack of tapetum and reduced pigmentation giving a reddish fundus coloration. In some areas the white of sclera can be seen.

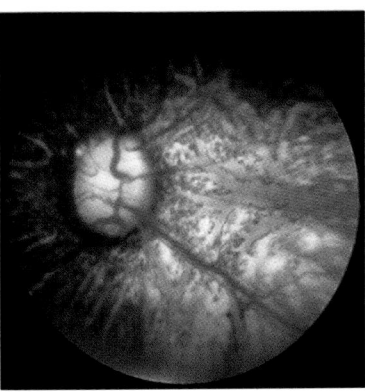

Fig. 105.8 Collie eye anomaly. Choroidal hypoplasia is present lateral to the disc. There are abnormally shaped choroidal vessels against a background of sclera.

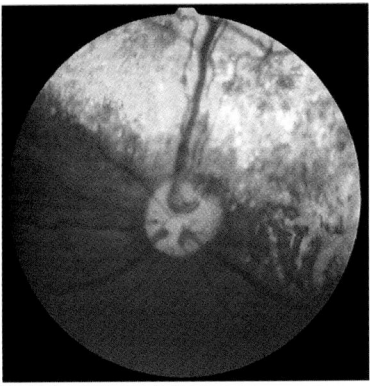

Fig. 105.7 Collie eye anomaly. Left eye of a collie puppy. An area of choroidal hypoplasia can be seen lateral to the disc. The affected area lacks tapetum and there is reduced pigmentation. Abnormally shaped choroidal vessels can be seen as can sclera in some areas.

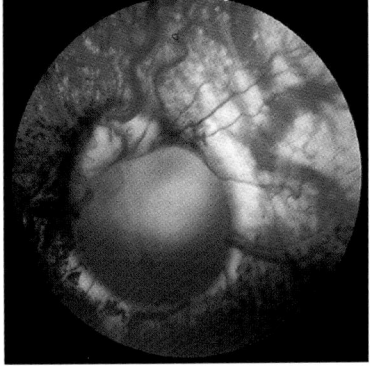

Fig. 105.9 Collie eye anomaly. In addition to the area of choroidal hypoplasia lateral to the disc there is a large coloboma affecting the disc.

obviously still genetically affected but may appear ophthalmoscopically normal. The incidence of 'go normal' is unknown but some authors report a high incidence (Bjerkås 1991).
- *Coloboma* – this is a defect which is only present in a proportion of CEA affected dogs. It is a lack of tissue which results in the occurrence of a pit of variable size involving the optic disc or adjacent fundus (Fig. 105.9). Large colobomas may, if they involve the disc, be associated with reduced vision or may predispose to retinal detachment.

- *Blindness* – due to *intra-ocular haemorrhage* and/or *retinal detachment* develop in a low percentage of affected dogs. It is unusual for this to be bilateral.

There are difficulties in diagnosing CEA in colour-dilute animals which have reduced fundus pigmentation making recognition of mild choroidal hypoplasia difficult. The 'go normal' can also lead to misdiagnosis.

Clinical Presentation

Affected dogs range from having apparently normal vision to being blind in one or occasionally both eyes. Vision loss affects a small percentage of dogs with CEA and results from either retinal detachment and/or intra-ocular haemorrhage. These occur most commonly in the first year of life.

Management

There is no treatment for CEA. The incidence can be reduced by participating in hereditary eye screening schemes and ensuring that puppies are screened at 6–8 weeks thus avoiding problems in diagnosis due to pigment masking the choroidal hypoplasia lesions.

Vitreoretinal Dysplasia (Total Retinal Dysplasia)

Retinal dysplasia may be inherited or result from an *in utero* insult. Vitreoretinal dysplasia leads to blindness in young puppies due to retinal non-attachment or detachment (Ashton *et al.* 1968; Rubin 1968; Blair *et al.* 1985). In some forms there are also other ocular abnormalities such as microphthalmos and cataracts, or abnormalities elsewhere in the body, e.g. cardiac or skeletal abnormalities as described in affected Labrador Retrievers (Barnett *et al.* 1970; Carrig *et al.* 1977).

Multifocal Retinal Dysplasia (MRD)

This is by far the commonest form of retinal dysplasia. Lesions vary from focal areas with duplication of one or more layers of the retina to larger areas of retinal degeneration with choroidal involvement. Focal or complete retinal detachment occurs in a small percentage of the more severely affected dogs. Autosomal recessive inheritance has been proven in some breeds. Breeds most commonly affected in the UK include English Springer Spaniel, American Cocker Spaniel and Cavalier King Charles Spaniel.

Lesions of MRD are most commonly situated in the tapetal fundus among the dorsal superficial retinal blood vessels. They may appear as bars, vermiform streaks or linear branching lesions which are darker than the surrounding tapetal area and may themselves be surrounded by a zone of hyper-reflectivity (Fig. 105.10). English Springer Spaniels have a potentially more serious form of retinal dysplasia in which areas of retinal degeneration develop (Lavach *et al.* 1978; O'Toole *et al.* 1983). These areas are characterised by zones of retinal thinning and resultant tapetal hyper-reflectivity and pigment proliferation, looking not dissimilar to post-inflammatory lesions (Fig. 105.11). Retinal detachment may occur in the more severely affected Springer Spaniels as may secondary cataract.

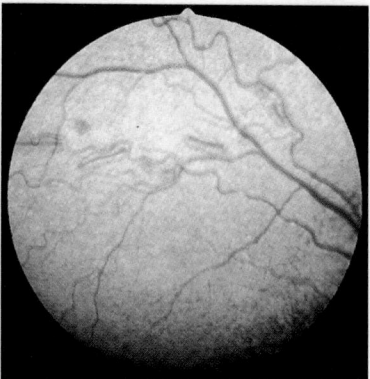

Fig. 105.10 Multifocal retinal dysplasia in a Cavalier King Charles Spaniel. The lesions appear as dark blue bars with a reflective peripheral zone and are positioned among the dorsal retinal blood vessels.

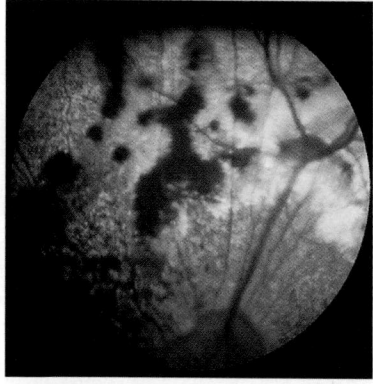

Fig. 105.11 Multifocal retinal dysplasia in an English Springer Spaniel. There are extensive areas of tapetal hyper-reflectivity with change in tapetal colour and dark pigment deposition. The lesions are typically positioned among the retinal blood vessels dorsal to the disc.

Clinical Presentation

Affected animals typically have no detectable visual deficits unless larger areas of retinal degeneration develop or the retina detaches.

Management

Treatment is not possible, but hereditary eye disease screening schemes should be used to try and avoid breeding from affected animals and relatives which may be potential carriers. The possible presence of retinal dysplasia should be remembered in English Springer Spaniels presenting for cataract extraction as retinal detachment appears to be common following cataract surgery in such cases.

Generalised Progressive Retinal Atrophy (gPRA)

gPRA is a common hereditary cause of blindness in pedigree dogs. Over 100 breeds are reported to suffer from it world-wide (Whitley *et al.* 1995) but in only a few of these has it been studied in any detail. Investigations have shown that there are several distinct genetic forms of gPRA all of which, with the exception of one X-linked form (Acland *et al.* 1994), are inherited in an autosomal recessive manner. The clinical signs and ophthalmoscopic changes are similar between the forms, although the age of onset and rate of progression vary both between and within the different forms.

Clinical Signs

The condition is bilateral and symmetrical.

- *Visual loss.* Deteriorating vision under dim lighting conditions (nyctalopia) is usually the first detectable sign. As the disease progresses day vision also deteriorates and eventual blindness is inevitable.
- *Reduced pupillary light responses.* The pupillary responses are reduced and as the disease progresses the pupils appear relatively dilated and poorly responsive. This may be noted by observant owners.
- *Secondary cataract formation.* Progressive cortical cataracts commonly develop secondary to gPRA. In some of the later-onset forms this may be the first change that the owner notices and is often thought by them to be the cause of the loss of vision.
- *Ophthalmoscopic changes* (Figs 105.12 & 105.13) – usually bilaterally symmetrical.
  - *Tapetal hyper-reflectivity.* A generalised hyper-reflectivity over the tapetal fundus due to retinal thinning is a typical finding. Initial changes are of a granular appearance of the tapetal fundus particularly adjacent to the peripheral tapetal border. This progresses to result in a uniform tapetal hyper-reflectivity. Some forms of gPRA have been described where a more prominent band of hyper-reflectivity above the ventral tapetal/ non-tapetal junction is a feature (Kommonen *et al.* 1995).

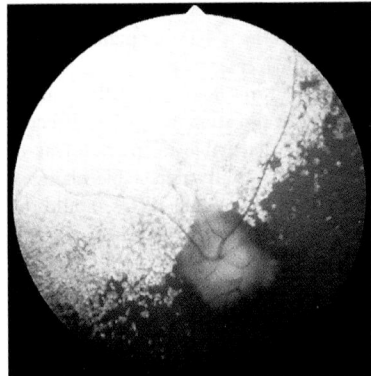

Fig. 105.12 Generalised progressive retinal atrophy in a Toy Poodle. There is tapetal hyper-reflectivity, superficial retinal blood vessel attenuation and optic atrophy.

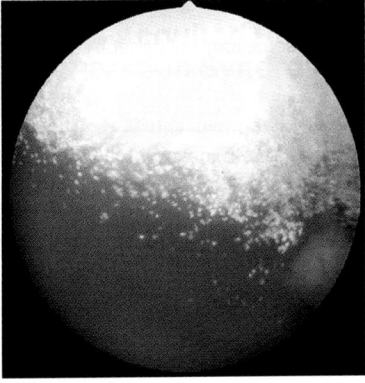

Fig. 105.13 Generalised progressive retinal atrophy in a Toy Poodle. There is very pronounced tapetal hyper-reflectivity, the superficial retinal blood vessels are no longer visible and there is marked optic atrophy.

Owners sometimes notice an increased reflection from their pet's eyes which is due to a combination of abnormally dilated pupils and tapetal hyper-reflectivity.
  - *Superficial retinal blood vessel attenuation.* The reduced requirements of the dying retina for a blood supply are reflected in the attenuation of retinal blood vessels. Small blood vessels are lost from view first and as the disease advances larger vessels appear noticeably thinned.
  - *Pigmentary changes in non-tapetal fundus.* As the retinal atrophy continues some pigmentary changes develop in the non-tapetal fundus giving a

Table 105.7   Aetiology of posterior segment haemorrhage.

Condition	Features
Congenital lesions	Collie eye anomaly Anomalous blood vessels PHPV/PHTVL
Retinal detachment	Tearing of retinal blood vessels at the time of detachment
Inflammatory disease	Posterior uveitis may be accompanied by haemorrhage, particularly when caused by fungal or rickettsial infections or parasitic infestations
Trauma	
Neoplasia or proliferative disease	Lymphoma probably the commonest neoplastic cause of haemorrhage Granulomatous meningioenecephalitis involving optic disc and adjacent retina
Systemic disorders	Coagulopathies (including poisoning) Hypertension Gammaglobulinopathy Severe anaemia Systemic causes of posterior uveitis

PHPV/PHTVL, persistent hyperplastic primary vitreous/persistent tonica vasculosa leutis.

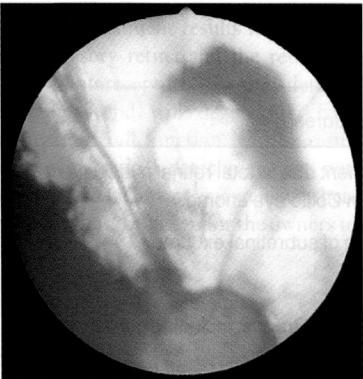

Fig. 105.19   Hypertensive retinopathy in a West Highland White Terrier with chronic renal failure. Extensive retinal and preretinal haemorrhages can be seen through a rather hazy vitreous.

- subretinal and retinal haemorrhages varying from focal to widespread,
- retinal detachment,
- papilloedema.

Early recognition and treatment of the hypertension is required to prevent progression of the ocular changes.

Lipaemia Retinalis (Lane *et al*. 1993)

The appearance of pale creamy coloured retinal vasculature due to gross abnormalities in circulating lipids.

Gammaglobulinopathies (Lane *et al*. 1993)

Serum hyperviscosity syndrome resulting from conditions such as multiple myelomas are reflected in the retinal vasculature. The following changes may result (Fig. 105.20):

- dilation of retinal vasculature (sludging of blood in veins),
- retinal haemorrhage,
- retinal oedema,
- serous retinal detachments.

Posterior Segment Neoplasia

Primary tumours are rare although choroidal melanomas have been reported.

Metastatic spread to the eye of a number of different tumour types has been reported and may involve the posterior segment. Lymphoma is the commonest metastatic tumour involving the eye. The anterior segment is most commonly affected with hyphaema and hypopyon.

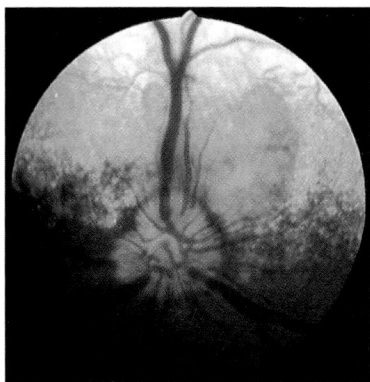

Fig. 105.20   Hyperviscosity syndrome in a dog with multiple myeloma. Note the dilated retinal blood vessels and the area of retinal detachment dorsal to the optic disc.

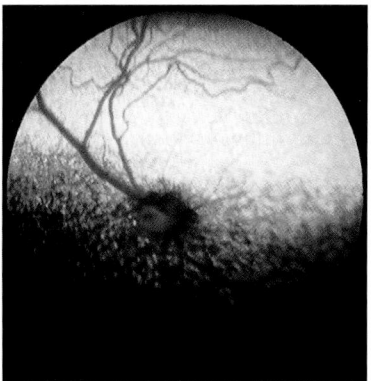

Fig. 105.21   Optic nerve hypoplasia in a Miniature Poodle. The affected eye was blind, but the other eye appeared normal.

Posterior involvement may result in retinal and pre-retinal haemorrhage.

Ultrasonography can be useful for investigating an eye where ophthalmoscopic examination of the posterior segment is hampered by anterior changes.

Conditions Involving the Optic Nerve Head

Congenital Conditions

Optic Nerve Colobomas
These appear as pits involving part or all of the optic nerve head. They are seen most commonly as part of Collie eye anomaly (Fig. 105.9). There may be an accompanying adjacent retinal detachment or in some instances there are associated anomalous blood vessels which may haemorrhage.

Optic Nerve Hypoplasia (Kern & Riis 1981)
Hypoplasia of the optic nerve is reflected in the optic nerve head which appears abnormally small, making the superficial retinal blood vessels look large in comparison (Fig. 105.21). The condition may be unilateral or bilateral and the affected eye is usually blind with an absence of direct pupillary light response. Some less severely affected dogs may just have abnormally small discs, visual impairment and reduced pupillary light responses.

Acquired Conditions

Papillitis
Papillitis is the result of an optic neuritis which extends to involve the optic nerve head. Optic neuritis can also occur

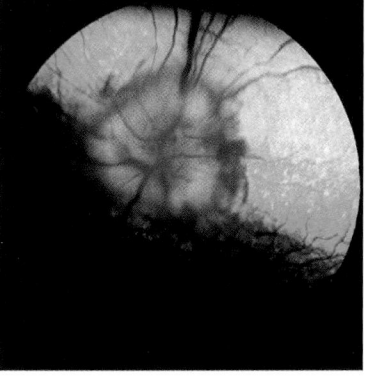

Fig. 105.22   Papillitis. There is swelling of the affected disc accompanied by haemorrhages. The peripapillary retina is also affected.

at sufficient distance from the optic nerve head to leave it grossly unaffected in which case the diagnosis can be more difficult (see Chapter 106).

Clinical Presentation and Signs of Papillitis (Fig. 105.22)

- Often bilateral
- Sudden-onset blindness
- Dilated fixed or sluggish pupils
- Disc enlarged and elevated
- Vascular engorgement of disc, possibly accompanied by haemorrhages

- Peripapillary retinal oedema (reduced fundus reflection) and possibly haemorrhages

Aetiology of Papillitis

- Infections (prevalence of the fungal agents varies from area to area):
  - distemper
  - cryptococcosis
  - blastomycosis
  - histoplasmosis
  - toxoplasmosis
- Non-infective causes:
  - granulomatous meningioencephalitis
  - idiopathic

Despite a complete blood screen and serology the aetiology of many cases remains obscure.

Management of Papillitis

- Initially give high level of systemic corticosteroids.
- Monitor vision and pupillary light reflex.
- Reduce corticosteroids gradually after one week to maintenance dose.
- Monitor for recurrence as medication is reduced – may need to keep on maintenance therapy.

Papilloedema

True papilloedema is a non-inflammatory swelling of the optic disc (Fig. 105.23) which does not affect vision. Most commonly in dogs it is seen as a result of a CNS tumour, for example impinging on the chiasm or involving the retrobulbar portion of the optic nerve. In such cases the presence of the tumour may cause a loss of vision. Papilloedema has also been described in dogs suffering from pancreatitis. Differences in ocular blood supply between humans and dogs means that in dogs papilloedema is not necessarily indicative of raised cerebrospinal fluid pressure as it is in man. Management is aimed at identifying the causal lesion and treating if possible.

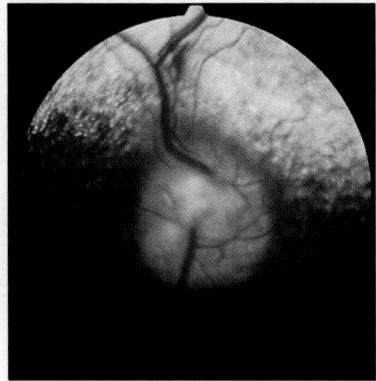

Fig. 105.23   Papilloedema. The optic disc was very swollen and could be seen on indirect ophthalmoscopy to be protruding into the vitreous. There is a small retinal haemorrhage dorsal to the disc. Both eyes were affected but the dog was visual. A CNS CT scan was unremarkable. The dog had pancreatitis.

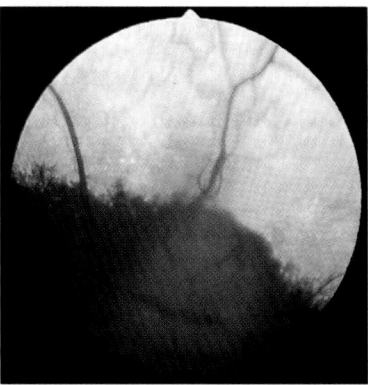

Fig. 105.24   Optic atrophy. The disc is very grey and flat as a result of demyelination and has a rather indistinct outline. This followed optic neuritis and was accompanied by retinal degeneration.

Condition	Features
Extensive retinal disease	Generalised progressive retinal atrophy (PRA) Sudden acquired retinal degeneration syndrome (SARDS) Extensive inflammation
Other intraocular disease	Chronic glaucoma (causes cupping and atrophy)
Optic nerve disease	Inflammation Trauma Neoplasia

Table 105.8   Aetiology of optic atrophy.

Optic Atrophy

Atrophy of the optic nerve head has several potential causes (see Table 105.8). The atrophied optic nerve head appears a pallid grey-colour, is flatter, smaller and possibly more rounded than before (Fig. 105.24). This appearance is due to a reduced blood supply and a loss of myelinated nerve fibres.

REFERENCES

Acland, G.M. (1988). Diagnosis and differentiation of retinal disease in small animals by electroretinography. *Seminars in Veterinary Medicine and Surgery (Small Animal)*, 3, 15–27.

Acland, G.M., Blanton, S.H., Hershfield, B. & Aguirre, G.D. (1994). Xlpra: a canine retinal degeneration inherited as an x-linked trait. *American Journal of Medical Genetics*, 52, 27–33.

Aguirre, G.D. & Acland, G.M. (1983). Progressive retinal atrophy in the English cocker spaniel. *Transactions of the American College of Veterinary Ophthalmologists*, 14, 104.

Aguirre, G.D. & Acland, G.M. (1988). Variation in retinal degeneration phenotype inherited at the prcd locus. *Experimental Eye Research*, 46, 663–687.

Aguirre, G.D. & Acland, G.M. (1989). Progressive retinal atrophy in the Labrador retriever is a progressive rod–cone degeneration (PRCD). *Transactions of the American College of Veterinary Ophthalmologists*, 20, 150.

Aguirre, G.D., Alligood, J., O'Brien, P. & Buyukmihci, N. (1982). Pathogenesis of progressive rod–cone degeneration in miniature poodles. *Investigative Ophthalmology and Visual Science*, 23, 610–630.

Ashton, N., Barnett, K.C. & Sachs, D.D. (1968). Retinal dysplasia in the Sealyham terrier. *Journal of Pathology and Bacteriology*, 96, 269–272.

Barnett, K.C. (1965). Canine retinopathies, II. The miniature and toy poodle. *Journal of Small Animal Practice*, 6, 93–109.

Barnett, K.C. (1969). Central progressive retinal atrophy in the Labrador retriever. *Veterinary Annual*, 17, 142–144.

Barnett, K.C., Bjorck, G.R. & Kock, E. (1970). Hereditary retinal dysplasia in the Labrador retriever in England and Sweden. *Journal of Small Animal Practice*, 10, 755–759.

Bedford, P.G.C. (1982). Collie eye anomaly in the United Kingdom. *Veterinary Record*, 111, 263–270.

Bjerkås, E. (1991). Collie eye anomaly in the rough collie in Norway. *Journal of Small Animal Practice*, 32, 89–92.

Blair, N.P., Dodge, J.T. & Schmidt, G.M. (1985). Rhegmatogenous retinal detachment in Labrador retrievers I. Development of retinal tears and detachment. *Archives of Ophthalmology*, 103, 842–847.

Bussanich, M.N., Rootman, J. & Dolman, C.L. (1982). Granulomatous pan uveitis and dermal depigmentation in dogs. *Journal of the American Animal Hospital Association*, 18, 131–138.

Carrig, C.B., MacMillan, A., Brundage, S., Pool, R.R. & Morgan, J.P. (1977). Retinal dysplasia associated with skeletal abnormalities in Labrador retrievers. *Journal of the American Veterinary Medical Association*, 170, 49–57.

Clements, P.J.M., Gregory, C.Y., Petersen-Jones, S.M., Sargan, D.R. & Bhattacharya, S.S. (1993). Confirmation of the rod cGMP phosphodiesterase beta-subunit (PDEbeta) nonsense mutation in affected rcd-1 Irish setters in the UK and development of a diagnostic test. *Current Eye Research*, 12, 861–866.

Curtis, R. & Barnett, K.C. (1993). Progressive retinal atrophy in miniature longhaired dachshund dogs. *British Veterinary Journal*, 149, 71–85.

Dziezyc, J., Wolf, E.D. & Barrie, K.P. (1986). Surgical repair of rhegmatogenous detachments in dogs. *Journal of the American Veterinary Medical Association*, 188, 902–904.

Håkanson, N. & Forrester, S.D. (1990). Uveitis in the dog and cat. *Veterinary Clinics of North America (Small Animal Practice)*, 20, 715–735.

Hendrix, D.V., Nasisse, M.P., Cowen, P. & Davidson, M.G. (1993). Clinical signs, concurrent diseases, and risk factors associated with retinal detachment in dogs. *Progress in Veterinary and Comparative Ophthalmology*, 3, 87–91.

Kern, T.J. & Riis, R.C. (1981). Optic nerve hypoplasia in three miniature poodles. *Journal of the American Veterinary Medical Association*, 178, 49–54.

Kommonen, B., Karhunen, U., Kylmä, T., Dawson, W.W. & Penn, J.S. (1995). Impaired retinal function in young Labrador retrievers heterozygous for late-onset rod–cone degeneration. *Investigative Ophthalmology and Visual Science (Supplement)*, 36, 4263.

Lane, I., Roberts, S.M. & Lappin, M.R. (1993). Ocular manifestations of vascular disease: hypertension, hyperviscosity, and hyperlipidemia. *Journal of the American Animal Hospital Association*, 29, 28–36.

Lavach, J.D., Murphy, J.M. & Severin, G.A. (1978). Retinal dysplasia in the English springer spaniel. *Journal of the American Animal Hospital Association*, 14, 192–199.

Miller, P.E. & Murphy, C.J. (1995). Vision in dogs. *Journal of the American Veterinary Medical Association*, 207, 1623–1634.

Millichamp, N.J., Curtis, R. & Barnett, K.C. (1988). Progressive retinal atrophy in Tibetan terriers. *Journal of the American Veterinary Medical Association*, 192, 769–776.

Narfström, K., Andersson, B-E., Andreasson, S. & Gouras, P. (1995). Clinical electroretinography in the dog using Ganzfeld stimulation: A practical method of examining rod and cone function. *Documenta Ophthalmologica*, 90, 279–290.

O'Toole, D.O., Young, S., Severin, G.A. & Neuman, S. (1983). Retinal dysplasia of English springer spaniels dogs: Light microscopy of the postnatal lesions. *Veterinary Pathology*, 20, 298–311.

O'Toole, D., Roberts, S. & Nunamaker, C. (1992). Sudden acquired retinal degeneration ('silent retina syndrome') in two dogs. *Veterinary Record*, 130, 157–161.

Parshall, C.J., Wyman, M., Nitroy, S., Acland, G. & Aguirre, G. (1991). Photoreceptor dysplasia: An inherited progressive retinal atrophy of miniature schnauzer dogs. *Progress in Veterinary and Comparative Ophthalmology*, **1**, 187–203.

Petersen-Jones, S.M., Clements, P.J.M., Barnett, K.C. & Sargan, D.R. (1995). Incidence of the gene mutation causal for rod-cone dysplasia type 1 in Irish setters in the UK. *Journal of Small Animal Practice*, **36**, 310–314.

Riis, R.C. (1990). EM observations of a SARD case. *Transactions of the American College of Veterinary Ophthalmologists*, **21**, 112–113.

Riis, R.C., Sheffy, B.E., Loew, E., Kern, T.J. & Smith, J.S. (1981). Vitamin E deficiency retinopathy in dogs. *American Journal of Veterinary Research*, **42**, 74–86.

Rubin, L.F. (1968). Heredity of retinal dysplasia in Bedlington terriers. *Journal of the American Veterinary Medical Association*, **152**, 260–262.

Suber, M.L., Pittler, S.J., Quin, N., *et al.* (1993). Irish setter dogs affected with rod-cone dysplasia contain a nonsense mutation in the rod cGMP phosphodiesterase beta-subunit gene. *Proceedings of the National Academy of Science of the USA*, **90**, 3968–3972.

Whitley, R.D., McLaughlin, S.A. & Gilger, B.C. (1995). Update on eye disorders among purebred dogs. *Veterinary Medicine*, **90**, 574–592.

Wilkie, D.A. (1990). Control of ocular inflammation. *Veterinary Clinics of North America (Small Animal Practice)*, **20**, 693–713.

van der Woerdt, A., Nasisse, M.P. & Davidson, M.G. (1991). Sudden acquired retinal degeneration in the dog: Clinical and laboratory findings in 36 cases. *Progress in Veterinary and Comparative Ophthalmology*, **1**, 11–18.

Wrigstad, A., Nilsson, S.E.G., Dubielzig, R. & Narfström, K. (1995). Neuronal ceroid lipofuscinosis in the Polish Owczarek Nizinny (PON) dog. *Documenta Ophthalmologica*, **91**, 33–47.

Yakely, W.L., Wyman, M., Donovan, E.F. & Fechheimer, N. (1968). Genetic transmission of an ocular fundus anomaly in collies. *Journal of the American Veterinary Medical Association*, **152**, 457–461.

Chapter 106

Neuro-Ophthalmology

S. Petersen-Jones

CENTRAL BLINDNESS

Central blindness results from lesions of the central visual pathways and the visual cortex. In addition to loss of vision, pupillary light reflexes may or may not be affected and ophthalmoscopically detectable fundus changes may develop in time. The presence or absence of these additional signs depends on the region of the visual pathway affected and the type of lesion present.

The following facts about the central visual pathway (CVP) (Fig. 106.1) and pupillary light reflex (PLR) (Fig. 106.2) should be appreciated:

- *The PLR is not an indicator of the ability to 'see'*. The nerve fibres that form the afferent portion of the PLR pathway diverge from the nerve fibres for conscious perception of vision before the lateral geniculate nucleus. Lesions distal to this divergence can affect one pathway without involving the other. The PLR will not be affected by lesions of the CVP at or distal to the lateral geniculate nucleus so it is possible for an animal to be blind and yet have a normal PLR. Conversely an absent PLR does not necessarily mean that the affected dog is blind.
- *Visual input from one side of the body projects to the contralateral visual cortex*, i.e. the lateral visual field of the left eye and medial field of the right eye project to the right visual cortex.
- *Unilateral lesions of the optic tract and more distal portions of the CVP cause a loss of vision to one side of the body and a greater loss of vision from the eye contralateral to the lesion*. This is because the majority of fibres in the optic nerve (75%) cross at the chiasm to form the major portion of the contralateral optic tract. The remaining 25% project to the ipsilateral visual cortex.

Investigation of a Dog Presenting with Apparent Central Blindness
(Scagliotti 1991; Petersen-Jones 1993)

Following the mandatory history taking, a full ophthalmoscopic examination should be performed; including vision testing (see page 955) and an assessment of pupillary function. Additionally a complete neurological examination is required.

Assessing the PLRs

When assessing the PLR the following facts should be remembered:

- On initial examination pupillary constriction is often sluggish. This is quite normal and is probably due to circulating adrenaline. Once the animal relaxes the pupillary responses should become brisker.
- It is normal to see some slight alterations in pupil size when a constant light is shone into an eye.

The first investigation of pupillary function involves even illumination of both eyes and is followed by differential illumination (Table 106.1).

Ophthalmoscopic Examination

Funduscopic changes may be apparent at the time of presentation or may develop later. Lesions resulting in ophthalmoscopically detectable changes at the time of presentation are considered in Chapter 105, e.g. optic nerve hypoplasia, coloboma of the optic disc, papillitis and papilloedema.

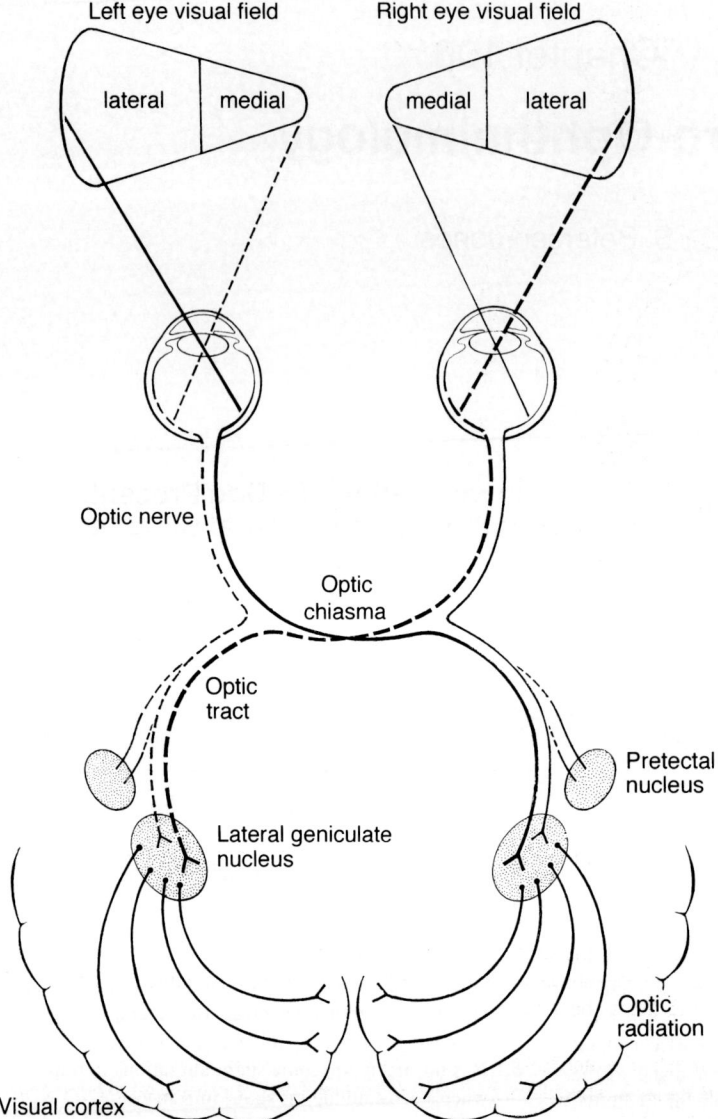

Fig. 106.1 Schematic representation of the central visual pathways (from Petersen-Jones 1993).

Extensive destruction of optic nerve or optic tract results in axonal death, eventually detectable as optic atrophy. The atrophied optic nerve head appears a pallid grey-colour, and is flatter and smaller than normal.

Electrodiagnostic Investigations

Electroretinography (ERG) is useful for assessing retinal function (see Chapter 105) and the cortical activity resulting from retinal stimulation may be investigated by measuring visual evoked potentials (VEPs). While ERG is a commonly used investigative tool in veterinary ophthalmology VEPs are more difficult to obtain and interpret therefore this technique has not achieved wide usage. In neuro-ophthalmology ERG is of particular use in investigating sudden-onset blindness and distinguishing between retinal and central causes.

Imaging

Imaging techniques may be useful (Table 106.2).

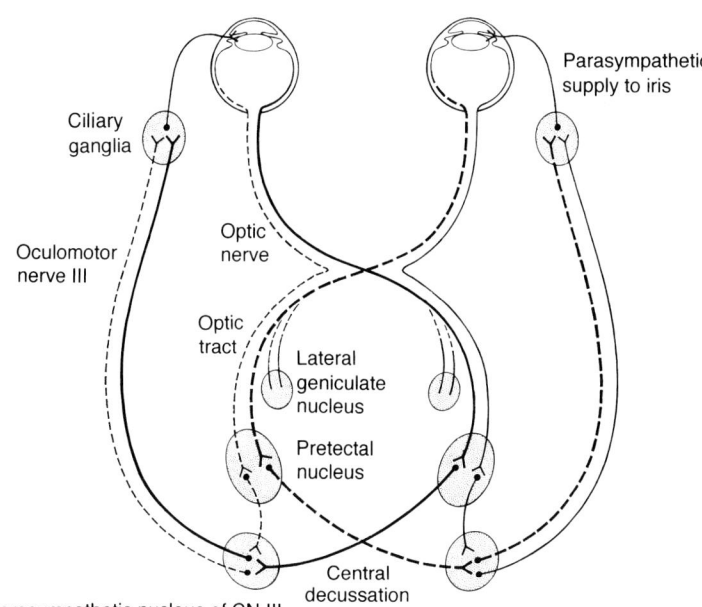

Fig. 106.2 Neuronal pathways for pupillary light reflex (from Petersen-Jones 1993).

Table 106.1 Assessment of pupillary function.

Pupil sizes under even illumination
- Do the pupils dilate fully and evenly in the dark?
- Are the pupils similar sizes when both eyes are evenly illuminated? (check this over a range of lighting intensities)

Pupil responses to differential illumination

Direct and consensual pupillary responses

In a darkened room shine a bright light into one eye, note the speed and extent of the pupillary constriction, also observe the response in the contralateral eye (consensual). The consensual response may be observed if there is sufficient background illumination, alternatively the swinging flashlight test may be used

Swinging flashlight test

(1) Shine light into first eye – note pupillary reaction (direct PLR)

(2) Quickly swing light across to the second eye, pupil should already be constricted (the consensual reflex) it will constrict slightly more under direct illumination (direct reflex)

(3) Finally swing light back to the original eye to observe consensual response from the contralateral eye, followed by the direct response again

---

Note: in dogs it is usual for the direct pupillary reflex to be slightly greater than the consensual reflex.

Laboratory Investigations

Depending on the possible differentials a variety of laboratory investigations may be indicated including haematology, blood biochemistry and serology.

Cerebrospinal fluid sampling may be useful for the investigation of certain CNS disorders.

Localising and Identifying Lesions Causing Central Blindness (Fig. 106.3)

The result of vision testing and the PLRs need to be considered together when trying to localise the lesion. When the PLR is absent and the pupils are dilated and non-responsive the lesion is likely to involve either retina, optic nerve or optic tract.

Retinal Disease

Sudden acquired retinal degeneration syndrome (SARDS) results in a rapid loss of vision (from overnight to over several days). The fundus initially looks normal. The presence of a 'flat' ERG is indicative of SARDS and distinguishes it from lesions of the optic nerves or tracts. SARDS is considered in more detail in Chapter 105.

Table 106.2 Imaging to investigate central blindness.

Radiography: limited to cases with bony involvement. Various contrast techniques designed to demonstrate soft tissue changes have been described but are of limited use

Ultrasonography: useful for orbital lesions

Advanced imaging: CT scan can be useful for detection of intracranial lesions. MRI gives even better soft tissue resolution. These techniques are becoming more widely available

Optic Nerve Lesions

Total lesions of the optic nerve result in blindness of the affected eye and a lack of direct and consensual PLR on the affected side. Bilateral lesions result in dilated non-responsive pupils. Possible causes include optic nerve hypoplasia, optic neuritis, trauma or neoplasia (Table 106.3). Neoplasia within the orbit will often result in exophthalmos. Orbital ultrasound, CT or MRI are useful for demonstrating the presence of a space-occupying lesion. Hypoplasia of the

Table 106.3 Retrobulbar optic neuritis (also see optic neuritis, Chapter 105).

Usually a bilateral condition
Results in sudden-onset blindness
Aetiology: idiopathic in many cases, although canine distemper virus is a possible cause
Differential diagnosis: main differential is SARDS, although animals with tumours in the region of the chiasm may present with a history of sudden loss of vision
Treatment: high levels of systemic steroids, initial response may be good but recurrences are likely

SARDS, sudden acquired retinal degeneration syndrome.

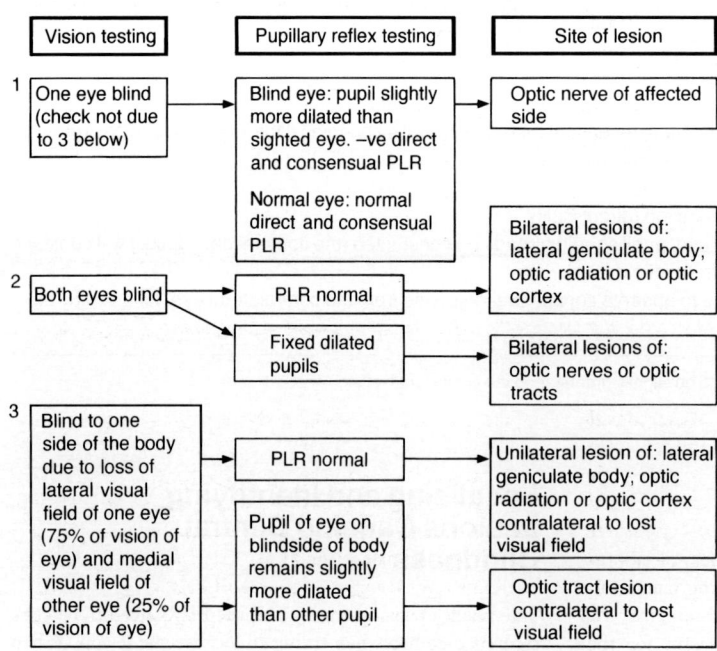

Fig. 106.3 Combining the results of vision testing and pupillary light reflex testing to localise lesions of the central visual pathways.

optic nerves is reflected by hypoplasia of the optic nerve head (see Chapter 105).

Optic Chiasm Lesions

Total destruction of the chiasm leads to complete blindness, the effect of partial destruction depends on the axons affected. Neoplasia and inflammatory reactions are the commonest cause of chiasmal damage.

Lesions of the Optic Tracts before Divergence of the Nerve Fibres Involved in the PLR

Bilateral optic tract lesions result in the same presentation as bilateral optic nerve lesions. Unilateral lesions result in a more severe visual impairment in the eye contralateral to the lesion. This renders the dog blind to one side of the body (loss of lateral visual field of one eye and medial visual field of other). The pupil of the eye contralateral to the lesion remains slightly more dilated than the other pupil. Potential causes include inflammatory lesions and space-occupying lesions.

Lesions Involving the Lateral Geniculate Nucleus, Optic Radiation or Optic cortex

The PLR is unaffected. Bilateral lesions result in blindness but subcortical reflexes, such as the dazzle reflex (blinking when a bright light is suddenly shone in the eye) may be maintained. Unilateral lesions result in visual impairment similar to that described for optic tract lesions.

The conditions above are summarised in Table 106.4.

PUPILLARY ABNORMALITIES

Lesions of the CVP that also involve the PLR are considered in the previous section. The pupil sizes and responses are also affected by lesions involving the nerve supply to the iridal musculature. The iris musculature consists of circular constrictor muscle innervated by the parasympathetic nerve supply via the oculomotor nerve, and radial dilator musculature under control of the sympathetic nervous system. The efferent arm of the PLR comprises the parasympathetic supply to the iris.

Table 106.4 Summary of sudden-onset blindness with no ophthalmoscopically detectable lesions.

Poor or absent PLR
- *Differentials*: sudden acquired retinal degeneration syndrome (SARDS); lesions of proximal portion of central visual pathway (CVP) (e.g. retrobulbar optic neuritis; inflammatory lesion of optic tracts; space-occupying lesion impinging on visual pathways)
- *Further investigations*: Electroretinography – unrecordable = SARDS; normal = lesion of visual pathways. If ERG was relatively normal an advanced imaging technique would be indicated to localise the problem

Normal PLR
- *Differentials*: lesions involving CVP from lateral geniculate nucleus to visual cortex, e.g. inflammatory process, ischaemia, cerebral anoxia, hydrocephalus
- *Investigation*: history may suggest a cause; other neurological signs may be present and help localise the site of the lesion. Advanced imaging techniques may be useful

Dilated, Fixed or Poorly Responsive Pupil(s)

Poorly responding pupils may result from one of the following:

- fear – circulating adrenaline,
- iridal disease,
  - ○ iris hypoplasia,
  - ○ iris adhesions (synechiae),
  - ○ glaucoma,
  - ○ iris atrophy,
- lesion of parasympathetic supply to pupil.

Anisocoria – Difference in Pupil Size (Neer and Carter 1987)

There are a number of possible causes of anisocoria:

- intraocular disease (as described above),
- unilateral lesion of parasympathetic supply to pupil (other components of the oculomotor nerve may be involved depending on the site of the lesion),
- unilateral lesion of optic tracts (see above),
- Horner's syndrome – this is a common cause of anisocoria in dogs.

HORNER'S SYNDROME

The clinical signs of Horner's syndrome are as follows (Fig. 106.4):

- miosis (pupil is more constricted than the fellow normal pupil),
- ptosis (drooping of upper and lower lids),
- enophthalmos,
- third eyelid protrusion,
- slight conjunctival congestion.

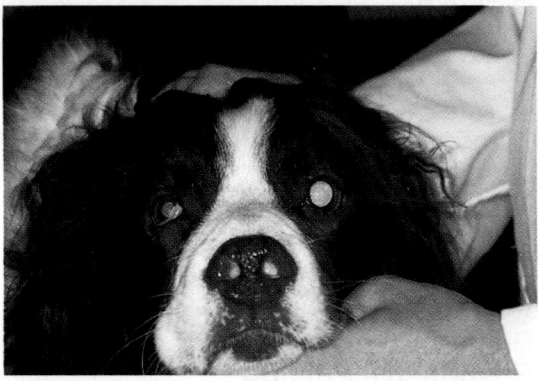

Fig. 106.4 Horner's syndrome. Note the upper eyelid ptosis, third eyelid protrusion and constricted pupil.

Horner's syndrome results from a lesion affecting the sympathetic nerve supply to the head (Table 106.5). The sympathetic nerve supply originates in the hypothalamus, passes via the spinal cord (first order neurones), exits to pass through the brachial plexus and join the vagosympathetic trunk in the musculature of the neck (second order neurones) and finally synapses in the cranial cervical ganglion. Third order neurones from the ganglion pass via the middle ear cavity to be distributed to the structures of the head. The sympathetic nerves supply the pupillary dilator muscle as well as smooth muscle in the eyelids and orbit. Denervation hypersensitivity is a feature of Horner's syndrome that can be used to try and localise the lesion to first, second or third order lesions. Topical 10% phenylephrine is applied to the affected and the normal eye and the time taken for pupillary dilation noted. The pupils denervated by third order lesions dilate rapidly (in about 20 min) whereas with second order lesions this takes approximately 45 min and in first order lesions 60+ min (Bistner *et al.* 1970). Indications as to the cause of the sympathetic nerve lesion should be sought, although in the majority of instances the lesion appears to be idiopathic.

Treatment

There is no specific treatment for Horner's syndrome, although if a causal lesion is identified it should be treated. If the third eyelid protrusion is sufficient to obscure vision application of topical phenylephrine drops will keep it retracted.

Table 106.5 Aetiology of Horner's syndrome.

Cause	Comments
Idiopathic	Commonest category of canine Horner's syndrome cases in the UK
	Most appear to be second order (pharmacological testing)
	The breed most commonly presented with Horner's syndrome in the UK is the Golden Retriever
	The signs gradually resolve
Middle ear disease	Otitis media
	Middle ear neoplasia
	Iatrogenic – after aural surgery
Injury to musculature of neck	Puncture wounds
	Iatrogenic – surgical damage
Brachial plexus (+other neurological signs)	Brachial plexus avulsion
	Brachial plexus neoplasm

EYE POSITION AND MOVEMENT

Active movement of the globes normally occurs in unison and is a complicated process controlled by the mid-brain with input from the higher visual centres, subcortical visual reflex centres and the vestibular system. The extra-ocular muscles and their actions were considered in Chapter 98.

Examination of Eye Position and Movement

The ability of the eyes to have a full range of movement and to move in unison should always be checked as part of a neuro-ophthalmological examination. The oculocephalic, or 'dolls-head' reflex can be invoked for this purpose. This involves moving the head to the left or right, or up and down and seeing the resulting ocular movement. This technique should invoke nystagmus. Nystagmus is a rhythmical eye movement consisting of a slow phase in which the eyes move away from the primary gaze (straight ahead) position followed by a fast phase which rapidly recentres them. The fast phase of nystagmus occurs in the direction of rotation. These repeated slow phase movements followed by fast phase corrections are induced by the vestibular system and will continue while there is a change in velocity (acceleration or deceleration) of head movements. A fixation nystagmus also occurs due to the action of higher centres, this allows visual fixation on moving objects.

Abnormalities in Eye Position

Abnormal deviation in the direction of gaze is known as strabismus or a squint (Table 106.6). It may be congenital or acquired. Acquired lesions of the nerves supplying the extra-ocular muscles result in different directions of squint depending on the actions of the muscles denervated. Surgical correction of a squint is rarely indicated in dogs.

Abnormalities in Eye Movement

Nystagmus which occurs spontaneously (spontaneous nystagmus) or when the dog's head is held in a different position by the examiner (positional nystagmus) is abnormal and can be readily differentiated from the normal nystag-

Table 106.6 Differential diagnosis of strabismus.

Congenital or juvenile onset disorder	Brachycephalics – due to conformation of skull and orbit
	Congenital anomaly of extraocular muscles or their innervation
	Hydrocephalus – strabismus secondary to the resulting skull deformity
	Gross congenital ocular abnormality leading to a lack of visual influence on the development of control centres for eye movement
Acquired disease	Orbital disease (see Chapter 98)
	Extraocular muscle disease (see Chapter 98)
	After proptosis (see Chapter 98)
	Lesion affecting the oculomotor, trochlear or abducens nerves or the mid-brain region containing the nuclei of these nerves and their connections

Table 106.7 Abnormal nystagmus.

Congenital nystagmus – rotatory, oscillatory or random eye movements (searching nystagmus)	Associated with severe congenital ocular malformations such as microphthalmos and associated multi-ocular disorders
Spontaneous horizontal nystagmus	May indicate peripheral vestibular disease (fast phase away from the affected side) – other signs of vestibular disease are likely to be present
Vertical nystagmus, spontaneous nystagmus	May indicate central vestibular disease – other signs of vestibular disease are likely to be present

mus induced by the oculocephalic reflex. The commonly occurring forms of abnormal nystagmus are listed in Table 106.7

ABNORMALITIES OF EYELID CLOSURE

Normal blinking is important in keeping the ocular surface healthy. The impetus to blink comes from corneal sensation and requires normal trigeminal innervation. Denervation results in a reduced blink rate, inadequate spreading of the tear film and the development of a neurogenic keratitis affecting the cornea exposed within the palpebral opening. Denervation of the facial musculature (supplied by the facial nerve) will result in a lack of blink, although corneal sensation is unaffected (Kern & Erb 1987). When the affected dog attempts to blink the globe is retracted and the third eyelid sweeps across the cornea. In many dogs this third eyelid movement will adequately spread the tear film and keep the cornea healthy, however in dogs where the third eyelid does not adequately cross the cornea (e.g. brachycephalic breeds) an exposure keratitis will develop.

REFERENCES

Bistner, S., Rubin, L., Cox, T.A. & Condon, W.E. (1970). Pharmacological diagnosis of Horner's syndrome in the dog. *Journal of the American Veterinary Medical Association*, **157**, 1220–1224.

Kern, T.J. & Erb, H.N. (1987). Facial neuropathy in dogs and cats: 95 cases (1975–1985). *Journal of the American Veterinary Medical Association*, **157**, 1604–1609.

Neer, T.M. & Carter, J.D. (1987). Anisocoria in dogs and cats: ocular and neurological causes. *Compendium on Continuing Education for the Practicing Veterinarian*, **9**, 817–823.

Petersen-Jones, S.M. (1993). Neuro-ophthalmology. In: *Manual of Small Animal Ophthalmology*, (eds S.M. Petersen-Jones & S.M. Crispin), pp. 267–281. BSAVA, Cheltenham.

Scagliotti, R.H. (1991). Neuro-ophthalmology. In: *Veterinary Ophthalmology*, (ed. K.N. Gelatt), 2nd edn. pp. 706–743. Lea & Febiger, Philadelphia.

Section 14

Poisons

Edited by Katie Dunn

Chapter 107

Poisons

K. Dunn

INTRODUCTION

Dogs, despite having a well developed protective vomiting reflex are at high risk of poisoning because of their tendency to scavenge indiscriminately. Poisoning should be suspected particularly in young dogs with an acute onset of clinical signs or sick dogs with neurological, gastrointestinal or respiratory signs. A high index of suspicion for poisoning should be retained in all cases of sudden onset status epilepticus. Seizures induced by poisoning are usually generalised and acute in onset. A diagnosis is usually based on a combination of clinical signs (Table 107.1) and circumstantial evidence.

Route of Intoxication

The route of toxin exposure affects not only the likelihood of systemic absorption (absorption is greater following parenteral exposure than oral or topical) but also the clinical signs and method of treatment. The potential routes of intoxication are:

- ingestion,
- cutaneous/topical,
- inhalation,
- injection,
- ocular.

In the dog most toxicoses arise from ingestion.

Although there is a huge range of poisons the most frequently reported poisonings in dogs are rodenticides closely followed by human medicines. In addition to the common poisons there are thousands of other potential poisons and if further information is required then a Poisons Information Centre should be contacted. It is now a requirement that a registration fee is paid by practices before information is given by these centres.

MANAGEMENT OF A CASE OF SUSPECTED POISONING (TABLE 107.2)

Instructions to Owner

Initial instructions given to the owner over the telephone in cases of suspected or known poisoning are important to minimise the risk to the owner and also as a first line in treatment of the dog.

- The dog should be protected and removed from potential sources of further intoxication.
- People in contact with the dog should take precautions since:
  - disorientated or frightened animals may become aggressive and
  - handlers may also be at risk from contamination with noxious substances.
- In cases of topical exposure the dog may be washed with water to reduce further absorption. Protective clothing must be worn to avoid human contamination.
- Water may act as a diluent for ingested poisons and oral consumption should be encouraged.
- If the dog is convulsing or unconscious no attempt should be made to administer anything by mouth.
- Emetics should be avoided particularly if the agent or timing of exposure is questionable.
- The owner should be requested to bring a sample of suspected poison or packaging to the practice/veterinary surgery where possible.

Emergency Care

On arrival at the veterinary surgery the dog must be assessed immediately and its condition should be stabilised before any other treatments are instigated. Emergency

Depression	Excitement	**Table 107.1** Common clinical signs associated with poisoning.

Depression
  Amitraz
  Ethylene glycol
  Achloralose
  Paraquat
  Lead
  Acrolein
  Street drugs
  ANTU (alpha-naphthyl urea)
  Nicotine

Excitement
  Metaldehyde
  Lead
  Organophosphates
  Strychnine
  Pyrethrins
  Methylxanthines

Vomiting
  Pyrethrins
  Ethylene glycol
  Methylxanthine
  Blue-green algae
  Lead
  Paraquat
  Paracetamol
  Nicotine
  Phenolics

Tachycardia
  Nicotine
  Methylxanthines
  Drug therapy
    Adrenaline
    Aminophylline
    Amphetamines
    Atropine
  Metaldehyde

Seizures
  Carbamates
  Metaldehyde
  Organophosphates
  Strychnine
  Lead
  Caffeine
  Toad toxin

Bradycardia
  Drug therapy
    Opiates
    Digitalis
    Cardiac glycosides
  Amitraz

Respiratory
  Acrolein
  Paraquat
  ANTU
  Organophosphates
  Chlorates
  Coumarins
  Carbon monoxide

Hepatotoxicity
  Paracetamol
  Phenolics
  Blue-green algae
  Lead

Coagulopathy
  Coumarins
  Sulphonamides
  Aflatoxin
  Aspirin

Nephrotoxicity
  Ethylene glycol
  Cholecalciferol
  Phenol
  Drug therapy
    Gentamicin/neomycin
    Amphotericin B
    Paracetamol
    Polymixin B
    Sulphonamides

Aim	Action
Stabilise animal	
Respiratory function	Intubate if required, manual ventilation/oxygen
Cardiovascular support	Fluid therapy
Control CNS signs	Administer anticonvulsants
Control body temperature	Heat pads or cold water/alcohol baths
Obtain history and further evaluate patient	
Prevent further absorption of toxin	
Dilution	Allow water to drink/wash off skin contamination
Emetics	Apomorphine, syrup of ipecac
Gastric lavage	Intubate and wash out stomach with water
Adsorbents/cathartics	Activated charcoal/sodium bisulphate
Facilitate removal of toxin	Diuresis, urinary pH manipulation, peritoneal dialysis, cathartics
Continue supportive care	i.v. fluids, pain relief, respiration

Table 107.2 Management of a case of suspected poisoning.

treatment as outlined below should be administered before investigating suspected toxicoses:

- If the animal is unconscious, respiratory and cardiovascular function should be assessed and support provided if necessary.
  - Intranasal catheters or endotracheal intubation will allow increased oxygenation of air supplied to animal.
  - In some cases a tracheostomy may need to be performed.
  - An intravenous catheter for fluid administration should be placed early in the course of the management.
- Seizures should be controlled by the use of benzodiazepines or induction of general anaesthesia with pentobarbitone if required.
- Core body temperature may be elevated or depressed and variation from normal should be corrected appropriately.
- Once the animal's condition is stable a detailed history can be obtained:
  - known access to possible intoxicants,
  - timing of exposure,
  - how much ingested,
  - previous administration of any drugs.

- A full clinical examination should be performed.
- If clinical signs do not concur with suspected poisoning the signs should be treated and *not* the suspected toxicosis.

General treatment is indicated during the first 6 hours after exposure to a potential toxin. This includes removal from the source, reduction of the amount of absorption followed by supportive care and an attempt to increase the rate of toxin excretion.

Managing the Toxicosis

As most toxins have a dose dependent toxicity it is vital to try to limit the total body dose of toxin.

Treatment of Topical Exposure

The animal may need to be clipped or bathed. If the coat is heavily contaminated with tar or oil, vegetable oil may be used as a solvent. The use of detergents and soaps may be contraindicated as these may enhance the percutaneous absorption of some toxins.

Treatment of Ingested Poisons

Following ingestion the primary aim is to remove the toxin from the gastrointestinal tract, to prevent further absorption or minimise local damage. If this is not possible, or where the process of removal might cause further trauma (e.g. if the substance ingested is an irritant), the toxin should be diluted and, if possible, bound to inert substances so that absorption is minimised. These aims can be achieved in a number of ways:

Reduction of Toxin Absorption

Induction of Emesis

- Should be attempted if ingestion occurred within 2 h of presentation.
- Aspirin and chocolate are more slowly cleared from the stomach and emesis may be induced usefully up to 6 h after ingestion.
- May be more successful if liquid food is given before administration of emetic.

Contraindications:

- Already vomiting
- Absence of gag reflex
- Unconscious or depressed dogs
- Ingestion of highly corrosive substances such as acids/bases or petroleum based products where aspiration into lungs must be avoided
- Ingestion of any irritant that may cause further damage to the oesophagus if vomited.

Techniques:

(1) Oral administration of 'syrup of ipecac' (ipecacuanha emetic draught)
   - Dose rate of 1–2 ml/kg up to maximum of 15 ml.
   - Induces vomiting within 15 min and can be repeated after 20 min if no vomiting occurs.
   - However, gastric lavage must be performed if the dog fails to vomit as the syrup may be cardiotoxic if absorbed.
   - Only effective in 50% of cases.
(2) Systemic administration of apomorphine
   - Dose rate of 0.04 mg/kg i.v. or 0.08 mg/kg s.c. or i.m.
   - Can result in protracted vomiting and should be avoided if additional CNS depression is undesirable, i.e. where toxin is likely to produce marked CNS depression (although naloxone at a dose rate of 0.04 mg/kg i.v. can be used to reverse this).

- Part of a tablet can be put into the conjunctival sac until vomiting occurs but there is a risk of overdose by this route.
- After vomition the tablet should be removed and the eye flushed with water.

The effectiveness and safety of table salt, washing soda, xylazine and hydrogen peroxide are questionable.

If vomitus is obtained this should be retained for possible identification of intoxicant.

Gastric Lavage. A useful technique if less than 2 h have elapsed since ingestion.

Techniques:

- Can be performed in unconscious animal or under light anaesthesia.
- A cuffed endotracheal tube must be placed to prevent aspiration.
- The head and thorax should be slightly lowered with respect to the stomach to facilitate retrieval of washings.
- A stomach tube of the same diameter as the endotracheal tube is used.
- Warm water (5–10 ml/kg) washed in and aspirated with 50 ml syringe.
- High pressure lavage should be avoided as this may force the toxin into duodenum.
- Particular care is required if the stomach wall is likely to be weakened.
- The lavage is repeated 10–15 times, until the lavage fluid is returning clear.
- Activated charcoal may be added to the lavage fluid which is then left *in situ* for 10 min before aspiration to assist in reclamation of the toxin.

Adsorbents

- The most commonly used adsorbent is activated charcoal at 2–8 g/kg.
- If activated charcoal is unavailable, burnt toast provides a good alternative.
- Particularly useful in cases of ingestion of:
   - strychnine,
   - alkaloids (morphine and atropine),
   - ethylene glycol,
   - barbiturates,
   - chocolate.

Techniques

- Make up slurry of 1 g charcoal to 5–10 ml water.
- Administer by stomach tube via funnel.

- This can be followed 30 min later with cathartic such as sodium sulphate.
- Bismuth in Pepto–Bismol™ is a weak adsorbent and can be given at a rate of 1 ml/kg but should not be used in cases of poisoning with antiprostaglandin agents, e.g. NSAIDs and aspirin.
- Alternatively an adsorbent may be administered 3–4 times daily for 3–4 days after intoxication.

Cathartics

- Useful to speed gastrointestinal elimination of substances.
- Sodium sulphate 40% solution administered at 1 g/kg orally.
- Mineral oil (liquid paraffin 5–15 ml per dog).
- A warm saline enema may be given at the same time.

Hasten Clearance of Absorbed Toxin

Diuresis. Diuresis helps in elimination of many toxins but is obviously of vital importance in those which are renally excreted in an unchanged form such as salicylates, barbiturates. Manipulation of urine pH will ensure that these substances, which are freely filtered at the glomerulus, are efficiently excreted in the urine rather than resorbed from the tubule (see below).

Contraindications

- Shock
- Reduced renal function
- Pre-existing heart disease.

Technique

- Intravenous fluids usually crystalloid (lactated Ringer's) given at a rate of 2–3 times maintenance will produce diuresis.
- It is essential to monitor urine output and it is safer to catheterise the dog so that urine production can be monitored.
- Diuretics should only be administered if intravenous fluid therapy is given and urine output is greater than 1 ml/kg per minute.
- Loop diuretics (frusemide 5 mg/kg every 6–8 h) or hyperosmolar diuretics (20% mannitol 2 g/kg per hour) may be used.

Peritoneal Dialysis

- If renal output is insufficient then peritoneal dialysis may be employed.

- Warm sterile saline is instilled into the peritoneal cavity until mild abdominal distension occurs and removed 30 min later.
- Repeat hourly as necessary.

Manipulation of Urine pH

- *Alkalinisation* for ethylene glycol, salicylates, phenobarbitone (weak acids) 1–2 mmol sodium bicarbonate/kg i.v. every 3–6 h.
- *Acidification* for amphetamines, quinine, strychnine (weak bases) 100 mg/kg ammonium chloride p.o. b.i.d. Contraindicated with hepatic/renal insufficiency or in severe cases of haemolysis as nephrotoxicity of haemoglobin and myoglobin are increased in acid urine.

Administer Antidote

If the toxin has been identified, an antidote may be available (see Table 107.3). However, there are few specific antidotes and they should only be used if toxicosis is severe as many antidotes themselves have severe side-effects. In most cases, treatment relies on supportive therapy while toxin is eliminated.

Provide Supportive Care and Monitor

Body Temperature

Hypothermia

- Keep wrapped up in blankets.
- Metabolism may be slow and therefore often need active warming with heat pads, warm i.v. fluids or baths.
- Care must be exercised in rewarming shocked animals as peripheral vasodilation can result in a fatal hypotension.
- Rewarming of comatose animals with central depression due to toxicosis may result in initial recovery followed by lapse of consciousness as temperature increase resolves paralytic ileus and further toxin is absorbed. It is important to take steps to limit toxin absorption before rewarming in these cases.

Hyperthermia

- Measures to reduce pyrexia should be instituted if the temperature rises above 40.5°C
- Alcohol cooling is the safest method as it is difficult to overchill animals this way.
- Ice bags or cold water baths may also be used.

Table 107.3 Specific toxins and antidotes.

Poison	Source	Specific treatment
Organophosphates	Veterinary drugs	Atropine 0.25–0.5 mg/kg quarter i.v., rest s.c. Pralidoxime 5% solution 20–50 mg/kg i.m. or slow i.v.
Lead	Old paint/putty, metallic objects, car batteries	Calcium Na$_2$EDTA 100 mg/kg per day divided q.i.d. s.c. up to maximum daily dose 2 g Na$_2$CaEDTA. D-penicillamine 100 mg/kg per day divided t.i.d. for 1–4 weeks Remove foreign body

Coumarins	Anticoagulant rat baits	Vitamin K$_1$ 5 mg/kg i.v. or i.m.
		2.5–10 mg/kg p.o. t.i.d. >5 days
		Blood transfusions
		
		Short acting coumarins
		  Warfarin
		  Vitamin K$_1$ 1 mg/kg for 10–14 days
		
		Intermediate acting
		  Fumarin/pindone/valone
		  Vitamin K$_1$ 1 mg/kg for 4–6 days
		
		Long acting
		  Diphacinone/chlorophacinone/bromodialone
		  Vitamin K$_1$ 2.5–5 mg/kg for 3–4 weeks
		  Brodifacoum
		  Vitamin K$_1$ 2.5–5 mg/kg for 4 weeks

Ethylene glycol	Antifreeze	Ethanol 1.1 g/kg i.v. or 5.5 ml/kg of 20% solution i.v. every 4 h for 5 treatments then every 6 h for 5 treatments Sodium bicarbonate 4-methylpyrazole
Metaldehyde	Slug bait	Diazepam 2–5 mg/kg Triflupromazine 0.2–2.0 mg/kg i.v.
Paracetamol	Human medicine	N-acetylcysteine 140–280 mg/kg p.o. then 70 mg/kg q.i.d. p.o. 2 days Sodium sulphate 50 mg/kg as 1.6% solution i.v. every 4 h for 4 treatments Ascorbic acid
Chlorate	Weedkillers	Methylene blue 2% 10 mg/kg i.v.

Respiratory Support

- While unconscious the dog must remain intubated with a cuffed endotracheal tube.
- Manual ventilation may be necessary in cases of respiratory depression and is much more effective than the use of analeptic drugs.

Cardiovascular Support

- If the dog is hypovolaemic as a result of haemorrhage give whole blood transfusion (try to raise PCV to 0.25–0.301/l).
- If fluid loss is the main problem then give plasma expanders or crystalloids (Hartmann's solution).

- If facilities are available, monitor for acidosis or alkalosis, correct acid–base disturbances as necessary. In clinical poisonings acidosis is the most likely acid–base disturbance, e.g. ethylene glycol, metaldehyde, aspirin.

Pain Relief

- Many poisonings result in severe pain and may require narcotic analgesia.
- Although this may cause some respiratory depression, ventilation is frequently better in a calm dog than in an animal in distress.
- Opiate analgesia is preferred but pethidine or buprenorphine may be used. (see Table 107.4).
- Non-steroidals and carprophen should be avoided, particularly if the animal is hypotensive and shocked, however, carprophen may be safer than flunixin in a shocked animal.

CNS Disturbances

Depression/Coma

- Most problems are due to respiratory depression therefore respiration should be monitored and supported as appropriate.

- 'Street drugs' show dose dependent clinical signs from ataxia through depression to coma.
- Terminal coma may develop with many other toxins with fixed, dilated pupils and irregular respiration. Calculation of a coma score may be helpful in monitoring progression of clinical signs particularly if the animal is being examined by a number of different clinicians (Kirk & Ford 1995).

Hyperactivity

- In cases of convulsion or excitement, diazepam may be given initially (2.5–100 mg i.v. to effect) – its effects are short-lived in the dog.
- Pentobarbitone (see Table 107.4) may be required but since this causes respiratory depression intubation with ventilation is often indicated.
- Avoid treatment of excitement associated with alphachloralose toxicity if possible, as animals subsequently become centrally depressed and sedation will exacerbate this effect.
- Dogs with CNS signs caused by hepatic encephalopathy are very sensitive to depressant effects of barbiturates and benzodiazepines.

Table 107.4 Dose rates of drugs used in management of poisonings.

Reason for use	Dose rate
Induction of vomiting	Ipecac syrup 1–2 ml/kg (maximum 15 ml) Apomorphine 0.04 mg/kg i.v. or 0.08 mg/kg s.c./i.m.
Seizures	Pentobarbitone (Sagatal™) 3–15 mg/kg i.v. slowly to effect – repeat every 4–8 h. Phenobarbitone 10–30 mg/kg i.v. Diazepam 0.5–1.5 mg/kg i.v. to effect
Induction of diuresis	Frusemide 2–5 mg/kg every 6–8 h Mannitol 20% 1–2 g/kg per hour
Analgesia	Morphine 1–2 mg/kg every 6 h Pethidine 2–5 mg/kg every 4 h Buprenorphine (Temgesic™) 0.06 mg/kg every 8 h
Gastrointestinal bleeding	Misoprostol (Cytotec™) 2–5 µg/kg every 8 h
Bradycardia (only if signs of syncope)	Atropine 0.04 mg/kg up to 0.2 mg/kg i.v.
Tachycardia	Propranolol 0.02–0.15 mg/kg i.v. over 2–3 min 0.2–1 mg/kg p.o.
Ventricular premature contractions (treat if clinical signs, more than 20–30 per min, in runs, or multifocal)	Lidocaine 2–4 mg/kg i.v. bolus slowly up to max. 8 mg/kg Procainamide 6–8 mg/kg i.v. over 5 min
Apnoea	Doxapram 1–10 mg/kg i.v. every 20–30 min
To reverse opiate effects	Naloxone 0.04 mg/kg i.v.

Nutritional Support

If an irritant or caustic substance has been ingested, a pharyngostomy or percutaneous endoscopic gastrostomy (PEG) tube may need to be placed to allow nutritional support.

If the animal is unable/unwilling to eat for other reasons, feeding via a nasogastric tube may be simpler.

Take Samples Required to Make Diagnosis

Diagnosis is unlikely to be achieved in time to aid therapy unless the ingested substance was identified. However, retrospective diagnosis may be important in some cases of dispute. All samples taken should be split into two aliquots, one of which is sent to a laboratory for analysis and the other retained in case of legal dispute.

Useful samples include:

- urine (50 ml) stored frozen,
- vomit or stomach/gastrointestinal contents stored frozen,
- sample of medication or commercial product suspected,
- blood (serum 20 ml stored frozen).

Post-mortem specimens should include brain, liver, kidney, and stomach contents which should all be divided and half stored frozen with the remainder fixed in formalin.

Hair samples are of limited use.

In addition, baseline samples of blood and urine should be taken to assess:

- renal function and evidence of tubular damage;
- hepatic function and evidence of hepatocellular damage;
- red blood cell mass;
- hydration status, electrolyte balance, acid–base status.

These samples will provide the baseline data from which the patient can be monitored for signs of improvement/deterioration in response to treatment.

MECHANISMS OF POISONING

The four principle methods of toxicity are neurotoxicity, respiratory effects, nephrotoxicity and hepatotoxicity (see Table 107.5).

Table 107.5   The four principle methods of toxicity.

Neurotoxicity
Toxins may produce neurological signs in a variety of ways.
- Specific neuronal tissue damage – lesions may be peripheral or central (brain and spinal cord) if toxin is able to cross blood brain barrier.
- Acute damage may be followed by necrosis and permanent loss of function.
- Interference with neurotransmission.
- Seizures secondary to uraemia or hepatic encephalopathy.

Respiratory problems
Reduced haemoglobin oyxgen binding capacity
- Binding of other substances to haemoglobin, e.g. carbon monoxide to form methaemoglobin.
Reduction of gaseous exchange mechanisms
- Toxins causing pulmonary damage or fibrosis reduce ability of lung to exchange gases.
Functional dyspnoea
- Haemorrhage into pleural space or pulmonary haemorrhage/oedema will cause dyspnoea.

Nephrotoxicity
There is often a lag phase between exposure of renal cells to toxin and cell death.
- The signs may not be seen for hours to days after ingestion of toxin.
- Frequently toxin has been eliminated before damage is recognised.
- Damage can manifest as oliguria or polyuria.
- Active urine sediment, e.g. the presence of casts is indicative of acute tubular necrosis.
- The reversibility should be assessed and the animal supported to allow healing.

Hepatotoxicity
- Short term exposure may cause acute hepatic damage but return to full liver function is often possible.
- Supportive therapy is indicated to allow hepatic regeneration.
- Chronic exposure may lead to cirrhosis.

Haematological Problems

Clinical signs are usually related to effects on the red cell series but there are a number of mechanisms by which this occurs:

Coagulopathy

- Usually the result of intoxication with coumarins which results in haemorrhage.

Marrow aplasia (leucopenia or anaemia)

- Direct cytotoxic effect or immunological damage to marrow.
- The reversibility of the condition should be assessed and blood transfusion will be required in the short term to allow regeneration to occur.

Haemolysis

- May be a direct result of the toxin or due to secondary immune-mediated destruction.
- If haemolysis can be stopped before administration of blood products the prognosis is better.

Miscellaneous Mechanisms

- Hypothermia

POISONINGS PRODUCING NEUROLOGICAL SIGNS

The information on specific poisons has been classified according to the predominant clinical sign in most cases of clinical poisoning. The same clinical sign may be manifested by a number of different underlying toxic mechanisms, e.g dyspnoea due to reduced oxygen carrying capacity, gaseous exchange or functional problems.

Excitatory Toxins

Organophosphates (OPs)/Carbamates

Source

- Insecticidal sprays, dips, collars, spot-ons (OPs).
- Fungicides, molluscicides and flea collars (carbamates).
- Toxicity may be enhanced by simultaneous or sequential exposure to different cholinesterase inhibitors or the use of certain drugs which compete for target esterases or have neuromuscular blocking activity, e.g. antibacterial drugs such as aminoglycosides, see Chapter 4 and phenothiazines, see Chapter 1.

Action

- Inhibit function of acetylcholinesterase and butyryl-cholinesterase.

- Carbamates have a rapidly and spontaneously reversible effect.
- The effect of OPs may be prolonged.

Signs
The signs are the results of actions on three sites:

(1) Muscarinic effects
  - gastrointestinal hypermotility/vomiting
  - bradycardia
  - salivation/lacrimation
  - dyspnoea/pallor
  - miosis
(2) Nicotinic effects
  - muscle fasciculations
  - followed by skeletal muscle weakness/paralysis
(3) Central nervous system
  - CNS depression

- In most cases signs are mild with rapid onset over minutes to hours.
- Delayed onset neuropathy (7–21 days after exposure) is rare but has been reported in dogs (only in association with OPs and not carbamates).
- Weakness, ataxia and proprioceptive deficits develop 7–21 days after exposure.
- If death occurs it is usually due to hypoxia from bronchoconstriction and erratic bradycardia.

Clinicopathological Changes
Diagnosis can be confirmed by measurement of whole blood or plasma cholinesterase activity (which is commonly less than 25% of normal activity in cases of poisoning with OPs).

Treatment

- Wash off contamination with mild detergent or water or remove source.
- Pralidoximine chloride (see Table 107.3) may be cautiously used to accelerate reversal of inhibition of cholinesterase.
- Atropine (see Table 107.3) counteracts muscarinic effects and can be given until the mouth is dry.
- Hypoxia should be corrected before atropine administration to avoid ventricular fibrillation.
- Response should be seen within 3–5 min of atropine administration (development of tachycardia implies atropine overdosage).
- Supportive care and oxygen therapy is important.
- Management and support of respiratory function greatly reduces fatalities.

Lead

Source

- Relatively common poisoning in dogs especially puppies.
- Ingestion of lead is necessary to cause poisoning as hydrochloric acid in stomach is needed to make it soluble.
- Often from licking lead paints or putty or eating lead shot.

Action

- The mechanism by which lead causes its toxic effects is incompletely understood.
- Lead has adverse biochemical effects in nearly all tissues in the body.

Signs

- Often slow in onset and hard to recognise.
- Gastrointestinal signs are prominent often vomiting, diarrhoea and abdominal cramps.
- Neurological signs, often hysteria or aggression, are also frequently seen.
- Limb radiographs may show 'lead line' on distal extremities.

Clinicopathological Changes

- Mild non-regenerative anaemia is common with nucleated red blood cells, basophillic stippling, anisocytosis seen on blood smear.
- Blood levels of lead are assayed for diagnosis >60 μg/100 ml (60 ppm) positive.
- Equivocal levels (30–60 μg/100 ml) are difficult to interpret as animal may have high background levels.
- Some animals have low blood levels of lead but show clinical signs of toxicity.
- Diagnosis is therefore based on clinical suspicion, history and blood samples in combination.

Treatment

- Prevent further exposure (remove foreign body if present).
- Calcium disodium ethylenediaminotetra-acetate (CaNa$_2$EDTA) diluted to 1–2% in 5% dextrose saline i.v. or s.c. (see Table 107.3). When given subcutaneously the duration of effective plasma concentration is prolonged and lead elimination is enhanced.
- Treat for up to 5 days.
- Clinical improvement should be seen within 24–48 h.

- If lead levels have not fallen to normal wait 5 days before retreating for a further 5 days to avoid CaNa$_2$EDTA induced nephrotoxicity.
- D-penicillamine is the only effective oral chelating agent (see Table 107.3).
- This is given on an empty stomach and if repeated courses are required these should be separated by weekly intervals.
- Side-effects include vomiting, listlessness, inappetance.
- Prognosis is poor if neurological signs are severe.

Pyrethrins and Pyrethroids

Source

- Insecticidal aerosols, sprays, dips, e.g. cypermethrin, permethrin, fenvalerate.
- These compounds are generally less toxic than OPs and toxicity not common in dogs.

Action

- Effect gating kinetics of sodium channels causing repetitive discharges or membrane depolarisation.

Signs

- Usually seen within a few hours of exposure but may be delayed.
- Hypersalivation, vomiting and diarrhoea, hyperaesthesia and hyperexcitability.
- Occasional severe skin reaction.

Clinicopathological Changes
Laboratory diagnosis is not routinely available.

Treatment

- Recover within 24 h in most cases but may be affected for up to 3 days.
- Signs are not responsive to atropine.
- Diazepam to effect to control neurological signs.

Methylxanthines

Source

- Chocolate (theobromine), coffee and theophylline as human and animal drug.
- Lethal dose of theobromine is 250–500 mg/kg achieved by eating 28 g of unsweetened baking choco-

late per kilogram. Milk chocolates contain much lower levels and virtually none in white chocolates. Poisoning is most common after eating cocoa powder.
- Caffeine is found in coffees, teas, some soft drinks and some chocolates. A lethal dose is 140 mg/kg, expresso coffee contains 100 mg/oz (3.52 g/kg).

Action

- Increase cAMP by inhibition of cellular phophodi-esterase as well as causing release of catecholamines.
- Stimulate release of calcium from intracellular stores in high concentrations.

Signs

- Vomiting, diarrhoea, hyperactivity/seizures, ataxia, hyperthermia followed by coma and death.
- Tachycardia may be the result of ventricular arrhythmias so electrocardiographic examination is indicated in all cases.
- Death is uncommon but can occur due to cardiovascular collapse.

Treatment

- Gastric emptying is often slow following chocolate ingestion and gastric lavage may be beneficial up to 6 h after ingestion.
- Activated charcoal 0.5 g/kg p.o. every 3 h for 72 h (due to long half-life of drug).
- Diazepam or phenobarbitone for seizures (see Table 107.4).
- Lignocaine for ventricular arrhythmias and propranolol for supraventricular tachycardias (see Table 107.4).
- Regular bladder emptying or catheterisation may help to reduce reabsorption through urinary tract mucosa.

Blue-Green Algae

Source
Poisonings are usually seen after hot dry spells and often where there is increased nitrate level in water.

Action

- Anatoxins produced can act as neuromuscular blockers, and microcystins are hepatotoxic.
- Saxitoxin mimicking toxins inhibit nerve conduction of action potentials and reduce acetylcholine release at motor end plates.

Signs

- Occur acutely and many dogs will be dead within a few minutes to hours.
- Severe vomiting, diarrhoea and loss of motor co-ordination.
- Muscle tremors, hyperaesthesia, dullness and flaccid paralysis may be seen.
- Dogs that survive acutely often die of hepatic damage.

Treatment

- Suspected water should be collected immediately for diagnosis as bloom may not survive long.
- Intravenous injection of sodium nitrate and sodium thiosulphate has been suggested but is unlikely to be effective.
- Supportive treatment only in most cases.

Strychnine

Source

- Naturally occurring alkaloid from seeds of a tree which grows naturally in India, Australia.
- Found in mole and fox bait (now illegal).
- Rare cause of toxicosis as sources of access are limited.
- Intoxication can arise from eating carcase of a poisoned animal as well as from bait.

Action

- Competitive antagonist at glycine receptors.
- Interferes with postsynaptic inhibition in medulla and spinal cord resulting in signs of central nervous system stimulation.

Signs

- Initial signs of excitement, apprehension and stiffness within 15–60 min.
- Progression to convulsions on stimulation.
- May develop acute renal failure.

Treatment

- General anaesthesia and gastric lavage (with a weakly acidic solution) recommended.
- Convulsions should be controlled with barbiturates (see Table 107.4).
- Keep in environment free of sensory stimulation (quiet, darkened room).
- Takes 6–12 h to metabolise toxic dose so prolonged nursing may be required.

Metaldehyde

Source

- Condensation product of acetaldehyde.
- Common constituent of slug baits (may be combined with carbamate).

Action

- Hydrolysed in stomach acid to acetaldehyde.
- Acetaldehyde and different sized fragments of the acetaldehyde polymer are absorbed.
- Both metaldehyde and acetaldehyde have pathological effects, crossing the blood–brain barrier and affecting neurotransmission in the brain.

Signs

- Hyperaesthesia, convulsions, tremors and inco-ordination precede opisthotonus, nystagmus and tachycardia.
- Liver damage and cirrhosis may result in delayed death of those animals which survive the acute neurotoxicity.

Treatment

- Intravenous fluids with bicarbonate for acidosis if required.
- Emesis or gastric lavage recommended in early stage.
- Liquid paraffin may help to reduce absorption.
- Anticonvulsants (diazepam, triflupromazine see Table 107.4) to control seizures.

Depressant Poisons

Cannabis Sativa (Marijuana)

Source

- Access to owners supply.
- Severe toxicosis usually by ingestion but can be affected by inhaling smoke from owner's supply.
- Signs usually seen in police 'sniffer dogs'.

Action

The active ingredient tetrahydrocannibol causes CNS depression, derangement and visual hallucinations.

Signs

- Muscle weakness, tremors, inco-ordination.
- Increased pulse rate, low blood pressure and hypothermia.
- Compulsive eating and dissociative behaviour.

Treatment

- Remove from gastrointestinal tract with adsorbents and cathartics.
- If ingested in bags can remove intact bags by enterotomy.
- Supportive care if necessary.
- Treatment of ingestion of other drugs such as cocaine is similar but needs to be more aggressive.

Alphachloralose

Sources
Rodenticide and bird poison.

Action

- Stimulatory and depressive actions on the CNS.
- Metabolised to chloroethanol which is a CNS depressant and excreted in urine as an inactive form.

Signs

- Initial excitement phase and ataxia then depression/coma.
- Salivation is an inconsistent feature.
- Low metabolic rate may result in hypothermia (with reduction in body temperature by up to 3.5°C) but fatal poisoning rare.

Treatment

- Emetics given early on (care if sedation already present) or gastric lavage if necessary.
- Sedation contraindicated due to CNS depressant summation effect.
- Animals should be kept warm as hypothermia contributes to fatalities.
- Respiratory support may be required.
- Sensory stimulation should be avoided.

Tobacco (Nicotine)

Source

- Ingestion of a single packet of cigarettes can cause signs of toxicity.
- Ingestion of cigar ends by puppies is not uncommon.

Action

- Binds to nicotinic cholinergic receptors.
- Small doses stimulate nicotinic receptors and larger doses block these.

Signs

- General activation of both divisions of the autonomic nervous system.
- Excitement, rapid respiration, salivation and vomiting/diarrhoea.
- Then depression, inco-ordination with coma and tachycardia.
- Terminally flaccid paralysis develops and death may result from respiratory muscle paralysis.
- Death often occurs during convulsive seizure.
- Dogs ingesting sublethal doses recover within 3 h.

Treatment
Gastric lavage and artificial respiration if required.

Amitraz

Source
Derasect™ demodectic mange wash available only through veterinary surgeon.

Action
α_2 adrenoreceptor agonist.

Signs

- Sedation is common (seen in 80% of dogs following first treatment).
- Hypotension, mydriasis, bradycardia, ataxia, vomiting/diarrhoea.

Treatment

- Intravenous fluids to counteract hypotension.
- Yohimbine an α_2-adrenoreceptor antagonist 0.1 mg/kg intravenously to reverse signs (atropine will reverse some signs but antagonises others).
- Atipamezole (Antisedan™) may be used.

Also consider severe ethylene glycol toxicity (page 1060) and toad poisoning (page 1063).

POISONINGS PRODUCING RESPIRATORY SIGNS

Poisons Affecting Oxygenation

Coumarins

Source

- Anticoagulant rodenticides.
- A single dose of warfarin bait 1 g/kg can kill.
- Second generation anticoagulants are only really toxic after repeated administration and in general repeated small doses are more toxic than single large doses.

Action
Antagonise action of vitamin K_1 in synthesis of clotting factors synthesised by the liver (prevent recycling of vitamin K_1, which is a co-enzyme in this process, from its oxidised form back to the reduced form which is necessary for this process).

Signs

- Dogs remain asymptomatic until clotting factors are depleted.
- Clinical signs are not present for up to 1–2 days following ingestion of poison.
- Signs can vary depending on the site of bleeding but often include depression, weakness, dyspnoea, and prolonged bleeding from venepuncture sites.
- Dyspnoea is common as a result of pulmonary or intrathoracic haemorrhage.

Clinicopathological Changes
Whole blood clotting time (WBCT), one stage prothrombin time (OSPT), activated partial thromboplastin time (APTT) are all increased, The OSPT is affected first as Factor VII has the shortest half-life within the circulation (approximately 7 h).

Treatment

- Cage rest and minimal handling are essential to minimise further bleeding.
- Synthesis of clotting factors takes 6–8 h and therefore the dog will need supportive care in the meantime.

- In severe cases fresh, whole blood administration and oxygen therapy may be required for anaemia or fresh frozen plasma transfusions to replace clotting factors. This may need to be repeated every 24 h due to the short half-lives of the clotting factors.
- Vitamin K_1 (phytomenadione) (see Table 107.3) administration until dog is able to resynthesise own factors.
- The vitamin itself *does not* have any effect on clotting time.
- Vitamin K_1 can be administered by
  ○ intramuscular route which may cause further severe haemorrhage,
  ○ subcutaneous route from where it is only slowly absorbed,
  ○ intravenous route which is associated with an increased risk of anaphylaxis,
  ○ Konakion™ contains polyethoxylate castor oil which may increase risk of anaphylaxis,
  ○ Konakion™ MM is in a mixed miselles vehicle for i.v. use but should not be used i.m.
- Vitamin K_1-induced Heinz body formation has been reported but is rare.
- In most cases intravenous therapy is given acutely followed by oral doses once the clotting time has been reduced.
- Absorption following oral administration is often poor but may be increased if given with a fatty meal.
- Newer coumarins have prolonged half-lives and duration of replacement therapy depends upon the type of coumarin ingested (see Table 107.3). If in any doubt the company manufacturing the rodenticide should be contacted for information.
- In all cases the clotting time (OSPT would be most sensitive test) must be re-evaluated after the end of treatment and therapy continued if necessary.

Poisons Affecting Gaseous Exchange

Bipyridyls

Source
Paraquat and diquat are constituents of some weedkillers.

Action

- Diquat is poorly absorbed from the gastrointestinal tract and the mechanism of action is unknown.
- Paraquat is accumulated in lung tissue, so it rapidly reaches sufficient concentration to cause toxic effects.

- Toxicity is the result of free radical formation so oxygen levels in the lung contribute to pathology of pulmonary lesions.
- Pulmonary oedema and haemorrhage progresses to fibrosis over days to weeks.
- Acute tubular necrosis.

Signs

- Following paraquat ingestion these include stomatitis/ulceration of the lips, depression, vomiting, diarrhoea and respiratory distress.
- Often associated with the presence of an oily substance on the coat and skin irritation.
- Pulmonary congestion and oedema develop over days to weeks with terminal fibrosis, leading to signs of dyspnoea and cyanosis.
- Oxygen therapy is contraindicated as this potentiates toxic effects.
- Diquat causes severe loss of body water into the gastrointestinal tract, animals that don't die of dehydration develop CNS signs and renal failure.

Clinicopathological Changes
Acute renal failure is often seen, with biochemical evidence of azotaemia.

Treatment

- In early stages induce emesis and use adsorbents and forced diuresis. If toxins removed from body in first 24 h recovery is possible.
- The prognosis is usually hopeless and euthanasia should be considered once a diagnosis is made.
- Diagnosis is based on history and clinical signs (sequence of vomiting followed by dyspnoea is distinctive).

ANTU (Alpha-Naphthylurea)

Sources

Rare rodenticide not used in UK any more but very toxic to dogs.

Action

- Biotransformed by dog to reactive intermediate.
- Most dangerous if ingested on a full stomach as emesis usually occurs if stomach empty.

Signs

- Signs include vomiting, diarrhoea, abdominal pain, inco-ordination, dyspnoea and death.
- Pleural fluid and pulmonary oedema also seen.

Treatment

- Symptomatic treatment with morphine for sedation.
- Frusemide and oxygen therapy for dyspnoea.
- Prognosis usually hopeless once dyspnoea develops.

Acrolein

Source
Poisoning from cooking fat fumes usually overheated chip fat.

Action
Cholinergic stimulation causes bronchodilation.

Signs

- Initial signs enlarged tonsils, epistaxis, respiratory distress and severe lacrimation.
- Progress to cyanosis 24 h later.
- Poisoning frequently fatal.

Poisons Affecting Oxygen Carrying Capacity

Onion Poisoning

Action
Oxidative intoxicants can cause intravascular haemolysis and Heinz body anaemia.

Signs
Haemoglobinuria, anaemia, icterus.

Treatment

- Avoid source.
- Supportive care, blood transfusions and fluid therapy.

Paracetamol/Acetaminophen

Sources
Household paracetamol 150–200 mg/kg needed for signs of toxicosis.

Action

- Paracetamol when given at low doses is glucuronidated, at high doses a greater proportion of the drug is metabolised by cytochrome P450 to form a reactive metabolite.
- The active metabolite is initially conjugated with glutathione but as concentrations of this become depleted the metabolite is free to cause damage to liver and red blood cells in particular, by binding covalently to cellular proteins.
- Depletion of red cell glutathione results in methaemoglobin formation.

Signs

- Seen 1–4 h after ingestion.
- Vomiting, abdominal pain, cyanosis (caused by methaemoglobinaemia) and depression.
- Progression to hepatic failure with jaundice and weight loss.

Clinicopathological Changes
Haemoglobinuria and haematuria frequently seen.

Treatment

- If less than 2 h since ingestion induce emesis.
- Gastric lavage is *not* recommended but can use cathartic.
- If antidote is being administered do *not* use activated charcoal.
- Administer antidote (*N*-acetylcysteine 140 mg/kg see Table 107.3) or sodium sulphate.
- Fluid therapy (lactated Ringer's solution) if required, monitor for acidosis and treat if present, and cimetidine to reduce hepatic metabolism of acetaminophen.
- Ascorbic acid can be used to reduce the methaemoglobinaemia.
- If cyanosis is severe give oxygen therapy.

Carbon Monoxide

Source
Incomplete combustion of solid fuel or natural gas, e.g. blocked flue.

Action
Formation of carboxyhaemoglobin which prevents oxygen binding to haemoglobin.

Signs

- Weakness and blindness with low level poisoning.
- Progresses to deafness, dyspnoea and coma.
- Mucous membranes are bright pink and blood is cherry red.

Clinicopathological Changes

Arterial blood gas will have a high normal Pa_{O_2} but a low percentage saturation of haemoglobin.

Treatment

- Give oxygen and 5% carbon dioxide (to stimulate respiration).
- Consider blood transfusion, but probably not necessary.
- Analeptics may be indicated in some cases.

Chlorates

Source
Found in non-selective weedkillers for paths.

Action

- Direct irritant to gastrointestinal tract.
- Produces methaemoglobin and subsequent tissue anoxia.
- Causes haemolysis by an action on the erythrocyte membrane.

Signs

- Vomiting usually occurs if ingested as concentrated solid form.
- If diluted solution is drunk, toxin acts as direct irritant and systemic poison.
- Signs of abdominal pain with cyanosis and brown mucous membranes due to methaemoglobinaemia.
- Dyspnoea may be apparent.

Treatment

- Methylene blue 2% solution see (Table 107.3) may help.
- Gastric lavage with 1% sodium thiosulphate.

Consider also toad poisoning (see page 1063).

POISONINGS CAUSING RENAL DAMAGE

Ethylene Glycol

Source
Antifreeze

- One of the most common causes of poisoning in dogs.
- The solution is highly palatable and dogs will readily drink it.
- Lethal dose is only 4–5 ml/kg
- Toxicity depends on the rapidity of uptake (which is slowed by the presence of food in the stomach).

Action

- Acts as a gastric irritant and metabolites have a cytotoxic effect.
- The agent is metabolised in the liver in a stepwise fashion to gluteraldehyde, glycolate, glycoxylate and oxalate.
- Ethylene glycol and its metabolites are excreted via the kidneys and can be measured in urine for 48 h following ingestion.
- CNS toxicity results from the effects of the aldehydes on the brain.
- Renal damage possibly due to oxalate crystal formation and acidosis.
- The metabolites are cytotoxic to renal tubular cells.

Signs

- Classically divided into three phases:
  - 6–12 h CNS signs predominate
  - 12–24 h cardiopulmonary signs appear
  - 24–72 h oliguric renal failure
- Occur within 1 h of ingestion, serum levels peak at 3 h and urinary excretion is evident at 6 h.
- CNS effects lead to vomiting, ataxia/weakness, dehydration, primary polydipsia with secondary polyuria initially.
- Hypothermia due to depression and sedation.
- Mild cases get oliguric renal failure, more severe toxicoses progress to CNS depression, convulsions or coma.

Clinicopathological Changes

- Diagnosis is difficult in the early stages. The presence of calcium oxalate crystalluria and cellular casts may raise the index of suspicion but it is not detectable in urine for 24–48 h.

- Serum osmolality markedly increased for 1–3 h after intoxication.
- Metabolic acidosis occurs within 3 h, with an increased anion gap.
- Blood samples show azotaemia, increased phosphate and hypocalcaemia (which is a rare finding in the veterinary world, therefore be suspicious of toxicoses).

Treatment

- Stop absorption and metabolism by the use of emetics, activated charcoal and cathartics.
- Correct fluid balance and metabolic acidosis and monitor urine output (see Chapter 62 for management of acute renal fature (ARF).
- Administration of alcohol (20% ethanol in saline) blocks alcohol dehydrogenase enzymes and metabolism of ethylene glycol to more toxic products.
- Sodium bicarbonate.
- Once rehydrated continue intravenous fluids until elimination is complete.
- Peritoneal dialysis to:
  ○ remove the toxic metabolites
  ○ support the animal through the ARF crisis.
- In addition 4-methylpyrazole may be given (see Table 107.3).
- Prognosis poor due to late diagnosis and treatment in most cases.

Cholecalciferol

Source

- Recently introduced rodenticide.
- Doses of 13 mg calciferol/kg have proved fatal despite the manufacturer's claim of 88 mg/kg LD_{50}.
- Ingestion of as little as 2 g of bait can be associated with clinical signs of toxicity.

Action

Metabolised to 25-hydroxycholecalciferol in liver and 1,25-dihydroxycholecalciferol in renal tubules which enhance calcium uptake from intestine and bone and increases calcium resorption by kidneys resulting in hypercalcaemia.

Signs

- Usually not seen for 18 h after ingestion.
- Anorexia, depression, constipation or diarrhoea, polyuria, polydipsia.

- In some cases ventricular fibrillation is a problem.
- Soft tissue calcification with hypercalcaemic nephropathy.

Clinicopathological Changes

- Laboratory findings include hyperphosphataemia, azotemia, hypercalcaemia.
- Hyperphosphataemia in hypercalcaemic animals which are not azotaemic or only mildly azotaemic, would be highly suggestive of vitamin D toxicity.
- Can measure vitamin D 1,25 dihydrocholecalciferol and 24,25 dihydrocholecalciferol at Guy's Hospital in London.

Treatment

- Emetics and activated charcoal administered acutely may help to reduce absorption.
- Intravenous saline (at 1.5 times maintenance), prednisolone (up to 1 mg/kg s.i.d.) should only be given if diagnosis is certain otherwise occult lymphoma may be missed, and frusemide (2–4 mg/kg t.i.d.) acutely to reduce hypercalcaemia.
- Avoid sunlight.
- High salt, low calcium diet.
- If hypercalcaemia is refractory give salmon calcitonin 4–6 IU/kg s.c. every 2–3 h until calcium levels stabilise.
- Since cholecalciferol is fat soluble treatment may be required for at least 2 weeks and it can take up to 4–6 weeks for the calciferol to be cleared from the body.

Salicylates/Ibuprofen

Very common causes of poisoning in the dog.

Source

- Aspirin (doses of 15 mg/kg t.i.d. have caused toxicoses).
- Ibuprofen (Brufen™) (doses of 50–125 mg/kg have caused toxicoses).
  8 mg/kg daily is likely to cause gastrointestinal ulceration.

Action

- Interfere with cyclo-oxygenase step of prostaglandin synthesis. This action is reversible following ibuprofen administration but irreversible after aspirin, which acetylates the enzyme.
- Ibuprofen has a narrow safety margin in the dog as it is excreted slowly.

- Inhibition of cyclo-oxygenase results in loss of production of:
  - cytoprotective PGI_2 and PGE_2 in the gastric mucosa
  - PGE_2 and PGI_2 which maintain renal blood flow in the face of vasoconstrictor mediators such as noradrenaline, angiotensin II and ADH.

Signs

- Signs are commonly seen in dogs with ibuprofen toxicity and develop 4–6 h after acute intoxication.
- Low doses tend to cause gastrointestinal signs, higher doses can also cause organ damage.
- Nausea, abdominal pain, respiratory stimulation due to metabolic acidosis, and occasionally seizures or coma.
- Dogs which are hypotensive and dehydrated when treated with non-steroidals can develop acute papillary necrosis leading to acute renal failure.
- Chronic therapy may result in gastric ulceration, bone marrow toxicity (reported for phenylbutazone, oxyphenbulzizone, dipyrone, sudoxicam), hepatopathy or nephrosis.

Treatment

- Gastric lavage with activated charcoal followed by cathartic if acute ingestion.
- Intravenous fluids with sodium bicarbonate for metabolic acidosis and alkalinisation of the urine encourages renal excretion.
- Sucralfate if ulcers present.
- Cimetidine to reduce gastric acid production.
- Misoprostol for preventing gastrointestinal ulceration and haemorrhage (see Table 107.4).
- In chronic cases stop drug and provide supportive care.

Consider also strychnine (see page 1055) and bipyridyls (see page 1058).

POISONINGS PRODUCING HEPATOTOXICITY

Phenolics

Sources

- Found in pitch, tar, creosote and some disinfectants.
- Phenol containing disinfectants may be applied topically by owner and licked off by dog.

Action

- Denatures and precipitates cellular proteins therefore cytotoxic.
- Caustic and hepatotoxic.

Signs

- Include vomiting/diarrhoea and inco-ordination.
- Convulsions, abdominal pain and jaundice are also common.
- Cutaneous burns seen if exposure is topical.

Treatment

- Do *not* induce emesis but gastric lavage may be employed.
- Oral administration of large volumes of water or milk to dilute toxin.
- Nil by mouth for 2–5 days with supportive care and intravenous fluid therapy.
- Glucose saline infusions may increase rate of elimination.

Consider also paracetamol (see page 1059) and blue-green algae and metaldehyde (see pages 1055 and 1056).

POISONINGS CAUSING CORROSIVE EFFECTS

Household Cleaners

Sources

- Cationics, e.g. fabric softener (primary quaternary ammonium compounds).
- Anionics, e.g. washing powder and some shampoos (sulphonated hydrocarbons).

Actions

- Mainly cause corrosive damage but can have systemic effects.
- Quaternary ammonium compounds may have cholinesterase blocking activity.

Signs

- Few severe signs with anionics.
- Cationics may cause vomiting, depression, collapse and corrosive damage to oesophagus.

Treatment

- Anionics, just neutralise alkalinity with milk, water or vinegar.
- Cationics are very toxic.
- Milk and activated charcoal should be administered immediately to dilute poison.
- Analgesia for pain.
- Supportive therapy as required.

Corrosives

Sources
Bleach (alkali) and acids.

Actions
Direct corrosive effect.

Treatment

- Use of emetics and gastric lavage is contraindicated.
- Diluents such as water or milk may be helpful.
- Charcoal is a poor absorbent for acid.

POISONINGS WITH CARDIOTOXIC EFFECTS

Plants with Cardiotoxic Effects

Glycoside Containing Plants

Source
Laurel, azaleas, oleander, foxglove.

Action
Induce arrhythmias including tachycardias, bradycardias or heart blocks.

Signs

- Vomiting/diarrhoea develop within 3 h.
- Arrhythmia development causes weakness, cyanosis or depression.

Treatment

- Stabilise cardiac arrhythmias.
- Activated charcoal and cathartic to minimise further absorption.
- If hypokalaemic supplement potassium provided no atrioventricular block.

- Treat sinus bradycardia with atropine.
- Tachycardias or ventricular premature contractions managed with lidocaine (see Table 107.4)

Labernum (Labernum Anagyroides)

Source
Seed pods can cause fatal intoxication.

Action
Reduction in intracellular potassium results in high atrioventricular block.

Signs
Muscle tremors and vomiting/diarrhoea.

Treatment
Supportive care and antiarrhythmic therapy.

MISCELLANEOUS POISONINGS

Toad Poisoning

Source

- Toads have glands in the skin which secrete noxious substances
- The common toad (*Bufo bufo*) is relatively harmless.

Action
Toad venom contains a number of potentially toxic substances:

- cardiotoxic steroid derivate,
- indole derivates,
- catecholamines.

Signs

- Effects include salivation and pawing at the mouth but resolution occurs without treatment (only requires the mouth to be washed out with a hose).
- In more severe poisonings signs include cyanosis, weakness, oedema and convulsions.

Treatment

- Propranolol and anesthesia induced with pentobarbitone (see Table 107.4).

- The animal should be intubated and the mouth thoroughly irrigated with water.
- ECG monitoring is important to identify arrhythmias and repeated doses of propranolol (see Table 107.4) may be required.

Snake Bites

Source

In the UK the common adder (*Vipera berus*) is the likely source.

Action

Haemotoxic venom produces local damage as well as systemic effects.

Signs

- Three factors affect seriousness of snake bite
  - size of dog,
  - location of bite,
  - type of snake.
- Signs include swelling at site, haemorrhagic oedema, dilated pupils, collapse and death.
- Vomiting, dehydration, haemolysis and icterus may also occur.

Treatment

- Clip hair and clean wounds.
- Broad-spectrum antibiotics.
- Tetanus antitoxin.
- Specific antivenom should be administered if available (dogs need a proportionately larger dose than humans).

FURTHER READING

Beasley, V.R. (guest ed.). (1990). Toxicology of selected pesticides drugs and chemicals. *Veterinary Clinics of North America*, **20**(2).

Humphreys, D.J. (1988). *Veterinary Toxicology*, 3rd edn. Baillière Tindall, London.

Kirk, R.W. & Ford, R. (eds) (1995). Poisoning. In: *Handbook of Veterinary Procedures and Emergency Treatment*. 6th edn. W.B. Saunders, Philadelphia.

MAFF/HSE (1995). *Pesticides 1995*. Reference. Book 500. HMSO, London.

Oehme, F. (ed.) (1975). Clinical toxicology for the small animal practioner. *Veterinary Clinics of North America*, **5**(4), 737–748.

Oehme, F. (1983). Chemical and physical disorders. In: *Current Veterinary Therapy VIII*, (ed. R.W. Kirk), pp. 76–189. W.B. Saunders, Philadelphia.

Osweiler, G. (1989). Chemical and physical disorders In: *Current Veterinary Therapy X*, (ed. R.W. Kirk), pp. 97–177. W.B. Saunders, Philadelphia.

Paton, P. (1989). Ethylene glycol poisoning in small animals. In: *Veterinary Annual*, pp. 189–194. Wright, London.

Index of Featured Conditions Related to Breeds in this Edition

Index